Lecture Notes in Arti~~ficial~~

Subseries of Lecture Notes i~~n Computer Sc~~

Edited by J. G. Carbonell and J. Siekmann

Lecture Notes in Computer Science

Edited by G. Goos, J. Hartmanis and J. van Leeuwen

Springer
Berlin
Heidelberg
New York
Barcelona
Hong Kong
London
Milan
Paris
Singapore
Tokyo

John Lloyd   Veronica Dahl   Ulrich Furbach
Manfred Kerber   Kung-Kiu Lau
Catuscia Palamidessi   Luís Moniz Pereira
Yehoshua Sagiv   Peter J. Stuckey (Eds.)

Computational
Logic – CL 2000

First International Conference
London, UK, July 24-28, 2000
Proceedings

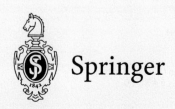 Springer

Series Editors

Jaime G. Carbonell, Carnegie Mellon University, Pittsburgh, PA, USA
Jörg Siekmann, University of Saarland, Saabrücken, Germany

Volume Editors

John Lloyd, The Australian National University
E-mail: jwl@csl.anu.edu.au

Veronica Dahl, Simon Fraser University, Canada
E-mail: veronica@cs.sfu.ca

Ulrich Furbach, Universität Koblenz, Germany
E-mail: uli@mailhost.uni-koblenz.de

Manfred Kerber, The University of Birmingham, UK
E-mail: M.Kerber@cs.bham.ac.uk

Kung-Kiu Lau, University of Manchester, UK
E-mail: kung-kiu@cs.man.ac.uk

Catuscia Palamidessi, The Pennsylvania State University, USA
E-mail: catuscia@cse.psu.edu

Luís Moniz Pereira, Universidade Nova de Lisboa, Portugal
E-mail: lmp@di.fct.unl.pt

Yehoshua Sagiv, The Hebrew University of Jerusalem, Israel
E-mail: sagiv@cs.huji.ac.il

Peter J. Stuckey, The University of Melbourne, Australia
E-mail: pjs@cs.mu.oz.au

Cataloging-in-Publication Data applied for

Die Deutsche Bibliothek - CIP-Einheitsaufnahme

Computational logic : first international conference ; proceedings /
CL 2000, London, UK, July 24 - 28, 2000. John Lloyd ... (ed.). -
Berlin ; Heidelberg ; New York ; Barcelona ; Hong Kong ; London ;
Milan ; Paris ; Singapore ; Tokyo : Springer, 2000
  (Lecture notes in computer science ; Vol. 1861 : Lecture notes in
  artificial intelligence)
  ISBN 3-540-67797-6

CR Subject Classification (1998): I.2.3, F.4, F.3, I.2, D.1-3, H.2

ISBN 3-540-67797-6 Springer-Verlag Berlin Heidelberg New York

Springer-Verlag Berlin Heidelberg New York
a member of BertelsmannSpringer Science+Business Media GmbH
© Springer-Verlag Berlin Heidelberg 2000
Printed in Germany

Typesetting: Camera-ready by author, data conversion by Christian Grosche, Hamburg
Printed on acid-free paper   SPIN: 10722222   06/3142   5 4 3 2 1 0

Preface

These are the proceedings of the First International Conference on Computational Logic (CL 2000) which was held at Imperial College in London from 24th to 28th July, 2000. The theme of the conference covered all aspects of the theory, implementation, and application of computational logic, where computational logic is to be understood broadly as the use of logic in computer science. The conference was collocated with the following events:

- 6th International Conference on Rules and Objects in Databases (DOOD 2000)
- 10th International Workshop on Logic-based Program Synthesis and Transformation (LOPSTR 2000)
- 10th International Conference on Inductive Logic Programming (ILP 2000).

CL 2000 consisted of seven streams:

- Program Development (LOPSTR 2000)
- Logic Programming: Theory and Extensions
- Constraints
- Automated Deduction: Putting Theory into Practice
- Knowledge Representation and Non-monotonic Reasoning
- Database Systems (DOOD 2000)
- Logic Programming: Implementations and Applications.

The LOPSTR 2000 workshop constituted the program development stream and the DOOD 2000 conference constituted the database systems stream. Each stream had its own chair and program committee, which autonomously selected the papers in the area of the stream. Overall, 176 papers were submitted, of which 86 were selected to be presented at the conference and appear in these proceedings. The acceptance rate was uniform across the streams. In addition, LOPSTR 2000 accepted about 15 extended abstracts to be presented at the conference in the program development stream. (These do not appear in these proceedings.) CL 2000 also had eight invited speakers, 12 tutorial speakers, and seven workshops held in-line with the conference.

ILP 2000 was held as a separate conference with its own proceedings, but shared invited speakers and tutorial speakers with CL 2000.

The unusual structure of CL 2000 relied for its success on the cooperation of various subcommunities inside computational logic. We would like to warmly thank members of the automated deduction, constraints, database, knowledge representation, logic programming, and program development communities who contributed so much to the technical program. In particular, we would like to thank everyone who submitted a paper, the members of the stream program committees, the other reviewers, the invited speakers, the tutorial speakers, the workshop organisers, and those who submitted papers to the workshops. Thanks to Vladimiro Sassone for allowing us to use his excellent software for electronic submission and reviewing of papers. We would also like to thank the members of the Executive Committee of the Association of Logic Programming for their support throughout the preparations for the conference.

May 2000

John Lloyd
Veronica Dahl
Ulrich Furbach
Manfred Kerber
Kung-Kiu Lau
Catuscia Palamidessi
Luís Moniz Pereira
Yehoshua Sagiv
Peter J. Stuckey

Organisation

Conference Organisation

Conference Chair
Marek Sergot (Imperial College of Science, Technology and Medicine, UK)

Program Chair
John Lloyd (The Australian National University)

Local Organisers
Frank Kriwaczek (Imperial College of Science, Technology and Medicine, UK)
Francesca Toni (Imperial College of Science, Technology and Medicine, UK)

Publicity Chair
Femke van Raamsdonk (Vrije Universiteit, The Netherlands)

Workshop Chair
Sandro Etalle (Universiteit Maastricht, The Netherlands)

Stream Chairs

Program Development (LOPSTR)
Kung-Kiu Lau (University of Manchester, UK)

Logic Programming: Theory and Extensions
Catuscia Palamidessi (The Pennsylvania State University, USA)

Constraints
Peter J. Stuckey (The University of Melbourne, Australia)

Automated Deduction: Putting Theory into Practice
Ulrich Furbach (Universität Koblenz, Gemany)
Manfred Kerber (The University of Birmingham, UK)

Knowledge Representation and Non-monotonic Reasoning
Luís Moniz Pereira (Universidade Nova de Lisboa, Portugal)

Database Systems (DOOD)
Yehoshua Sagiv (The Hebrew University of Jerusalem, Israel)

Logic Programming: Implementations and Applications
Veronica Dahl (Simon Fraser University, Canada)

Stream Program Committees

Program Development (LOPSTR)

David Basin (Albert-Ludwigs-Universität Freiburg, Germany)
Annalisa Bossi (Università di Venezia "Ca Foscari", Italy)
Antonio Brogi (Università di Pisa, Italy)
Maurice Bruynooghe (Katholieke Universiteit Leuven, Belgium)
Mireille Ducassé (IRISA/INSA, France)
Sandro Etalle (Universiteit Maastricht, The Netherlands)
Pierre Flener (Uppsala Universitet, Sweden)
Michael Hanus (Christian-Albrechts-Universität zu Kiel, Germany)
Ian Hayes (The University of Queensland, Australia)
Manuel Hermenegildo (Universidad Politécnica de Madrid, Spain)
Patricia Hill (University of Leeds, UK)
Baudouin Le Charlier (Facultés Universitaires Notre-Dame de la Paix, Belgium)
Michael Leuschel (University of Southampton, UK)
Michael Lowry (NASA Ames Research Center, USA)
Ali Mili (West Virginia University, USA)
Torben Mogensen (University of Copenhagen, Denmark)
Alberto Pettorossi (Università di Roma "Tor Vergata", Italy)
Don Sannella (University of Edinburgh, UK)
Douglas R. Smith (Kestrel Institute, USA)
Zoltan Somogyi (The University of Melbourne, Australia)

Logic Programming: Theory and Extensions

Sergio Antoy (Portland State University, USA)
Krzysztof R. Apt (CWI, The Netherlands)
Michele Bugliesi (Università di Venezia "Ca Foscari", Italy)
Amy Felty (University of Ottawa, Canada)
Gérard Ferrand (Université d'Orléans, France)
Maurizio Gabbrielli (Università di Udine, Italy)
Joshua S. Hodas (Harvey Mudd College, USA)
Joxan Jaffar (National University of Singapore)
Jan Maluszynski (Linköpings Universitet, Sweden)
Mario Rodríguez-Artalejo (Universidad Complutense de Madrid, Spain)
Harald Søndergaard (The University of Melbourne, Australia)
Robert F. Stärk (ETH Zürich, Switzerland)

Constraints

Frédéric Benhamou (Université de Nantes, France)
Alan Borning (University of Washington, USA)
Alex Brodsky (George Mason University, USA)
Yves Caseau (Bouygues, France)
Joxan Jaffar (National University of Singapore)

Andreas Podelski (Max-Planck-Institut für Informatik, Germany)
Patrick Prosser (University of Strathclyde, UK)
Francesca Rossi (Università di Padova, Italy)
Christian Schulte (Universität des Saarlandes, Germany)
Bart Selman (Cornell University, USA)
Helmut Simonis (Cosytec, France)
Barbara Smith (University of Leeds, UK)
Divesh Srivastava (AT&T Labs Research, USA)
Edward Tsang (University of Essex, UK)
Pascal Van Hentenryck (Université Catholique de Louvain, Belgium)
Mark Wallace (IC-PARC, UK)

Automated Deduction: Putting Theory into Practice

Alessandro Armando (Università di Genova, Italy)
Peter Baumgartner (Universität Koblenz, Germany)
Nikolaj Bjørner (Stanford University, USA)
François Bry (Ludwig-Maximilians-Universität München, Germany)
Bruno Buchberger (Johannes Kepler Universität Linz, Austria)
Ricardo Caferra (IMAG Grenoble, France)
Jürgen Dix (University of Maryland, USA)
Michael Fisher (Manchester Metropolitan University, UK)
Fausto Giunchiglia (IRST Trento, Italy)
Mateja Jamnik (The University of Birmingham, UK)
Christoph Kreitz (Cornell University, USA)
Ilkka Niemelä (Helsinki University of Technology, Finland)
Wolfgang Reif (Universität Ulm, Germany)
Julian Richardson (Heriot-Watt University, UK)
Maarten de Rijke (Universiteit van Amsterdam, The Netherlands)
Erik Sandewall (Linköpings Universitet, Sweden)
Bart Selman (Cornell University, USA)
Jörg Siekmann (DFKI Saarbrücken, Germany)
Toby Walsh (University of York, UK)

Knowledge Representation and Non-monotonic Reasoning

José J. Alferes (Universidade Nova de Lisboa, Portugal)
Gerhard Brewka (Universität Leipzig, Germany)
Jürgen Dix (Universität Koblenz, Germany)
Michael Gelfond (Texas Tech University, USA)
Katsumi Inoue (Kobe University, Japan)
Antonis Kakas (University of Cyprus)
Nicola Leone (Technischen Universität Wien, Austria)
Vladimir Lifschitz (University of Texas at Austin, USA)
Jack Minker (University of Maryland, USA)
Ilkka Niemelä (Helsinki University of Technology, Finland)

Teodor Przymusinski (University of California, Riverside, USA)
Chiaki Sakama (Wakayama University, Japan)
Terrance Swift (State University of New York at Stony Brook, USA)
Mirosław Truszczyński (University of Kentucky, USA)

Database Systems (DOOD)

Paolo Atzeni (Università di Roma Tre, Italy)
Alex Brodsky (George Mason University, USA)
Tiziana Catarci (Università di Roma "La Sapienza", Italy)
Sophie Cluet (INRIA, France)
Richard Hull (Bell Laboratories, USA)
Laks Lakshmanan (Concordia University, Canada)
Georg Lausen (Albert-Ludwigs-Universität Freiburg, Germany)
Werner Nutt (DFKI, Germany)
Kenneth Ross (Columbia University, USA)
Divesh Srivastava (AT&T Labs Research, USA)
Dan Suciu (AT&T Labs Research, USA)
S. Sudarshan (IIT Bombay, India)
Victor Vianu (University of California, San Diego, USA)
Gottfried Vossen (Westfälische Wilhelms-Universität Münster, Germany)
Ke Wang (Simon Fraser University, Canada)
Masatoshi Yoshikawa (NAIST, Japan)

Logic Programming: Implementations and Applications

Hassan Aït-Kaci (Simon Fraser University, Canada)
Maria Alpuente (Universidad Politécnica de Valencia, Spain)
Jamie Andrews (University of Western Ontario, Canada)
Phillipe Codognet (Université Paris 6, France)
Saumya Debray (University of Arizona, USA)
Bart Demoen (Katholieke Universiteit Leuven, Belgium)
Robert Demolombe (ONERA Toulouse, France)
Juliana Freire (Bell Laboratories, USA)
María García de la Banda (Monash University, Australia)
Fergus Henderson (The University of Melbourne, Australia)
Bharat Jayaraman (State University of New York at Buffalo, USA)
Guy Lapalme (University of Montreal, Canada)
Jorge Lobo (Bell Laboratories, USA)
José Gabriel P. Lopes (Universidade Nova de Lisboa, Portugal)
Fariba Sadri (Imperial College of Science, Technology and Medicine, UK)
Kostis Sagonas (Uppsala Universitet, Sweden)
Camilla Schwind (Laboratoire d'Informatique de Marseille, France)
Paul Tarau (University of North Texas, USA)
David Scott Warren (State University of New York at Stony Brook, USA)

Reviewers

The following reviewers were in addition to the members of the Stream Program Committees.

Program Development (LOPSTR)

Jamie Andrews
Robert Colvin
Bart Demoen

Elvira Pino
Maurizio Proietti

David Robertson
Paul Tarau

Logic Program: Theory and Extensions

Elvira Albert
Marc Bezem
Annalisa Bossi
Nicoletta Cocco
Agostino Cortesi
Giorgio Delzanno
Pierre Deransart
Włodzimierz Drabent
Rachid Echahed
Patrice Enjalbert
A. Gavilanes-Franco
Benjamin Grosof
Irène Guessarian
Gerhard Jäger
Beata Konikowska
Arnaud Lallouet

Francisco López-Fraguas
Bernard Malfon
Narciso Martí-Oliet
Bart Massey
Maria Chiara Meo
Eric Monfroy
Lee Naish
Stanislas Nanchen
Paliath Narendran
Ulf Nilsson
Manuel Núñez-García
Nicola Olivetti
Stephen Omohundro
Yolanda Ortega-Mallén
Prakash Panangaden
Dino Pedreschi

Avi Pfeffer
Carla Piazza
Alberto Policriti
Christian Prehofer
Femke van Raamsdonk
Francesca Rossi
Peter Schachte
Jan-Georg Smaus
Terrance Swift
Andrew Tolmach
Germán Vidal
Christel Vrain
Herbert Wiklicky
David Wolfram
Limsoon Wong
Roland Yap

Constraints

Alan Frisch
Nevin Heintze
Martin Henz
Andrew Lim

Tobias Müller
Rafael Ramirez
Vincent Tam
Peter Van Roy

Roland Yap
Yuanlin Zhang

Automated Deduction: Putting Theory into Practice

Carlos Areces
Christoph Benzmüller
Claudio Castellini
Henry Chinaski
Hubert Comon

Ingo Dahn
David Espinosa
Klaus Fischer
Reinhold Letz
Christof Monz

Silvio Ranise
Mark D. Ryan
Renate Schmidt
Frieder Stolzenburg
Michael Thielscher

Knowledge Representation and Non-monotonic Reasoning

Chandrabose Aravindan
Chitta Baral
Carlos Viegas Damásio
Alexander Dekhtyar
Yannis Dimopoulos
Thomas Eiter
Esra Erdem
Wolfgang Faber
Peter Flach
Enrico Giunchiglia
Sergio Greco

Keijo Heljanko
Koji Iwanuma
Tomi Janhunen
Elpida Keravnou
João Alexandre Leite
Fangzhen Lin
Rob Miller
Luigi Palopoli
Gerald Pfeifer
Alexandro Provetti
Halina Przymusinska

Paulo Quaresma
Riccardo Rosati
Pasquale Rullo
Ken Satoh
Francesco Scarcello
Eugenia Ternovskaia
Michael Thielscher
Richard Watson
Jia-Huai You

Database Systems (DOOD)

Toshiyuki Amagasa
Diego Calvanese
Jan Chomicki
Giuseppe De Giacomo

Kenji Hatano
Hiroyuki Kato
Hiroko Kinutani
Maurizio Lenzerini

Riccardo Rosati
Takeshi Sannomiya
Giuseppe Santucci

Logic Programming: Implementations and Applications

Matilde Celma
Michael Codish
Frédéric Cuppens
Gopal Gupta

Robert Kowalski
Ludwig Krippahl
Salvador Lucas
Lidia Moreno

David Toman
Henk Vandecasteele

Sponsoring Institutions

Association for Logic Programming
ESPRIT Network of Excellence in Computational Logic

Table of Contents

Invited Papers

Program Development (LOPSTR)

Logic Programming: Theory and Extensions

Constraints

Automated Deduction: Putting Theory into Practice

Knowledge Representation and Non-monotonic Reasoning

Logic Programming: Implementations and Applications

Computational Logic: Memories of the Past
and Challenges for the Future

John Alan Robinson

Highland Institute, 96 Highland Avenue, Greenfield, MA 01301, USA.

Abstract. The development of computational logic since the introduction of Frege's modern logic in 1879 is presented in some detail. The rapid growth of the field and its proliferation into a wide variety of subfields is noted and is attributed to a proliferation of subject matter rather than to a proliferation of logic itself. Logic is stable and universal, and is identified with classical first order logic. Other logics are here considered to be first order theories, syntactically sugared in notationally convenient forms. From this point of view higher order logic is essentially first order set theory. The paper ends by presenting several challenging problems which the computational logic community now faces and whose solution will shape the future of the field.

1   Introduction

Although logic and computing are each very old subjects, going back very much more than a mere hundred years, it is only during the past century that they have merged and become essentially one subject. As the logican Quine wrote in 1960, "The basic notions of proof theory converge with those of machine computing. ... The utterly pure theory of mathematical proof and the utterly technological theory of machine computation are thus at bottom one, and the basic insights of each are henceforth insights of the other" ([1], p. 41).

The aptly-named subject of computational logic - no pun intended - subsumes a wide variety of interests and research activities. All have something to do with both logic and computation. Indeed, as the declaration of scope of the new ACM journal Transactions on Computational Logic says, computational logic reflects all uses of logic in computer science. If things are no longer as simple as they seemed to be when logic and computing first came together, it is not because logic has become more complex, but because computing has.

Computational logic seemed simple enough when first order logic and electronic computing first met, in the 1950s. There was just one thing to know: the proof procedure for first order logic. It was clear that now at last it could be implemented on the fantastic new computers that were just becoming available. The proof procedure itself had of course been invented a generation earlier in 1930. It had waited patiently in the literature, supported by beautiful correctness and completeness proofs, for twenty five years until the first electronic digital computers were made available for general research. Then, in the first wave of

J. Lloyd et al. (Eds.): CL 2000, LNAI 1861, pp. 1-24, 2000.
© Springer-Verlag Berlin Heidelberg 2000

euphoria, it seemed possible that there would soon be proof-finding software which could serve as a computational assistant for mathematicians, in their regular work. Even though that still has not quite happened, there has been remarkable progress. Such automated deduction aids are now in use in developing and verifying programs.

Our small niche within general computer science was at first known simply as "mechanical theorem proving". It really was a small niche. In 1960 only a handful of researchers were working seriously on mechanical theorem proving. Theirs was a minority interest, which hardly counted as "real" computing. The numerical analysts, coding theorists, electronic engineers and circuit designers who ruled mainstream computer conferences and publications tended to be suspicious of our work. It was not so easy to find funding or places to publish. Most people in the computing mainstream considered logic to be boolean algebra, and logical computations to be what you had to do in order to optimize the design of digital switching circuits.

A half century later, our small niche has grown into a busy international federation of associations of groups of small niches housing thousands of researchers. At meetings like the present one the topics cover a broad range of theory and applications reaching into virtually every corner of computer science and software engineering. Such fertile proliferation is gratifying, but brings with it not a little bemusement. No one person can hope any more to follow closely everything going on in the whole field. Each of us now knows more and more about less and less, as the saying goes. Yet there is, after all, a unity under all this diversity: logic itself. We all speak essentially the same language, even if we use many different dialects and a variety of accents. It is just that nowadays logic is used to talk about so many different things.

1.1   First Order Predicate Calculus: All the Logic We Have and All the Logic We Need

By logic I mean the ideas and notations comprising the classical first order predicate calculus with equality (FOL for short). FOL is all the logic we have and all the logic we need. It was certainly all the logic Gödel needed to present all of general set theory, defining in the process the "higher order" notions of function, infinite cardinals and ordinals, and so on, in his classic monograph on the consistency of the axiom of choice and the continuum hypothesis with the other axioms of set theory [2]. Within FOL we are completely free to postulate, by formulating suitably axiomatized first order theories, whatever more exotic constructions we may wish to contemplate in our ontology, or to limit ourselves to more parsimonious means of inference than the full classical repertoire. The first order theory of combinators, for example, provides the semantics of the lambda abstraction notation, which is thus available as syntactic sugar for a deeper, first-order definable, conceptual device. Thus FOL can be used to set up, as first order theories, the many "other logics" such as modal logic, higher order logic, temporal logic, dynamic logic, concurrency logic, epistemic logic, nonmonotonic logic, relevance logic, linear logic, fuzzy logic, intuitionistic logic, causal logic, quantum logic; and so on and so on.   The idea that FOL is just one among many "other logics" is an unfortunate source of confusion and apparent complexity.   The "other logics" are simply notations reflecting syntactically sugared definitions of notions or limitations which can be formalized within FOL.   There are certain universal reasoning patterns, based on the way that our minds actually work, and these are captured in FOL.   In any given use it is simply a matter of formulating suitable axioms and definitions (as Gödel did in his monograph) which single out the subject matter to be dealt with and provide the notions to deal with it.   The whole sprawling modern landscape of computational logic is simply the result of using this one flexible, universal formal language FOL, in essentially the same way, to talk about a host of different subject matters. All those "other logics", including higher-order logic, are thus theories formulated, like general set theory and indeed all of mathematics, within FOL.

There are, of course, many different ways to present FOL. The sequent calculi, natural deduction systems, resolution-based clausal calculi,   tableaux systems, Hilbert-style formulations, and so on, might make it seem that there are many logics, instead of just one, but these differences are just a matter of style, convenience and perspicuity.

2   Hilbert's 1900 Address

On this occasion it is natural to think of David Hilbert's famous 1900 Paris address to the International Congress of Mathematicians [3].   When he looked ahead at the future of his field, he actually determined, at least partially, what that future would be. His list of twenty three leading open problems in mathematics focussed the profession's attention and steered its efforts towards their solutions. Today, in wondering about the future of computational logic we have a much younger, and much more untidy and turbulent subject to deal with. It would be very surprising if we could identify a comparable set of neat open technical problems which would represent where computational logic should be trying to go next.   We have no Hilbert to tell us what to do next (nor, these days, does mathematics).   In any case computational logic is far less focussed than was mathematics in 1900. So instead of trying to come up with a Hilbertian list of open problems, we will do two things: first we will reflect on the historical developments which have brought computational logic this far, and then we will look at a representative sampling of opinion from leaders of the field, who kindly responded to an invitation to say what they thought the main areas of interest will, or should, be in its future.

3   The Long Reign of the Syllogistic Logic

In the long history of logic we can discern only one dominating idea before 1879, and it was due to Aristotle. People had certainly begun to reason verbally, before Aristotle, about many things, from physical nature, politics, and law to metaphysics and aesthetics. For example, we have a few written fragments, composed about 500 B.C, of an obviously detailed and carefully reasoned philosophical position by Parmenides. Such thinkers surely used logic, but if they had any thoughts about logic, we now have no written record of their ideas. The first written logical ideas to have survived are those of Aristotle, who was active about 350 B.C. Aristotle's analysis of the class of inference patterns known as *syllogisms* was the main, and indeed the only, logical paradigm for well over two millennia. It became a fundamental part of education and culture along with arithmetic and geometry. The syllogism is still alive in our own day, being a proper and valid part of basic logic. Valid forms of inference remain valid, just as 2 plus 2 remains 4. However, the view that the syllogistic paradigm exhausts all possible logical forms of reasoning was finally abandoned in 1879, when it was subsumed by Frege's vastly more general and powerful modern scheme.

Before Frege, there had also been a few ingenious but (it seems today) hopeless attempts to automate deductive reasoning. Leibniz and Pascal saw that syllogistic analysis could be done by machines, analogous to the arithmetical machines which were feasible even in the limited technology of their time. Leibniz even dreamed of fully automatic deduction engines like those of today. Even now we have still not quite completed his dream – we cannot yet settle any and all disputes merely by powering up our laptops and saying to each other: calculemus. We still have to do the difficult job of formalizing the dispute as a proof problem in FOL. It may not be long, however, before computational conflict resolution turns out to be one more successful application of computational logic.

As modern mathematics grew in sophistication, the limitations of the syllogistic framework became more and more obvious. From the eighteenth century onwards mathematicians were routinely making proofs whose deductive patterns fell outside the Aristotelian framework. Nineteenth-century logicians such as Boole, Schroeder, de Morgan, Jevons, and Peirce tried to expand the repertoire of logical analysis accordingly, but with only partial success. As the end of the nineteenth century approached, it was clear that a satisfactory general logical theory was needed that would cover all possible logical inferences. Such a theory finally arrived, in 1879.

4   Frege's Thought Notation

The new logic was Frege's *Begriffschrifft*, alias (in a weird graphical notation) FOL ([4], pp. 5 - 82). One can reasonably compare the historical significance of its arrival on the scientific scene with that of the integral and differential calculus. It opened up an entirely new world of possibilities by identifying and modelling the way the mind works when reasoning deductively. Frege's German name for FOL means something like *Thought Notation*.

Frege's breakthough was followed by fifty years of brilliant exploration of its strengths and limitations by many mathematicians. The heroic efforts of Russell and Whitehead (following the lead of Peano, Dedekind, Cantor, Zermelo, and Frege himself) to express all of mathematics in the new notation showed that it could in principle be done. In the course of this investigation, new kinds of foundational problems appeared. The new logical tool had made it possible not only to detect and expose these foundational problems, but also to analyze them and fix them.

It soon became evident that the syntactic concepts comprising the notation for predicates and the rules governing inference forms needed to be supplemented by appropriate *semantic* ideas. Frege himself had discussed this, but not in a mathematically useful way. Russell's theory of types was also an attempt to get at the basic semantic issues. The most natural, intuitive and fruitful approach turned out to be the axiomatization, in the predicate calculus notation, of the concept of a set. Once this was done the way was cleared for a proper semantic foundation to be given to FOL itself. The rigorous mathematical concept of an interpretation, and of the denotation of a formula within an interpretation, was introduced by Alfred Tarski, who thus completed, in 1929, the fundamentals of the semantics of FOL ([5], p. 277). From the beginning FOL had come with the syntactic property, ascribable to sentences, of being formally derivable. Now it was possible to add to it the semantic properties, ascribable to sentences, of being true (in a given interpretation) and logically true (true in all interpretations). The notion of logical consequence could now be defined by saying that a sentence S logically follows from a sentence P if there is no interpretation in which P is true and S is false.

5   Completeness: Herbrand and Gödel

This now made it possible to raise the following fundamental question about FOL: is the following Completeness Theorem provable: for all sentences S and P, S is formally derivable from P if and only if S logically follows from P?

The question was soon positively answered, independently, in their respective doctoral theses, by two graduate students. Kurt Gödel received his degree on February 6, 1930 at the University of Vienna, aged 23, and Jacques Herbrand received his at the Sorbonne on 11 June, 1930, aged 22 ([4], pp. 582 ff., and pp 525 ff.). Today's graduate students can be forgiven for thinking of these giants of our field as wise old greybeards who made their discoveries only after decades of experience. In fact they had not been around very long, and were relatively inexperienced and new to FOL.

The theorem is so important because the property of formal derivability is semidecidable: there is an algorithm by means of which, if a sentence S is in fact formally derivable from a sentence P, then this fact can be mechanically detected. Indeed, the detection procedure is usually organized in such a way that the detection consists of actually constructing a derivation of S from P. In other words, when looked at semantically, the syntactic detection algorithm becomes a proof procedure.

Herbrand did not live to see the power of the completeness theorem exploited usefully in modern implementations. He was killed in a climbing accident on July 27, 1931.

Gödel, however, lived until 1978, well into the era in which the power of the completeness theorem was widely displayed and appreciated. It is doubtful, however, whether he paid any attention to this development. Already by 1931, his interest had shifted to other areas of logic and mathematical foundations. After stunning the mathematical (and philosophical) world in 1931 with his famous incompleteness theorems ([4], pp. 592 ff.), he went off in yet another direction to prove (within FOL) the consistency of the axiom of choice and the generalized continuum hypothesis with each other and with the remaining axioms of set theory ([2]), leading to the later proof (by Paul Cohen) of their independence both from each other and from the remaining axioms ([6]).

Interestingly, it was also Gödel and Herbrand who played a major role in the computational part of computational logic. In the course of his proof of the incompletness theorems, Gödel introduced the first rigorous characterization of computability, in his definition of the class of the primitive recursive functions. In 1934 (reprinted in [7]) he broadened and completed his characterization of computability by defining the class of general recursive functions, following up a suggestion made to him by Herbrand in "a private communication".

6   Computation: Turing, Church, and von Neumann

In this way Gödel and Herbrand not only readied FOL for action, but also opened up the field of universal digital computation. Soon there were others. At the time of the proof of the completeness theorem in 1930, the 18-year-old Alan Turing was about become a freshman mathematics student at Cambridge University. Alonzo Church was already, at age 28, an instructor in the mathematics department at Princeton. John von Neumann had just emigrated, at age 27, to Princeton, where he was to spend the rest of his life. By 1936 these five had essentially laid the basis for the modern era of computing, as well as its intimate relationship with logic.

Turing's 1936 paper (reprinted in [7]) on Hilbert's Decision Problem was crucial. Ostensibly it was yet another attempt to characterize with mathematical precision the concept of computability, which he needed to do in order to show that there is no fixed computation procedure by means of which every definite mathematical assertion can be decided (determined to be true or determined to be false).

Alonzo Church independently reached the same result at essentially the same time, using his own quite different computational theory (reprinted in [7]) of lambda-definability. In either form, its significance for computational logic is that it proved the impossibility of a decision procedure for FOL. The semidecision procedure reflecting the deductive completeness of FOL is all there is, and we have to be content to work with that.

Remarkable as this theoretical impossibility result was, the enormous practical significance of Turing's paper came from a technical device he introduced into his argument. This device turned out to be the theoretical design of the modern universal digital computer. The concept of a Turing machine, and in particular of a universal Turing machine, which can simulate the behavior of any individual Turing machine when supplied with a description of it, may well be the most important conceptual discovery of the entire twentieth century. Computability by the universal Turing machine became virtually overnight the criterion for absolute computability. Church's own criterion, lambda-definability, was shown by Turing to be equivalent to Turing computability. Other notions (e.g., Kleene's notion of deducibility in his equational-substitutional calculus, Post's notion of derivability within a Post production system) were similarly shown to be equivalent to Turing's notion. There was obviously a fundamental robustness here in the basic concept of computability, which led Alonzo Church to postulate that any function which was found to be effectively computatble would in fact be computable by a Turing machine ("Church's Thesis").

During the two years from 1936 to 1938 that Turing spent in Princeton, working on a Ph.D. with Church as supervisor, he and von Neumann became friends. In 1938 von Neumann offered Turing a job as his assistant at the Institute for Advanced Study, and Turing might well have accepted the offer if it had not been for the threat of World War 2. Turing was summoned back to Britain to take part in the famous Bletchley Park code-breaking project, in which his role has since become legendary.

Von Neumann had been enormously impressed by Turing's universal machine concept and continued to ponder it even as his wide-ranging interests and national responsibilities in mathematics, physics and engineering occupied most of his attention and time. He was particularly concerned to improve computing technology, to support the increasingly more complex numerical computing tasks which were crucial in carrying out wartime weapons development. His knowledge of Turing's idea was soon to take on great practical significance in the rapid development of the universal electronic digital computer throughout the 1940s. He immediately saw the tremendous implications of the electronic digital computing technology being developed by Eckert and Mauchly at the University of Pennsylvania, and essentially assumed command of the project. This enabled him to see to it that Turing's idea of completely universal computing was embodied in the earliest American computers in 1946.

The work at Bletchley Park had also included the development of electronic digital computing technology, and it was used in devices designed for the special purposes of cryptography. Having been centrally involved in this engineering development, Turing came out of the war in 1945 ready and eager to design and build a full-fledged universal electronic digital computer based on his 1936 ideas, and to apply it to a wide variety of problems. One kind of problem which fascinated him was to write programs which would carry out intelligent reasoning and engage in interesting conversation. In 1950 he published his famous essay in the philosophical journal *Mind* discussing artificial intelligence and computing. In this essay he did not deal directly with automated deduction as such, but there can be little doubt that he was very much aware of the possibilities. He did not live to see computational logic take off. His death in 1954 occurred just as things were getting going.

7   Computational Logic

In that very same year, 1954, Martin Davis (reprinted in [8]) carried out one of the earliest computational logic experiments by programming and running, on von Neumann's Institute for Advanced Study computer in Princeton, Presburger's Decision Procedure for the first order theory of integer addition. The computation ran only very slowly, as well it might, given the algorithm's worse than exponential complexity. Davis later wryly commented that its great triumph was to prove that the sum of two even numbers is itself an even number.

Martin Davis and others then began in earnest the serious computational applications of FOL. The computational significance of the Gödel-Herbrand completeness theorem was tantalizingly clear to them. In 1955 a particularly attractive and elegant version of the basic proof procedure – the semantic tableau method – was described (independently) by Evert Beth [9] and Jaakko Hintikka [10]. I can still remember the strong impression made on me, as a graduate student in philosophy, when I first read their descriptions of this method. They pointed out the intimate relationship of the semantic or analytic tableau algorithm to the natural deductive framework of the sequent calculi pioneered in the mid-1930s by Gerhard Gentzen [11]. Especially vivid was the intuitive interpretation of a growing, ramifying semantic tableau as the on-going record of an organized systematic search, with the natural diagrammatic structure of a tree, for a counterexample to the universally quantified sentence written at the root of the tree. The closure of the tableau then signified the failure of the search for, and hence the impossibility of, such a counterexample. This diagrammatic record of the failed search (the closed tableau) itself literally becomes a proof, with each of its steps corresponding to an inference sanctioned by some sequent pattern in the Gentzen-style logic. One simply turns it upside-down and reads it from the tips back towards the root. A most elegant concept as well as a computationally powerful technique!

8   Heuristics and Algorithms: The Dartmouth and Cornell Meetings

In the 1950's there occurred two meetings of major importance in the history of computational logic. The first was the 1956 Dartmouth conference on Artificial Intelligence, at which Herbert Simon and Allen Newell first described their heuristic theorem-proving work. Using the RAND Corporation's von Neumann computer JOHNNIAC, they had programmed *a heuristic search* for proofs in the version of the propositional calculus formulated by Russell and Whitehead. This pioneering experiment in computational logic attracted wide attention as an attempt to reproduce computationally the actual human proof-seeking behavior of a person searching for a proof of a given formula in that system. In their published accounts (reprinted in [8], Volume 1) of this experiment they claimed that the only alternative algorithmic proof-seeking technique offered by logic was the so-called "British Museum" method of enumerating all possible proofs in the hope that one would eventually turn up that proved the theorem being considered.

This was of course both unfair and unwise, for it simply advertised their lack of knowledge of the proof procedures already developed by logicians. Hao Wang showed in 1960 how easy the search for these proofs became if one used a semantic tableau method (reprinted in [8], Volume 1, pp. 244-266).

The other significant event was the 1957 Cornell Summer School in Logic. Martin Davis, Hilary Putnam, Paul Gilmore, Abraham Robinson and IBM's Herbert Gelernter were among those attending. The latter gave a talk on his heuristic program for finding proofs of theorems in elementary geometry, in which he made use of ideas very similar to those of Simon and Newell. Abraham Robinson was provoked by Gelernter's advocacy of heuristic, psychological methods to give an extempore lecture (reprinted in [8], Volume 1) on the power of logical methods in proof seeking, stressing the computational significance of Herbrand's version of the FOL completeness theorem and especially of the technique of elimination of existential quantifiers by introducing Skolem function sysmbols. One can see now how this talk in 1957 must have motivated Gilmore, Davis and Putnam to write their Herbrand-based proof procedure programs. Their papers are reprinted in [8], Volume 1, and were based fundamentally on the idea of systematically enumerating the Herbrand Universe of a proposed theorem – namely, the (usually infinite) set of all terms constructible from the function symbols and individual constants which (after its Skolemization) the proposed theorem contained.   This technique is actually the computational version of Herbrand's so-called Property B method. It did not seem to be realized (as in retrospect it perhaps ought to have been) that this Property B method, involving a systematic enumeration of all possible instantiations over the Herbrand Universe, is really a version of the British Museum method so rightly derided by Simon and Newell.

9   Combinatorial Explosions with Herbrand's Property B

These first implementations of the Herbrand FOL proof procedure thus revealed the importance of trying to do better than merely hoping for the best as the exhaustive enumeration forlornly ground on, or than guessing the instantiations that might be the crucial ones in terminating the process. In fact, Herbrand himself had already in 1930 shown how to avoid this enumerative procedure, in what he called the Property A method. The key to Herbrand's Property A method is the idea of unification.

Herbrand's writing style in his doctoral thesis was not, to put it mildly, always clear. As a consequence, his exposition of the Property A method is hard to follow, and is in fact easily overlooked. At any rate, it seems to have attracted no attention except in retrospect, after the independent discovery of unification by Prawitz thirty years later.

In retrospect, it is nevertheless quite astonishing that this beautiful, natural and powerful idea was not immediately taken up in the early 1930s by the theoreticians of first order logic.

10   Prawitz's Independent Rediscovery of Unification Ushers in Resolution

In 1960 an extraordinary thing happened. The Swedish logician Dag Prawitz independently rediscovered unification, the powerful secret which had been buried for 30 years in the obscurity of the Property A section of Herbrand's thesis. This turned out to be an important moment in the history of computational logic. Ironically, Prawitz' paper (reprinted in [8], Volume 1) too was rather inaccessible. William Davidon, a physicist at Argonne, drew my attention to Prawitz' paper in 1962, two years after it had first appeared. I wish I had known about it sooner. It completely redirected my own increasingly frustrated efforts to improve the computational efficiency of the Davis-Putnam Herbrand Property B proof procedure. Once I had managed to recast the unification algorithm into a suitable form, I found a way to combine the Cut Rule with unification so as to produce a rule of inference of a new machine-oriented kind. It was machine-oriented because in order to obtain the much greater deductive power than had hitherto been the norm, it required much more computational effort to apply it than traditional human-oriented rules typically required. In writing this work up for publication, when I needed to think of a name for my new rule, I decided to call it "resolution", but at this distance in time I have forgotten why. This was in 1963. The resolution paper took more than another year to reach print, finally coming out in January 1965 (it is reprinted in [8], Volume 1).

The trick of combining a known inference rule with unification can of course be applied to many other rules besides the cut rule. At Argonne, George Robinson and Larry Wos quickly saw this, and they applied it to the rule of Equality Substitution, producing another powerful new machine-oriented rule which they subsequently exploited with much success.   They called their new rule "paramodulation". Their paper is reprinted in [8], Volume 2.   It and resolution have been mainstays of the famous Argonne theorem provers, such as McCune's OTTER, ever since. See, for example, the 1991 survey ([12], pp. 297 ff.) by Larry Wos.

After 1965 there ensued a somewhat frenetic period of exploration of what could now be done with the help of these new unification-based rules of inference. They were recognized as a big boost in the development of an efficient, practical automated deduction technology.   People quite rapidly came up with ways to adapt them to other computational applications quite different from their original application, mechanical theorem-proving.

11   Computational Logic in Edinburgh: The A.I. Wars

Some of my memories of this period are still vivid. In 1965 Bernard Meltzer spent a three-month study leave at Rice University, where I was then a member of the Philosophy Department.   Bernard rapidly assimilated the new resolution technique, and on his return to Edinburgh immediately organized a new research group which he called the Metamathematics Unit, with the aim of pursuing full-time mechanical theorem-proving research. This turned out to be an important event. Edinburgh was already making its mark in Artificial Intelligence. Donald Michie, Christopher Longuet-Higgins, and Rod Burstall, in addition to Bernard Meltzer, were realigning their scientific careers in order to pursue AI full-time. Over the next few years Bernard's group became a lively, intense critical mass of graduate students who would go on to become leaders in computational logic: Bob Kowalski, Pat Hayes, Frank Brown, Donald Kuehner, Bob Boyer, J Strother Moore. Next door, in Donald Michie's Machine Intelligence group, were Gordon Plotkin, David Warren, Maarten van Emden and John Darlington. I spent a sabbatical year with these groups, from May 1967 to September 1968, and thereafter visited them for several extended study periods. Edinburgh was, at that time, the place to be. It was a time of great excitement and intellectual ferment. There was a pervasive feeling of optimism, of pioneering, of great things to come. We had fruitful visits from people in other AI centers: John McCarthy, Bert Raphael, Nils Nilsson, Cordell Green, Keith Clark, Carl Hewitt, Seymour Papert, Gerald Sussman. The last three were advocates of the MIT view (championed by Marvin Minsky) that computational logic was not at all the AI panacea some people thought it was. The MIT view was that the engineering of machine intelligence would have to be based on heuristic, procedural, associative organization of knowledge. The "logic" view (championed by John McCarthy) was that for AI purposes knowledge should be axiomatized declaratively using FOL, and mechanized thinking should consist of theorem-proving computation. This was, at that time, the view prevailing in Edinburgh and Stanford. The two opposing views gave rise to some stimulating debates with the MIT visitors.

Cordell Green's question-answering system in 1969 ([13], pp. 219 ff.) demonstrated the possibilities of intelligent deductive datebases and automatic robot planning using a resolution theorem prover as the reasoning engine. He showed how John McCarthy's 1959 scheme of a deductive Advice Taker (reprinted in [14]) could be implemented.

12   The Colmerauer-Kowalski Encounter

The possibilities of resolution logic for computational linguistics were immediately seen by Alain Colmerauer, who had been working in Grenoble since 1963 on parsing and syntactic analysis ([15]). By 1968 he was working for an Automatic Translation Project in Montreal, where he developed what later could be seen as a precursor of Prolog (the Q-systems formalism). Returning to France in 1970 he took up the theme of making deductions from texts instead of just parsing them, and began to study the resolution principle. This brought him into contact with Edinburgh's Bob Kowalski, who had, in collaboration with Donald Kuehner ([16]), recently devised a beautiful refinement of resolution (SL-resolution) which permitted linear deductions and which could be implemented with great efficiency, as Boyer and Moore soon showed ([17], pp.101 ff.) by the first of their many programming masterpieces, the Edinburgh Structure-Sharing Linear Resolution Theorem Prover.

The result of this Colmerauer-Kowalski encounter was the birth of Prolog and of logic programming.   Colmerauer's colleague Philippe Roussel, following discussions with Boyer and Moore, designed the first modern Prolog interpreter using Boyer-Moore's shared data structures. Implemented in Fortran by Meloni and Battani, this version of Prolog was widely disseminated and subsequently improved, in Edinburgh, by David Warren.

13   Computational Logic Officially Recognized: Prolog's Spectacular Debut

By 1970 the feeling had grown that Bernard Meltzer's Metamathematics Unit might be better named, considering what what was going on under its auspices. At the 1970 Machine Intelligence Workshop in Edinburgh, in a paper ([18], pp. 63-72) discussing how to program unification more efficiently, I suggested that "computational logic" might be better than "theorem proving" as a description of the new field we all seemed now to be working in. By December 1971 Bernard had convinced the university administration to sign on to this renaming. From that date onwards, his official stationery bore the letterhead: University of Edinburgh: Department of Computational Logic.

During the 1970s logic programming moved to the center of the stage of computational logic, thanks to the immediate applicability, availability, and attractiveness of the Marseille - Edinburgh Prolog implementation, and to Bob Kowalski's eloquent and tireless advocacy of the new programming paradigm. In 1977, I was present at the session of the Lisp and Functional Programming Symposium in Rochester, New York, when David Warren awed a partisan audience of LISP devotees with his report of the efficiency of the Edinburgh Prolog system, compared with that of Lisp ([19]). A little later, in [20], Bob Kowalski spelled out the case for concluding that, as Prolog was showing in practice, the Horn clause version of resolution was the ideal programming instrument for all Artificial Intelligence research, in that it could be used to represent knowledge declaratively in a form that, without any modification, could then be run procedurally on the computer. Knowledge was both declarative and procedural at once: the "nothing buttery" of the contending factions in the Great A.I. War now could be seen as mere partisan fundamentalist fanaticism.

14   The Fifth Generation Project

These were stirring times indeed. In Japan, as the 1970s drew to a close, there were bold plans afoot which would soon startle the computing world. The 10-year Fifth Generation Project was three years (1979 to 1981) in the planning, and formally began in April 1982. A compact retrospective summary of the project is given by Hidehiko Tanaka in his Chairman's message in [21]. It was a pleasant surprise to learn around 1980 that this major national research and development effort was to be a large-scale concerted attempt to advance the state of the art in computer technology by concentrating on knowledge information processing using Logic Programming as a central concept and technique.

The decade of the 1980s was dominated by the Fifth Generation Project. It was gratifying for the computational logic community to observe the startled response of the authorities in the United States and Europe to such an unexpectedly sophisticated and powerful challenge from a country which had hitherto tended to be viewed as a follower rather than a leader. One of the splendid features of the Fifth Generation Project was its wise and generous provision for worldwide cooperation and interaction between Japanese researchers and researchers from every country where logic programming was being studied and developed.

In 1984 the first issue of The Journal of Logic Programming appeared. In the Editor's Introduction I noted [22] that research activity in logic programming had grown rapidly since 1971, when the first Prolog system introduced the idea, and that a measure of the extent of this growth was the size of the comprehensive bibliography of logic programming compiled by Michael Poe of Digital Equipment Corporation, which contains over 700 entries. The substantial length of Poe's bibliography in [22] was only one sign of the explosion of interest in logic programming. Another sign was the size and frequency of international conferences and workshops devoted to the subject, and the increasing number of people attending them from all over the world. It was inevitable that enthusiastic and in some respects overoptimistic expectations for the future of the new programming paradigm would eventually be followed by a more sober realism, not to say a backlash.

15   The Aftermath: Pure Logic Programming not a Complete Panacea

There is no getting around the fact that a purely declarative programming language, with a purely evaluative deductive engine, lacks the capability for initiating and controlling events: what should happen, and where, when, and how. If there are no side effects, then there are no side effects, and that is that. This applies both to internal events in the steps of execution of the deduction or evaluation computation, and to external events in the outside world, at a minimum to the input and output of data, but (for example if the program is functioning as an operating system) to the control of many other external sensors and actuators besides. One wants to create and manipulate objects which have states.

So although the pure declarative logic programming paradigm may be a thing of beauty and a joy forever, it is a practically useless engineering tool. To be useful, its means of expression must be augmented by imperative constructs which will permit the programmer to design, and oblige the computer to execute, happenings – side effects.

There was a tendency (there still may be, but I am a little out of touch with the current climate of opinion on this) to deplore side effects, in the spirit of Edsger Dijkstra's famous "GO TO considered harmful" letter to the Editor of the Communications of the ACM. There is no denying that one can get into a terrible mess by abusing imperative constructs, often creating (as Dijkstra wrote elsewhere) a "disgusting mass of undigested complexity" on even a single page of code. The remedy, however, is surely not to banish imperative constructs from our programming languages, but to cultivate a discipline of programming which even when using imperative constructs will aim at avoiding errors and promoting intelligibility.

So the Prolog which looked as if it might well sweep the computing world off its feet was not simply the pure embodiment of Horn clause resolution, but a professional engineering tool crucially incorporating a repertoire of imperative constructs: sequential execution of steps (namely a guaranteed order in which the subgoals would be tried), cut (for pruning the search on the fly), assert and retract (for changing the program during the computation) and (of course) read, print, and so on.

Bob Kowalski's equation ALGORITHM = LOGIC + CONTROL summarized the discipline of programming needed to exploit the new paradigm - strict separation of the declarative from the imperative aspects. One must learn how to keep the denotation (the presumably intended declarative meaning, as specified by the clauses) of a program fixed while purposefully varying the process by which it is computed (the pragmatic meaning, as specified by the sequence of the clauses and, within each clause, the sequence of the literals, together with the other imperative constructs). Versions of Prolog began to reflect this ideal strict separation, by offering the programmer the use of such features as modes and various other pragmatic comments and hints.

16   Realism: Side   Effects,   Concurrency,   Software Engineering

Others were less concerned with declarative purism and the holy grail of dispensing with all imperative organization of explicit control. In some sense they went to the opposite extreme and explored how far one could go by making the most intelligent use of the clausal formalism as a means of specifying computational events.

Ehud Shapiro, Keith Clark, Kazunori Ueda and others followed this direction and showed how concurrency could be specified and controlled within the new idiom. If you are going into the business of programming a system whose purpose is to organize computations as complexes of interacting events evolving over time, you have to be able not only to describe the processes you want to have happen but also to start them going, maintain control over them once they are under way, and stop them when they have gone far enough, all the while controlling their interaction and communication with each other, and managing their consumption of system resources. An operating system is of course just such a system. It was therefore a triumph of the concurrent logic programming methodology when the Fifth Generation Project in 1992 successfully concluded a decade of work having designed, built and successfully run the operating system of the ICOT knowledge processing parallel computation system entirely in the Flat Guarded Horn Clause programming language [21].

Much had been achieved technologically and scientifically at ICOT by 1994, when the project (which with a two-year extension had lasted twelve years) finally closed down, but there continued (and continues) to be a splendid spinoff in the form of a worldwide community of researchers and entrepreneurs who were drawn together by the ICOT adventure and remain linked by a common commitment to the future of logic programming. Type "logic programming" into the search window of a search engine. There emerges a cornucopia of links to websites all over the world dealing either academically or commercially (or sometimes both) with LP and its applications.

17   Robbins' Conjecture Proved by Argonne's Theorem Prover

Although logic programming had occupied the center of the stage for fifteen years or so, the original motivation of pursuing improved automatic deduction techniques for the sake of proof discovery was still alive and well. In 1996 there occurred a significant and exciting event which highlighted this fact. Several groups have steadily continued to investigate the application of unification-based inference engines, term-rewriting systems, and proof-finding search strategies to the classic task of discovering proofs for mathematical theorems. Most notable among these has been the Argonne group under the leadership of Larry Wos. Wos has continued to lead Argonne's tightly focussed quest for nontrivial machine-generated proofs for over thirty-five years. In 1984 his group was joined by William McCune, who quickly made his mark in the form of the highly successful theorem proving program OTTER, which enabled the Argonne group to undertake a large-scale pursuit of computing real mathematical proofs. The spirit of the Argonne program was similar to that of Woody Bledsoe, who at the University of Texas headed a research group devoted to automating the discovery of proofs in what Woody always referred to as "real" mathematics. At the symposium celebrating Woody's seventieth birthday in November 1991 [12] Larry Wos reviewed the steady progress in machine proof-finding made with the help of McCune's OTTER, reporting that already copies of that program were at work in several other research centers in various parts of the world. Sadly, Woody did not live to relish the moment in 1996 when Argonne's project paid off brilliantly in the machine discovery of what was undoubtedly a "real" mathematical proof.

The Argonne group's achievement is comparable with that of the program developed by the IBM Deep Blue group which famously defeated the world chess champion Kasparov. Both events demonstrated how systematic, nonhuman combinatorial search, if organized sufficiently cleverly and carried out at sufficiently high speeds, can rival even the best human performance based heuristically and associatively on expertise, intuition, and judgment. What the Argonne program did was to find a proof of the Robbins conjecture that a particular set of three equations is powerful enough to capture all of the laws of

Boolean algebra. This conjecture had remained unproved since it was formulated in the 1930s by Herbert Robbins at Harvard. It had been tackled, without success, by many "real" matheticians, including Alfred Tarski. Argonne attacked the problem with a new McCune-designed program EQP embodying a specialized form of unification in which the associative and commutative laws were integrated. After 20 hours of search on a SPARC 2 workstation, EQP found a proof. Robbins' Conjecture may not be Fermat's Last Theorem, but it is certainly "real" mathematics. Woody Bledsoe would have been delighted, as we all were, to see the description of this noteworthy success for computational logic written up prominently in the science section of the New York Times on December 10, 1996.

18   Proliferation of Computational Logic

By now, logic programming had completed a quarter-century of fruitful scientific and technological ferment. The new programming paradigm, exploding in 1971 following the original Marseille-Edinburgh interaction, had by now proliferated into an array of descendants. A diagram of this genesis would look like the cascade of elementary particle tracks in a high-energy physics experiment. We are now seeing a number of interesting and significant phenomena signalling this proliferation.

The transition from calling our field "logic programming" to calling it "computational logic" is only one such signal. It was becoming obvious that the former phrase had come to mean a narrower interest within a broader framework of possible interests, each characterized by some sort of a connection between computing and logic.

As we noted earlier, the statement of scope of the new ACM journal TOCL points out that the field of computational logic consists of all uses of logic in computer science. It goes on to list many of these explicitly: artificial intelligence; computational complexity; database systems; programming languages; automata and temporal logic; automated deduction; automated software verification; commonsense and nonmonotonic reasoning; constraint programming; finite model theory; complexity of logical theories; functional programming and lambda calculus; concurrency calculi and tools; inductive logic programming and machine learning; logical aspects of computational complexity; logical aspects of databases; logic programming; logics of uncertainty; modal logics, including dynamic and epistemic logics; model checking; program development; program specification; proof theory; term rewriting systems; type theory and logical frameworks.

19   A Look at the Future: Some Challenges

So the year 2000 marks a turning point. It is the closing of the opening eventful chapter in a story which is still developing. We all naturally wonder what will happen next. David Hilbert began his address to the International Congress of

Mathematicians by asking: who of us would not be glad to lift the veil behind which the future lies hidden; to cast a glance at the next advances of our science and at the secrets of its development during future centuries? The list of open problems he then posed was intended to – and certainly did – help to steer the course of mathematics over the next decades. Can we hope to come up with a list of problems to help shape the future of computational logic? The program committee for this conference thought that at least we ought to try, and its chairman John Lloyd therefore set up an informal email committee to come up with some ideas as to what the main themes and challenges are for computational logic in the new millennium. The following challenges are therefore mainly distilled from communications I have received over the past three months or so from members of this group: Krzysztof Apt, Marc Bezem, Maurice Brynooghe, Jacques Cohen, Alain Colmerauer, Veronica Dahl, Marc Denecker, Danny De Schreye, Pierre Flener, Koichi Furukawa, Gopal Gupta, Pat Hill, Michael Kifer, Bob Kowalski, Kung-Kiu Lau, Jean-Louis and Catherine Lassez, John Lloyd, Kim Marriott, Dale Miller, Jack Minker, Lee Naish, Catuscia Palamidessi, Alberto Pettorossi, Taisuke Sato, and Kazunori Ueda. My thanks to all of them. I hope they will forgive me for having added one or two thoughts of my own. Here are some of the challenges we think worth pondering.

19.1   To Shed Further Light on the P = NP Problem

The field of computational complexity provides today's outstanding challenge to computational logic theorists. Steve Cook was originally led to formulate the P = NP problem by his analysis of the complexity of testing a finite set S of clauses for truth-functional satisfiability. This task certainly seems exponential: if S contains n distinct atoms and is unsatisfiable then every one of the 2^n combinations of truth values must make all the clauses in S come out false simultaneously. All the ways we know of for checking S for satisfiability thus boil down to searching this set of combinations. So why are we are still unable to prove what most people now strongly believe, that this problem is exponentially complex? We not only want to know the answer to the problem, but we also want to understand why it is such a hard problem.

This challenge was only one of several which call for an explanation of one or another puzzling fact. The next one is another.

19.2   To Explain the Intelligibility/Efficiency Trade-off

This trade-off is familiar to all programmers and certainly to all logic programmers. Why is it that the easier a program is to understand, the less efficient it tends to be? Conversely, why do more computationally efficient programs tend to be more difficult to reason about? It is this curious epistemological reciprocity which forces us to develop techniques for program transformations, program verification, and program synthesis. It is as though there is a deep mismatch between our brains and our computing devices. One of the big advantages claimed for logic programming – and more generally for declarative programming – is the natural intelligibility of programs which are essentially just declarations - sets of mutually recursive definitions of predicates and functions. But then we have to face the fact that "naive" programs written in this way almost always need to be drastically reformulated so as to be made computationally efficient. In the transformation they almost always become more obscure. This is a price we have become used to paying. But why should we have to pay this price? It surely must have something to do with the peculiar constraints under which the human mind is forced to work, as well as with objective considerations of the logical structure and organization of the algorithms and data structures. An explanation, if we ever find one, will presumably therefore have to be partly psychological, partly physiological, partly logical.

The nature of our brains, entailing the constraints under which we are forced to perceive and think about complex structures and systems, similarly raises the next challenge.

19.3   To Explain Why Imperative Constructs are Harmful to a Program's Intelligibility

This is obviously related to the previous challenge.   It has become the conventional wisdom that imperative programming constructs are at best an unpleasaant necessity. We are supposed to believe that while we apparently can't do without them, they are a deplorable source of confusion and unintelligibility in our programs. In Prolog the notorious CUT construct is deployed masterfully by virtuoso logic programmers but regretted by those who value the elegance and clarity of "pure" Prolog. Why? The sequential flow of control is counted on by programmers to obtain the effects they want. If these features are indispensible to writing effective programs, in practice, then why does our theory, not to say our idealogy, treat them as pariahs? This is a kind of intellectual hypocrisy. It may well be that imperative constructs are dangerous, but we are acting as though it is impossible that our programming methodology should ever be able to manage them safely. If true, this is extremely important, but it has to be proved rather than just assumed.   The same issue arises, of course, in the case of functional programming.   "Pure" declarativeness of a program is promoted as an ideal stylistic desideratum but (as, e.g., in classical Lisp) hardly ever a feature of practical programs.   The imperative features of "real" Lisp are in practice indispensible. The dominance of unashamedly imperative languages like C, C++, and Java in the "outside world" is rooted in their frank acceptance of the imperative facts of computational life. But this is precisely what earns them the scorn of the declarative purists. Surely this is an absurd situation. It is long overdue to put this issue to rest and to reconcile lofty but unrealistic ideals with the realities of actual software engineering practice.

A similar issue arises within logic itself, quite apart from computation. If logic is to be a satisfactory science of reasoning, then it must face the following challenge.

19.4   To Explain the (Informal, Intuitive) / (Formal, Rigorous) Trade-off in Proofs

Why is it that intuitive, easy-to-understand proofs tend to become more complex, less intelligible and less intuitive, when they are formalized in order to make them more rigorous? This is suspiciously like the trade-offs in the previous three challenges. What, anyway, is rigor? What is intuition? These concepts are epistemological rather than logical. We all experience this trade-off in our everyday logical experience, but we lack an explanation for it. It is just something we put up with, but at present it is a mystery. If logic cannot explain it, then logic is lacking something important.

The prominence of constraint logic programming in current research raises the following challenge.

19.5   To Understand the Limits of Extending Constraint Logic Programming

As constraint solving is extended to even richer domains, there is a need to know how far automatic methods of constraint satisfaction can in fact feasibly be extended. It would appear that directed combinatorial search is at the bottom of most constraint solution techniques, just as it is in the case of systematic proof procedures. There must then be ultimate practical limits imposed on constraint-solving searches by sheer computational complexity. It would certainly seem to be so in the classic cases, for example, of Boolean satisfiability, or the Travelling Salesman Problem. The concept of constraint logic programming is open-ended and embarrassingly general. The basic problem is simply to find, or construct, an entity X which satisfies a given property P. Almost any problem can be thrown into this form. For example the writing of a program to meet given specifications fits this description. So does dividing one number Y by another number Z: it solves the problem to find a number R such that $R = Y/Z$. So does composing a fugue for four voices using a given theme.

It is illuminating, as a background to this challenge, to recall the stages by which the increasingly rich versions of constraint logic programming emerged historically. Alain Colmerauer's reformulation of unification for Prolog II originally led him to consider constraint programming [15]. Just as had Herbrand in 1930, and Prawitz in 1960, Colmerauer in 1980 saw unification itself as a constraint problem, of satisfying a system of equations in a domain of terms. After loosening the constraints to permit cyclic (infinite) terms as solutions of equations like $x = f(x)$, which had the virtue of eliminating the need for an occur check, he also admitted inequations as well as equations. It became clear that unification was just a special case of the general concept of constraint solving in a given domain with given operations and relations, which led him to explore constraint solving in richer domains. Prolog III could also handle two-valued Boolean algebra and a numerical domain, involving equations, inequalities and infinite precision arithmetical operations. Thus logic programming morphed by stages into the more general process of finding a satisfying assignment of values to a set of unknowns subjected to a constraint (i.e., a sentence) involving operations and relations defined over a given domain. The computer solves the constraint by finding or somehow computing values which, when assigned to its free variables, make it come out true. Later in the 1980s Joxan Jaffar and Jean-Louis Lassez further elaborated these ideas, thus deliberately moving logic programming into the general area of mathematical programming which had formed the heart of Operations Research since the 1940s. Constraint solving of course is an even older mathematical idea, going back to the classical methods of Gauss and Fourier, and to Lagrange, Bernouilli and the calculus of variations. In its most general form it is extremely ancient: it is nothing other than the fundamental activity of mathematics itself: to write down an open sentence of some kind, and then to find the values of its free variables, if any, which make it true.

In summary: the challenge is to pull together all the diversity within the general notion of constraint satisfaction programming, and to try to develop a unified theory to support, if possible, a single formalism in which to formulate all such problems and a single implementation in which to compute the solutions to the solvable ones.

It has not escaped the notice of most people in our field that despite our better mousetrap the world has not yet beaten a path to our door. We are challenged not just to try to make our mousetrap even better but to find ways of convincing outsiders. We need applications of existing LP and CLP technology which will attract the attention and enthusiasm of the wider computing world. Lisp has had an opportunity to do this, and it too has fallen short of perhaps over-hyped expectations of wide adoption. Logic programming still has vast unrealized potential as a universal programming tool. The challenge is to apply it to real problems in ways that outdo the alternatives.

Kazunori Ueda and Catuscia Palamidessi both stress the importance of Concurrent Constraint Programming. Catuscia maintains that concurrency itself poses a fundamental challenge, whether or not it is linked to constraint programming. She even suggests that the notion of concurrent computation may require an extension or a reformulation of the theory of computability, although she notes that this challenge is of course not specific to computational logic. It is interesting to note that the early computing models of Turing and Post avoided the issue of concurrency entirely.

19.6   To Find New Killer Applications for LP

This challenge has always been with us and will always be with us. In general, advances and evolution in the methodology and paradigms of logic programming have repeatedly been stimulated and driven by demands imposed by applications. The first such application was the parsing of natural languages (Alain Colmerauer and Veronica Dahl both say this is still the most natural LP application). Future applications to natural language processing could well be killers. Jack Minker points out that the deductive retrieval of information from databases was one of the earliest applications and today still has an enormous unrealized potential.

Following the example of Burstall and Darlington in functional programming, Ehud Shapiro and others soon demonstrated the elegance and power of the paradigm in the specification, synthesis, transformation, debugging and verification of logic programs. Software engineering is a hugely promising application area. Kung-Kiu Lau and Dale Miller emphasize the need for software engineering applications dealing with programming in the large - the high level organization of modules in ways suitable for re-use and component-based assembly by users other than the original composers.

Shapiro, Clark, Ueda and others then opened up the treatment of concurrency, shedding new light on the logic of message-passing and the nature of parallel processes through the remarkable properties of partial binding of logic variables. Shapiro and Takeuchi showed how the LP paradigm could embody the object-oriented programming style, and of course LP came to the fore in the representation of knowledge in the programming and control of robots and in other artificial intelligence systems. Already there are signs of further development in the direction of parallel and high-performance computing, distributed and network computing, and real-time and mobile computing. The challenge is to anticipate and stay ahead of these potential killer applications by enriching the presentation of the basic LP methodology to facilitate the efficient and smooth building-in of suitable special concepts and processes to deal with them. This may well (as it has in the past) call for the design of special purpose languages and systems, each tailored to a specific class of applications. Whatever form it takes, the challenge is to demonstrate the power of LP by actual examples, not just to expound its virtues in the abstract.

Examples of killer applications will help, but it is better to teach people to fish for themselves rather than simply to throw them an occasional salmon or halibut. The challenge is to provide the world with an irresistably superior set of programming tools and accompanying methodology, which will naturally replace the existing status quo.

19.7   To Enhance and Propagate the Declarative Programming Paradigm

Major potential growth areas within CL include the development of higher order logic programming. Higher order logic has already been applied (by Peter Andrews and Dale Miller, for example) to the development of higher order theorem provers. The functional programming community has for years been preaching and illustrating the conceptual power of higher order notions in writing elegantly concise programs and making possible the construction and encapsulation of large, high level computational modules. The consequences for software engineering are many, but as yet the software engineers, even the more theoretically inclined among them, have not responded to these attractions by adopting the higher-order paradigm and incorporating it into their professional repertoire.

The computational logic community should feel challenged to carry out the necessary missionary work here too, as well as to develop the necessary programming tools and technical infrastructure.   Dale Miller points out that mechanical theorem provers for higher order logics have already been successfully applied experimentally in many areas including hardware verification and synthesis; verification of security and communications protocols; software verification, transformation and refinement; compiler construction; and concurrency. The higher order logics used to reason about these problems and the underlying theorem prover technology that support them are also active areas of research.   Higher order logic is however still a relatively esoteric corner of computational logic. Its conceptual basis has perhaps been unduly obscured in the past by an over-formal theoretical approach and by unnecessarily metaphysical conceptual foundations.   The computational formalisms based on the elegant Martin-Löf theory of types are not yet ready to be launched on an industrial scale. It is a challenge to bring higher order methods and ideas down to earth, and to demonstrate to the computing world at large that the rewards are great and the intellectual cost is reasonable.   Lambda-calculus computing has a simple operational rationale based on an equality logic of term rewriting.   Its essential idea is that of the normalization of a given expression.   Namely, a directed search is made for an equivalent expression which is in a form suitable as an answer. This process is also thought of as evaluation of the given expression.   Under suitable patterns of rewriting (e.g., by so-called lazy evaluation) a successful search for a normal form is guaranteed to succeed if a normal form exists.   In constraint satisfaction the essential idea is instantiation of a given expression: a directed search is made for an instance which is in a form suitable as an answer (e.g., if the given expression is a sentence, then the instance should be true). Both these ideas are simple yet powerful, and are extremely suitable as the basis for a pedagogical account of high level computation.

It has been a source of weakness in logic programming that there have been two major paradigms needlessly pitted against each other, competing in the same marketplace of ideas. The challenge is to end the segregation and merge the two. There is in any case, at bottom, only one idea.   So our final challenge is the following one.

19.8   To Integrate Functional Programming with Logic Programming

These are two only superficially different dialects of computational logic. It is inexplicable that the two idioms have been kept apart for so long within the computational logic repertory. We need a single programming language in which both kinds of programming are possible and can be used in combination with each other.   There have been a number of attempts to devise programming formalisms which integrate the two. None have so far been taken up seriously by users. This may well be because the systems offered so far have been only experimental and tentative. Some experiments have grafted evaluation on to a logic programming host, as for example, in the form of the limited arithmetical expressions allowed in Prolog. Others have grafted constraint satisfying onto a functional programming host in the form of the "setof" construct. More recently there have been attempts to subsume both idioms within a unified system based on term rewriting, for example, Michael Hanus's integrated functional logic programming language

Curry [25], the Vesper formalism of Robinson and Barklund (in [23]), the Escher system of Lloyd (in [23]) and the Alma system of Apt and Bezem [24]. These unified systems have hitherto been mere experiments, and have attracted few if any actual users. The system of Hanus is the currently most promising one. May its momentum increase and its user community thrive. The challenge is to create a usable unified public LP language which will attract every kind of user by its obvious superiority over the alternatives.

Those are only some of the challenges which await us.

20   Hilbert Has the Last Word

Hilbert's ending for his 1900 address was a stirring declaration of faith in the continuing unity of his field. If we substitute "computational logic" for "mathematics", what he said on that occasion becomes exactly what we should be telling ourselves now. So let us borrow and re-use his words to end this address on a similar note.

> The problems mentioned are merely samples of problems, yet they will suffice to show how rich, how manifold and how extensive the [computational logic] of today is, and the question is urged upon us whether [computational logic] is doomed to the fate of those other sciences that have split up into separate branches, whose representatives scarcely understand one another and whose connection becomes ever more loose. I do not believe this nor wish it. [Computational logic] is in my opinion an indivisible whole, an organism whose vitality is conditioned upon the connection of its parts. For ... we are still clearly conscious of the similarity of the logical devices, the relationship of the ideas in [computational logic] as a whole and the numerous analogies in its different departments. ... So it happens that, with the extension of [computational logic], its organic character is not lost but only manifests itself the more clearly.   But, we ask, with the extension of [computational logic] will it not finally become impossible for the single investigator to embrace all departments of this knowledge?   In answer let me point out how thoroughly it is ingrained in [computational logic] that every real advance goes hand in hand with the invention of sharper tools and simpler methods which at the same time assist in understanding earlier theories and cast aside older more complicated developments. ... The organic unity of [computational logic] is inherent in the nature of this science ... . That it may completely fulfil [its] high mission, may the new century bring it gifted masters and many zealous and enthusiastic disciples!

References

1. Quine, W.V. The Ways of Paradox and Other Essays, Random House, 1966.
2. Gödel, K. The Consistency of the Axiom of Choice and of the Generalized Continuum Hypothesis with the Axioms of Set Theory. Princeton, 1940.
3. Hilbert, D. Mathematical Problems. Bulletin of the American Mathematical Society, Volume 8, 1902, pp. 437 - 479. (Engish translation of original German version).
4. Heijenoort, J. van (editor). From Frege to Gödel; A source Book in Mathematical Logic, 1879 - 1931. Harvard, 1967.
5. Tarski, A. Logic, Semantics, Metamathematics. Oxford, 1956.
6. Cohen, P. J. Set Theory and the Continuum Hypothesis. Benjamin, 1966.
7. Davis, M. (editor). The Undecidable. Raven Press, 1965.
8. Siekmann, J. and Wrightson, G. (editors). The Automation of Reasoning: Classical Papers on Computational Logic. 2 Volumes, Springer, 1983.
9. Beth, E. Semantic Entailmentand Formal Derivability, North Holland, 1955.
10. Hintikka, J. Form and Content in Quantification Theory. Acta Philosophica Fennica 8, 1955, pp. 7-55.
11. Gentzen, G. Untersuchungen über das logische Schliessen. Mathematische Zeitschrift 39, 1934, pp. 176-210, 405-431.
12. Boyer, R. S. (editor). Automated Reasoning. Essays in Honor of Woody Bledsoe. Kluwer, 1991.
13. Walker, D. and Norton, L. (editors). Proceedings of the International Joint Conference on Artificial Intelligence, Washington D.C., 1969.
14. Brachman, R. and Levesque, H. (editors). Readings in Knowledge Representation. Morgan Kaufmann, 1985.
15. Colmerauer, A. Curriculum Vitae, January 1999. Private communication.
16. Kowalski, R. and Kuehner, D. Linear Resolution with Selection Function. Artificial Intelligence 2, 1971, pp. 227-260.
17. Meltzer, B. and Michie, D. Machine Intelligence 7, Edinburgh, 1972.
18. Meltzer, B. and Michie, D. Machine Intelligence 6, Edinburgh, 1971.
19. Warren, D. and Pereira, L. PROLOG: The Language and Its Implementation Compared with LISP. SIGPLAN Notices 12, No 8, August 1977, pp. 109 ff.
20. Kowalski, R. Logic for Problem Solving. North Holland, 1979.
21. International Conference on Fifth Generation Computer Systems 1992, Proceedings, ICOT, Tokyo, 1992.
22. The Journal of Logic Programming, 1, 1984.
23. Furukawa, K., Michie, D. and Muggleton, S. Machine Intelligence 15, Oxford University Press, 1999.
24. Apt, K. and Bezem, M. Formulas as Programs. Report PNA-R9809, CWI, Amsterdam, October 1998.
25. Hanus, M. A Unified Computation Model for Functional and Logic Programming. 24th Annual SIGPLAN-SIGACT Symposium on Principles of Programming Languages (POPL'97), 1997.

ILP: Just Do It

David Page

Dept. of Biostatistics and Medical Informatics
and Dept. of Computer Sciences
University of Wisconsin
1300 University Ave., Rm 5795 Medical Sciences
Madison, WI 53706, U.S.A.
page@biostat.wisc.edu

Abstract. Inductive logic programming (ILP) is built on a foundation laid by research in other areas of computational logic. But in spite of this strong foundation, at 10 years of age ILP now faces a number of new challenges brought on by exciting application opportunities. The purpose of this paper is to interest researchers from other areas of computational logic in contributing their special skill sets to help ILP meet these challenges. The paper presents five future research directions for ILP and points to initial approaches or results where they exist. It is hoped that the paper will motivate researchers from throughout computational logic to invest some time into "doing" ILP.

1 Introduction

Inductive Logic Programming has its foundations in computational logic, including logic programming, knowledge representation and reasoning, and automated theorem proving. These foundations go well beyond the obvious basis in definite clause logic and SLD-resolution. In addition ILP has heavily utilized such theoretical results from computational logic as Lee's Subsumption Theorem [18], Gottlob's Lemma linking implication and subsumption [12], Marcinkowski and Pacholski's result on the undecidability of implication between definite clauses [22], and many others. In addition to utilizing such theoretical results, ILP depends crucially on important advances in logic programming implementations. For example, many of the applications summarized in the next brief section were possible only because of fast deductive inference based on indexing, partial compilation, etc. as embodied in the best current Prolog implementations. Furthermore, research in computational logic has yielded numerous important lessons about the art of knowledge representation in logic that have formed the basis for applications. Just as one example, definite clause grammars are central to several ILP applications within both natural language processing and bioinformatics.

ILP researchers fully appreciate the debt we owe to the rest of computational logic, and we are grateful for the foundation that computational logic has provided. Nevertheless, the goal of this paper is not merely to express gratitude, but

J. Lloyd et al. (Eds.): CL 2000, LNAI 1861, pp. 25–40, 2000.

also to point to the present and future needs of ILP research. More specifically, the goal is to lay out future directions for ILP research and to attract researchers from the various other areas of computational logic to contribute their unique skill sets to some of the challenges that ILP now faces.[1] In order to discuss these new challenges, it is necessary to first briefly survey some of the most challenging application domains of the future. Section 2 provides such a review. Based on this review, Section 3 details five important research directions and concomitant challenges for ILP, and Section 4 tries to "close the sale" in terms of attracting new researchers.

2   A Brief Review of Some Application Areas

One of the most important application domains for machine learning in general is bioinformatics, broadly interpreted. This domain is particularly attractive for (1) its obvious importance to society, and (2) the plethora of large and growing data sets. Data sets obviously include the newly completed and available DNA sequences for *C. elegans* (nematode), *Drosophila* (fruitfly), and (depending on one's definitions of "completed" and "available") man. But other data sets include gene expression data (recording the degree to which various genes are expressed as protein in a tissue sample), bio-activity data on potential drug molecules, x-ray crystallography and NMR data on protein structure, and many others. Bioinformatics has been a particularly strong application area for ILP, dating back to the start of Stephen Muggleton's collaborations with Mike Sternberg and Ross King [29, 16]. Application areas include protein structure prediction [29, 37], mutagenicity prediction [17], and pharmacophore discovery [7] (discovery of a 3D substructure responsible for drug activity that can be used to guide the search for new drugs with similar activity). ILP is particularly well-suited for bioinformatics tasks because of its abilities to take into account background knowledge and structured data and to produce human-comprehensible results. For example, the following is a potential pharmacophore for ACE inhibition (a form of hypertension medication), where the spacial relationships are described through pairwise distances.[2]

```
Molecule A is an ACE inhibitor if:
    molecule A contains a zinc binding site B, and
    molecule A contains a hydrogen acceptor C, and
    the distance between B and C is 7.9 +/- .75 Angstroms, and
    molecule A contains a hydrogen acceptor D, and
    the distance between B and D is 8.5 +/- .75 Angstroms, and
    the distance between C and D is 2.1 +/- .75 Angstroms, and
    molecule A contains a hydrogen acceptor E, and
    the distance between B and E is 4.9 +/- .75 Angstroms, and
```

---

[1] Not to put too fine a point on the matter, this paper contains unapologetic proselytizing.

[2] Hydrogen acceptors are atoms with a weak negative charge. Ordinarily, zinc-binding would be irrelevant; it is relevant here because ACE is one of several proteins in the body that typically contains an associated zinc ion. This is an automatically generated translation of an ILP-generated clause.

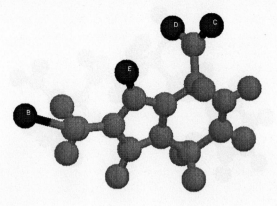

Fig. 1. ACE inhibitor number 1 with highlighted 4-point pharmacophore.

```
the distance between C and E is 3.1 +/- .75 Angstroms, and
the distance between D and E is 3.8 +/- .75 Angstroms.
```

Figures 1 and 2 show two different ACE inhibitors with the parts of pharmacophore highlighted and labeled.

A very different type of domain for machine learning is natural language processing (NLP). This domain also includes a wide variety of tasks such as part-of-speech tagging, grammar learning, information retrieval, and information extraction. Arguably, natural language translation (at least, very rough-cut translation) is now a reality—witness for example the widespread use of Altavista's Babelfish. Machine learning techniques are aiding in the construction of information extraction engines that fill database entries from document abstracts (e.g., [3]) and from web pages (e.g., WhizBang! Labs, http://www.whizbanglabs.com). NLP became a major application focus for ILP in particular with the ESPRIT project ILP^2. Indeed, as early as 1998 the majority of the application papers at the ILP conference were on NLP tasks.

A third popular and challenging application area for machine learning is knowledge discovery from large databases with rich data formats, which might contain for example satellite images, audio recordings, movie files, etc. While Dzeroski has shown how ILP applies very naturally to knowledge discovery from ordinary relational databases [6], advances are needed to deal with multimedia databases.

ILP has advantages over other machine learning techniques for all of the preceding application areas. Nevertheless, these and other potential applications also highlight the following shortcomings of present ILP technology.

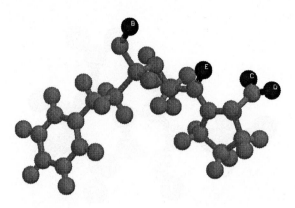

Fig. 2. ACE inhibitor number 2 with highlighted 4-point pharmacophore.

- Other techniques such as hidden Markov models, Bayes Nets and Dynamic Bayes Nets, and bigrams and trigrams can expressly represent the probabilities inherent in tasks such as part-of-speech tagging, alignment of proteins, robot maneuvering, etc. Few ILP systems are capable of representing or processing probabilities.[3]
- ILP systems have higher time and space requirements than other machine learning systems, making it difficult to apply them to large data sets. Alternative approaches such as stochastic search and parallel processing need to be explored.
- ILP works well when data and background knowledge are cleanly expressible in first-order logic. But what can be done when databases contain images, audio, movies, etc.? ILP needs to learn lessons from constraint logic programming regarding the incorporation of special-purpose techniques for handling special data formats.
- In scientific knowledge discovery, for example in the domain of bioinformatics, it would be beneficial if ILP systems could collaborate with scientists rather than merely running in batch mode. If ILP does not take this step, other forms of collaborative scientific assistants will be developed, supplanting ILP's position within these domains.

---

[3] It should be noted that Stephen Muggleton and James Cussens have been pushing for more attention to probabilities in ILP. Stephen Muggleton initiated this direction with an invited talk at ILP'95 and James Cussens has a recently-awarded British EPSRC project along these lines. Nevertheless, litte attention has been paid to this shortcoming by other ILP researchers, myself included.

In light of application domains and the issues they raise, the remainder of this paper discusses five directions for future research in ILP. Many of these directions require fresh insights from other areas of computational logic. The author's hope is that this discussion will prompt researchers from other areas to begin to explore ILP.[4]

3   Five Directions for ILP Research

Undoubtedly there are more than five important directions for ILP research. But five directions stand out clearly at this point in time. They stand out not only in the application areas just mentioned, but also when examining current trends in AI research generally. These areas are

- Incorporating explicit probabilities into ILP,
- Stochastic search,
- Building special-purpose reasoners into ILP,
- Enhancing human-computer interaction to make ILP systems true *collaborators* with human experts,
- Parallel execution using commodity components.

Each of these research directions can contribute substantially to the future widespread success of ILP. And each of these directions could benefit greatly from the expertise of researchers from other areas of computational logic. This section discusses these five research directions in greater detail.

3.1   Probabilistic Inference: ILP and Bayes Nets

Bayesian Networks have largely supplanted traditional rule-based expert systems. Why? Because in task after task we (AI practitioners) have realized that probabilities are central. For example, in medical diagnosis few universally true rules exist and few entirely accurate laboratory experiments are available. Instead, probabilities are needed to model the task's inherent uncertainty. Bayes Nets are designed specifically to model probability distributions and to reason about these distributions accurately and (in some cases) efficiently. Consequently, in many tasks including medical diagnosis [15], Bayes Nets have been found to be superior to rule-based systems. Interestingly, inductive inference, or machine learning, has turned out to be a very significant component of Bayes Net reasoning. Inductive inference from data is particularly important for developing or adjusting the conditional probability tables (CPTs) for various network nodes, but also is used in some cases even for developing or modifying the structure of the network itself.

---

[4] It is customary in technical papers for the author to refer to himself in the third person. But because the present paper is an invited paper expressing the author's opinions, the remainder will be much less clumsy if the author dispenses with that practice, which I now will do.

But not all is perfection and contentment in the world of Bayes Nets. A Bayes Net is less expressive than first-order logic, on a par with propositional logic instead. Consequently, while a Bayes Net is a graphical representation, it cannot represent relational structures. The only relationships captured by the graphs are conditional dependencies among probabilities. This failure to capture other relational information is particularly troublesome when using the Bayes Net representation in learning. For a concrete illustration, consider the task of pharmacophore discovery. It would be desirable to learn probabilistic predictors, e.g., what is the probability that a given structural change to the molecule fluoxetine (Prozac) will yield an equally effective anti-depressant (specifically, serotonin reuptake inhibitor)? To build such a probabilistic predictor, we might choose to learn a Bayes Net from data on serotonin reuptake inhibitors. Unfortunately, while a Bayes Net can capture the probabilistic information, it cannot capture the structural properties of a molecule that are predictive of biological activity.

The inability of Bayes Nets to capture relational structure is well known and has led to attempts to extend the Bayes Net representation [8, 9] and to study inductive learning with such an extended representation. But the resulting extended representations are complex and yet fall short of the expressivity of first-order logic. An interesting alternative for ILP researchers to examine is learning clauses with probabilities attached. It will be important in particular to examine how such representations and learning algorithms compare with the extended Bayes Net representations and learning algorithms. Several candidate clausal representations have been proposed and include probabilistic logic programs, stochastic logic programs, and probabilistic constraint logic programs; Cussens provides a nice survey of these representations [5]. Study already has begun into algorithms and applications for learning stochastic logic programs [27], and this is an exciting area for further work. In addition, the first-order representation closest to Bayes Nets is that of Ngo and Haddawy. The remainder of this subsection points to approaches for, and potential benefits of, learning these clauses in particular.

Clauses in the representation of Ngo and Haddawy may contain random variables as well as ordinary logical variables. A clause may contain at most one random variable in any one literal, and random variables may appear in body literals only if a random variable appears in the head. Finally, such a clause also has a Bayes Net fragment attached, which may be thought of as a constraint. This fragment has a very specific form. It is a directed graph of node depth two (edge depth one), with all the random variables from the clause body as parents of the random variable from the clause head.[5] Figure 3 provides an example of such a clause as might be learned in pharmacophore discovery (CPT not shown). This clause enables us to specify, through a CPT, how the probability of a molecule being active depends on the particular values assigned to the distance variables

---

[5] This is not exactly the definition provided by Ngo and Haddawy, but it is an equivalent one. Readers interested in deductive inference with this representation are encouraged to see [31, 30].

D1, D2, and D3. In general, the role of the added constraint in the form of a Bayes net fragment is to define a conditional probability distribution over the random variable in the head, conditional on the values of the random variables in the body. When multiple such clauses are chained together during inference, a larger Bayes Net is formed that defines a joint probability distribution over the random variables.

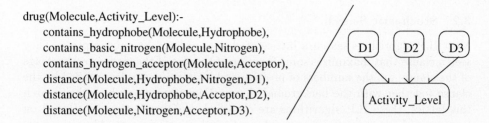

```
drug(Molecule,Activity_Level):-
    contains_hydrophobe(Molecule,Hydrophobe),
    contains_basic_nitrogen(Molecule,Nitrogen),
    contains_hydrogen_acceptor(Molecule,Acceptor),
    distance(Molecule,Hydrophobe,Nitrogen,D1),
    distance(Molecule,Hydrophobe,Acceptor,D2),
    distance(Molecule,Nitrogen,Acceptor,D3).
```

Fig. 3. A clause with a Bayes Net fragment attached (CPT not included). The random variables are *Activity_Level*, D1, D2, and D3. Rather than using a hard range in which the values of D1, D2, and D3 must fall, as the pharmacophores described earlier, this new representation allows us to describe a probability distribution over *Activity_Level* in terms of the values of D1, D2, and D3. For example, we might assign higher probabilities to high *Activity_Level* as D1 gets closer to 3 Angstroms from either above or below. The CPT itself might be a linear regression model, i.e. a linear function of D1, D2, and D3 with some fixed variance assumed, or it might be a discretized model, or other.

I conjecture that existing ILP algorithms can effectively learn clauses of this form with the following modification. For each clause constructed by the ILP algorithm, collect the positive examples covered by the clause. Each positive example provides a value for the random variable in the head of the clause, and because the example is covered, the example together with the background knowledge provides values for the random variables in the body. These values, over all the covered positive examples, can be used as the data for constructing the conditional probability table (CPT) that accompanies the attached Bayes Net fragment. When all the random variables are discrete, a simple, standard method exists for constructing CPTs from such data and is described nicely in [14]. If some or all of the random variables are continuous, then under certain assumptions again simple, standard methods exist. For example, under one set of assumptions linear regression can be used, and under another naive Bayes can be used. In fact, the work by Srinivasan and Camacho [35] on predicting levels of mutagenicity and the work by Craven and colleagues [4, 3] on information extraction can be seen as special cases of this proposed approach, employing linear regression and naive Bayes, respectively.

While the approach just outlined appears promising, of course it is not the only possible approach and may not turn out to be the best. More generally, ILP and Bayes Net learning are largely orthogonal. The former handles relational domains well, while the latter handles probabilities well. And both Bayes Nets and ILP have been applied successfully to a variety of tasks. Therefore, it is reasonable to hypothesize the existence and utility of a representation and learning algorithms that effectively capture the advantages of both Bayes net learning and ILP. The space of such representations and algorithms is large, so combining Bayes Net learning and ILP is an area of research that is not only promising but also wide open for further work.

3.2   Stochastic Search

Most ILP algorithms search a lattice of clauses ordered by subsumption. They seek a clause that maximizes some function of the size of the clause and coverage of the clause, i.e. the numbers of positive and negative examples entailed by the clause together with the background theory. Depending upon how they search this lattice, these ILP algorithms are classified as either bottom-up (based on least general generalization) or top-down (based on refinement). Algorithms are further classified by whether they perform a greedy search, beam search, admissible search, etc. In almost all existing algorithms these searches are deterministic. But for other challenging logic/AI tasks outside ILP, stochastic searches have consistently outperformed deterministic searches. This observation has been repeated for a wide variety of tasks, beginning with the 1992 work of Kautz, Selman, Levesque, Mitchell, and others on satisfiability using algorithms such as GSAT and WSAT (WalkSAT) [34,33]. Consequently, a promising research direction within ILP is the use of stochastic search rather than deterministic search to examine the lattice of clauses. A start has been made in stochastic search for ILP and this section describes that work. Nevertheless many issues remain unexamined, and I will mention some of the most important of these at the end of this section.

ILP algorithms face not one but two difficult search problems. In addition to the search of the lattice of clauses, already described, simply testing the coverage of a clause involves repeated searches for proofs—"if I assume this clause is true, does a proof exist for that example?" The earliest work on stochastic search in ILP (to my knowledge) actually addressed this latter search problem. Sebag and Rouveirol [32] employed stochastic matching, or theorem proving, and obtained efficiency improvements over Progol in the prediction of mutagenicity, without sacrificing predictive accuracy or comprehensibility. More recently, Botta, Giordana, Saitta, and Sebag have pursued this approach further, continuing to show the benefits of replacing deterministic matching with stochastic matching [11, 2].

But at the center of ILP is the search of the clause lattice, and surprisingly until now the only stochastic search algorithms that have been tested have been genetic algorithms. Within ILP these have not yet been shown to significantly outperform deterministic search algorithms. I say it is surprising that only GAs have been attempted because for other logical tasks such as satisfiability and planning almost every other approach outperforms GAs, including simulated annealing, hill-climbing with random restarts and sideways moves (e.g. GSAT), and directed random walks (e.g. WSAT) [33]. Therefore, a natural direction for ILP research is to use these alternative forms of stochastic search to examine the lattice of clauses. The remainder of this section discusses some of the issues involved in this research direction, based on my initial foray in this direction with Ashwin Srinivasan that includes testing variants of GSAT and WSAT tailored to ILP.

The GSAT algorithm was designed for testing the satisfiability of Boolean CNF formulas. GSAT randomly draws a truth assignment over the n propositional variables in the formula and then repeatedly modifies the current assignment by flipping a variable. At each step all possible flips are tested, and the flip that yields the largest number of satisfied clauses is selected. It may be the case that every possible flip yields a score no better (in fact, possibly even worse) than the present assignment. In such a case a flip is still chosen and is called a "sideways move" (or "downward move" if strictly worse). Such moves turn out to be quite important in GSAT's performance. If GSAT finds an assignment that satisfies the CNF formula, it halts and returns the satisfying assignment. Otherwise, it continues to flip variables until it reaches some pre-set maximum number of flips. It then repeats the process by drawing a new random truth assignment. The overall process is repeated until a satisfying assignment is found or a pre-set maximum number of iterations is reached.

Our ILP variant of this algorithm draws a random clause rather than a random truth assignment. Flips involve adding or deleting literals in this clause. Applying the GSAT methodology to ILP in this manner raises several important points. First, in GSAT scoring a given truth assignment is very fast. In contrast, scoring a clause can be much more time consuming because it involves repeated theorem proving. Therefore, it might be beneficial to combine the "ILP-GSAT" algorithm with the type of stochastic theorem proving mentioned above. Second, the number of literals that can be built from a language often is infinite, so we cannot test all possible additions of a literal. Our approach has been to base any given iteration of the algorithm on a "bottom clause" built from a "seed example," based on the manner in which the ILP system PROGOL [26] constrains its search space. But there might be other alternatives for constraining the set of possible literals to be added at any step. Or it might be preferable to consider changing literals rather than only adding or deleting them. Hence there are many alternative GSAT-like algorithms that might be built and tested.

Based on our construction of GSAT-like ILP algorithms, one can imagine analogous WSAT-like and simulated annealing ILP algorithms. Consider WSAT in particular. On every flip, with probability p (user-specified) WSAT makes an randomly-selected efficacious flip instead of a GSAT flip. An efficacious flip is a flip that satisfies some previously-unsatisfied clause in the CNF formula, even if the flip is not the highest-scoring flip as required by GSAT. WSAT outperforms GSAT for many satisfiability tasks because the random flips make it less likely to get trapped in local optima. It will be interesting to see if the benefit of WSAT over GSAT for satisfiability carries over to ILP. The same issues mentioned above for ILP- GSAT also apply to ILP-WSAT.

It is too early in the work to present concrete conclusions regarding stochastic ILP. Rather the goal of this section has been to point to a promising direction and discuss the space of design alternatives to be explored. Researchers with experience in stochastic search for constraint satisfaction and other logic/AI search tasks will almost certainly have additional insights that will be vital to the exploration of stochastic search for ILP.

3.3   Special-Purpose Reasoning Mechanisms

One of the well-known success stories of computational logic is constraint logic programming. And one of the reasons for this success is the ability to integrate logic and special purpose reasoners or constraint solvers. Many ILP applications could benefit from the incorporation of special-purpose reasoning mechanisms. Indeed, the approach advocated in Section 3.1 to incorporating probabilities in ILP can be thought of as invoking special purpose reasoners to construct constraints in the form of Bayes Net fragments. The work by Srinivasan and Camacho mentioned there uses linear regression to construct a constraint, while the work by Craven and Slattery uses naive Bayes techniques to construct a constraint. The point that is crucial to notice is that ILP requires a "constraint constructor," such as linear regression, in addition to the constraint solver required during deduction. Let's now turn to consideration of tasks where other types of constraint generators might be useful.

Consider the general area of knowledge discovery from databases. Suppose we take the standard logical interpretation of a database, where each relation is a predicate, and each tuple in the relation is a ground atomic formula built from that predicate. Dzeroski and Lavrac show how ordinary ILP techniques are very naturally suited to this task, if we have an "ordinary" relational database. But now suppose the database contains some form of complex objects, such as images. Simple logical similarities may not capture the important common features across a set of images. Instead, special-purpose image processing techniques may be required, such as those described by Leung and colleagues [20, 19]. In addition to simple images, special-purpose constraint constructors might be required when applying ILP to movie (e.g. MPEG) or audio (e.g. MIDI) data, or other data forms that are becoming ever more commonplace with the growth of multimedia. For example, a fan of the Bach, Mozart, Brian Wilson, and Elton John would love to be able to enter her/his favorite pieces, have ILP with a constraint generator build rules to describe these favorites, and have the rules suggest other pieces or composers s/he should access. As multimedia data becomes more commonplace, ILP can remain applicable only if it is able to incorporate special-purpose constraint generators.

Alan Frisch and I have shown that the ordinary subsumption ordering over formulas scales up quite naturally to incorporate constraints [10]. Nevertheless, that work does not address some of the hardest issues, such as how to ensure the efficiency of inductive learning systems based on this ordering and how to design the right types of constraint generators. These questions require much further research involving real-world applications such as multimedia databases.

One final point about special purpose reasoners in ILP is worth making. Constructing a constraint may be thought of as inventing a predicate. Predicate invention within ILP has a long history [28, 39, 40, 25]. General techniques for predicate invention encounter the problem that the space of "inventable" predicates is unconstrained, and hence allowing predicate invention is roughly equivalent to removing all bias from inductive learning. While removing bias may sound at first to be a good idea, inductive learning in fact requires bias [23, 24]. Special purpose techniques for constraint construction appear to make it possible to perform predicate invention in way that is limited enough to be effective [35, 3].

3.4 Interaction with Human Experts

To discover new knowledge from data in fields such as telecommunications, molecular biology, or pharmaceuticals, it would be beneficial if a machine learning system and a human expert could act as a team, taking advantage of the computer's speed and the expert's knowledge and skills. ILP systems have three properties that make them natural candidates for collaborators with humans in knowledge discovery:

Declarative Background Knowledge. ILP systems can make use of declarative background knowledge about a domain in order to construct hypotheses. Thus a collaboration can begin with a domain expert providing the learning system with general knowledge that might be useful in the construction of hypotheses. Most ILP systems also permit the expert to define the hypothesis space using additional background knowledge, in the form of a *declarative bias*.

Natural Descriptions of Structured Examples. Feature-based learning systems require the user to begin by creating features to describe the examples. Because many knowledge discovery tasks involve complex structured examples, such as molecules, users are forced to choose only composite features such as molecular weight—thereby losing information—or to invest substantial effort in building features that can capture structure (see [36] for a discussion in the context of molecules). ILP systems allow a structured example to be described naturally in terms of the objects that compose it, together with relations between those objects. The 2-dimensional structure of a molecule can be represented directly using its atoms as the objects and bonds as the relations; 3-dimensional structure can be captured by adding distance relations.

Human-Comprehensible Output. ILP systems share with propositional-logic learners the ability to present a user with declarative, comprehensible rules as output. Some ILP systems can return rules in English along with visual aids. For example, the pharmacophore description and corresponding figures in Section 2 were generated automatically by PROGOL.

Despite the useful properties just outlined, ILP systems—like other machine learning systems—have a number of shortcomings as collaborators with humans in knowledge discovery. One shortcoming is that most ILP systems return a single theory based on heuristics, thus casting away many clauses that might be interesting to a domain expert. But the only currently existing alternative is the version space approach, which has unpalatable properties that include inefficiency, poor noise tolerance, and a propensity to overwhelm users with too large a space of possible hypotheses. Second, ILP systems cannot respond to a human expert's questions in the way a human collaborator would. They operate in simple batch mode, taking a data set as input, and returning a hypothesis on a take-it-or-leave-it basis. Third, ILP systems do not question the input data in the way a human collaborator would, spotting surprising (and hence possibly erroneous) data points and raising questions about them. Some ILP systems will flag mutually inconsistent data points but to my knowledge none goes beyond this. Fourth, while a human expert can provide knowledge-rich forms of hypothesis justification, for example relating a new hypothesis to existing beliefs, ILP systems merely provide accuracy estimates as the sole justification.

To build upon ILP's strengths as a technology for human-computer collaboration in knowledge discovery, the above shortcomings should be addressed. ILP systems should be extended to display the following capabilities.

1. Maintain and summarize alternative hypotheses that explain or describe the data, rather than providing a single answer based on a general-purpose heuristic;
2. Propose to human experts practical sequences of experiments to refine or distinguish between competing hypotheses;
3. Provide non-numerical justification for hypotheses, such as relating them to prior beliefs or illustrative examples (in addition to providing numerical accuracy estimates);
4. Answer an expert's questions regarding hypotheses;
5. Consult the expert regarding anomalies or surprises in the data.

Addressing such human-computer interface issues obviously requires a variety of logical and AI expertise. Thus contributions from other areas of computational logic, such as the study of logical agents, will be vital. While several projects have recently begun that investigate some of these issues,[6] developing collaborative systems is an ambitious goal with more than enough room for many more researchers. And undoubtedly other issues not mentioned here will become apparent as this work progresses.

3.5 Parallel Execution

While ILP has numerous advantages over other types of machine learning, including advantages mentioned at the start of the previous section, it has two

---

[6] Stephen Muggleton has a British EPSRC project on closed-loop learning, in which the human is omitted entirely. While this seems the reverse of a collaborative system, it raises similar issues, such as maintaining competing hypotheses and automatically proposing experiments. I am beginning a U.S. National Science Foundation project on collaborative systems with (not surprisingly) exactly the goals above.

particularly notable disadvantages—run time and space requirements. Fortunately for ILP, at the same time that larger applications are highlighting these disadvantages, parallel processing "on the cheap" is becoming widespread. Most notable is the widespread use of "Beowulf clusters" [1] and of "Condor pools" [21], arrangements that connect tens, hundreds, or even thousands of personal computers or workstations to permit parallel processing. Admittedly, parallel processing cannot change the order of the time or space complexity of an algorithm. But most ILP systems already use broad constraints, such as maximum clause size, to hold down exponential terms. Rather, the need is to beat back the large constants brought in by large real-world applications.

Yu Wang and David Skillicorn recently developed a parallel implementation of PROGOL under the Bulk Synchronous Parallel (BSP) model and claim superlinear speedup from this implementation [38]. Alan Wild worked with me at the University of Louisville to re-implement on a Beowulf cluster a top-down ILP search for pharmacophore discovery, and the result was a linear speedup [13]. The remainder of this section described how large-scale parallelism can be achieved very simply in a top-down complete search ILP algorithm. This was the approach taken in [13]. From this discussion, one can imagine more interesting approaches for other types of top-down searches such as greedy search.

The ideal in parallel processing is a decrease in processing time that is a linear function, with a slope near 1, of the number of processors used. (In some rare cases it is possible to achieve superlinear speed-up.) The barriers to achieving the ideal are (1) overhead in communication between processes and (2) competition for resources between processes. Therefore, a good parallel scheme is one where the processes are relatively independent of one another and hence require little communication or resource sharing. The key observation in the design of the parallel ILP scheme is that two competing hypotheses can be tested against the data completely independently of one another. Therefore the approach advocated here is to distribute the hypothesis space among different processors for testing against the data. These processors need not communicate with one another during testing, and they need not write to a shared memory space.

In more detail, for complete search a parallel ILP scheme can employ a master-worker design, where the master assigns different segments of the hypothesis space to workers that then test hypotheses against the data. Workers communicate back to the master all hypotheses achieving a pre-selected minimum valuation score (e.g. 95 % accuracy) on the data. As workers become free, the master continues to assign new segments of the space until the entire space has been explored. The only architectural requirements for this approach are (1) a mechanism for communication between the master and each worker and (2) read access for each worker to the data. Because data do not change during a run, this scheme can easily operate under either a shared memory or message passing architecture; in the latter, we incur a one-time overhead cost of initially communicating the data to each worker. The only remaining overhead, on either architecture, consists of the time spent by the master and time for master-worker communication. In "needle in a haystack" domains, which are the motivation for complete search, one expects very few hypotheses to be communicated from workers to the master, so overhead for the communication of results will be low. If it also is possible for the master to rapidly segment the hypothesis space in such a way that the segments can be communicated to the workers succinctly, then overall overhead will be low and the ideal of linear speed-up can be realized.

4   Conclusions

ILP has attracted great interest within the machine learning and AI communities at large because of its logical foundations, its ability to utilize background knowledge and structured data representations, and its comprehensible results. But most of all, the interest has come from ILP's application successes. Nevertheless, ILP needs further advances to maintain this record of success, and these advances require further contributions from other areas of computational logic. System builders and parallel implementation experts are needed if the ILP systems of the next decade are to scale up to the next generation of data sets, such as those being produced by Affymetrix's (TM) gene expression microarrays and Celera's (TM) shotgun approach to DNA sequencing. Researchers on probability and logic are required if ILP is to avoid being supplanted by the next generation of extended Bayes Net learning systems. Experts on constraint satisfaction and constraint logic programming have the skills necessary to bring successful stochastic search techniques to ILP and to allow ILP techniques to extend to multimedia databases. The success of ILP in the next decade (notice I avoided the strong temptation to say "next millennium") depends on the kinds of interactions being fostered at Computational Logic 2000.

Acknowledgements

This work was supported in part by NSF grant 9987841 and by grants from the University of Wisconsin Graduate School and Medical School.

References

1. D. Becker, T. Sterling, D. Savarese, E. Dorband, U. Ranawake, and C. Packer. Beowulf: A parallel workstation for scientific computation. In *Proceedings of the 1995 International Conference on Parallel Processing (ICPP)*, pages 11–14, 1995.
2. M. Botta, A. Giordana, L. Saiita, and M. Sebag. Relational learning: Hard problems and phase transitions. 2000.
3. M. Craven and J. Kumlien. Constructing biological knowledge bases by extracting information from text sources. In *Proceedings of the Seventh International Conference on Intelligent Systems for Molecular Biology*, Heidelberg, Germany, 1999. AAAI Press.
4. M. Craven and S. Slattery. Combining statistical and relational methods for learning in hypertext domains. In *Proceedings of the Eighth International Conference on Inductive Logic Programming (ILP-98)*, pages 38–52. Springer Verlag, 1998.

5. J. Cussens. Loglinear models for first-order probabilistic reasoning. In *Proceedings of the 15th Conference on Uncertainty in Artificial Intelligence*. Stockholm, Sweden, 1999.

6. S. Dzeroski. Inductive logic programming and knowledge discovery in databases. In U. Fayyad, G. Piatetsky-Shapiro, P. Smyth, and R. Uthurusamy, editors, *Advances in Knowledge Discovery and Data Mining*. 1996.

7. P. Finn, S. Muggleton, D. Page, and A. Srinivasan. Discovery of pharmacophores using Inductive Logic Programming. *Machine Learning*, 30:241–270, 1998.

8. N. Friedman, L. Getoor, D. Koller, and A. Pfeffer. Learning probabilistic relational models. In *Proceedings of the 16th International Joint Conference on Artificial Intelligence*. Stockholm, Sweden, 1999.

9. N. Friedman, D. Koller, and A. Pfeffer. Structured representation of complex stochastic systems. In *Proceedings of the 15th National Conference on Artificial Intelligence*. AAAI Press, 1999.

10. A. M. Frisch and C. D. Page. Building theories into instantiation. In *Proceedings of the Fourteenth International Joint Conference on Artificial Intelligence (IJCAI-95)*, 1995.

11. A. Giordana and L. Saitta. Phase transitions in learning with fol languages. Technical Report 97, 1998.

12. G. Gottlob. Subsumption and implication. *Information Processing Letters*, 24(2):109–111, 1987.

13. J. Graham, D. Page, and A. Wild. Parallel inductive logic programming. In *Proceedings of the Systems, Man, and Cybernetics Conference (SMC-2000)*, page To appear. IEEE, 2000.

14. D. Heckerman. A tutorial on learning with bayesian networks. Microsoft Technical Report MSR-TR-95-06, 1995.

15. D. Heckerman, E. Horvitz, and B. Nathwani. Toward normative expert systems: Part i the pathfinder project. *Methods of Information in Medicine*, 31:90–105, 1992.

16. R. King, S. Muggleton, R. Lewis, and M. Sternberg. Drug design by machine learning: The use of inductive logic programming to model the structure-activity relationships of trimethoprim analogues binding to dihydrofolate reductase. *Proceedings of the National Academy of Sciences*, 89(23):11322–11326, 1992.

17. R. King, S. Muggleton, A. Srinivasan, and M. Sternberg. Structure-activity relationships derived by machine learning: the use of atoms and their bond connectives to predict mutagenicity by inductive logic programming. *Proceedings of the National Academy of Sciences*, 93:438–442, 1996.

18. C. Lee. *A completeness theorem and a computer program for finding theorems derivable from given axioms*. PhD thesis, University of California, Berkeley, 1967.

19. T. Leung, M. Burl, and P. Perona. Probabilistic affine invariants for recognition. In *Proceedings IEEE Conference on Computer Vision and Pattern Recognition*, 1998.

20. T. Leung and J. Malik. Detecting, localizing and grouping repeated scene elements from images. *IEEE Transactions on Pattern Analysis and Machine Intelligence*, page To appear, 2000.

21. M. Litzkow, M. Livny, and M. Mutka. Condor—a hunter of idle workstations. In *Proceedings of the International Conference on Distributed Computing Systems*, pages 104–111, 1988.

22. J. Marcinkowski and L. Pacholski. Undecidability of the horn-clause implication problem. In *Proceedings of the 33rd IEEE Annual Symposium on Foundations of Computer Science*, pages 354–362. IEEE, 1992.

23. T.M. Mitchell. The need for biases in learning generalizations. Technical Report CBM-TR-117, Department of Computer Science, Rutgers University, 1980.

24. T.M. Mitchell. Generalisation as search. *Artificial Intelligence*, 18:203–226, 1982.

25. S. Muggleton. Predicate invention and utilization. *Journal of Experimental and Theoretical Artificial Intelligence*, 6(1):127–130, 1994.

26. S. Muggleton. Inverse entailment and Progol. *New Generation Computing*, 13:245–286, 1995.

27. S. Muggleton. Learning stochastic logic programs. In *Proceedings of the AAAI2000 Workshop on Learning Statistical Models from Relational Data*. AAAI, 2000.

28. S. Muggleton and W. Buntine. Machine invention of first-order predicates by inverting resolution. In *Proceedings of the Fifth International Conference on Machine Learning*, pages 339–352. Kaufmann, 1988.

29. S. Muggleton, R. King, and M. Sternberg. Protein secondary structure prediction using logic-based machine learning. *Protein Engineering*, 5(7):647–657, 1992.

30. L. Ngo and P. Haddawy. Probabilistic logic programming and bayesian networks. *Algorithms, Concurrency, and Knowledge: LNCS 1023*, pages 286–300, 1995.

31. L. Ngo and P. Haddawy. Answering queries from context-sensitive probabilistic knowledge bases. *Theoretical Computer Science*, 171:147–177, 1997.

32. M. Sebag and C. Rouveirol. Tractable induction and classification in fol. In *Proceedings of the 15th International Joint Conference on Artificial Intelligence*, pages 888–892. Nagoya, Japan, 1997.

33. B. Selman, H. Kautz, and B. Cohen. Noise strategies for improving local search. In *Proceedings of the Twelfth National Conference on Artificial Intelligence*. AAAI Press, 1994.

34. B. Selman, H. Levesque, and D. Mitchell. A new method for solving hard satisfiability problems. In *Proceedings of the Tenth National Conference on Artificial Intelligence*, pages 440–446. AAAI Press, 1992.

35. A. Srinivasan and R.C. Camacho. Numerical reasoning with an ILP system capable of lazy evaluation and customised search. *Journal of Logic Programming*, 40:185–214, 1999.

36. A. Srinivasan, S. Muggleton, R. King, and M. Sternberg. Theories for mutagenicity: a study of first-order and feature based induction. *Artificial Intelligence*, 85(1,2):277–299, 1996.

37. M. Turcotte, S. Muggleton, and M. Sternberg. Application of inductive logic programming to discover rules governing the three-dimensional topology of protein structures. In *Proceedings of the Eighth International Conference on Inductive Logic Programming (ILP-98)*, pages 53–64. Springer Verlag, 1998.

38. Y. Wang and D. Skillicorn. Parallel inductive logic for data mining. http://www.cs.queensu.ca/home/skill/papers.html#datamining, 2000.

39. R. Wirth and P. O'Rorke. Constraints on predicate invention. In *Proceedings of the 8th International Workshop on Machine Learning*, pages 457–461. Kaufmann, 1991.

40. J. Zelle and R. Mooney. Learning semantic grammars with constructive inductive logic programming. In *Proceedings of the Eleventh National Conference on Artificial Intelligence*, pages 817–822, San Mateo, CA, 1993. Morgan Kaufmann.

Databases and Higher Types

Melvin Fitting

Dept. Mathematics and Computer Science
Lehman College (CUNY), Bronx, NY 10468
fitting@alpha.lehman.cuny.edu
http://comet.lehman.cuny.edu/fitting

Abstract. Generalized databases will be examined, in which attributes can be sets of attributes, or sets of sets of attributes, and other higher type constructs. A precise semantics will be developed for such databases, based on a higher type modal/intensional logic.

1 Introduction

In some ways this is an eccentric paper—there are no theorems. What I want to do, simply stated, is present a semantics for relational databases. But the semantics is rich, powerful, and oddly familiar, and applies to databases that are quite general. It is a topic whose exploration I wish to recommend, rather than a finished product I simply present.

Relational databases generally have entities of some kind as values of attributes, though it is a small stretch to allow sets of entities as well. I want to consider databases that stretch things further, allowing attributes to have as values sets of sets of entities, and so on, but further, I also want to allow sets of attributes, sets of sets of attributes, and so on. There are quite reasonable examples showing why one might find such things desirable, at least at low levels, and a very simple one will be given below.

It is not enough to just allow eccentric attribute values—a semantics must also be supplied to give them meaning. And rather than looking to some version of classical logic, I will show that modal logic provides a very natural tool. Of course it must be higher type modal logic, to encompass the kinds of things I have been talking about. I will use the one presented in [3], which mildly generalizes work of Montague [8–10] and Gallin [5].

This paper is a sequel to [2], in which a modal/intensional approach to databases is developed in some detail at the first-order level. Once a full hierarchy of types is introduced things become complex, and no more than a sketch can be presented here. In particular, though a tableau system exists for the modal logic I use, it will not be discussed in this paper.

It may be of interest that I did not get into this line of work from the database side. I began with attempts to treat various classic philosophical problems as simply as possible in a modal context—work culminating in [4]. This, in turn, led to an interest in higher type modal logics, connected with a desire to understand Gödel's ontological argument, [6]. My work on this can be found in [3]. Databases

J. Lloyd et al. (Eds.): CL 2000, LNAI 1861, pp. 41–52, 2000.

came in, unnoticed, by a side door. But they are at the party, and it may be they will have a good time.

2   A Sample Database

In order to illustrate the higher-type constructs, I'll create a miniature database of some complexity. I will take ground-level entities to be strings. Let's say the Locomobile Company[1] still exists, and manufactures cars, motorcycles, and pianos. Table 1 shows the start of a database—more attributes will be added later.

Table 1. Locomobile Sales List

IDNumber	Item	Cylinders	Engine	Colors	Air	Config
1	automobile	2	{A, B}	{red, green, black}	{no}	$\perp$
2	automobile	4	{A}	{green, black}	{yes, no}	$\perp$
3	motorcycle	2	{C, D}	{blue, black}	$\perp$	$\perp$
4	piano	$\perp$	$\perp$	$\perp$	$\perp$	{upright, grand}

Notice that in Table 1 some of the attributes have values that are ground objects—Cylinders, say—while some are sets of ground objects—Engine types, for instance. An entry of $\perp$ indicates an attribute that is not relevant to the particular item.

In the table above, let us say that for the 2 cylinder automobile the choice of engine type, A or B, is not up to the buyer, since both are functionally equivalent. But the choice of Colors, naturally, would be up to the customer. Similarly for the 4 cylinder. But let's say that for the motorcycle, the engine type is something the customer chooses. Then let us have an additional attribute telling us, for each record, which (other) attributes are customer chosen. Rather than repeating the whole table, I'll just give this single additional attribute in Table 2.

Notice that in Table 2, the Customer attribute has as values sets of attributes. Finally, many of the attributes for an item can be irrelevant, as has been indicated by $\perp$. Rather than explicitly having an 'undefined' value in our semantics, instead let us add additional attributes telling us which of the other attributes are relevant.

Values of the Relevant0 attribute, in Table 3, are sets of attributes whose values are ground level objects, values of Relevant1 are sets of attributes whose values are sets of ground level objects, and values of Relevant2 are sets of

---

[1] The actual company was founded in 1899 to manufacture steam powered cars. It moved to luxury internal combustion automobiles in 1902, and went into receivership in 1922. When active, they manufactured four cars a day.

Table 2. Locomobile Customer Attribute

IDNumber	Customer
1	{Colors}
2	{Colors, Air}
3	{Engine, Colors}
4	{Configuration}

Table 3. Locomobile Relevancy Attribute

IDNumber	Relevant0	Relevant1	Relevant2
1	{IDNumber, Item, Cylinders}	{Engine, Colors, Air}	{Customer}
2	{IDNumber, Item, Cylinders}	{Engine, Colors, Air}	{Customer}
3	{IDNumber, Item, Cylinders}	{Engine, Colors}	{Customer}
4	{IDNumber, Item}	{Configuration}	{Customer}

attributes whose values are sets of attributes whose values are sets of ground level objects.

Finally, all this is really an instance of a relation schema, and that schema has a few constraints which I've implicitly been obeying. Clearly **IDNumber** is a key attribute. Also, an attribute belongs to the **Relevant0**, **Relevant1**, or **Relevant2** attribute of a record if and only if the attribute is defined for that record, that is, has a value other than $\bot$. I'll come back to the notion of constraint later on.

3   Higher Order Modal Logic

Shifting gears abruptly (something the Locomobile did smoothly) I now present a sketch of a higher order modal logic, taken from [3], and derived from [11] via [5]. The machinery is somewhat complex, and space here is limited. See [3] for a fuller discussion of underlying ideas.

I'll start with the notion of types. The key feature here is that there are both intensional and extensional types.

Definition 1. *The notion of a type, extensional and intensional, is given as follows.*

1. *0 is an* extensional *type.*
2. *If $t_1, \ldots, t_n$ are types, extensional or intensional, $\langle t_1, \ldots, t_n \rangle$ is an extensional type.*
3. *If t is an extensional type, $\Uparrow t$ is an intensional type.*

A type is an intensional or an extensional type.

As usual, 0 is the type of ground-level objects, unanalyzed "things." The type $\langle t_1, \ldots, t_n \rangle$ is for n-ary relations in the conventional sense, where the components are of types $t_1, \ldots, t_n$ respectively. The type $\Uparrow t$ is the unfamiliar piece of machinery—it will be used as the type of an intensional object which, in a particular context, determines an extensional object of type t. All this will be clearer once models have been presented.

For each type t I'll assume there are infinitely many variable symbols of that type. I'll also assume there is a set C constant symbols, containing at least an equality symbol $=^{\langle t,t \rangle}$ for each type t. I denote the higher-order language built up from C by $L(C)$. I'll indicate types, when necessary, by superscripts, as I did with equality above.

In formulating a higher order logic one can use comprehension axioms, or one can use explicit term formation machinery, in effect building comprehension into the language. I'll follow the later course, but this means terms cannot be defined first, and then formulas. Instead they must be defined in a mutual recursion. Most of the items below are straightforward, but a few need comment. First, concerning the term formation machinery mentioned above, predicate abstraction, it should be noted that $\langle \lambda \alpha_1, \ldots, \alpha_n.\Phi \rangle$ is taken to be a term of *intensional* type. Its meaning can vary from world to world, simply because the behavior of the formula Φ changes from world to world. Second, there is a new piece of machinery, $\downarrow$, mapping intensional terms to extensional ones. Think of it as the "extension of" operator—at a possible world it supplies the extension there for an intensional term.

Definition 2. *Terms and formulas of $L(C)$ are defined as follows.*

1. *A constant symbol or variable of $L(C)$ of type t is a term of $L(C)$ of type t. If it is a constant symbol, it has no free variable occurrences. If it is a variable, it has one free variable occurrence, itself.*

2. *If Φ is a formula of $L(C)$ and $\alpha_1, \ldots, \alpha_n$ is a sequence of distinct variables of types $t_1, \ldots, t_n$ respectively, then $\langle \lambda \alpha_1, \ldots, \alpha_n.\Phi \rangle$ is a term of $L(C)$ of the intensional type $\Uparrow \langle t_1, \ldots, t_n \rangle$. It is called a predicate abstract, and its free variable occurrences are the free variable occurrences of Φ, except for occurrences of the variables $\alpha_1, \ldots, \alpha_n$.*

3. *If τ is a term of $L(C)$ of type $\Uparrow t$ then $\downarrow \tau$ is a term of type t. It has the same free variable occurrences that τ has.*

4. *If τ is a term of either type $\langle t_1, \ldots, t_n \rangle$ or type $\Uparrow \langle t_1, \ldots, t_n \rangle$, and $\tau_1, \ldots, \tau_n$ is a sequence of terms of types $t_1, \ldots, t_n$ respectively, then $\tau(\tau_1, \ldots, \tau_n)$ is a formula (atomic) of $L(C)$. The free variable occurrences in it are the free variable occurrences of $\tau, \tau_1, \ldots, \tau_n$.*

5. *If Φ is a formula of $L(C)$ so is $\neg \Phi$. The free variable occurrences of $\neg \Phi$ are those of Φ.*

6. *If Φ and Ψ are formulas of $L(C)$ so is $(\Phi \wedge \Psi)$. The free variable occurrences of $(\Phi \wedge \Psi)$ are those of Φ together with those of Ψ.*

7. *If Φ is a formula of $L(C)$ and α is a variable then $(\forall \alpha)\Phi$ is a formula of $L(C)$. The free variable occurrences of $(\forall \alpha)\Phi$ are those of Φ, except for occurrences of α.*

8. *If Φ is a formula of $L(C)$ so is $\Box\Phi$. The free variable occurrences of $\Box\Phi$ are those of Φ.*

Other connectives, quantifiers, and modal operators have the usual definitions.

The next thing is semantics. Actually, the only modal logic I'll need will be **S5**, for which the accessibility relation, $\mathcal{R}$, is an equivalence relation, but it does no harm to present the general case now. Note that the ground-level domain, $\mathcal{D}$, is not world dependent—in effect, type-0 quantification is *possibilist* and not *actualist*.

Definition 3. *An augmented Kripke frame is a structure $\langle\mathcal{G}, \mathcal{R}, \mathcal{D}\rangle$ where $\mathcal{G}$ is a non-empty set (of possible worlds), $\mathcal{R}$ is a binary relation on $\mathcal{G}$ (called accessibility) and $\mathcal{D}$ is a non-empty set, the (ground-level) domain.*

Next I say what the objects of each type are, relative to a choice of ground-level domain and set of possible worlds. In classical higher order logic, *Henkin models* are standard. In these, rather than having all objects of higher types, one has "enough" of them. It is well-known that a restriction to "true" higher order classical models gives a semantics that is not axiomatizable, while Henkin models provide an axiomatizable version. A similar thing happens here, but the definition of the modal analog of Henkin models is fairly complex, because saying what it means to have "enough" objects requires serious effort. I will just give the "true" model version—the Henkin generalization can be found in [3]. But I also note that, in applications to databases, ground level domains will often be finite.

Definition 4. *Let $\mathcal{G}$ be a non-empty set (of possible worlds) and let $\mathcal{D}$ be a non-empty set (the ground-level domain). For each type t, the collection $[\![t, \mathcal{D}, \mathcal{G}]\!]$, of objects of type t with respect to $\mathcal{D}$ and $\mathcal{G}$, is defined as follows ($\mathcal{P}$ is the powerset operator).*

1. $[\![0, \mathcal{D}, \mathcal{G}]\!] = \mathcal{D}$.
2. $[\![\langle t_1, \ldots, t_n\rangle, \mathcal{D}, \mathcal{G}]\!] = \mathcal{P}([\![t_1, \mathcal{D}, \mathcal{G}]\!] \times \cdots \times [\![t_n, \mathcal{D}, \mathcal{G}]\!])$.
3. $[\![\Uparrow t, \mathcal{D}, \mathcal{G}]\!] = [\![t, \mathcal{D}, \mathcal{G}]\!]^{\mathcal{G}}$.

O is an object of type t *if $O \in [\![t, \mathcal{D}, \mathcal{G}]\!]$. O is an* intensional *or* extensional *object according to whether its type is intensional or extensional.*

Now the terminology should be a little clearer. If O is extensional, it is a relation in the conventional sense. If O is intensional, it is a mapping that assigns an object to each possible world, that is, its designation can vary from state to state. Next we move to models, and remember, these are "true" models, and not a Henkin version. Much of this looks quite technical, but it reflects reasonable intuitions and, in fact, an intuitive understanding will be sufficient for this paper.

Definition 5. *A model for the language $L(C)$ is a structure $\mathcal{M} = \langle\mathcal{G}, \mathcal{R}, \mathcal{D}, \mathcal{I}\rangle$, where $\langle\mathcal{G}, \mathcal{R}, \mathcal{D}\rangle$ is an augmented frame and $\mathcal{I}$ is an interpretation, which meets the following conditions.*

1. If A is a constant symbol of type t, $\mathcal{I}(A)$ is an object of type t.
2. If $=^{\langle t,t\rangle}$ is an equality constant symbol, $\mathcal{I}(=^{\langle t,t\rangle})$ is the equality relation on $[\![t,\mathcal{D},\mathcal{G}]\!]$.

Definition 6. A mapping v is a valuation in the model $\mathcal{M} = \langle \mathcal{G},\mathcal{R},\mathcal{D},\mathcal{I}\rangle$ if v assigns to each variable α of type t some object of type t, that is, $v(\alpha) \in [\![t,\mathcal{D},\mathcal{G}]\!]$. An α variant of v is a valuation that agrees with v on all variables except α. Similarly for $\alpha_1, \ldots, \alpha_n$ variant.

Finally, designation of a term, and truth of a formula, are defined by a simultaneous recursion.

Definition 7. Let $\mathcal{M} = \langle \mathcal{G},\mathcal{R},\mathcal{D},\mathcal{I}\rangle$ be a model, let v be a valuation in it, and let $\Gamma \in \mathcal{G}$ be a possible world. A mapping $(v*\mathcal{I}*\Gamma)$, assigning to each term an object that is the designation of that term at Γ is defined, and a relation $\mathcal{M},\Gamma \Vdash_v \Phi$ expressing truth of Φ at possible world Γ are characterized as follows.

1. If A is a constant symbol of $L(C)$ then $(v*\mathcal{I}*\Gamma)(A) = \mathcal{I}(A)$.
2. If α is a variable then $(v*\mathcal{I}*\Gamma)(\alpha) = v(\alpha)$.
3. If τ is a term of type $\Uparrow t$ then $(v*\mathcal{I}*\Gamma)(\downarrow\tau) = (v*\mathcal{I}*\Gamma)(\tau)(\Gamma)$
4. If $\langle\lambda\alpha_1,\ldots,\alpha_n.\Phi\rangle$ is a predicate abstract of $L(C)$ of type $\Uparrow\langle t_1,\ldots,t_n\rangle$, then $(v*\mathcal{I}*\Gamma)(\langle\lambda\alpha_1,\ldots,\alpha_n.\Phi\rangle)$ is an intensional object; it is the function that assigns to an arbitrary world Δ the following member of $[\![\langle t_1,\ldots,t_n\rangle,\mathcal{D},\mathcal{G}]\!]$:

$$\{\langle w(\alpha_1),\ldots,w(\alpha_n)\rangle \mid w \text{ is an } \alpha_1,\ldots,\alpha_n \text{ variant of } v \text{ and } \mathcal{M},\Delta \Vdash_w \Phi\}$$

5. For an atomic formula $\tau(\tau_1,\ldots,\tau_n)$,
    (a) If τ is of an intensional type, $\mathcal{M},\Gamma \Vdash_v \tau(\tau_1,\ldots,\tau_n)$ provided $\langle(v*\mathcal{I}*\Gamma)(\tau_1),\ldots,(v*\mathcal{I}*\Gamma)(\tau_n)\rangle \in (v*\mathcal{I}*\Gamma)(\tau)(\Gamma)$.
    (b) If τ is of an extensional type, $\mathcal{M},\Gamma \Vdash_v \tau(\tau_1,\ldots,\tau_n)$ provided $\langle(v*\mathcal{I}*\Gamma)(\tau_1),\ldots,(v*\mathcal{I}*\Gamma)(\tau_n)\rangle \in (v*\mathcal{I}*\Gamma)(\tau)$.
6. $\mathcal{M},\Gamma \Vdash_v \neg\Phi$ if it is not the case that $\mathcal{M},\Gamma \Vdash_v \Phi$.
7. $\mathcal{M},\Gamma \Vdash_v \Phi\wedge\Psi$ if $\mathcal{M},\Gamma \Vdash_v \Phi$ and $\mathcal{M},\Gamma \Vdash_v \Psi$.
8. $\mathcal{M},\Gamma \Vdash_v (\forall\alpha)\Phi$ if $\mathcal{M},\Gamma \Vdash_{v'} \Phi$ for every α-variant v' of v.
9. $\mathcal{M},\Gamma \Vdash_v \Box\Phi$ if $\mathcal{M},\Delta \Vdash_v \Phi$ for all $\Delta \in \mathcal{G}$ such that $\Gamma\mathcal{R}\Delta$.

4   A Modal Interpretation

So far two separate topics, databases and modal logic, have been discussed. It is time to bring them together. I'll show how various database concepts embed naturally into a modal setting. Think of the database as having an informal semantics, and the embedding into modal logic as supplying a precise, formal version.

First of all, think of a record in a database as a possible world in a modal model. This is not at all far-fetched—conceptually they play similar roles. When dealing with databases, records are behind the scenes but are not first-class objects. That is, an answer to a query might be a record *number*, but it will not be a record. In a modal logic possible worlds have a similar role—they are present in the semantics, but a modal language does not refer to them directly.

There is no reason to assume some records outrank others, whatever that might mean, so I'll take the accessibility relation to be the one that always holds. This means our modal operators are those of **S5**.

In the little Locomobile database considered earlier, ground-level objects were strings. I'll carry that over to the modal setting now—the ground level domain will consist of strings. Clearly this choice is not a critical issue.

Attributes are a key item in interpreting a database modally. Fortunately there is a natural counterpart. An attribute assigns to each record some entity of an appropriate kind. In a modal model, an interpreted constant symbol of intensional type assigns to each possible world an object of an appropriate type. I'll simply provide an intensional constant symbol for each attribute, and interpret it accordingly.

By way of illustration, let's create a modal language and model corresponding to the particular database presented in Section 2. It is an example that is sufficiently general to get all the basic ideas across.

To specify the language, it is enough to specify the set C of constant symbols, and their respective types. These will be ground level strings, which give us type 0 constant symbols, and various attributes, which give us intensional constant symbols of various types. The strings from the Locomobile example are 1, 2, 3, 4, automobile, motorcycle, piano, A, B, C, D, red, green, black, blue, yes, no, upright, grand, all of which are taken as type 0 constant symbols. The attributes provide the following higher type constant symbols: IDNumber, Item, and Cylinders, all of type $\uparrow 0$; Engine, Colors, Air, and Config, all of type $\uparrow\langle 0\rangle$; Customer, of type $\uparrow\langle\uparrow\langle 0\rangle\rangle$; Relevant0, of type $\uparrow\langle\uparrow 0\rangle$; Relevant1, of type $\uparrow\langle\uparrow\langle 0\rangle\rangle$; and Relevant2, of type $\uparrow\langle\uparrow\langle\uparrow\langle 0\rangle\rangle\rangle$.

Now that we have our modal language, $L(C)$, the next job is to create a specific modal model, corresponding to the Locomobile tables.

Let $\mathcal{G}$ be the set $\{\Gamma_1, \Gamma_2, \Gamma_3, \Gamma_4\}$, where the intention is that each of these corresponds to one of the four records in the database given in Section 2. Specifically, Γ_i corresponds to the record with an IDNumber of i. As noted above, I'll use an **S5** logic, so $\mathcal{R}$ simply holds between any two members of $\mathcal{G}$.

Let $\mathcal{D}$ be the set of strings used in the Table entries of Section 2, specifically, $\{$1, 2, 3, 4, automobile, motorcycle, piano, A, B, C, D, red, green, black, blue, yes, no, upright, grand$\}$ (thus these are treated as both constant symbols of the language and as members of the ground level domain).

Finally the interpretation $\mathcal{I}$ is specified. On constant symbols of type 0, $\mathcal{I}$ is the identity function—such constant symbols designate themselves. For instance, $\mathcal{I}(\text{piano}) = \text{piano}$. And for the intensional constant symbols, we make them behave as the Locomobile tables of Section 2 specify. For instance, $\mathcal{I}(\text{IDNumber})$ is the function that maps Γ_1 to $\mathcal{I}(1) = 1$, Γ_2 to $\mathcal{I}(2) = 2$, and so on. $\mathcal{I}(\text{Engine})$ is the function that maps Γ_1 to $\{\mathcal{I}(\text{A}), \mathcal{I}(\text{B})\} = \{\text{A}, \text{B}\}$, Γ_2 to $\{\mathcal{I}(\text{A})\} = \{\text{A}\}$, Γ_3 to $\{\mathcal{I}(\text{C}), \mathcal{I}(\text{D})\} = \{\text{C}, \text{D}\}$, and has some arbitrary value on Γ_4. Likewise

$\mathcal{I}(\texttt{Relevant0})$ is the function that maps Γ_1, Γ_2 and Γ_3 to $\{\mathcal{I}(\texttt{IDNumber}), \mathcal{I}(\texttt{Item}),$ $\mathcal{I}(\texttt{Cylinders})\}$, and maps Γ_4 to $\{\mathcal{I}(\texttt{IDNumber}), \mathcal{I}(\texttt{Item})\}$

This completes the definition of a language and a model corresponding to the database of Section 2. I'll call the model $\mathcal{M}_L$ from now on.

5   Queries

Databases exist to be queried. With higher type constructs present, a careful specification of behavior is needed to determine how queries behave. Modal models take care of this very simply, since we have a precise definition of truth available. The question is how to translate queries into the modal language. I'll give some natural language examples of queries for the Locomobile database, and then I'll provide formal versions in the modal language $L(C)$ specified in Section 4. For each I'll consider how the formal version behaves in the model $\mathcal{M}_L$ that was constructed in Section 4. It will be seen that the formal behavior matches intuition quite nicely.

Example 1. Query: Which items have 2 cylinders? Here and in the other examples, I'll use an item's IDNumber to uniquely identify it. As a first attempt at formalizing this query, we might ask for the value of the attribute `IDNumber` in worlds where the value of `Cylinders` is 2. In effect, the modal operators $\square$ and $\Diamond$ act like quantifiers over possible worlds, or records. And we can ask for the value of an attribute at a world by using the extension-of operator, $\downarrow$. This leads us to the following type $\uparrow\langle 0 \rangle$ predicate abstract, in which α is a variable of type 0, and $=$ is the equality symbol of type $\langle 0, 0 \rangle$.

$$\langle \lambda\alpha.\Diamond[(\downarrow\texttt{IDNumber} = \alpha) \wedge (\downarrow\texttt{Cylinders} = 2)]\rangle \tag{1}$$

The problem with this is that the `Cylinders` attribute is undefined for pianos in Table 1. In [2] I specifically allowed partially defined objects, but with a full hierarchy of higher types available, I thought better of that approach here. Instead I introduced "relevancy" attributes. An entry of $\perp$ in a table indicates an irrelevant attribute; no value can have a meaning for the record. In a modal model constant symbols of intensional type are total, but values corresponding to $\perp$ are entirely arbitrary, and should not be considered in queries. Consequently, (1) must be revised to the following.

$$\langle \lambda\alpha.\Diamond[(\downarrow\texttt{IDNumber} = \alpha) \wedge \texttt{Relevant0}(\texttt{Cylinders}) \wedge (\downarrow\texttt{Cylinders} = 2)]\rangle \tag{2}$$

Since this is the first example, I'll do it in some detail, beginning with a verification that (2) is well-formed. For later examples, things will be more abbreviated.

The constant symbol `IDNumber` is of type $\uparrow 0$, so $\downarrow\texttt{IDNumber}$ is of type 0, by part 3 of Definition 2. The variable α is of type 0 and $=$ is of type $\langle 0, 0 \rangle$, so

$=$ (IDNumber, α) is an atomic formula by part 4 of Definition 2. This we write more conventionally as ($\downarrow$IDNumber $= \alpha$). In a similar way ($\downarrow$Cylinders $= 2$) is an atomic formula. Finally, Relevant0 is of type $\uparrow\langle\uparrow 0\rangle$ and Cylinders is of type $\uparrow 0$, so Relevant0(Cylinders) is an atomic formula by part 4 of Definition 2 again. It follows that $\Diamond[(\downarrow$IDNumber $= \alpha) \wedge$ Relevant0(Cylinders) $\wedge (\downarrow$Cylinders $= 2)]$ is a formula. Then (2) is a predicate abstract of type $\uparrow\langle 0\rangle$, by part 2 of Definition 2.

Now if τ is a constant of type 0, by part 4 of Definition 2,

$$\langle\lambda\alpha.\Diamond[(\downarrow\text{IDNumber} = \alpha) \wedge$$
$$\text{Relevant0(Cylinders)} \wedge (\downarrow\text{Cylinders} = 2)]\rangle(\tau) \tag{3}$$

is a formula. The claim is, it is valid in the model $\mathcal{M}_L$ if and only if τ is 1 or 3, which is exactly what we would expect intuitively. (Valid in the model means it is true at each world of it.) I'll check this in some detail for 3.

Let Γ be an arbitrary world of the model, and let v be an arbitrary valuation. I want to verify the following.

$$\mathcal{M}_L, \Gamma \Vdash_v \langle\lambda\alpha.\Diamond[(\downarrow\text{IDNumber} = \alpha) \wedge$$
$$\text{Relevant0(Cylinders)} \wedge (\downarrow\text{Cylinders} = 2)]\rangle(3)$$

By part 5a of Definition 7, this is equivalent to

$$(v * \mathcal{I} * \Gamma)(3) \in (v * \mathcal{I} * \Gamma)(\langle\lambda\alpha.\Diamond[(\downarrow\text{IDNumber} = \alpha) \wedge$$
$$\text{Relevant0(Cylinders)} \wedge (\downarrow\text{Cylinders} = 2)]\rangle)(\Gamma)$$

Now, $(v * \mathcal{I} * \Gamma)(3) = \mathcal{I}(3) = 3$, so by part 4 of Definition 7 we must show

$$\mathcal{M}_L, \Gamma \Vdash_w \Diamond[(\downarrow\text{IDNumber} = \alpha) \wedge \text{Relevant0(Cylinders)} \wedge (\downarrow\text{Cylinders} = 2)]$$

where w is the α-variant of v such that $w(\alpha) = 3$. And this is so because we have the following.

$$\mathcal{M}_L, \Gamma_3 \Vdash_w (\downarrow\text{IDNumber} = \alpha) \wedge \text{Relevant0(Cylinders)} \wedge (\downarrow\text{Cylinders} = 2)$$

I'll check two of the components. To verify that

$$\mathcal{M}_L, \Gamma_3 \Vdash_w (\downarrow\text{IDNumber} = \alpha)$$

we need

$$\langle(w * \mathcal{I} * \Gamma_3)(\downarrow\text{IDNumber}), (w * \mathcal{I} * \Gamma_3)(\alpha)\rangle \in (w * \mathcal{I} * \Gamma_3)(=).$$

But $(w*\mathcal{I}*\Gamma_3)(\downarrow\text{IDNumber}) = (w*\mathcal{I}*\Gamma_3)(\text{IDNumber})(\Gamma_3) = \mathcal{I}(\text{IDNumber})(\Gamma_3) = 3$, and $(w * \mathcal{I} * \Gamma_3)(\alpha) = w(\alpha) = 3$. And equality symbols are always interpreted as equality on extensional objects.

Finally I'll verify that

$$\mathcal{M}_L, \Gamma_3 \Vdash_w \text{Relevant0(Cylinders)}.$$

This will be the case provided we have the following, by part $5a$ of Definition 7.

$$(w * \mathcal{I} * \Gamma_3)(\texttt{Cylinders}) \in (w * \mathcal{I} * \Gamma_3)(\texttt{Relevant0})(\Gamma_3)$$

Now, $(w*\mathcal{I}*\Gamma_3)(\texttt{Cylinders}) = \mathcal{I}(\texttt{Cylinders})$, and $(w*\mathcal{I}*\Gamma_3)(\texttt{Relevant0})(\Gamma_3) = \mathcal{I}(\texttt{Relevant0})(\Gamma_3) = \{\mathcal{I}(\texttt{IDNumber}), \mathcal{I}(\texttt{Item}), \mathcal{I}(\texttt{Cylinders})\}$, and we are done.

Equation (3) has been verified in the case where τ is 1. The case where it is 3 is similar. If τ is 2, it fails because of the ($\downarrow\texttt{Cylinders} = 2$) clause. And the case where τ is 4 fails because of the $\texttt{Relevant0}(\texttt{Cylinders})$ clause.

I'll conclude the section with a few more examples of somewhat greater complexity. There will be no detailed analysis for these.

Example 2. Query: what choices does a customer have when purchasing a four-cylinder car? This turns into the following predicate abstract, where α is of type $\uparrow\langle 0 \rangle$ and β is of type 0. (I've omitted relevancy clauses because $\texttt{Item}$ is always relevant, and for $\texttt{automobile}$ items $\texttt{Cylinders}$ is always relevant. These will be among the various constraints discussed in the next section.)

$$\langle \lambda\alpha, \beta.\Diamond[(\downarrow\texttt{Item} = \texttt{automobile}) \wedge (\downarrow\texttt{Cylinders} = 4) \\ \wedge \texttt{Customer}(\alpha) \wedge \alpha(\beta)]\rangle \tag{4}$$

Abbreviating (4) by τ, we have $\tau(\tau_1, \tau_2)$ is valid in $\mathcal{M}_L$ just in case $\langle \tau_1, \tau_2 \rangle$ is one of

$$\langle\texttt{Colors}, \texttt{green}\rangle \\ \langle\texttt{Colors}, \texttt{black}\rangle \\ \langle\texttt{Air}, \texttt{yes}\rangle \\ \langle\texttt{Air}, \texttt{no}\rangle$$

Example 3. Query: what features can a customer choose, that are available for more than one product? This gives us the following predicate abstract, in which α is of type $\uparrow\langle 0 \rangle$, and β, γ, and δ are of type 0.

$$\langle \lambda\alpha, \beta.\texttt{Customer}(\alpha) \wedge \\ (\exists\gamma)(\exists\delta)\{\neg(\gamma = \delta) \wedge \\ \Diamond[(\uparrow\texttt{IDNumber} = \gamma) \wedge \alpha(\beta)] \wedge \\ \Diamond[(\uparrow\texttt{IDNumber} = \delta) \wedge \alpha(\beta)]\}\rangle \tag{5}$$

Equation (5) validly applies, in $\mathcal{M}_L$, to just the following.

$$\langle\texttt{Colors}, \texttt{green}\rangle \\ \langle\texttt{Colors}, \texttt{black}\rangle$$

6   Constraints

The Locomobile example is really an instance of a database scheme. In order to qualify as an instance, certain constraints must be met. So far, these have been implicit, but now it is time to state them precisely. This provides additional examples of the modal machinery at work.

I've been treating IDNumber as a key attribute. I now want to make this a formal requirement. Ordinarily, to say something is a key is to say there cannot be two records that have a common value on this attribute. In a modal setting, this means the constant symbol IDNumber cannot be interpreted to have the same value at two possible worlds. But possible worlds cannot be referred to directly in our modal language. What we can say instead is that, in any model, worlds agreeing on a value for IDNumber must agree on every attribute. Since we have a full type theory here, this cannot be said with a single formula—we need an infinite family of them, one for each intensional type. Consider the following formula, where α is of type $\uparrow t$, x is of type 0 and y is of type t.

$$(\forall \alpha)\langle \lambda x, y. \Box[(x = \downarrow \text{IDNumber}) \supset (y = \downarrow \alpha)]\rangle(\downarrow \text{IDNumber}, \downarrow \alpha) \qquad (6)$$

Requiring validity of (6) in a model is equivalent to requiring that two worlds where IDNumber is interpreted identically are worlds that agree on values of all intensional attributes of type $\uparrow t$. For the Locomobile example, we only need 5 instances: for types $\uparrow 0$, $\uparrow\langle 0\rangle$, $\uparrow\langle\uparrow 0\rangle$, $\uparrow\langle\uparrow\langle 0\rangle\rangle$, and $\uparrow\langle\uparrow\langle\uparrow\langle 0\rangle\rangle\rangle$.

Formula (6) is actually of more general interest than would appear at first glance. In [2] I noted that such a formula is a *relative rigidity* expression—it requires that all intensional objects of type $\uparrow t$ be rigid relative to IDNumber. Such requirements can be more elaborate, requiring rigidity relative to some combination of attributes. They can also be less elaborate, requiring absolute rigidity. As such, they relate to Kripke's notion of *rigid designator* in [7], but a further discussion would take us too far afield here.

In Example 2 I noted that Item should always be relevant. Clearly so should IDNumber. I also noted that Cylinders should be relevant for items that were automobiles. This means we should require validity of the following.

> Relevant0(Item)
> Relevant0(IDNumber)
> ($\downarrow$Item = automobile) $\supset$ Relevant0(Cylinders)

To be precise, for a modal model to be considered as an instance of the Locomobile scheme, the various constraints above must be valid formulas in it.

This can be turned into a proof-theoretic condition as well. Consider the tables of Section 2 again. It is not hard to see that the first line of Table 1 corresponds to the following formula.

$$\Diamond[(\downarrow \text{IDNumber} = 1) \wedge (\downarrow \text{Item} = \text{automobile}) \wedge (\downarrow \text{Cylinders} = 2) \wedge$$
$$\text{Engine}(A) \wedge \text{Engine}(B) \wedge$$
$$\text{Colors}(\text{red}) \wedge \text{Colors}(\text{green}) \wedge \text{Colors}(\text{black}) \wedge$$
$$\text{Air}(\text{no})]$$

Similarly for the other lines, and tables. Now, to say we have presented an instance of the Locomobile database scheme amounts to saying the constraint formulas given earlier, combined with the various formulas derived from the tables and representing individual records, make up a consistent set.

Consistency can, of course, be checked using a proof procedure, and the higher type modal logic used here does have a tableau system, see [3]. But that system is complete relative to a Henkin model version of our semantics, and is not complete relative to the "true" semantics given in Section 3. Also, a tableau procedure is not a decision method. I leave it as an open problem whether, for formulas of the particular forms that arise in database applications, a decision procedure can be extracted from the tableau method.

7   Conclusion

As promised, I have not proved any theorems. I have, however, provided a precise modal semantics that can be applied naturally to databases containing higher type constructs. Issues of practicability of implementation have been ignored. Issues of decidability for fragments directly applicable to databases have been ignored. I wanted to present the basics with the hope that others would find the subject of sufficient interest to pursue questions like these. I hope I have succeeded, at least a little.

References

1. S. Feferman, J. John W. Dawson, W. Goldfarb, C. Parsons, and R. N. Solovay, editors. *Kurt Gödel Collected Works, Volume III, Unpublished Essays and Lectures.* Oxford University Press, New York, 1995.
2. M. C. Fitting. Modality and databases. Forthcoming, LNCS, Tableaux 2000, 2000.
3. M. C. Fitting. *Types, Tableaus, and Gödel's God.* 2000. Available on my web site: http://comet.lehman.cuny.edu/fitting.
4. M. C. Fitting and R. Mendelsohn. *First-Order Modal Logic.* Kluwer, 1998. Paperback, 1999.
5. D. Gallin. *Intensional and Higher-Order Modal Logic.* North-Holland, 1975.
6. K. Gödel. Ontological proof. In Feferman et al. [1], pages 403–404.
7. S. Kripke. *Naming and Necessity.* Harvard University Press, 1980.
8. R. Montague. On the nature of certain philosophical entities. *The Monist*, 53:159–194, 1960. Reprinted in [11], 148–187.
9. R. Montague. Pragmatics. pages 102–122. 1968. In *Contemporary Philosophy: A Survey*, R. Klibansky editor, Florence, La Nuova Italia Editrice, 1968. Reprinted in [11], 95–118.
10. R. Montague. Pragmatics and intensional logic. *Synthèse*, 22:68–94, 1970. Reprinted in [11], 119–147.
11. R. H. Thomason, editor. *Formal Philosophy, Selected Papers of Richard Montague.* Yale University Press, New Haven and London, 1974.

A Denotational Semantics for First-Order Logic

Krzysztof R. Apt[1,2]

[1] CWI, P.O. Box 94079, 1090 GB Amsterdam, The Netherlands
[2] University of Amsterdam, The Netherlands
http://www.cwi.nl/~apt

Abstract. In Apt and Bezem [AB99] we provided a computational interpretation of first-order formulas over arbitrary interpretations. Here
we complement this work by introducing a denotational semantics for
first-order logic. Additionally, by allowing an assignment of a non-ground
term to a variable we introduce in this framework logical variables.
The semantics combines a number of well-known ideas from the areas of
semantics of imperative programming languages and logic programming.
In the resulting computational view conjunction corresponds to sequential composition, disjunction to "don't know" nondeterminism, existential quantification to declaration of a local variable, and negation to the
"negation as finite failure" rule. The soundness result shows correctness
of the semantics with respect to the notion of truth. The proof resembles
in some aspects the proof of the soundness of the SLDNF-resolution.

1 Introduction

Background

To explain properly the motivation for the work here discussed we need to go
back to the roots of logic programming and constraint logic programming. *Logic
programming* grew out of the seminal work of Robinson [Rob65] on the *resolution method* and the *unification method*. First, Kowalski and Kuehner [KK71]
introduced a limited form of resolution, called linear resolution. Then Kowalski
[Kow74] proposed what we now call *SLD-resolution*. The SLD-resolution is both
a restriction and an extension of the resolution method. Namely, the clauses are
restricted to Horn clauses. However, in the course of the resolution process a
substitution is generated that can be viewed as a result of a computation. Right
from the outset the SLD-resolution became then a crucial example of the *computation as deduction* paradigm according to which the computation process is
identified with a constructive proof of a formula (a query) from a set of axioms
(a program) with the computation process yielding the witness (a substitution).

This lineage of logic programming explains two of its relevant characteristics:

1. the queries and clause bodies are limited to the conjunctions of atoms,
2. the computation takes place (implicitly) over the domain of all ground terms
   of a given first-order language.

J. Lloyd et al. (Eds.): CL 2000, LNAI 1861, pp. 53–69, 2000.

The restriction in item 1. was gradually lifted and through the works of Clark [Cla78] and Lloyd and Topor [LT84] one eventually arrived at the possibility of using as queries and clause bodies arbitrary first-order formulas. This general syntax is for example available in the language Gödel of Lloyd and Hill [HL94].

A way to overcome the restriction in item 2. was proposed in 1987 by Jaffar and Lassez in their influential CLP(X) scheme that led to *constraint logic programming*. In this proposal the computation takes place over an arbitrary interpretation and the queries and clause bodies can contain constraints, i.e., atomic formulas interpreted over the chosen interpretation. The unification mechanism is replaced by a more general process of constraint solving and the outcome of a computation is a sequence of constraints to which the original query reduces.

This powerful idea was embodied since then in many constraint logic programming languages, starting with the CLP($\mathcal{R}$) language of Jaffar, Michaylov, Stuckey, and Yap [JMSY92] in which linear constraints over reals were allowed, and the CHIP language of Dincbas et al. [DVS+88] in which linear constraints over finite domains, combined with constraint propagation, were introduced. A theoretical framework for CHIP was provided in van Hentenryck [Van89].

This transition from logic programming to constraint logic programming introduced a new element. In the CLP(X) scheme the test for satisfiability of a sequence of constraints was needed, while a proper account of the CHIP computing process required an introduction of constraint propagation into the framework. On some interpretations these procedures can be undecidable (the satisfiability test) or computationally expensive (the "ideal" constraint propagation). This explains why in the realized implementations some approximation of the former or limited instances of the latter were chosen for.

So in both approaches the computation (i.e., the deduction) process needs to be parametrized by external procedures that for each specific interpretation have to be provided and implemented separately. In short, in both cases the computation process, while parametrized by the considered interpretation, also depends on the external procedures used. In conclusion: constraint logic programming did not provide a satisfactory answer to the question of how to lift the computation process of logic programming from the domain of all ground terms to an arbitrary interpretation without losing the property that this process is effective.

Arbitrary interpretations are important since they represent a declarative counterpart of data types. In practical situations the selected interpretations would admit sorts that would correspond to the data types chosen by the user for the application at hand, say terms, integers, reals and/or lists, each with the usual operations available. It is useful to contrast this view with the one taken in typed versions of logic programming languages. For example, in the case of the Gödel language (polymorphic) types are provided and are modeled by (polymorphic) sorts in the underlying theoretic model. However, in this model the computation still implicitly takes place over one fixed domain, that of all ground terms partitioned into sorts. This domain properly captures the built-in types but does not provide an account of user defined types. Moreover, in this approach different (i.e., not uniform) interpretation of equality for different types is needed, a feature present in the language but not accounted for in the theoretical model.

Formulas as Programs

The above considerations motivated our work on a computational interpretation of first-order formulas over arbitrary interpretations reported in Apt and Bezem [AB99]. This allowed us to view first-order formulas as executable programs. That is why we called this approach *formulas as programs*. In our approach the computation process is a search of a satisfying valuation for the formula in question. Because the problem of finding such a valuation is in general undecidable, we had to introduce the possibility of partial answers, modeled by an existence of run-time errors.

This ability to compute over arbitrary interpretations allowed us to extend the computation as deduction paradigm to arbitrary interpretations. We noted already that the SLD-resolution is both a restriction and an extension of the resolution method. In turn, the formulas as programs approach is both a restriction and an extension of the logic programming. Namely, the unification process is limited to an extremely simple form of matching involving variables and ground terms only. However, the computation process now takes place over an arbitrary structure and full-first order syntax is adopted.

The formulas as programs approach to programming has been realized in the programming language Alma-0 [ABPS98] that extends imperative programming by features that support declarative programming. In fact, the work reported in Apt and Bezem [AB99] provided logical underpinnings for a fragment of Alma-0 that does not include destructive assignment or recursive procedures and allowed us to reason about non-trivial programs written in this fragment.

Rationale for this Paper

The computational interpretation provided in Apt and Bezem [AB99] can be viewed as an operational semantics of first-order logic. The history of semantics of programming languages has taught us that to better understand the underlying principles it is beneficial to abstract from the details of the operational semantics. This view was put forward by Scott and Strachey [SS71] in their proposal of *denotational semantics* of programming languages according to which, given a programming language, the meaning of each program is a mathematical function of the meanings of its direct constituents.

The aim of this paper is to complement the work of [AB99] by providing a denotational semantics of first-order formulas. This semantics combines a number of ideas realized in the areas of (nondeterministic) imperative programming languages and the field of logic programming. It formalizes a view according to which conjunction can be seen as sequential composition, disjunction as "don't know" nondeterminism, existential quantification as declaration of a local variable, and it relates negation to the "negation as finite failure" rule.

The main result is that the denotational semantics is sound with respect to the truth definition. The proof is reminiscent in some aspects of the proof of the soundness of the SLDNF-resolution of Clarke [Cla78]. The semantics of equations allows matching involving variables and non-ground terms, a feature not present in [AB99] and in Alma-0. This facility introduces logical variables in this framework but also creates a number of difficulties in the soundness proof because bindings to local variables can now be created.

First-order logic is obviously a too limited formalism for programming. In [AB99] we discussed a number of extensions that are convenient for programming purposes, to wit sorts (i.e., types), arrays, bounded quantification and non-recursive procedures. This leads to a very expressive and easy to program in subset of Alma-0. We do not envisage any problems in incorporating these features into the denotational semantics here provided. A major problem is how to deal with recursion.

The plan of the paper is as follows. In the next section we discuss the difficulties encountered when solving arbitrary equations over algebras. Then, in Section 3 we provide a semantics of equations and in Section 4 we extend it to the case of first-order formulas interpreted over an arbitrary interpretation. The resulting semantics is denotational in style. In Section 5 we relate this semantics to the notion of truth by establishing a soundness result. In Section 6 we draw conclusions and suggest some directions for future work.

2   Solving Equations over Algebras

Consider some fixed, but arbitrary, *language of terms* L and a fixed, but arbitrary *algebra* $\mathcal{J}$ for it (sometimes called a *pre-interpretation*). A typical example is the language defining arithmetic expressions and its standard interpretation over the domain of integers.

We are interested in solving equations of the form $s = t$ over an algebra, that is, we seek an instantiation of the variables occurring in s and t that makes this equation true when interpreted over $\mathcal{J}$. By varying L and $\mathcal{J}$ we obtain a whole array of specific decision problems that sometimes can be solved efficiently, like the unification problem or the problem of solving linear equations over reals, and sometimes are undecidable, like the problem of solving Diophantine equations.

Our intention is to use equations as a means to assign values to variables. Consequently, we wish to find a natural, general, situation for which the problem of determining whether an equation $s = t$ has a solution in a given algebra is decidable, and to exhibit a "most general solution", if one exists. By using most general solutions we do not lose any specific solution.

This problem cannot be properly dealt with in full generality. Take for example the polynomial equations over integers. Then the equation $x^2 - 3x + 2 = 0$ has two solutions, $\{x/1\}$ and $\{x/2\}$, and none is "more general" than the other under any reasonable definition of a solution being more general than another.

In fact, given an arbitrary interpretation, the only case that seems to be of any use is that of comparing a variable and an arbitrary term. This brings us to equations of the form $x = t$, where x does not occur in t. Such an equation has obviously a most general solution, namely the instantiation $\{x/t\}$.

A dual problem is that of finding when an equation $s = t$ has no solution in a given algebra. Of course, non-unifiability is not a rescue here: just consider the already mentioned equation $x^2 - 3x + 2 = 0$ the sides of which do not unify.

Again, the only realistic situation seems to be when both terms are ground and their values in the considered algebra are different. This brings us to equations $s = t$ both sides of which are ground terms.

3 Semantics of Equations

After these preliminary considerations we introduce specific "hybrid" objects in which we mix the syntax and semantics.

Definition 1. *Consider a language of terms L and an algebra $\mathcal{J}$ for it. Given a function symbol f we denote by $f_{\mathcal{J}}$ the interpretation of f in $\mathcal{J}$.*

- *Consider a term of L in which we replace some of the variables by the elements of the domain D. We call the resulting object a* generalized term.
- *Given a generalized term t we define its $\mathcal{J}$-evaluation as follows:*
  - *replace each constant occuring in t by its value in $\mathcal{J}$,*
  - *repeatedly replace each sub-object of the form $f(d_1, \ldots, d_n)$ where f is a function symbol and $d_1, \ldots, d_n$ are the elements of the domain D by the element $f_{\mathcal{J}}(d_1, \ldots, d_n)$ of D.*

  We call the resulting generalized term a $\mathcal{J}$-term and denote it by $[\![t]\!]_{\mathcal{J}}$. Note that if t is ground, then $[\![t]\!]_{\mathcal{J}}$ is an element of the domain of $\mathcal{J}$.
- *By a $\mathcal{J}$-substitution we mean a finite mapping from variables to $\mathcal{J}$-terms which assigns to each variable x in its domain a $\mathcal{J}$-term different from x. We write it as $\{x_1/h_1, \ldots, x_n/h_n\}$.*   □

The $\mathcal{J}$-substitutions generalize both the usual substitutions and the valuations, which assign domain values to variables. By adding to the language L constants for each domain element and for each ground term we can reduce the $\mathcal{J}$-substitutions to the substitutions. We preferred not to do this to keep the notation simple.

In what follows we denote the empty $\mathcal{J}$-substitution by ε and arbitrary $\mathcal{J}$-substitutions by θ, η, γ with possible subscripts.

A more intuitive way of introducing $\mathcal{J}$-terms is as follows. Each ground term of s of L evaluates to a unique value in $\mathcal{J}$. Given a generalized term t replace each maximal ground subterm of t by its value in $\mathcal{J}$. The outcome is the $\mathcal{J}$-term $[\![t]\!]_{\mathcal{J}}$.

We define the notion of an application of a $\mathcal{J}$-substitution θ to a generalized term t in the standard way and denote it by $t\theta$. If t is a term, then $t\theta$ does not have to be a term, though it is a generalized term.

Definition 2.

 – A composition of two $\mathcal{J}$-substitutions θ and η, written as $\theta\eta$, is defined as the unique $\mathcal{J}$-substitution γ such that for each variable x

$$x\gamma = [\![(x\theta)\eta]\!]_{\mathcal{J}}.$$

$\square$

Let us illustrate the introduced concepts by means of two examples.

Example 1. Take an arbitrary language of terms L. The *Herbrand algebra* Her for L is defined as follows:

 – its domain is the set HU_L of all ground terms of L (usually called the *Herbrand universe*),
 – if f is an n-ary function symbol in L, then its interpretation is the mapping from $(HU_L)^n$ to HU_L which maps the sequence $t_1, \ldots, t_n$ of ground terms to the ground term $f(t_1, \ldots, t_n)$.

Consider now a term s. Then $[\![s]\!]_{Her}$ equals s because in Her every ground term evaluates to itself. So the notions of a term, a generalized term and a Her-term coincide. Consequently, the notions of substitutions and Her-substitutions coincide. $\square$

Example 2. Take as the language of terms the language AE of *arithmetic expressions*. Its binary function symbols are the usual $\cdot$ ("times"), $+$ ("plus") and $-$ ("minus"), and its unique binary symbol is $-$ ("unary minus"). Further, for each integer $\mathbf{k}$ there is a constant k.

As the algebra for AE we choose the standard algebra Int that consists of the set of integers with the function symbols interpreted in the standard way. In what follows we write the binary function symbols in the usual infix notation.

Consider the term $s \equiv x + (((3+2) \cdot 4) - y)$. Then $[\![s]\!]_{AE}$ equals $x + (20 - y)$. Further, given the AE-substitution $\theta := \{x/6 - z, y/3\}$ we have $s\theta \equiv (6 - z) + (((3 + 2) \cdot 4) - \mathbf{3})$ and consequently, $[\![s\theta]\!]_{AE} = (6 - z) + \mathbf{17}$. Further, given $\eta := \{z/4\}$, we have $\theta\eta = \{x/2, y/3, z/4\}$. $\square$

To define the meaning of an equation over an algebra $\mathcal{J}$ we view $\mathcal{J}$-substitutions as states and use a special state

 – *error*, to indicate that it is not possible to determine effectively whether a solution to the equation $s\theta = t\theta$ in $\mathcal{J}$ exists.

We now define the semantics $[\![\cdot]\!]$ of an equation between two generalized terms as follows:

$$[\![s = t]\!](\theta) := \begin{cases} \{\theta\{s\theta/[\![t\theta]\!]_{\mathcal{J}}\}\} & \text{if } s\theta \text{ is a variable that does not occur in } t\theta, \\ \{\theta\{t\theta/[\![s\theta]\!]_{\mathcal{J}}\}\} & \text{if } t\theta \text{ is a variable that does not occur in } s\theta \\ & \text{and } s\theta \text{ is not a variable,} \\ \{\theta\} & \text{if } [\![s\theta]\!]_{\mathcal{J}} \text{ and } [\![t\theta]\!]_{\mathcal{J}} \text{ are identical,} \\ \emptyset & \text{if } s\theta \text{ and } t\theta \text{ are ground and } [\![s\theta]\!]_{\mathcal{J}} \neq [\![t\theta]\!]_{\mathcal{J}}, \\ \{error\} & \text{otherwise.} \end{cases}$$

It will become clear in the next section why we collect here the unique outcome into a set and why we "carry" θ in the answers.

Note that according to the above definition we have $[\![s = t]\!](\theta) = \{error\}$ for the non-ground generalized terms $s\theta$ and $t\theta$ such that the $\mathcal{J}$-terms $[\![s\theta]\!]_{\mathcal{J}}$ and $[\![t\theta]\!]_{\mathcal{J}}$ are different. In some situations we could safely assert then that $[\![s = t]\!](\theta) = \{\theta\}$ or that $[\![s = t]\!](\theta) = \emptyset$. For example, for the standard algebra Int for the language of arithmetic expressions we could safely assert that $[\![x + x = 2 \cdot x]\!](\theta) = \{\theta\}$ and $[\![x + 1 = x]\!](\theta) = \emptyset$ for any AE-substitution θ.

The reason we did not do this was that we wanted to ensure that the semantics is uniform and decidable so that it can be implemented.

4   A Denotational Semantics for First-Order Logic

Consider now a first-order language with equality $\mathcal{L}$. In this section we extend the semantics $[\![\cdot]\!]$ to arbitrary first-order formulas from $\mathcal{L}$ interpreted over an arbitrary interpretation. $[\![\cdot]\!]$ depends on the considered interpretation but to keep the notation simple we do not indicate this dependence. This semantics is denotational in the sense that meaning of each formula is a mathematical function of the meanings of its direct constituents.

Fix an interpretation $\mathcal{I}$. $\mathcal{I}$ is based on some algebra $\mathcal{J}$. We define the notion of an application of a $\mathcal{J}$-substitution θ to a formula ϕ of $\mathcal{L}$, written as $\phi\theta$, in the usual way.

Consider an atomic formula $p(t_1, \ldots, t_n)$ and a $\mathcal{J}$-substitution θ. We denote by $p_{\mathcal{I}}$ the interpretation of p in $\mathcal{I}$.

We say that

- $p(t_1, \ldots, t_n)\theta$ is *true* if $p(t_1, \ldots, t_n)\theta$ is ground and $([\![t_1\theta]\!]_{\mathcal{J}}, \ldots, [\![t_n\theta]\!]_{\mathcal{J}}) \in p_{\mathcal{I}}$,
- $p(t_1, \ldots, t_n)\theta$ is *false* if $p(t_1, \ldots, t_n)\theta$ is ground and $([\![t_1\theta]\!]_{\mathcal{J}}, \ldots, [\![t_n\theta]\!]_{\mathcal{J}}) \notin p_{\mathcal{I}}$.

In what follows we denote by $Subs$ the set of $\mathcal{J}$-substitutions and by $\mathcal{P}(A)$, for a set A, the set of all subsets of A.

For a given formula ϕ its semantics $[\![\phi]\!]$ is a mapping

$$[\![\phi]\!] : Subs \to \mathcal{P}(Subs \cup \{error\}).$$

The fact that the outcome of $[\![\phi]\!](\theta)$ is a set reflects the possibility of a nondeterminism here modeled by the disjunction.

To simplify the definition we extend $[\![\cdot]\!]$ to deal with subsets of $Subs \cup \{error\}$ by putting

$$[\![\phi]\!](error) := \{error\},$$

and for a set $X \subseteq Subs \cup \{error\}$

$$[\![\phi]\!](X) := \bigcup_{e \in X} [\![\phi]\!](e).$$

Further, to deal with the existential quantifier, we introduce an operation $DROP_x$, where x is a variable. First we define $DROP_x$ on the elements of $Subs \cup \{error\}$ by putting for a $\mathcal{J}$-substitution θ

$$DROP_x(\theta) := \begin{cases} \theta \text{ if } x \text{ is not in the domain of } \theta, \\ \eta \text{ if } \theta \text{ is of the form } \eta \uplus \{x/s\}, \end{cases}$$

and

$$DROP_x(error) := error.$$

Then we extend it element-wise to subsets of $Subs \cup \{error\}$, that is, by putting for a set $X \subseteq Subs \cup \{error\}$

$$DROP_x(X) := \{DROP_x(e) \mid e \in X\}.$$

$[\![\cdot]\!]$ is defined by structural induction as follows, where A is an atomic formula different from $s = t$:

- $[\![A]\!](\theta) := \begin{cases} \{\theta\} & \text{if } A\theta \text{ is true}, \\ \emptyset & \text{if } A\theta \text{ is false}, \\ \{error\} & \text{otherwise, that is if } A\theta \text{ is not ground}, \end{cases}$
- $[\![\phi_1 \wedge \phi_2]\!](\theta) := [\![\phi_2]\!]([\![\phi_1]\!](\theta))$,
- $[\![\phi_1 \vee \phi_2]\!](\theta) := [\![\phi_1]\!](\theta) \cup [\![\phi_2]\!](\theta)$,
- $[\![\neg\phi]\!](\theta) := \begin{cases} \{\theta\} & \text{if } [\![\phi]\!](\theta) = \emptyset, \\ \emptyset & \text{if } \theta \in [\![\phi]\!](\theta), \\ \{error\} & \text{otherwise}, \end{cases}$
- $[\![\exists x\, \phi]\!](\theta) := DROP_y([\![\phi\{x/y\}]\!](\theta))$, where y is a fresh variable.

To better understand this definition let us consider some simple examples that refer to the algebras discussed in Examples 1 and 2.

Example 3. Take an interpretation $\mathcal{I}$ based on the Herbrand algebra Her. Then

$$[\![f(x) = z \wedge g(z) = g(f(x))]\!](\{x/g(y)\}) = [\![g(z) = g(f(x))]\!](\theta) = \{\theta\},$$

where $\theta := \{x/g(y), z/f(g(y))\}$. On the other hand

$$[\![g(f(x)) = g(z)]\!](\{x/g(y)\}) = \{error\}.$$

$\square$

Example 4. Take an interpretation $\mathcal{I}$ based on the standard algebra AE for the language of arithmetic expressions. Then

$$[\![y = z - 1 \wedge z = x + 2]\!](\{x/1\}) = [\![z = x + 2]\!](\{x/1, y/z - 1\}) = \{x/1, y/2, z/3\}.$$

Further,

$$[\![y + 1 = z - 1]\!](\{y/1, z/3\}) = \{y/1, z/3\}$$

and even

$$\llbracket x \cdot (y + 1) = (v + 1) \cdot (z - 1) \rrbracket(\{x/v + 1,\ y/1,\ z/3\}) = \{x/v + 1,\ y/1,\ z/3\}.$$

On the other hand

$$\llbracket y - 1 = z - 1 \rrbracket(\varepsilon) = \{error\}.$$

□

The first example shows that the semantics given here is weaker than the one provided by the logic programming. In turn, the second example shows that our treatment of arithmetic expressions is more general than the one provided by Prolog.

This definition of denotational semantics of first-order formulas combines a number of ideas put forward in the area of semantics of imperative programming languages and the field of logic programming.

First, for an atomic formula A, when $A\theta$ is ground, its meaning coincides with the meaning of a Boolean expression given in de Bakker [dB80, page 270]. In turn, the meaning of the conjunction and of the disjunction follows [dB80, page 270] in the sense that the conjunction corresponds to the sequential composition operation ";" and the disjunction corresponds to the "don't know" nondeterministic choice, denoted there by $\cup$.

Next, the meaning of the negation is inspired by its treatment in logic programming. To be more precise we need the following observations the proofs of which easily follow by structural induction.

Note 1.

(i) If $\eta \in \llbracket \phi \rrbracket(\theta)$, then $\eta = \theta\gamma$ for some $\mathcal{J}$-substitution γ.
(ii) If $\phi\theta$ is ground, then $\llbracket \phi \rrbracket(\theta) \subseteq \{\theta\}$.   □

First, we interpret $\llbracket \phi \rrbracket(\theta) \cap Subs \neq \emptyset$ as the statement "the query $\phi\theta$ succeeds". More specifically, if $\eta \in \llbracket \phi \rrbracket(\theta)$, then by Note 1(i) for some γ we have $\eta = \theta\gamma$.

In general, γ is of course not unique: take for example $\theta := \{x/0\}$ and $\eta = \theta$. Then both $\eta = \theta\varepsilon$ and $\eta = \theta\theta$. However, it is easy to show that if η is less general than θ, then in the set $\{\gamma \mid \eta = \theta\gamma\}$ the $\mathcal{J}$-substitution with the smallest domain is uniquely defined. In what follows given $\mathcal{J}$-substitutions η and θ such that η is less general than θ, when writing $\eta = \theta\gamma$ we always refer to this uniquely defined γ.

Now we interpret $\theta\gamma \in \llbracket \phi \rrbracket(\theta)$ as the statement "γ is the computed answer substitution for the query $\phi\theta$". In turn, we interpret $\llbracket \phi \rrbracket(\theta) = \emptyset$ as the statement "the query $\phi\theta$ finitely fails".

Suppose now that $\llbracket \phi \rrbracket(\theta) \cap Subs \neq \emptyset$, which means that the query $\phi\theta$ succeeds. Assume additionally that $\phi\theta$ is ground. Then by Note 1(ii) $\theta \in \llbracket \phi \rrbracket(\theta)$ and consequently by the definition of the meaning of negation $\llbracket \neg\phi \rrbracket(\theta) = \emptyset$, which means that the query $\neg\phi\theta$ finitely fails.

In turn, suppose that $[\![\phi]\!](\theta) = \emptyset$, which means that the query $\phi\theta$ finitely fails. By the definition of the meaning of negation $[\![\neg\phi]\!](\theta) = \{\theta\}$, which means that the query $\neg\phi\theta$ succeeds with the empty computed answer substitution.

This explains the relation with the "negation as finite failure" rule according to which for a ground query Q:

- if Q succeeds, then $\neg Q$ finitely fails,
- if Q finitely fails, then $\neg Q$ succeeds with the empty computed answer substitution.

In fact, our definition of the meaning of negation corresponds to a generalization of the negation as finite failure rule already mentioned in Clark [Cla78], according to which the requirement that Q is ground is dropped and the first item is replaced by:

- if Q succeeds with the empty computed answer substitution, then $\neg Q$ finitely fails.

Finally, the meaning of the existential quantification corresponds to the meaning of the block statement in imperative languages, see, e.g., de Bakker [dB80, page 226], with the important difference that the local variable is not initialized. From this viewpoint the existential quantifier $\exists x$ corresponds to the declaration of the local variable x. The $DROP_x$ operation was introduced in Clarke [Cla79] to deal with the declarations of local variables.

We do not want to make the meaning of the formula $\exists x\ \phi$ dependent on the choice of y. Therefore we postulate that for *any* fresh variable y the set $DROP_y([\![\phi\{x/y\}]\!](\theta))$ is a meaning of $\exists x\ \phi$ given a $\mathcal{J}$-substitution θ. Consequently, the semantics of $\exists x\ \phi$ has many outcomes, one for each choice of y. This "multiplicity" of meanings then extends to all formulas containing the existential quantifier. So for example for any variable y different from x and z the $\mathcal{J}$-substitution $\{z/f(y)\}$ is the meaning of $\exists x\ (z = f(x))$ given the empty $\mathcal{J}$-substitution ε.

5   Soundness

To relate the introduced semantics to the notion of truth we first formalize the latter using the notion of a $\mathcal{J}$-substitution instead of the customary notion of a valuation.

Consider a first-order language $\mathcal{L}$ with equality and an interpretation $\mathcal{I}$ for it based on some algebra $\mathcal{J}$. Let θ be a $\mathcal{J}$-substitution. We define the relation $\mathcal{I} \models_\theta \phi$ for a formula ϕ by structural induction. First we assume that θ is defined on all free variables of ϕ and put

- $\mathcal{I} \models_\theta s = t$ iff $[\![s\theta]\!]_{\mathcal{J}}$ and $[\![t\theta]\!]_{\mathcal{J}}$ coincide,
- $\mathcal{I} \models_\theta p(t_1,\ldots,t_n)$ iff $p(t_1,\ldots,t_n)\theta$ is ground and $([\![t_1\theta]\!]_{\mathcal{J}},\ldots,[\![t_n\theta]\!]_{\mathcal{J}}) \in p_{\mathcal{I}}$.

In other words, $\mathcal{I} \models_\theta p(t_1, \ldots, t_n)$ iff $p(t_1, \ldots, t_n)\theta$ is true. The definition extends to non-atomic formulas in the standard way.

Now assume that θ is not defined on all free variables of ϕ. We put

- $\mathcal{I} \models_\theta \phi$ iff $\mathcal{I} \models_\theta \forall x_1, \ldots, \forall x_n \phi$ where $x_1, \ldots, x_n$ is the list of the free variables of ϕ that do not occur in the domain of θ.

Finally,

- $\mathcal{I} \models \phi$ iff $\mathcal{I} \models_\theta \phi$ for all $\mathcal{J}$-substitutions θ.

To prove the main theorem we need the following notation. Given a $\mathcal{J}$-substitution $\eta := \{x_1/h_1, \ldots, x_n/h_n\}$ we define $\langle \eta \rangle := x_1 = h_1 \wedge \ldots \wedge x_n = h_n$.

In the discussion that follows the following simple observation will be useful.

Note 2. For all $\mathcal{J}$-substitutions θ and formulas ϕ

$$\mathcal{I} \models_\theta \phi \text{ iff } \mathcal{I} \models \langle \theta \rangle \to \phi.$$

$\square$

The following theorem now shows correctness of the introduced semantics with respect to the notion of truth.

Theorem 1 (Soundness).

Consider a first-order language $\mathcal{L}$ with equality and an interpretation $\mathcal{I}$ for it based on some algebra $\mathcal{J}$. Let ϕ be a formula of $\mathcal{L}$ and θ a $\mathcal{J}$-substitution.

(i) For each $\mathcal{J}$-substitution $\eta \in [\![\phi]\!](\theta)$

$$\mathcal{I} \models_\eta \phi.$$

(ii) If error $\notin [\![\phi]\!](\theta)$, then

$$\mathcal{I} \models \phi\theta \leftrightarrow \bigvee_{i=1}^{k} \exists \mathbf{y}_i \langle \eta_i \rangle,$$

where $[\![\phi]\!](\theta) = \{\theta\eta_1, \ldots, \theta\eta_k\}$, and for $i \in [1..k]$ $\mathbf{y}_i$ is a sequence of variables that appear in the range of η_i.

Note that by *(ii)* if $[\![\phi]\!](\theta) = \emptyset$, then

$$\mathcal{I} \models_\theta \neg\phi.$$

In particular, if $[\![\phi]\!](\varepsilon) = \emptyset$, then

$$\mathcal{I} \models \neg\phi.$$

Proof. The proof proceeds by simultaneous induction on the structure of the formulas.

ϕ is $s = t$.

If $\eta \in [\![\phi]\!](\theta)$, then three possibilities arise.

1. $s\theta$ is a variable that does not occur in $t\theta$.

Then $[\![s = t]\!](\theta) = \{\theta\{s\theta/[\![t\theta]\!]_{\mathcal{J}}\}\}$ and consequently $\eta = \theta\{s\theta/[\![t\theta]\!]_{\mathcal{J}}\}$. So $\mathcal{I} \models_\eta (s = t)$ holds since $s\eta = [\![t\theta]\!]_{\mathcal{J}}$ and $t\eta = t\theta$.

2. $t\theta$ is a variable that does not occur in $s\theta$ and $s\theta$ is not a variable.

Then $[\![s = t]\!](\theta) = \{\theta\{t\theta/[\![s\theta]\!]_{\mathcal{J}}\}\}$. This case is symmetric to 1.

3. $[\![s\theta]\!]_{\mathcal{J}}$ and $[\![t\theta]\!]_{\mathcal{J}}$ are identical.

Then $\eta = \theta$, so $\mathcal{I} \models_\eta (s = t)$ holds.

If $error \notin [\![\phi]\!](\theta)$, then four possibilities arise.

1. $s\theta$ is a variable that does not occur in $t\theta$.

Then $[\![s = t]\!](\theta) = \{\theta\{s\theta/[\![t\theta]\!]_{\mathcal{J}}\}\}$. We have $\mathcal{I} \models (s = t)\theta \leftrightarrow s\theta = [\![t\theta]\!]_{\mathcal{J}}$.

2. $t\theta$ is a variable that does not occur in $s\theta$ and $s\theta$ is not a variable.

Then $[\![s = t]\!](\theta) = \{\theta\{t\theta/[\![s\theta]\!]_{\mathcal{J}}\}\}$. This case is symmetric to 1.

3. $[\![s\theta]\!]_{\mathcal{J}}$ and $[\![t\theta]\!]_{\mathcal{J}}$ are identical.

Then $[\![s = t]\!](\theta) = \{\theta\}$. We have $[\![s = t]\!](\theta) = \{\theta\varepsilon\}$ and $\mathcal{I} \models_\theta s = t$, so $\mathcal{I} \models (s = t)\theta \leftrightarrow \langle\varepsilon\rangle$, since $\langle\varepsilon\rangle$ is vacuously true.

4. $s\theta$ and $t\theta$ are ground $\mathcal{J}$-terms and $[\![s\theta]\!]_{\mathcal{J}} \neq [\![t\theta]\!]_{\mathcal{J}}$.

Then $[\![s = t]\!](\theta) = \emptyset$ and $\mathcal{I} \models_\theta \neg(s = t)$, so $\mathcal{I} \models (s = t)\theta \leftrightarrow falsum$, where $falsum$ denotes the empty disjunction.

ϕ is an atomic formula different from $s = t$.

If $\eta \in [\![\phi]\!](\theta)$, then $\eta = \theta$ and $\phi\theta$ is true. So $\mathcal{I} \models_\theta \phi$, i.e., $\mathcal{I} \models_\eta \phi$.

If $error \notin [\![\phi]\!](\theta)$, then either $[\![\phi]\!](\theta) = \{\theta\}$ or $[\![\phi]\!](\theta) = \emptyset$. In both cases the argument is the same as in case 3. and 4. for the equality $s = t$.

Note that in both cases we established a stronger form of (ii) in which each list $\mathbf{y}_i$ is empty, i.e., no quantification over the variables in $\mathbf{y}_i$ appears.

ϕ is $\phi_1 \wedge \phi_2$. This is the most elaborate case.

If $\eta \in [\![\phi]\!](\theta)$, then for some $\mathcal{J}$-substitution γ both $\gamma \in [\![\phi_1]\!](\theta)$ and $\eta \in [\![\phi_2]\!](\gamma)$. By induction hypothesis both $\mathcal{I} \models_\gamma \phi_1$ and $\mathcal{I} \models_\eta \phi_2$. But by Note 1(i) η is less general than γ, so $\mathcal{I} \models_\eta \phi_1$ and consequently $\mathcal{I} \models_\eta \phi_1 \wedge \phi_2$.

If $error \notin [\![\phi]\!](\theta)$, then for some $X \subseteq Subs$ both $[\![\phi_1]\!](\theta) = X$ and $error \notin [\![\phi_2]\!](\eta)$ for all $\eta \in X$.

By induction hypothesis

$$\mathcal{I} \models \phi_1\theta \leftrightarrow \bigvee_{i=1}^{k} \exists \mathbf{y}_i \langle \eta_i \rangle,$$

where $X = \{\theta\eta_1, \ldots, \theta\eta_k\}$ and for $i \in [1..k]$ $\mathbf{y}_i$ is a sequence of variables that appear in the range of η_i. Hence

$$\mathcal{I} \models (\phi_1 \wedge \phi_2)\theta \leftrightarrow \bigvee_{i=1}^{k} (\exists \mathbf{y}_i \langle \eta_i \rangle \wedge \phi_2 \theta),$$

so by appropriate renaming of the variables in the sequences $\mathbf{y}_i$

$$\mathcal{I} \models (\phi_1 \wedge \phi_2)\theta \leftrightarrow \bigvee_{i=1}^{k} \exists \mathbf{y}_i (\langle \eta_i \rangle \wedge \phi_2 \theta).$$

But for any $\mathcal{J}$-substitution δ and a formula ψ

$$\mathcal{I} \models \langle \delta \rangle \wedge \psi \leftrightarrow \langle \delta \rangle \wedge \psi \delta,$$

so

$$\mathcal{I} \models (\phi_1 \wedge \phi_2)\theta \leftrightarrow (\bigvee_{i=1}^{k} \exists \mathbf{y}_i (\langle \eta_i \rangle \wedge \phi_2 \theta \eta_i)). \tag{1}$$

Further, we have for $i \in [1..k]$

$$[\![\phi_2]\!](\theta\eta_i) = \{\theta\eta_i\gamma_{i,j} \mid j \in [1..\ell_i]\}$$

for some $\mathcal{J}$-substitutions $\gamma_{i,1}, \ldots, \gamma_{i,\ell_i}$. So

$$[\![\phi_1 \wedge \phi_2]\!](\theta) = \{\theta\eta_i\gamma_{i,j} \mid i \in [1..k], j \in [1..\ell_i]\}.$$

By induction hypothesis we have for $i \in [1..k]$

$$\mathcal{I} \models \phi_2\theta\eta_i \leftrightarrow \bigvee_{j=1}^{\ell_i} \exists \mathbf{v}_{i,j} \langle \gamma_{i,j} \rangle,$$

where for $i \in [1..k]$ and $j \in [1..\ell_i]$ $\mathbf{v}_{i,j}$ is a sequence of variables that appear in the range of $\gamma_{i,j}$.

Using (1) by appropriate renaming of the variables in the sequences $\mathbf{v}_{i,j}$ we now conclude that

$$\mathcal{I} \models (\phi_1 \wedge \phi_2)\theta \leftrightarrow \bigvee_{i=1}^{k} \bigvee_{j=1}^{\ell_i} \exists \mathbf{y}_i \exists \mathbf{v}_{i,j} (\langle \eta_i \rangle \wedge \langle \gamma_{i,j} \rangle),$$

so

$$\mathcal{I} \models (\phi_1 \wedge \phi_2)\theta \leftrightarrow \bigvee_{i=1}^{k} \bigvee_{j=1}^{\ell_i} \exists \mathbf{y}_i \exists \mathbf{v}_{i,j} \langle \eta_i \gamma_{i,j} \rangle,$$

since the domains of η_i and $\gamma_{i,j}$ are disjoint and for any $\mathcal{J}$-substitutions γ and δ with disjoint domains we have

$$\mathcal{I} \models \langle \gamma \rangle \wedge \langle \delta \rangle \leftrightarrow \langle \gamma\delta \rangle.$$

ϕ is $\phi_1 \lor \phi_2$.

If $\eta \in [\![\phi]\!](\theta)$, then either $\eta \in [\![\phi_1]\!](\theta)$ or $\eta \in [\![\phi_2]\!](\theta)$, so by induction hypothesis either $\mathcal{I} \models_\eta \phi_1$ or $\mathcal{I} \models_\eta \phi_2$. In both cases $\mathcal{I} \models_\eta \phi_1 \lor \phi_2$ holds.

If $error \notin [\![\phi]\!](\theta)$, then for some $\mathcal{J}$-substitutions $\eta_1, \ldots, \eta_k$

$$[\![\phi_1]\!](\theta) = \{\theta\eta_1, \ldots, \theta\eta_k\},$$

where $k \geq 0$, for some $\mathcal{J}$-substitutions $\eta_{k+1}, \ldots, \eta_{k+\ell}$,

$$[\![\phi_2]\!](\theta) = \{\theta\eta_{k+1}, \ldots, \theta\eta_{k+\ell}\},$$

where $\ell \geq 0$, and

$$[\![\phi_1 \lor \phi_2]\!](\theta) = \{\theta\eta_1, \ldots, \theta\eta_{k+\ell}\}.$$

By induction hypothesis both

$$\mathcal{I} \models \phi_1\theta \leftrightarrow \bigvee_{i=1}^{k} \exists \mathbf{y}_i \langle \eta_i \rangle$$

and

$$\mathcal{I} \models \phi_2\theta \leftrightarrow \bigvee_{i=k+1}^{k+\ell} \exists \mathbf{y}_i \langle \eta_i \rangle$$

for appropriate sequences of variables $\mathbf{y}_i$. So

$$\mathcal{I} \models (\phi_1 \lor \phi_2)\theta \leftrightarrow \bigvee_{i=1}^{k+\ell} \exists \mathbf{y}_i \langle \eta_i \rangle.$$

ϕ is $\neg\phi_1$.

If $\eta \in [\![\phi]\!](\theta)$, then $\eta = \theta$ and $[\![\phi_1]\!](\theta) = \emptyset$. By induction hypothesis $\mathcal{I} \models_\theta \neg\phi_1$, i.e., $\mathcal{I} \models_\eta \neg\phi_1$.

If $error \notin [\![\phi]\!](\theta)$, then either $[\![\phi]\!](\theta) = \{\theta\}$ or $[\![\phi]\!](\theta) = \emptyset$. In the former case $[\![\phi]\!](\theta) = \{\theta\varepsilon\}$, so $[\![\phi_1]\!](\theta) = \emptyset$. By induction hypothesis $\mathcal{I} \models_\theta \neg\phi_1$, i.e., $\mathcal{I} \models (\neg\phi_1)\theta \leftrightarrow \langle\varepsilon\rangle$, since $\langle\varepsilon\rangle$ is vacuously true. In the latter case $\theta \in [\![\phi_1]\!](\theta)$, so by induction hypothesis $\mathcal{I} \models_\theta \phi_1$, i.e., $\mathcal{I} \models (\neg\phi_1)\theta \leftrightarrow falsum$.

ϕ is $\exists x\, \phi_1$.

If $\eta \in [\![\phi]\!](\theta)$, then $\eta \in DROP_y([\![\phi_1\{x/y\}]\!](\theta))$ for some fresh variable y. So either (if y is not in the domain of η) $\eta \in [\![\phi_1\{x/y\}]\!](\theta)$ or for some $\mathcal{J}$-term s we have $\eta \uplus \{y/s\} \in [\![\phi_1\{x/y\}]\!](\theta)$. By induction hypothesis in the former case $\mathcal{I} \models_\eta \phi_1\{x/y\}$ and in the latter case $\mathcal{I} \models_{\eta\uplus\{y/s\}} \phi_1\{x/y\}$. In both cases $\mathcal{I} \models \exists y\, (\phi_1\{x/y\}\eta)$, so, since y is fresh, $\mathcal{I} \models (\exists y\, \phi_1\{x/y\})\eta$ and consequently $\mathcal{I} \models (\exists x\, \phi_1)\eta$, i.e., $\mathcal{I} \models_\eta \exists x\, \phi_1$.

If $error \notin [\![\phi]\!](\theta)$, then $error \notin [\![\phi_1\{x/y\}]\!](\theta)$, as well, where y is a fresh variable. By induction hypothesis

$$\mathcal{I} \models \phi_1\{x/y\}\theta \leftrightarrow \bigvee_{i=1}^{k} \exists \mathbf{y}_i \langle \eta_i \rangle, \tag{2}$$

where

$$[\![\phi_1\{x/y\}]\!](\theta) = \{\theta\eta_1, \ldots, \theta\eta_k\} \tag{3}$$

and for $i \in [1..k]$ $\mathbf{y}_i$ is a sequence of variables that appear in the range of η_i.

Since y is fresh, we have $\mathcal{I} \models \exists y\,(\phi_1\{x/y\}\theta) \leftrightarrow (\exists y\,\phi_1\{x/y\})\theta$ and $\mathcal{I} \models (\exists y\,\phi_1\{x/y\})\theta \leftrightarrow (\exists x\,\phi_1)\theta$. So (2) implies

$$\mathcal{I} \models (\exists x\,\phi_1)\theta \leftrightarrow \bigvee_{i=1}^{k} \exists y \exists \mathbf{y}_i \langle \eta_i \rangle.$$

But for $i \in [1..k]$

$$\mathcal{I} \models \exists y\langle \eta_i \rangle \leftrightarrow \exists y \langle DROP_y(\eta_i) \rangle,$$

since if $y/s \in \eta_i$, then the variable y does not appear in s. So

$$\mathcal{I} \models (\exists x\,\phi_1)\theta \leftrightarrow \bigvee_{i=1}^{k} \exists \mathbf{y}_i \exists y \langle DROP_y(\eta_i) \rangle. \tag{4}$$

Now, by (3)

$$[\![\exists x\,\phi_1]\!](\theta) = \{DROP_y(\theta\eta_1), \ldots, DROP_y(\theta\eta_k)\}.$$

But y does not occur in θ, so we have for $i \in [1..k]$

$$DROP_y(\theta\eta_i) = \theta DROP_y(\eta_i)$$

and consequently

$$[\![\exists x\,\phi_1]\!](\theta) = \{\theta DROP_y(\eta_1), \ldots, \theta DROP_y(\eta_k)\}.$$

This by virtue of (4) concludes the proof. □

Informally, (i) states that every computed answer substitution of $\phi\theta$ validates it. It is useful to point out that (ii) is a counterpart of Theorem 3 in Clark [Cla78]. Intuitively, it states that a query is equivalent to the disjunction of its computed answer substitutions written out in an equational form (using the $\langle \eta \rangle$ notation). In our case this property holds only if $error$ is not a possible outcome. Indeed, if $[\![s = t]\!](\theta) = \{error\}$, then nothing can be stated about the status of the statement $\mathcal{I} \models (s = t)\theta$.

Note that in case $error \notin [\![\phi]\!](\theta)$, (ii) implies (i) by virtue of Note 2. On the other hand, if $error \in [\![\phi]\!](\theta)$, then (i) can still be applicable while (ii) not.

Additionally existential quantifiers have to be used in an appropriate way. The formulas of the form $\exists \mathbf{y}\langle \eta \rangle$ also appear in Maher [Mah88] in connection with a study of the decision procedures for the algebras of trees. In fact, there are some interesting connections between this paper and ours that could be investigated in a closer detail.

6   Conclusions and Future Work

In this paper we provided a denotational semantics to first-order logic formulas. This semantics is a counterpart of the operational semantics introduced in Apt and Bezem [AB99]. The important difference is that we provide here a more general treatment of equality according to which a non-ground term can be assigned to a variable. This realizes logical variables in the framework of Apt and Bezem [AB99]. This feature led to a number of complications in the proof of the Soundness Theorem 1.

One of the advantages of this theorem is that it allows us to reason about the considered program simply by comparing it to the formula representing its specification. In the case of operational semantics this was exemplified in Apt and Bezem [AB99] by showing how to verify non-trivial Alma-0 programs that do not include destructive assignment.

Note that it is straightforward to extend the semantics here provided to other well-known programming constructs, such as destructive assignment, **while** construct and recursion. However, as soon as a destructive assignment is introduced, the relation with the definition of truth in the sense of Soundness Theorem 1 is lost and the just mentioned approach to program verification cannot be anymore applied. In fact, the right approach to the verification of the resulting programs is an appropriately designed Hoare's logic or the weakest precondition semantics.

The work here reported can be extended in several directions. First of all, it would be useful to prove equivalence between the operational and denotational semantics. Also, it would interesting to specialize the introduced semantics to specific interpretations for which the semantics could generate less often an error. Examples are Herbrand interpretations for an arbitrary first-order language in which the meaning of equalities could be rendered using most general unifiers, and the standard interpretation over reals for the language defining linear equations; these equations can be handled by means of the usual elimination procedure. In both cases the equality could be dealt with without introducing the *error* state at all.

Other possible research directions were already mentioned in Apt and Bezem [AB99]. These involved addition of recursive procedures, of constraints, and provision of a support for automated verification of programs written in Alma-0. The last item there mentioned, relation to dynamic predicate logic, was in the meantime extensively studied in the work of van Eijck [vE98] who, starting with Apt and Bezem [AB99], defined a number of semantics for dynamic predicate logic in which the existential quantifier has a different, dynamic scope. This work was motivated by applications in natural language processing.

Acknowledgments

Many thanks to Marc Bezem for helpful discussions on the subject of this paper.

References

[AB99]   K. R. Apt and M. A. Bezem. Formulas as programs. In K.R. Apt, V.W. Marek, M. Truszczyński, and D.S. Warren, editors, *The Logic Programming Paradigm: A 25 Year Perspective*, pages 75–107, 1999. Available via http://xxx.lanl.gov/archive/cs/.

[ABPS98] K. R. Apt, J. Brunekreef, V. Partington, and A. Schaerf. Alma-0: An imperative language that supports declarative programming. *ACM Toplas*, 20(5):1014–1066, 1998.

[Cla78]   K. L. Clark. Negation as failure. In H. Gallaire and J. Minker, editors, *Logic and Databases*, pages 293–322. Plenum Press, New York, 1978.

[Cla79]   E. M. Clarke. Programming language constructs for which it is impossible to obtain good Hoare axiom systems. *J. of the ACM*, 26(1):129–147, January 1979.

[dB80]   J. W. de Bakker. *Mathematical Theory of Program Correctness*. Prentice-Hall International, Englewood Cliffs, N.J., 1980.

[DVS⁺88] M. Dincbas, P. Van Hentenryck, H. Simonis, A. Aggoun, T. Graf, and F. Berthier. The Constraint Logic Programming Language CHIP. In *FGCS-88: Proceedings International Conference on Fifth Generation Computer Systems*, pages 693–702, Tokyo, December 1988. ICOT.

[HL94]   P. M. Hill and J. W. Lloyd. *The Gödel Programming Language*. The MIT Press, 1994.

[JMSY92] J. Jaffar, S. Michayov, P. Stuckey, and R. Yap. The CLP($\mathcal{R}$) language and system. *ACM Transactions on Programming Languages and Systems*, 14(3):339–395, July 1992.

[KK71]   R.A. Kowalski and D. Kuehner. Linear resolution with selection function. *Artificial Intelligence*, 2:227–260, 1971.

[Kow74]   R.A. Kowalski. Predicate logic as a programming language. In *Proceedings IFIP'74*, pages 569–574. North-Holland, 1974.

[LT84]   J. W. Lloyd and R. W. Topor. Making Prolog more expressive. *Journal of Logic Programming*, 1:225–240, 1984.

[Mah88]   M.J. Maher. Complete axiomatizations of the algebras of finite, rational and infinite trees. In *Proceedings of the Fifth Annual Symposium on Logic in Computer Science*, pages 348–357. The MIT Press, 1988.

[Rob65]   J.A. Robinson. A machine-oriented logic based on the resolution principle. *J. ACM*, 12(1):23–41, 1965.

[SS71]   D. S. Scott and C. Strachey. Towards a mathematical semantics for computer languages. Technical Report PRG–6, Programming Research Group, University of Oxford, 1971.

[Van89]   P. Van Hentenryck. *Constraint Satisfaction in Logic Programming*. Logic Programming Series. MIT Press, Cambridge, MA, 1989.

[vE98]   J. van Eijck. Programming with dynamic predicate logic. Technical Report INS-R9810, CWI, Amsterdam, 1998.

Logic, Knowledge Representation, and Bayesian Decision Theory

David Poole

Department of Computer Science
University of British Columbia
2366 Main Mall, Vancouver, B.C., Canada V6T 1Z4
poole@cs.ubc.ca
http://www.cs.ubc.ca/spider/poole/

Abstract. In this paper I give a brief overview of recent work on uncertainty in AI, and relate it to logical representations. Bayesian decision theory and logic are both normative frameworks for reasoning that emphasize different aspects of intelligent reasoning. Belief networks (Bayesian networks) are representations of independence that form the basis for understanding much of the recent work on reasoning under uncertainty, evidential and causal reasoning, decision analysis, dynamical systems, optimal control, reinforcement learning and Bayesian learning. The independent choice logic provides a bridge between logical representations and belief networks that lets us understand these other representations and their relationship to logic and shows how they can extended to first-order rule-based representations. This paper discusses what the representations of uncertainty can bring to the computational logic community and what the computational logic community can bring to those studying reasoning under uncertainty.

> *"It is remarkable that a science which began with the consideration of games of chance should become the most important object of human knowledge...The most important questions of life are, for the most part, really only problems of probability."*
> *"The theory of probabilities is at bottom nothing but common sense reduced to calculus."*

— Pierre Simon de Laplace (1794–1827)

1 Introduction

There are good normative arguments for using logic to represent knowledge (Nilsson, 1991; Poole, Mackworth and Goebel, 1998). These arguments are usually based on reasoning with symbols with an explicit denotation, allowing relations amongst individuals, and permitting quantification over individuals. This is often translated as needing (at least) the first-order predicate calculus. Unfortunately, the first-order predicate calculus has very primitive mechanisms for handling uncertainty, namely, the use of disjunction and existential quantification.

J. Lloyd et al. (Eds.): CL 2000, LNAI 1861, pp. 70–86, 2000.

There are also good normative reasons for using Bayesian decision theory for decision making under uncertainty (Von Neumann and Morgenstern, 1953; Savage, 1972). These arguments can be intuitively interpreted as seeing decision making as a form of gambling, and that probability and utility are the appropriate calculi for gambling. These arguments lead to the assignment of a single probability to a proposition; thus leading to the notion of probability of a measure of subjective belief. The probability of a proposition for an agent is a measure of the agent's belief in the truth of the proposition. This measure of belief is a function of what the agent knows. Probability theory can be seen as the study of how knowledge affects belief.

It is important to note that decision theory has nothing to say about representations. Adopting decision theory doesn't mean adopting any particular representation. While there are some representations that can be directly extracted from the theory, such as the explicit reasoning over the state space or the use of decision trees, these become intractable as the problem domains become large; it is like theorem proving by enumerating the interpretations. Adopting logic doesn't mean you have to enumerate interpretations or generate the semantic tree (Chang and Lee, 1973), nor does adopting decision theory mean you have to use analogous representations.

First, I will talk about knowledge representation, in which tradition this representation is built. Then I will introduce belief networks. The ICL will then be presented from three alternate viewpoints: as a semantic framework in terms of choices made by agents, in terms of first-order belief networks (Bayesian networks) and as a framework for a abduction and argumentation. I then discuss work on diagnosis, dynamical systems and learning from the uncertainty point of view and relate it to logical representations.

1.1 Knowledge Representation

In order to understand where this work fits in, Figure 1 (from (Poole et al., 1998)) shows the knowledge representation (KR) view. Given a problem we want a solution to, we find a representation for the problem; using this representation we can do computation to find an answer that can then be interpreted as a solution to the problem.

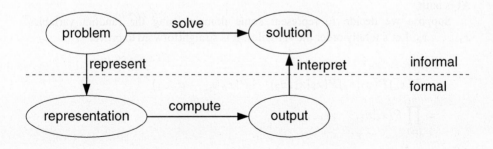

Fig. 1. Knowledge Representation Framework

When considering representations, there are a number of often competing considerations:

- The representation should be rich enough to be able to contain enough information to actually solve the problem.
- The representation should be as close to the problem as possible. We want the representation to be as "natural" as possible, so that a small changes in the problem result in small changes in the representation.
- We want the representation to be amenable to efficient computation. This does not necessarily mean that the representation needs to be efficient in the worst case (because that usually invalidates the first consideration). Rather we would like to be able to exploit features of the problem for computational gain. This means that the representation must be capable of expressing those features of the problem that can be exploited computationally.
- We want to be able to learn the representation from data and from past experiences in solving similar problems.

Belief networks (or Bayesian networks) (Pearl, 1988) are of interest because they provide a language that is represents the sort of knowledge a person may have about a domain, because they are rich enough for many applications, because features of the representation can be exploited for computational gain, and because they can be learned from data. Unfortunately, the underlying logic of belief networks is propositional. We cannot have relations amongst individuals as we can, for example, in the first-order predicate calculus.

2   Belief Networks

Probability specifies a semantic construction and not a representation of knowledge. A belief network (Pearl, 1988) is a way to represent probabilistic knowledge. The idea is to represent a domain in terms of random variables and to explicitly model the interdependence of the random variables in terms of a graph. This is useful when a random variable only depends on a few other random variables, as occurs in many domains. Belief networks form the foundation from which much of the work on uncertainty in AI is built.

Suppose we decide to represent some domain using the random variables[1] $x_1, \ldots, x_n$. Let's totally order the variables. It is straightforward to prove:

$$P(x_1, \ldots, x_n)$$
$$= P(x_1)P(x_2|x_1)P(x_3|x_1, x_2) \cdots P(x_n|x_1 \cdots x_{n-1})$$
$$= \prod_{i=1}^{n} P(x_i|x_1, \ldots, x_{i-1})$$

For each variable x_i suppose there is some minimal set $\pi_{x_i} \subseteq \{x_1, \ldots, x_{i-1}\}$ such that

$$P(x_i|x_1, \ldots, x_{i-1}) = P(x_i|\pi_{x_i})$$

---

[1] Or in terms of propositions. A proposition is a random variable with two possible values *true* and *false* (these are called Boolean random variables). In examples, I will often write $x = true$ as x and $x = false$ as $\neg x$.

That is, once you know the values of the variables in π_{x_i}, knowing the values of other predecessors of x_i in the total ordering will not change your belief in x_i. The elements of the set π_{x_i} are known as the **parents** of variable x_i. We say x_i is **conditionally independent** of its predecessors given its parents. We can create a graph where there is an arc from each parent of a node into that node. Such a graph, together with the conditional probabilities for $P(x_i|\pi_{x_i})$ for each variable x_i is known as a **belief network** or a **Bayesian network** (Pearl, 1988; Jensen, 1996).

Example 1. An example belief network is given in Figure 2. The parents of *projec-*

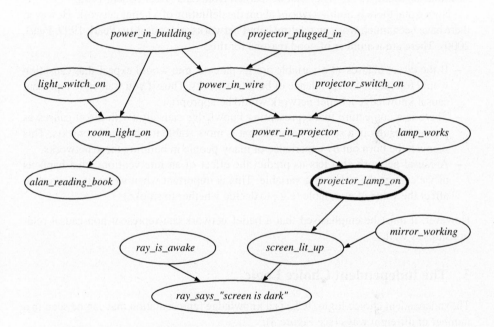

Fig. 2. A belief network for an overhead projector (we discuss the node in bold)

tor_lamp_on are *power_in_projector* and *lamp_works*. Note that this graph does not specify how *power_in_projector* depends on *projector_lamp_on* and *lamp_works*. It does, however, specify that *power_in_projector* is independent of *power_in_building*, *alan_reading_book* and the other non-descendent given these parents. Separately we need a specification of how each variable depends on its parents.

There are a few important points to notice about a Bayesian network:

- By construction, the graph defining a Bayesian network is acyclic.
- Different total orderings of the variables can result in different Bayesian networks for the same underlying distribution.
- The size of a conditional probability table for $P(x_i|\pi_{x_i})$ is exponential in the number of parents of x_i.

Typically we try to build belief networks so that the total ordering results in few parents and a sparse graph. Belief networks can be constructed taking into account just local information, the information that has to be specified is reasonably intuitive, and there are many domains that have concise representations as belief networks. There are algorithms that can exploit the sparseness of the graph for computational gain (Lauritzen and Spiegelhalter, 1988; Dechter, 1996; Zhang and Poole, 1996), exploit the skewness of distributions (Poole, 1996a), use the structure for stochastic simulation (Henrion, 1988; Pearl, 1987; Dagum and Luby, 1997) or exploit special features of the conditional probabilities (Zhang and Poole, 1996; Poole, 1997b; Jordan, Ghahramani, Jaakkola and Saul, 1997). They can be learned from data (Heckerman, 1995).

Notice that there is nothing *causal* about the definition of a belief network. However, there have been much work on relating belief networks and causality (Pearl, 1999; Pearl, 2000). There are a number of good reasons for this:

- If the direct clauses of a variable are its parents, one would expect that causation would follow the independence of belief networks. Thus if you wanted to represent causal knowledge a belief network would be appropriate.
- There is a conjecture that representing knowledge causally (with direct causes as parents) results in a sparser network that is more stable to changing contexts. This seems to be born out by experience of many people in building these networks.
- A causal network also lets us predict the effect of an intervention: what happens of we change the value of a variable. This is important when we want an agent to affect the value of a variable (e.g., to decide whether to smoke).

However, it must be emphasised that a belief network can represent non-causal relationships as well.

3   The Independent Choice Logic

The independent choice logic (ICL) is a knowledge representation that can be seen in a number of different ways (see Figure 3):

- It is a way to add Bayesian probability to the predicate logic. In particular we want to have all uncertainty to be handled by probabilities (or for decision problems, as choices of various agents). So we start with logic programs, which can be seen as predicate logic with no uncertainty (no disjunctive assertions), and have independent choices that have associated probability distributions. A logic program specifies what follows from the choices made.
- It is a way to lift Bayesian networks into a first-order language. In particular a Bayesian network can be seen as a deterministic system with "noise" (independent stochastic) inputs (Pearl, 1999; Pearl, 2000). In the ICL, the deterministic system is modelled as a logic program. Thus we write the conditional probabilities in rule form. The noise inputs are given in terms of independent choices.
- It is a sound way to have probabilities over assumptions. Explaining observations means that we use abduction; we find the explanations (set of hypotheses) that imply the observations, and from these we make predictions. This reasoning is sound probabilistic inference in the ICL.

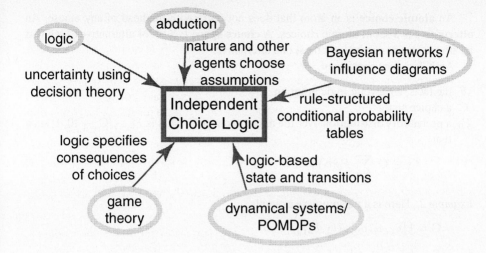

Fig. 3. ICL Influences

The ICL started off as Probabilistic Horn Abduction (Poole, 1991a; Poole, 1991b; Poole, 1993a; Poole, 1993b) (the first three had a slightly different language). The independent choice logic extends probabilistic Horn abduction in allowing for multiple agents making choices (Poole, 1997a) (where nature is a special agent who makes choices probabilistically) and in allowing negation as failure in the logic (Poole, 2000a).

3.1 The Language

In this section we give the language and the semantics of the ICL. This is simplified slightly; the general ICL allows for choices by various agents (Poole, 1997b) which lets us model decisions in a decision-theoretic (single agent) or game-theoretic (multiple agents) situation.

We assume that we have atomic formulae as in a normal logical language (Lloyd, 1987). We use the Prolog convention of having variables in upper case, and predicate symbol and function symbols in lower case.

A **clause** is either an atom or is of the form

$$h \leftarrow a_1 \land \cdots \land a_k$$

where h is an atom and each a_i is an atom or the negation of an atom.

A **logic program** is a set of clauses. We assume the logic program is acyclic[2] (Apt and Bezem, 1991).

---

[2] All recursions for variable-free queries eventually halt. We disallow programs such as $\{a \leftarrow \neg a\}$ and $\{a \leftarrow \neg b, b \leftarrow \neg a\}$. We want to ensure that there is a unique model for each logic program.

An **atomic choice** is an atom that does not unify with the head of any clause. An **alternative** is a set of atomic choices. A **choice space** is a set of alternatives such that an atomic choice can be in at most one alternative.

An ICL theory consists of

F the facts, an acyclic logic program
C a choice space
P_0 a probability distribution over the alternatives in C. That is $P_0 : \cup C \to [0, 1]$ such that

$$\forall \chi \in \mathbf{C} \sum_{\alpha \in \chi} P_0(\alpha) = 1$$

Example 2. Here is a meaningless example:

$$C = \{\{c_1, c_2, c_3\}, \{b_1, b_2\}\}$$

$$\mathbf{F} = \{ f \leftarrow c_1 \wedge b_1, \; f \leftarrow c_3 \wedge b_2,$$
$$\quad d \leftarrow c_1, \qquad d \leftarrow \neg c_2 \wedge b_1,$$
$$\quad e \leftarrow f, \qquad e \leftarrow \neg d\}$$

$$P_0(c_1) = 0.5 \; P_0(c_2) = 0.3 \; P_0(c_3) = 0.2$$
$$P_0(b_1) = 0.9 \; P_0(b_2) = 0.1$$

3.2 Semantics

The semantics is defined in terms of possible worlds. Here we present the semantics for the case of a finite choice space, where there are only finitely many possible worlds. The more general case is considered in other places (Poole, 1997b; Poole, 2000a).

A **total choice** for choice space C is a selection of exactly one atomic choice from each alternative in C.

There is a **possible world** for each total choice. What is **true** in a possible world is defined by the atoms chosen by the total choice together with the logic program. In particular an atom is true if it in in the (unique) stable model[3] of the total choice together with the logic program (Poole, 2000a). The measure of a possible world is the product of the values $P_0(\alpha)$ for each α selected by the total choice.

The probability of a proposition is the sum of the measures of the possible worlds in which the proposition is true.

Example 3. In the ICL theory of example 2, there are six possible worlds:

$$w_1 \models c_1 \; b_1 \quad f \quad d \quad e \qquad P(w_1) = 0.45$$
$$w_2 \models c_2 \; b_1 \; \neg f \; \neg d \quad e \qquad P(w_2) = 0.27$$
$$w_3 \models c_3 \; b_1 \; \neg f \quad d \; \neg e \qquad P(w_3) = 0.18$$
$$w_4 \models c_1 \; b_2 \; \neg f \quad d \; \neg e \qquad P(w_4) = 0.05$$
$$w_5 \models c_2 \; b_2 \; \neg f \; \neg d \quad e \qquad P(w_5) = 0.03$$
$$w_6 \models c_3 \; b_2 \quad f \; \neg d \quad e \qquad P(w_6) = 0.02$$

---

[3] The acyclicity of the logic program and the restriction that atomic choices don't unify with the head of clauses guarantees there there is a single model for each possible world.

The probability of any proposition can be computed by summing the measures of the worlds in which the proposition is true. For example

$$P(e) = 0.45 + 0.27 + 0.03 + 0.02 = 0.77$$

3.3 ICL and Belief Networks

It may seem that, with independent alternatives, that the ICL is restricted in what it can represent. This is not the case; in particular it can represent anything the is representable by a Belief network. Moreover the translation is local, and (if all variables and alternatives are binary) there is the same number of alternatives as there are free parameters in the belief network.

Example 4. If we had Boolean variables a, b and c, where b and c are the parents of a, we will have rules such as

$a \leftarrow b \wedge \neg c \wedge aifbnc$

where *aifbnc* is an atomic choice where $P_0(aifbnc)$ has the same value as the conditional probability as $P(a|b, \neg c)$ in the belief network. This generalizes to arbitrary discrete belief networks in the analogous way (Poole, 1993b).

This representation lets us naturally specify context-specific independence (Boutilier, Friedman, Goldszmidt and Koller, 1996; Poole, 1997b), where, for example, a may be independent of c when b is false but be dependent when b is true. Context-specific independence is often specified in terms of a tree for each variable; the tree has probabilities at the leaves and parents of the variable on the internal nodes. It is straightforward to translate these into the ICL.

Example 5. In the belief network of Figure 2, we can axiomatize how *power_in_projector* depends on *projector_lamp_on* and *lamp_works*:

$projector\_lamp\_on \leftarrow$

$power\_in\_projector \wedge$

$lamp\_works \wedge$

$projector\_working\_ok.$

$projector\_lamp\_on \leftarrow$

$power\_in\_projector \wedge$

$\neg lamp\_works \wedge$

$working\_with\_faulty\_lamp.$

We also have the alternatives:

$\{projector\_working\_ok, projector\_broken\}$

$\{working\_with\_faulty\_lamp, not\_working\_with\_faulty\_lamp\}$

The ICL lets us see the relationship of Belief networks to logical languages. The logic programs are standard logic programs (they can even have negation as failure (Poole, 2000a)). Viewing them as logic programs gives us a natural way to lift belief networks to the first-order case (i.e., with logical variables universally quantified over individuals).

3.4   ICL, Abduction, and Logical Argumentation

The ICL can also be seen as a language for abduction. In particular, if all of the atomic choices are assumable (they are abducibles or possible hypotheses). An **explanation**[4] for g is a consistent set of assumables that implies g. A set of atomic choices is consistent if there is at most one element in any alternative.

An explanation can be seen as an argument based on explicit assumptions about what is true. Each of these explanations has an associated probability obtained by computing the product of the probabilities of the atomic choices that make up the explanation. The probability of g can be computed by summing[5] the probabilities of the explanations for g (Poole, 1993b; Poole, 2000a).

If we want to do evidential reasoning and observe obs, we compute

$$P(g|obs) = \frac{P(g \wedge obs)}{P(obs)}$$

In terms of explanations, we can first find the explanations for obs (which would give us $P(obs)$) and then try to extend these explanations to also explain g (this will give us $P(g \wedge obs)$). Intuitively, we explain all of the observations and see what these explanations also predict. This is similar to proposals in the nonmonotonic reasoning community to mix abduction and default reasoning (Poole, 1989; Shanahan, 1989; Poole, 1990).

We can also bound the prior and posterior probabilities by generating only a few of the most plausible explanations (either top-down (Poole, 1993a) or bottom-up (Poole, 1996b)). Thus we can use inference to the best explanations to do sound (approximate) probabilistic reasoning.

3.5   Reasoning in the ICL

To do reasoning in the ICL we can either do

- variable elimination (marginalization) to simplify the model (Poole, 1997b). We sum out variables to reduce the detail of the representation. This is similar to partial evaluation in logic programs.
- Generating some of the explanations to bound the probabilities (Poole, 1993a; Poole, 1996a). If we generated all of the explanations we could compute the probabilities exactly, but there are combinatorially many explanations.
- Stochastic simulation; generating the needed atomic choices stochastically, and estimating the probabilities by counting the resulting proportions.

---

[4] We need to extend the definition of explanation to account for negation as failure. The explanation of $\neg a$ are the duals of the explanations of a (Poole, 2000a).

[5] This assumes the bodies for the rules for each atom a are mutually exclusive. This is a common practice in logic programming and the rules obtained from the translation from belief networks have this property. We need to do something a bit more sophisticated if the rules are not disjoint (Poole, 2000a).

4 Relating Work in Other Fields

4.1 Reasoning about Actions

In this section I will review some of the work about actions outside of the logic camp. See Shanahan (1997) for a review of the logicist approach to representing actions; I do not have the space to review this here.

Much work in AI, dynamical systems, stochastic control, and operations research is built on the motion of a Markov process (see for example (Luenberger, 1979; Bertsekas, 1995; Boutilier, Dean and Hanks, 1999)), where there is a state variable that depends on the previous state and the action being carried out. In general, we don't observe the state, but only get to observe what our sensors provide. When an agent makes a decision the only information available is the history of observations and actions.

One case with no control is the hidden Markov model (HMM); this can be seen as a simple belief network as in Figure 4. In this figure s_t is random variable representing the

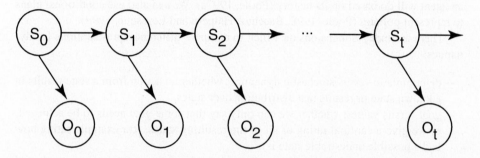

Fig. 4. Belief network corresponding to a hidden Markov model

state at time[6] t and o_t is a random variable representing the observation at time t. The probabilities we need to specify are $P(s_0)$, $P(s_t|s_{t-1})$ and $P(o_t|s_t)$. These represent the initial state, the system dynamics and the observation model respectively.

We can use the general mechanism to convert this to a logic program. The result looks like:

$$state(S, T) \leftarrow T > 0 \land state(S1, T - 1) \land trans(S1, S)$$

where there is an alternative for each state si

$$\{trans(si, s0), trans(si, s1), \ldots, trans(si, sn)\}$$

where the states are $s0, s1, \ldots, sn$. We only need to include those transitions that have a non-zero probability. Omitting the zero probabilities can be exploited in sparse matrix computations.

---

[6] This is either fixed time steps or is based on the times of interesting events. In the latter case $T + 1$ is the time of the next interesting event (or the state that results from the action). There is also a large body of work on continuous time dynamical systems that I won't review.

We don't want to specify each state by name, but would rather describe the properties of states. That is we describe the states in terms of random variables (or propositions). In the probabilistic literature this is known as dynamic belief networks (or dynamic Bayes networks) (Dean and Kanazawa, 1989; Dean and Wellman, 1991). In a dynamic belief network we divide the state into a number of random variables and then specify how each variable depends on values at the same[7] and previous times.

In the ICL, the direct translation results in rules like:

$$a(T) \leftarrow a_1(T-1) \wedge \ldots \wedge a_k(T-1) \wedge b_1(T) \wedge \ldots b_r(T) \wedge n(T)$$

where the a_i and b_i are literal fluents and $n(T)$ is an atomic choice (there is a different atomic choice for each combinations of the a_i and b_j).

When we have a control problem, (such as in Markov decision processes) we have to choose the actions based on the information available (the history of actions of and observations). In this case, using the same representation as we used for conditional probabilities, a policy in the ICL is represented as a logic program that specifies what an agent will do based on its history (Poole, 1997a). We can also use conditional plans to represent policies (Poole, 1998; Bacchus, Halpern and Levesque, 1999).

There are many dimensions on which to compare different representations for dynamics:

- deterministic versus stochastic dynamics; whether an action from a state results in a known state or results in a distribution over states.
- goal versus values; whether we can only say that some goal needs to be achieved, or we give a cardinal rating of all of the resulting states, (for example rating how bad a possible undesirable state is).
- finite stage versus infinite stage; whether we plan for a specific given number of future actions or for an indeterminate number of future actions.
- fully observable versus partial observability; whether the agent gets to observe (or knows) the actual state it is in when it has to decide what to do, or whether it has only limited and noisy sensors of the state.
- explicit state space versus states described in terms of properties (using random variables or propositions); whether there is a single state variable or the state is factored into a number of random variables.
- zeroth-order versus first-order; whether we can quantify over individuals or not.
- given dynamics and rewards versus dynamics and rewards acquired through interaction with the world; whether we must learn through trial and error the dynamics and the value or whether the dynamics is provided.
- single agent versus multiple agents
- perfect rationality versus bounded rationality; whether we can assume that the agent has unbounded computation or whether it must act within time and space limitations (Simon, 1996; Horvitz, 1989; Russell and Subramanian, 1995; Russell, 1997).

---

[7] We need to be able to specify how variables depend on other variables at the same time to account for correlated action effects. This could also be achieved by inventing new variables (that represent a common cause that makes two effects correlated). Of course, we still must maintain the acyclicity of the resulting belief network.

For each of these choices, the left-hand alternative is simpler than the right-hand one. We know how to build agents that only have a few of the right-hand sides. However, when we have more of the right-hand sides, we know that the problems are much more computationally difficult.

For example, when there stochastic dynamics, values, infinite stages and partially observable, we get partially observable Markov decision processes (POMDPs) (Cassandra, Kaelbling and Littman, 1994). Even the most efficient exact algorithms known (Cassandra, Littman and Zhang, 1997) can only work for a few hundred states[8]. Interestingly, these exact algorithms are essentially backward conditional planning algorithms, where multiple conditional plans are maintained. The difficult problem is to determine which plans stochastically dominate others (see Poole, 1998, for a review).

Similarly, where there are multiple agents, determining locally optimal solutions for each agent (Nash equilibria) is exponentially more difficult than the corresponding single-agent case (Koller and Megiddo, 1992).

	(a) CP	(b) DTP	(c) IDs	(d) RL	(e) HMM	(f) GT
Stochastic dynamics		✔	✔	✔	✔	✔
Values		✔	✔	✔		✔
infinite stage	✔	✔		✔	✔	
partially observable			✔		✔	✔
random variables	✔	✔	✔	✔		✔
first-order	✔					
dynamics not given				✔	✔	
multiple agents						✔
bounded rationality						

- (a) classical planning (e.g., Strips (Fikes and Nilsson, 1971) or the Situation Calculus (McCarthy and Hayes, 1969))
- (b) decision-theoretic planning (Boutilier, Dearden and Goldszmidt, 1995; Boutilier et al., 1999)
- (c) influence diagrams (Howard and Matheson, 1984)
- (d) reinforcement learning (Sutton and Barto, 1998; Kaelbling, Littman and Moore, 1996; Bertsekas and Tsitsiklis, 1996)
- (e) hidden Markov models (Jurafsky and Martin, 2000; Rabiner, 1989)
- (f) game theory: the extensive form of a game (Von Neumann and Morgenstern, 1953; Ordeshook, 1986; Myerson, 1991; Fudenberg and Tirole, 1992)

Fig. 5. Comparing Models of Dynamics

---

[8] There are excellent online resources on POMDPs by Tony Cassandra (http://www.cs.brown.edu/research/ai/pomdp/index.html) and Michael Littman (http://www.cs.duke.edu/~mlittman/topics/pomdp-page.html).

Figure 5 shows various representations and how they differ on the dimensions above. What is important to notice is that they share the same underlying notion of dynamics and the translation into belief networks (and ICL) is like that of the HMMs).

Reinforcement learning (Sutton and Barto, 1998; Kaelbling et al., 1996; Bertsekas and Tsitsiklis, 1996) is an interesting case of the general paradigm of understanding dynamics under uncertainty. While there has been much work with states described in terms of properties, virtually all of this learns the the value function (or the state transition function and the reward function) in terms of neural networks. There is one notable exception; Chapman and Kaelbling (1991) use decision trees (which can easily be converted into rules) to represent value functions (Q-functions).

One other interesting comparison is with hidden Markov models that have been used extensively in speech recognition (Rabiner, 1989; Jurafsky and Martin, 2000). In other work, Hobbs, Stickel, Appelt and Martin (1993) use a language similar to the independent choice logic (but with "costs" that are added; these costs can be seen a log-probabilities) to represent a way to combine syntax, semantic and pragmatic preferences into a coherent framework. The ICL show a way how these two, seemingly unrelated pieces of work can be combined into a coherent framework.

4.2   Model-Based Diagnosis

There is a large body of work on model-based diagnosis using belief networks and decision analysis tools based on these such as influence diagrams (Henrion, Breese and Horvitz, 1991). Essentially we write a forward simulation of the system, making explicit the possible faults and the uncertainty involved in the working of normal and faulty components. In terms of the ICL, we write a logic program that implies the outputs from the inputs, the status of the components and the stochastic mechanisms. There is a strong relationship between the search methods for belief networks and the traditional methods for model-based diagnosis (Poole, 1996a).

4.3   Bayesian Leaning

There is a large body of work on learning and belief networks. This means either:

- Using the belief network as a representation for the problem of Bayesian learning of models (Buntine, 1994). In Bayesian learning, we want the posterior distribution of hypotheses (models) given the data. To handle multiple cases, Buntine uses the notion of plates that corresponds to the use of logical variables in the ICL (Poole, 2000b). Poole (2000b) shows the tight integration of abduction and induction. These papers use belief networks to learn various representations including decision trees and neural networks, as well us unsupervised learning.
- Learning the structure and probabilities of belief networks (Heckerman, 1995). We can use Bayesian learning or other learning techniques to learn belief networks. One of the most successful methods is to learn a decision tree for each variable given its predecessors in a total ordering (Friedman and Goldszmidt, 1996; Chickering, Heckerman and Meek, 1997), and then search over different total orderings. It is straightforward to translate from these decision trees to the ICL.

The ICL can also be compared to the stochastic logic programs of Muggleton (1995). Stochastic logic programs allow for annotated logic programs of the form:

$$p : h \leftarrow a_1 \wedge \ldots \wedge a_k$$

This can be seen as similar to the ICL rule:

$$h \leftarrow a_1 \wedge \ldots \wedge a_k \wedge n_p$$

where n_p is an atomic choice with $P_0(n_p) = p$. The definition of stochastic logic programs has problems with programs such as:

$$1.0 : a \leftarrow b \wedge c$$
$$0.5 : b$$
$$1.0 : c \leftarrow b$$

Intuitively a should have probability one half (as it is true whenever b is true, and b is true half the time). Stochastic logic programs double-count b, which is used in the proof for a twice. The use of atomic choices lets us not double count, as we keep track of the assumptions used (and only use them once in the set of assumptions for a goal). The semantics of the ICL is simpler than the semantics for stochastic logic programs; all of the clauses in the ICL have their standard meaning.

The ICL has the potential to form the basis for an integration of inductive logic programming (Muggleton and De Raedt, 1994; Quinlan and Cameron-Jones, 1995; Muggleton, 1995) with reinforcement learning and leaning of belief networks.

5   Conclusion

This paper has provided a too-brief sketch of work in uncertainty in AI. I aimed to show that belief networks provide a way to understand much of the current work in stochastic dynamical systems, diagnosis and learning under uncertainty. The ICL provides a bridge between that work and the work in the logic community. Eventually we will need to build systems with first-order representations and reason about uncertainty, dynamics and learning. Hopefully I have provided some idea of how this could be achieved. There is still much work to be done.

Acknowledgements

This work was supported by Institute for Robotics and Intelligent Systems and the Natural Sciences and Engineering Research Council of Canada Operating Grant OG-POO44121.

References

Apt, K. R. and Bezem, M. (1991). Acyclic programs, *New Generation Computing* **9**(3-4): 335–363.

Bacchus, F., Halpern, J. Y. and Levesque, H. J. (1999). Reasoning about noisy sensors and effectors in the situation calculus, *Artificial Intelligence* **111**(1–2): 171–208.
http://www.lpaig.uwaterloo.ca/~fbacchus/on-line.html

Bertsekas, D. P. (1995). *Dynamic Programming and Optimal Control*, Athena Scientific, Belmont, Massachusetts. Two volumes.

Bertsekas, D. P. and Tsitsiklis, J. N. (1996). *Neuro-Dynamic Programming*, Athena Scientific, Belmont, Massachusetts.

Boutilier, C., Dean, T. and Hanks, S. (1999). Decision-theoretic planning: Structual assumptions and computational leverage, *Journal of Artificial Intelligence Research* **11**: 1–94.

Boutilier, C., Dearden, R. and Goldszmidt, M. (1995). Exploiting structure in policy construction, *Proc. 14th International Joint Conf. on Artificial Intelligence (IJCAI-95)*, Montréal, Québec, pp. 1104–1111.

Boutilier, C., Friedman, N., Goldszmidt, M. and Koller, D. (1996). Context-specific independence in Bayesian networks, *in* E. Horvitz and F. Jensen (eds), *Proc. Twelfth Conf. on Uncertainty in Artificial Intelligence (UAI-96)*, Portland, OR, pp. 115–123.

Buntine, W. L. (1994). Operations for learning with graphical models, *Journal of Artificial Intelligence Research* **2**: 159–225.

Cassandra, A., Littman, M. and Zhang, N. (1997). Incermental pruning: A simple, fast, exact mehtod for partially observable markov decision processes, *in* D. Geiger and P. Shenoy (eds), *Proc. Thirteenth Conf. on Uncertainty in Artificial Intelligence (UAI-97)*, pp. ??–??

Cassandra, A. R., Kaelbling, L. P. and Littman, M. L. (1994). Acting optimally in partially observable stochastic domains, *Proc. 12th National Conference on Artificial Intelligence*, Seattle, pp. 1023–1028.

Chang, C. L. and Lee, R. C. T. (1973). *Symbolic Logical and Mechanical Theorem Proving*, Academic Press, New York.

Chapman, D. and Kaelbling, L. P. (1991). Input generrlization in delayed reinforcement learning: An algorithm and performance comparisons, *Proc. 12th International Joint Conf. on Artificial Intelligence (IJCAI-91)*, Sydney, Australia.

Chickering, D. M., Heckerman, D. and Meek, C. (1997). A bayesian approach to learning bayesian networks with local structure, *Proc. Thirteenth Conf. on Uncertainty in Artificial Intelligence (UAI-97)*, pp. 80–89.

Dagum, P. and Luby, M. (1997). An optimal approximation algorithm for Bayesian inference, *Artificial Intelligence* **93**(1–2): 1–27.

Dean, T. and Kanazawa, K. (1989). A model for reasoning about persistence and causation, *Computational Intelligence* **5**(3): 142–150.

Dean, T. L. and Wellman, M. P. (1991). *Planning and Control*, Morgan Kaufmann, San Mateo, CA.

Dechter, R. (1996). Bucket elimination: A unifying framework for probabilistic inference, *in* E. Horvitz and F. Jensen (eds), *Proc. Twelfth Conf. on Uncertainty in Artificial Intelligence (UAI-96)*, Portland, OR, pp. 211–219.

Fikes, R. E. and Nilsson, N. J. (1971). STRIPS: A new approach to the application of theorem proving to problem solving, *Artificial Intelligence* **2**(3-4): 189–208.

Friedman, N. and Goldszmidt, M. (1996). Learning Bayesian networks with local structure, *Proc. Twelfth Conf. on Uncertainty in Artificial Intelligence (UAI-96)*, pp. 252–262.
http://www2.sis.pitt.edu/~dsl/UAI/UAI96/Friedman1.UAI96.html

Fudenberg, D. and Tirole, J. (1992). *Game Theory*, MIT Press, Cambridge, MA.

Heckerman, D. (1995). A tutorial on learning with Bayesian networks, *Technical Report MSR-TR-95-06*, Microsoft Research. (Revised November 1996).
http://www.research.microsoft.com/research/dtg/heckerma/heckerma.html

Henrion, M. (1988). Propagating uncertainty in Bayesian networks by probabilistic logic sampling, *in* J. F. Lemmer and L. N. Kanal (eds), *Uncertainty in Artificial Intelligence 2*, Elsevier Science Publishers B.V., pp. 149–163.

Henrion, M., Breese, J. and Horvitz, E. (1991). Decision analysis and expert systems, *AI Magazine* **12**(4): 61–94.

Hobbs, J. R., Stickel, M. E., Appelt, D. E. and Martin, P. (1993). Interpretation as abduction, *Artificial Intelligence* **63**(1–2): 69–142.

Horvitz, E. J. (1989). Reasoning about beliefs and actions under computational resource constraints, *in* L. Kanal, T. Levitt and J. Lemmer (eds), *Uncertainty in Artificial Intelligence 3*, Elsevier, New York, pp. 301–324.

Howard, R. A. and Matheson, J. E. (1984). Influence diagrams, *in* R. A. Howard and J. E. Matheson (eds), *The Principles and Applications of Decision Analysis*, Strategic Decisions Group, Menlo Park, CA.

Jensen, F. V. (1996). *An Introduction to Bayesian Networks*, Springer Verlag, New York.

Jordan, M. I., Ghahramani, Z., Jaakkola, T. S. and Saul, L. K. (1997). An introduction to variational methods for graphical models, *Technical report*, MIT Computational Cognitive Science.
http://www.ai.mit.edu/projects/jordan.html

Jurafsky, D. and Martin, J. (2000). *Speech and Language Processing*, Prentice Hall.

Kaelbling, L. P., Littman, M. L. and Moore, A. W. (1996). Reinforcement learning: A survey, *Journal of Artificial Intelligence Research* **4**: 237–285.

Koller, D. and Megiddo, N. (1992). The complexity of two-person zero-sum games in extensive form, *Games and Economic Behavior* **4**: 528–552.

Lauritzen, S. L. and Spiegelhalter, D. J. (1988). Local computations with probabilities on graphical structures and their application to expert systems, *Journal of the Royal Statistical Society, Series B* **50**(2): 157–224.

Lloyd, J. W. (1987). *Foundations of Logic Programming*, Symbolic Computation Series, second edn, Springer-Verlag, Berlin.

Luenberger, D. G. (1979). *Introduction to Dynamic Systems: Theory, Models and Applications*, Wiley, New York.

McCarthy, J. and Hayes, P. J. (1969). Some philosophical problems from the standpoint of artificial intelligence, *in* M. Meltzer and D. Michie (eds), *Machine Intelligence 4*, Edinburgh University Press, pp. 463–502.

Muggleton, S. (1995). Inverse entailment and Progol, *New Generation Computing* **13**(3,4): 245–286.

Muggleton, S. and De Raedt, L. (1994). Inductive logic programming: Theory and methods, *Journal of Logic Programming* **19,20**: 629–679.

Myerson, R. B. (1991). *Game Theory: Analysis of Conflict*, Harvard University Press, Cambridge, MA.

Nilsson, N. J. (1991). Logic and artificial intelligence, *Artificial Intelligence* **47**: 31–56.

Ordeshook, P. C. (1986). *Game theory and political theory: An introduction*, Cambridge University Press, New York.

Pearl, J. (1987). Evidential reasoning using stochastic simulation of causal models, *Artificial Intelligence* **32**(2): 245–257.

Pearl, J. (1988). *Probabilistic Reasoning in Intelligent Systems: Networks of Plausible Inference*, Morgan Kaufmann, San Mateo, CA.

Pearl, J. (1999). Reasoning with cause and effect, *Proc. 16th International Joint Conf. on Artificial Intelligence (IJCAI-99)*, pp. 1437–1449.

Pearl, J. (2000). *Causality: Models, Reasoning and Inference*, Cambridge University Press.

Poole, D. (1989). Explanation and prediction: An architecture for default and abductive reasoning, *Computational Intelligence* **5**(2): 97–110.

Poole, D. (1990). A methodology for using a default and abductive reasoning system, *International Journal of Intelligent Systems* **5**(5): 521–548.

Poole, D. (1991a). Representing diagnostic knowledge for probabilistic Horn abduction, *Proc. 12th International Joint Conf. on Artificial Intelligence (IJCAI-91)*, Sydney, pp. 1129–1135.

Poole, D. (1991b). Search-based implementations of probabilistic Horn abduction, *Technical report*, Department of Computer Science, University of British Columbia, Vancouver, B.C., Canada.

Poole, D. (1993a). Logic programming, abduction and probability: A top-down anytime algorithm for computing prior and posterior probabilities, *New Generation Computing* **11**(3–4): 377–400.

Poole, D. (1993b). Probabilistic Horn abduction and Bayesian networks, *Artificial Intelligence* **64**(1): 81–129.

Poole, D. (1996a). Probabilistic conflicts in a search algorithm for estimating posterior probabilities in Bayesian networks, *Artificial Intelligence* **88**: 69–100.

Poole, D. (1996b). Probabilistic conflicts in a search algorithm for estimating posterior probabilities in Bayesian networks, *Artificial Intelligence* **88**: 69–100.

Poole, D. (1997a). The independent choice logic for modelling multiple agents under uncertainty, *Artificial Intelligence* **94**: 7–56. special issue on economic principles of multi-agent systems. http://www.cs.ubc.ca/spider/poole/abstracts/icl.html

Poole, D. (1997b). Probabilistic partial evaluation: Exploiting rule structure in probabilistic inference, *Proc. 15th International Joint Conf. on Artificial Intelligence (IJCAI-97)*, Nagoya, Japan, pp. 1284–1291. http://www.cs.ubc.ca/spider/poole/abstracts/pro-pa.html

Poole, D. (1998). Decision theory, the situation calculus and conditional plans, *Electronic Transactions on Artificial Intelligence* **2**(1–2). http://www.etaij.org

Poole, D. (2000a). Abducing through negation as failure: stable models in the Independent Choice Logic, *Journal of Logic Programming* **44**(1–3): 5–35. http://www.cs.ubc.ca/spider/poole/abstracts/abnaf.html

Poole, D. (2000b). Learning, bayesian probability, graphical models, and abduction, *in* P. Flach and A. Kakas (eds), *Abduction and Induction: essays on their relation and integration*, Kluwer.

Poole, D., Mackworth, A. and Goebel, R. (1998). *Computational Intelligence: A Logical Approach*, Oxford University Press, New York.

Quinlan, J. R. and Cameron-Jones, R. M. (1995). Induction of logic programs: FOIL and related systems, *New Generation Computing* **13**(3,4): 287–312.

Rabiner, L. (1989). A tutorial on hidden Markov models and selected applications in speech recognition, *Proceedings of the IEEE* **77**(2): 257–286.

Russell, S. (1997). Rationality and intelligence, *Artificial Intelligence* **94**: 57–77.

Russell, S. J. and Subramanian, D. (1995). Provably bounded-optimal agents, *Journal of Artificial Intelligence Research* **2**: 575–609.

Savage, L. J. (1972). *The Foundation of Statistics*, 2nd edn, Dover, New York.

Shanahan, M. (1989). Prediction is deduction, but explanation is abduction, *Proc. 11th International Joint Conf. on Artificial Intelligence (IJCAI-89)*, Detroit, MI, pp. 1055–1060.

Shanahan, M. (1997). *Solving the Frame Problem: A Mathematical Investigation of the Common Sense Law of Inertia*, MIT Press, Cambridge, MA.

Simon, H. (1996). *The Sciences of the Artificial*, third edn, MIT Press, Cambridge, MA.

Sutton, R. S. and Barto, A. G. (1998). *Reinforcement Learning: An Introduction*, MIT Press, Canbridge, MA.

Von Neumann, J. and Morgenstern, O. (1953). *Theory of Games and Economic Behavior*, third edn, Princeton University Press, Princeton, NJ.

Zhang, N. and Poole, D. (1996). Exploiting causal independence in Bayesian network inference, *Journal of Artificial Intelligence Research* **5**: 301–328.

Logic Program Synthesis in a Higher-Order Setting

David Lacey[1], Julian Richardson[2], and Alan Smaill[1]

[1] Division of Informatics, University of Edinburgh
[2] Dept. of Computing & Electrical Engineering, Heriot-Watt University, Edinburgh

Abstract. We describe a system for the synthesis of logic programs from specifications based on higher-order logical descriptions of appropriate refinement operations. The system has been implemented within the proof planning system $\lambda Clam$. The generality of the approach is such that its extension to allow synthesis of higher-order logic programs was straightforward. Some illustrative examples are given. The approach is extensible to further classes of synthesis.

1 Introduction

Earlier work on the synthesis of logic programs has taken the approach of constructing a program in the course of proving equivalence to a specification, which is written in a richer logic than the resulting program.

Typically, quantifiers and thus binding of variables are present in the specification, and have to be manipulated correctly. We extend earlier work using as far as possible a declarative reading in a higher-order logic. The higher-order proof planning framework which we employ provides a more expressive language for writing methods, allows some methods to be entirely replaced by higher-order rewrite rules, and automatically takes care of variable scoping. While allowing first-order examples to be dealt with more easily than is possible in a less powerful proof planning language, we can also synthesise higher-order logic programs with minimal change to the underlying machinery.

The paper is organised as follows. §2 covers earlier work in the area; §3 describes the proof planning framework used here. §4 explains the methods used in the synthesis task, §5 shows how these methods apply for synthesis of higher-order programs, and §6 presents discussion and future work. We concentrate in this paper on the proof planning level, and omit technical details of the logic. The code and examples are available at:

http://dream.dai.ed.ac.uk/software/systems/lambda-clam/lpsynth/

2 Background

Our starting point is work on program synthesis via automatic proofs of equivalence between a specification in predicate calculus, and an implementation in a restricted, executable, subset of the logic. The work in [13, 14, 1, 12] gives the

J. Lloyd et al. (Eds.): CL 2000, LNAI 1861, pp. 87–100, 2000.

general principles, and following this work, we also aim to automate and control the synthesis process using *proof planning* (see §3).

The specifications of a program we will be working with are complete specifications of the form:

$$\forall \overline{x}. \; pred(\overline{x}) \leftrightarrow spec(\overline{x}) \tag{1}$$

$pred(\overline{x})$ is the predicate whose definition we wish to synthesise. $spec(\overline{x})$ is a logical formula describing the program. The aim is to prove an equivalence with a synthesised program, in a restricted logic, initially that of *horn programs* (Horn programs translate straightforwardly into pure Prolog programs) in the terminology of [1], i.e. to find a *horn body*: $horn(\overline{x})$ such that the specification will follow from the following program definition:

$$\forall \overline{x}. \; pred(\overline{x}) \leftrightarrow horn(\overline{x}) \tag{2}$$

The program is normally initially completely undetermined, and is therefore represented by a meta-variable.[1]

Unifications which are carried out (for example during rewriting) as the proof of this equivalence is constructed instantiate the (initially only one) meta-variables in the program. This technique of successive instantiation of meta-variables during the construction of a proof is known as *middle-out reasoning* [2]. Refinement operators in the form of derived inference rules allow the problem to be decomposed, while partially instantiating the synthesised program.

We are also interested in a more general problem, *parameterised synthesis*, which allows a much more flexible representation for the syntax of specification. It adds conditions to the synthesis of programs. So a specification is of the form:

$$\forall \overline{x}. \; cond(\overline{x}) \rightarrow \forall \overline{y}. \; pred(\overline{x}, \overline{y}) \leftrightarrow spec(\overline{x}, \overline{y}) \tag{3}$$

Additional kinds of specifications such as those described in [15] could also be considered.

Various aspects of this work suggest that a higher-order logical description is appropriate for the task, and that indeed a formulation in a higher-order metalogic would provide a better foundation for this approach – see for example [10]. A higher-order formulation gives us a direct treatment of quantification and variable binding, respecting α-conversion of bound variables, and scoping restrictions on variable instantiations that occur in the synthesis process. In addition both first-order logic and higher-order logic can be represented.

Thus the instantiation of higher-order variables standing for as yet undetermined program structure is given a declarative treatment. The higher-order approach also extends easily to synthesis of programs in a higher-order logic.

Unification of higher-order terms is provided by λProlog, which uses a version of Huet's algorithm. There may therefore be more than one higher-order unifier, and unification may not terminate. In practice, this does not seem to hinder the

---

[1] Meta-variables are not variables of the specification/proof calculus, but instead variables of the proof system we use to reason about this calculus, i.e. they are variables at the metalevel. They may be instantiated to terms in this calculus.

synthesis process, but this is a topic which should be investigated further. In contrast, Kraan restricts unification to *higher-order patterns* [18].

Although we use a language with full higher-order unification many of its uses are for higher-order matching of a pattern to a sub-term of a specification. Higher-order matching appears in existing work on functional program transformation and synthesis, for example in [11].

3   Proof Planning

A proof of a theorem can be attained by applying sound derivation rules to certain axioms until the theorem is reached. Alternatively, one can start with a theorem and back-chain through the rules until axioms are reached. The search space defined by these rules, however, is too large to be exhaustively searched for anything except the most trivial theorems. So some heuristic search control must be used to guide the search.

Certain sequences of steps following schematic patterns are commonly used to prove theorems. These sequences of steps are called *tactics*. When to apply certain tactics can be recognised from the syntactic form of the current goal to be proved and the outcome of applying these tactics can be easily derived from the goal. The $\lambda Clam$ system [20] uses objects called methods which detail the conditions and results of applying such tactics. The stated preconditions of applying a tactic allow methods to encode heuristic control knowledge about planning a proof.

So, instead of searching the space of applying derivation rules, $\lambda Clam$ searches the space of methods at the meta-level. On succeeding with the search it produces a proof plan which details which tactics have to be applied. This plan can then be used to construct a proof of the theorem in terms of the original derivation rules. Further search control can be added by linking the methods together via *methodicals*, the planning analogue of *tacticals*.

The methods in $\lambda Clam$ are compound data structures consisting of:

- The name of the method.
- The syntactic form of a goal to which the method can be applied.
- The preconditions that goals must meet for the method to be applied.
- The effects that hold of subgoals after the method is applied.
- The form of the subgoal(s) after the method is applied.
- The tactic which implements the method.

Methodicals link the methods together to control search. They are functions which take methods as arguments and return a new method.

4   Controlling the Synthesis Process

4.1   Example 1: Symbolic Evaluation

For an example method used in $\lambda Clam$ to prove theorems, we consider symbolic evaluation. This method rewrites a term in the goal formula to an equivalent term. An example rewrite rule is:

$$plus(s(X), Y) :\Rightarrow s(plus(X, Y))$$

where X, Y are meta-level variables. The left hand side of the rewrite is matched with a term in the goal and rewritten to the right hand side.

The soundness of a rewrite is usually based on an underlying equivalence, or equality, such as:

$$\forall x, \forall y. \ plus(s(x), y) = s(plus(x), y)$$

With such underlying equivalences we can soundly replace a term in a goal matching the left hand side of a rewrite with the right hand side. The resultant goal with the rewritten term will be equivalent to the previous goal. Therefore, proving the new goal will also prove the old goal. Rewriting with implications is also carried out, with appropriate checking of polarity.

The use of higher-order rewrite rules can reduce the amount of special-purpose machinery needed by the theorem prover since some proof steps which would normally be implemented using separate machinery can be expressed as higher-order rewrite rules (in the style of [4]), for example:

$$\exists x. \ Q(x) \wedge (x = Y) \wedge P(x) :\Rightarrow Q(Y) \wedge P(Y).$$

This rewrite cannot be stated as a first order rewrite and proved useful in several synthesis proofs. Many such rewrites need to be duplicated to cope with associative and commutative permutations of a pattern and A-C matching could have been useful but was not implemented in $\lambda Clam$.

Thus the method **sym_eval** is specified as follows.

Input Goal:	Any.
Output Goal:	The same as the input goal with any sub-term of the goal rewritten if it matches the left hand side of a rewrite in a prestored list. The rewriting is done exhaustively so no rewritable sub-term will exist in the output goal.
Precondition:	The goal must contain a subterm that matches the left hand side of a stored rewrite.
Postcondition:	None
Tactic:	A rewrite can be taken as a simple proving step or as a compound step consisting of reasonings about equalities in the hypothesis or background theory.

4.2   Example 2: Induction

The method of induction splits a goal containing a universally quantified variable into base case and step case goals. The splitting of the goal is performed by matching the goal to one of a prestored set of *induction schemes*. The induction scheme used is important since it determines the recursive structure of the program.

To illustrate, here is the goal in the synthesis of *subset*:

$$\forall i, j.\ subset(i, j) \leftrightarrow H(i, j)$$
$$\vdash$$
$$\forall i, j.\ subset(i, j) \leftrightarrow \forall x.\ member(x, i) \rightarrow member(x, j)$$

Here, the capitalised H represents a meta-variable to be instantiated to the program body.

Applying the induction method on variable i will split the goal into two subgoals:[2]

Base Case
$$\forall j.\ subset(nil, j) \leftrightarrow H(nil, j)$$
$$\vdash$$
$$\forall i, j.\ subset(nil, j) \leftrightarrow \forall x.\ member(nil, i) \rightarrow member(x, j)$$

Step Case
$$\forall j.\ subset(t, j) \leftrightarrow H(t, j)$$
$$\vdash$$
$$\forall j.\ subset(h :: t, j) \leftrightarrow \forall x.\ member(x, h :: t) \rightarrow member(x, j)$$

The program meta-variable H is now partially instantiated with a recursive structure matching the induction scheme:

$$H = \lambda x.\ \lambda y.\ (x = nil) \wedge B(x, y)\ \vee$$
$$\exists x', xs.\ x = x' :: xs \wedge S(x', xs, y)$$

Where B and S are new higher-order meta-variables. B will be instantiated during the proof of the base case goal and S during the step case. This illustrates the parallel between induction in the proof and recursion in the program.

4.3   Example 3: Unrolling

An example of a method added to specifically aid logic program synthesis is unrolling. This is a technique for eliminating existential quantifiers. It performs a structural case split based on the type of the variable quantified. For example the following rewrite could be used:

$$\exists x : nat.\ P(x) :\Rightarrow P(0) \vee \exists x' : nat.\ P(s(x'))$$

This performs a structural case split on the variable x into its base case and a constructor case. Many inductive function definitions are defined for either side of a structural split such as this, for example this definition of list append:

$$app(nil, Y) :\Rightarrow Y \qquad app(H :: T, Y) :\Rightarrow H :: app(T, Y)$$

---

[2] h and t are newly introduced constants.

So unrolling an existential quantifier in this way can often allow a rewrite rule to be applied. This method comes up reasonably often in synthesis of logic programs since logic programs often include existential quantifiers. For example, during an induction in the synthesis of *backn*:

$$\forall n, x.backn(n, x, h :: z) \leftrightarrow \exists k.\ app(k, x) = h :: z \wedge length(x) = n^3$$

the existential quantifier can be unrolled to give term:

$$app(nil, x) = h :: z \vee \exists k', k''.\ app(k' :: k'', x) = h :: z$$

This can be rewritten into the goal and the proof can continue since the definition of *app* can be used.

The technique is applied when directed to by rippling [3], a heuristic which restricts the application of rewriting in order to successively reduce the differences between an induction hypothesis and conclusion.

One problem with unrolling is that it does not terminate. In fact, any application of an unrolling step can be immediately followed by another unrolling step so it easily causes looping. A heuristic is needed to decide when to apply it. The one chosen was that an unrolling step can only be applied once per inductive step case proof. This ensures termination but may limit the number of programs that can be synthesised.

The method **unroll** is specified as follows.

Input Goal:	A goal containing an existential quantifier.
Output Goal:	The same as the input goal with the existentially quantified subterm replaced with its structural case split.
Precondition:	A rewrite must exist that will be applicable only after the split. This is directed by rippling. The unrolling method cannot have been used previously in the proof of the current step case goal.
Postcondition:	None
Tactic:	This is a higher-order rewrite. So the appropriate tactic for rewriting can be used.

4.4   Methods Used by the System

A brief description of the different proof planning methods used is given in Table 1. The methods are tried in the following order: symbolic evaluation, tautology check, induction, appeal to program, auxiliary synthesis. If a method succeeds then the the methods are tried again in the same order on the resultant goal(s). The exception to this is step case goal(s) of induction where the methods of rippling, unrolling, shared variable introduction and case splitting are repeatedly tried in that order. The resulting planning engine was successfully tested on a number of synthesis examples, including all those from [12].

---

[3] *backn* is the relation between a number n, a list and the suffix of the same list of length n

Table 1. Methods used by $\lambda Clam$

Method	Description
symbolic evaluation	Performs rewriting. See Section 4.1
conditional rewriting	Performs rewriting depending on whether a condition attached to the rewrite rule is fulfilled.
case split	Splits a goal into several goals with different sides of a case split in their hypotheses. This is applied so that a conditional rewrite can be applied.
tautology checking	Completes the proof plan if the goal is a tautology i.e. true by virtue of its logical connectives.
induction	Splits a universally quantified goal into base case and step case goals as in mathematical induction.
rippling	Annotates the goal so the rippling heuristic can be used. Rippling is a heuristic that only allows rewriting steps that reduce the difference between the conclusion and the hypothesis of a step case goal of induction.
unrolling	Performs a structural case split on an existential quantifier. See Section 4.3.
shared variable introduction	This method introduces an existentially quantified variable that is shared across an equality i.e. it performs the rewrite: $P(Q) = R :\Rightarrow \exists z.P(z) = R \wedge Q = z$. This is directed by rippling.
appeal to the program	This method tries to finish the proof plan by unifying the program body in the hypothesis with the specification in the goal. For this to succeed the specification must have been transformed to the executable logic subset we are interested in.
auxiliary synthesis	This method tries to synthesise a predicate that is equivalent to a sub-formula of the current goal. This auxiliary predicate can then be used to produce a full synthesis.

5 Synthesising Higher-Order Logic Programs

Given our approach, it is natural to consider the synthesis of programs that are themselves in higher-order logic; in particular, programs in λProlog [19]. We were also interested in parameterised synthesis. Surprisingly, both of these were successfully carried out with only minor modifications to the system developed for the first-order case, supporting our case that higher-order proof planning provides a good framework for program synthesis. Section 5.1 gives some examples of how $\lambda Clam$ encodes and manipulates the logic while Sections 5.2 and 5.3 describe the results of higher-order program synthesis and parameterised synthesis.

5.1 Encoding of the Object Logic

The proof planner $\lambda Clam$ reasons about formulae in a generic typed higher-order logic. First-order terms in this logic are represented by objects of λProlog type `oterm` and formulas are represented by objects of λProlog type `form`.

Functions in the object logic are represented in λProlog as terms of function type. Stored within the system are predicates describing the object level type of the function and its arity. For example the function *plus* is represented by the λProlog function `plus`. The object level type and arity of this function are stored as predicates describing `plus`. Quantifiers are represented as higher-order functions, taking as arguments an object type and a function to a formula and returning a function.

This leads to a very neat representation of formulae. For example, below is a formula stating the commutativity of *plus* (note that functions are curried and x\ is λProlog syntax for lambda abstraction of variable x):[4]

```
forall nat x\ (forall nat y\ (eq (x plus y) (y plus x)))
```

One advantage of this representation is that the bound variables x and y are bound by lambda abstraction. The programming language takes care of some of the reasoning of the proof planner. For example, equality modulo α-conversion is handled by λProlog.

This representation can be extended to handle higher-order quantifiers needed to reason about higher-order logic programs.[5] For example we can have a quantifier `forallp1` to quantify over first order predicates and can represent statements about them, for example:

```
forallp1 p\ (exists nat x\ (p x)) or (forall nat x\ (not (p x)))
```

5.2 Higher-Order Program Synthesis

Synthesising higher-order programs is different from synthesising first-order programs in the following way:

- The specification of the programs involves quantification over higher-order objects.
- The program definition contains quantification over higher-order objects.
- The program may not be restricted to horn clauses, so it becomes harder to know when a program is synthesised.

---

[4] `forall`,`nat` and `eq` are all terms defined in λProlog, not part of the programming language itself.

[5] Functions of the object-level logic are represented by functions in the meta-level logic; a consequence of this simple encoding is that there is one quantifier for each arity of function/predicate over which we wish to quantify. A less direct encoding could avoid this inconvenience.

The last point is relevant when trying to synthesise programs in a language such as λProlog where the executable subset of logic is large but the notion of consequence is different to that in the logic we are proof planning in (in particular when proving in λProlog there is no inductive consequence).

In order to synthesise higher-order programs, $\lambda Clam$ needs to be extended to recognise $\forall$ quantifiers over higher-order objects, such as the `forallp1` predicate mentioned in the previous section.

Significantly, this was the only change needed to the code in $\lambda Clam$ to do higher-order program synthesis. An example specification of a higher-order logic program is the all_hold predicate:

$$\forall p, l.\ all\_hold(p, l) \leftrightarrow \forall x.\ member(x, l) \rightarrow p(x)$$

Which yields synthesised program:

$$\forall p, l.\ all\_hold(p, l) \leftrightarrow l = nil\ \lor\ (\exists h, t.\ l = h :: t \land p(h) \land all\_hold(p, t))$$

This synthesis uses the methods of symbolic evaluation, tautology checking, induction, rippling and shared variable introduction (see table 1).

5.3   Parameterised Synthesis

Parameterised synthesis performs synthesis where the specification holds under a certain condition. Specifications are of the form (3) in Section 2, which effectively allows synthesis proofs to be parameterised and capture a group of syntheses in one go. Two examples which show the parameterisation were successfully synthesised.

The examples capture the type of synthesis that converts a function into a relation where we know how to recursively evaluate a function. Example syntheses of this type were the syntheses of $rapp$ and $rplus$. Two parameterised syntheses can be done (one for lists and one for natural numbers). Here is the (higher-order) natural number specification (note that the meta-predicate $prog$ is to indicate that its argument is allowed to appear in the final synthesised program body):

$$\forall f, f1, f2.\ (\ prog(f1)\ \land\ prog(f2)$$
$$f(zero) = f1\ \land\ \forall x.\ f(s(x)) = f2(f(x))$$
$$\rightarrow$$
$$\forall y, z.\ rnat(f, f1, f2, y, z) \leftrightarrow f(y) = z)$$

This yields the synthesised (higher-order) program :

$$\forall f, f1, f2, y, z.\ rnat(f, f1, f2, y, z) \leftrightarrow (y = zero \land z = f1)\ \lor$$
$$(\exists y', z'.\ y = s(y') \land z = f2(z') \land$$
$$rnat(f, f1, f2, y', z'))$$

Parameterised syntheses promise to provide a framework for more sophisticated synthesis. The programs that can be synthesised using this method needs investigation. The type of syntheses that could be achieved include:

Synthesis Based on Assumptions. Some programs are based on assumptions about the input data (in the case of logic programming on assumptions about one or more of the arguments of a relation). For example, some sorting algorithms are based on assumptions about the data distribution of the elements of the list being sorted, multiplication in the case where one of the arguments in a power of two is often handled with a different program than general multiplication. Such programs can be synthesised from conditional specifications.

General Classes of Synthesis. Many syntheses follow the same pattern of proof. Parameterised synthesis allows these general syntheses to be performed. One example is given in the results of this project but other general patterns will exist.

The advantage of performing these general syntheses is that they are much more likely to match future specifications and be reused as components (see Section 6.2).

Examples of higher-order and parameterised synthesis are in §A.2.

6   Discussion

6.1   Comparison with Other Systems

Synthesis in *Clam*, Kraan. A similar system to the one presented is given in [12]. The $\lambda Clam$ implementation can synthesise all the examples given in this work. However, in [12] a method is given to automatically obtain certain lemmas based on the properties of propositional logic; these were hand-coded into our system. The same technique would work with the more recent proof-planner.

The advantage of the $\lambda Clam$ (implemented in λProlog) over the *Clam* (implemented in Prolog) system is the ease with which one can move to higher-order programs. Using λProlog as a meta-logic we can assure that code written for the first-order case will be compatible with the higher-order case. This is due to the fact that higher-order quantification can be raised to the programming language level and does not need to be dealt with at the level of the actual program except in relatively few areas.

Lau and Prestwich. In [16], Lau and Prestwich present a synthesis system based on the analysis of folding problems. The system is similar to synthesis by proof planning in that both systems apply transformation steps in a top down fashion.

The system presented here is different from Lau and Prestwich's system is several ways. Firstly, Lau and Prestwich's system only synthesises partially correct programs and not necessarily complete ones, whereas $\lambda Clam$ synthesises totally correct programs.

Secondly, Lau and Prestwich's work requires user interaction in the specification of the recursive calls of the program before synthesis and in the choosing of strategies during synthesis. We aim at fully automated synthesis. The recursive form of a program synthesised by proof planning is decided by the choice of induction scheme and which variable the induction is performed on. The amount of user interaction in Lau and Prestwich's system does allow more control over the type of program synthesis and can synthesise certain programs which are beyond this work (in [17], several types of sorting algorithms are synthesised, for example).

Higher-order program synthesis has not been tried by Lau and Prestwich's methods.

Schema-Based Synthesis. In schema-based synthesis (or transformation) common programming patterns are encoded as pairs $\langle P_1, P_2 \rangle$, where the P_i are program patterns which contain meta-variables. Synthesis proceeds recursively by finding a schema whose first element matches part of the specification. This part is then replaced by the appropriately instantiated second element of the schema. The majority of schema-based synthesis systems are either mostly manually guided (for example [6]), or apply schemas exhaustively (for example [21]). In order to achieve automation, we can associate applicability heuristics to program synthesis schemas, which then become much like proof planning methods [7].

Higher-order program synthesis has not been covered by schema based approaches. [8] represents schemas in λProlog to make them more extensible. It is feasible that this approach could be adapted to higher-order program schemas. In [9], an approach is given for synthesising definite-clause grammars which could represent higher-order schemas. The synthesis process depends on sample input/output pairs and so is more like *in*ductive program synthesis rather than the *de*ductive approach given here.

One way of viewing parameterised synthesis is the synthesis of program schemas.

6.2   Further Work

Empirical Testing. We have successfully synthesised many examples from the existing literature. However, as in many AI systems, the extent of the system is only obtainable by empirical investigation. More work is needed to fully discover which kinds of algorithm we can synthesise given the current heuristic techniques encoded in the proof planner.

Further Heuristic Control. The proof planning framework of methods and methodicals can be extended to enlarge the class of programs that can be synthesised. For example, searching and sorting algorithms along with certain more complicated higher order programs such as filtering a list could not be synthesised given current work. Progress is likely to involve analyzing the techniques used to create certain types of program. In particular, the choice of induction and induction variable in a proof determine the structure of recursion in a program. Increasing the planner's ability to find and choose induction schemes will doubtless lead to greater power of synthesis.

Component Based Synthesis. When people write programs, they often reuse a lot of existing code. In contrast, our system can synthesise programs from specifications but each synthesis is individual and synthesised programs are not reused. This is clearly a limitation, which we would like to address in the future.

One form of program reuse can be achieved by deriving rewrite rules from previously synthesised programs, and using these during the synthesis of new programs.

As pointed out in [5], however, exact matches between specifications and specifications of stored program fragments are rare, and a specialised matching system is required.

6.3   Summary

We have provided a higher-order formulation of logic program synthesis that subsumes earlier work in the area. To implement this work some general features needed to be added to $\lambda Clam$ and also some methods particular for synthesis were created.

The extended flexibility allowed higher-order programs to be synthesised as well as other first-order programs that were beyond other approaches. We believe the use of λProlog and the $\lambda Clam$ system were key to allowing these extensions with practically no change to the code. Some questions remain on judging the correctness of higher-order program syntheses. However, the extensions indicate the system is capable of being developed to achieve quite powerful and flexible fully automated syntheses.

Acknowledgements

The authors gratefully acknowledge the anonymous referees for their comments on this paper. The research was supported by EPSRC grant GR/M45030, and EPSRC funding for David Lacey's MSc in Artificial Intelligence.

References

1. David Basin, Alan Bundy, Ina Kraan, and Sean Matthews. A framework for program development based on schematic proof. In *Proceedings of the 7th International Workshop on Software Specification and Design (IWSSD-93)*, 1993. Also available as Max-Planck-Institut für Informatik Report MPI-I-93-231 and Edinburgh DAI Research Report 654.
2. A. Bundy, A. Smaill, and J. Hesketh. Turning eureka steps into calculations in automatic program synthesis. In S. L.H. Clarke, editor, *Proceedings of UK IT 90*, pages 221–6. IEE, 1990. Also available from Edinburgh as DAI Research Paper 448.
3. A. Bundy, A. Stevens, F. van Harmelen, A. Ireland, and A. Smaill. Rippling: A heuristic for guiding inductive proofs. *Artificial Intelligence*, 62:185–253, 1993. Also available from Edinburgh as DAI Research Paper No. 567.

4. A. Felty. A logic programming approach to implementing higher-order term rewriting. In L-H Eriksson et al., editors, *Second International Workshop on Extensions to Logic Programming*, volume 596 of *Lecture Notes in Artificial Intelligence*, pages 135–61. Springer-Verlag, 1992.

5. Bernd Fischer and Jon Whittle. An integration of deductive retrieval into deductive synthesis. In *Proceedings of the 14th IEEE International Conference on Automated Software Engineering (ASE'99)*, pages 52–61, Cocoa Beach, Florida, USA, October 1999.

6. P. Flener and Y. Deville. Logic program synthesis from incomplete specifications. *Journal of Symbolic Computation: Special Issue on Automatic Programming*, 1993.

7. P. Flener and J. D. C. Richardson. A unified view of programming schemas and proof methods. In *LOPSTR '99: Preproceedings of the Ninth International Workshop on Logic Program Synthesis and Transformation, Venice, Italy, September 1999*, 1999.

8. T. Gegg-Harrison. Representing logic program schemata in lambdaprolog. Technical report, Dept Computer Science, Winona State University, 1995.

9. J. Haas and B. Jayaraman. From context-free to definite-clause grammars: A type-theoretic approach. *Journal of Logic Programming*, 30, 1997.

10. J. Hannan and D. Miller. Uses of higher-order unification for implementing program transformers. In R. A. Kowalski and K. A. Bowen, editors, *Proceedings of the Fifth International Conference and Symposium*, pages 942–59. MIT Press, 1988.

11. G. Huet and B. Lang. Proving and applying program transformation expressed with second order patterns. *Acta Informatica*, 11:31–55, 1978.

12. I. Kraan. *Proof Planning for Logic Program Synthesis*. PhD thesis, Department of Artificial Intelligence, University of Edinburgh, 1994.

13. I. Kraan, D. Basin, and A. Bundy. Logic program synthesis via proof planning. In K. K. Lau and T. Clement, editors, *Logic Program Synthesis and Transformation*, pages 1–14. Springer-Verlag, 1993. Also available as Max-Planck-Institut für Informatik Report MPI-I-92-244 and Edinburgh DAI Research Report 603.

14. I. Kraan, D. Basin, and A. Bundy. Middle-out reasoning for logic program synthesis. In D. S. Warren, editor, *Proceedings of the Tenth International Conference on Logic Programming*. MIT Press, 1993. Also available as Max-Planck-Institut für Informatik Report MPI-I-93-214 and Edinburgh DAI Research Report 638.

15. K.-K. Lau and M. Ornaghi. Forms of logic specifications. A preliminary study. In J. Gallagher, editor, *LOPSTR '96*, number 1207 in Lecture Notes in Computer Science, pages 295–312. Springer-Verlag, 1996.

16. K.-K. Lau and S.D. Prestwich. Top-down synthesis of recursive logic procedures from first-order logic specifications. In D.H.D. Warren and P. Szeredi, editors, *Proc. 7th Int. Conf. on Logic Programming*, pages 667–684. MIT Press, 1990.

17. K.-K. Lau and S.D. Prestwich. Synthesis of a family of recursive sorting procedures. In V. Saraswat and K. Ueda, editors, *Proc. 1991 Int. Logic Programming Symposium*, pages 641–658. MIT Press, 1991.

18. D. Miller. A logic programming language with lambda abstraction, function variables and simple unification. Technical Report MS-CIS-90-54, Department of Computer and Information Science, University of Pennsylvania, 1990. Appeared in *Extensions of Logic Programming*, edited by P. Schröder-Heister, Lecture Notes in Artificial Intelligence, Springer-Verlag.

19. D. Miller and G. Nadathur. An overview of λProlog. In R. Bowen, K. & Kowalski, editor, *Proceedings of the Fifth International Logic Programming Conference/ Fifth Symposium on Logic Programming*. MIT Press, 1988.

20. J.D.C Richardson, A. Smaill, and Ian Green. System description: proof planning in higher-order logic with lambdaclam. In Claude Kirchner and Hélène Kirchner, editors, *15th International Conference on Automated Deduction*, volume 1421 of *Lecture Notes in Artificial Intelligence*, Lindau, Germany, July 1998.
21. W. W. Vasconcelos and N.E. Fuchs. An opportunistic approach for logic program analysis and optimisation using enhanced schema-based transformations. In *Proceedings of LoPSTr'95, Fifth International Workshop on Logic Program Synthesis and Transformation, Utrecht, Netherlands*, volume 1048 of *Lecture Notes in Computer Science*, pages 175–188. Springer Verlag, 1996.

A   Sample Example Synthesis Results

Here is a sample of some of the specifications from which $\lambda Clam$ can successfully synthesis programs.

A.1   First-Order Programs

Name	Specification
subset	$\forall i, j.\ subset(i, j) \leftrightarrow \forall x.\ member(x, i) \rightarrow member(x, j)$
max	$\forall x, l.\ max(x, l) \leftrightarrow member(x, l) \wedge \forall y.\ (member(y, l) \rightarrow leq(y, x))$
add3	$\forall w, x, y, z.\ add3(x, y, z, w) \leftrightarrow w + (x + y) = z$
replicate	$\forall x, y.\ replicate(x, y) \leftrightarrow \forall z.member(z, y) \rightarrow z = x$
front	$\forall x, y.\ front(x, y) \leftrightarrow \exists k.\ app(x, k) = y$
frontn	$\forall x, y, n.\ frontn(x, y, n) \leftrightarrow (\exists k.\ app(x, k) = y) \wedge (length(x) = n)$

A.2   Higher-Order Horn Clause Examples

Name	Specification
listE	$\forall p, x, y.\ (listE\ p\ x\ y) \leftrightarrow (p\ x) \wedge (member\ x\ y)$
all_hold	$\forall f, l.\ (all\_hold\ f\ l) \leftrightarrow \forall x.\ (member\ x\ l) \rightarrow (f\ x)$
takep	$\forall p, x, y.\ (takep\ p\ x\ y) \leftrightarrow \begin{array}{l}(\exists z, k.\quad (app\ x\ z :: k) = y \\ \qquad \wedge\ \forall n.\ (member\ n\ x) \rightarrow (p\ n) \\ \qquad \wedge\ \neg(p\ z))\end{array}$
subsetp	$\forall p, x, y.\ (subsetp\ p\ x\ y) \leftrightarrow \begin{array}{l}(\forall z.\ (member\ z\ x) \rightarrow (member\ z\ y)) \wedge \\ (\forall z.\ (member\ z\ x) \rightarrow (p\ z))\end{array}$

A.3   Parameterised Synthesis

Name	Specification
rnat	$\forall f, f1, f2.(\begin{array}{l}(prog\ f1) \wedge \\ (prog\ f2) \wedge \\ (f\ zero) = f1 \wedge \\ (\forall x.\ (f\ (s\ x)) = (f2\ (f\ x)))\end{array}) \rightarrow \begin{array}{l}\forall x, y.\ (rnat\ f\ f1\ f2\ x\ y) \leftrightarrow \\ \qquad (f\ x) = y\end{array}$
rlst	$\forall f, f1, f2.(\begin{array}{l}(prog\ f1) \wedge \\ (prog\ f2) \wedge \\ (f\ nil) = f1 \wedge \\ (\forall h, t.\ (f\ h :: t) = (f2\ h\ (f\ t)))\end{array}) \rightarrow \begin{array}{l}\forall x, y.\ (rlst\ f\ f1\ f2\ x\ y) \leftrightarrow \\ \qquad (f\ x) = y\end{array}$

Coverability of Reset Petri Nets and Other Well-Structured Transition Systems by Partial Deduction

Michael Leuschel and Helko Lehmann

Department of Electronics and Computer Science
University of Southampton, Highfield, Southampton, SO17 1BJ, UK
{mal,hel99r}@ecs.soton.ac.uk
http://www.ecs.soton.ac.uk/~mal

Abstract. In recent work it has been shown that infinite state model checking can be performed by a combination of partial deduction of logic programs and abstract interpretation. It has also been shown that partial deduction is powerful enough to mimic certain algorithms to decide coverability properties of Petri nets. These algorithms are *forward* algorithms and hard to scale up to deal with more complicated systems. Recently, it has been proposed to use a *backward* algorithm scheme instead. This scheme is applicable to so–called well–structured transition systems and was successfully used, e.g., to solve coverability problems for reset Petri nets. In this paper, we discuss how partial deduction can mimic many of these backward algorithms as well. We prove this link in particular for reset Petri nets and Petri nets with transfer and doubling arcs. We thus establish a surprising link between algorithms in Petri net theory and program specialisation, and also shed light on the power of using logic program specialisation for infinite state model checking.

1   Introduction

Recently there has been interest in applying logic programming techniques to model checking. Table-based logic programming and set-based analysis can be used as an efficient means of performing explicit model checking [29][4]. Despite the success of model checking, most systems must still be substantially simplified and considerable human ingenuity is required to arrive at the stage where the push button automation can be applied [31]. Furthermore, most *software* systems cannot be modelled directly by a *finite* state system. For these reasons, there has recently been considerable interest in *infinite model checking*. This, by its very undecidable nature, is a daunting task, for which *abstraction* is a key issue.

Now, an important question when attempting infinite model checking in practice is: How can one *automatically* obtain an abstraction which is finite, but still as precise as required? A solution to this problem can be obtained by using existing techniques for the *automatic* control of *logic program specialisation* [19]. More precisely, in program specialisation and partial evaluation, one faces a very

J. Lloyd et al. (Eds.): CL 2000, LNAI 1861, pp. 101–115, 2000.

similar (and extensively studied) problem: To be able to produce efficient specialised programs, *infinite* computation trees have to be abstracted in a *finite*
but also as *precise* as possible way. To be able to apply this existing technology
we simply have to model the system to be verified as a logic program (by means
of an interpreter). This obviously includes finite LTS, but also allows to express
infinite state systems. This translation is often very straightforward, due to the
built-in support of logic programming for non-determinism and unification. First
successful steps in that direction have been taken in [12,24]. [22] gave a first formal answer about the power of the approach and showed that when we encode
ordinary Petri nets as logic programs and use existing program specialisation algorithms, we can decide the so-called "coverability problems" (which encompass
quasi-liveness, boundedness, determinism, regularity,...). This was achieved by
showing that the Petri net algorithms by Karp–Miller [15] and Finkel [8] can be
exactly mimicked. Both algorithms are *forward* algorithms, i.e. they construct
an abstracted representation of the whole reachability tree of a Petri net starting
from the initial marking. However, to decide many coverability problems, such a
complete abstraction is not necessary or even not precise enough for more complicated systems. To decide coverability problems for a wider class of transition
systems, namely well structured transition systems, in [1, 9, 10] a backward algorithm scheme was proposed instead. This scheme has been successfully applied,
e.g., to *reset Petri nets*.

In this paper we discuss how partial deduction can mimic these backward
algorithms as well. We prove this correspondence in particular for reset Petri
nets, since for many problems they lie on the "border between decidability and
undecidability" [6]. Thus, in addition to establishing a link between algorithms
in Petri net theory and program specialisation, our results also shed light on the
power of using logic program analysis and specialisation techniques for infinite
state model checking.

2   (Reset) Petri Nets and the Covering Problem

In this paper we want to study the power of partial deduction based approaches
for model checking of infinite state systems. To arrive at precise results, it makes
sense to focus on a particular class of infinite state systems and properties which
are known to be decidable. One can then examine whether the partial deduction approach provides a decision procedure and how it compares to existing
algorithms. In this section, we describe such a decidable class of properties and
systems, namely covering problems for Petri nets, reset Petri nets, and well-
structured transition systems. We start out by giving definitions of some important concepts in Petri net theory [30].

Definition 1. *A Petri net Π is a tuple (S, T, F, M_0) consisting of a finite set of
places S, a finite set of transitions T with $S \cap T = \emptyset$ and a flow relation F which
is a function from $(S \times T) \cup (T \times S)$ to $\mathbb{N}$. A marking M for Π is a mapping
$S \to \mathbb{N}$. M_0 is a marking called* initial.

A transition $t \in T$ is enabled *in a marking M iff $\forall s \in S : M(s) \geq F(s,t)$. An enabled transition can be* fired, *resulting in a new marking M' defined by $\forall s \in S : M'(s) = M(s) - F(s,t) + F(t,s)$. We will denote this by $M[t\rangle M'$. By $M[t_1,\ldots,t_k\rangle M'$ we denote the fact that for some intermediate markings $M_1,\ldots,M_{k-1}$ we have $M[t_1\rangle M_1, \ldots, M_{k-1}[t_k\rangle M'$.*

We define the reachability tree *$RT(\Pi)$ inductively as follows: Let M_0 be the label of the root node. For every node n of $RT(\Pi)$ labelled by some marking M and for every transition t which is enabled in M, add a node n' labelled M' such that $M[t\rangle M'$ and add an arc from n to n' labelled t. The set of all labels of $RT(\Pi)$ is called the* reachability set *of Π, denoted $RS(\Pi)$. The set of words given by the labels of finite paths of $RT(\Pi)$ starting in the root node is called* language *of Π, written $L(\Pi)$.*

For convenience, we denote $M \geq M'$ iff $M(s) \geq M'(s)$ for all places $s \in S$. We also introduce *pseudo-markings*, which are functions from S to $I\!N \cup \{\omega\}$ where we also define $\forall n \in I\!N : \omega > n$ and $\omega + n = \omega - n = \omega + \omega = \omega$. Using this we also extend the notation $M_{k-1}[t_1,\ldots,t_k\rangle M'$ for such markings.

Reset Petri Nets and WSTS's. One can extend the power of Petri nets by adding a set of *reset arcs* $R \subseteq (S \times T)$ from places to transitions: when the associated transition fires the number of tokens in the originating place is reset to zero. Such nets were first introduced in [2], and we adapt all of the above concepts and notations in the obvious way.

Well-structured transition systems (WSTS) [9, 10] are a further generalisation of Petri nets. They cover reset Petri nets but also Petri nets with transfer arcs, post self-modifying nets, as well as many formalisms not directly related to Petri nets (Basic Process Algebras, Context-free grammars, Timed Automata,...). To define WSTS we first need the concept of a well-quasi order:

Definition 2. *A sequence $s_1, s_2, \ldots$ of elements of S is called* admissible wrt a *binary relation $\leq_S$ on $S \times S$ iff there are no $i < j$ such that $s_i \leq_S s_j$. We say that $\leq_S$ is a* well-quasi relation *(wqr) iff there are no infinite admissible sequences wrt $\leq_S$. A* well quasi order *(wqo) is a reflexive and transitive wqr.*

A well-structured transition system (WSTS) [9, 10] is a structure $\langle S, \rightarrow, \leq \rangle$ where S is a (possibly infinite) set of states, $\rightarrow \subseteq S \times S$ a set of transitions, and:
(1) $\leq \subseteq S \times S$ is a wqo and
(2) $\leq$ is (upward) compatible wrt $\rightarrow$: for all $s_1 \leq t_1$ and $s_1 \rightarrow s_2$ there exists a sequence $t_1 \rightarrow^* t_2$ such that $s_2 \leq t_2$.
Reset Petri nets can be modelled as a WSTS $\langle S, \rightarrow, \leq \rangle$ with S being the set of markings, $M \rightarrow M'$ if for some t we have $M[t\rangle M'$ and using the corresponding $\leq$ order on markings seen as vectors of numbers (this order is a wqo).

Coverability Analysis. The *covering problem* is a classical problem in Petri net theory and is also sometimes referred to as the *control-state reachability problem*. The question is: given a marking M is there a marking M' in $RS(\Pi)$

which covers M, i.e., $M' \geq M$. This problem can be analysed using the so-called Karp-Miller-tree $KM(\Pi)$ [15], which is computed as follows:
1.start out from a tree with a single node labelled by the initial marking M_0; **2.** repeatedly pick an unprocessed leaf labelled by some M; for every transition t such that $M[t\rangle M'$ and such that there is no ancestor $M'' = M'$ do: **a.** generalise M' by replacing all $M'(p)$ by ω such that there is an ancestor $M'' < M'$ and $M''(p) < M'(p)$ **b.** create a child of M labelled by M'.

The intuition behind step 2a. is that if from M'' we can reach the strictly larger marking M' we then extrapolate the growth by inserting ω's. For example for $M'' = \langle 0, 1, 1 \rangle$ and $M' = \langle 1, 2, 1 \rangle$ we will produce $\langle \omega, \omega, 1 \rangle$. This is sufficient to ensure termination of the procedure and thus finiteness of $KM(\Pi)$.

Some of the properties of ordinary Petri nets decidable by examining $KM(\Pi)$ are:[1] boundedness, place-boundedness, quasi-liveness of a transition t (i.e. is there a marking in $RT(\Pi)$ where t is enabled), and regularity of $L(\Pi)$ (cf. [8],[15], [35]).

The quasi-liveness question is a particular instance of the covering problem, which can be decided using the Karp-Miller tree simply by checking whether there is a pseudo-marking M' in $KM(\Pi)$ such that $M' \geq M$. For example if there is a marking $\langle \omega, \omega, 1 \rangle$ in $KM(\Pi)$ then we know that we can, e.g., reach a marking greater or equal to $\langle 10, 55, 1 \rangle$.

The reason why this approach is correct is the monotonicity of ordinary Petri nets: if $M[t_1, \ldots, t_k\rangle M'$ and $M'' > M$ (the condition to introduce ω) then $M''[t_1, \ldots, t_k\rangle M'''$ for some $M''' > M'$ (i.e., we can repeat the process and produce ever larger markings and when an ω is generated within $KM(\Pi)$ for a particular place s we can generate an arbitrarily large number of tokens in s^2).

Unfortunately, this monotonicity criterion is no longer satisfied for Petri nets with reset arcs! More precisely, when we have $M[t_1, \ldots, t_k\rangle M'$ with $M' > M$ (the condition to introduce ω) we still have that $M'[t_1, \ldots, t_k\rangle M''$ for some M'' but we no longer have $M'' > M'$ (we just have $M'' \geq M'$). This means that, when computing the Karp-Miller tree, the generation of ω places is sound but no longer "precise," i.e., when we generate an ω we are no longer guaranteed that an unbounded number of tokens can actually be produced. The Karp-Miller tree can thus no longer be used to decide boundedness or coverability.

Example 1. Take for example a simple reset Petri net with two transitions t_1, t_2 and two places s_1, s_2 depicted in Fig. 1. Transition t_1 takes one token in s_1 and putting one token in s_2 and resetting s_1. Transition t_2 takes one token from s_2 and producing 2 tokens in s_1. Then we have $\langle 1, 0 \rangle [t_1\rangle \langle 0, 1 \rangle [t_2\rangle \langle 2, 0 \rangle$ and the Karp-Miller procedure generates a node labelled with $\langle \omega, 0 \rangle$ even though the net is bounded!

---

[1] It was shown in [8] that these problems can also be decided using minimal coverability graphs, which are often significantly smaller.

[2] However, it does not guarantee that we can generate *any* number of tokens. To decide whether we can, e.g., reach *exactly* the marking $\langle 10, 55, 1 \rangle$ the Karp-Miller tree is not enough.

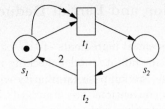

Fig. 1. Reset Petri from Ex. 1

It turns out that boundedness (as well as reachability) is actually undecidable for Petri nets with reset arcs [6]. However, the covering problem (and thus, e.g., quasi-liveness) is still decidable using a backwards algorithm [1, 9, 10], which works for any WSTS for which $\leq$ and $pb(.)$ (see below) can be computed.

Given a WSTS $\langle S, \rightarrow, \leq \rangle$ and a set of states $I \in S$ we define:

- the upwards-closure $\uparrow I = \{y \mid y \geq x \wedge x \in I\}$
- the immediate predecessor states of I: $Pred(I) = \{y \mid y \rightarrow x \wedge x \in I\}$
- all predecessor states of I, $Pred^*(I) = \{y \mid y \rightarrow^* x \wedge x \in I\}$
- $pb(I) = \bigcup_{x \in I} pb(x)$ where $pb(x)$ is a finite basis of $\uparrow Pred(\uparrow \{x\})$ (i.e., $pb(x)$ is a finite set such that $\uparrow pb(x) = \uparrow Pred(\uparrow \{x\})$).

The *covering problem* for WSTS is as follows: given two states s and t can we reach $t' \geq t$ starting from s. Provided that $\leq$ is decidable and $pb(x)$ exists and can be effectively computed, the following algorithm [1, 9, 10] can be used to decide the covering problem:

1. Set $K_0 = \{t\}$ and $j = 0$
2. $K_{j+1} = K_j \cup pb(K_j)$
3. if $\uparrow K_{j+1} \neq \uparrow K_j$ then increment j and goto 2.
4. return true if $\exists s' \in K_j$ with $s' \leq s$ and false otherwise

This procedure terminates and we also have the property that $\uparrow \bigcup_i K_i = Pred^*(\uparrow \{t\})$ [10]. At step 4. we test whether $s \in \uparrow K_j$, which thus corresponds to $s \in Pred^*(\uparrow \{t\})$ (because we have reached the fixpoint), i.e., we indeed check whether $s \rightarrow^* t'$ for some $t' \geq t$.

$pb(M)$ can be effectively computed for Petri nets and reset Petri nets by simply executing the transitions backwards and setting a place to the minimum number of tokens required to fire the transition if it caused a reset on this place:

$$pb(M) = \{ P' \mid \exists t \in T : (P[t\rangle M \wedge \\ \forall s \in S : P'(s) = (F(s,t) \text{ if } (s,t) \in R \text{ else } P(s))) \}$$

We can thus use the above algorithm to decide the covering problem. In the remainder of the paper we will show that, surprisingly, the exact same result can be obtained by encoding the (reset) Petri net as a logic program and applying a well-established program specialisation technique!

3   Partial Evaluation and Partial Deduction

We will now present the essential ingredients of the logic program specialisation techniques that were used for infinite model checking in [12, 24].

Throughout this article, we suppose familiarity with basic notions in logic programming. Notational conventions are standard. In particular, we denote variables through (strings starting with) an uppercase symbol, while constants, functions, and predicates begin with a lowercase character.

In logic programming full input to a program P consists of a goal $\leftarrow Q$ and evaluation corresponds to constructing a complete SLD-tree for $P \cup \{\leftarrow Q\}$, i.e., a tree whose root is labeled by $\leftarrow Q$ and where children of nodes are obtained by first selecting a literal of the node and then resolving it with the clauses of P. For partial evaluation, static input takes the form of a *partially instantiated* goal $\leftarrow Q'$ and the specialised program should be correct for all runtime instances $\leftarrow Q'\theta$ of $\leftarrow Q'$. A technique which achieves this is known under the name of *partial deduction*, which we present below.

3.1   Generic Algorithm for Partial Deduction

The general idea of partial deduction is to construct a finite number of finite but possibly incomplete[3] trees which "cover" the possibly infinite SLD-tree for $P \cup \{\leftarrow Q'\}$ (and thus also all SLD-trees for all instances of $\leftarrow Q'$). The derivation steps in these SLD-trees are the computations which have been pre-evaluated and the clauses of the specialised program are then extracted by constructing one specialised clause (called a *resultant*) per branch. These incomplete SLD-trees are obtained by applying an unfolding rule:

Definition 3. *An* unfolding rule *is a function which, given a program P and a goal $\leftarrow Q$, returns a non-trivial[4] and possibly incomplete SLD-tree τ for $P \cup \{\leftarrow Q\}$. We also define the set of leaves, leaves(τ), to be the leaf goals of τ.*

Given *closedness* (all leaves are an instance of a specialised atom) and *independence* (no two specialised atoms have a common instance), correctness of the specialised program is guaranteed [25]. Independence is usually (e.g. [23, 5]) ensured by a *renaming* transformation. Closedness is more difficult to ensure, but can be satisfied using the following generic algorithm based upon [27, 23]. This algorithm structures the atoms to be specialised in a *global tree*: i.e., a tree whose nodes are labeled by atoms and where A is a descendant of B if specialising B lead to the specialisation of A. Apart from the missing treatment of conjunctions [5] the following is basically the algorithm implemented in the ECCE system [23, 5] which we will employ later on.

---

[3] An *incomplete* SLD-tree is a SLD-tree which, in addition to success and failure leaves, also contains leaves where no literal has been selected for a further derivation step.

[4] A trivial SLD-tree has a single node where no literal has been selected for resolution.

Algorithm 3.1 (*Generic Partial Deduction Algorithm*)

Input: a program P and a goal $\leftarrow A$
Output: a set of atoms or conjunctions $\mathcal{A}$ and a global tree γ
Initialisation: $\gamma :=$ a "global" tree with a single unmarked node, labelled by A
repeat
    pick an unmarked leaf node L in γ
    if $covered(L, \gamma)$ **then**   mark L as processed
    else
        $W = whistle(L, \gamma)$
        if $W \neq fail$ **then**
            $label(L) := abstract(L, W, \gamma)^5$
        else
            mark L as processed
            for all atoms $A \in leaves(U(P, label(L)))$ **do**
                add a new unmarked child C of L to γ
                $label(C) := A$
until all nodes are processed
output $\mathcal{A} := \{label(A) \mid A \in \gamma\}$ and γ

The above algorithm is parametrised by an unfolding rule U, a predicate $covered(L, \gamma)$, a whistle function $whistle(L, \gamma)$ and an abstraction function $abstract(L, W, \gamma)$. Intuitively, $covered(L, \gamma)$ is a way of checking whether L or a generalisation of L has already been treated in the global tree γ. Formally, $covered(L, \gamma) = true$ must imply that $\exists M \in \gamma$ such that M is processed or abstracted and for some substitution θ: $label(M)\theta = label(L)$. A particular implementation could be more demanding and, e.g., return true only if there is another node in γ labelled by a variant of L.

The other two parameters are used to ensure termination. Intuitively, the $whistle(L, \gamma)$ is used to detect whether the branch of γ ending in L is "dangerous", in which case it returns a value different from $fail$ (i.e., it "blows"). This value should be an ancestor W of L compared to which L looked dangerous (e.g., L is bigger than W in some sense). The abstraction operation will then compute a generalisation of L and W, less likely to lead to non-termination. Formally, $abstract(L, W, \gamma)$ must be an atom which is more general than both L and W. This generalisation will replace the label of W in the global tree γ.

If the Algorithm 3.1 terminates then the closedness condition of [25] is satisfied, i.e., it is ensured that *together* the SLD-trees $\tau_1, \ldots, \tau_n$ form a *complete description* of all possible computations that can occur for all concrete instances $\leftarrow A\theta$ of the goal of interest [20, 18]. We can then produce a *totally correct* specialised program. On its own, Algorithm 3.1 does not ensure termination (so its strictly speaking not an algorithm but a procedure). To ensure termination, we have to use an unfolding rule that builds finite SLD-trees only. We also have to guarantee that infinite branches in the global tree γ will be spotted by the *whistle* and that the abstraction can not be repeated infinitely often.

---

^{5} Alternatively one could remove all descendants of W and change the label of W. This is controlled by the *parent_abstraction* switch in ECCE.

3.2 Concrete Algorithm

We now present a concrete partial deduction algorithm, which is *online* (as opposed to *offline*) in the sense that control decisions are taken *during* the construction of γ and not beforehand. It is also rather naïve (e.g., it does not use characteristic trees [23]; also the generic Algorithm 3.1 does not include recent improvements such as conjunctions [5], constraints [21,16] or abstract interpretation [18]). However, it is easier to comprehend (and analyse) and will actually be sufficiently powerful for our purposes (i.e., decide covering problems of reset Petri nets and other WSTS's).

Unfolding Rule. In this paper we will use a very simple method for ensuring that each individual SLD-tree constructed by U is finite: we ensure that we unfold every predicate at most once in any given tree!

Whistle. To ensure that no infinite global tree γ is being built-up, we will use a more refined approach based upon well-quasi orders: In our context we will use a wqo to ensure that no infinite tree γ is built up in Algorithm 3.1 by setting *whistle* to true whenever the sequence of labels on the current branch is not admissible. A particularly useful wqo (for a finite alphabet) is the pure homeomorphic embedding [33,23]:

Definition 4. *The* (pure) *homeomorphic embedding relation* $\trianglelefteq$ *on expressions is inductively defined as follows (i.e.* $\trianglelefteq$ *is the least relation satisfying the rules):*

   1. $X \trianglelefteq Y$ *for all variables* X, Y
   2. $s \trianglelefteq f(t_1, \ldots, t_n)$ *if* $s \trianglelefteq t_i$ *for some* i
   3. $f(s_1, \ldots, s_n) \trianglelefteq f(t_1, \ldots, t_n)$ *if* $\forall i \in \{1, \ldots, n\} : s_i \trianglelefteq t_i$.

Notice that n is allowed to be 0 and we thus have $c \trianglelefteq c$ for all constant and proposition symbols. The intuition behind the above definition is that $A \trianglelefteq B$ iff A can be obtained from B by "striking out" certain parts, or said another way, the structure of A reappears within B. We have $f(a, b) \trianglelefteq p(f(g(a), b))$.

Abstraction. Once the *whistle* has identified a potential non-termination one will usually compute generalisations which are as precise as possible (for partial deduction): The *most specific generalisation* of a finite set of expressions S, denoted by $msg(S)$, is the most specific expression M such that all expressions in S are instances of M. E.g., $msg(\{p(0, s(0)), p(0, s(s(0)))\}) = p(0, s(X))$. The msg can be computed [17].

Algorithm 3.2 We define an instance of Algorithm 3.1 as follows:
  – U unfolds every predicate just once
  – $covered(L, \gamma) = true$ if there exists a processed node in γ whose label is *more general than* L
  – $whistle(L, \gamma) = M$ iff M is an ancestor of L such that $label(M) \trianglelefteq label(L)$ and $whistle_{\trianglelefteq}(L, \gamma) = fail$ if there is no such ancestor.
  – $abstract(L, W, \gamma) = msg(L, W)$.

Algorithm 3.2 terminates for any program P and goal $\leftarrow Q$ (this can be proven by simplified versions of the proofs in [23] or [32]).

4 Encoding (Reset) Petri Nets as Logic Programs

It is very easy to implement (reset) Petri nets as (non-deterministic) logic programs (see also [11]). Figure 2 contains a particular encoding of the reset Petri Net from Ex. 1 and a simple predicate `reachable` searching for reachable markings in $RS(\Pi)$. To model a reset arc (as opposed to an ordinary arc), one simply allows the `trans/3` facts to carry a 0 within the post-marking. Other nets can be encoded by changing the `trans/3` facts and the `initial_marking` fact.

Based upon such a translation, [12,24] pursued the idea that model checking of safety properties amounts to showing that there exists no trace which leads to an invalid state, i.e., exploiting the fact that $\forall\Box safe \equiv \neg\exists\Diamond(\neg safe)$. Proving that no trace leads to a state where $\neg safe$ holds is then achieved by a *semantics-preserving program specialisation and analysis technique*. For this, an instance of Algorithm 3.1 was applied to several systems, followed by an abstract interpretation based upon [26] (we will return to [26] later in the paper).

```
reachable(R) :- initial_marking(M), reachable(Tr,R,M).
reachable([],State,State).
reachable([Action|As],Reach,InState) :-
    trans(Action,InState,NewState),reachable(As,Reach,NewState).
trans(t1, [s(S1),S2],[0,s(S2)]).
trans(t2, [S1,s(S2)],[s(s(S1)),S2]).
initial_marking([s(0),0]).
```

Fig. 2. Encoding a Reset Petri net as a logic program

As was shown in [22], this approach actually gives a decision procedure for coverability, (place-)boundedness, regularity of ordinary Petri nets. One can even establish a one-to-one correspondence between the Karp-Miller tree $KM(\Pi)$ and the global tree produced by (an instance of) partial deduction [22].

As we have seen, boundedness is undecidable for Petri nets with reset arcs [6] so the partial deduction approach, although guaranteed to terminate, will no longer give a decision procedure. (However, using default settings, ECCE can actually prove that the particular Reset net of Fig. 1 is bounded.)

But let us turn towards the covering problem which is decidable, but using the backwards algorithm we presented in Section 2. To be able to use partial deduction on this problem it seems sensible to write an "inverse" interpreter for reset Petri nets. This is not very difficult, as shown in Fig. 3, exploiting the fact that logic programs can be run backwards.

We can use this program in Prolog to check whether a particular marking such as $\langle 2, 0 \rangle$ can be reached from the initial marking:

```
| ?- search_initial(T,[s(s(0)),0]).
T = [t2,t1]
```

Unfortunately, we cannot in general solve covering problems using Prolog or even XSB-Prolog due to their inability of detecting infinite failures. For example,

```
search_initial([],State) :- initial_marking(State).
search_initial([Action|As],InState) :-
    trans(Action,PredState,InState),search_initial(As,PredState).
trans(t1,[s(P1),P2],[0,s(P2)]).
trans(t2,[P1,s(P2)],[s(s(P1)),P2]).
initial_marking([s(0),0]).
```

Fig. 3. Backwards Interpreter for Reset Petri nets

the query ?-search_initial(T,[s(s(s(_X1))),_X2]), checking whether $\langle 3, 0 \rangle$ can be covered from the initial situation will loop in both Prolog or XSB-Prolog. However, the logic program and query is still a correct encoding of the covering problem: indeed, no instance of search_initial(T,[s(s(s(_X1))),_X2]) is in the least Herbrand model. Below, we will show how this information can be extracted from the logic program using partial deduction, even to the point of giving us a decision procedure.

We will denote by $C(\Pi, M_0)$ the variation of the logic program in Fig. 3 encoding the particular (reset) Petri net Π with the initial marking M_0.[6]

5 Coverability of Reset Petri Nets by Partial Deduction

We will now apply our partial deduction algorithm to decide the covering problem for reset Petri nets. For this we need to establish a link between markings and atoms produced by partial deduction.

First, recall that an atom for partial deduction denotes all its instances. So, if during the partial deduction we encounter search_initial(T,[M1,...,Mk]) this represents all markings $\langle m_1, ..., m_k \rangle$ such that for some substitution θ we have $\forall i$: Mi$\theta = \lceil m_i \rceil$. For example the term $s(s(s(X)))$ corresponds to the set represented by the number 3 in Section 2 (where a number n represents all numbers $m \geq n$). The following is a formalisation of the encoding of natural numbers as terms that will occur when specialising $C(\Pi, M_0)$:

- $\lceil i \rceil = X$ if $i = 0$ and where X is a fresh variable
- $\lceil i \rceil = s(\lceil i - 1 \rceil)$ otherwise

From now on, we also suppose that the order of the places in M_0 is the same as in the encoding in Figures 2, 3 and define $\lceil \langle m_1, ..., m_k \rangle \rceil = [\lceil m_1 \rceil, ..., \lceil m_k \rceil]$.

Lemma 1. *Let M and M' be two markings. Then:*
1. $M \leq M'$ *iff* $\lceil M \rceil$ *is more general than* $\lceil M' \rceil$.
2. $M \leq M'$ *iff* $\lceil M \rceil \trianglelefteq \lceil M' \rceil$.
3. $M < M'$ *iff* $\lceil M \rceil$ *is strictly more general than* $\lceil M' \rceil$.
4. $\uparrow \{M\} = \{M' \mid \exists \theta \text{ with } \lceil M' \rceil = \lceil M \rceil \theta\}$.

---

[6] To keep the presentation as simple as possible, contrary to [22], we do not perform a preliminary compilation. We compensate this by using a slightly more involved unfolding rule (in [22] only a single unfolding step is performed).

We can now establish a precise relationship between the computation of $pb(.)$ and SLD-derivations of the above logic program translation:

Lemma 2. *Let Π be Petri Net with reset arcs, and M be a marking for Π. Then $M_i \in pb(M)$ iff there exists an incomplete SLD-derivation of length 2 for $C(\Pi, M_0) \cup \{\leftarrow search\_initial(T, \lceil M \rceil)\}$ leading to $\leftarrow search\_initial(T', \lceil M_i \rceil)$. Also, $M_0 \in\uparrow \{M\}$ iff there exists an SLD-refutation of length 2 for $C(\Pi, M_0) \cup \{\leftarrow search\_initial(T, \lceil M \rceil)\}$.*

However, partial deduction atoms are more expressive than markings: e.g., we can represent all $\langle m_1, m_2, m_3 \rangle$ such that $m_1 > 0$, $m_2 = m_1 + 1$, and $m_3 = 1$ by: search_initial(T,[s(X),s(s(X)),s(0)]). In other words, we can establish a link between the number of tokens in several places via shared variables and we can represent exact values for places.[7] However, such information will never appear, because a) we start out with a term which corresponds exactly to a marking, b) we only deal with (reset) Petri nets and working backwards will yield a new term which corresponds exactly to a marking (as proven in Lemma 2) c) the generalisation will never be needed, because if our whistle based upon $\trianglelefteq$ blows then, by Lemma 1, the dangerous atom is an instance of an already processed one.[8]

Theorem 1. *Let Π be Petri Net with reset arcs with initial marking M_0 and let P be the residual program obtained by Algorithm 3.2 applied to $C(\Pi, M_0)$ and $\leftarrow search\_initial(T', \lceil M_c \rceil)$. Then P contains facts iff there exists a marking M' in $RT(\Pi)$ which covers M_c, i.e., $M' \geq M_c$.*

The above theorem implies that when we perform a bottom-up abstract interpretation after partial deduction using, e.g., [26] (as done in [24]), we will be able to deduce failure of $\leftarrow search\_initial(T', \lceil M_c \rceil)$ if and only if $RT(\Pi)$ does not cover M_c! The following example illustrates this. When applying Algorithm 3.2 (using the ECCE system) to specialise the program in Fig. 3 for $\leftarrow search\_initial(T', \lceil \langle 3, 0 \rangle \rceil)$ we get:

```
/* Specialised Predicates:
search_initial__1(A,B,C) :- search_initial(C,[s(s(s(B))),A]).
search_initial__2(A,B) :- search_initial(B,[s(A),s(C1)]).
search_initial__3(A,B) :- search_initial(B,[A,s(s(C1))]).     */

search_initial(A,[s(s(s(B))),C]) :- search_initial__1(C,B,A).
search_initial__1(A,B,[t2|C]) :- search_initial__2(B,C).
search_initial__2(s(A),[t2|B]) :- search_initial__3(A,B).
search_initial__3(0,[t1|A]) :- search_initial__2(B,A).
search_initial__3(s(s(A)),[t2|B]) :- search_initial__3(A,B).
```

---

[7] More precisely, each atom represents a linear set $L \subseteq I\!N^k$ of markings $L = \{b + \sum_{i=1}^{r} n_i p^i \mid n_i \in I\!N\}$ with $b, p^i \in I\!N^k$ and the restriction that $\sum_{i=1}^{r} p^i \leq \langle 1, \ldots, 1 \rangle$.
[8] This also implies that a similar result to Theorem 1, for reset Petri nets, might be obtained by using OLDT abstract interpretation in place of partial deduction.

After which the most specific version abstract interpretation [26] implemented in ECCE will produce:

```
search_initial(A,[s(s(s(B))),C]) :-  fail.
```

It turns out that Algorithm 3.2, when expanding the global tree γ in a breadth-first manner, can actually mimic an improved version of the backwards algorithm from [10] (see Section 2): provided that we improve the backwards algorithm to not compute $pb(.)$ of markings which are already covered, we obtain that the set of labels in $\gamma = \{search\_initial(T, \lceil M \rceil) \mid M \in K_j\}$, where K_j is the set obtained by the improved backwards algorithm.

6   Other Well-Structured Transition Systems

Let us now turn to another well-known Petri net extension which does not violate the WSTS character [10]: *transfer arcs* [13, 6] which enable transitions to transfer tokens from one place to another, *doubling arcs* which double the number of tokens in a given place, or any mixture thereof. Take for example the following simple fact:

```
trans(t3,[P1,s(P2)],[P2,P2]).
```

This transition employs a combination of a reset arc (removing the number of tokens $P1$ present in place 1) and a kind of transfer arc (transferring all but one token from place 2 to place 1). Transitions like these will not pose a problem to our partial deduction algorithm: it can be used as is as a decision procedure for the covering problem and Theorem 1 holds for this extended class of Petri nets as well. In fact, a similar theorem should hold for any *post self-modifying net* [34, 10] and even *Reset Post G-nets* [6]. (However, the theorem is not true for Petri nets with inhibitor arcs.)

Another class of WSTS are basic process algebras (BPP's) [7], a subset of CCS without synchronisation. Below, we try to analyse them using our partial deduction approach. Plugging the following definitions into the code of Fig. 3 we encode a process algebra with action prefix ., choice +, and parallel composition $\|$, as well as a process starting from $(a.stop + b.stop)\|c.stop)$:

```
trans(A,pre(A,P),P).
trans(A,or(X,_Y),XA) :- trans(A,X,XA).
trans(A,or(_X,Y),YA) :- trans(A,Y,YA).
trans(A,par(X,Y),par(XA,Y)) :- trans(A,X,XA).
trans(A,par(X,Y),par(X,YA)) :- trans(A,Y,YA).
initial_marking(par(or(pre(a,stop),pre(b,stop)),pre(c,stop))).
```

Compared to the WSTS's we have studied so far, the term representation of states gets much more complex (we no longer have lists of fixed length of natural numbers but unbounded process expressions). Our $\trianglelefteq$ relation is of course still a wqo on processes in this algebra, and it is also upwards compatible. Unfortunately we no longer have the nice correspondence between $\trianglelefteq$ and the instance-of relation (as in Lemma 1 for reset nets). For instance, we have $pre(a, stop) \trianglelefteq stop$, but $pre(a, stop)$ is not more general than $stop$ and partial deduction will not realise that it does not have to analyse $stop$ if has already analysed $pre(a, stop)$ (indeed, in general it would be unsound not to examine $stop$). This means that the partial deduction approach will contain some "redundant" nodes. It also means that we cannot in general formulate covering problems as queries; although we can formulate reachability questions (for reset Petri nets we could do both). Nonetheless, specialising the above code using Algorithm 3.2 and [26], e.g., for the reachability query search_initial(A,stop), we get:

```
search_initial(A,stop) :- fail.
```

This is correct: we can reach $stop||stop$ but not $stop$ itself. However, despite the success on this particular example, we believe that to arrive at a full solution we will need to move to an abstract partial deduction [18] algorithm: this will enable us to re-instate the correspondence between the wqo of the WSTS and the instance-of relation of the program specialisation technique, thus arriving at a full-fledged decision procedure.

7   Future Work and Conclusion

One big advantage of the partial deduction approach to model checking is it scales up to any formalism expressible as a logic program. More precisely, proper instantiations of Algorithm 3.1 will terminate for any system and will provide safe approximations of properties under consideration. However, as is to be expected, we might no longer have a decision procedure.

[24] discusses how to extend the model checking approach to liveness properties and full CTL. Some simple examples are solved. E.g., the approach was applied to the manufacturing system used in [3] and it was able to prove absence of deadlocks for parameter values of, e.g., 1,2,3. When leaving the parameter unspecified, the system was unable to prove the absence of deadlocks and produced a residual program with facts. And indeed, for parameter value ≥ 9 the system can actually deadlock. The timings compare favourably with HyTech [14].

Reachability can be decided in some but not all cases using the present partial deduction algorithm. In future we want to examine the relationship to Mayr's algorithm [28] for ordinary Petri nets and whether it can be mimicked by abstract partial deduction [18].

Finally, an important aspect of model checking of finite state systems is the complexity of the underlying algorithms. We have not touched upon this issue in the present paper, but plan to do so in future work.

Conclusion. We have examined the power of partial deduction (and abstract interpretation) for a particular class of infinite state model checking tasks, namely covering problems for reset Petri nets. The latter are particularly interesting as they lie on the "border between decidability and undecidabilty" [6]. We have proven that a well-established partial deduction algorithm based upon $\trianglelefteq$ can be used as a decision procedure for these problems and we have unveiled a surprising correspondence with an existing algorithm from the Petri net area.

We have also shown that this property of partial deduction holds for other Petri net extensions which can be viewed as WSTS's. We have also studied other WSTS's from the process algebra arena. For these we have shown that, to arrive at a full-fledged decision procedure, we will need to move to the more powerful abstract partial deduction [18].

References

1. P. A. Abdulla, K. Čerāns, B. Jonsson, and Y.-K. Tsay. General decidability theorems for infinite-state systems. In *Proceedings LICS'96*, pages 313–321, July 1996. IEEE Computer Society Press.

2. T. Araki and T. Kasami. Some decision problems related to the reachability problem for Petri nets. *Theoretical Computer Science*, 3:85–104, 1977.

3. B. Bérard and L. Fribourg. Reachability analysis of (timed) petri nets using real arithmetic. In *Proceedings Concur'99*, LNCS 1664, pages 178–193. Springer-Verlag, 1999.

4. W. Charatonik and A. Podelski. Set-based analysis of reactive infinite-state systems. In B. Steffen, editor, *Proceedings TACAS'98*, LNCS 1384, pages 358–375. Springer-Verlag, March 1998.

5. D. De Schreye, R. Glück, J. Jørgensen, M. Leuschel, B. Martens, and M. H. Sørensen. Conjunctive partial deduction: Foundations, control, algorithms and experiments. *J. Logic Progam.*, 41(2 & 3):231–277, November 1999.

6. C. Dufourd, A. Finkel, and P. Schnoebelen. Reset nets between decidability and undecidability. In *Proceedings ICALP'98*, LNCS 1443, pages 103–115. Springer-Verlag, 1998.

7. J. Ezparza. Decidability of model-checking for infinite-state concurrent systems. *Acta Informatica*, 34:85–107, 1997.

8. A. Finkel. The minimal coverability graph for Petri nets. *Advances in Petri Nets 1993*, LNCS 674, pages 210–243, 1993.

9. A. Finkel and P. Schnoebelen. Fundamental structures in well-structured infinite transition systems. In *Proceedings LATIN'98*, LNCS 1380, pages 102–118. Springer-Verlag, 1998.

10. A. Finkel and P. Schnoebelen. Well-structured transition systems everywhere ! *Theoretical Computer Science*, 2000. To appear.

11. L. Fribourg and H. Olsen. Proving Safety Properties of Infinite State Systems by Compilation into Presburger Arithmtic. In *Proceedings Concur'97*, LNCS 1243, pages 213–227. Springer-Verlag, 1997.

12. R. Glück and M. Leuschel. Abstraction-based partial deduction for solving inverse problems – a transformational approach to software verification. In *Proceedings PSI'99*, LNCS 1755, pages 93–100, 1999. Springer-Verlag.

13. B. Heinemann. Subclasses of self-modifying nets. In *Applications and Theory of Petri Nets*, pages 187–192. Springer-Verlag, 1982.

14. T. A. Henzinger and P.-H. Ho. HYTECH: The Cornell HYbrid TECHnology tool. *Hybrid Systems II*, LNCS 999:265–293, 1995.

15. R. M. Karp and R. E. Miller. Parallel program schemata. *Journal of Computer and System Sciences*, 3:147–195, 1969.

16. L. Lafave and J. Gallagher. Constraint-based partial evaluation of rewriting-based functional logic programs. In N. Fuchs, editor, *Proceedings LOPSTR'97*, LNCS 1463, pages 168–188, July 1997.

17. J.-L. Lassez, M. Maher, and K. Marriott. Unification revisited. In J. Minker, editor, *Foundations of Deductive Databases and Logic Programming*, pages 587–625. Morgan-Kaufmann, 1988.

18. M. Leuschel. Program specialisation and abstract interpretation reconciled. In J. Jaffar, editor, *Proceedings JICSLP'98*, pages 220–234, Manchester, UK, June 1998. MIT Press.

19. M. Leuschel. Logic program specialisation. In J. Hatcliff, T. Æ. Mogensen, and P. Thiemann, editors, *Partial Evaluation: Practice and Theory*, LNCS 1706, pages 155–188 and 271–292, 1999. Springer-Verlag.

20. M. Leuschel and D. De Schreye. Logic program specialisation: How to be more specific. In H. Kuchen and S. Swierstra, editors, *Proceedings PLILP'96*, LNCS 1140, pages 137–151, September 1996. Springer-Verlag.

21. M. Leuschel and D. De Schreye. Constrained partial deduction and the preservation of characteristic trees. *New Gen. Comput.* , 16:283–342, 1998.

22. M. Leuschel and H. Lehmann. Solving Coverability Problems of Petri Nets by Partial Deduction. Submitted.

23. M. Leuschel, B. Martens, and D. De Schreye. Controlling generalisation and polyvariance in partial deduction of normal logic programs. *ACM Transactions on Programming Languages and Systems*, 20(1):208–258, January 1998.

24. M. Leuschel and T. Massart. Infinite state model checking by abstract interpretation and program specialisation. In A. Bossi, editor, *Proceedings LOPSTR'99*, LNCS 1817, pages 63–82, Venice, Italy, September 1999.

25. J. W. Lloyd and J. C. Shepherdson. Partial evaluation in logic programming. *J. Logic Progam.*, 11(3& 4):217–242, 1991.

26. K. Marriott, L. Naish, and J.-L. Lassez. Most specific logic programs. *Annals of Mathematics and Artificial Intelligence*, 1:303–338, 1990.

27. B. Martens and J. Gallagher. Ensuring global termination of partial deduction while allowing flexible polyvariance. In L. Sterling, editor, *Proceedings ICLP'95*, pages 597–613, June 1995. MIT Press.

28. E. W. Mayr. An algorithm for the general Petri net reachability problem. *Siam Journal on Computing*, 13:441–460, 1984.

29. Y. S. Ramakrishna, C. R. Ramakrishnan, I. V. Ramakrishnan, S. A. Smolka, T. Swift, and D. S. Warren. Efficient model checking using tabled resolution. In *Proceedings CAV'97*, LNCS 1254, pages 143–154. Springer-Verlag, 1997.

30. W. Reisig. *Petri Nets - An Introduction*. Springer Verlag, 1982.

31. J. Rushby. Mechanized formal methods: Where next? In *Proceedings of FM'99*, LNCS 1708, pages 48–51, Sept. 1999. Springer-Verlag.

32. M. H. Sørensen. Convergence of program transformers in the metric space of trees. In *Proceedings MPC'98*, LNCS 1422, pages 315–337. Springer-Verlag, 1998.

33. M. H. Sørensen and R. Glück. An algorithm of generalization in positive supercompilation. In J. W. Lloyd, editor, *Proceedings ILPS'95*, pages 465–479, December 1995. MIT Press.

34. R. Valk. Self-modifying nets, a natural extension of Petri neets. In *Proceedings ICALP'78*, LNCS 62, pages 464–476. Springer-Verlag, 1978.

35. R. Valk and G. Vidal-Naquet. Petri nets and regular languages. *Journal of Computer and System Sciences*, 23(3):299–325, Dec. 1981.

Binary Speed Up for Logic Programs

Jan Hrůza and Petr Štěpánek

Charles University, Department of Theoretical Computer Science
Malostranské nám. 25, 118 00 Praha 1, Czech Republic
hruza@kti.mff.cuni.cz, stepanek@ksi.mff.cuni.cz

Abstract. Binary logic programs can be obtained from ordinary logic programs by a binarizing transformation. In most cases, binary programs obtained by this way are less efficient than the original programs. Demoen [2] showed an interesting example of a logic program whose computational behavior was improved if it was transformed to a binary program and then specialized by partial deduction.

The class of so called B-stratifiable logic programs is defined. It is shown that for every B-stratifiable logic program, binarization and subsequent partial deduction produce a binary program which usually has a better computational behavior than the original one. Both binarization and partial deduction can be automated.

1 Introduction

Binary clauses appear quite naturally when simulating computations of Turing machines by logic programs. Tärnlund (1977) [20] introduced the concept of binary clauses. Šebelík and Štěpánek (1982) [16] constructed logic programs for recursive functions. It turned out that these programs were stratifiable. Moreover, it was possible to transform every such program to a binary logic program computing the same function, the length of computations of the resulting binary program being the same on every input.

Since then various binarizing transformations have been defined by Maher [8], Štěpánková and Štěpánek [17], Sato and Tamaki [15] and by Tarau and Boyer [19]. It is not difficult to show that the last three transformations produce programs with identical computational behavior.

While in the beginning, binarization was a rather theoretical issue, later, with the advent of Prolog compilers for programs consisting of binary clauses, it found important applications. Paul Tarau [18] built a PROLOG system called BinProlog that makes use of binarization. In a preprocessing phase, the Prolog program is binarized (see [19]) and the binary program is compiled using BinWAM, a specialized version of the Warren Abstract Machine for binary programs. BinWAM is simpler than WAM and the size of the code of the binary program is reduced.

Hence, it is of practical use to investigate transformations changing a logic program to an equivalent binary logic program.

J. Lloyd et al. (Eds.): CL 2000, LNAI 1861, pp. 116–130, 2000.

The paper is organized as follows. Section 2 presents the above mentioned transformation of logic programs to binary logic programs. Section 3 deals with the problem of computational efficiency of binarized programs. In section 4, B-stratifiable programs are introduced and it is proved that the transformation consisting of binarization and partial evaluation succeeds on these programs. This transformation usually leads to a computationally more efficient program.

We shall adopt the terminology and notation of [1]. Let H be an atom,

$$\boldsymbol{A} \equiv A_1, A_2, \ldots, A_m \text{ and } \boldsymbol{B} \equiv B_1, B_2, \ldots B_n, \; n, m \geq 0$$

be (possibly empty) sequences of atoms. We restrict our attention to definite logic programs, hence programs consisting of clauses $H \leftarrow \boldsymbol{B}$ with the atom H in the head and a sequence $\boldsymbol{B}$ of atoms in the body. If $\boldsymbol{B}$ is empty, we write simply $H \leftarrow$. A clause is called binary if it has at most one atom in the body. A program consisting of binary clauses is called binary.

A query is a sequence of atoms. Queries are denoted by Q with possible subscripts. Computation of a logic program starts by a non-empty query and generate a possibly infinite sequence of queries by SLD-resolution steps. Maximal sequences of queries generated by this way are called SLD-derivations. Finite SLD-derivations are successful if they end with the empty query, otherwise they are failed.

In what follows, by an LD-resolvent we mean an SLD-resolvent with respect to the leftmost selection rule and by an LD-derivation we mean an SLD-derivation w.r.t. the leftmost selection rule. Similarly, an LD-tree is an SLD-tree w.r.t. the leftmost selection rule. A *continuation* is a data structure representing the rest of the computation to be performed [18].

2   A Transformation to Binary Logic Programs

We shall describe the transformation [17] of definite logic programs to programs consisting of binary clauses. We define the functor B_S transforming the queries and the clauses of the input program. The resulting binary program is completed by an additional clause c_S.

Let q be a new unary predicate symbol. Given a logic program P,

(i) for a query

$$Q \equiv A_1, A_2, \ldots, A_n$$

to P, let

$$B_S(Q) \equiv q([A_1, A_2, \ldots, A_n])$$

in particular, for the empty query, we put $B_S(\square) \equiv q([\,])$.

(ii) for a clause

$$C \equiv H \leftarrow B_1, B_2, \ldots, B_n$$

let

$$B_S(C) \equiv q([H|Cont]) \leftarrow q([B_1, B_2, \ldots, B_n|Cont])$$

where $Cont$ is a continuation variable. In particular, if C is a unit clause, then $B_S(C) \equiv q([H|Cont]) \leftarrow q(Cont)$.

(iii) the clause c_S is $q([])$,

(iv) for a program P, we put

$$B_S(P) \equiv \{B_S(C)|C \in P\} \cup \{c_S\}$$

Note that c_S, is the only unit clause of the binarized program, that provides the step $B_S(\square) \Rightarrow \square$ in successful SLD-derivations.

2.1 Example. Transformation of a program by clauses

```
a <- b,c.          q([a|Cont]) <- q([b,c|Cont]).
b <- d.            q([b|Cont]) <-  q([d|Cont]).
c <-.              q([c|Cont]) <-  q([Cont]).
d <-.              q([d|Cont]) <-  q([Cont]).

                   q([]).
```

3   Transformations and Binarization

3.1   Binarization Can Lead to More Efficient Programs

Contrary to what could be expected, that binarization can only slow down the computations of a program because extra arguments and extra computation steps are involved in the transformed program, binarization followed by partial deduction can in some cases speed up the computations of a program significantly. Demoen [2] was the first to present a case study of such behavior.

We will discuss why this transformation gives more efficient programs when applied to programs with certain syntactical features and why it leads to identical or worse programs if applied to other programs. Then, we will describe a class of programs on which this transformation succeeds .

It was shown in [17] that binarization transforms logic programs to stratified logic programs. It turns out that a sufficient condition for a logic program to be transformed into a computationally more efficient binary program can be stated in terms of the concept of stratifiability due to Šebelík, Štěpánek [16].

3.1 Transformation Steps. Demoen [2] introduced the following steps of transformation of the SAMELEAVES program:

- binarization
- specialization w.r.t. continuation `true`
- unfolding with some final optimization steps such as removing duplicate variables

In our work, the second and the third steps were performed by the Mixtus partial evaluator [13]. This procedure gave the same result as that of Demoen, and, in some other cases it produced programs which were both binary and more efficient than the original program.

We are going to investigate programs with the binary speed up behavior. First, we shall recall the SAMELEAVES program.

3.2 Example. Program SAMELEAVES tests whether two binary trees have the same sequence of leaves disregarding the structure of the compared trees. The trees with the same sequence of leaves need not be isomorphic.

Program. SAMELEAVES

```
sameleaves(leaf(L),leaf(L)).
sameleaves(tree(T1,T2),tree(S1,S2)):-
        getleaf(T1,T2,L,T),
        getleaf(S1,S2,L,S),
        sameleaves(S,T).
getleaf(leaf(A),C,A,C).
getleaf(tree(A,B),C,L,O):-getleaf(A,tree(B,C),L,O).
```

As the first step of transformation, we apply the binarizing functor B_S from Section 2. The resulting program reads as follows

```
q([sameleaves(leaf(L),leaf(L))|V]):-q(V).
q([sameleaves(tree(T1,T2),tree(S1,S2))|V]):-
        q([getleaf(T1,T2,L,T),
           getleaf(S1,S2,L,S),
           sameleaves(S,T)|V]).

q([getleaf(leaf(A),C,A,C)|V]):-q(V).
q([getleaf(tree(A,B),C,L,O)|V]):-
        q([getleaf(A,tree(B,C),L,O)|V]).

q([]).
```

3.3. Now we perform the steps 2 and 3. Using Mixtus, the automated partial evaluator (Sahlin [13]), we partially evaluate the binarized program with the goal

```
q([sameleaves(Tree1,Tree2)])
```

where the continuation is the empty query [], hence **true**.

Alternatively, we could perform the partial deduction step by step as Demoen did.

3.4. By these steps, we obtain the following program

```
sameleaves1(leaf(A), leaf(A)).
sameleaves1(tree(A,B), tree(C,D)) :-
        getleaf1(A,B,C,D).

getleaf1(leaf(C),D,A,B) :-
        getleaf2(A,B,C,D).
getleaf1(tree(A,D),E,B,C) :-
        getleaf1(A,tree(D,E),B,C).

getleaf2(leaf(C),A,C,B) :-
        sameleaves1(A,B).
getleaf2(tree(A,D),E,B,C) :-
        getleaf2(A,tree(D,E),B,C).
```

It was shown by Demoen that the resulting program is faster by approx. 40%.

3.5. The transformation is interesting for yet another reason. If we skip binarization and perform only partial deduction on the original non-binary program, we get only an identical copy of the logic program. On the other hand, by binarization and specialization w.r.t. continuation **true**, hence by adding no information, we get a computationally more efficient binary program by partial deduction .

The program **FRONTIER** below computes the frontier, i.e. list of leaves of a binary tree. It gives an example that the above described steps of binarization, specialization and partial deduction need not give any reasonable improvement. In this case, the automated partial deduction after binarization leads to a clearly worse program.

3.6 Example. FRONTIER

```
frontier(leaf(X),[X]).
frontier(nil,[]).
frontier(tree(Left,Right,Label),Res):-
        frontier(Left,L1),
        frontier(Right,R1),
        append(L1,R1,Res).
```

```
append([],X,X).
append([H|T],X,[H|Y]):-
          append(T,X,Y).
```

If we perform the above steps on this program, we do not get a computationally more efficient program. We present below part of the output of the Mixtus partial evaluator:

3.6' Example. FRONTIER

```
q([frontier(A,B)]) :-
          'q.frontier1'(A, B).

'q.frontier1'(tree(A,E,_), D) :-
          'q.frontier1'(A,B,frontier(E,C),[append(B,C,D)]).
'q.frontier1'(leaf(C), [C], A, B) :-
          'q.1'(A, B).
'q.frontier1'(nil, [], A, B) :-
          'q.1'(A, B).
'q.frontier1'(tree(A,G,_), F, C, D) :-
          'q.frontier1'(A,B,frontier(G,E),[append(B,E,F),C|D]).
'q.1'(frontier(leaf(B),[B]), A) :-
          q1(A).
 q.1'(append([],B,B), A) :-
          q1(A).
q1([frontier(leaf(B),[B])|A]) :-
          q1(A).
q1([frontier(nil,[])|A]) :-
          q1(A).
q1([frontier(tree(F,E,_),D)|A]) :-
          q1([frontier(F,B),frontier(E,C),append(B,C,D)|A]).
q1([append([],B,B)|A]) :-
          q1(A).
q1([append([E|B],C,[E|D])|A]) :-
          q1([append(B,C,D)|A]).
...
```

The length of the output program is growing significantly during the partial deduction. It turns out that as the partial deduction system tries to specialize w.r.t. the continuations, it can never remove calls with a free continuation variable such as

```
q1([append([],B,B)|A]) :-
          q1(A).
```

This is due to the fact that the size and structure of continuation in this program depends on inputs of the program .

Efficiency of Programs.

Pettorossi and Proietti [11], [12] pointed out that inefficient computations of programs may be caused by presence of so called unnecessary variables. They define several types of such variables and describe a method of eliminating them by means of unfold/fold transformations. We shall refine the definition of unnecessary variables and describe methods to eliminate some of them.

3.7 Definition. Given a program P, H an atom, $\boldsymbol{A}$ a sequence of atoms such that $H \leftarrow \boldsymbol{A}$ be a clause of P. Let

$$q(H|Cont) \leftarrow q([\boldsymbol{A}|Cont])$$

be the binarized version in $B_S(P)$ of the above clause. We call

(i) *an existential variable* a variable that occurs in the body and not in the head of the clause,

(ii) *a body-multiple variable* a variable occuring in several terms in the body of the clause,

(iii) *an argument-multiple variable* a variable that occurs more then once in a term in the body,

(iv) *a continuation variable* a variable that is introduced by binarization to hold a continuation, occuring e.g. in the contexts of $call(X)$, $q(X)$ or $q([\ldots|X])$ at the last argument position.

We call *unnecessary* all existential, body-multiple, argument-multiple and continuation variables.

Now we can analyze what happens during transformation and can see these stages:

1. the original program possibly contains some existential, body-multiple, argument-multiple variables causing inefficiency

2. the program is binarized. Hence body-multiple variables are converted into argument-multiple variables and continuation variables are introduced. The program may become even less efficient.

3. the program is specialized and continuation variables are removed

4. it may be possible to remove other unnecessary variables, often up to the point where no unnecessary variables are left.

We say that the binarization + partial deduction transformation was successful if it eliminated continuation variables. In fact, it has been observed that when the continuation variables of the binarized program are eliminated, the resulting program was as fast as the original one, or faster.

4   B-Stratifiable Programs

In this Section, we will define a class of B-stratifiable programs, prove that for this class of programs the transformation succeeds (i.e. it eliminates continuation variables) and claim that by further specialization some more unnecessary variables can be removed that cannot be eliminated by partial deduction alone.

The notion of a B-stratifiable program is stated in terms of the concept of stratifiable logic programs from [16].

4.1 Definition. We say that a program P is B-stratifiable if there is a partition of the set of all predicates of P into disjunctive sets

$$S_0, S_1, \ldots, S_n \tag{2}$$

called strata, such that

(i) if a predicate p, $p \in S_i$ calls a predicate q, $q \in S_j$ in the same clause, then $i \geq j$, and

(ii) in any clause $H \leftarrow \mathbb{B}$ of P, the predicate symbol p from the head H calls at most one predicate q from the same stratum in the body $\mathbb{B}$. In this case, q is the predicate symbol of the rightmost atom in $\mathbb{B}$.

Then the partition (2) is called the stratification of P.   □

4.2 Example. Program

$$
\begin{aligned}
&\texttt{p :- q,p.}\\
&\texttt{q :- r,r.}\\
&\texttt{r.}\\
&\texttt{r :- q.}
\end{aligned}
\tag{3}
$$

$$\tag{4}$$

is not B-stratifiable because q, r are mutually dependent and hence in the same stratum, but in the body of (3) there are two calls to r. If we remove the clause (4), the program becomes B-stratifiable. It suffices to take the stratification $S_1 = \{r\}$, $S_2 = \{q\}$, $S_3 = \{p\}$.

It is easy to check that the program SAMELEAVES is B-stratifiable while the program FRONTIER is not.

4.3. On B-stratifiable programs, the transformation consisting of binarization and partial deduction succeeds. B-stratifiable programs can be transformed with binarization and partial deduction into programs that are usually more efficient. This is due to the fact that the number of atoms in continuations is bounded. To prove this we shall need some definitions.

4.4 Definition. Let P be a logic program, A an atom and let

$$\mathbf{A} \equiv A_1, \ldots, A_n$$

be a sequence of atom. Let

$$A, \; \mathbb{B} \Rightarrow \boldsymbol{A}, \; \mathbb{B}\theta$$

be an LD-resolution step of $P \cup \{A\}$. We say that each atom $A_i \in \boldsymbol{A}$, $1 \le i \le n$ is an immediate successor of A and write $A \succ A_i$. Let $\succeq$ be the reflexive and transitive closure of the immediate successor relation $\succ$. If $A \succeq B$, we say that B is a successor of A. $\qquad\square$

4.5 Lemma. Let P be a B-stratifiable logic program, let

$$S_0, S_1, \ldots, S_n \tag{5}$$

be a stratification of P and let A be an atom with a predicate symbol from the highest stratum S_n. Let m be the maximum number of atoms in the body of a clause from P and let ξ be an arbitrary LD-derivation of $P \cup \{A\}$.

Then A has at most $n*m$ successors in every LD-resolvent of ξ. In general, if A is an atom with a predicate symbol from a stratum S_k, $1 \le k \le n$ then A has at most $k*m$ successors in every LD-resolvent in ξ. Hence $n*m$ is a bound on the number of successors of an arbitrary atom in every LD-resolvent in ξ. $\quad\square$

4.6 Corollary. Let P be a B-stratifiable program with a B-stratification (5). Let Q be a query to P and ξ an arbitrary LD-derivation of $P \cup \{Q\}$. Let A be an atom in Q with a predicate symbol from the k-th stratum S_k, $0 \le k \le n$. The A has at most $k*m$ successors in every LD-resolvent in ξ. $\qquad\square$

4.7 Claim. The length of a continuation in any LD-resolvent of the binarized program $B_S(P) \cup \{B_S(Q)\}$ is equal to the length of the corresponding LD-resolvent of $P \cup \{Q\}$ minus 1. $\qquad\square$

Proof. It is easy to see that for any LD-resolvent $A_1, A_2, \ldots A_n$ of $P \cup \{Q\}$, the corresponding continuation in the binarized program is $[A_2, \ldots, A_n]$. $\qquad\square$

4.8 Theorem. Let P be a program A an atom. Assume that there is a bound on the number of atoms in all continuations in computations of $B_S(P) \cup \{B_S(A)\}$, then there is a bound on the number of sequences of predicate symbols in continuations that occur in any computation of $B_S(P) \cup \{B_S(A)\}$, too. $\qquad\square$

4.9 Lemma. Let P be a program A an atom. Assume that there is a bound on the number of sequences of predicate symbols in continuations that occur in any computation of $B_S(P) \cup \{B_S(A)\}$. Then it is possible to partially evaluate $B_S(P)$ w.r.t. $B_S(A)$ so that the resulting program will not contain any continuation variables.

Proof. In order to prove this lemma, we will compute a partial evaluation of $B_S(P)$ w.r.t. a set A to eliminate continuation variables. Later on, another specialization will be performed. (This splitting of specialization to 2 stages is needed only for the proof of the lemma.)

Elimination of Continuation Variables

We can eliminate the continuation variables by specializing the program $B_S(P)$ to the value $[]$ (true) of the variable $Cont$. As the program $B_S(P)$ is binary, we can use an instance of the Lloyd and Shepherdson [7] general partial deduction to remove the continuation variables. To this purpose, it is sufficient to compute (incomplete) SLD^--trees to the depth one.

To make sure that the condition of so called $A-$closedness which makes sure that the specialized program computes the same set of answers is guaranteed, we use a generalization operator in the construction of the set A.

4.10 Definition. Let

$$Q \equiv p_1(t_1, t_2, \ldots), p_2(t_{j_2}, t_{j_2+1}, \ldots), \ldots p_n(t_{j_n}, \ldots) \tag{7}$$

be a general (non-binary) query. We define a generalization operator Gen which replaces each term t_i by a new variable X_i. We put

$$Gen(Q) = p_1(X_1, X_2, \ldots), p_2(X_{j_2}, X_{j_2+1}, \ldots), \ldots p_n(X_{j_n}, \ldots)$$

We say that $Gen(Q)$ is a sequence of pure atoms. For a binarized query

$$Q_1 \equiv B_S(Q) \equiv q([p_1(t_1, t_2, \ldots), p_2(t_{j_2}, t_{j_2+1}, \ldots), \ldots p_n(t_{j_n}, \ldots)])$$

we put

$$\begin{aligned} G(Q_1) \equiv G(B_S(Q)) &:= B_S(Gen(Q)) \\ &= q([p_1(X_1, X_2, \ldots), p_2(X_{j_2}, X_{j_2+1}, \ldots), \ldots p_n(X_{j_n}, \ldots)]) \end{aligned}$$

in particular, $G(q([])) = q([])$.

4.11 Algorithm 1.

Input: Binarized program $B_S(P)$ and the top-level query $q([p(X_1, \ldots, X_n)])$
Output: A program New_Prog with no continuation variables

I. $A := \{\}$,
   $To\_be\_evaluated := \{q([p(X_1, X_2, \ldots, X_n)])\}$,
   $Prog := \{\}$

II. **While.** $To\_be\_evaluated \neq \{\}$ **do**

   a) take an atom $a \in To\_be\_evaluated$;
      $A := A \cup \{a\}$;

   b) compute partial deduction of $B_S(P) \cup \{a\}$ obtaining an incomplete SLD^--tree of depth 1 (i. e. perform one unfolding step)

      $R :=$ the set of resultants.
      $B :=$ the set of bodies of resultants from R.

   It follows from the fact that the program $B_S(P)$ is binary, that all elements of B are atoms.

   c) $Prog := Prog \cup R$;

$$To\_be\_evaluated := (To\_be\_evaluated \cup G(B)) - A;$$

III. **Renaming.** We shall define a functor Ren which renames each atom

$$q([p_1(t_1, t_2, \ldots), p_2(t_{j_2}, t_{j_2+1}, \ldots), \ldots, p_n(t_{j_n}, \ldots)]) \tag{8}$$

in $Prog$ to

$$q\_p_1\_p_2\_\ldots\_p_n(t_1, t_2, \ldots, t_{j_2}, t_{j_2+1}, \ldots, t_{j_n}, \ldots) \tag{8'}$$

obtaining the program New_Prog.

As (8) is obtained from (7) by the binarizing functor B_S, we can define a functor R that transforms the sequences of atoms in the language of P (the queries to P) to the atoms in the language of New_Prog as follows. For a query Q to P, we put

$$R(Q) := Ren(B_S(Q))$$

Hence

$$R(p_1(t_1, t_2, \ldots), p_2(t_{j_2}, t_{j_2+1}, \ldots), \ldots p_n(t_{j_n}, \ldots)) =$$
$$= q\_p_1\_p_2\_\ldots\_p_n(t_1, t_2, \ldots, t_{j_2}, t_{j_2+1}, \ldots, t_{j_n}, \ldots)$$

4.12 Theorem. If P is a B-stratifiable program, Q a pure atom, then Algorithm 1 terminates on the input $B_S(P) \cup \{B_S(Q)\}$. The LD-derivations of $New\_Prog \cup \{R(Q)\}$ give the same set of computed answer substitutions as the LD-derivations of $P \cup \{Q\}$.

Proof. *Termination.* Algorithm 1 terminates if the set $To\_be\_evaluated$ of goals for partial deduction is empty. The elements of this set are pure atoms obtained by application of the generalization functor G. To guarantee the so called $A-$closedness condition of partial deduction (see [7]), each goal evaluated by partial deduction is removed from $To\_be\_evaluated$ and is put to A. The goals from the set $G(B) - A$ are added to $To\_be\_evaluated$, where B is the set of goals from the bodies of resultants obtained by partial deduction. It follows from the definition of G that it maps any two goals with the same sequence of predicate symbols to the same atom. We assumed that P is a $B-$stratifiable program, hence it follows from Lemma 4.5 and Theorem 4.8 that there is a bound on the number of sequences of predicate symbols in continuations that occur in any resultant obtained by partial deduction of $B_S(P) \cup \{Q\}$, where Q is a goal from $To\_be\_evaluated$. It turns out that after a finite number of steps, $To\_be\_evaluated$ is empty and the computation of the algorithm terminates.

Equivalence of computed answer substitutions holds due to Lloyd, Shepherdson [7]. □

4.13. Some redundant occurrences of unnecessary variables of a B-stratifiable program P program can be eliminated during partial evaluation after binarization. □

This is done by a renaming operation. The body–multiple variables of a program become argument–multiple variables during binarization and then, their redundant occurrences can be eliminated by renaming. This operation is performed by standard partial deduction systems. Then further elimination can be performed by the FAR procedure [3] [6].

Example: Consider a clause of the FRONTIER1 program

```
front1(tree(Left,Right),[L|Ls]):-
    getleaf(Left,Right,NewTree,L),
    front1(NewTree,Ls).
```

In this clause, variable NewTree is both *body-multiple* and *existential*. After binarization and partial deduction, the clause becomes

```
front1(tree(Left,Right),[L|Ls]):-
    gf(Left,Right,NewTree,L,Ls).
```

Here, NewTree has become an argument multiple variable and one of its occurrences has been eliminated by renaming. Then, using the FAR procedure, even the last occurrence of NewTree can be eliminated:

```
front1(tree(Left,Right),[L|Ls]):-
    gf(Left,Right,L,Ls).
```

5   Results and Comparison

We have shown that binarization + partial deduction *succeeds* when applied to B-stratifiable programs, and produces programs that are usually more efficient than the original programs. It might seem that the class of B-stratifiable programs is relatively small. However, it turns out that it is possible to transform some programs to a B-stratifiable form. The program FRONTIER served us as an example of a program that is not B-stratifiable. It is possible, though, to write another program, FRONTIER1 with equivalent semantics, which is B-stratifiable

```
front1(leaf(X),[X]).
front1(tree(Left,Right),[L|Ls]):-
    getleaf(Left,Right,NewTree,L),
    front1(NewTree,Ls).
```

```
getleaf(leaf(A),Tree,Tree,A).
getleaf(tree(Left,Right),Rest_tree,Out_tree,L):-
    getleaf(Left,tree(Right,Rest_tree),Out_tree,L).
```

We have experimented with a set of programs taken from [5], [6], [2], [11] and [1]. Some of them were B-stratifiable, some of them had a B-stratifiable companion. Listings of the programs can be found at
`http://kti.ms.mff.cuni.cz/~hruza/binarization`.
The results are presented in the table below.

	run time			speed up		
program	orig	B-strat	bin-pd	Bstrat/orig	bin-pd/orig	bin-pd/B-strat
sameleaves	990	-	756	-	1.31	-
frontier	1575	690	477	2.28	3.32	1.45
permutation	2800	-	2304	-	1.22	-
double-append	1453	-	1407	-	1.03	-
rotate-leftdepth	408	518	526	0.79	0.78	0.99
rotate-prune	232	266	320	0.87	0.73	0.83

The first columne gives the name of the program, the next three columns give the run times (in miliseconds) for the original program, for its B-stratifiable companion, if the original itself is not B-stratifiable, and for the binarized and partially deduced version of the program. The run times are computed as an average from 5 runs on different data. The last three columns present the speed ups of the B-stratifiable companion w.r.t. to the original program, of the binarized and partially deduced program w.r.t to the original one and of the binarized and partial deduced program w.r.t. the B-stratifiable companion of the original program.

The transformation of the FRONTIER program gives the best results of the presented programs. The transformation to the B-stratifiable companion program FRONTIER1 removed the calls to the APPEND program and this resulted in a reasonable speed up. Then, further speed up is achieved by binarization, partial deduction and unnecessary variable elimination. The SAMELEAVES program contained an unnecessary variable that was eliminated by binarization and partial deduction, which improved the computational behavior of the program. There have also been not B–stratifiable programs the computational behaviour of which deteriorated after a transformation to a B–stratifiable program and binarization with partial deduction (e.g. ROTATE_PRUNE and ROTATE_LEFTDEPTH). It seems that it was so due to the fact that during transformation to a B–stratifiable program, new data structures such as a stack were introduced which could not be later eliminated from these programs. Neither did we succeed to eliminate unnecessary variables. The methods of transformation of logic programs to the B-stratifiable form and the corresponding methods of elimination of variables are a matter of further research.

Binarization and Partial Deduction and Other Approaches

It turns out that the reason why binarized and partially evaluated programs are more efficient is elimination of unnecessary variables. It is useful to compare this approach with other two approaches eliminating unnecessary variables.

1) *unfold/fold transformations* to remove unnecessary variables from a program were introduced by Pettorossi and Proietti in [11]. They consist in repeated applications of unfolding, definition and folding on clauses that contain unnecessary variables. This approach is general and applicable to all programs, however, it is difficult to control. Binarization + partial evaluation is applicable only to B-stratifiable programs, but is more straightforward and can be easily automated. Both binarization and partial deduction can be expressed in terms of unfold/fold transformations.

2) Another, more recent approach to elimination of unnecessary variables is *conjunctive partial deduction* [3]. Unlike traditional partial deduction which considers only atoms for partial deduction, conjunctive partial deduction attempts to specialize entire conjunctions of atoms. This approach is closely related to binarization + partial deduction. There is a difference, however. In the present approach, a program is first binarized and hence does not contain any conjunctions. Then standard partial deduction can be used. Unlike that, in conjunctive partial deduction the conjunctions are left and the system decides on splitting conjunctions into appropriate subconjunctions. This approach may be somewhat more difficult to control but it gives greater flexibility and applicability.

It seems that binarization + partial deduction and conjunctive partial deduction yield similar results when applied to some B-stratifiable programs.

References

1. K. R. Apt, From Logic Programming to Prolog, Prentice Hall International, NJ 1996
2. B. Demoen, *On the Transformation of a Prolog Program to a More Efficient Binary Program*, in: Logic Program Synthesis and Transformation 1992, Kung-Kiu Lau and Tim Clement (editors),Lecture Notes in Computer Science Vol. Springer-Verlag 1993 pp. 242 – 252
3. D. De Schreye, R. Gluck, J. Jorgensen, M. Leuschel, B. Martens, M. H. Sorensen, *Conjunctive partial deduction: foundations, control, algorithms and experiments*, The Journal of Logic Programming 41 (1999), 231 - 277
4. M. Falaschi, G. Levi, M. Martelli, C. Palamidessi, *Declarative Modeling of the Operational Behavior of Logic Languages*, Theoretical Comp. Sci. 69(3):289-318 (1989)
5. M. Leuschel, *Dozen Problems for Partial Deduction (A Set of Benchmarks)* http://www.ecs.soton.ac.uk/~mal/systems/dppd/
6. M. Leuschel, M. H. Sorensen, *Redundant Arguments Filtering of Logic Programs*, in John Gallagher (ed.), Logic Programm Synthesis and Transformation, Proceedings of the 6th International Workshop, LOPSTR'96, LCNS 1207, 83–103, Stockholm, 1996.
7. J. W. Lloyd and J. C. Shepherdson, *Partial Evaluation in Logic Programming*, J. Logic Programming 11(1991), 217–242

8. M. J. Maher, *Equivalences of Logic Programs,* in: Proc. Third Int. Conference on Logic Programming, London 1986, E. Shapiro (editor), Lecture Notes in Comp. Sci. Vol 225, Springer – Verlag, Berlin 1986, pp. 410 – 424

9. U. W. Neumerkel, *Specialization of Prolog Programs with Partially Static Goals and Binarization,* PhD Thesis, Technical University, Wien, 1993

10. M. Proietti, A. Pettorossi, *Tranformation of logic programs: Foundations and Techniques,* Journal of Logic Programming, 19,20:261-320, 1994

11. M. Proietti, A. Pettorossi, *Unfolding - definition - folding, in this order, for avoiding unnecessary variables in logic programs,* Theoretical Computer Science 142 (1995), 98 - 124

12. A. Pettorossi, M. Proietti, *Synthesis and Transformation of Logic Programs Using Unfold/Fold Proofs,* Tech. Rep. 457, Dipartimento di Informatica, Sistemi e Produzione, Universita di Roma, Tor Vergata, Giugno 1997,

13. D. Sahlin, *An Automatic Partial Evaluator for Full Prolog,* PhD Dissertation, The Royal Institute of Technology, Dept. of Telecommunication and Computer Science, Stockholm, March 1991

14. T. Sato, H. Tamaki, *Unfold/Fold Transformation of Logic Programs* in: Proc. of the 2nd Int. Logic Programming Conference, Uppsala 1984, S. Å. Tärnlund (editor), pp. 127 – 138

15. T. Sato, H. Tamaki, *Existential Continuation,* New Generation Computing 6 (1989), 421 – 438

16. J. Šebelík and P. Štěpánek, *Horn Clause Programs for Recursive Functions,* in: Logic Programming, K. J. Clark and S. Å. Tärnlund (editors), ACADEMIC PRESS, London 1982, pp. 325 - 240

17. O. Štěpánková and P. Štěpánek, *Stratification of Definite Clause Programs and of General Logic Programs,* in: Proc. CSL '89, Third Workshop on Computer Science Logic, Kaiserslautern, Germany, 1989, Lect. Notes in Comp. Sci. Vol 440, Springer-Verlag, Berlin 1989, pp. 396 – 408

18. P. Tarau, *A Continuation Passing Style Prolog Engine,* Lecture Notes in Computer Science, Vol. 631, pp. 479-480, Springer-Verlag, Berlin 1992

19. P. Tarau and M. Boyer, *Elementary Logic Programs,* in: Proc. PLILP'90, P. Deransart and J. Maluzsyński (editors), Lecture Notes in Comp. Sci. Vol. Springer-Verlag, Berlin
1990, pp. 159 – 173

20. S. Å. Tärnlund, *Horn Clause Computability,* BIT 17 (1977), 215 – 226

21. K. Ueda, *Making Exhaustive Search Programs Deterministic,* New Generation Computing 5 (1987), 317 – 326

A New Module System for Prolog*

Daniel Cabeza and Manuel Hermenegildo

Department of Computer Science, Technical U. of Madrid (UPM)
dcabeza@fi.upm.es, herme@fi.upm.es

Abstract. It is now widely accepted that separating programs into modules is useful in program development and maintenance. While many Prolog implementations include useful module systems, we argue that these systems can be improved in a number of ways, such as, for example, being more amenable to effective global analysis and transformation and allowing separate compilation or sensible creation of standalone executables. We discuss a number of issues related to the design of such an improved module system for Prolog and propose some novel solutions. Based on this, we present the choices made in the Ciao module system, which has been designed to meet a number of objectives: allowing separate compilation, extensibility in features and in syntax, amenability to modular global analysis and transformation, enhanced error detection, support for meta-programming and higher-order, compatibility to the extent possible with official and de-facto standards, etc.

Keywords: Modules, Modular Program Processing, Global Analysis and Transformation, Separate Compilation, Prolog, Ciao-Prolog.

1 Introduction

Modularity is a basic notion in modern computer languages. Modules allow dividing programs into several parts, which have their own independent name spaces and a clear interface with the rest of the program. Experience has shown that there are at least two important advantages to such program modularization. The first one is that being able to look at parts of a program in a more or less isolated way allows a divide-and-conquer approach to program development and maintenance. For example, it allows a programmer to develop or update a module at a time or several programmers to work on different modules in parallel. The second advantage is in efficiency: tools which process programs can be more efficient if they can work on a single module at a time. For example, after a change to a program module the compiler needs to recompile only that module (and perhaps a few related modules). Another example is a program

---

* This work was supported in part by the "EDIPIA" (CICYT TIC99-1151) and "EC-COSIC" (Fulbright 98059) projects. The authors would like to thank Francisco Bueno and the anonymous referees for their useful comments on previous versions of this document. The Ciao system is a collaborative international effort and includes contributions from members of several institutions, which are too many to mention here: a complete list can be found in the Ciao system documentation.

J. Lloyd et al. (Eds.): CL 2000, LNAI 1861, pp. 131–148, 2000.
© Springer-Verlag Berlin Heidelberg 2000

verifier which is applied to one module at a time and does its job assuming some properties of other modules. Also, modularity is also one of the fundamental principles behind object-oriented programming.

The topic of modules and logic programming has received considerable attention (see, for example, [23, 9, 34, 13, 21, 22]). Currently, many popular Prolog systems such as Quintus [28] and SICStus [8] include module systems which have proved very useful in practice.[1] However, these practical module systems also have a series of shortcomings, specially with respect to effectively supporting separate program compilation, debugging, and optimization.

Our objective is to discuss from a practical point of view a number of issues related to the design of an improved module system for Prolog and, based on this, to present the choices made in the module system of Ciao Prolog [2].[2] Ciao Prolog is a next-generation logic programming system which, among other features, has been designed with modular incremental compilation, global analysis, debugging, and specialization in mind. The module system has been designed to stay as similar as possible to the module systems of the most popular Prolog implementations and the ISO-Prolog module standard currently being finished [20], but with a number of crucial changes that achieve the previously mentioned design objectives. We believe that it would not be difficult to incorporate these changes in the ISO-Prolog module standard or in other module systems. The rest of the paper proceeds as follows: Section 2 discusses the objectives of the desired module system and Section 3 discusses some of the issues involved in meeting these objectives. Section 4 then describes the Ciao Prolog module system. Within this section, Subsection 4.5 discusses some enhancements to standard Prolog syntax extension facilities. Finally, Section 5 describes the notion of packages, a flexible mechanism for implementing modular language extensions and restrictions, which emerges naturally from the module system design. An example of a package is provided which illustrates some of the advantages of this design. Because of space restrictions and because the focus is on the motivations behind the choices made, the presentation is informal.

2   Objectives in the Design of the Ciao Module System

We start by stating the main objectives that we have had in mind during the design of the Ciao module system:

- *Allowing modular (separate) and efficient compilation.* This means that it should be possible to compile (or, in general, process) a module without having to compile the code of the related modules. This allows for example having pre-compiled (pre-processed, in general) system or user-defined libraries. It also allows the incremental and parallel development of large software projects.

---

[1] Surprisingly, though, it is also true that a number of Prolog systems do not have any module system at all.

[2] The Ciao system can be downloaded from http://www.clip.dia.fi.upm.es/Software.

- *Local extensibility/restriction, in features and in syntax.* This means that it should be possible to define syntactic and semantic extensions and restrictions of the language in a local way, i.e., so that they affect only selected modules. This is very important in the context of Ciao, since one of its objectives is to serve as an experimental workbench for new extensions to logic programming (provided that they can be translated to the core language).
- *Amenability to modular global analysis.* We foresee a much larger role for global analysis of logic programs, not only in the more traditional application of optimization [35, 33, 31, 4], but also in new applications related to program development, such as automated debugging, validation, and program transformation [3, 10, 5, 16, 17]. This is specially important in Ciao because the program development environment already includes a global analysis and transformation tool (`ciaopp`, the Ciao preprocessor [17, 15]) which performs these tasks and which in our experience to date has shown to be an invaluable help in program development and maintenance.
- *Amenability to error detection.* This means that it should be possible to check statically the interfaces between the modules and detect errors such as undefined predicates, incompatible arities and types, etc.
- *Support for meta-programming and higher-order.* This means that it should be possible to do meta- and higher-order programming across modules without too much burden on the programmer. Also, in combination with the previous point, it should be possible to detect errors (such as calls to undefined predicates) on sufficiently determined higher-order calls.
- *Compatibility with official and de-facto standards.* To the extent possible (i.e., without giving up other major objectives to fulfill this one) the module system should be compatible with those of popular Prolog systems (e.g., Quintus/SICStus) and official standards, such as the core ISO-Prolog standard [19, 12] and the current drafts of the ISO-Prolog module standards [20]. This is because it is also a design objective of Ciao that it be (thanks to a particular set of libraries which is loaded by default) a standard Prolog system. This is in contrast to systems like Mercury [30] or Goedel [18] which are more radical departures from Prolog. This means that the module system will be (at least by default) *predicate-based* rather than *atom-based* (as in XSB [29] and BIM [32]), i.e., it will provide separation of predicate symbols, but not of atom names. Also, the module system should not require the language to become strongly typed, since traditional Prologs are untyped.[3]

3   Discussion of the Main Issues Involved

None of the module systems used by current Prolog implementations fulfill all of the above stated objectives, and some include characteristics which are in clear

---

[3] Note however, that this does not prevent having voluntary type declarations or more general assertions, as is indeed done in Ciao [25, 26].

opposition to such objectives.[4] Thus, we set out to develop an improved design. We start by discussing a number of desirable characteristics of the module system in order to fulfill our objectives. Amenability to global analysis and being able to deal with the core ISO-Prolog standard features were discussed at length in [3], where many novel solutions to the problems involved were proposed. However, the emphasis of that paper was not on modular analysis. Herein, we will choose from some of the solutions proposed in [3] and provide further solutions for the issues that are more specific to modular analysis and to separate compilation.[5]

- *Syntax, flags, etc. should be local to modules.* The syntax or mode of compilation of a module should not be modified by unrelated modules, since otherwise separate compilation and modular analysis would be impossible. Also, it should be possible to use different syntactic extensions (such as operator declarations or term expansions) in different modules without them interacting. I.e., it should be possible to use the same operator in different modules with different precedences and meanings. In most current module systems for Prolog this does not hold because syntactic extensions and compilation parameters (e.g., Prolog flags) are global. As a result, a module can be compiled in radically different ways depending on the operators, expansions, Prolog flags, etc. set by previously loaded modules or simply typed into the top level. Also, using a syntactic extension in a module prevents the use of, e.g., the involved operators in other modules in a different way, making the development of optional language extensions very complicated. In conclusion, we feel that directives such as `op/3` and `set_prolog_flag/2` must be local to a module.

- *The entry points of a module should be statically defined.* Thus, the only external calls allowed from other modules should be to exported predicates. Note that modules contain code which is usually related in some way to that of other modules. A good design for a modular program should produce a set of modules such that each module can be understood independently of the rest of the program and such that the communication (dependencies) among the different modules is as reduced as possible. By a *strict* module system we refer to one in which a module can only communicate with other modules via its *interface* (this interface usually contains data such as the names of the *exported* predicates). Other modules can only use predicates which are among the ones exported by the considered module. Predicates which are not exported are not visible outside the module. Many current module systems for Prolog are not strict and allow calling a procedure of a module even if it is not exported by the module. This clearly defeats the purpose of the module system and, in addition, has a catastrophic impact

---

[4] Unfortunately, lack of space prevents us from making detailed comparisons with other individual module systems. Instead, we discuss throughout the paper advantages and disadvantages of particular solutions present in different current designs.

[5] We concentrate here on the design on the module system. The issue of how this module system is applied to modular analysis is addressed in more detail in [27].

on the precision of global analysis, precluding many program optimizations. Thus, we feel that the module system should be strict.

- *Module qualification is for disambiguating predicate names, not for changing naming context.* This a requirement of separate compilation (processing) since otherwise to compile (process) a module it may be necessary to know the imports/exports of all other modules. As an example, given a call m:p ("call p in module m"), with the proposed semantics the compiler only needs to know the exports of module m. If qualification meant changing naming context, since module m can import predicate p from another module, and that module from another, the interfaces of all those modules would have to be read. Furthermore, in some situations changing naming context could invalidate the strictness of the module system.
- *Module text should not be in unavailable or unrelated parts.* This means that all parts of a module should be within the module itself or directly accessible at the time of compilation, i.e., the compiler must be able to automatically and independently access the complete source of the module being processed.[6]
- *Dynamic parts should be isolated as much as possible.* Dynamic code modification, such as arbitrary runtime clause addition (by the use of assert-like predicates), while very useful in some applications, has the disadvantage that it adds new entry points to predicates which are not "visible" at compile-time and are thus very detrimental to global analysis [3]. One first idea is to relegate such predicates to a library module, which has to be loaded explicitly.[7] In that way, only the modules using those functionalities have to be specially handled, and the fact that such predicates are used can be determined statically. Also, in our experience, dynamic predicates are very often used only to implement "global variables", and for this purpose a facility for adding facts to the program suffices. This simpler feature, provided that this kind of dynamic predicates are declared as such explicitly in the source, pose no big problems to modular global analysis. To this end, Ciao provides a set of builtins for adding and deleting facts to a special class of dynamic predicates, called "data predicates" (asserta_fact/1, retract_fact/1, etc), which are declared as ":- data ..." (similar kinds of dynamic predicates are mentioned in [11]). Furthermore, the implementation of such data predicates can be made much more efficient than that of the normal dynamic predicates, due to their restricted nature.
- *Most "built-ins" should be in libraries which can be loaded and/or unloaded from the context of a given module.* This is a requirement related to extensibility and also to more specific needs, such as those of the previous point, where it was argued that program modification "built-ins" should be

---

[6] Note that this is not the case with the classical *user files* used in non-modular Prolog systems: code used by a user file may be in a different user file with no explicit relation with the first one (there is no usage declaration that allows relating them).

[7] Note, however, that in Ciao, to preserve compatibility for older programs, a special case is implemented: if no library modules are explicitly loaded, then all the modules containing the ISO predicates are loaded by default.

relegated to a library. The idea is to have a core language with very few pre-defined predicates (if any) and which should be a (hopefully pure) subset of ISO-Prolog. This makes it possible to develop alternative languages defining, for example, alternative I/O predicates, and to use them in a given module while others perhaps use full ISO-Prolog. It also makes it easier to produce small executables.

- *Directives should not be queries.* Traditionally, directives (clauses starting with ":-") were executed by the Prolog interpreter as queries. While this makes some sense in an interpretative environment, where program compilation, load (linking), and startup are simultaneous, is does not in other environments (and, specially, in the context of separate compilation) in which program compilation, linking, and startup occur at separate times. For example, some of the directives used traditionally are meant as instructions for the compiler while, e.g., others are used as initialization goals. Fortunately, this is well clarified in the current ISO standard [19, 12], where declarations are clearly separated from initialization goals.
- *Meta-predicates should be declared, at least if they are exported, and the declaration must reflect the type of meta-information handled in each argument.* This is needed in order to be able to perform a reasonable amount of error checking for meta-predicates and also to be able to statically resolve meta-calls across modules in most cases.

4   The Ciao Module System

Given the premises of previous sections, we now proceed to present their concretization in the Ciao module system.

4.1   General Issues

Defining Modules: The source of a Ciao module is typically contained in a single file, whose name must be the same as the name of the module, except that it may have an optional .pl extension. Nevertheless, the system allows inclusion of source from another file at a precise point in the module, by using the ISO-Prolog [19, 12] :- include declaration. In any case, such included files must be present at the time of processing the module and can for all purposes be considered as an integral part of the module text. The fact that the file contains a module (as opposed to, e.g., being a user file –see below) is flagged by the presence of a ":- module(..." declaration at the beginning of the file.

For the reasons mentioned in Section 2 the Ciao module system is, as in most logic programming system implementations, predicate-based (but only by default, see below). This means that non-exported predicate names are local to a module, but all functor and atom names in data are shared. We have found that this choice does provide the needed capabilities most of the time, without imposing too much burden on the user or on the implementation. The advantage of this, other than compatibility, and probably the reason why this option has been chosen traditionally, is that it is more concise for typical Prolog programs in which many atoms and functors are shared (and would thus have to be exported in an atom-based system). On the other hand, it forces having to deal specially with meta-programming, since in that case functors can become predicate names and vice-versa. It can also complicate having truly abstract data types in modules. The meta-predicate problem is solved in Ciao through suitable declarations (see Section 4.4). Also, in order to allow defining truly abstract data types in Ciao, it is possible to *hide* atom/functor names, i.e., make them local to a module, by means of ":- hide ..." declarations, which provide an automatic renaming of such symbols. This does not prevent a program from creating data *of that type* if meta-predicates such as "=.." are loaded and used, but it does prevent creating and matching such data using unification. Thus, in contrast to predicate names, which are local unless explicitly exported, functor and atom names are exported by default unless a :- hide declaration is used.[8]

Imports, Exports, and Reexports: A number of predicates in the module can be *exported*, i.e., made available outside the module, via explicit :- export declarations or in an export list in the :- module(... declaration. It is also possible to state that *all* predicates in the module are exported (by using '_').

It is possible to *import* a number of individual predicates or also all predicates from another module, by using :- use_module declarations. In any case it is only possible to import from a module predicates that it exports. It is possible to import a predicate which has the same name/arity as a local predicate. It is also possible to import several predicates with the same name from different modules. This applies also to predicates belonging to *implicitly-imported modules*, which play the role of the built-ins in other logic programming systems. In Ciao there are really no "built-ins": all system predicates are (at least conceptually) defined in libraries which have to be loaded for these predicates to be accessible to the module. However, for compatibility with ISO, a set of these libraries implementing the standard set of ISO builtins is loaded by default.

A module m1 can *reexport* another module, m2, via a :- reexport declaration. The effect of this is that m1 exports all predicates of m2 as if they had been defined in m1 in the same way as they are defined in m2. This allows implementing modules which *extend* other modules (or, in object-oriented terms, classes which inherit from other classes [24]). It is also possible to reexport only some of the predicates of another module, by providing an explicit list in the :- reexport declaration, *restricting* that module.

In Ciao it is possible to mark certain predicates as being *properties*. Examples of properties are *regular types*, *pure properties* (such as sorted), *instantiation properties* (such as var, indep, or ground), *computational properties* (such as det or fails), etc. Such properties, since they are actually predicates, can be exported or imported using the same rules as any other predicate. Imported properties can be used in assertions (declarations stating certain characteristics

---

[8] This feature of being able to hide functor and atom names is not implemented in the distribution version of Ciao as of the time of writing of this paper (Vers. 1.4).

of the program, such as, e.g., preconditions and postconditions) in the same
way as locally defined ones. This allows defining, e.g., the abstract data types
mentioned above. This is discussed in more detail in the descriptions of the Ciao
assertion language [2, 25] and the Ciao preprocessor [17, 15].

Visibility Rules: The predicates which are *visible* in a module are the predicates defined in that module plus the predicates imported from other modules. It is possible to refer to predicates with or without a *module qualification.* A module-qualified predicate name has the form *module:predicate* as in the
call `lists:append(A,B,C)`. We call *default module* for a given predicate name
the module which contains the definition of the predicate which will be called
when using the predicate name without module qualification, i.e., when calling
`append(A,B,C)` instead of `lists:append(A,B,C)`. Module qualification makes
it possible to refer to a predicate from a module which is not the default for that
predicate name.

We now state the rules used to determine the default module of a given
predicate name. If the predicate is defined in the module in which the call occurs,
then this module is the default module. I.e., local definitions have priority over
imported definitions. Otherwise, the default module is the *last module* from
which the predicate is imported in the module text. Also, predicates which are
explicitly imported (i.e. listed in the importation list of a `:- use_module`) have
priority over those which are imported implicitly (i.e. imported when importing
all predicates of a module). As implicitly-imported modules are considered to
be imported first, the system allows the redefinition of "builtins". By combining
implicit and explicit calls it is also possible not only to redefine builtins, but
also to *extend* them, a feature often used in the implementation of many Ciao
libraries. Overall, the rules are designed so that it is possible to have a similar
form of inheritance to that found in object-oriented programming languages
(in Ciao this also allows supporting a class/object system naturally as a simple
extension of the module system [24]). It is not possible to access predicates which
are not imported from a module, even if module qualification is used and even
if the module exports them. It is also not possible to define clauses of predicates
belonging to other modules, except if the predicate is defined as dynamic and
exported by the module in which it is defined.

Additional rules govern the case when a module redefines predicates that it
also reexports, which allows making specialized modules which are the same as
a reexported module but with some of the predicates redefined as determined by
local predicate definitions (i.e., *instances* of a module/class, in object-oriented
terms –see the Ciao manual [2] for details).

4.2   User Files and Multifile Predicates

For reasons mainly of backwards compatibility with non-modular Prolog systems, there are some deviations from the visibility rules above which are common to other modular logic programming systems [28, 8]: the "`user`" module
and *multifile* predicates.

User Files: To provide backwards compatibility with non-modular code, all code belonging to files which have no module declaration is assumed to belong to a single special module called "`user`". These files are called "user files", as opposed to calling them modules (or packages –see later). All predicates in the user module are "exported". It is possible to make unrestricted calls from any predicate defined in a user file to any other predicate defined in another user file. However, and differently to other Prolog systems, predicates imported from a normal module into a user file are not visible in the other user files unless they are explicitly imported there as well. This at least allows performing separate static compilation of each user file, as all static predicate calls in a file are defined by reading only that file. Predicates defined in user files can be visible in regular modules, but such modules must explicitly import the "user" module, stating explicitly which predicates are imported from it.

The use of user files is discouraged because, apart from losing the separation of predicate names, their structure makes it impossible to detect many errors that the compiler detects in modules by looking at the module itself (and perhaps the interfaces of related modules). As an example, consider detecting undefined predicates: this is not possible in user files because a missing predicate in a user file may be defined in another user file and used without explicitly importing it. Thus, it is only possible to detect a missing predicate by examining all user files of a project, which is itself typically an unknown (and, in fact, not even in this way, since that predicate could even be meant to be typed in at the top level after loading the user files!). Also, global analysis of user files typically involves considerable loss of precision because all predicates are possible entry points [3]. Note that it is often just as easy and flexible to use modules which export all predicates in place of user files (by simply adding a `:- module(_,_).` header to the file), while being able to retain many of the advantages of modules.

Multifile Predicates: Multifile predicates are a useful feature (also defined in ISO-Prolog) which allows a predicate to be defined by clauses belonging to different files (modules in the case of Ciao). To fit this in with the module system, in Ciao these predicates are implemented as if belonging to a special module `multifile`. However, calls present in a clause of a multifile predicate are always to visible predicates of the module where that clause resides. As a result, multifile predicates do not pose special problems to the global analyzer (which considers them exported predicates) nor to code processing in general.

4.3   Dynamic Modules

The module system described so far is quite flexible but it is *static*, i.e., except in user files, it is possible to determine statically the set of imports and exports of a given module and the set of related modules, and it is possible to statically resolve to which module each call in the program refers to. This has many advantages: modular programs can be implemented with no run-time overhead with respect to a non-modular system and it is also possible to perform extensive static analysis for optimization and error detection. However, in practice it is sometimes very useful to be able to load code dynamically and call it. In Ciao this is fully supported, but only if the special library **dynmods** which defines the appropriate builtins (e.g., **use_module**) is explicitly loaded (**dynmods** actually reexports a number of predicates from the compiler, itself another library). This can then be seen by compile-time tools which can act more conservatively if needed. Also, the adverse effects are limited to the module which imports the compiler.

4.4   Dealing with Meta-calls

As mentioned before, the fact that the Ciao module system is predicate-based forces having to deal specially with meta-programming, since in that case functors can become predicate names and vice-versa. This problem is solved in Ciao, as in similar systems [28, 8] through **meta_predicate** declarations which specify which arguments of predicates contain meta-data. However, because of the richer set of higher-order facilities and predicate types provided by Ciao [6], there is a correspondingly richer set of types of meta-data (this also allows more error detection):

goal: denotes a goal (either a simple or a complex one) which will be called.

clause: denotes a clause, of a dynamic predicate, which will be asserted/ retracted.

fact: denotes a fact (a head-only clause), of a **data** predicate.

spec: denotes a predicate name, given as *Functor/Arity* term (this kind of meta-term is used somewhat frequently in builtin predicates, but seldom in user-defined predicates).

pred(N): denotes a predicate construct to be called by means of a **call/N** predicate call. That is, it should be an atom equal to the name of a predicate of arity N, a structure with functor the name of a predicate of arity M (greater than N) and with M-N arguments, or a predicate abstraction with N arguments.[9]

addmodule:

this in fact is not a real meta-data specification. Rather, it is used to pass, along with the predicate arguments, the calling module, to allow handling more involved meta-data (e.g., lists of goals) by using conversion builtins.[10]

   The compiler, by knowing which predicates have meta-arguments, can verify if there are undetermined meta-calls (which for example affect the processing when performing global analysis), or else can determine (or approximate) the calls that these meta-arguments will produce.

---

[9] A full explanation of this type of meta-term is outside the scope of this paper. See [6] for details.

[10] This a "low-level" solution, which can be a reasonable overall solution for systems without a type system. The higher-level solution in Ciao involves the combination of the type and meta-data declarations (currently in progress).

4.5   Modular Syntax Enhancements

Traditionally (and also now in the ISO standard [19, 12]) Prolog systems have included the possibility of changing the syntax of the source code by the use of the op/3 builtin/directive. Furthermore, in many Prolog systems it is also possible to define *expansions* of the source code (essentially, a very rich form of "macros") by allowing the user to define (or extend) a predicate typically called term_expansion/2 [28, 8]. This is usually how, e.g., definite clause grammars (DCG's) are implemented.

However, these features, in their original form, pose many problems for modular compilation or even for creating sensible standalone executables. First, the definitions of the operators and expansions are global, affecting a number of files. Furthermore, which files are affected cannot be determined statically, because these features are implemented as a side-effect, rather than a declaration, and they are meant to be active after they are read by the code processor (top-level, compiler, etc.) and remain active from then on. As a result, it is impossible by looking at a source code file to know if it will be affected by expansions or definitions of operators, which may completely change what the compiler really sees. Furthermore, these definitions also affect how a compiled program will read terms (when using the term I/O predicates), which will also be affected by operators and expansions. However, in practice it is often desirable to use a set of operators and expansions in the compilation process (which are typically related to source language enhancements) and a completely different set for reading or writing data (which can be related to data formatting or the definition of some application-specific language that the compiled program is processing). Finally, when creating executables, if the compile-time and run-time roles of expansions are not separated, then the code that defines the expansions must be included in the executable, even if it was only meant for use during compilation.

To solve these problems, in Ciao we have redesigned these features so that it is still possible to define source translations and operators but they are local to the module or user file defining them. Also, we have implemented these features in a way that has a well defined behavior in the context of a stand-alone compiler (the Ciao compiler, ciaoc [7]). In particular, the directive load_compilation_module/1 allows separating code that will be used at compilation time from code which will be used at run-time. It loads the module defined by its argument *into the compiler* (if it has not been already loaded). It differs from the use_module/1 declaration in that the latter defines a use by the module being compiled, but does not load the code into the compiler itself. This distinction also holds in the Ciao interactive top-level, in which the compiler (which is the same library used by ciaoc) is also a separate module.

In addition, in order to make the task of writing expansions easier,[11] the effects usually achieved through term_expansion/2 can be obtained in Ciao by means of four different, more specialized directives, which, again, *affect only the current module*. Each one defines a different target for the translations, the first

---

[11] Note that, nevertheless, writing interesting and powerful translations is not necessarily a trivial task.

being equivalent to the **term_expansion/2** predicate which is most commonly
included in Prolog implementations. The argument for all of them is a predicate
indicator of arity 2 or 3. When reading a file, the compiler (actually, the general
purpose module processing library –see [7]) invokes these translation predicates
at the appropriate times, instantiating their first argument with the item to be
translated (whose type varies from one kind of predicate to the other). If the
predicate is of arity 3, the optional third argument is also instantiated with the
name of the module where the translation is being done, which is sometimes
needed during certain expansions. If the call to the expansion predicate is successful, the term returned by the predicate in the second argument is used to
replace the original. Else, the original item is kept. The directives are:

add_sentence_trans/1 : Declares a translation of the terms read by the compiler which affects the rest of the current text (module or user file). For each
subsequent term (directive, fact, clause, ...) read by the compiler, the translation predicate is called to obtain a new term which will be used by the
compiler in place of the term present in the file. An example of this kind of
translation is that of DCG's.

add_term_trans/1 : Declares a translation of the terms and sub-terms read by
the compiler which affects the rest of the current text. This translation is
performed after all translations defined by add_sentence_trans/1 are done.
For each subsequent term read by the compiler, and recursively any subterm
included in such a term, the translation predicate is called to possibly obtain
a new term to replace the old one. Note that this is computationally intensive,
but otherwise very useful to define translations which should affect any term
read. For example, it is used to define *records* (feature terms [1]), in the Ciao
standard library argnames (see 5.1).

add_goal_trans/1 : Declares a translation of the goals present in the clauses
of the current text. This translation is performed after all translations defined by **add_sentence_trans/1** and **add_term_trans/1** are done. For each
clause read by the compiler, the translation predicate is called with each goal
present in the clause to possibly obtain another goal to replace the original
one, and the translation is subsequently applied to the resulting goal. Note
that this process is aware of meta_predicate definitions. In the Ciao system,
this feature is used for example in the **functions** library which provides
functional syntax, as functions inside a goal add new goals before that one.

add_clause_trans/1 : Declares a translation of the clauses of the current text.
The translation is performed before **add_goal_trans/1** translations but after **add_sentence_trans/1** and **add_term_trans/1** translations. This kind
of translation is defined for more involved translations and is related to the
compiling procedure of Ciao. The usefulness of this translation is that information on the interface of related modules is available when it is performed,
but on the other hand it must maintain the predicate defined by each clause,
since the compiler has already made assumptions regarding which predicates
are defined in the code. For example, the object-oriented extension of Ciao
(O'Ciao) uses this feature [24].

```
c(D,B) :- findall(l(S,D), cf(B,D,S), Ls), cl(0, Ls).
```

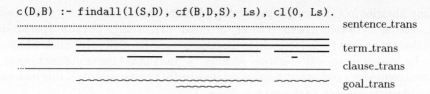

Fig. 1. Subterms to which each translation type is applied in a clause

Figure 1 shows, for an example clause of a program, to which subterms each type of translation would be applied, and also the order of translations. The principal functor of the head in the clause translation is dashed because the translation cannot change it.

Finally, there is another directive in Ciao related to syntax extension, whose raison d'être is the parametric and extensible nature of the compiler framework: `new_declaration/1` (there is also a /2 variant). Note that in ISO-Standard Prolog declarations cannot be arbitrary Prolog goals. Thus, the Ciao compiler flags an error if a declaration is found which is not in a predefined set. A declaration `new_declaration(Decl)` can be used to declare that `Decl` is a valid declaration *in the rest of the current text* (module or user file). Such declarations are simply ignored by the compiler or top level, but can be used by other code processing programs. For example, in the Ciao system, program assertions and machine-readable comments are defined as new declarations and are processed by the `ciaopp` preprocessor and the `lpdoc` [14] automatic documenter.

5 Packages

Experience using the Ciao module system shows that the local nature of syntax extensions and the distinction between compile-time and run-time work results in the libraries defining extensions to the language having a well defined and repetitive structure. These libraries typically consist of a main source file which defines only some declarations (operator declarations, declarations loading other modules into the compiler or the module using the extension, etc.). This file is meant to be *included* as part of the file using the library, since, because of their local effect, such directives must be part of the code of the module which uses the library. Thus, we will call it the "include file". Any auxiliary code needed at compile-time (e.g., translations) is included in a separate module which is to be loaded into the compiler via a `load_compilation_module` directive which is placed in the include file. Also, any auxiliary code to be used at run-time is placed in another module, and the corresponding `use_module` declaration is also placed in the include file. Note that while this run-time code could also be inserted in the include file itself, it would then be replicated in each module that uses the library. Putting it in a module allows the code to be shared by all modules using the library.

Libraries constructed in this manner are called "packages" in Ciao. The main file of such a library is a file which is to be *included* in the importing module.

Many libraries in Ciao are packages: dcg (definite clause grammars), functions (functional syntax), class (object oriented extension), persdb (persistent database), assertions (to include assertions –see [25, 26]), etc. Such libraries can be loaded using a declaration such as :- include(library(functions)). For convenience (and other reasons related to ISO compatibility), this can also be written as :- use_package(functions).[12]

There is another feature which allows defining modules which do not start with a :- module declaration, and which is useful when defining language extensions: when the first declaration of a file is unknown, the declared library paths are browsed to find a package with the same name as the declaration, and if it is found the declaration is treated as a module declaration plus a declaration to use that package. For example, the package which implements the object oriented capabilities in Ciao is called "class": this way, one can start a class (a special module in Ciao) with the declaration ":- class(myclass)", which is then equivalent to defining a module which loads the class package. The class package then defines translations which transform the module code so that it can be used as a class, rather than as a simple module.

5.1   An Example Package: argnames

To clarify some of the concepts introduced in the paper, we will describe as an example the implementation of the Ciao library package "argnames".[13] This library implements a syntax to access term arguments by name (also known as *records*). For example, Fig. 2 shows a fragment of the famous "zebra" puzzle written using the package. The declaration :- argnames (where argnames is defined as an operator with suitable priority) assigns a name to each of the arguments of the functor house/5. From then on, it is possible to write a term with this functor by writing its name (house), then the infix operator '$', and then, between brackets (which are as in ISO-Prolog), the arguments one wants to specify, using the infix operator '=>' between the name and the value. For example, house${} is equivalent in that code to house(_,_,_,_,_) and house${nation=>Owns_zebra,pet=>zebra} to house(_,Owns_zebra,zebra, _,_).

The library which implements this feature is composed of two files, one which is the package itself, called argnames, and an auxiliary module which implements the code translations required, called argnames_trans (in this case no run-time code is necessary). They are shown in Appendix A (the transformation has been simplified for brevity by omitting error checking code).

The contents of package argnames are self-explanatory: first, it directs the compiler to load the module argnames_trans (if not already done before), which

---

[12] We are also considering adding a feature to allow loading packages using normal :- use_module declarations, which saves the user from having to determine whether what is being loaded is a package or an ordinary module.

[13] This package uses only a small part of the functionality described. Space restrictions do not allow adding a longer example or more examples. However, many such examples can be found in the Ciao system libraries.

```
:- use_package([argnames]).
:- argnames house(color, nation, pet, drink, car).
zebra(Owns_zebra, Drinks_water, Street) :-
    Street = [house${},house${},house${},house${},house${}],
    member(house${nation=>Owns_zebra,pet=>zebra}, Street),
    member(house${nation=>Drinks_water,drink=>water}, Street),
    member(house${drink=>coffee,color=>green}, Street),
    left_right(house${color=>ivory}, house${color=>green}, Street),
    member(house${car=>porsche,pet=>snails}, Street),
    ...
```

Fig. 2. "zebra" program using argnames

contains the code to make the required translations. Then, it declares a sentence translation, which will handle the argnames declarations, and a term translation, which will translate any terms written using the argnames syntax. Finally, it declares the operators used in the syntax. Recall that a module using this package is in fact including these declarations into its code, so the declarations are local to the module and will not affect the compilation of other modules.

The auxiliary module `argnames_trans` is also quite straightforward: it exports the two predicates which the compiler will use to do the translations. Then, it declares a data predicate (recall that this is a simplified dynamic predicate) which will store the declarations made in each module. Predicate `argnames_def/3` is simple: if the clause term is an `argnames` declaration, it translates it to nothing but stores its data in the above mentioned data predicate. Note that the third argument is instantiated by the compiler to the module where the translation is being made, and thus is used so that the declarations of a module are not mixed with the declarations in other modules. The second clause is executed when the end of the module is reached. It takes care of deleting the data pertaining to the current module. Then, predicate `argnames_use/3` is in charge of making the translation of argname'd-terms, using the data collected by the other predicate. Although more involved, it is a simple Prolog exercise.

Note that the argnames library only affects the modules that load it. Thus, the operators involved (`argnames`, `$`, `=>`) can be used in other modules or libraries for different purposes. This would be very difficult to do with the traditional model.

6   Conclusions

We have presented a new module system for Prolog which achieves a number of fundamental design objectives such as being more amenable to effective global analysis and translation, allowing separate compilation and sensible creation of standalone executables, extensibility/restriction in features and in syntax, etc. We have also shown in other work that this module system can be implemented easily [7] and can be applied successfully in several modular program processing tasks, from compilation to debugging to automatic documentation generation [7, 27, 17, 14]. The proposed module system has been designed to stay as similar as possible to the module systems of the most popular Prolog implementations and the ISO-Prolog module standard currently being finished, but with a number of crucial changes that achieve the previously mentioned design objectives. We believe that it would not be difficult to incorporate these changes in the ISO-Prolog module standard or in other module systems. In the latter case, the cost would be some minor backward-incompatibility with some of the existing modular code, but which could generally be fixed easily with a little rewriting. We argue that the advantages that we have pointed out clearly outweigh this inconvenience.

References

1. H. Aït-Kaci, A. Podelski, and G. Smolka. A feature-based constraint system for logic programming with entailment. In *Proc. Fifth Generation Computer Systems 1992*, pages 1012–1021, 1992.
2. F. Bueno, D. Cabeza, M. Carro, M. Hermenegildo, P. López-García, and G. Puebla. The Ciao Prolog System. Reference Manual. TR CLIP3/97.1, School of Computer Science, Technical University of Madrid (UPM), August 1997.
3. F. Bueno, D. Cabeza, M. Hermenegildo, and G. Puebla. Global Analysis of Standard Prolog Programs. In *European Symposium on Programming*, number 1058 in LNCS, pages 108–124, Sweden, April 1996. Springer-Verlag.
4. F. Bueno, M. García de la Banda, and M. Hermenegildo. Effectiveness of Abstract Interpretation in Automatic Parallelization: A Case Study in Logic Programming. *ACM Trans. on Programming Languages and Systems*, 21(2):189–238, March 1999.
5. F. Bueno, P. Deransart, W. Drabent, G. Ferrand, M. Hermenegildo, J. Maluszynski, and G. Puebla. On the Role of Semantic Approximations in Validation and Diagnosis of Constraint Logic Programs. In *Int'l WS on Automated Debugging–AADEBUG'97*, pages 155–170, Sweden, May 1997. U. of Linköping Press.
6. D. Cabeza and M. Hermenegildo. Higher-order Logic Programming in Ciao. TR CLIP7/99.0, Facultad de Informática, UPM, September 1999.
7. D. Cabeza and M. Hermenegildo. The Ciao Modular Compiler and Its Generic Program Processing Library. In *ICLP'99 WS on Parallelism and Implementation of (C)LP Systems*, pages 147–164. N.M. State U., December 1999.
8. M. Carlsson and J. Widen. *Sicstus Prolog User's Manual*. Po Box 1263, S-16313 Spanga, Sweden, April 1994.
9. W. Chen. A theory of modules based on second-order logic. In *Proc. 4th IEEE Internat. Symposium on Logic Programming*, pages 24–33, San Francisco, 1987.
10. M. Comini, G. Levi, M. C. Meo, and G. Vitiello. Proving properties of logic programs by abstract diagnosis. In M. Dams, editor, *Analysis and Verification of Multiple-Agent Languages, 5th LOMAPS Workshop*, number 1192 in Lecture Notes in Computer Science, pages 22–50. Springer-Verlag, 1996.
11. S.K. Debray. Flow analysis of dynamic logic programs. *Journal of Logic Programming*, 7(2):149–176, September 1989.
12. P. Deransart, A. Ed-Dbali, and L. Cervoni. *Prolog: The Standard*. Springer, 1996.
13. J.A. Goguen and J. Meseguer. Eqlog: equality, types, and generic modules for logic programming. In *Logic Programming: Functions, Relations, and Equations*, Englewood Cliffs, 1986. Prentice-Hall.
14. M. Hermenegildo. A Documentation Generator for (C)LP Systems. In this volume: Proceedings of CL2000, LNCS, Springer-Verlag.
15. M. Hermenegildo, F. Bueno, G. Puebla, and P. López-García. Program Analysis, Debugging and Optimization Using the Ciao System Preprocessor. In *Proc. of ICLP'99*, pages 52–66, Cambridge, MA, November 1999. MIT Press.

16. M. Hermenegildo and The CLIP Group. Programming with Global Analysis. In *Proc. of ILPS'97*, pages 49–52, October 1997. MIT Press. (Invited talk abstract).

17. M. Hermenegildo, G. Puebla, and F. Bueno. Using Global Analysis, Partial Specifications, and an Extensible Assertion Language for Program Validation and Debugging. In K. R. Apt, V. Marek, M. Truszczynski, and D. S. Warren, editors, *The Logic Programming Paradigm: a 25-Year Perspective*, pages 161–192. Springer-Verlag, July 1999.

18. P. Hill and J. Lloyd. *The Goedel Programming Language*. MIT Press, 1994.

19. International Organization for Standardization. *PROLOG. ISO/IEC DIS 13211 — Part 1: General Core*, 1994.

20. International Organization for Standardization. *PROLOG. Working Draft 7.0 X3J17/95/1 — Part 2: Modules*, 1995.

21. D. Miller. A logical analysis of modules in logic programming. *Journal of Logic Programming*, pages 79–108, 1989.

22. L. Monteiro and A. Porto. Contextual logic programming. In *Proc. of ICLP'89*, pages 284–299. MIT Press, Cambridge, MA, 1989.

23. R.A. O'Keefe. Towards an algebra for constructing logic programs. In *IEEE Symposium on Logic Programming*, pages 152–160, Boston, Massachusetts, July 1985. IEEE Computer Society.

24. A. Pineda and M. Hermenegildo. O'ciao: An Object Oriented Programming Model for (Ciao) Prolog. TR CLIP 5/99.0, Facultad de Informática, UPM, July 1999.

25. G. Puebla, F. Bueno, and M. Hermenegildo. An Assertion Language for Debugging of Constraint Logic Programs. In *ILPS'97 WS on Tools and Environments for (C)LP*, October 1997. Available as TR CLIP2/97.1 from ftp://clip.dia.fi.upm.es/pub/papers/assert_lang_tr_discipldeliv.ps.gz.

26. G. Puebla, F. Bueno, and M. Hermenegildo. An Assertion Language for Debugging of Constraint Logic Programs. In *Analysis and Visualization Tools for Constraint Programming*, LNCS. Springer-Verlag, 2000. To appear.

27. G. Puebla and M. Hermenegildo. Some Issues in Analysis and Specialization of Modular Ciao-Prolog Programs. In *ICLP'99 WS on Optimization and Implementation of Declarative Languages*, pages 45–61. U. of Southampton, U.K, Nov. 1999.

28. *Quintus Prolog User's Guide and Reference Manual—Version 6*, April 1986.

29. K. Sagonas, T. Swift, and D.S. Warren. The XSB Programming System. In *ILPS WS on Programming with Logic Databases*, TR #1183, pages 164–164. U. of Wisconsin, October 1993.

30. Z. Somogyi, F. Henderson, and T. Conway. The execution algorithm of Mercury: an efficient purely declarative LP language. *JLP*, 29(1–3), October 1996.

31. A. Taylor. High performance prolog implementation through global analysis. Slides of the invited talk at PDK'91, Kaiserslautern, 1991.

32. P. Van Roy, B. Demoen, and Y. D. Willems. Improving the Execution Speed of Compiled Prolog with Modes, Clause Selection, and Determinism. In *Proceedings of TAPSOFT '87*, LNCS. Springer-Verlag, March 1987.

33. P. Van Roy and A.M. Despain. High-Performace Logic Programming with the Aquarius Prolog Compiler. *IEEE Computer Magazine*, pages 54–68, January 1992.

34. D.S. Warren and W. Chen. Formal semantics of a theory of modules. TR 87/11, SUNY at Stony Brook, 1987.

35. R. Warren, M. Hermenegildo, and S. K. Debray. On the Practicality of Global Flow Analysis of Logic Programs. In *Fifth International Conference and Symposium on Logic Programming*, pages 684–699. MIT Press, August 1988.

CLIP WS papers, TRs and manuals available at
http://www.clip.dia.fi.upm.es

A   Code for the Package argnames

The package argnames:

```
:- load_compilation_module(library(argnames_trans)).
:- add_sentence_trans(argnames_def/3).
:- add_term_trans(argnames_use/3).
:- op(150, xfx, [$]).
:- op(950, xfx, (=>)).
:- op(1150, fx, [argnames]).
```

The translation module argnames_trans:

```
:- module(argnames_trans, [argnames_def/3, argnames_use/3]).
:- data argnames/4.

argnames_def((:- argnames(R)), [], M) :-
        functor(R, F, N),
        assertz_fact(argnames(F,N,R,M)).
argnames_def(end_of_file, end_of_file, M) :-
        retractall_fact(argnames(_,_,_,M)).

argnames_use($(F,TheArgs), T, M) :-
        atom(F),
        argnames_args(TheArgs, Args),
        argnames_trans(F, Args, M, T).

argnames_args({}, []).
argnames_args({Args}, Args).

argnames_trans(F, Args, M, T) :-
        argnames(F, A, R, M),
        functor(T, F, A),
        insert_args(Args, R, A, T).

insert_args([], _, _, _).
insert_args('=>'(F,A), R, N, T) :-
        insert_arg(N, F, A, R, T).
insert_args(('=>'(F,A), As), R, N, T) :-
        insert_arg(N, F, A, R, T),
        insert_args(As, R, N, T).

insert_arg(N, F, A, R, T) :-
        N > 0,
        (   arg(N, R, F)
        -> arg(N, T, A)
        ; N1 is N-1,
            insert_arg(N1, F, A, R, T) ).
```

Partial Models of Extended Generalized Logic Programs

José J. Alferes[1,3], Heinrich Herre[2], and Luís Moniz Pereira[3]

[1] Departamento de Matemàtica, Universidade de Évora
jja@di.fct.unl.pt
[2] Institute of Informatics, University of Leipzig, Augustusplatz 10-11
herre@informatik.uni-leipzig.de
[3] Centro de Inteligência, Universidade Nova de Lisboa, 2825 Monte da Caparica
{jja,lmp}@di.fct.unl.pt

Abstract. In recent years there has been an increasing interest in extensions of the logic programming paradigm beyond the class of normal logic programs motivated by the need for a satisfactory respresentation and processing of knowledge. An important problem in this area is to find an adequate declarative semantics for logic programs. In the present paper a general preference criterion is proposed that selects the 'intended' partial models of extended generalized logic programs which is a conservative extension of the stationary semantics for normal logic programs of [13], [14] and generalizes the WFSX-semantics of [12]. The presented preference criterion defines a partial model of an extended generalized logic program as intended if it is generated by a stationary chain. The GWFSX-semantics is defined by the set-theoretical intersection of all stationary generated models, and thus generalizes the results from [9] and [1].

1 Introduction

Declarative semantics provides a mathematical precise definition of the meaning of a program in a way, which is independent of procedural considerations. Finding a suitable declarative or intended semantics is an important problem in logic programming and deductive databases. Logic programs and deductive databases should be as easy to write and comprehend and as close to natural discourse as possible.

Standard logic programs are not sufficiently expressive for comprehensible representation of large classes of knowledge bases and of informal descriptions. Formalisms admitting more complex formulas, as extended generalized logic programs, are more expressive and natural to use since they permit in many cases easier translation from natural language expressions and from informal specifications. The expressive power of generalized logic programs also simplifies the problem of translation of non-monotonic formalisms into logic programs, as shown in [4], [5], and consequently facilitates using logic programming as an inference engine for non-monotonic reasoning. We assume that a reasonable extension of logic programs should satisfy the following conditions:

J. Lloyd et al. (Eds.): CL 2000, LNAI 1861, pp. 149–163, 2000.
© Springer-Verlag Berlin Heidelberg 2000

1. The proposed syntax of rules in such programs resembles the syntax of logic programs but it applies to a significantly broader class of programs.
2. The proposed semantics of such programs constitute a natural extension of the semantics of normal logic programs;
3. There is a natural relationship between the proposed class of programs and their semantics and broader classes of non-monotonic formalisms.

We believe that the class of extended generalized logic programs and the stationary generated semantics, introduced in this paper, presents an extension of logic programming for which the above mentioned principles 1. and 2. can be realized. There are also results in [4] and [5] partially realizing principle 3, where relations to temporal logic and default logic are studied.

A set of facts can be viewed as a database whose semantics is determined by its minimal models. In the case of logic programs, where there are rules, minimal models are not adequate because they are not able to capture the directedness of rules. Therefore, *partial stable* models in the form of certain fixpoints have been proposed by [13] , [14], and [12]. We generalize this notion by presenting a definition which is neither fixpoint-based nor dependent on any specific rule syntax. We call our preferred models *stationary generated* because they are generated by a *stationary chain*, i.e. a stratified sequence of rule applications where all applied rules satisfy certain persistence properties. We show the partial stable models of an extended normal programs coincide with its stationary generated models. Hence, our semantics generalizes the WFSX-semantics.

The paper has the following structure. After introducing some basic notation in section 2, we recall some facts about Herbrand model theory and sequents in section 3. In section 4, we define the general concept of a stationary generated model[1] and introduce the GWFSX-semantics. In section 5 we investigate the relationship of the stationary generated models to the original fixpoint-based definitions for normal programs. In particular, we relate the stationary semantics to the WFSX-semantics for extended normal logic programs. It turns out that, for extended normal logic programs, the stationary generated models and the partial stable models coincide.

2   Preliminaries

A *signature* $\sigma = \langle Rel, ExRel, Const, Fun \rangle$ consists of a set Rel of relation symbols, a set of it exact relations symbols $ExRel \subseteq Rel$, a set $Const$ of constant symbols, and a set Fun of function symbols. U_σ denotes the set of all ground terms of σ. The logical functors are $not, \neg, \wedge, \vee, \rightarrow, \forall, \exists$, and the functors $\mathbf{t}, \mathbf{f}, \mathbf{u}$ of arity zero. $L(\sigma)$ is the smallest set containing the constants $\mathbf{t}, \mathbf{f}, \mathbf{u}$ and the atomic first order formulas of σ, and being closed with respect to the following conditions: if $F, G \in L(\sigma)$, then $\{ not\, F, \neg F, F \wedge G, F \vee G, F \rightarrow G, \exists x F, \forall x F \} \subseteq L(\sigma)$. $L^0(\sigma)$ denotes the corresponding set of sentences (closed formulas), where the constants

---

[1] The term "stationary" is borrowed from [14], but the concept of a stationary generated model differs essentially from the stationary model as introduced in [14].

$\mathbf{t}$ (true) , $\mathbf{f}$ (false) , $\mathbf{u}$ (undefined) are considered as sentences. For sublanguages of $L(\sigma)$ formed by means of a subset $\mathcal{F}$ of the logical functors, we write $L(\sigma; \mathcal{F})$. Let $L_1(\sigma) = L(\sigma; \{\, not, \neg, \wedge, \vee, \mathbf{t}, \mathbf{f}, \mathbf{u}\})$, $L_2(\sigma) = L(\sigma; \{\, not, \neg, \wedge, \vee\})$, $L_p(\sigma) = L_1(\sigma) \cup \{F \rightarrow G : F \in L_1(\sigma), G \in L_2(\sigma)\}$; $L_p(\sigma)$ is the set of program formulas over σ. Program formulas are equivalently denoted by expressions of the form $G \leftarrow F$ using the left-directed arrow. With respect to a signature σ we define the following sublanguages: $\mathrm{At}(\sigma) = L(\sigma; \{\mathbf{t}, \mathbf{f}, \mathbf{u}\})$, the set of all atomic formulas (also called *atoms*). The set $\mathrm{GAt}(\sigma)$ of all ground atoms over σ is defined as $\mathrm{GAt}(\sigma) = \mathrm{At}(\sigma) \cap L^0(\sigma)$. $\mathrm{Lit}(\sigma) = L(\sigma; \{\neg, \mathbf{t}, \mathbf{f}, \mathbf{u}\})$, the set of all *objective literals*; we identify the literal $\neg\neg l$ with l. The set $\mathrm{OL}(\sigma)$ of all objective ground literals over σ is defined as $\mathrm{OL}(\sigma) = \mathrm{Lit}(\sigma) \cap L^0(\sigma)$. For a set X of formulas let $not\,X = \{\, not\,F | F \in X\}$. The set $\mathrm{XLit}(\sigma)$ of all extended literals over σ is defined by $\mathrm{XLit}(\sigma) = \mathrm{Lit}(\sigma) \cup not\,\mathrm{Lit}(\sigma)$. Finally, $\mathrm{XG}(\sigma) = \mathrm{OL}(\sigma) \cup not\,\mathrm{OL}(\sigma)$ is the set of all extended grounds literals.

We introduce the following conventions. When $L \subseteq L(\sigma)$ is some sublanguage, L^0 denotes the corresponding set of sentences. If the signature σ does not matter, we omit it and write, e.g., L instead of $L(\sigma)$. If Y is a set and $\leq$ a partial ordering on Y then $\mathrm{Min}_\leq(Y)$ denotes the set of all minimal elements of $(Y, \leq)$. $\mathrm{Pow}(X) = \{Y \mid Y \subseteq X\}$ denotes the power set of X.

Definition 1 (Partial Interpretation).   *Let $\sigma = \langle Rel, Const, Fun\rangle$ be a signature. A partial interpretation I of signature σ is defined by a function $I : \mathrm{OL}(\sigma) \longrightarrow \{0, \frac{1}{2}, 1\}$ satisfying the conditions $I(\mathbf{t}) = 1, I(\neg \mathbf{f}) = 1$, $I(\mathbf{u}) = I(\neg \mathbf{u}) = \frac{1}{2}$. I is said to be coherent if the following coherence principles are satisfied: $I(\neg a) = 1$ implies $I(a) = 0$, and $I(a) = 1$ implies $I(\neg a) = 0$ for every ground atom a.*

A partial σ-interpretation I can equivalently be represented by a set of extended ground literals $I^* \subseteq \mathrm{OL}(\sigma) \cup not\,\mathrm{OL}(\sigma)$ by the following stipulation: $I^* = \{l \mid I(l) = 1\} \cup \{\, not\,l \mid I(l) = 0\}$. Then, I^* satisfies the following conditions:

1. *$\{\mathbf{t}, \neg \mathbf{f}\} \subseteq I^*$, $\{\mathbf{u}, \neg \mathbf{u}\} \cap I^* = \emptyset$.*
2. *There is no objective ground literal $l \in \mathrm{OL}$
   such that $\{l, not\,l\} \subseteq I$ (consistency).
   If I is coherent then I^* satisfies the additional conditions:*
3. *$\neg a \in I^*$ implies $not\,a \in I^*$ for every ground atom a.*
4. *$a \in I^*$ implies $not\,\neg a \in I^*$ for every ground atom a.*

Conversely, every set J of extended ground literals satisfying the conditions 1.and 2. defines a function $I : \mathrm{OL}(\sigma) \longrightarrow \{0, \frac{1}{2}, 1\}$ being an interpretation by the following conditions: $I(l) = 1$ iff $l \in J$, $I(l) = 0$ iff $not\,l \in J$, $I(l) = \frac{1}{2}$ iff $\{l, not\,l\} \cap J = \emptyset$. If J satisfies conditions 3. and 4., then I is coherent.

Remark: In the sequel we use both descriptions of an interpretation (the functional or the literal version), and it should be clear from the context which kind of representation is meant.

For a partial interpretation I let $Pos(I) = I \cap OL$ and $Neg(I) = I \cap not\,OL$. A partial interpretation I is two-valued (or total) if for every $l \in OL$ the condition $\{l, not\,l\} \cap I \neq \emptyset$ is satisfied. A *generalized partial interpretation* is a (arbitrary) set $I \subseteq OL(\sigma) \cup not\,OL(\sigma)$ of extended ground literals. A generalized partial interpretation is said to be *consistent* if conditions 1) and 2) in definition 1 are satisfied, and it is called *coherent* if the conditions 3) and 4) from definition 1 are fulfilled. The class of all generalized partial σ-interpretations is denoted by $I_{gen}(\sigma)$, and the class of all consistent partial σ-interpretations is denoted by $I(\sigma)$, and the class of all consistent coherent interpretations by $I_{coh}(\sigma)$. In the sequel we shall also simply say 'interpretation' instead of 'consistent partial interpretation'. A *valuation* over an interpretation I is a function ν from the set of all variables *Var* into the Herbrand universe U_σ, which can be naturally extended to arbitrary terms by $\nu(f(t_1, \ldots, t_n)) = f(\nu(t_1), \ldots, \nu(t_n))$. Analogously, a valuation ν can be canonically extended to arbitrary formulas F, where we write $F\nu$ instead of $\nu(F)$. The model relation $\models \subseteq I(\sigma) \times L^0(\sigma)$ between an interpretation and a sentence from $L_p(\sigma)$ is defined inductively as follows; it generalizes the definition 4.1.4 in [1] to arbitrary formulas from L_p.

Definition 2 (Model Relation). *Let I be an interpretation of signature σ. Then I can be naturally expanded to a function $\overline{I}$ from the set of all sentences of $L_p(\sigma)$ into the set $\{0, \frac{1}{2}, 1\}$.*

1. $\overline{I}(l) = I(l)$ *for every $l \in OL$.*
2. $\overline{I}(not\,F) = 1 - \overline{I}(F)$;
3. $\overline{I}(F \wedge G) = min\{\overline{I}(F), \overline{I}(G)\}$.
4. $\overline{I}(F \vee G) = max\{\overline{I}(F), \overline{I}(G)\}$
5. $\overline{I}(\neg\neg F) = \overline{I}(F)$;
6. $\overline{I}(\neg\,not\,F) = \overline{I}(F)$;
7. $\overline{I}(\neg(F \wedge G)) = \overline{I}(\neg F \vee \neg G)$;
8. $\overline{I}(\neg(F \vee G)) = \overline{I}(\neg F \wedge \neg G)$;
9. $\overline{I}(F \rightarrow G) = 1$ *if* $\overline{I}(F) \leq \overline{I}(G)$ *or* $\overline{I}(\neg G) = 1$ *and* $\overline{I}(F) = \frac{1}{2}$.
10. $\overline{I}(F \rightarrow G) = 0$ *if condition 9. is not satisfied.* [2]
11. $\overline{I}(\exists x F(x)) = sup\{\overline{I}(F(x/t))|t \in U_\sigma\}$
12. $\overline{I}(\forall x F(x)) = inf\{\overline{I}(F(x/t))|t \in U_\sigma\}$.

To simplify the notation we don't distinguish between I and $\overline{I}$. A sentence F is true in I, denoted by $I \models F$, iff $I(F) = 1$. For arbitrary formulas F we write $I \models F \iff I \models F\nu$ for all $\nu : Var \rightarrow U_\sigma$. For a set X of formulas we write $I \models X$ iff for all $F \in X$ it holds $I \models F$. I is said to be model of a set X of formulas if $I \models X$, and we use the notation $\mathrm{Mod}(X) = \{I \mid I \models X\}$.

Remark: If the conditions 9. and 10. of definition 2 are replaced by 9a. $\overline{I}(F \rightarrow G) = 1$ if $\overline{I}(F) \leq \overline{I}(G)$ and 10a. $\overline{I}(F \rightarrow G) = 0$ if $\overline{I}(F) \not\leq \overline{I}(G)$, then we get the truth-relation considered in [13] which we denote by $I \models_{pr} F$.

---

[2] The condition "not 9." is equivalent to $\overline{I}(F) \not\leq \overline{I}(G)$ and $(\overline{I}(\neg G) < 1$ or $\overline{I}(F) = 1)$.

A coherent consistent interpretation I is called a *AP-model* of a set X of formulas if and only if for all $F \in X$ it holds $I \models F$. An interpretation I is called a *Pr-model* of X iff $I \models_{pr} X$.

Example 1 (AP-Models and Pr-Models). *Let P be the following program:*
$\{\neg b;\ c \leftarrow not\,\neg c;\ a \leftarrow not\,a,\,not\,c;\ \neg a \leftarrow not\,c;\ b \leftarrow a\}.$
P has following AP-models:

$M_1 = \{\neg b,\ not\,b\}$

$M_2 = \{\neg b,\ not\,b,\,c,\ not\,\neg c\}$

$M_3 = \{\neg b,\ not\,b,\,c,\ not\,\neg c,\ not\,a\}$

$M_4 = \{\neg b,\ not\,b,\,not\,c,\,\neg c\}$

$M_5 = \{\neg b,\ not\,b,\,\neg a,\ not\,a\}$

$M_6 = \{\neg b,\ not\,b,\,\neg a,\ not\,a,\,c,\ not\,\neg c\}$

$M_7 = \{\neg b,\ not\,b,\ not\,\neg a\}$

$M_8 = \{\neg b,\ not\,b,\,c,\ not\,\neg c,\ not\,\neg a\}$

$M_9 = \{\neg b,\ not\,b,\,c,\ not\,\neg c,\ not\,a,\ not\,\neg a\}$

$M_{10} = \{\neg b,\ not\,b,\,not\,c,\,\neg c,\ not\,\neg a\}$

Only the models M_3, M_6, M_9 are Pr-models.

Remark: The relevance of AP-models wrt. to Pr-models is that the former impose coherence on interpretations while the latter not. So, take for instance the set $P = \{a \leftarrow \neg a, b;\ b \leftarrow not\,b\}$. Now $\{\neg a,\ not\,a,\ not\,\neg b\}$ is an AP-model but not an Pr-model of P. While $\{\neg a,\ not\,\neg b\}$ is a Pr-model of P but not an AP-model because it is not an coherent interpretation. In this case, coherence imposes "$not\,a$" true on the basis of the truth of $\neg a$, if "$not\,a$" is otherwise undefined as in P. That is, explicit negation $\neg$ overrides undefinedness. Pr-models do not impose coherence they allow the unnatural result that though "a" is explicitly false "$not\,a$" remains undefined. In our opinion, the truth relation $\models$ of definition 2 is better suited to treat coherent interpretations.

Definition 3 (Partial Orderings between Interpretations). *Let $I, I_1 \in \boldsymbol{I}_{gen}$ be two generalized interpretations.*

1. *Let $I \preceq I_1$ if and only if $Pos(I) \subseteq Pos(I_1)$ and $Neg(I_1) \subseteq Neg(I)$. $\preceq$ is called the truth-ordering between interpretations, and I_1 is said to be a truth-extension (briefly t-extension) of I.*
2. *I_1 is informationally greater or equal to I if and only if $I \subseteq I_1$. The partial ordering $\subseteq$ between interpretations is called information-ordering. I_1 is said to be an information-extension (briefly i-extension) of I.*

Proposition 1. *The system $\mathcal{C} = (\boldsymbol{I}_{coh}, \preceq)$ of coherent and consistent generalized partial interpretations is a complete lower semi-lattice.*

Proof: Let $\Omega \subseteq \boldsymbol{I}$ an arbitrary subset. We show that there exists a greatest lower bound for Ω with respect to $\preceq$. Let I be defined by $Pos(I) = \bigcap\{Pos(J) : J \in \Omega\}$, and $Neg(I) = \bigcup\{Neg(J) : J \in \Omega\}$. Obviously, $I \preceq J$ for every $J \in J \in \Omega$, and I is the greatest lower bound within $(\boldsymbol{I}_{gen}, \preceq)$. I is consistent. Assume there are $l \in \mathrm{OL}$ such that $\{l, not\, l\} \subseteq I$. Then $l \in I$. From $not\, l \in I$ there follows the existence of a $J \in \Omega$ such that $not\, l \in J$, a contradiction. The coherency of I is immediate. Hence $I \in \boldsymbol{I}_{coh}$. $\square$

Remark: $\mathcal{C}$ is not a lattice, there are elements $I, J \in \boldsymbol{I}$ having no least upper bound. Take, for example: $I = \{\neg a, not\, a\}$, $J = \{\neg b, not\, b\}$. Every upper bound K of I, J has to contain $\{\neg a, \neg b\}$, and because of coherence also $\{not\, a, not\, b\}$. But this violates the condition $I \preceq K$ because $Neg(K) \not\subseteq Neg(I)$. The set of (consistent) interpretations $(\boldsymbol{I}, \preceq)$ is a complete lattice.

Let $I_1 \preceq I_2 \preceq \ldots \preceq I_\alpha \preceq \ldots$ be a t-increasing sequence of interpretations. The supremum $J = sup\{I_\alpha : \alpha < \kappa\}$ of this sequence is defined by $Pos(J) = \bigcup_\alpha < \kappa : Pos(I_\alpha)$ and $Neg(J) = \bigcap_\alpha < \kappa : Neg(I_\alpha$. For a t-decreasing sequence of interpretations $I_1 \succeq I_2 \succeq \ldots \succeq I_\alpha \succeq \ldots$ its infimum $J = inf\{I_\alpha : \alpha < \kappa\}$ is defined by the following conditions $Neg(J) = \bigcup_{\alpha<\kappa} Neg(I_\alpha)$, and $Pos(J) = \bigcap_{\alpha<\kappa} Pos(I_\alpha)$. An interpretation I is called a *t-minimal* model of X if $I \in Min_\preceq(Mod(X))$, it is called *i-minimal* if $I \in Min_\subseteq(Mod(X))$. The following version of proposition 1 is true: for any t-increasing sequence $\{I_\alpha \mid \alpha < \kappa\}$ of coherent interpretations the interpretation $sup_{\alpha<\kappa} I_\alpha$ is itself coherent.

3   Sequents and Programs

Here, we propose to use sequents for the purpose of representing rule knowledge.[3] A sequent, then, is a concrete expression representing some piece of knowledge.

Definition 4 (Sequent). *A sequent s is an expression of the form*

$$F_1, \ldots, F_m \Rightarrow G_1, \ldots, G_n$$

where $F_i, G_j \in L(\sigma, \{\wedge, \vee, \neg, not\})$ for $i = 1, \ldots, m$ and $j = 1, \ldots, n$. The body of s, denoted by $B(s)$, is given by $\{F_1, \ldots, F_m\}$, and the head of s, denoted by $H(s)$, is given by $\{G_1, \ldots, G_n\}$. $Seq(\sigma)$ denotes the class of all sequents s such that $Hs, Bs \subseteq L(\sigma; \wedge, \vee, \neg, not)$, and for a given set $S \subseteq Seq(\sigma)$, $[S]$ denotes the set of all ground instances of sequences from S. Sometimes, we write a sequent in the following rule-form: $G_1 \vee \ldots \vee G_n \leftarrow F_1, \ldots, F_m$.

Definition 5 (Model of a Sequent). *Let $I \in \boldsymbol{I}$. Then,*

$$I \models F_1, \ldots, F_m \Rightarrow G_1, \ldots, G_n$$

if and only if for all ground substitutions the condition

$$I \models \bigwedge_{i \leq m} F_i \nu \to \bigvee_{j \leq n} G_j \nu$$

is satisfied. In this case, I is said to be model of $F_1, \ldots, F_m \Rightarrow G_1, \ldots, G_n$.

---

[3] The motivation for choosing sequents is to get a connection to Gentzen-like proof systems. Furthermore, the sequent-arrow $\Rightarrow$ and the material implication $\to$ have different properties.

We define the following classes of sequents corresponding to different types of logic programs.

- $\text{EPLP}^*(\sigma) = \{s \in \text{Seq}(\sigma) : H(s) \in \text{Lit}(\sigma),\ B(s) \subseteq \text{Lit}(\sigma) \cup \{\mathbf{t}, \mathbf{u}, \mathbf{f}\}\}$.
- $\text{EPLP}(\sigma) = \{s \in \text{Seq}(\sigma) : H(s) \in \text{Lit}(\sigma),\ B(s) \subseteq \text{Lit}(\sigma)\}$.
- $\text{ENLP}(\sigma) = \{s \in \text{Seq}(\sigma) : H(s) \in \text{Lit}(\sigma),\ B(s) \subseteq \text{XLit}(\sigma)\}$.
- $\text{EDLP}(\sigma) = \{s \in \text{Seq}(\sigma) : H(s) \subseteq \text{Lit}(\sigma),\ B(s) \subseteq \text{XLit}(\sigma), H(s) \neq \emptyset\}$.
- $\text{EGLP}(\sigma) = \{s \in \text{Seq}(\sigma) : H(s), B(s) \subseteq L(\sigma;\ not, \neg, \wedge, \vee)\}$.

Subsets of EPLP^* are called *non-negative extended* logic programs, programs associated to EPLP are called *extended positive* programs, ENLP relates to *extended normal* programs, EDLP to *extended disjunctive programs*, and EGLP to *extended generalized* logic programs. The following lemma is an important tool for analyzing the structure of the partial models of a generalized logic program.

Lemma 1. [4]

1. *Let $J_0 \succeq J_1 \succeq \ldots J_n \succeq \ldots$ be an infinite t-decreasing sequence of partial interpretations and $J = inf\{J_n \mid n < \omega\}$. Let $F \in L_p^0(\sigma)$. Then there exists a number k such that for all $s > k$ the condition $J(F) = J_s(F)$ is satisfied.*
2. *Let $J_0 \preceq J_1 \preceq \ldots J_n \preceq \ldots$ be an infinite t-increasing sequence of partial interpretations and $J = sup\{J_n \mid n < \omega\}$. Let $F \in L_p^0(\sigma)$. Then there exists a number k such that for all $s > k$ the condition $J(F) = J_s(F)$ is satisfied.*

Proposition 2. *Let P be a set of formulas from L_p and K an interpretation. Let I be a model of P such that $K \preceq I$. Then there exists a model $J \models P$ satisfying the following conditions:*

1. *$K \preceq J \preceq I$;*
2. *for every interpretation J_1 the conditions $K \preceq J_1 \preceq J$ and $J_1 \models P$ imply $J = J_1$.*

Proof: Let be $I \models P$ and $\Omega(K, I) = \{K | K \preceq M \preceq I$ and $M \models P\}$. Assume $I = J_0 \succeq J_1 \succeq \ldots \succeq J_n \ldots$, and $J_n \in \Omega(K, I)$. Let be $J = inf_{n<\omega} J_n$. We show that $J \models P$; then, by Zorn's lemma, the set $\Omega(K, I)$ contains a $\preceq$-minimal element satisfying the conditions 1. and 2. Let $r : B(r) \Rightarrow H(r) \in [P]$, and $F := \bigwedge B(r)$, $G := \bigvee H(r)$. It is sufficient to show $J \models F \rightarrow G$. Assume this is not the case, then $J \not\models F \rightarrow G$, and by definition $J(F \rightarrow G) = 0$. By lemma 1 there is a number $k < \omega$ such that for all $s > k$ we have $J_s(F \rightarrow G) = 0$, this is a contradiction, because $J_s \models P$. $\square$

Corollary 3. *Let P be an extended generalized logic program. Every partial model of P is an t-extension of a t-minimal partial model of P and can be t-extended to a t-maximal partial model of P.*

Proposition 4. *Every non-negative extended logic program P having a partial Pr-model has a t-least partial Pr-model.*

---

[4] Complete proofs will be published in the full paper [2].

Remark: Proposition 4 is not true for AP-models as the following example shows.

Example 2. *Let* $P = \{c \leftarrow \mathbf{f}; \ a \leftarrow b; \ b \leftarrow \mathbf{u}; \ \neg a; \ d \leftarrow b\}$.
Let $I = \{\neg a, \ not\, a, \ not\, c, \ not\, \neg b, \ not\, \neg c, \ not\, \neg d\}$. *Obviously,* I *is a t-minimal AP-model of* P. *Take* $I_1 = (I - \{not\, \neg d\}) \cup \{\neg d, \ not\, d\}$. *Then* $I_1 \not\preceq I$ *and* $I \not\preceq I_1$. *It is easy to see that* I_1 *is a t-minimal model of* P.

Example 3. *The following program P has AP-models but no coherent Pr-model.*
$$P = \{a \leftarrow b; \ \neg a; \ b \leftarrow \mathbf{u}\}.$$
Then $\{\neg a, \ not\, a, \ not\, \neg b\}$ *is an AP-model.*

4   Stationary Generated Models and GWFX-Semantics

A preferential semantics is given by a preferred model operator $\Phi : Pow(Seq) \rightarrow Pow(\mathbf{I})$ satisfying the condition $\Phi(P) \subseteq \mathrm{Mod}(P)$ for $P \subseteq Seq$, and determining the associated preferential entailment relation defined by $P \models_\Phi F$ iff $\Phi(P) \subseteq \mathrm{Mod}(F)$. The definition of a stationary chain uses certain persistence properties of formulas which are based on the following notion of truth intervals.

Definition 6 (Truth Interval of Interpretations). *Let* $I_1, I_2 \in \mathbf{I}$. *Then,* $[I_1, I_2] = \{I \in \mathbf{I} : I_1 \preceq I \preceq I_2\}$. *Let P be an extended generalized logic program, for $r \in P$ let $H(r) :=$ head of r, $B(r) :=$ body if r, $[P] :=$ set of all ground instantiations of rules of P. We introduce the following notions and sets:*

- $[I, J](F) \geq \frac{1}{2} =_{df}$ *for all* $K \in [I, J] : K(F) \geq \frac{1}{2}$
- $[I, J](F) = 1 =_{df}$ *for all* $K \in [I, J] : K(F) = 1$
- $P_{[I,J]} = \{r | r \in [P] \text{ and } [I, J](\wedge B(r)) \geq \frac{1}{2}\}$
- $\overline{P}_{[I,J]} = \{r | r \in [P] \text{ and } [I, J](\wedge B(r)) = 1\}$.

The following notion of a *stationary generated* is an essential refinement of the notion of a stable generated (two-valued) model which was introduced in [9].

Definition 7 (Stationary Generated Model). *Let* $P \subseteq EGLP(\sigma)$ *an extended generalized logic program. Let I be an AP-model of P. I is a stationary generated model of P, symbolically $I \in \mathrm{Mod}_{statg}(S)$, if there is a sequence* $\{I_\alpha : \alpha < \kappa\}$ *of coherent interpretations satisfying following conditions:*

1. $I_0 = not\,\mathrm{OL}$ *(is the t-least interpretation).*
2. $I_\alpha \preceq I_{\alpha+1}$ *and* $I_\alpha \preceq I$ *for all* $\alpha < \kappa$.
3. $sup_{\alpha < \kappa} I_\alpha = I$.
4. $I_{\alpha+1} \in Min_{\preceq}\{J | I_\alpha \preceq J \preceq I$ *and*
   (a) for all $r \in \overline{P}_{[I_\alpha, I]}$ *it holds* $J(\vee H(r)) = 1$ *and*
   (b) for all $r \in P_{[I_\alpha, I]} : J(\vee H(r)) \geq \frac{1}{2}$ *or* $I(\neg \vee H(r)) = 1\}$.
5. $I_\lambda = sup_{\alpha < \lambda} I_\alpha$, λ *a limit ordinal.*

The sequence $\{I_\alpha : \alpha < \kappa\}$ *is called a stationary AP-chain (or briefly a stationary chain) generating I. I is called a stationary generated Pr-model if I is a Pr-model,* I_α *are consistent interpretations, and in condition 4. the Pr-truth-relation* $\models_{Pr}$ *is used and if the condition (b) is replaced by* $\forall r \in P_{[I_\alpha, I]} : I_{\alpha+1}(\vee H(r)) \geq \frac{1}{2}$. *In this case* $\{I_\alpha : \alpha < \kappa\}$ *is called a stationary Pr-chain generating I.*

By using proposition 2 one may prove that the set $\text{Min}_{\preceq}\{J \mid I_\alpha \preceq J \preceq I \ \& \ (a) \ \& \ (b)\}$ in condition 4. of definition 7 is non-empty. Hence, for every model $I \models P$, we may construct, according to definition 7, chains of interpretations satisfying the conditions 1.,2.,4. (but not neccessarily 3.). Such chains are called stationary chains in I. A stationary chain $\{I_\alpha \mid \alpha < \kappa\}$ in I is said to be maximal if for $K = sup\{I_\alpha\}$ we have $\text{Min}_{\preceq}\{J \mid K \preceq J \preceq I \ \& \ (a) \ \& \ (b)\} = \{K\}$, i.e. if K cannot be further extended. The set of stationary generated models of S is denoted by $\text{Mod}_{statg}(S)$. The associated entailment relation is defined as follows:

$$S \models_{statg} F \quad \text{iff} \quad \text{Mod}_{statg}(S) \subseteq \text{Mod}(F)$$

Notice that our definition of stationary generated models also accommodates

1. Negation in the head of a rule, such as in

$$\Rightarrow not\,(nationality(x, German) \wedge nationality(x, US))$$

   expressing the integrity constraint that it is not possible to have both the German and the US nationality.
2. Nested negations, such as in $p(x) \wedge not\,(q(x) \wedge not\,r(x)) \Rightarrow s(x)$ which would be the result of folding $p(x) \wedge not\,ab(x) \Rightarrow s(x)$ and $q(x) \wedge not\,r(x) \Rightarrow ab(x)$.

We continue this section with the investigations of some fundamental properties of the introduced concepts. What can be said about the length of the stationary chains?

Proposition 5. *Let* $P \subseteq EGLP$ *and let I be a stationary generated model of P generated by the sequence* $\{I_\alpha : \alpha < \kappa\}$, $\kappa \geq \omega$. *Then there is an ordinal* $\beta \leq \omega$ *such that* $I_\beta = I$ *and* $I_\beta = I_{\beta+1}$. *We say that this sequence stabilizes at* β.

Definition 8 (Rank of a Stationary Generated Model). *Given a program P and let I be a stationary generated AP- model of P. Let* $St(I) = \{\alpha \mid there\ is\ a\ stationary\ chain\ for\ I\ stabilizing\ at\ \alpha\}$. *Then* $Rk\ (I) = infimum\ St(I)$ *is called the rank of I.*

Corollary 6. *If M is a stationary generated AP-model of* $P \subseteq EGLP$, *then there is either a finite P-stationary chain, or a P-stationary chain of length* ω, *generating M.*

Example 4. *Consider the following program* $P = \{a \leftarrow not\,b; \ b \leftarrow not\,a; \ \neg a\}$. *The following interpretation* $\{\neg a, \ not\,a, \ b, \ not\,\neg b\} = K$ *is a stationary generated AP-model of P. It is* $I_0 = \{not\,a, \ not\,b, \ not\,\neg a, \ not\,\neg b\}$, *and* $P_{[I_0,K]} = \{b \leftarrow not\,a; \ \neg a\}$, *and* $\overline{P}_{[I_0,K]} = P_{[I_0,K]}$. *Then K is a minimal extension of* I_0 *such that for all* $r \in \overline{P}_{[I_0,K]}$ *it holds that* $K(H(r)) = 1$. *Hence,* $\{I_0, K\}$ *is a stationary sequence generating K. Obviously,* $Rk(K) = 1$.

Example 5. *Consider the program* $P = \{a \vee b; \; \neg b \leftarrow a; \; a \leftarrow not\,a\}$. *The following interpretation is a stationary generated model of P:* $K = \{a, \; \neg b, \; not\,b, \; not\,\neg a\}$. $I_0 = \{not\,a, \; not\,\neg a, \; not\,b, \; not\,\neg b\}$. *Then* $P_{[I_0, K]} = \{a \vee b\} = \overline{P}_{[I_0, K]}$. *Then* $I_1 = \{a, \; not\,\neg a, \; not\,b, \, not\,\neg b\}$ *is a t-minimal extension of* I_0. *It is* $P_{[I_1, K]} = \{a \vee b, \; \neg b \leftarrow a\} = \overline{P}_{[I_1, K]}$. *Then* K *is a minimal t-extension of* I_1, *hence* $\{I_0, I_1, K\}$ *is a stationary sequence generating* K. *Obviously,* $Rk(K) = 2$.

The GWFSX-semantics can be introduced as follows.

Definition 9 (Generalized Wellfounded Semantics). *Let P be an extended generalized logic program and* $GWFSX(P) = \bigcap \text{Mod}_{statg}(P) = \{l \mid l \in XG \;\&\; P \models_{statg} l\}$. $GWFSX(P)$ *is said to be the generalized well-founded semantics of P.*

Let $QF = L^0(\,not, \neg, \wedge, \vee)$ be denote the set of quantifier-free sentences (not containing $\rightarrow$) and $C_{statg}(P) = \{F \mid P \models_{statg} F\}$. An inference operation $C : Pow(EGLP) \rightarrow Pow(QF)$ is said to be cumulative iff for every $X \subseteq C(P), X \subseteq QF$ holds $C(P \cup X) = C(P)$. Unfortunately, the operation C_{statg} is not cumulative on the set of all generalized logic programs, thus the important task remains to find natural cumulative approximations of C_{statg} (cf section 6).

5   Extended Normal Logic Programs and WFSX-Semantics

In this section we present the result that for extended normal logic programs the $WFSX$-semantics models introduced in [12] coincides with the partial stationary generated semantics. To make the paper self-contained we recall the main notions. Let $P \subseteq$ ENLP a normal logic program, i.e. the rules r have the form: $r := a_1, \ldots, a_m, not\,b_1, \ldots, not\,b_n \Rightarrow c$, where a_i, b_j, c are objective literals. Such a rule is denoted in the following also by $c \leftarrow a_1, \ldots, a_m, not\,b_1, \ldots, not\,b_n$. Let $I \subseteq \text{OL} \cup not\,\text{OL}$ be a (consistent) partial interpretation.

Definition 10. *Let I be an interpretation and P a (instantiated) program,* $r \in P$. *The I-transformation of r, denoted by* $tr_I(r)$, *is defined as follows:*

- *if* $not\,l \in B(r)$ *and* $l \in I$ *then* $not\,l$ *is replaced by* $tr_I(\,not\,l) = \mathbf{f}$;
- *if* $l \in B(r)$, l *objective and* $\neg l \in I$, *then* l *is replaced by* $tr_I(l) = \mathbf{f}$;
- *if* $l \in B(r)$, l *objective and* $\neg l \notin I$ *then* $tr_I(l) = l$;
- *if* $not\,l \in I$ *then* $tr_I(\,not\,l) = \mathbf{t}$;
- *the remaining default literals* $not\,l$ *are replaced by* $tr_I(\,not\,l) = \mathbf{u}$.

Let be $tr_I(B(r)) = \{tr_I(l) | l \in B(r)\}$, $tr_I(r) = H(r) \leftarrow tr_I(B(r))$, and $tr_I(P) = \{tr_I(r) | r \in P\}$. *Obviously,* $tr_I(P)$ *is a non-negative logic program, also denoted by* P/I.

We now investigate a semi-constructive description of a special AP-model of a non-negative logic program; note that there are consistent non-negative logic programs without a t-least AP-model.

Definition 11. *Let P be a instantiated non-negative normal program. The operator $\Gamma_P : \boldsymbol{I} \to \boldsymbol{I}$ is defined as follows:*
$\Gamma_P(I) = \{l \mid \text{ there is a rule } l \leftarrow B(r) \in [P] \text{ such that } I(\wedge B(r)) = 1\} \cup \{\, not\, l \mid \text{for every rule } r \in [P] \text{ satisfying } H(r) = l \text{ it is } I(\wedge B(r)) = 0\}.$

The operator Γ_P is monotonic with respect to the truth-ordering $\preceq$. We construct a sequence $\{I_n\}_{n<\omega}$ of interpretations as follows. Let $I_0 = \{\, not\, a \mid a \in \text{OL}\}$, i.e. I_0 is the t-least interpretation (it is the least element in the semi-lattice $\mathcal{C} = (\boldsymbol{I}, \preceq)$), and $I_{n+1} = \Gamma_P(I_n)$. Obviously, $I_n \preceq I_{n+1}$, for $n < \omega$. Let be $I_\omega = \Gamma_P^\omega = sup\{I_n : n < \omega\}$. Define $Coh(I) = \{\, not\, \neg l \mid l \in Pos(I)\} \cup I$, $Coh(I)$ is called the coherency-closure of I.

Proposition 7. *Let P be a non-negative normal logic program and I_ω defined as above. If $Coh(I_\omega) = K$ is a consistent interpretation then K is a AP-model of P.*

Proof: Obviously, K is coherent. Let $l \leftarrow B(r) \in [P]$. We have to show that $K(l \leftarrow B(r)) = 1$, by definition: $K(B(r)) \leq K(l)$ or $(K(\neg l) = 1$ and $K(B(r)) = \frac{1}{2})$. We may assume that $K(B(r)) \geq \frac{1}{2}$ (the case $K(B(r)) = 0$ is trivial.)
1) $K(B(r)) = \frac{1}{2}$. If $K(H(r)) \geq \frac{1}{2}$ we are ready. Assume that for $l = H(r)$ we have $K(l) = 0$, i.e. $not\, l \in K$. By the definition of the sequence $\{I_n\}_{n<\omega}$ follows that $not\, l \notin I_\omega$. This implies $\neg l \in I_\omega$ and this verifies $K(r) = 1$.
2) $K(B(r)) = 1$, $B(r) = l_1, \ldots, l_m$. We may assume that $\{l_1, \ldots, l_m\} \subseteq \text{OL}$. By lemma 1 there is a k such that for all $n > k$ we have $\{l_1, \ldots, l_m\} \subseteq I_n$, hence $l \in I_\omega$ and this implies $K(r) = 1$. $\square$

Remark: If $Coh(I_\omega) = K$ is consistent then K is a t-minimal AP-model of P. In general, K is no Pr-model.

Example 6. *Let $P = \{a \leftarrow b;\ \neg a;\ b \leftarrow \mathbf{u}\}$. Then $Coh(I_\omega) = \{\neg a, not\, a, not\, \neg b\}$ is a AP-model, but P has no coherent Pr-model.*

The interpretations $I_1, I_2, \ldots, I_n, \ldots$ are (in general) not coherent. We define a new sequence $J_n = I_n \cup Ch(I_\omega)$, where $Ch(I_\omega) = \{\, not\, \neg l \mid l \in Pos(I)\}$. Obviously, the following conditions are satisfied

- $J_1 \preceq J_2 \preceq \ldots \preceq J_n \preceq \ldots$
- every J_n is coherent
- $I_\omega = sup_{n<\omega} J_n$.

$\{I_n\}_{n<\omega}$ is said to be the *standard sequence with respect to* P, and $\{J_n\}_{n<\omega}$ is called the *coherent standard sequence with respect to* P. We show now that the stationary generated models coincides with the partial stable models in the sense of [1].

Definition 12. *[1] Let be $P \subseteq ENLP$. A coherent interpretation I is a partial stable model of P if $I = Coh(\Gamma_{P/I}^\omega(I_0))$.*

We use the following technical lemma to prove the main result in this section.

Lemma 2. *Let P be a normal extended logic program, I an interpretation. Let be $\{I_n\}_{n<\omega}$ resp. $\{J_n\}_{n<\omega}$ be the standard resp. coherent standard sequence with respect to P/I, and $l \leftarrow B(r) \in [P]$. Then the following conditions are equivalent:*
(1) $I_n(\wedge tr_I(B(r))) \geq \frac{1}{2}$;
(2) $[J_n, I](\wedge B(r)) \geq \frac{1}{2}$ (i.e. $r \in P_{[J_n,I]}$).

Remark: Lemma 2 remains true if in condition 1) and 2) the relation "$\geq \frac{1}{2}$" is replaced by "$=1$".

Proposition 8. *Let P be an extended normal logic program and I a model of P. Then I is a stationary generated AP-model if and only if I is a partial stable model of P.[5]*

Sketch of the Proof: We sketch only one direction. Let I be a partial stable model. By definition we have $I = Coh(\Gamma_{P/I}^\omega(I_0))$, I_0 is the t-least interpretation. Let $I_0 \preceq I_1 \preceq \ldots \preceq I_n \preceq$ be the standard sequence associated to $\Gamma_{P/I}$ and $I_\omega = \Gamma_{P/I}^\omega(I_0)$. Let $J_0 \preceq J_1 \preceq \ldots J_n \preceq$ be the coherent standard sequence defined by $J_n = I_n \cup Coh(Pos(I_\omega))$. We show that $\{J_n | n < \omega\}$ is a stationary chain. One has to show that for every $n < \omega$ the interpretation J_{n+1} is a minimal t-extension of J_n satisfying the following two condition of stationary generatedness:

1. $\forall r(r \in \overline{P}_{[J_n,I]} \rightarrow J_{n+1}(H(r)) = 1)$ and
2. $\forall r(r \in P_{[J_n,I]} \rightarrow J_{n+1}(H(r)) \geq \frac{1}{2}$ or $I(\neg H(r)) = 1)$.

By definition is
$$(*) : J_{n+1} = \{l | l \leftarrow B(r) \in [P/I] \wedge I_n(\wedge tr(B(r)) = 1\} \cup$$
$$\{\, not\, l | \forall (l \leftarrow B(r)) \in [tr_I(P)] : I_n(\wedge B(r)) = 0\} \cup Coh(Pos(I_\omega)).$$

1. Let $l \leftarrow B(r) \in \overline{P}_{[J_n,I]}$, then $[J_n, I](B(r)) = 1$. Let $B(r) = l_1, \ldots, l_s$, $not\, m_1$, $\ldots$, $not\, m_t$. By 1. it is $I(\wedge B(r)) = 1$, hence $tr_I(not\, m_j) = 1$ which yields $I_n(tr_I(B(r))) = 1$, by definition $(*)$ it is $l \in I_{n+1}$ and this implies $l \in J_{n+1}$, hence $J_{n+1}(l) = 1$, $l = H(r)$.

2. Let $l \leftarrow B(r) \in P_{[J_n,I]}$. We have to show that the condition
$$(**): (J_{n+1}(l) \geq \tfrac{1}{2} \vee I(\neg l) = 1)$$
is satisfied. Since $[J_n, I](B(r)) \geq \frac{1}{2}$ this implies $I_n(tr(B(r))) \geq \frac{1}{2}$ for all $r \in P_{[J_n,I]}$. Assume there is a rule $l \leftarrow B(r) \in P_{[J_n,I]}$ such that $(**)$ is not satisfied. Then $J_{n+1} = 0$ and $I(\neg L) < 1$. Then $not\, l \in Neg(\Gamma_P(I_n))$ (if $not\, l \notin Neg(\Gamma_P(I_n))$ this would imply $not\, l \in Coh(Pos(I_\omega))$, which is impossible since $I(\neg l) < 1$). $not\, l \in Neg(\Gamma_P(I_n))$ implies for all $l \leftarrow B(s) \in [P/I]$ the condition $I_n(B(s)) = 0$. But, there is one rule $l \leftarrow B(r) \in P_{[J_n,I]}$. i.e. $[J_n, I](B(r)) \geq \frac{1}{2}$, $B(r) = l_1, \ldots, l_s$, $not\, m_1, \ldots$, $not\, m_t$. It is sufficient to show that $I_n(tr(B(r))) \geq \frac{1}{2}$ which gives a contradiction. The condition $I_n(tr(B(r))) \geq \frac{1}{2}$ follows from lemma 2.

We finally show that for all J such that $J_n \preceq J \preceq J_{n+1}$ satisfying the conditions 1. and 2. it follows $J = J_{n+1}$ (i.e. J_{n+1} is a minimal extension satisfying 1. and

---

[5] A similar proposition may be proved for Pr-models of P.

2.). Assume that J satisfies 1. and 2. From 1. follows that $Pos(J_{n+1}) \subseteq Pos(J)$, hence $Pos(J_{n+1}) = Pos(J)$. It remains to show that $Neg(J_{n+1}) = Neg(J)$ and since $Neg(J_{n+1}) \subseteq Neg(J)$ it is sufficient to show that $Neg(J) \subseteq Neg(J_{n+1})$. From 2. follows for all $r \in P_{[J_n, I]}$ the condition $(J(H(r)) \geq \frac{1}{2} \vee I(\neg H(r)) = 1)$. Assume, by contradiction $Neg(J) \not\subseteq Neg(J_{n+1})$. Then there is a default literal $not\, l \in Neg(J)$ such that $not\, l \notin Neg(J_{n+1})$. Obviously, $not\, l \notin Coh(I_\omega)$, otherwise we would have $not\, l \in Neg(J_{n+1})$ since $Coh(I_\omega)$ is contained in any $Neg(J_n)$. The condition $not\, l \notin Coh(I_\omega)$ implies $I(\neg l) \neq 1$. By assumption $J(l) = 0$; also $not\, l \notin Neg(I_{n+1})$, and by definition of I_{n+1} there is a rule $r \in tr_I(P)$ such that $I_n(B(r)) \geq \frac{1}{2}$ and $H(r) := l$. Let $tr_I(B(s)) = B(r)$. Then, by lemma 2 we have $[J_n, I](B(s)) \geq \frac{1}{2}$; hence $s \in P_{[J_n, I]]}$. Since J satisfies the condition 1. and $I(\neg l) \neq 1$ this implies $J(l) \geq \frac{1}{2}$, which yields a contradiction.$\square$

Let be $P \subseteq ENLP$ and I be a coherent and consistent set of extended literals. We may test whether I is partial stable AP-Model or a partial stable Pr-model by using proposition 8. Let be $\kappa \leq \omega$ and $\{I_n : n < \kappa\}$ a sequence of interpretations satisfying the conditions 1., 2. , and 4. of definition 7 with respect to I. Such a sequence is said to be a successful AP-sequence for (P, I) if $I = sup_{n < \kappa} I_n$ and one of the following conditions is satisfied:

(1) $k = \omega$ and $\{I_n : n < \kappa\}$ does not stabilize at any $m < \kappa$;

(2) $\kappa < \omega$ and $\{I_n : n < \kappa\}$ stabilizes at a number $m < \kappa$.

From proposition 8 and corollary 6 follows:

Proposition 9. *Let P be an extended normal logic program and I be a coherent and consistent interpretation. I is a stationary generated AP-model of P if and only if there exists a successful AP-sequence for (P,I).*

An analogous proposition holds for stationary generated Pr-models.

Example 7. *Let be $P = \{c \leftarrow a; \; a \leftarrow b; \; b \leftarrow not\, b; \; \neg a\}$ and*
$I = \{\neg a, not\, a, not\, c, not\, \neg b, not\, \neg c\}$.
Then there exists a successful AP-sequence for (P,I):
Take $I_0 = \{ not\, a, not\, \neg a, not\, c, not\, \neg c, not\, b, not\, \neg b\}$.
Then $\overline{P}_{[I_0, I]} = \{\neg a\}$ and $P_{[I_0, I]} = \{\neg a, \; b \leftarrow not\, b\}$. Take $I_1 := I$, then I_1 is a minimal t-extension of I_0 such that $I_1(\neg a) = 1$ and $I_1(b) \geq \frac{1}{2}$.
Now consider $\overline{P}_{[I_1, I]} = \{\neg a\}$, and $P_{[I_1, I]} = \{\neg a, \; a \leftarrow b, \; b \leftarrow not\, b\}$. There is a minimal t-extension I_2 of I_1, namely $I_2 = I_1$, such that $I_2(\neg a) = 1$, $I_2(b) \geq \frac{1}{2}$ and $(I_2(a) \geq \frac{1}{2} \vee I(\neg a) = 1)$. Hence, the sequence $\{I_0, I_1, I_2\}$ is a successful AP-sequence for (P, I) of length 2 which stabilizes at 1; it is $I_1 = I_2 = I$.
It is easy to see that there is no successful Pr-sequence for (P, I).

6 Conclusion

By introducing a new general definition of stationary generated models, we have sketched the idea of a *stationary model theory* for logic programs. The conceptual tools presented may be useful for a systematic study of partial models of extended logic programs. One interesting invariant of a model I of P is the set $StatC(I)$ of its stationary chains constructed according to definition 7. Evidently, I is stationary generated if there is a chain in $StatC(I)$ reaching I. Furthermore, it seems to be possible to analyze further extensions of normal logic programs, such as quantifiers in bodies and heads of rules. An interesting task is to find natural cumulative approximations of the inference operation C_{statg}. An inference operation $C : Pow(EGLP) \rightarrow Pow(QF)$ is a cumulative approximation of C_{stat} iff the following conditions are fulfilled:

1. For all $P \subseteq EGLP$ it is $C(P) \subseteq C_{statg}(P)$;
2. for extended normal logic programs P it is $C(P) = C_{statg}(P)$;
3. C is cumulative for arbitrary extended generalized logic programs P, i.e. for for all $X \subseteq C(P) \cap QF$ holds $C(P) = C(P \cup X)$.

Recently, several kinds of semantics were studied beyond the class of normal logic programs. Gelfond and Lifschitz [8], and Przymusinski [13] expand the stable model semantics to the class of disjunctive logic programs admitting two kinds of negation, classical negation $\neg$ and default negation not. Their semantics do not assume coherency, a condition that we consider as very natural.

Super logic programs were introduced in [16], they present a proper subclass of generalized logic programs. The semantics is based on the notion of minimal belief operator which is a part of the *Autoepistemic Logic of Beliefs*, [15]. This approach does not include strong negation and the coherency principle.

Brass and Dix investigate in [3] the so-called D-WFS-semantics for normal disjunctive logic programs. This semantics is defined by an abstract inference operation satisfying certain structural properties of proof-theoretical type. The D-WFS semantics does not determine a proper model theory, furthermore it is not clear how to expand it to generalized logic programs.

Lifschitz, Tang and Turner propose in [10] a semantics for logic programs allowing nested expressions in the heads and the body of the rules. The syntax of these programs is similar to ours, but the semantics differs.

Pearce presents in [11] an elegant characterization of the non-monotonic inference relation associated with the stable model semantics by using intuitionistic logic.

Acknowledgments

The support of the German INIDA and the Portuguese ICCTI organizations is thankfully acknowledged, as well as the Praxis programme MENTAL project 2/2.1/TIT/1593/95. Thanks due to the anonymous referees for their criticism and useful comments.

References

1. J.J.Alferes, L.M.Pereira. Reasoning with Logic Programming, LNAI vol. 1111, 1996, Springer Lecture Notes in Artificial Intelligence
2. J. J. Alferes, H. Herre, L.M. Pereira. Partial Models of Extended Generalized Logic Programs, Report Nr. (2000), University of Leipzig
3. S. Brass and J. Dix. Characterizing D-WFS. Confluence and Iterated GCWA. *Logics in Artificial Intelligence, Jelia'96*, p.268–283,1996, Srpinger LNCS 1121
4. J. Engelfriet and H. Herre. Generated Preferred Models and Extensions of Nonmonotonic Systems; *Logic Programming*, p. 85-99, Proc. of the 1997 International Symposium on LP, J. Maluszinski (ed.), The MIT Press, 1997
5. J. Engelfriet and H. Herre. Stable Generated Models, Temporal Logic and Disjunctive Defaults, *Journal of Logic Programming* 41: 1-25 (1999)
6. M. Gelfond and V. Lifschitz. The stable model semantics for logic programming. In R. A. Kowalski and K. A. Bowen, editors, *Proc. of ICLP*, pages 1070–1080. MIT Press, 1988.
7. M. Gelfond and V. Lifschitz. Logic programs with classical negation. *Proc. of ICLP'90*, pages 579–597. MIT Press, 1990.
8. M. Gelfond and V. Lifschitz. Classical negation in logic programs and disjunctive databases. *New Generation Computing*, 9:365–385, 1991.
9. H. Herre and G. Wagner. Stable Models are Generated by a Stable Chain. *Journal of Logic Programming*, 30 (2): 165-177, 1997
10. V. Lifschitz, L.R. Tang and H. Turner. Nested Expressions in Logic Programs, *Annals of Mathematics and A.I.*, to appear (1999)
11. D. Pearce. Stable inference as intuitionistic validity, *Journal of Logic Programming* 38, 79-91 (1999)
12. L.M.Pereira, J.J.Alferes. Wellfounded semantics for logic programs with explicit negation. In B. Neumann:(ed.) European Conference on AI, 102-106, Wien, 1992
13. T.C. Przymusinski. Stable semantics for disjunctive programs. *New Generation Computing*, 9:401–424, 1991.
14. T.C. Przymusinski. Autoepsitemic Logic of Knolwedge and Belief. *Proc. of the 12th Nat. Conf. on A.I.*, AAAI'94, 952-959
15. T.C. Przymusinski. Well-founded and Stationary Models of Logic Programs; *Annals of Mathematics and Artificial Intelligence*, 12 (1994), 141-187
16. T.C. Przymusinski. Super Logic Programs and Negation as Belief. In: R. Dyckhoff, H. Herre, P. Schroeder-Heister, editors, *Proc. of the 5th Int. Workshop on Extensions of Logic Programming*, Springer LNAI 1050, 229–236

Alternating Fixpoint Theory for Logic Programs with Priority

Kewen Wang[1], Lizhu Zhou[1], and Fangzhen Lin[2]

[1] Department of Computer Science and Technology
Tsinghua University, Beijing, 100084, China
{kewen,dcszlz}@tsinghua.edu.cn
[2] Department of Computer Science
Hong Kong University of Science and Technology
Clear Water Bay, Kowloon, Hong Kong
flin@cs.ust.hk

Abstract. van Gelder's alternating fixpoint theory has proven to be a very useful tool for unifying and characterizing various semantics for logic programs without priority. In this paper we propose an extension of van Gelder's alternating fixpoint theory and show that it can be used as a general semantic framework for logic programs with priority. Specifically, we define three declarative and model-theoretic semantics in this framework for prioritied logic programs: prioritized answer sets, prioritized regular extensions and prioritized well-founded model. We show that all of these semantics are natural generalizations of the corresponding semantics for logic programs without priority. We also show that these semantics have some other desirable properties. In particular, they can handle conflicts caused indirectly by the priorities.

Keywords: Logic programs; alternating fixpoints, priority, answer sets, well-founded model.

1 Introduction

Priorities play an important role in logic programming, and they arise in various applications for various purposes. For example, in inheritance hierarchies, it is generally assumed that more specific rules has precedence over less specific ones, and the exact axiomatization of this intuition has been attempted and investigated extensively by researchers in default reasoning. Other application domains include reasoning about actions and causality, where causal effect rules are considered to be preferred over inertia rules [4], and legal reasoning and diagnosis.

There have been some proposals for axiomatizing prioritized logic programs (for example, [1,5,6,8,12,14,15,19,28]), but as pointed out in [6],they are far from satisfactory. In particular, they cannot handle indirect conflicts. Consider the following program P:

$$
\begin{aligned}
R1 &: \quad p \leftarrow q_1 \\
R2 &: \neg p \leftarrow q_2 \\
R3 &: \quad q_1 \leftarrow \sim w_1 \\
R4 &: \quad q_2 \leftarrow \sim w_2
\end{aligned}
$$

J. Lloyd et al. (Eds.): CL 2000, LNAI 1861, pp. 164–178, 2000.

If a priority between $R1$ and $R2$ is specified, the situation is simple enough to be dealt with by many existing approaches. However, in many cases, we are only informed a priority between $R3$ and $R4$, say $R3 \prec R4$. Intuitively, $R1$ has precedence over $R2$, implicitly, and p should be derived from P rather than $\neg p$. Unfortunately, most of existing semantics for prioritized logic programs are unable to represent such domains.

In this paper, we shall propose an extension to van Gelder's alternative fixed point theory and use it as a uniform semantic framework to give three different semantics to logic programs with priorities. These three semantics have their correspondences for logic programs without priorities, and capture different intuitions about logic programs and are tailored for different application needs.

This paper is organized as follows. Motivated by van Gelder's alternating fixpoint theory [23] and the semi-constructive definition of extensions in default logic [3, 21], in section 3 we develop a semantic framework for prioritized logic programs, in which various semantics can be defined. In particular, we defined three semantics *prioritized answer sets*, *prioritized regular extensions* and *prioritized well-founded model* in section 4 and some demonstrating examples are given. In section 5, we prove some important semantic properties to justify the suitability of our semantics. We prove that these three semantics generalize the traditional well-known answer set semantics, regular extension semantics and well-founded semantics, respectively. The relation of our approach to some other semantics is compared in section 6. Section 7 is our conclusion.

2   Alternating Fixpoints without Priority

In this section, we briefly review the alternating fixpoint theory in [23] and related definitions.

An extended logic program P is a finite set of rules of the form

$$R : \quad l \leftarrow l_1, \ldots, l_r, \sim l_{r+1}, \ldots, \sim l_m$$

where ls with or without subscripts are literals, the symbol $\sim$ is default negation and the symbol $\neg$ is explicit negation. A literal is either an atom a or its explicit negation $\neg a$. The set of literals of P is denoted Lit.

A rule R of an extended logic program is also expressed as $head(R) \leftarrow pos(R), \sim neg(R)$, where $head(R) = l$, $pos(R) = \{l_1, \ldots, l_r\}$ and $neg(R) = \{l_{r+1}, \ldots, l_m\}$.

We assume all logic programs are propositional and each rule R is automatically interpreted into its "semi-normal" rule $head(R) \leftarrow pos(R), \sim neg(R), \sim \neg head(R)$. The reason will be explained later on.

The alternating fixpoint theory, introduced by van Gelder [23], is proven to be a very useful tool to unify and characterize different semantic intuitions for logic programs (without priority). This theory is based on an *immediate consequence mapping* [9].

Let P be an extended logic program and S a set of literals. S is *logically closed* if it is consistent or is Lit.

The GL-transformation P^S of P with respect to S is the logic program (without default negation) $P^S = \{head(R) \leftarrow pos(R) \mid R \in P, neg(R) \cap S = \emptyset\}$. The set $C_P(S)$ of consequences of P^S is the smallest set of literals which is both logically closed and closed under the rules of P^S.

For any set S of literals, $GR(P, S) = \{R \in P \mid pos(R) \subseteq S, neg(R) \cap S = \emptyset\}$ is said to be the generating set of S in P.

Notice that, if $C_P(S)$ is consistent, then $C_P(S) = T_{P^S} \uparrow \omega$, where T_{P^S} is the immediate consequence operator of P^S by considering each negative literal as a new atom. $C_P(S)$ is anti-monotonic, i. e. $C_P(S_1) \subseteq C_P(S_2)$ whenever $S_2 \subseteq S_1$.

The alternating operator $\mathcal{A}_P(S) = C_P^2(S)$ is defined through the immediate consequences $C_P(S)$. It is known that $\mathcal{A}_P$ is a monotonic operator. A fixpoint of $\mathcal{A}_P$ is said to be an *alternating fixpoint* of P. An alternating fixpoint S is normal if $S \subseteq C_P(S)$.

By the alternating fixpoint theory, many semantics for logic programs can be defined including the following three ones [23, 26]:

1. The well-founded model: the least alternating fixpoint.
2. The regular extensions: the maximal normal alternating fixpoints.
3. The answer sets: a special kind of the maximal normal alternating fixpoints (namely, $C_P(S) = S$).

3   Alternating Fixpoints with Priority

As noted in section 2, the existing alternating fixpoint approach considers only logic programs without priority. In this section, we will first define an intuitive generalization of the immediate consequence mapping for extended logic programs with priority, and then establish the corresponding alternating fixpoint theory.

Let P be an extended logic program and $\prec$ an irreflexive and transitive binary relation on rules of P. Then the pair $\mathcal{P} = (P, \prec)$ is said to be a *prioritized logic program*. By $R1 \prec R2$ we mean that $R1$ has precedence over $R2$.

Let S_1 and S_2 be two sets of literals in a prioritized logic program $\mathcal{P}$. A rule R in P is *active* with respect to the pair (S_1, S_2) if $pos(R) \subseteq S_1$ and $neg(R) \cap S_2 = \emptyset$. In particular, if $S_1 = S_2 = S$, then R is active with respect to (S, S) if and only if the body of R is satisfied by S (in the usual sense).

For two rules $R1$ and $R2$ such that $R1 \prec R2$ (i. e. $R1$ has precedence over $R2$), there are often two kinds of existing approaches to represent this preference relation. One is to reflect that $R2$ will not be applied provided that $R1$ is applicable. The other is to reflect that the rule that has higher priority is first applied: (1) if both $R1$ and $R2$ are applicable, $R1$ is first applied. (2) if $R1$ has been applied and $R2$ is applicable, then $R2$ can still be applied.

As argued by Delgrade and Schaub in [7], the second kind of approaches may be more general and thus can be used in wider application domains. The following definition is just designed to reflect the second intuition.

Definition 1. *Let $\mathcal{P} = (P, \prec)$ be a prioritized logic program and S be a set of literals. Set*

$S_0 = \emptyset$,

$S_{i+1} = S_i \cup \{l \mid$ *there exists a rule R of P such that (1) $head(R) = l$ and R is active with respect to (S_i, S) and, (2) no rule $R' \prec R$ is active with respect to (S, S_i) and $head(R') \notin S_i\}$.*

Then the reduct of $\mathcal{P}$ with respect to S is defined as the set of literals $C_{\mathcal{P}}(S) = \cup_{i \geq 0} S_i$ if $\cup_{i \geq 0} S_i$ is consistent. Otherwise, $C_{\mathcal{P}}(S) = Lit$.

The rule R is *accepted by stage $i+1$ with respect to S* if R satisfies the above two conditions in the definition of S_{i+1}. The sequence $S_0, S_1, \ldots, S_i, \ldots$ will be called the $\prec$-sequence of S in $\mathcal{P}$.

We may note that $C_{\mathcal{P}}$ and C_P are two quite different operators. This abusing of notions should cause no confusion in understanding this paper. The main difference of our definition from van Gelder's approach is that we obtain the consequences from $\mathcal{P}$ and S directly. The traditional approaches (i. e. without considering priority) first obtain a positive program from $\mathcal{P}$ with respect to S and then the consequences are derived from this positive program.

Another point on the above definition that should be addressed is why we do not replace the pair (S, S_i) by the pair (S_i, S) in the condition (2) of the definition of S_{i+1}. The reason for this can be explained by the following example.

Example 1. Let $\mathcal{P}$ be a prioritized logic program as follows:

$$
\begin{array}{ll}
R1 & p \leftarrow q \\
R2 & \neg p \leftarrow q'' \\
R3 & q'' \leftarrow q' \\
R4 & q \leftarrow \\
R5 & q' \leftarrow
\end{array}
$$

Here $R2 \prec R1 \prec R3$. We should not infer p since $R2 \prec R1$. Though $R2 \prec R1$, we can not infer p because $R2$ depends on the rule $R3$ and $R1 \prec R3$.

This means that we should assign both p and $\neg p$ the truth value 'undefined'.

However, if we replace (S, S_i) by (S_i, S) in Definition 1, then p is inferred. As a semantics for general purpose, we do not expect such a conclusion, though there also exist some domains that need a more credulous interpretation. Thus, we adopt a skeptical approach in our Definition 1 to treat the conflicts among rules.

The transformation $C_{\mathcal{P}}$ is not a monotonic operator in general, but we can prove its anti-monotonicity.

Lemma 1. *$C_{\mathcal{P}}$ is an anti-monotonic operator. That is, for any two sets S and S' of literals such that $S \subseteq S'$, $C_{\mathcal{P}}(S') \subseteq C_{\mathcal{P}}(S)$.*

Proof. If $S \subseteq S'$, it suffices to prove that, for any number $i \geq 0$,

$$S_i' \subseteq S_i, \qquad\qquad (\star)$$

where S_i and S_i' are defined as Definition 1.

The proof of $(\star)$ is a direct induction on i and thus, we omit it here.

Definition 2. *Let* $\mathcal{P} = (P, \prec)$ *be a prioritized logic program. The* alternating transformation *of* $\mathcal{P}$ *is defined as, for any set* S *of literals,*

$$\mathbf{A}_{\mathcal{P}}(S) = C_{\mathcal{P}}(C_{\mathcal{P}}(S)).$$

Proposition 1. *The operator* $\mathbf{A}_{\mathcal{P}}$ *is monotonic and thus possesses the least fixpoint.*

Proof. It follows from Lemma 1 and Tarski's Theorem.

– A fixpoint of $\mathbf{A}_{\mathcal{P}}$ is called an *alternating fixpoint* of $\mathcal{P}$.

By now, we establish the basic semantic framework for prioritized logic programs by using alternating fixpoint approach, in which a semantics of prioritized logic programs can be defined as a subset of the alternating fixpoints.

4   Semantics for Prioritized Logic Programs

In this section we will define three semantics in the framework established in section 3: *prioritized answer sets, prioritized regular extensions* and *prioritized well-founded model.* Like the traditional answer set semantics and well-founded model without priority, our new semantics are also to represent two intuitions in AI, i.e. maximalism and minimalism. It should be noted that we will omit the adjective 'prioritized' or add an adjective 'unprioritized' when we mention a semantics for logic programs without priority.

To characterize credulous reasoning, it is natural to choose all the maximal alternating fixpoints as the intended models of a prioritized logic program. If S is a maximal alternating fixpoint of prioritized program $\mathcal{P} = (P, \prec)$, it may be the case that $S \nsubseteq C_{\mathcal{P}}(S)$. This case is not what we want since every literal in S should be derived from $\mathcal{P}$ with respect to S for an intended model S.

Definition 3. *Let* $\mathcal{P} = (P, \prec)$ *be a prioritized logic program.* S *is a prioritized regular extension of* $\mathcal{P}$ *if it is a maximal normal alternating fixpoint of* $\mathcal{P}$*: for any normal alternating fixpoint* S' *of* $\mathcal{P}$ *such that* $S \subseteq S'$, $S' = S$.

The prioritized semantics PRE *(i. e. prioritized regular extension semantics) for P is defined as the set of its prioritized regular extensions.*

This definition has the same form as the characterization of the regular extensions without priority in [26].

Example 2. Consider the following prioritized logic program:

$$R1 : q \leftarrow \sim p$$
$$R2 : w \leftarrow \sim w$$

The rule R1 has precedence over R2: $R1 \prec R2$. This prioritized program has the unique prioritized regular extension $S = \{q\}$. Notice that S is not a fixpoint of $C_{\mathcal{P}}$ since $C_{\mathcal{P}}(S) = \{w, q\}$.

Example 3. [3] If we have a knowledge base as follows:

$$R'_1 : \qquad \neg Fly(x) \leftarrow Peguin(x), \sim Fly(x)$$
$$R'_2 : \qquad Winged(x) \leftarrow Bird(x), \sim \neg Winged(x)$$
$$R'_3 : \qquad Fly(x) \leftarrow Winged(x), \sim \neg Fly(x)$$
$$R'_4 : \qquad Bird(x) \leftarrow Peguin(x)$$
$$R'_5 : Peguin(Tweety) \leftarrow$$

By the principle of specificity, $R'_1 \prec R'_2$.

The difference of this example from the classical *Bird-Fly* example is that there is no explicit priority between R'_1 and R'_3 but there is an implicitly specified priority between R'_1 and R'_3: R'_1 has precedence over R'_3 since R'_3 depends on R'_2 and $R'_1 \prec R'_2$.

Intuitively, a suitable semantics for this knowledge base should infer $\neg Fly(Tweety)$ and $Winged(Tweety)$. In particular, any semantics suitable should not contain the set $\{Peguin(Tweety), Bird(Tweety), Fly(Tweety), \{Winged(Tweety)\}$ as a model.

For simplicity, we rewrite the above rules as the following prioritized logic program $\mathcal{P} = (P, \prec)$:

$$R1 : \qquad \neg Fly \leftarrow Peguin, \sim Fly$$
$$R2 : Winged \leftarrow Bird, \sim \neg Winged$$
$$R3 : \qquad Fly \leftarrow Winged, \sim \neg Fly$$
$$R4 : \qquad Bird \leftarrow Peguin$$
$$R5 : \quad Peguin \leftarrow$$

$$R1 \prec R2.$$

Let $S = \{Peguin, Bird, \neg Fly, Winged\}$ and $S' = \{Peguin, Bird, Fly, \{Winged\}$. It can be verified that S is the unique prioritized regular extension but S' is not. However, the prioritized semantics in [6] and [28] admit S' as an intended model.

Another interesting credulous semantics for $\mathcal{P}$ is defined by the set of all fixpoints of $C_{\mathcal{P}}$ (this set is also a set of alternating fixpoints).

Definition 4. *S is said to be a* prioritized answer set *of $\mathcal{P}$ if S is a fixpoint of $C_{\mathcal{P}}$: $C_{\mathcal{P}}(S) = S$.*

The semantics PAS (i. e. prioritized answer set semantics) of $\mathcal{P}$ is defined by the set of all prioritized answer sets of $\mathcal{P}$.

In Example 3, $S = \{Peguin, Bird, \neg Fly, Winged\}$ is also a prioritized answer set of $\mathcal{P}$. In general, each prioritized answer set is a prioritized regular extension. But a prioritized regular extension may not be a prioritized answer set as Example 2 has shown.

Proposition 2. *If S is a prioritized answer set of $\mathcal{P}$, then S is also a prioritized regular extension of $\mathcal{P}$.*

However, it should be noted that our definition of prioritized answer sets can not 'tolerate' too unreasonable ordering. For instance, if P has three rules $R1 : q \leftarrow w$, $R2 : p \leftarrow\sim v$ and $R3 : w \leftarrow$. Suppose $R1 \prec R2 \prec R3$, then, intuitively, $R1$ should not have precedence over $R3$ since $R1$ depends on $R3$. It is not hard to verify that $\mathcal{P} = (P, \prec)$ has no prioritized answer set though P has the unique answer set $\{w, p, q\}$.

The third semantics that will be defined in our semantic framework is named the *prioritized well-founded model*, which is to characterize skeptical reasoning in artificial intelligence as the traditional well-founded semantics does.

Definition 5. *The prioritized well-founded model of $\mathcal{P} = (P, \prec)$ is defined as the least alternating fixpoint of $\mathcal{P} = (P, \prec)$.*

The semantics PWF *(i. e. prioritized well-founded semantics) of $\mathcal{P}$ is defined by the prioritized well-founded model of $\mathcal{P}$.*

Proposition 3. *Every prioritized logic program has the unique prioritized well-founded model.*

Proof. It follows directly from Proposition 1.

This proposition shows that our prioritized well-founded semantics also possesses an important semantic property: *completeness*.

One often criticized deficiency of the well-founded model without priority is that it is too skeptical that, in many cases, nothing useful can be derived from programs under the well-founded semantics. In certain degree, our prioritized well-founded semantics may overcome this problem as the following two examples demonstrate. This will also be shown theoretically in the next section.

Example 4.

$$R1 : p \leftarrow \sim q$$
$$R2 : q \leftarrow \sim p$$

$R1 \prec R2$. Then the prioritized well-founded model of $\mathcal{P} = (P, \prec)$ is $\{p\}$. Notice that the well-founded model of P is $\emptyset$.

The next example further shows how to resolve conflicts with the prioritized well-founded model.

Example 5. Imagine such a scenario: when a train is approaching a bridge, the robot driver is told that a bomb may be put under the bridge and thus, he stops the train. He is also told that he cannot pass the bridge if this reported bomb is not found. Afterwards, he is told again that enough evidence proves that there is no such a bomb under the bridge. According to our commonsense, at this moment, the train can pass the bridge. This knowledge can be represented as an extended logic program P as follows:

$$
\begin{aligned}
R1 : &\quad \neg pass \leftarrow \sim bombFound, \sim pass \\
R2 : &\quad pass \leftarrow \neg bomb, \sim \neg pass \\
R3 : &\ \neg bombFound \leftarrow \neg bomb \\
R4 : &\quad \neg bomb \leftarrow
\end{aligned}
$$

$R2 \prec R1$ because the rule $R2$ is newer than $R1$.

It can be verified that the prioritized well-founded model of $\mathcal{P} = (P, \prec)$ is $\{\neg bomb, \neg bombFound, pass\}$, which is just our intuition on this program. But the ordinary well-founded semantics can not say 'yes' or 'no' about 'pass'. Notice that $\neg pass$ cannot be added to S_1 since $R2 \prec R1$ and $R2$ is active with respect to (S, S_0) (though $R1$ is active with respect to (S, S_0)).

As mentioned before, if both rules $R1$ and $R2$ appear in $\mathcal{P}$ and their heads are complementary literals, then we understand these rules as their corresponding semi-normal counterparts. For example, if P consists of two rules $R1 : p \leftarrow\sim q$ and $R2 : \neg p \leftarrow\sim q$, and let $R1 \prec R2$. Then P is actually understood as $\{p \leftarrow\sim q, \sim \neg q; \neg p \leftarrow\sim q, \sim p\}$. Under this assumption, the prioritized program $\mathcal{P}$ has the unique intended model $\{p\}$. Otherwise, $\mathcal{P}$ will be inconsistent.

5   Properties of Prioritized Semantics

Currently there are many different proposals about the semantics of logic programs with priorities ([5, 6, 8, 14, 15, 19, 28]). It is too early to say which one will eventually prevail. In the meantime, it may be useful to look at reasonable "postulates" that a sound semantics should satisfy. Recently, Brewka and Eiter [6] proposed two such postulates:

P1. Let B_1 and B_2 be two belief sets of a prioritized theory $(T, <)$ generated by the (ground) rules $R \cup \{d_1\}$ and $R \cup \{d_2\}$, where $d_1, d_2 \notin R$, respectively. If d_1 is preferred over d_2, then B_2 is not an intended belief set of T.

P2. Let B be an intended belief set of a prioritized theory $(T, <)$ and r a (ground) rule such that at least one prerequisite of r is not in B. Then B is an intended belief set of $(T \cup \{r\}, <')$ whenever $<'$ agrees with $<$ on priorities among rules in T.

Unfortunately, many of the existing prioritized semantics do not satisfy their postulates as pointed out by Brewka and Eiter [6], and it is not clear whether the fault is with most of the current semantics or that their postulates are too strict. However, at least the following example shows that *P1* is not so intuitive. Let $(P, <)$ be the following logic programs with $r_1 < d_1 < d_2$:

$$r_1 \quad bird \leftarrow$$
$$d_1 \quad \neg fly \leftarrow peguin$$
$$d_2 \quad fly \leftarrow not\ peguin, bird$$

We observe that: (1) $\neg peguin$ and $bird$ should be included in the intended belief set; and (2) the rule d_1 is defeated by r_1; and thus (3) d_2 could be used to derive further beliefs. Accordingly, the intended belief set should be $B = \{bird, \neg peguin, fly\}$. But, if we take $R = \{r_1\}$, *P1* does not allow d_2 is used in the case that d_1 is defeated.

In this paper, we are going to play on the safe side and consider some relationships between semantics for logic programs with priorities and those without. In this direction, we notice that for logic programs without priorities, there are some well understood semantics such as the well-founded model and answer set semantics. It seems to us reasonable then that proposed new semantics for logic programs with priorities should be an extension of one of the semantics for logic programs without priorities. Since, as is well-known, all major semantics for logic programs without priorities agree on logic programs that are stratified, this means that for any stratified logic program, if the priorities associated with the rules are consistent with the stratification, then any semantics for this prioritied logic program should agree as well. In particular, they should agree with the perfect model semantics, which is indeed the case for our three semantics, as we shall show in this section. It should be noted that many semantics for prioritized logic programs are only defined for total orderings and thus, these semantics do not possess the above mentioned properties.

We start with the following lemma which will be very crucial in proving the results of this section. In the following, we assume that all programs are finite propositional programs.

Lemma 2. *Let S be a set of literals in $\mathcal{P} = (P, \prec)$. Then*

1. *$C_{\mathcal{P}}(S) \subseteq C_P(S)$.*
2. *if $S \subseteq C_{\mathcal{P}}(S)$, then $C_{\mathcal{P}}(S) = C_P(S)$.*
3. *if $\prec$ is empty, then $C_{\mathcal{P}}(S) = C_P(S)$.*

Proposition 4. *For any prioritized logic program $\mathcal{P} = (P, \prec)$, each prioritized regular extension of $\mathcal{P}$ is contained in a regular extension of P. In particular, if the relation $\prec$ is empty, then S is a prioritized regular extension of $\mathcal{P}$ if and only if S is a regular extension of P.*

This proposition reveals two connections between prioritized regular extension and unprioritized regular extension: (1) the adding of some priority makes the information represented by the logic program without priority more concrete (the number of 'models' and the number of elements in each 'model' are all reduced in general). (2) when the priority relation is empty (i. e. there is no preferences among rules), the prioritized regular extension semantics is the same as the unprioritized regular extension semantics. These two properties seem to be natural.

The next proposition convinces that our prioritized answer sets generalize Gelfond and Lifschitz's answer sets [10].

Proposition 5. *A prioritized answer set of $\mathcal{P} = (P, \prec)$ is also an answer set of P. In particular, if $\prec$ is empty, S is a prioritized answer set of $\mathcal{P} = (P, \prec)$ iff S is an answer set of P.*

Like the well-founded model without priority, the prioritized well-founded model also possesses the property of completeness.

Proposition 6. *Every prioritized logic program has a prioritized well-founded model.*

Proof. It follows directly from Proposition 1.

The relationship between the well-founded model and the prioritized well-founded model can be stated as follows.

Proposition 7. *Let M_p be the prioritized well-founded model of $\mathcal{P} = (P, \prec)$ and M the well-founded model of P. Then $M \subseteq M_p$. In particular, if $\prec = \emptyset$, then $M = M_p$.*

Proof. If $M_p = Lit$, then $M = Lit$, the conclusion is obvious. We need only consider the case when M_p is consistent. Since M_p is a normal alternating fixpoint of $\mathcal{P}$, it follows that M_p is a normal alternating fixpoint of P by Lemma 2. Since the well-founded model M is the least alternating fixpoint of P, we have $M \subseteq M_p$.

The last part is obvious from Lemma 2.

Proposition 7 and Example 4 show that the prioritized well-founded semantics is less skeptical than the traditional well-founded semantics in general. This proposition also makes it possible to overcome the drawback (i. e. too skeptical) of the traditional well-founded model by adding preferences to rules of logic programs.

In the rest of this section, we study the relation of our three prioritized semantics to the perfect model [2, 20]. The perfect model semantics of stratified logic programs has already been well-accepted. Moreover, a stratification of a stratified program P actually determines a priority on rules of the program and thus a prioritized logic program $\mathcal{P}$ is obtained. Intuitively, a suitable semantics for priority should be consistent with the perfect model. Namely, $\mathcal{P}$ should has the unique 'model' M and M is exactly the perfect model of P for any stratified logic program.

The following proposition will convince that the prioritized regular extensions, prioritized answer sets and prioritized well-founded model exactly reflect the semantic intuition above.

Definition 6. *A logic program P (without explicit negation) is said to be stratified if P has a partition (i. e. stratification) $P = P_1 \cup \cdots \cup P_t$ such that the following conditions are satisfied:*

1. *$P_i \cap P_j = \emptyset$ for $i \neq j$.*
2. *If a rule R is in P_i, then the atoms in $pos(R)$ can appear only in $\cup_{j=1}^{i} P_j$ and the atoms in $neg(R)$ can appear only in $\cup_{j=1}^{i-1} P_j$.*

We recall that $pos(R)$ is the set of atoms that appear positively in the body of R; $neg(R)$ is the set of atoms that appear negatively in the body of R.

The perfect model of the stratified logic program P is recursively defined as follows.

- $P_1' := P_1$ and $M_1 := T_{P_1'} \uparrow \omega$.
- $P_{i+1}' := \{p \leftarrow \ | \ p \in M_i\} \cup \{head(R) \leftarrow pos(R) \ | \ R \in P_{i+1}, neg(R) \cap M_i = \emptyset\}$, and $M_{i+1} := T_{P_{i+1}'} \uparrow \omega$.

Let P be a stratified logic program and $P = P_1 \cup \cdots \cup P_t$ a stratification of P. A natural priority relation $\prec_s$ on P can be defined as:

for any $R1$ and $R2$ in P, $R1 \prec_s R2$ if and only if $R1 \in P_i$ and $R2 \in P_j$ such that $i < j$.

Thus, we obtain a prioritized logic program $\mathcal{P} = (P, \prec_s)$ for any given stratified logic program P and a stratification.

Proposition 8. *Let the prioritized logic program* $\mathcal{P} = (P, \prec_s)$ *be defined as above and the perfect model of P is M_t. Then*

1. *$\mathcal{P}$ has the unique prioritized answer set M_t.*
2. *$\mathcal{P}$ has the unique prioritized regular extension M_t.*
3. *$\mathcal{P}$ has the unique prioritized well-founded model M_t.*

Proposition 5 states that each prioritized answer set of a prioritized logic program $\mathcal{P} = (P, \prec)$ is also an answer set of P. In turn, we will show that, for each answer set S of a logic program P, there is an ordering $\prec$ on rules of P such that S is the unique prioritized answer set of $\mathcal{P} = (P, \prec)$.

Proposition 9. *Let P be a logic program and S an answer set of P. Then there is a well-order $\prec$ such that S is the unique prioritized answer set of the prioritized program $\mathcal{P} = (P, \prec)$.*

As noted previously, a totally ordered $\mathcal{P}$ may have no prioritized answer set. But we will prove that, when the rules in P are totally ordered, $\mathcal{P} = (P, \prec)$ has at most one prioritized answer set.

Proposition 10. *Let $\prec$ is a total ordering on the rules of logic program P. If $\mathcal{P} = (P, \prec)$ has prioritized answer set, then it has the unique one.*

The two results above illustrate that, for any prioritized program $\mathcal{P} = (P, \prec)$ such that $\prec$ is a total ordering, its prioritized answer set semantics $PAS(\mathcal{P})$ always outputs either nothing or the unique prioritized answer set (i. e. an answer set of P).

6   Comparison to Related Approaches

Several approaches treating priorities in the setting of logic programming have been described in the literature. In this section, we summarize their relationships to our approach.

Both preferred answer sets in [6] and prioritized answer sets in [28] extend Gelfond and Lifschitz's answer sets to handle rules with priority. Like our approach, they assume a priority among rules of logic program. The basic idea behind their approaches (though very different) is to transform a prioritized logic program $\mathcal{P}$ into a unprioritized program and the answer sets of $\mathcal{P}$ are defined through the GL-answer sets of the obtained program. As shown in Example 3, these semantics cannot correctly resolve conflicts caused by indirectly or implicitly specified priorities.

Another interesting definition of preferred answer sets was defined in [22]. This approach assumes a preference among the set of atoms of program and bears a similar idea as the perfect model of stratified programs [2, 20].

Brewka's preferred well-founded model in [5] extends the well-founded model to treat logic programs with priority. His approach is different from our prioritized well-founded model in at least two aspects: (1) he represents priority in object level; (2) given a set of literals S, he first gradually extends the empty set to a set of rules and then obtains a set of literals as the transformation of S. But we directly extend the empty set and obtain the transformation of S. Though the precise relationship between Brewka's and ours is not clear, we still believe these two semantics have some close connection.

Two argumentation-based semantics for prioritized logic programs are defined in [27, 19]. These approaches are also semantic frameworks for logic programs with priority. Clearly, their intuition is quite different from ours and they also obtain different semantics from ours. The approach in [27] is to characterize the first kind of semantic intuition mentioned in section 1. For example, let P consists two rules: $R1 : bird \leftarrow peguin$ and $R2 : peguin \leftarrow$. If $R1$ has precedence over $R2$, our semantics allows to derive $peguin$ and $bird$. But theirs allows to derive only $peguin$. The difference between the semantics in [19] and our approach can be illustrated by Example 2. According to our and Brewka's approaches, P has the unique model $\{p\}$, but under Prakken and Sartor's semantics, the priority between $R1 : p \leftarrow \sim q$ and $R2 : q \leftarrow \sim p$ has not effect on the reasoning in P. Namely, this prioritized program has two models $\{p\}$ and $\{q\}$ under their semantics.

Both our approach and BH-prioritized default logic [3] employ the semi-constructive definition of default extensions [21] and our prioritized answer sets correspond to the BH-extensions. But they are different semantics as shown in the following example.

Example 6. Let P consist of the following rules:

$$R1 : \quad p \leftarrow w, \sim q, \sim \neg p$$
$$R2 : \neg p \leftarrow \sim q, \sim p$$
$$R3 : \quad w \leftarrow$$

Here, $R1 \prec R2$.

It can be verified that $\mathcal{P} = (P, \prec)$ has the unique prioritized answer set $S = \{w, p\}$. This set should be the intended semantics. But if we regard P as a set of defaults and take $W = \emptyset$, then the prioritized default theory $(P, W, \prec)$ has the unique BH-extension S' and S' contains $\neg p$ rather than p.

Marek, Nerode and Remmel [15] propose a bottom-up procedure for computing the answer sets of a logic program P when the rules of P are totally ordered. For each stable model S of P, there is a total ordering on P such that their procedure outputs S. This procedure is not sound with respect to our prioritized answer sets.

Example 7. Let P consist of the following rules:

$$R1 : q \leftarrow \sim p$$
$$R2 : w \leftarrow \sim v$$
$$R3 : p \leftarrow w$$

Here, $R1 \prec R2 \prec R3$. Then the procedure proposed in [14] outputs the set $\{q\}$ which is not a stable model of P. Under our semantics, $\mathcal{P}$ has the unique prioritized answer set $\{w.p\}$.

There are also some other approaches about treating priority in default logic and logic programming, such as [7, 8, 11], we will not discuss them here.

7 Conclusion

We have proposed a framework for studying logic programs with priorities based on van Gelder's alternating fixpoint theory for logic programs without priorities. To illustrate the usefulness of this framework, we have proposed three different semantics: PAS (the prioritized answer sets), PWF (the prioritized well-founded model) and PRE (prioritized regular extensions), all of which have counterparts for logic programs without priorities, and have some additional properties. We believe that this framework is simple and intuitive. In the full version of this paper (see [25]), we shall show that the semantics defined by our prioritized answer sets can also be used to represent defeasible causal theories. Hopefully, this theory might provide a unifying framework for different semantics with priority. Currently, we are also working on extending the augmentation-theoretic framework in [24] to disjunctive logic programs with priority.

Recently, Marek, Truszczynski [16] and Niemelä [18] discussed the stable model semantics (answer set semantics) as the foundation of a computational logic programming system (i.e. SLP). This system differs from standard logic programming systems in several aspects including the following two important points:

- In the SLP, each program is assigned a collection of intended models rather than a single model.
- In the SLP, the rules of a program are interpreted as *constraints* on objects to be computed.

Similar to the methods of solving constraint satisfaction problems, there are two steps to develop an SLP program for a given application domain: (1) to specify an SLP program whose set of answer sets encodes the general domain of candidate objects. (2) to add to this program more rules representing *constraints* that must be enforced.

As shown in [16, 18], many constraint satisfaction problems can be solved in SLP. However, if the preferences among rules are also enforced as constraints to the program obtained in the first step, the task of representing and solving application domains will most probably become simpler and more powerful. Thus, the semantics with priority may provide a suitable framework for SLP.

Acknowledgments

We would like to thank the anonymous referees for their useful comments. This work was supported in part by the Natural Science Foundation of China (No. 69883008, 69773027), the National Foundation Research Program of China (No. G1999032704), and the IT School of Tsinghua University.

References

1. A. Analyti, S. Pramanik. Reliable semantics for extended logic programs with rule prioritization. *Journal of Logic and Computation*, 303-325, 1995.
2. K. Apt, H. Blair and A. Walker. Towards a theory of declarative knowledge. In: J. Minker ed. *Foundations of Deductive Databases and Logic Programming*, Morgan Kaufmann, Washington, pages 89-148, 1988.
3. F. Badder, B. Hollunder. Priorities on defaults with prerequisites, and their application in treating specificity in terminological default logic. *Journal of Automated Reasoning*, 15(1), 41-68, 1995.
4. C. Baral, J. Lobo. Defeasible specifications in action theories. In: *Proceedings of IJCAI'97*, Morgan Kaufmann, pages 1441-1446, 1997.
5. G. Brewka. Well-founded semantics for extended logic programs with dynamic preferences. *J. AI Research*, 4: 19-36, 1996.
6. G. Brewka, T. Either. Preferred answer sets for extended logic programs, *Artificial Intelligence*, 109(1-2), 295-356, 1999.
7. J. Delgrade, T. Schaub. Compiling reasoning with and about preferences in default logic. In: *Proc. IJCAI'97*, pages 168-174, 1997.
8. D. Gabbay, E. Laenens and D. Vermeir. Credulous vs. skeptical semantics for ordered logic programs. In: *Proc. KR'92*, pages 208-217, 1992.
9. M. Gelfond, V. Lifschitz. The stable model semantics for logic programming, in *Logic Programming: Proc. Fifth Intl Conference and Symposium*, pages 1070-1080, MIT Press, 1988.
10. M. Gelfond, V. Lifschitz. Classical negation in logic programs and disjunctive databases. *New Generation Computing*, 9: 365-386, 1991.
11. M. Gelfond, T. Son. Reasoning with prioritized defaults. In: *Proc. LPKR'97 (LNAI1471)*, Springer, pages 164-233, 1998.
12. E. Laenens, D. Vermeir. A fixpoint semantics for ordered logic. *Journal of Logic and Computation*, 1:159-185, 1990.
13. F. Lin. Embracing causality in specifying the indirect effects of actions. In: *Proc. IJCAI'95*, pages 1985-1991, 1995.
14. W. Marek, A. Nerode and J. B. Remmel. Basic forward chaining construction for logic programs. In *Logic Foundations of Computer Science* (LNCS 1234), Springer, 1997.
15. W. Marek, A. Nerode and J. B. Remmel. Logic programs, well-ordering, and forward chaining. *Journal of Pure and Applied Logic*, 96(1-3):231-76, 1999.
16. W. Marek, M. Truszczynski. Stable models and an alternative logic programming paradigm. In: *The Logic Programming Paradigm: a 25-Year Perspective*, Springer, pages 375-398, 1999.
17. J. McCarthy, P. Hayes. Some philosophical problems from the standpoint of artificial intelligence. In: B. Meltzer and D. Michie eds. *Machine Intelligence*, vol.4, pages 463-502, 1969.

18. I. Niemelä. Logic programs with stable model semantics as a constraint programming paradigm. In: *Proc. the Workshop on Computational Aspects of Nonmonotonic Reasoning*, pages 72-79, 1998.

19. H. Prakken, G. Sartor. Argument-based logic programming with defeasible priorities. *J. Applied Non-Classical Logics*, 7: 25-75, 1997.

20. T. Przymusinski. On the declarative semantics of deductive databases and logic programming. In: J. Minker ed. *Foundations of Deductive Databases and Logic Programming*, Morgan Kaufmann, Washington, pages 193-216, 1988.

21. R. Reiter. A logic for default reasoning. *Artificial Intelligence*, 13(1-2), 81-132, 1980.

22. C. Sakama, K. Inoue. Representing priorities in logic programs. In: *Proc. IJC-SLP'96*, MIT Press, pages 82-96, 1996.

23. A. van Gelder. The alternating fixpoint of logic programs with negation. *Journal of Computer and System Science*, 47: 185-120, 1993.

24. K. Wang. Argumentation-based abduction in disjunctive logic programming. *Journal Logic Programming* (47 pages, to appear), 2000.

25. K. Wang, L. Zhou and F. Lin. A semantic framework for prioritized logic programs and its application to causal theories. Tech. report TUCS-9906, 1999.

26. J. You, L. Yuan. Three-valued semantics of logic programming: is it needed? In *Proc. the 9th ACM PODS*, pages 172-182, 1990.

27. J. You, X. Wang and L. Yuan. Disjunctive logic programming as constrained inferences. In: *Proc. ICLP'97*, MIT Press, 1997.

28. Y. Zhang, N. Foo. Answer sets for prioritized logic programs. In: *Proc. the 1997 International Symposium on Logic Programming*, MIT Press, pages 69-83, 1997.

Proving Failure in Functional Logic Programs*

Francisco J. López-Fraguas and Jaime Sánchez-Hernández

Dep. Sistemas Informáticos y Programación, Univ. Complutense de Madrid
{fraguas,jaime}@sip.ucm.es

Abstract. How to extract negative information from programs is an important issue in logic programming. Here we address the problem for functional logic programs, from a proof-theoretic perspective. The starting point of our work is *CRWL* (Constructor based ReWriting Logic), a well established theoretical framework for functional logic programming, whose fundamental notion is that of non-strict non-deterministic function. We present a proof calculus, *CRWLF*, which is able to deduce negative information from *CRWL*-programs. In particular, *CRWLF* is able to prove 'finite' failure of reduction within *CRWL*.

1 Introduction

We address in this paper the problem of extracting negative information from functional logic programs. The question of negation is a main topic of research in the logic programming field, and the most common approach is *negation as failure*, as an easy effective approximation to the *CWA* (*closed world assumption*), which is a simple, but uncomputable, way of deducing negative information from positive programs (see e.g. [1] for a survey on negation in logic programming).

On the other hand, functional logic programming (*FLP* for short) is a powerful programming paradigm trying to combine the nicest properties of functional and logic programming (see [4] for a now 'classical' survey on *FLP*). *FLP* subsumes *pure* logic programming: predicates can be defined as functions returning the value 'true', for which definite clauses can be written as conditional rewrite rules. In some simple cases it is enough, to handle negation, just to define predicates as two-valued boolean functions returning the values 'true' or 'false'. But negation as failure is far more expressive, and it is then of clear interest to investigate a similar notion for the case of *FLP*. Failure in logic programs, when seen as functional logic programs, corresponds to failure of reduction to 'true'. This generalizes to a natural notion of failure in *FLP*, which is 'failure of reduction'.

As technical setting for our work we have chosen *CRWL* [3], a well established theoretical framework for *FLP*. The fundamental notion in *CRWL* is that of non-strict non-deterministic function, for which *CRWL* provides a firm logical basis, as mentioned for instance in [5]. Instead of equational logic, *CRWL* considers a Constructor based ReWriting Logic, presented by means of a proof calculus,

---

* The authors have been partially supported by the Spanish CICYT (project TIC 98-0445-C03-02 'TREND').

J. Lloyd et al. (Eds.): CL 2000, LNAI 1861, pp. 179–193, 2000.

which determines what statements can be deduced from a given program. In addition to the proof-theoretic semantics, [3] develop a model theoretic semantics for $CRWL$, with existence of distinguished free term models for programs, and a sound and complete lazy narrowing calculus as operational semantics. The $CRWL$ framework (with many extensions related to types, HO and constraints) has been implemented in the system $\mathcal{TOY}$ [8].

Here we are interested in extending the proof-theoretic side of $CRWL$ to cope with failure. More concretely, we look for a proof calculus, which will be called $CRWLF$ ('$CRWL$ with failure'), which is able to prove failure of reduction in $CRWL$. Since reduction in $CRWL$ is expressed by proving certain statements, our calculus will provide proofs of unprovability within $CRWL$. As for the case of CWA, unprovability is not computable, which means that our calculus can only give an approximation, corresponding to cases which can be intuitively described as 'finite failures'.

There are very few works about negation in FLP. In [10] the work of Stuckey about *constructive negation* [12] is adapted to the case of FLP with strict functions and innermost narrowing as operational mechanism. In [11] a similar work is done for the case of non-strict functions and lazy narrowing. The approach is very different of the proof-theoretic view of our work. The fact that we also consider non-deterministic functions makes a significant difference.

The proof-theoretic approach, although not very common, has been followed sometimes in the logic programming field, as in [6], which develops for logic programs (with negation) a framework which resembles, in a very general sense, $CRWL$: a program determine a deductive system for which deducibility, validity in a class of models, validity in a distinguished model and derivability by an operational calculus are all equivalent. Our work attempts to be the first step of what could be a similar program for FLP extended with the use of failure as a programming construct.

The rest of the paper is organized as follows. In Section 2 we give the essentials of $CRWL$ which are needed for our work. Section 3 presents the $CRWLF$-calculus, preceded by some illustrative examples. Section 4 contains the results about $CRWLF$. Most of the results are technically involved, and their proofs have been skipped because of the lack of space (full details can be found in [9]). Section 5 contains some conclusions.

2   The $CRWL$ Framework

We give here a short summary of $CRWL$, in its proof-theoretic face. Model theoretic semantics and lazy narrowing operational semantics are not considered here. Full details can be found in [3].

2.1   Technical Preliminaries

We assume a signature $\Sigma = DC_\Sigma \cup FS_\Sigma$ where $DC_\Sigma = \bigcup_{n \in \mathbb{N}} DC_\Sigma^n$ is a set of *constructor* symbols and $FS_\Sigma = \bigcup_{n \in \mathbb{N}} FS_\Sigma^n$ is a set of *function* symbols, all of them with associated arity and such that $DC_\Sigma \cap FS_\Sigma = \emptyset$. We also assume a countable set $\mathcal{V}$ of *variable* symbols. We write $Term_\Sigma$ for the set of (total) *terms* (we say also *expressions*) built up with Σ and $\mathcal{V}$ in the usual way, and we distinguish the subset $CTerm_\Sigma$ of (total) constructor terms or (total) *c-terms*, which only make use of DC_Σ and $\mathcal{V}$. The subindex Σ will usually be omitted. Terms intend to represent possibly reducible expressions, while c-terms represent data values, not further reducible.

We will need sometimes to use the signature $\Sigma_\perp$ which is the result of extending Σ with the new constant (0-arity constructor) $\perp$, that plays the role of the undefined value. Over $\Sigma_\perp$, we can build up the sets $Term_\perp$ and $CTerm_\perp$ of (partial) terms and (partial) c-terms respectively. Partial c-terms represent the result of partially evaluated expressions; thus, they can be seen as approximations to the value of expressions.

As usual notations we will write $X, Y, Z, \ldots$ for variables, $c, d, \ldots$ for constructor symbols, $f, g, \ldots$ for functions, $e, e', \ldots$ for terms and $s, t, \ldots$ for c-terms.

We will use the sets of substitutions $CSubst = \{\theta : \mathcal{V} \to CTerm\}$ and $CSubst_\perp = \{\theta : \mathcal{V} \to CTerm_\perp\}$. We write $e\theta$ for the result of applying θ to e.

Given a set of constructor symbols S we say that the terms t and t' have an S-clash if they have different constructor symbols of S at the same position.

2.2   The Proof Calculus for *CRWL*

A *CRWL*-program $\mathcal{P}$ is a set of conditional rewrite rules of the form:

$$\underbrace{f(t_1, \ldots, t_n)}_{head} \to \underbrace{e}_{body} \Leftarrow \underbrace{C_1, \ldots, C_n}_{condition}$$

where $f \in FS^n$; $(t_1, \ldots, t_n)$ is a linear tuple (each variable in it occurs only once) with $t_1, \ldots, t_n \in CTerm$; $e \in Term$ and each C_i is a constraint of the form $e' \bowtie e''$ (*joinability*) or $e' \diamondsuit e''$ (*divergence*) where $e', e'' \in Term$. The reading of the rule is: $f(t_1, \ldots, t_n)$ reduces to e if the conditions $C_1, \ldots, C_n$ are satisfied. We write $\mathcal{P}_f$ for the set of defining rules of f in $\mathcal{P}$.

From a given program $\mathcal{P}$, the proof calculus for *CRWLF* can derive three kinds of statements:

- *Reduction or approximation statements*: $e \to t$, with $e \in Term_\perp$ and $t \in CTerm_\perp$. The intended meaning of such statement is that e can be reduced to t, where reduction may be done by applying rewriting rules of $\mathcal{P}$ or by replacing subterms of e by $\perp$. If $e \to t$ can be derived, t represents one of the possible values of the denotation of e.
- *Joinability statements*: $e \bowtie e'$, with $e, e' \in Term_\perp$. The intended meaning in this case is that e and e' can be both reduced to some common totally defined value, that is, we can prove $e \to t$ and $e' \to t$ for some $t \in CTerm$.
- *Divergence statements*: $e \diamondsuit e'$, with $e, e' \in Term_\perp$. The intended meaning now is that e and e' can be reduced to some (possibly partial) c-terms t and t' such that they have a DC-clash.

Table 1. Rules for $CRWL$-provability

$$(1) \quad \frac{}{e \to \bot}$$

$$(2) \quad \frac{}{X \to X} \qquad X \in \mathcal{V}$$

$$(3) \quad \frac{e_1 \to t_1, ..., e_n \to t_n}{c(e_1, ..., e_n) \to c(t_1, ..., t_n)} \qquad c \in DC^n, \quad t_i \in CTerm_\bot$$

$$(4) \quad \frac{e_1 \to s_1, ..., e_n \to s_n \quad C \quad e \to t}{f(e_1, ..., e_n) \to t} \qquad \begin{array}{l} \text{if } t \not\equiv \bot, R \in \mathcal{P}_f \\ (f(s_1, ..., s_n) \to e \Leftarrow C) \in [R]_\bot \end{array}$$

$$(5) \quad \frac{e \to t \quad e' \to t}{e \bowtie e'} \qquad \text{if } t \in CTerm$$

$$(6) \quad \frac{e \to t \quad e' \to t'}{e \diamondsuit e'} \qquad \text{if } t, t' \in CTerm_\bot \text{ and have a } DC-\text{clash}$$

It must be mentioned that the $CRWL$ framework as presented in [3] does not consider divergence conditions. They have been incorporated to $CRWL$ in [7] as a useful and expressive resource for programming.

When using function rules to derive statements, we will need to use what are called *c-instances* of such rules: the set of c-instances of a program rule R is defined as $[R]_\bot = \{R\theta | \theta \in CSubst_\bot\}$. This allows, in particular, to express parameter passing.

Table 1 shows the proof calculus for $CRWL$. We write $\mathcal{P} \vdash_{CRWL} \varphi$ for expressing that the statement φ is provable from the program $\mathcal{P}$.

The rule 4 allows to use c-instances of program rules to prove approximations. These c-instances may contain $\bot$ and rule (1) allows to reduce any expression to $\bot$. This reflects a non-strict semantics.

A distinguished feature of $CRWL$ is that functions can be *non-deterministic*. For example, assuming the constructors z (zero) and s (successor) for natural numbers, a non-deterministic function $coin$ can defined by the rules $coin \to z$ and $coin \to s(z)$. The use of c-instances in rule (4) instead of general instances corresponds to *call time choice* semantics for non-determinism (see [3]). As an example, if in addition to $coin$ we consider the function definition $mkpair(X) \to pair(X,X)$ ($pair$ is a constructor), it is possible to build a $CRWL$-proof for $mkpair(coin) \to pair(z,z)$ and also for $mkpair(coin) \to pair(s(z),s(z))$, but not for $mkpair(coin) \to pair(z,s(z))$.

Observe that $\diamondsuit$ is not the logical negation of $\bowtie$. They are not even incompatible: due to non-determinism, two expressions e, e' can satisfy both $e \bowtie e'$ and $e \diamondsuit e'$ (although this cannot happen if e, e' are c-terms). In the 'coin' example, we can derive both $coin \bowtie z$ and $coin \diamondsuit z$.

We can define the *denotation* of an expression e as the set of c-terms to which e can be reduced according to this calculus: $[\![e]\!] = \{t \in CTerm_\bot | \mathcal{P} \vdash_{CRWL} e \to t\}$

3 The *CRWLF* Framework

We now address the problem of failure in *CRWL*. Our primary interest is to obtain a calculus able to prove that a given expression fails to be reduced. Since reduction corresponds in *CRWL* to approximation statements $e \rightarrow t$, we can reformulate our aim more precisely: we look for a calculus able to prove that a given expression e has no possible reduction (other than the trivial $e \rightarrow \perp$) in *CRWL*, i.e., $\llbracket e \rrbracket = \{\perp\}$.

Of course, we cannot expect to achieve that with full generality since, in particular, the reason for having $\llbracket e \rrbracket = \{\perp\}$ can be non-termination of the program as rewrite system, which is uncomputable. Instead, we look for a suitable computable approximation to the property $\llbracket e \rrbracket = \{\perp\}$, corresponding to cases where failure of reduction is due to 'finite' reasons, which can be constructively detected and managed.

Previous to the formal presentation of the calculus, which will be called *CRWLF* (for '*CRWL* with failure') we give several simple examples for a preliminary understanding of some key aspects of it, and the reasons underlying some of its technicalities.

3.1 Some Illustrative Examples

Consider the following functions, in addition to *coin* , defined in Sect. 2:

$$f(z) \rightarrow f(z) \qquad g(s(s(X))) \rightarrow z \qquad \begin{array}{l} h \rightarrow s(z) \\ h \rightarrow s(h) \end{array} \qquad k(X) \rightarrow z \Leftarrow X \bowtie s(z)$$

The expressions $f(z)$ and $f(s(z))$ fail to be reduced, but for quite different reasons. In the first case $f(z)$ does not terminate. The only possible proof accordingly to *CRWL* is $f(z) \rightarrow \perp$ (by rule 1); any attempt to prove $f(z) \rightarrow t$ with $t \neq \perp$ would produce an 'infinite derivation'. In the second case, the only possible proof is again $f(s(z)) \rightarrow \perp$, but if we try to prove $f(s(z)) \rightarrow t$ with $t \neq \perp$ we have a kind of '*finite failure*': rule 4 needs to solve the parameter passing $s(z) \rightarrow z$, that could be finitely checked as failed, since no rule of the *CRWL*-calculus is applicable. The *CRWLF*-calculus does not prove non-termination of $f(z)$, but will be able to detect and manage the failure for $f(s(z))$. In fact it will be able to perform a *constructive proof* of this failure.

Consider now the expression $g(coin)$. Again, the only possible reduction is $g(coin) \rightarrow \perp$ and it is intuitively clear that this is another case of finite failure. But this failure is not as simple as in the previous example for $f(s(z))$: in this case the two possible reductions for *coin* to defined values are $coin \rightarrow z$ and $coin \rightarrow s(z)$. Both of z and $s(z)$ fail to match the pattern $s(s(X))$ in the rule for g, but none of them can be used separately to detect the failure of $g(coin)$. A suitable idea is to collect the set of defined values to which a given expression can be reduced. In the case of *coin* that set is $\{z, s(z)\}$. The fact that $\mathcal{C}$ is the collected set of values of e is expressed in *CRWLF* by means of the statement $e \lhd \mathcal{C}$. In our example, *CRWLF* will prove $coin \lhd \{z, s(z)\}$. Statements $e \lhd \mathcal{C}$

generalize the approximation statements $e \to t$ of $CRWL$, and in fact can replace them. Thus, $CRWLF$ will not need to use explicit $e \to t$ statements.

How far should we go when collecting values? The idea of collecting all values (and to have them completely evaluated) works fine in the previous example, but there are problems when the collection is infinite. For example, according to its definition above, the expression h can be reduced to any positive natural number, so the corresponding set would be $\{s(z), s(s(z)), s(s(s(z))), ...\}$. Then, what if we try to reduce the expression $f(h)$?. From an intuitive point of view it is clear that the value z will not appear in this set, because all the values in it have the form $s(...)$. We can represent all this values by the set $\{s(\bot)\}$. Here we can understand $\bot$ as an *incomplete information*: we know that all the possible values for h are successor of 'something'; we do not know what is this 'something', but in fact, we do not need to know it. Anyway the set does not contain the value z, so $f(h)$ fails. Notice that all the possible values for h are represented (not present) in the set $\{s(\bot)\}$, and this information is sufficient to prove the failure of $f(h)$. The $CRWLF$-calculus will be able to prove the statement $h \lhd \{s(\bot)\}$, and we say that $\{s(\bot)\}$ is a *Sufficient Approximation Set* (*SAS*) for h.

In general, an expression will have multiple *SAS*'s. Any expression has $\{\bot\}$ as its simplest *SAS*. And, for example, the expression h has an infinite number of *SAS*'s: $\{\bot\}, \{s(\bot)\}, \{s(z), s(s(\bot))\}, ...$ The *SAS*'s obtained by the calculus for *coin* are $\{\bot\}, \{\bot, s(\bot)\}, \{\bot, s(z)\}, \{z, \bot\}, \{z, s(\bot)\}$ and $\{z, s(z)\}$. The $CRWLF$-calculus provides appropriate rules for working with *SAS*'s. The derivation steps will be guided by these *SAS*'s in the same sense that $CRWL$ is guided by approximation statements.

Failure of reduction is due in many cases to failure in proving the conditions in the program rules. The calculus must be able to prove those failures. Consider for instance the expression $k(z)$. In this case we would try to use the c-instance $k(z) \to z \Leftarrow z \bowtie s(z)$ that allows to perform parameter passing. But the condition $z \bowtie s(z)$ is clearly not provable, so $k(z)$ must fail. For achieving it we must be able to give a proof for '$z \bowtie s(z)$ *cannot be proved with respect to CRWL*'. For this purpose we introduce a new constraint $e \not\bowtie e'$ that will be true if we can build a *proof of non-provability* for $e \bowtie e'$. In our case, $z \not\bowtie s(z)$ is clear simply because of the clash of constructors. In general the proof for a constraint $e \not\bowtie e'$ will be guided by the corresponding *SAS*'s for e and e' as we will see in the next section. As our initial $CRWL$ framework also allows constraints of the form $e \diamond e'$, we need still another constraint $\not\diamond$ for expressing 'failure of $\diamond$'.

There is another important question to justify: we use an explicit representation for failure by means of the new constant symbol F. Let us examine some examples involving failures. First, consider the expression $g(s(f(s(z))))$; for reducing it we would need to do parameter passing, i.e., matching $s(f(s(z)))$ with some c-instance of the pattern $s(s(X))$ of the definition of g. As $f(s(z))$ fails to be reduced the parameter passing must also fail. If we take $\{\bot\}$ as an *SAS* for $f(s(z))$ we have not enough information for detecting the failure (nothing can be said about the matching of $s(s(X))$ and $s(\bot)$). But if we take $\{F\}$ as an *SAS* for $f(s(z))$, this provides enough information to ensure that $s(F)$ cannot match any c-instance of the pattern $s(s(X))$. Notice that we allow the value F to appear inside the term $s(\text{F})$. It could appear that the information $s(\text{F})$ is essentially the same of F (for instance, F also fails to match any c-instance of $s(s(X))$), but this is not true in general. For instance, the expression $g(s(s(f(s(z)))))$ is reducible to z. But if we take the *SAS* $\{\text{F}\}$ for $f(s(z))$ and we identify the expression $s(s(f(s(z))))$ with F, matching with the rule for g would not succeed, and the reduction of $g(s(s(f(s(z)))))$ would fail.

We can now proceed with the formal presentation of the *CRWLF*-calculus.

3.2   Technical Preliminaries

We introduce the new constant symbol F into the signature Σ to obtain $\Sigma_{\perp,\text{F}} = \Sigma \cup \{\perp, \text{F}\}$. The sets $Term_{\perp,\text{F}}, CTerm_{\perp,\text{F}}$ are defined in the natural way and we will use the set $CSubst_{\perp,\text{F}} = \{\theta : \mathcal{V} \to CTerm_{\perp,\text{F}}\}$.

A natural *approximation ordering* $\sqsubseteq$ over $Term_{\perp,\text{F}}$ can be defined as the least partial ordering over $Term_{\perp,\text{F}}$ satisfying the following properties:

- $\perp \sqsubseteq e$ for all $e \in Term_{\perp,\text{F}}$,
- $h(e_1, ..., e_n) \sqsubseteq h(e'_1, ..., e'_n)$, if $e_i \sqsubseteq e'_i$ for all $i \in \{1, ..., n\}$, $h \in DC \cup FS$

The intended meaning of $e \sqsubseteq e'$ is that e is less defined or has less information than e'. Two expressions $e, e' \in Term_{\perp,\text{F}}$ are *consistent* if they can be refined to obtain the same information, i.e., if there exists $e'' \in Term_{\perp,\text{F}}$ such that $e \sqsubseteq e''$ and $e' \sqsubseteq e''$.

Notice that the only relations satisfied by F are $\perp \sqsubseteq \text{F}$ and $\text{F} \sqsubseteq \text{F}$. In particular, F is maximal. This is reasonable, since F represents 'failure of reduction' and this gives a no further refinable information about the result of the evaluation of an expression. This contrasts with the status given to failure in [11], where F is chosen to verify $\text{F} \sqsubseteq t$ for any t different from $\perp$.

The class of programs that we consider in the following is less general than in the *CRWL* framework. Rules of functions have the same form, but they must not contain *extra variables*, i.e., for any rule $(f(\bar{t}) \to e \Leftarrow \overline{C}) \in \mathcal{P}$ all the variables appearing in e and $\overline{C}$ must also appear in the head $f(\bar{t})$, i.e., $var(e) \cup \mathcal{V}(\overline{C}) \subseteq var(\bar{t})$. In *FLP* with non-deterministic functions this is not *as* restrictive as it could appear: function nesting can replace the use (typical in logic programming) of variables as repositories of intermediate values, and in many other cases where extra variables represent unknown values to be computed by search, they can be successfully replaced by non-deterministic 'lazy generating' functions (see [3] for some examples).

We will frequently use the following notation: given $e \in Term_{\perp,\text{F}}$, $\hat{e}$ stands for the result of replacing by $\perp$ all the occurrences of F in e (notice that $\hat{e} \in Term_{\perp}$, and $e = \hat{e}$ iff $e \in Term_{\perp}$).

3.3   The Proof Calculus for $CRWLF$

In $CRWLF$ five kinds of statements can be deduced:

- $e \lhd \mathcal{C}$, intended to mean '$\mathcal{C}$ is an SAS for e'.
- $e \bowtie e'$, $e \Diamond e'$, with the same intended meaning as in $CRWL$.
- $e \not\bowtie e'$, $e \not\Diamond e'$, intended to mean failure of $e \bowtie e'$ and $e \Diamond e'$ respectively.

We will sometimes speak of $\bowtie, \Diamond, \not\bowtie, \not\Diamond$ as 'constraints', and use the symbol $\Diamond$ to refer to any of them. The constraints $\not\bowtie$ and $\bowtie$ are called the *complementary* of each other; the same holds for $\not\Diamond$ and $\Diamond$, and we write $\widetilde{\Diamond}$ for the complementary of $\Diamond$.

When proving a constraint $e\Diamond e'$ the calculus $CRWLF$ will evaluate an SAS for the expressions e and e'. These SAS's will consist of c-terms from $CTerm_{\bot,F}$, and provability of the constraint $e\Diamond e'$ depends on certain syntactic (hence decidable) relations between those c-terms. Actually, the constraints $\bowtie, \Diamond, \not\bowtie$ and $\not\Diamond$ can be seen as the result of generalizing to expressions the relations $\downarrow, \uparrow, \not\downarrow$ and $\not\uparrow$ on c-terms, which we define now.

Definition 1 (Relations over $CTerm_{\bot,F}$).

- $t \downarrow t' \Leftrightarrow_{def} t = t', t \in CTerm$
- $t \uparrow t' \Leftrightarrow_{def} t$ and t' have a DC-clash
- $t \not\downarrow t' \Leftrightarrow_{def} t$ or t' contain F as subterm or they have a DC-clash
- $\not\uparrow$ is defined as the least symmetric relation over $CTerm_{\bot,F}$ satisfying:
  - i) $X \not\uparrow X$, for all $X \in \mathcal{V}$
  - ii) $F \not\uparrow t$, for all $t \in CTerm_{\bot,F}$
  - iii) if $t_1 \not\uparrow t'_1, ..., t_n \not\uparrow t'_n$ then $c(t_1, ..., t_n) \not\uparrow c(t'_1, ..., t'_n)$ for all $c \in DC^n$

The relations $\downarrow$ and $\uparrow$ do not take into account the presence of F, which behaves in this case as $\bot$. The relation $\downarrow$ is *strict* equality, i.e., equality restricted to total c-terms. It is the notion of equality used in lazy functional or functional-logic languages as the suitable approximation to 'true' equality ($=$) over $CTerm_{\bot}$. The relation $\uparrow$ is a suitable approximation to '$\neg =$', and hence to '$\neg \downarrow$' (where $\neg$ stands for logical negation). The relation $\not\downarrow$ is also an approximation to '$\neg \downarrow$', but in this case using failure information ($\not\downarrow$ can be read as '$\downarrow$ fails'). Notice that $\not\downarrow$ does not imply '$\neg =$' anymore (we have, for instance, $F \not\downarrow F$). Similarly, $\not\uparrow$ is also an approximation to '$\neg \uparrow$' which can be read as '$\uparrow$ fails'.

The following proposition reflects these and more good properties of $\downarrow, \uparrow, \not\downarrow, \not\uparrow$.

Proposition 1. *The relations $\downarrow, \uparrow, \not\downarrow, \not\uparrow$ verify*

(a) *For all $t, t', s, s' \in CTerm_{\bot,F}$*
  - (i) $t \downarrow t' \Leftrightarrow \hat{t} \downarrow \hat{t}'$ and $t \uparrow t' \Leftrightarrow \hat{t} \uparrow \hat{t}'$
  - (ii) $t \uparrow t' \Rightarrow t \not\downarrow t' \Rightarrow \neg(t \downarrow t')$
  - (iii) $t \downarrow t' \Rightarrow t \not\uparrow t' \Rightarrow \neg(t \uparrow t')$

(b) $\downarrow, \uparrow, \not\downarrow, \not\uparrow$ *are monotonic, i.e., if $t \sqsubseteq s$ and $t' \sqsubseteq s'$ then: $t\Re t' \Rightarrow s\Re s'$, where $\Re \in \{\downarrow, \uparrow, \not\downarrow, \not\uparrow\}$. Furthermore $\not\downarrow_B$ and $\not\uparrow_B$ are the greatest monotonic approximations to $\neg \downarrow_B$ and $\neg \uparrow_B$ respectively, where $\Re_B$ is the restriction of $\Re$ to the set of basic (i.e., without variables) c-terms from $CTerm_{\bot,F}$.*

(c) $\downarrow$ *and* $\uparrow$ *are closed under substitutions from* $CSubst$; $\not\downarrow$ *and* $\uparrow$ *are closed under substitutions from* $CSubst_{\perp,F}$

By *(b)*, we can say that $\downarrow, \uparrow, \not\downarrow, \not\uparrow$ behave well with respect to the information ordering: if they are true for some terms, they remain true if we refine the information contained in the terms. Furthermore, *(b)* states that $\not\downarrow, \not\uparrow$ are defined in the best way, at least for basic c-terms. For c-terms with variables, we must take care: for instance, given the constructor z, we have $\neg(X \downarrow z)$, but not $X \not\downarrow z$. Actually, to have $X \not\downarrow z$ would violate a basic intuition about free variables in logical statements: if the statement is true, it should be true for any value (taken from an appropriate range) substituted for its free variables. The part *(c)* shows that the definitions of $\downarrow, \uparrow, \not\downarrow, \not\uparrow$ respect such principle. Propositions 2 and 3 of the next section show that monotonicity and closedness by substitutions are preserved when generalizing $\downarrow, \uparrow, \not\downarrow, \not\uparrow$ to $\bowtie, \diamondsuit, \not\bowtie, \not\diamondsuit$.

Table 2 contains the $CRWLF$-calculus. Some of the rules use a generalized notion of c-instances of a rule R: $[R]_{\perp,F} = \{R\theta \mid \theta \in CSubst_{\perp,F}\}$. We will use the notation $\mathcal{P} \vdash_{CRWLF} \varphi$ ($\mathcal{P} \not\vdash_{CRWLF} \varphi$ resp.) for expressing that the statement φ is provable (is not provable resp.) with respect to the calculus $CRWLF$ and the program $\mathcal{P}$.

The first three rules are analogous to those of the $CRWL$-calculus, now dealing with SAS's instead of simple approximations (notice the cross product of SAS's in rule 3). In rule 4, for evaluating an expression $f(\overline{e})$ we produce SAS's for the arguments e_i and then, for each combination of values in these SAS's and each program rule for f, a part of the whole SAS is produced; all of them are unioned to obtain the final SAS for $f(\overline{e})$. This is quite different from rule 4 in $CRWL$: there we could use any c-instance of any rule for f; here we need to consider simultaneously the contribution of each rule to achieve 'complete' information about the values to which the expression can be evaluated. We use the notation $f(\overline{t}) \lhd_R \mathcal{C}$ to indicate that only the rule R is used to produce $\mathcal{C}$.

Rules 5 to 8 consider all the possible ways in which a concrete rule R can contribute to the SAS of a call $f(\overline{t})$, where the arguments $\overline{t}$ are all in $CTerm_{\perp,F}$ (come from the evaluation of the arguments of a previous call $f(\overline{e})$). Rules 5 and 6 can be viewed as *positive* contributions. The first one obtains the trivial SAS and 6 works if there is a c-instance of the rule R with a head identical to the head of the call (parameter passing); in this case, if the constraints of this c-instance are provable, then the resulting SAS is generated by the body of the c-instance. Rules 7 and 8 consider the *negative* or *failed* contributions. Rule 7 applies when parameter passing can be done, but it is possible to prove the complementary $e_i \tilde{\diamond} e_i'$ of one of the constraints $e_i \diamond e_i'$ in the condition of the used c-instance. In this case the constraint $e_i \diamond e_i'$ (hence the whole condition in the c-instance) fails. Finally, rule 8 considers the case in which parameter passing fails because of a $DC \cup \{F\}$-clash between one of the arguments in the call and the corresponding pattern in R.

We remark that for given $f(\overline{t})$ and R, the rule 5 and exactly one of rules 6 to 8 are applicable. This fact, although intuitive, is far from being trivial to prove and constitutes in fact an important technical detail in the proofs of the

Table 2. Rules for $CRWLF$-provability

---

(1) $\dfrac{}{e \lhd \{\bot\}}$

(2) $\dfrac{}{X \lhd \{X\}} \qquad X \in \mathcal{V}$

(3) $\dfrac{e_1 \lhd \mathcal{C}_1 \quad \ldots \quad e_n \lhd \mathcal{C}_n}{c(e_1, \ldots, e_n) \lhd \{c(t_1, \ldots, t_n) \mid \bar{t} \in \mathcal{C}_1 \times \ldots \times \mathcal{C}_n\}} \qquad c \in DC^n \cup \{\mathsf{F}\}$

(4) $\dfrac{e_1 \lhd \mathcal{C}_1 \quad \ldots \quad e_n \lhd \mathcal{C}_n \quad \ldots \quad f(\bar{t}) \lhd_R \mathcal{C}_{R,\bar{t}} \quad \ldots}{f(e_1, \ldots, e_n) \lhd \bigcup_{R \in \mathcal{P}_f, \bar{t} \in \mathcal{C}_1 \times \ldots \times \mathcal{C}_n} \mathcal{C}_{R,\bar{t}}} \qquad f \in FS^n$

(5) $\dfrac{}{f(\bar{t}) \lhd_R \{\bot\}}$

(6) $\dfrac{e \lhd \mathcal{C} \quad \overline{C}}{f(\bar{t}) \lhd_R \mathcal{C}} \qquad (f(\bar{t}) \to e \Leftarrow \overline{C}) \in [R]_{\bot,\mathsf{F}}$

(7) $\dfrac{e_i \diamondsuit e_i'}{f(\bar{t}) \lhd_R \{\mathsf{F}\}} \qquad (f(\bar{t}) \to e \Leftarrow \ldots, e_i \diamondsuit e_i', \ldots) \in [R]_{\bot,\mathsf{F}}, \text{ where } i \in \{1, \ldots, n\}$

(8) $\dfrac{}{f(t_1, \ldots, t_n) \lhd_R \{\mathsf{F}\}} \qquad \begin{array}{l} R \equiv (f(s_1, \ldots, s_n) \to e \Leftarrow \overline{C}), t_i \text{ and } s_i \text{ have a} \\ DC \cup \{\mathsf{F}\}\text{-clash for some } i \in \{1, \ldots, n\} \end{array}$

(9) $\dfrac{e \lhd \mathcal{C} \quad e' \lhd \mathcal{C}'}{e \bowtie e'} \qquad \exists t \in \mathcal{C}, t' \in \mathcal{C}' \ t \downarrow t'$

(10) $\dfrac{e \lhd \mathcal{C} \quad e' \lhd \mathcal{C}'}{e \Diamond e'} \qquad \exists t \in \mathcal{C}, t' \in \mathcal{C}' \ t \uparrow t'$

(11) $\dfrac{e \lhd \mathcal{C} \quad e' \lhd \mathcal{C}'}{e \not\bowtie e'} \qquad \forall t \in \mathcal{C}, t' \in \mathcal{C}' \ t \not\downarrow t'$

(12) $\dfrac{e \lhd \mathcal{C} \quad e' \lhd \mathcal{C}'}{e \not\Diamond e'} \qquad \forall t \in \mathcal{C}, t' \in \mathcal{C}' \ t \not\uparrow t'$

---

results in the next section. We also remark that, for the sake of a better reading of rule 4, we have written ordinary set union for collecting SAS's. This could be modified in such a way that F is excluded from the union if it contains some other c-term different from F. For example, if we obtain the SAS's $\{z\}$ and $\{\mathsf{F}\}$ from two function rules, we could take $\{z\}$ as the final SAS for the call instead of $\{\mathsf{F}, z\}$. All the results of the next section are valid with this modification.

Rules 9 to 12 deal with constraints. With the use of the relations $\downarrow, \uparrow, \not\downarrow, \not\uparrow$ introduced in Sect. 3.3 the rules are easy to formulate. For $e \bowtie e'$ it is sufficient to find two c-terms in the SAS's verifying the relation $\downarrow$, what in fact is equivalent to find a common totally defined c-term such that both expressions e and e' can be reduced to it (observe the analogy with rule 5 of $CRWL$). For the complementary constraint $\not\bowtie$ we need to use all the information of SAS's in order to check the relation $\not\downarrow$ over all the possible pairs. The explanation of rules 11 and 12 is quite similar.

The next example shows a derivation of failure using the *CRWLF*-calculus.

Example 1. Let us consider a program $\mathcal{P}$ with the constructors z, s for natural numbers, $[]$ and ':' for lists (although we use Prolog-like notation for them, that is, $[z, s(z)|L]$ represents the list $(z : (s(z) : L))$) and also the constructors t, f that represent the boolean values *true* and *false*. Assume the functions *coin* and h defined in Sect. 2.2 and also the function *mb* (member) defined as:

$$mb(X, [Y|Ys]) \to t \Leftarrow X \bowtie Y$$
$$mb(X, [Y|Ys]) \to t \Leftarrow mb(X, Ys) \bowtie t$$

If we try to evaluate the expression $mb(coin, [s(h)])$ it will fail. Intuitively, from definition of h the list in the second argument can be reduced to lists of the form $[s(s(...))]$ and the possible values of *coin*, z and $s(z)$, will never belong to those lists. The *CRWLF*-calculus allows to build a proof for this fact, that is, $mb(coin, [s(h)]) \lhd \{f\}$, in the following way: by application of rule 4 the proof could proceed by generating *SAS*'s for the arguments

$$coin \lhd \{z, s(z)\} \quad (\varphi_1) \qquad [s(h)] \lhd \{[s(s(\bot))]\} \quad (\varphi_2)$$

and then collecting the contributions of rules of *mb* for each possible combination of values for the arguments; for the pair $(z, [s(s(\bot))])$ the contribution of rules for *mb* (here we write $\lhd_1$ to refer to the first rule of *mb* and $\lhd_2$ for the second) will be

$$mb(z, [s(s(\bot))]) \lhd_1 \{f\} \quad (\varphi_3) \qquad mb(z, [s(s(\bot))]) \lhd_2 \{f\} \quad (\varphi_4)$$

and for the pair $(s(z), [s(s(\bot))])$ we will have

$$mb(s(z), [s(s(\bot))]) \lhd_1 \{f\} \quad (\varphi_5) \qquad mb(s(z), [s(s(\bot))]) \lhd_2 \{f\} \quad (\varphi_6)$$

The following derivation shows the form of the full derivation, but we only give details of the proofs for φ_3 and φ_4. At each step, we indicate by a number on the left the rule of the calculus applied in each case:

$$
\cfrac{
  \cfrac{
    \cfrac{
      \cfrac{1}{\bot \lhd \{\bot\}}
    }{3 \; \cfrac{}{s(\bot) \lhd \{s(\bot)\}}}
    \quad
    {}^3\cfrac{z \lhd \{z\} \quad {}^3 s(s(\bot)) \lhd \{s(s(\bot))\}}{11 \; \cfrac{z \bowtie\!\!\!\!/ \; s(s(\bot))}{}}
  }{}
  \;\;
  \varphi_1 \; \varphi_2 \quad {}_7\cfrac{}{\varphi_3 \equiv mb(z, [s(s(\bot))]) \lhd_1 \{f\}}
  \quad
  \cfrac{
    {}^3 z \lhd \{z\} \quad {}^3 [] \lhd \{[]\} \quad {}^8 mb(z, []) \lhd_{1,2} \{f\}
  }{4 \; \cfrac{mb(z, []) \lhd \{f\}}{11 \; \cfrac{mb(z, []) \bowtie\!\!\!\!/ \; \{t\}}{{}_7 \varphi_4 \equiv mb(z, [s(s(\bot))]) \lhd_2 \{f\}}}}
  \quad {}^3\cfrac{}{t \lhd \{t\}}
  \;\; \varphi_5 \; \varphi_6
}{4 \; mb(coin, [s(h)]) \lhd \{f\}}
$$

In both φ_3 and φ_4 the failure is due to a failure in the constraints of rules, what requires to prove the complementary constraint $\bowtie\!\!\!\!/$ by rule 11. In the first case, $z \bowtie\!\!\!\!/ \; s(s(\bot))$, there is a clear clash of constructors. But in the second case it involves the failure for the expression $mb(z, [])$ that is proved again by rule 4 of the calculus. The *SAS*'s for the arguments only produce the combination $(z, [])$ and both rules of *mb* fails over it by rule 8 of the calculus. The notation $mb(z, []) \lhd_{1,2} \{f\}$ which appears on the top of the proof of φ_4 is an abbreviation for both statements $mb(z, []) \lhd_1 \{f\}$ and $mb(z, []) \lhd_2 \{f\}$.

All the contributions of $\varphi_3, \varphi_4, \varphi_5$ and φ_6 are $\{f\}$, and putting them together we obtain $\{f\}$ as an *SAS* for the original expression $mb(coin, [s(h)])$ as expected.

4   Properties of $CRWLF$

In this section we explore some properties of the $CRWLF$-calculus and its relation with $CRWL$. In the following we assume a fixed program $\mathcal{P}$.

The non-determinism of the $CRWLF$-calculus allows to obtain different SAS's for the same expression. As the SAS for an expression is a finite approximation to the denotation of the expression it is expected some kind of consistency between SAS's for the same expression. Given two of them, we cannot ensure that one SAS must be more defined than the other in the sense that all the elements of the first are more defined than all of the second. For instance, two SAS's for $coin$ are $\{\perp, s(z)\}$ and $\{z, \perp\}$. The kind of consistency for SAS's that we can expect is the following:

Definition 2 (Consistent Sets of c-Terms). *Two sets* $\mathcal{C}, \mathcal{C}' \subset CTerm_{\perp,F}$ *are consistent iff for all* $t \in \mathcal{C}$ *there exists* $t' \in \mathcal{C}'$ *(and vice versa, for all* $t' \in \mathcal{C}'$ *there exists* $t \in \mathcal{C}$*) such that* t *and* t' *are consistent.*

Our first result states that two different SAS's for the same expression must be consistent.

Theorem 1 (Consistency of SAS). *Given* $e \in Term_{\perp,F}$*, if* $\mathcal{P} \vdash_{CRWLF} e \lhd \mathcal{C}$ *and* $\mathcal{P} \vdash_{CRWLF} e \lhd \mathcal{C}'$*, then* $\mathcal{C}$ *and* $\mathcal{C}'$ *are consistent.*

This result is a trivial corollary of part $a)$ of the following lemma.

Lemma 1 (Consistency). *For any* $e, e', e_1, e_2, e_1', e_2' \in Term_{\perp,F}$

a) *If* e, e' *are consistent,* $\mathcal{P} \vdash_{CRWLF} e \lhd \mathcal{C}$ *and* $\mathcal{P} \vdash_{CRWLF} e' \lhd \mathcal{C}'$*, then* $\mathcal{C}$ *and* $\mathcal{C}'$ *are consistent.*

b) *If* e_1, e_1' *are consistent and* e_2, e_2' *are also consistent, then:* $\mathcal{P} \vdash_{CRWLF} e_1 \Diamond e_2 \Rightarrow$ $\mathcal{P} \not\vdash_{CRWLF} e_1' \tilde{\Diamond} e_2'$

As a trivial consequence of part $b)$ we have:

Corollary 1. $\mathcal{P} \vdash_{CRWLF} e \Diamond e' \Rightarrow \mathcal{P} \not\vdash_{CRWLF} e \tilde{\Diamond} e'$*, for all* $e, e' \in Term_{\perp,F}$

This supports our original idea about $\not\bowtie$ and $\tilde{\Diamond}$ as computable approximations to the negations of $\bowtie$ and $\Diamond$.

Another desirable property of our calculus is *monotonicity*, that we can informally understand in this way: the information that can be extracted from an expression can not decrease when we add information to the expression itself. This also reflects in the fact that if we can prove a constraint and we consider more defined terms in both sides of it, the resulting constraint must be also provable. Formally:

Proposition 2 (Monotonicity of $CRWLF$). *For* $e, e', e_1, e_2, e_1', e_2' \in Term_{\perp,F}$

a) *If* $e \sqsubseteq e'$ *and* $\mathcal{P} \vdash_{CRWLF} e \lhd \mathcal{C}$*, then* $\mathcal{P} \vdash_{CRWLF} e' \lhd \mathcal{C}$

b) *If* $e_1 \sqsubseteq e_1'$*,* $e_2 \sqsubseteq e_2'$ *and* $\mathcal{P} \vdash_{CRWLF} e_1 \Diamond e_2$ *then* $\mathcal{P} \vdash_{CRWLF} e_1' \Diamond e_2'$*, where* $\Diamond \in \{\bowtie, \not\bowtie, \Diamond, \tilde{\Diamond}\}$

Monotonicity, as stated here, refers to the degree of evaluation of expression, and does not contradict the well known fact that negation as failure is a non-monotonic reasoning rule. In our setting it is also clearly true that, if we 'define more' the functions (i.e, we refine the program, not the evaluation of a given expression), an expression can become reducible when it was previously failed.

The next property says that what is true for free variables is also true for any possible (totally defined) value, i.e., provability in $CRWLF$ is closed under total substitutions.

Proposition 3. *For any* $\theta \in CSubst$, $e, e' \in Term_{\perp,F}$

a) $\mathcal{P} \vdash_{CRWLF} e \lhd \mathcal{C} \Rightarrow \mathcal{P} \vdash_{CRWLF} e\theta \lhd \mathcal{C}\theta$
b) $\mathcal{P} \vdash_{CRWLF} e \lozenge e' \Rightarrow \mathcal{P} \vdash_{CRWLF} e\theta \lozenge e'\theta$

4.1 $CRWLF$ Related to $CRWL$

The $CRWLF$-calculus has been built as an extension of $CRWL$ for dealing with failure. Here we show that our aims have been achieved.

We recall that a $CRWLF$-program is a $CRWL$-program not containing extra variables in rules. The following results are all referred to $CRWLF$-programs.

The next result shows that the $CRWLF$-calculus indeed extends $CRWL$. Parts a) and b) show that statements $e \lhd \mathcal{C}$ generalize approximation statements $e \to t$ of $CRWL$. Parts c) and d) show that $CRWLF$ and $CRWL$ are able to prove exactly the same joinabilities and divergences (if F is ignored for the comparison).

Proposition 4. *For any* $e, e' \in Term_{\perp,F}$

a) $\mathcal{P} \vdash_{CRWLF} e \lhd \mathcal{C} \Rightarrow \forall t \in \mathcal{C}, \mathcal{P} \vdash_{CRWL} \hat{e} \to \hat{t}$
b) $\mathcal{P} \vdash_{CRWL} \hat{e} \to t \Rightarrow \exists \mathcal{C}$ *such that* $t \in \mathcal{C}$ *and* $\mathcal{P} \vdash_{CRWLF} e \lhd \mathcal{C}$
c) $\mathcal{P} \vdash_{CRWLF} e \bowtie e' \Leftrightarrow \mathcal{P} \vdash_{CRWL} \hat{e} \bowtie \hat{e}'$
d) $\mathcal{P} \vdash_{CRWLF} e \lozenge e' \Leftrightarrow \mathcal{P} \vdash_{CRWL} \hat{e} \lozenge \hat{e}'$

We can revise within $CRWLF$ the notion of denotation of an expression, and define $[\![e]\!]^F = \{t \in CTerm_{\perp,F} \mid e \lhd \mathcal{C}, t \in \mathcal{C}\}$, for any $e \in Term_{\perp,F}$. As a consequence of the previous proposition we have $[\![e]\!] \subseteq [\![e]\!]^F$ for any $e \in Term_{\perp}$ and $\widehat{[\![e]\!]^F} = [\![\hat{e}]\!]$ for any $e \in Term_{\perp,F}$, where, given a set S, $\hat{S}$ is defined in the natural way $\hat{S} = \{\hat{t} \mid t \in S\}$.

All the previous results make easy the task of proving that we have done things right with respect to failure. We will need a result stronger than Prop. 4, which does not provide enough information about the relation between the denotation of an expression and each of its calculable SAS's.

Proposition 5. *Given* $e \in Term_{\perp,F}$, *if* $\mathcal{P} \vdash_{CRWLF} e \lhd \mathcal{C}$ *and* $t \in [\![\hat{e}]\!]$, *then there exists* $s \in \mathcal{C}$ *such that* s *and* t *are consistent.*

Proof. Assume $\mathcal{P} \vdash_{CRWLF} e \lhd \mathcal{C}$. If we take $t \in CTerm_{\perp}$ such that $\mathcal{P} \vdash_{CRWL} \hat{e} \to t$, then by part b) of Prop. 4 there exists $\mathcal{C}'$ such that $\mathcal{P} \vdash_{CRWLF} e \lhd \mathcal{C}'$ with $t \in \mathcal{C}'$.

By Theorem 1 it follows that $\mathcal{C}$ and $\mathcal{C}'$ are consistent. By definition of consistent SAS's, as $t \in \mathcal{C}'$, then there exist $s \in \mathcal{C}$ such that t and s are consistent. $\square$

We easily arrive now at our final result.

Theorem 2. *Given* $e \in Term_{\perp,F}$, *if* $\mathcal{P} \vdash_{CRWLF} e \lhd \{F\}$ *then* $[\![\hat{e}]\!] = \{\perp\}$

Proof. If $t \in [\![\hat{e}]\!]$, we know from Prop. 5 that F and t must be consistent. As F is consistent only with $\perp$ and itself, and $t \in CTerm_{\perp}$, we conclude that $t = \perp$. $\square$

5   Conclusions and Future Work

We have proposed the proof calculus $CRWLF$ (Constructor based ReWriting Logic with Failure), which allows to deduce negative information from a wide class of functional logic programs. In particular, the calculus provides proofs of failure of reduction, a notion that can be seen as the natural FLP counterpart of negation as failure in logic programming.

The starting point for $CRWLF$ has been the proof calculus of $CRWL$ [3], a well established theoretical framework for FLP. The most remarkable insight has been to replace the statements $e \to t$ of $CRWL$ (representing a single reduction of e to an approximated value t) by $e \lhd \mathcal{C}$ (representing a whole, somehow complete, set $\mathcal{C}$ of approximations to e). With the aid of $\lhd$ we have been able to cover all the derivations in $CRWL$, as well as to prove failure of reduction and, as auxiliary notions, failure of joinability and divergence, the two other kinds of statements that $CRWL$ was able to prove.

It is interesting to remark that $\lhd$ provide, at the level of logical descriptions, a finer control over reduction than $\to$. Two examples: $e \lhd \{t\}, t \in CTerm$ expresses the property that e is reducible to the unique totally defined value t; $e \lhd \mathcal{C}, e' \lhd \mathcal{C}$, with $\mathcal{C}$ consisting only of total c-terms, expresses that e and e' reduce to exactly the same (totally defined) values. The same properties, if expressed by means of $\to$, would require the use of universal quantification, which is out of the scope of $CRWL$. Observe that, although the side conditions '$t \in CTerm$' and '$\mathcal{C}$ consisting only of total c-terms' of the examples are not statements of $CRWLF$, they are purely syntactical conditions.

The idea of collecting into an SAS values coming from different reductions for a given expression e presents some similarities with abstract interpretation which, within the FLP field, has been used in [2] for detecting unsatisfiability of equations $e = e'$ (something similar to failure of our $e \bowtie e'$). We can mention some differences between our work and [2]:

- Programs in [2] are much more restrictive: they must be confluent, terminating, satisfy a property of stratification on conditions, and define strict and total functions.
- In our setting, each SAS for an expression e consists of (down) approximations to the denotation of e, and the set of SAS's for e determines in a precise sense (Props. 4 and 5) the *exact* denotation of e. In the abstract interpretation approach one typically obtains, for an expression e, an abstract term representing a *superset* of the denotation of all the instances of e. But some of the rules of the $CRWLF$-calculus (like (9) or (10)) are not valid if we replace SAS's by such supersets. To be more concrete, if we adopt an abstract

interpretation view of our SAS's, it would be natural to see $\bot$ as standing for the set of all constructor terms (since $\bot$ is refinable to any value), and therefore to identify an SAS like $\mathcal{C} = \{\bot, z\}$ with $\mathcal{C}' = \{\bot\}$. But from $e \lhd \mathcal{C}$ we can deduce $e \bowtie z$, while it is not correct to do the same from $e \lhd \mathcal{C}'$. Therefore, the good properties of $CRWLF$ with respect to $CRWL$ are lost.

We see our work as the first step in the research of a whole framework for dealing with failure in FLP. Some natural (but not small!) future steps are: to enlarge the class of considered programs by allowing extra variables; to consider 'general' programs which make use of failure information, and to develop model theoretic and operational semantics for them.

Acknowledgments: We thank the anonymous referees for their useful comments.

References

[1] K.R. Apt and R. Bol. Logic programming and negation: A survey. *Journal of Logic Programming*, 19&20:9–71, 1994.

[2] D. Bert and R. Echahed. Abstraction of conditional term rewriting systems. In *Proc. ILPS'95*, pages 162–176. MIT Press, 1995.

[3] J.C. González-Moreno, T. Hortalá-González, F.J. López-Fraguas, and M. Rodríguez-Artalejo. An approach to declarative programming based on a rewriting logic. *Journal of Logic Programming*, 40(1):47–87, 1999.

[4] M. Hanus. The integration of functions into logic programming: From theory to practice. *Journal of Logic Programming*, 19&20:583–628, 1994.

[5] M. Hanus (ed.). Curry: An integrated functional logic language. Available at http://www-i2.informatik.rwth-aachen.de/~hanus/curry/report.html, February 2000.

[6] G. Jäger and R.F. Stärk. A proof-theoretic framework for logic programming. In S.R. Buss (ed.), *Handbook of Proof Theory*, pages 639–682. Elsevier, 1998.

[7] F.J. López-Fraguas and J. Sánchez-Hernández. Disequalities may help to narrow. In *Proc. APPIA-GULP-PRODE'99*, pages 89–104, 1999.

[8] F.J. López-Fraguas and J. Sánchez-Hernández. $\mathcal{TOY}$: A multiparadigm declarative system. In *Proc. RTA'99, Springer LNCS* 1631, pages 244–247, 1999.

[9] F.J. López-Fraguas and J. Sánchez-Hernández. Proving failure in functional logic programs (extended version). Tech. Rep. SIP 00/100-00, UCM Madrid, 2000.

[10] J.J. Moreno-Navarro. Default rules: An extension of constructive negation for narrowing-based languages. In *Proc. ICLP'95*, pages 535–549. MIT Press, 1994.

[11] J.J. Moreno-Navarro. Extending constructive negation for partial functions in lazy functional-logic languages. In *Proc. ELP'96*, pages 213–227. Springer LNAI 1050, 1996.

[12] P.J. Stuckey. Constructive negation for constraint logic programming. In *Proc. LICS'91*, pages 328–339, 1991.

Semantics of Input-Consuming Logic Programs

Annalisa Bossi[1], Sandro Etalle[2], and Sabina Rossi[1]

[1] Dipartimento di Informatica, Università di Venezia, Italy
{bossi,srossi}@dsi.unive.it
[2] Universiteit Maastricht, The Netherlands
etalle@cs.unimaas.nl

Abstract. Input-consuming programs are logic programs with an additional restriction on the selectability (actually, on the resolvability) of atoms. This class of programs arguably allows to model logic programs employing a dynamic selection rule and constructs such as *delay declarations*: as shown also in [5], a large number of them are actually input-consuming.

In this paper we show that – under some syntactic restrictions – the *S*-semantics of a program is correct and fully abstract also for input-consuming programs. This allows us to conclude that for a large class of programs employing delay declarations there exists a model-theoretic semantics which is equivalent to the operational one.

Keywords: Logic programming, dynamic scheduling, semantics.

1 Introduction

Most implementations of logic programming languages allow the possibility of employing a *dynamic selection rule*: a selection rule which is not bound to the fixed left-to-right order of PROLOG. While this allows for more flexibility, it can easily yield to nontermination or to an inefficient computation. For instance, if we consider the standard program APPEND

```
app([ ],Ys,Ys).
app([H|Xs],Ys,[H|Zs]) ← app(Xs,Ys,Zs).
```

we have that the query q1: app([1,2],[3,4],Xs), app(Xs,[5,6],Ys). might easily loop infinitely (one just has to keep resolving the rightmost atom together with the second clause). To avoid this, most implementations use constructs such as *delay declarations*. In the case of APPEND when used for concatenating two lists the natural delay declaration is

```
d1: delay app(Xs,_,_) until nonvar(Xs).
```

This statement forbids the selection of an atom of the form app(s,t,u) unless s is a non-variable term, which is precisely what we need in order to run the query q1 without overhead. Delay declarations, advocated by van Emden and de Lucena [16] and introduced explicitly in logic programming by Naish [13], provide the programmer with a better control over the computation and allow one to

J. Lloyd et al. (Eds.): CL 2000, LNAI 1861, pp. 194–208, 2000.
© Springer-Verlag Berlin Heidelberg 2000

improve the efficiency of programs (wrt unrestricted selection rule), to prevent run-time errors, to enforce termination and to express some degree of synchronization among different processes (i.e., atoms) in a program, which allows to model parallelism (coroutining).

This extra control comes at a price: Many crucial results of logic programming do not hold in this extended setting. In particular, the equivalence between the declarative and operational semantics does not apply any longer. For instance, while the Herbrand semantics of APPEND is non-empty, the query app(X,Y,Z) has no successful derivation, as the computation starting in it *deadlocks*[1].

In this paper we address the problem of providing a model-theoretic semantics to programs using dynamic scheduling. In order to do so, we need a declarative way of modeling construct such as delay declarations: for this we restrict our attention to *input-consuming programs*. The definition of input-consuming program employs the concept of *mode*: We assume that programs are *moded*, that is, that the positions of each atom are partitioned into *input* and *output* ones. Then, *input-consuming* derivation steps are precisely those in which the input arguments of the selected atom will not be instantiated by the unification with the clause's head. For example, the standard mode for the program APPEND when used for concatenating two lists is app(In,In,Out). Notice that in this case, for queries of the form app(ts,us,X) (X is variable disjoint from ts and us, which can be any possibly non-ground terms) the delay declaration d1 guarantees precisely that if an atom is selectable and resolvable, then it is so via an input-consuming derivation step; conversely, in every input-consuming derivation the resolved atom satisfies the d1, thus it would have been selectable also in presence of the delay declaration. This reasoning applies for a large class of queries (among which q1), and is actually not a coincidence: In the sequel we argue that in most situations delay declarations are employed precisely for ensuring that the derivation is input-consuming (modulo renaming, i.e. modulo ~, as explained later). Because of this, we are interested in providing a model-theoretic semantics for input-consuming programs. Clearly, most difficulties one has in doing this for programs with delay declarations apply to input-consuming programs as well. Intuitively speaking, the crucial problem here lies in the fact that computations may deadlock: i.e., reach a state in which no atom is resolvable (e.g., the query app(X,Y,Z)). Because of this the operational semantics is correct but not complete wrt the declarative one.

We prove that, if a program is well- and nicely-moded, then, for nicely-moded queries the operational semantics provided by the input-consuming resolution rule is correct and complete wrt the $\mathcal{S}$-semantics [11] for logic programs. The $\mathcal{S}$-semantics is a denotational semantics which – for programs without delay declarations – intuitively corresponds to the set of answer substitutions to the most general atomic queries, i.e., queries of the form $p(x_1, \ldots, x_n)$ where $x_1, \ldots, x_n$ are distinct variables. Moreover, the $\mathcal{S}$-semantics is compositional, it enjoys a

---

[1] A deadlock occurs when the current query contains no atom which can be selected for resolution.

model-theoretic reading, and it corresponds to the least fixpoint of a continuous operator.

Summarizing, we show that the $\mathcal{S}$-semantics of a program is compositional, correct and fully abstract also for input-consuming programs, provided that the programs considered are well- and nicely-moded, and that the queries are nicely-moded. It is important to notice that the queries we are considering don't have to be well-moded. Because of this, they might also deadlock. For instance, the query app(X,Y,Z) is nicely-moded, thus our results are applicable to it. One of the interesting aspects of the results we will present is that in some situations one can determine, purely from the declarative semantics of a program, that a query does (or does not) yield to deadlock.

This paper is organized as follows. The next section contains the preliminary notations and definitions. In the one which follows we introduce the $\mathcal{S}$-semantics together with the key concepts of moded and of input-consuming program. Section 4 contains the main results, and some examples of their applications. Section 5 concludes the paper. Some proofs are omitted for space reasons, and can be found in [7].

2   Preliminaries

The reader is assumed to be familiar with the terminology and the basic results of the semantics of logic programs [1, 2, 12]. Here we adopt the notation of [2] in the fact that we use boldface characters to denote sequences of objects; therefore t denotes a sequence of terms while B is a query (notice that – following [2] – queries are simply conjunctions of atoms, possibly empty). We denote atoms by $A, B, H, \ldots$, queries by $Q, A, B, C, \ldots$, clauses by $c, d, \ldots$, and programs by P.

For any syntactic object o, we denote by $Var(o)$ the set of variables occurring in o. We also say that o is *linear* if every variable occurs in it at most once. Given a *substitution* $\sigma = \{x_1/t_1, \ldots, x_n/t_n\}$ we say that $\{x_1, \ldots, x_n\}$ is its *domain* (denoted by $Dom(\sigma)$) and that $Var(\{t_1, \ldots, t_n\})$ is its *range* (denoted by $Ran(\sigma)$). Further, we denote by $Var(\sigma) = Dom(\sigma) \cup Ran(\sigma)$. If $\{t_1, \ldots, t_n\}$ consists of variables then σ is called a *pure variable substitution*. If, in addition, $t_1, \ldots, t_n$ is a permutation of $x_1, \ldots, x_n$ then we say that σ is a *renaming*. The *composition* of substitutions is denoted by juxtaposition $(\theta\sigma(X) = \sigma(\theta(X)))$. We say that a term t is an *instance* of t' iff for some σ, $t = t'\sigma$, further t is called a *variant* of t', written $t \approx t'$ iff t and t' are instances of each other. A substitution θ is a *unifier* of terms t and t' iff $t\theta = t'\theta$. We denote by $mgu(t, t')$ any *most general unifier* (*mgu*, in short) of t and t'. An mgu θ of terms t and t' is called *relevant* iff $Var(\theta) \subseteq Var(t) \cup Var(t')$. The definitions above are extended to other syntactic objects in the obvious way.

Computations are sequences of derivation steps. The non-empty query q : A, B, C and a clause $c : H \leftarrow B$ (renamed apart wrt q) yield the resolvent $(A, B, C)\theta$, provided that $\theta = mgu(B, H)$. A *derivation step* is denoted by $A, B, C \overset{\theta}{\Longrightarrow}_{P,c} (A, B, C)\theta$. c is called its *input clause*, and B is called the *selected atom* of q. A derivation is obtained by iterating derivation steps. A maximal sequence $\delta := Q_0 \overset{\theta_1}{\Longrightarrow}_{P,c_1} Q_1 \overset{\theta_2}{\Longrightarrow}_{P,c_2} \cdots Q_n \overset{\theta_{n+1}}{\Longrightarrow}_{P,c_{n+1}} Q_{n+1} \cdots$ of derivation steps is called an *SLD derivation of* $P \cup \{Q_0\}$ provided that for every step the standardization apart condition holds, i.e., the input clause employed at each step is variable disjoint from the initial query Q_0 and from the substitutions and the input clauses used at earlier steps. If the program P is clear from the context and the clauses $c_1, \ldots, c_{n+1}, \ldots$ are irrelevant, then we drop the reference to them. An SLD derivation in which at each step the leftmost atom is resolved is called a *LD derivation*. Derivations can be finite or infinite. If $\delta := Q_0 \overset{\theta_1}{\Longrightarrow}_{P,c_1} \cdots \overset{\theta_n}{\Longrightarrow}_{P,c_n} Q_n$ is a finite prefix of a derivation, also denoted $\delta := Q_0 \overset{\theta}{\longrightarrow} Q_n$ with $\theta = \theta_1 \cdots \theta_n$, we say that δ is a *partial derivation* of $P \cup \{Q_0\}$. If δ is maximal and ends with the empty query then the restriction of θ to the variables of Q is called its *computed answer substitution* (*c.a.s.*, for short). The length of a (partial) derivation δ, denoted by $len(\delta)$, is the number of derivation steps in δ.

We recall the notion of *similar* SLD derivations and some related properties.

Definition 1 (Similar Derivations). *We say that two SLD derivations δ and δ' are similar $(\delta \sim \delta')$ if (i) their initial queries are variants of each other; (ii) they have the same length; (iii) for every derivation step, atoms in the same positions are selected and the input clauses employed are variants of each other.*

Lemma 2. *Let $\delta := Q_1 \overset{\theta}{\longrightarrow} Q_2$ be a partial SLD derivation of $P \cup \{Q_1\}$ and Q_1' be a variant of Q_1. Then, there exists a partial SLD derivation $\delta' := Q_1' \overset{\theta'}{\longrightarrow} Q_2'$ of $P \cup \{Q_1'\}$ such that δ and δ' are similar.*

Lemma 3. *Consider two similar partial SLD derivations $Q \overset{\theta}{\longrightarrow} Q'$ and $Q \overset{\theta'}{\longrightarrow} Q''$. Then $Q\theta$ and $Q\theta'$ are variants of each other.*

3 Basic Definitions

In this section we introduce the basic definitions we need: The ones of input-consuming derivations and of the $\mathcal{S}$-semantics. Then we introduce the concepts of well- and nicely-moded programs.

Input-Consuming Derivations. We start by recalling the notion of *mode*, which is a function that labels as *input* or *output* the positions of each predicate in order to indicate how the arguments of a predicate should be used.

Definition 4 (Mode). *Consider an n-ary predicate symbol p. By a mode for p we mean a function m_p from $\{1, \ldots, n\}$ to $\{In, Out\}$.*

If $m_p(i) = In$ (resp. *Out*), we say that i is an *input* (resp. *output*) *position* of p (with respect to m_p). We assume that each predicate symbol has a unique mode associated to it; multiple modes may be obtained by simply renaming the predicates. We denote by $In(Q)$ (resp. $Out(Q)$) the sequence of terms filling in the input (resp. output) positions of Q. Moreover, when writing an atom as $p(\boldsymbol{s}, \boldsymbol{t})$, we are indicating with $\boldsymbol{s}$ the sequence of terms filling in its input positions and with t the sequence of terms filling in its output positions. The notion of input-consuming derivation was introduced in [14] and is defined as follows.

Definition 5 (Input-Consuming).

- A derivation step $\mathbf{A}, B, \mathbf{C} \stackrel{\theta}{\Longrightarrow}_c (\mathbf{A}, \mathbf{B}, \mathbf{C})\theta$ is called input-consuming iff $In(B)\theta = In(B)$.
- A derivation is called input-consuming iff all its derivation steps are input-consuming.

Thus, a derivation step is input consuming if the corresponding mgu does not affect the input positions of the selected atom. Clearly, because of this additional restriction, there exist queries in which no atom is resolvable via an input-consuming derivation step. In this case we say that the query *suspends*.

Example 6. Consider the following program REVERSE using an accumulator.

```
reverse(Xs,Ys) ← reverse_acc(Xs,Ys,[ ]).
reverse_acc([ ],Ys,Ys).
reverse_acc([X|Xs],Ys,Zs) ← reverse_acc(Xs,Ys,[X|Zs]).
```

When used for reversing a list, the natural mode for this program is[2] the following one: reverse(In,Out), reverse_acc(In,Out,In). Consider now the query reverse([X1,X2],Zs). The following derivation is input-consuming.

$$\text{reverse([X1,X2],Zs)} \quad \Rightarrow \text{reverse\_acc([X1,X2],Zs,[ ])} \Rightarrow$$
$$\Rightarrow \text{reverse\_acc([X2],Zs,[X1])} \Rightarrow \text{reverse\_acc([ ],Zs,[X2,X1])} \Rightarrow \square$$

As usual, $\square$ denotes the empty query. Notice also that a natural delay declaration for this program would be

```
delay reverse(X,_) until nonvar(X).
delay reverse_acc(X,_,_) until nonvar(X).
```

Now, it is easy to see that for queries of the form reverse(t,X), where t is *any* term and X any variable disjoint from t, the above delay declarations guarantee precisely that the resulting derivations are input-consuming (modulo $\sim$). Furthermore, for the same class of queries it holds that in any input-consuming derivation the selected atom satisfies the above delay declarations.   □

Delay Declarations vs. Input-Consuming Derivations. As suggested in the above example, and stated in the introduction, we believe that the concept of input-consuming program allows one to model programs employing delay declarations in a nice way: we claim that in most programs delay declarations are used to enforce that the derivations are input-consuming (modulo $\sim$). We have addressed this topic already in [5]. We now borrow a couple of arguments from it, and extend them.

---

[2] The other possible modes are reverse(Out,In) (which is symmetric and equivalent to the above one) and reverse(In,In) which might be used for checking if a list is a palindrome.

Generally, delay declarations are employed to guarantee that the interpreter will not use an "inappropriate" clause for resolving an atom (the other, perhaps less prominent use of delay declarations is to ensure absence of runtime errors, we don't address this issue in this paper). In fact, if the interpreter always selected the appropriate clause, by the independence from the selection rule one would not have to worry about the order of the selection of the atoms in the query. In practice, delay declarations prevent the selection of an atom until a certain degree of instantiation is reached. This degree of instantiation ensures that the atom is unifiable only with the heads of the "appropriate" clauses. In presence of modes, we can reasonably assume that this degree of instantiation is the one of the *input* positions. Now, take an atom $p(s, t)$, that it is resolvable with a clause c by means of an input-consuming derivation step. Then, for every instance s' of s, we have that the atom $p(s', t)$ is as well resolvable with c by means of an input-consuming derivation step. Thus, no further instantiation of the input positions of $p(s, t)$ can rule out c as a possible clause for resolving it, and c must then be one of the "appropriate" clauses for resolving $p(s, t)$ and we can say that $p(s, t)$ is "sufficiently instantiated" in its input positions to be resolved with c. On the other hand, following the same reasoning, if $p(s, t)$ is resolvable with c but not via an input-consuming derivation step, then there exists an instance s' of s, such that $p(s', t)$ is not resolvable with c. In this case we can say that $p(s, t)$ is not instantiated enough to know whether c is one of the "appropriate" clauses for resolving it.

We conclude this section with a result stating that also when considering input-consuming derivations, it is not restrictive to assume that all mgu's used in a derivation are relevant. The proof can be found in [7].

Lemma 7. *Let $p(s, t)$ and $p(u, v)$ be two atoms. If there exists an mgu θ of $p(s, t)$ and $p(u, v)$ such that $s\theta = s$ then there exists a relevant mgu ϑ of $p(s, t)$ and $p(u, v)$ such that $s\vartheta = s$.*

From now on, we assume that all mgu's used in the input-consuming derivation steps are relevant.

The S-Semantics. The aim of the S-semantics approach (see [8]) is modeling the observable behaviors for a variety of logic languages. The observable we consider here is the *computed answer substitutions*. The semantics is defined as follows:

$$S(P) = \{\ p(x_1, \ldots, x_n)\theta \mid x_1, \ldots, x_n \text{ are distinct variables and}$$
$$p(x_1, \ldots, x_n) \xrightarrow{\ \theta\ }_P \square \text{ is an SLD derivation}\}.$$

This semantics enjoys all the valuable properties of the least Herbrand model. Technically, the crucial difference is that in this setting an interpretation might contain non-ground atoms. To present the main results on the S-semantics we need to introduce two further concepts: Let P be a program, and I be a set of atoms. The immediate consequence operator for the S-semantics is defined as:

$$T_P^S(I) = \{\ H\theta \mid \exists\ H \leftarrow \boldsymbol{B} \in P$$
$$\exists\ \boldsymbol{C} \in I, \text{renamed apart}^3 \text{ wrt } H, \boldsymbol{B}$$
$$\theta = mgu(\boldsymbol{B}, \boldsymbol{C}) \qquad\qquad \}.$$

Moreover, a set of atoms I is called an $\mathcal{S}$-*model* of P if $T_P^{\mathcal{S}}(I) \subseteq I$. Falaschi et al. [11] showed that $T_P^{\mathcal{S}}$ is continuous on the lattice of term interpretations, that is sets of possibly non-ground atoms, with the subset-ordering. They proved the following:

- $\mathcal{S}(P) = $ least $\mathcal{S}$-model of $P = T_P^{\mathcal{S}} \uparrow \omega$.

Therefore, the $\mathcal{S}$-semantics enjoys a declarative interpretation and a bottom-up construction, just like the Herbrand one. In addition, we have that the $\mathcal{S}$-semantics reflects the observable behavior in terms of computed answer substitutions, as shown by the following well-known result.

Theorem 8. *[11] Let P be a program, $\boldsymbol{A}$ be a query, and θ be a substitution. The following statements are equivalent.*

- *There exists an SLD derivation $\boldsymbol{A} \xrightarrow{\vartheta}_P \square$, where $\boldsymbol{A}\vartheta \approx \boldsymbol{A}\theta$.*
- *There exists $\boldsymbol{A}' \in \mathcal{S}(P)$ (renamed apart wrt $\boldsymbol{A}$), such that $\sigma = mgu(\boldsymbol{A}, \boldsymbol{A}')$ and $\boldsymbol{A}\sigma \approx \boldsymbol{A}\theta$.*

Let us see this semantics applied to the programs so far encountered.

$$\mathcal{S}(\text{APPEND}) = \{ \text{ app}([\,],X,X),$$
$$\text{app}([X1],X,[X1|X]),$$
$$\text{app}([X1,X2],X,[X1,X2|X]), \qquad \dots \}.$$
$$\mathcal{S}(\text{REVERSE}) = \{ \text{ reverse}([\,],[\,]),$$
$$\text{reverse}([X1],[X1]),$$
$$\text{reverse}([X1,X2],[X2,X1]), \qquad \dots$$
$$\text{reverse\_acc}([\,],X,X),$$
$$\text{reverse\_acc}([X1],X,[X1|X]),$$
$$\text{reverse\_acc}([X1,X2],X,[X2,X1|X]), \dots \}.$$

Well and Nicely-Moded Programs. Even in presence of modes, the $\mathcal{S}$-semantics does not reflect the operational behavior of input-consuming programs (and thus of programs employing delay declarations). In fact, if we extend APPEND by adding to it the clause q $\leftarrow$ app(X,Y,Z). we have that q belongs to the semantics but the query q will not succeed (it suspends). In order to guarantee that the semantics is fully abstract (wrt the computed answer substitutions) we need to restrict the class of allowed programs and queries. To this end we introduce the concepts of well-moded [10] and of nicely-moded programs.

Definition 9 (Well-Moded).

- A *query* $p_1(\boldsymbol{s}_1, \boldsymbol{t}_1), \dots, p_n(\boldsymbol{s}_n, \boldsymbol{t}_n)$ is well-moded *if for all* $i \in [1, n]$

$$Var(\boldsymbol{s}_i) \subseteq \bigcup_{j=1}^{i-1} Var(\boldsymbol{t}_j).$$

---

[3] Here and in the sequel, when we write "$\boldsymbol{C} \in I$, renamed apart wrt some expression e", we naturally mean that I contains a set of atoms $C_1', \dots, C_n'$, and that $\boldsymbol{C}$ is a renaming of $C_1', \dots, C_n'$ such that $\boldsymbol{C}$ shares no variable with e and that two distinct atoms of $\boldsymbol{C}$ share no variables with each other.

- A *clause* $p(t_0, s_{n+1}) \leftarrow p_1(s_1, t_1), \ldots, p_n(s_n, t_n)$ *is* well-moded *if for all* $i \in [1, n+1]$

$$Var(s_i) \subseteq \bigcup_{j=0}^{i-1} Var(t_j).$$

- *A program is* well-moded *if all of its clauses are well-moded.*

Thus a query is well-moded if every variable occurring in an input position of an atom occurs in an output position of an earlier atom in the query. A clause is well-moded if (1) every variable occurring in an input position of a body atom occurs either in an input position of the head, or in an output position of an earlier body atom; (2) every variable occurring in an output position of the head occurs in an input position of the head, or in an output position of a body atom.

The concept of nicely-moded programs was first introduced by Chadha and Plaisted [9].

Definition 10 (Nicely-Moded).

- *A query* $p_1(s_1, t_1), \ldots, p_n(s_n, t_n)$ *is called* nicely-moded *if* $t_1, \ldots, t_n$ *is a linear sequence of terms and for all* $i \in [1, n]$

$$Var(s_i) \cap \bigcup_{j=i}^{n} Var(t_j) = \emptyset.$$

- *A clause* $p(s_0, t_0) \leftarrow p_1(s_1, t_1), \ldots, p_n(s_n, t_n)$ *is* nicely-moded *if its body is nicely-moded and*

$$Var(s_0) \cap \bigcup_{j=1}^{n} Var(t_j) = \emptyset.$$

- *A program P is* nicely-moded *if all of its clauses are nicely-moded.*

Note that an atomic query $p(s, t)$ is nicely-moded if and only if t is linear and $Var(s) \cap Var(t) = \emptyset$.

Example 11. Programs APPEND and REVERSE are both well- and nicely-moded. Furthermore, Consider now the following program PALINDROME

```
palindrome(Xs) ← reverse(Xs,Xs).
```

Together with REVERSE. With the mode palindrome(In), this program is well-moded but not nicely-moded (Xs occurs both in an input and in an output position of the same body atom). Nevertheless, it becomes both well-moded and nicely-moded if the adopted modes of REVERSE are the following ones: reverse(In,In), reverse_acc(In,In,In).   □

4   Semantics of Input-Consuming Programs

In this section we are going to make the link between input-consuming program-s, well- and nicely-moded programs and the $\mathcal{S}$-semantics: We show that the $\mathcal{S}$-semantics of a program is compositional, correct and fully abstract also for input-consuming programs, provided that the programs are well- and nicely-moded and that only nicely-moded queries are considered.

Properties of Well-Moded Programs. We start by demonstrating some important features of well-moded programs. For this, we need additional notations: First, the following notion of *renaming for a term t* from [2] will be used.

Definition 12. *A substitution* $\theta := \{x_1/y_1, \dots, x_n/y_n\}$ *is called a* renaming *for a term* t *if* $Dom(\theta) \subseteq Var(t)$, $y_1, \dots, y_n$ *are different variables, and* $(Var(t) - \{x_1, \dots, x_n\}) \cap \{y_1, \dots, y_n\} = \emptyset$ *(θ does not introduce variables which occur in t but are not in the domain of θ).*

Observe that terms s and t are variants iff there exists a renaming θ for s such that $t = s\theta$. Then, we need the following: Let $Q := p_1(s_1, t_1), \dots, p_n(s_n, t_n)$. We define

- $VIn^*(Q) = \bigcup_{i=1}^{n} \{x \mid x \in Var(s_i) \text{ and } x \notin \bigcup_{j=1}^{i-1} Var(t_j)\}$

Thus, $VIn^*(Q)$ denotes the set of variables occurring in an input position of an atom of Q but not occurring in an output position of an earlier atom. Note also that if Q is well-moded then $VIn^*(Q) = \emptyset$.

We now need the following technical result concerning well-moded programs. Because of lack of space, the proof is omitted, and can be found in [7].

Lemma 13. *Let P be a well-moded program, Q be a query and $\delta := Q \xrightarrow{\theta} Q'$ be a partial LD derivation of $P \cup \{Q\}$. If $\theta_{|VIn^*(Q)}$ is a renaming for Q then δ is similar to an input-consuming partial (LD) derivation.*

We can now prove our crucial result concerning well-moded programs. Basically, it states the *correctness* of the $\mathcal{S}$-semantics for well-moded, input-consuming programs. This can be regarded as "one half" of the main result we are going to propose.

Proposition 14. *Let P be a well-moded program, A be an atomic query and θ be a substitution.*

- *If there exists $A' \in \mathcal{S}(P)$ (renamed apart wrt A), and $\sigma = mgu(A, A')$ such that*
  (i) $In(A)\sigma \approx In(A)$,
  (ii) $A\sigma \approx A\theta$,
- *then there exists an input-consuming (LD) derivation $\delta := A \xrightarrow{\vartheta}_P \square$, such that $A\vartheta \approx A\theta$.*

Proof. Let $A' \in \mathcal{S}(P)$ (renamed apart wrt A) and σ be such that the hypothesis are satisfied. By Theorem 8, there exists a successful SLD derivation of $P \cup \{A\}$ with c.a.s. ϑ' such that $A\vartheta' \approx A\theta$. By the Switching Lemma [2], there exists a successful LD derivation δ' of $P \cup \{A\}$ with c.a.s. ϑ'. From the hypothesis, it follows that $\vartheta'_{|In(A)}$ is a renaming for A. By Lemma 13, there exists an input-consuming derivation $A \xrightarrow{\vartheta}_P \square$ similar to δ'. The thesis follows by Lemma 3. $\square$

Properties of Nicely-Moded Programs. Now, we need to establish some properties of nicely-moded programs. First, we recall the following from [5, 6].

Lemma 15. *Let the program P and the query Q be nicely moded. Let $\delta :=$ $Q \xrightarrow{\theta} Q'$ be a partial input-consuming derivation of $P \cup \{Q\}$. Then, for all $x \in Var(Q)$ and $x \notin Var(Out(Q))$, $x\theta = x$.*

Note that if Q is nicely-moded then $x \in Var(Q)$ and $x \notin Var(Out(Q))$ iff $x \in VIn^*(Q)$. Now, we can prove that the $\mathcal{S}$-semantics is *fully abstract* for input-consuming, nicely-moded programs and queries. This can be regarded as the counterpart of Proposition 14.

Proposition 16. *Let P be a nicely-moded program, A be a nicely-moded atomic query and θ be a substitution.*

- *If there exists an input-consuming SLD derivation $\delta := A \xrightarrow{\vartheta}_P \square$, such that $A\vartheta \approx A\theta$,*
- *then there exists $A' \in \mathcal{S}(P)$ (renamed apart wrt A), and $\sigma = mgu(A, A')$ such that*
  (i) $In(A)\sigma \approx In(A)$,
  (ii) $A\sigma \approx A\theta$.

Proof. By Theorem 8, there exist $A' \in \mathcal{S}(P)$ (renamed apart wrt A) and a substitution σ such that $\sigma = mgu(A, A')$ and (ii) holds. Since δ is an input-consuming derivation, by Lemma 15, it follows that $\vartheta_{|In(A)}$ is a renaming for A. Hence (i) follows by the hypothesis and (ii). $\square$

Semantics of Input-Consuming Derivations. We now put together the above propositions and extend them compositionally to arbitrary (non-atomic) queries. For this, we need the the following simple result.

Lemma 17. *Let the program P be well and nicely-moded and the query Q be nicely-moded. Then, there exists a well- and nicely-moded program P' and a nicely-moded atomic query A such that the following statements are equivalent.*

- *There exists an input-consuming successful derivation δ of $P \cup \{Q\}$ with c.a.s. θ.*
- *There exists an input-consuming successful derivation δ' of $P' \cup \{A\}$ with c.a.s. θ.*

Proof. (sketch). This is done in a straightforward way by letting P' be the program $P \cup \{c : new(\boldsymbol{x}, \boldsymbol{y}) \leftarrow Q\}$ where $\boldsymbol{x} = VIn^*(Q)$, $\boldsymbol{y} = Var(Out(Q))$, *new* is a fresh predicate symbol and $A = new(\boldsymbol{x}, \boldsymbol{y})$. □

We are now ready for the main result of this paper, which asserts that the declarative semantics $\mathcal{S}(P)$ is compositional and fully abstract for input-consuming programs, provided that programs are well- and nicely-moded and that queries are nicely-moded.

Theorem 18. *Let P be a well- and nicely-moded program, $\boldsymbol{A}$ be a nicely-moded query and θ be a substitution. The following statements are equivalent.*

(i) There exists an input-consuming derivation $\boldsymbol{A} \overset{\vartheta}{\longrightarrow}_P \square$, such that $\boldsymbol{A}\vartheta \approx \boldsymbol{A}\theta$.
(ii) There exists $\boldsymbol{A}' \in \mathcal{S}(P)$ (renamed apart wrt $\boldsymbol{A}$), and $\sigma = mgu(\boldsymbol{A}, \boldsymbol{A}')$ such that

    (a) $\sigma_{|VIn^*(\boldsymbol{A})}$ is a renaming for $\boldsymbol{A}$,
    (b) $\boldsymbol{A}\sigma \approx \boldsymbol{A}\theta$.

Proof. It follows immediately from Propositions 14, 16 and Lemma 17. □

Note that in case of an atomic query $\boldsymbol{A} := A$, we might substitute condition *(a)* above with the somewhat more attractive condition *(a')* $In(A)\sigma \approx In(A)$. Let us immediately see some examples.

Example 19.

- `app([X,b],Y,Z)` has an input-consuming successful derivation, with c.a.s. $\theta \approx \{Z/[X,b|Y]\}$. This can be concluded by just looking at $\mathcal{S}(\text{APPEND})$, from the fact that $A = \text{app}([X1,X2],X3,[X1,X2|X3]) \in \mathcal{S}(P)$. Notice that `app([X,b],Y,Z)` is – in its input position – an instance of A.
- `app(Y,[X,b],Z)` has no input-consuming successful derivations. This is because there is no $A \in \mathcal{S}(P)$ such that $In(\text{app}(Y, [X, b], Z)$ is an instance of A in the input position. This actually implies that in presence of delay declarations `app(Y,[X,b],Z)` will eventually either deadlock or run into an infinite derivation; we are going to talk more about this in the next section. □

Note that Theorem 18 holds also in the case that programs are *permutation well- and nicely-moded* and queries are *permutation nicely-moded* [15], i.e., programs which would be well- and nicely-moded after a permutation of the atoms in the bodies and queries which would be nicely-moded through a permutation of their atoms.

Deadlock. We now consider again programs employing delay declarations. An important consequence of Theorem 18 is that when the delay declarations imply that the derivations are input-consuming (modulo $\sim$), then one can determine from the model-theoretic semantics whether a query is bound to deadlock or not. Let us establish some simple notation. In this section we assume that programs are augmented with delay declarations, and we say that a derivation *respects* the delay declarations iff every selected atom satisfies the delay declarations.

Notation 20. Let P be a program and A be a query.

– We say that $P \cup \{A\}$ is *input-consuming correct* iff every SLD derivation of $P \cup \{A\}$ which respects the delay declarations is similar to an input-consuming derivation.
– We say that $P \cup \{A\}$ is *input-consuming complete* iff every input-consuming derivation of $P \cup \{A\}$ respects the delay declarations.
– We say that $P \cup \{A\}$ *is bound to deadlock* if
  (i) every SLD derivation of $P \cup \{A\}$ which respects the delay declarations either fails or deadlocks[4], and
  (ii) there exists at least one non-failing SLD derivation of $P \cup \{A\}$ which respects the delay declarations.   □

For example, consider the program REVERSE (including delay declarations).

– REVERSE ∪ reverse(s,Z) is input-consuming correct and complete provided that Z is a variable disjoint from s.

Consider now the program APPEND augmented with the delay declaration d1 of the introduction.

– APPEND ∪ app(s,t,Z) is input-consuming correct and complete provided that Z is a variable disjoint from the possibly non-ground terms s and t.
– Now, following up on Example 19, since APPEND ∪ app([X,b],Y,Z) is input-consuming complete, we can state that APPEND ∪ app([X,b],Y,Z) is not bound to deadlock.

In order to say something about the other query of Example 19 (app(Y,[X,b],Z)) we need a further reasoning: Consider for the moment the nicely-moded query app(X,Y,Z). Since $\mathcal{S}$(APPEND) contains instances of it, by Theorem 8, app(X,Y,Z) has at least one successful SLD derivation. Thus, it does not fail. On the other hand, every atom in $\mathcal{S}$(APPEND) is in its input positions a proper instance of app(X,Y,Z). Thus by Theorem 18, app(X,Y,Z) has no input-consuming successful derivations. Therefore, since APPEND ∪ app(X,Y,Z) is input-consuming correct, we can state that app(X,Y,Z) either has an infinite input-consuming derivation or it is bound to deadlock. This fact can be nicely combined with the fact that APPEND is *input-terminating* [5]: i.e., all its input-consuming derivations starting in a nicely-moded query are finite. In [5] we provided conditions which guaranteed that a program is input-terminating; these conditions easily allow one to show that APPEND in input-terminating. Because of this, we can conclude that the query app(X,Y,Z) is bound to deadlock.

By simply formalizing this reasoning, we obtain the following.

Theorem 21. *Let P be a well- and nicely-moded program, and A be a nicely-moded atomic query. If*

---
[4] A derivation deadlocks if its last query contains no selectable atom, i.e., no atom which satisfies the delay declarations

1. $\exists\ B \in \mathcal{S}(P)$, such that A unifies with B,
2. $\forall\ B \in \mathcal{S}(P)$, if A unifies with B, then $In(A)$ is not an instance of $In(B)$,
3. $P \cup \{A\}$ is input-consuming-correct,

then A either has an infinite SLD derivation respecting the delay declarations or it is bound to deadlock.
If in addition P is input-terminating then A is bound to deadlock.

This result can be immediately generalized to non-atomic queries, as done for our main result. Let us see more examples:

- APPEND $\cup$ app(Y,[X,b],Z) either has an infinite derivation or it is bound to deadlock.
- Since APPEND is input terminating, we have that APPEND $\cup$ app(Y,[X,b],Z) is bound to deadlock.

One might wonder why in order to talk about deadlock we went back to programs using delay declarations. The crucial point here lies in the difference between *resolvability* - via an input-consuming derivation step - (used in input-consuming programs) and *selectability* (used in programs using delay declarations). When resolvability does not reduce to selectability, we cannot talk about (the usual definition of) deadlocking derivation. Consider the following program, where all atom's positions are moded as *input*.

$$p(X) \leftarrow q(a). \qquad p(a). \qquad q(b).$$

The derivation starting in p(X) does not succeed, does not fail, but it also does not deadlock in the usual sense: in fact, p(X) can be resolved with the first clause, which however yields to failure. We can say that each input-consuming SLD tree starting in p(X) is incomplete, as it contains a branch which cannot be followed. In the moment that the program is input-consuming correct, we can refer to the usual definition of deadlocking derivation.

Counterexamples. The following examples demonstrate that the syntactic restrictions used in Theorem 18 are necessary. Consider the following program.

```
p(X,Y)   ← equal_lists(X,Y), list_of_zeroes(Y).
equal_lists([ ],[ ]).
equal_lists([H|T],[H|T']) ← equal_lists(T,T').
list_of_zeroes([ ]).
list_of_zeroes([0|T]) ← list_of_zeroes(T).
```

With the modes: p(In,Out), equal_lists(In,Out), list_of_zeroes(Out). The first clause is not nicely-moded because of the double occurrence of Y in the body's output positions. Here, there exists a successful input-consuming derivation starting in p([X1],Y), and producing the c.a.s. $\{X1/0, Y/[X1]\}$. Nevertheless, there exists no corresponding $A' \in \mathcal{S}(P)$ (in fact, $\mathcal{S}(P)|_p$ contains all and only all the atoms of the form p(list0, list0) where list0 is a list containing only zeroes). This shows that if the program is well-moded but not nicely-moded then the implication (i) $\Rightarrow$ (ii) in Theorem 18 does not hold. Now consider the following program:

```
p(X) ← list(Y), equal_lists(X,Y).
equal_lists([ ], [ ]).
equal_lists([H|T],[H|T']) ← equal_lists(T,T').
list([ ]).
list([HH|T]) ← list(T).
```

With the modes p(In), equal_lists(In, In), list(Out). This program is nicely-moded, but not well-moded: The variable HH in the output position of the head occurs neither in an output position of the body nor in an input position of the head. It is easy to check that there does not exist any successful input-consuming derivation for the query p([a]); at the same time, p([X1]) ∈ $\mathcal{S}(P)$. Thus, if the program is nicely-moded but not well-moded then the implication (ii) ⇒ (i) in Theorem 18 does not hold.

5 Concluding Remarks

We have shown that – under some syntactic restrictions – the $\mathcal{S}$-semantics reflects the operational semantics also when programs are *input-consuming*. The $\mathcal{S}$-semantics is a denotational semantics which enjoys a model-theoretical reading. The relevance of the results is due to the fact that input-consuming programs often allow to model the behavior of programs employing delay declarations; hence for a large part of programs employing dynamic scheduling there exists a declarative semantics which is equivalent to the operational one.

As related work we want to mention Apt and Luitjes [3]. The crucial difference with it is that in [3] conditions which ensure that the queries are *deadlock-free* are employed. Under these circumstances the equivalence between the operational and the Herbrand semantics follows. On the other hand, the class of queries we consider here (the nicely-moded ones) includes many which would "deadlock" (e.g., app(X,Y,Z)): Theorem 18 proves that in many cases one can tell by the declarative semantics for instance if a query is "sufficiently instantiated" to yield a success or if it is bound to deadlock.

Concerning the restrictiveness of the syntactic concepts we use here (well- and nicely-moded programs and nicely-moded queries) we want to mention that [4, 5] both contain mini-surveys of programs with the indication whether they are well- and nicely-moded or not. From them, it appears that most "usual" programs satisfy both definitions. It is important to stress that under this restriction one might still want to employ a dynamic selection rule. Consider for instance a query of the form read_tokens(X), modify(X,Y), write_tokens(Y), where the modes are read_tokens(Out), modify(In,Out), write_tokens(Out). If read_tokens cannot read the input stream all at once, it makes sense that modify and write_tokens be called in order to process and display the tokens that are available, even if read_tokens has not finished reading the input. This can be done by using dynamic scheduling, using either delay declarations or an input-consuming resolution rule in order to avoid nontermination and inefficiencies.

References

[1] K. R. Apt. Introduction to Logic Programming. In J. van Leeuwen, editor, *Handbook of Theoretical Computer Science*, volume B: Formal Models and Semantics, pages 495–574. Elsevier, Amsterdam and The MIT Press, Cambridge, 1990.

[2] K. R. Apt. *From Logic Programming to Prolog.* Prentice Hall, 1997.

[3] K. R. Apt and I. Luitjes. Verification of logic programs with delay declarations. In A. Borzyszkowski and S. Sokolowski, editors, *Proceedings of the Fourth International Conference on Algebraic Methodology and Software Technology, (AMAST'95)*, Lecture Notes in Computer Science, Berlin, 1995. Springer-Verlag.

[4] K. R. Apt and A. Pellegrini. On the occur-check free Prolog programs. *ACM Toplas*, 16(3):687–726, 1994.

[5] A. Bossi, S. Etalle, and S. Rossi. Properties of input-consuming derivations. *Electronic Notes in Theoretical Computer Science*, 30(1), 1999. http://www.elsevier.nl/locate/entcs, temporarily available at http://www.cs.unimaas.nl/~etalle/papers/index.htm.

[6] A. Bossi, S. Etalle, and S. Rossi. Properties of input-consuming derivations. Technical Report CS 99-06, Universiteit Maastricht, 1999.

[7] A. Bossi, S. Etalle, and S. Rossi. Semantics of input-consuming programs. Technical Report CS 00-01, Universiteit Maastricht, 2000.

[8] Annalisa Bossi, Maurizio Gabrielli, Giorgio Levi, and Maurizio Martelli. The S-semantics approach: Theory and applications. *The Journal of Logic Programming*, 19 & 20:149–198, May 1994.

[9] R. Chadha and D.A. Plaisted. Correctness of unification without occur check in Prolog. Technical report, Department of Computer Science, University of North Carolina, Chapel Hill, N.C., 1991.

[10] P. Dembinski and J. Maluszynski. AND-parallelism with intelligent backtracking for annotated logic programs. In *Proceedings of the International Symposium on Logic Programming*, pages 29–38, Boston, 1985.

[11] M. Falaschi, G. Levi, M. Martelli, and C. Palamidessi. Declarative modeling of the operational behavior of logic languages. *Theoretical Computer Science*, 69(3):289–318, 1989.

[12] J. W. Lloyd. *Foundations of Logic Programming.* Symbolic Computation – Artificial Intelligence. Springer-Verlag, Berlin, 1987. Second edition.

[13] L. Naish. An introduction to mu-prolog. Technical Report 82/2, The University of Melbourne, 1982.

[14] J. G. Smaus. Proving termination of input-consuming logic programs. In D. De Schreye, editor, *16th International Conference on Logic Programming*. MIT press, 1999.

[15] J.-G. Smaus, P. M. Hill, and A. M. King. Termination of logic programs with block declarations running in several modes. In C. Palamidessi, editor, *Proceedings of the 10th Symposium on Programming Language Implementations and Logic Programming*, LNCS. Springer-Verlag, 1998.

[16] M.H. van Emden and G.J. de Lucena. Predicate logic as a language for parallel programming. In K.L. Clark and S.-A. Tärnlund, editors, *Logic Programming*, London, 1982. Academic Press.

A Denotational Semantics of Defeasible Logic

Michael J. Maher

CIT, Griffith University
Nathan, QLD 4111, Australia
mjm@cit.gu.edu.au

Abstract. Defeasible logic is an efficient non-monotonic logic for defeasible reasoning. It is defined through a proof theory, and has no model theory. In this paper a denotational semantics is given for defeasible logic, as a step towards a full model theory. The logic is sound and complete wrt this semantics, but the semantics is not completely satisfactory as a model theory. We indicate directions for research that might resolve these issues.

1   Introduction

Defeasible logic is a logic designed for efficient defeasible reasoning. The logic was designed by Nute [19,20] with the intention that it be efficiently implementable. This intention has been realised in systems that can process hundreds of thousands of defeasible rules quickly [4]. Over the years, Nute and others have proposed many variants of defeasible logic [20,1]. In this paper we will address a particular defeasible logic, which we denote by DL. However, our work is easily modified to address other defeasible logics.

DL, and similar logics, have been proposed as the appropriate language for executable regulations [3], contracts [21], and business rules [11]. The logics are considered to have satisfactory expressiveness and the efficiency of the implementations supports real-time response in applications such as electronic commerce [11].

Defeasible reasoning is rather similar to default reasoning, but differs in the way rules are employed [20]. In default reasoning, if all the pre-conditions of a rule are satisfied then the consequent of the rule is established. In defeasible reasoning, however, such a consequent may be defeated by the action of other rules.

Default logic has a model-theoretic semantics through the use of extensions as a kind of model. This has proven a fruitful tool for the analysis of default theories [18].

On the other hand, neither DL nor any other variant of modern defeasible logic has a model theory. DL is defined purely in proof-theoretic terms [5]. Furthermore, a model theory based on the idea of extensions is likely to be inappropriate for defeasible logic, since the kind of scepticism that is developed from intersection of extensions in default logic is different from the kind of scepticism that occurs in defeasible logic [17].

J. Lloyd et al. (Eds.): CL 2000, LNAI 1861, pp. 209–222, 2000.

In early work on semantics for defeasible logics, Nute [19] defined a model theory for LDR, a substantially simpler precursor of DL, in terms of a minimal belief state for each theory. LDR defines defeat only in terms of definite provability; this limitation is the main reason why the approach is successful [19]. Recently, this approach has been extended [7] to a defeasible logic that is closer to DL, and more general in one respect. However, the semantics is based on the idea of intersection of extensions and consequently the logic is sound but not complete for this semantics.

There has been some work on providing a semantics for DL in other styles. In [16] we showed that DL can be defined in terms of a meta-program, defined to reflect the inference rules of the logic, and a semantics for the language of the meta-program. While this approach was successful in establishing a relationship between DL and Kunen's semantics of negation-as-failure, it does not directly address model-theoretic reasoning.

In recent work [10] we have described DL in argumentation-theoretic terms. Such a characterization is useful for the applications of the logic that we have in mind, but the resulting semantics is again a meta-level treatment of the proof theory: proof trees are grouped together as arguments, and conflicting arguments are resolved by notions of argument defeat that reflect defeat in defeasible logic. Thus this work also fails to address model theory.

In this paper a semantics for DL is defined in the denotational style. Denotational semantics was developed as a framework for defining non-operational semantics for programming languages. It was inspired by model-theoretic semantics for classical logic [22].

Nevertheless, we do not claim that the denotational semantics we present represents a completely satisfactory solution to the problem of finding a model theory for defeasible logic. In particular, our semantics is not fully abstract. There are defeasible rule sets that are assigned different denotational semantics, but are not observably different. However, the denotational semantics is a strong basis from which to obtain a fully abstract semantics, and we suggest research directions that could achieve a satisfactory semantics.

The structure of the paper is as follows. In the next section we introduce the constructs of defeasible logic, and part of the proof theory of DL. We then define a denotational semantics for DL. The next two sections address issues of correctness and full abstraction for this semantics. Finally, we discuss directions for further research.

2   The Defeasible Logic DL

We begin by presenting the basic ingredients of defeasible logic. A defeasible theory contains five different kinds of knowledge: facts, strict rules, defeasible rules, defeaters, and a superiority relation.

Facts are indisputable statements, for example, "Tweety is an emu". This might be expressed as $emu(tweety)$.

Strict rules are rules in the traditional sense: whenever the premises are indisputable (e.g. facts) then so is the conclusion. An example of a strict rule is "Emus are birds". Written formally:

$$emu(X) \to bird(X).$$

Defeasible rules are rules that can be defeated by contrary evidence. An example of such a rule is "Birds typically fly"; written formally:

$$bird(X) \Rightarrow flies(X)$$

The idea is that if we know that something is a bird, then we may conclude that it flies, *unless there is other evidence suggesting that it may not fly.*

Defeaters are rules that cannot be used to draw any conclusions. Their only use is to prevent some conclusions. In other words, they are used to defeat some defeasible rules by producing evidence to the contrary. An example is "If an animal is heavy then it might not be able to fly". Formally:

$$heavy(X) \rightsquigarrow \neg flies(X)$$

The main point is that the information that an animal is heavy is not sufficient evidence to conclude that it doesn't fly. It is only evidence that the animal *may* not be able to fly. In other words, we don't wish to conclude $\neg flies(tweety)$ if $heavy(tweety)$; we simply want to prevent a conclusion $flies(tweety)$.

The *superiority relation* among rules is used to define priorities among rules, that is, where one rule may override the conclusion of another rule. For example, given the defeasible rules

$$r: \qquad bird(X) \Rightarrow flies(X)$$
$$r': brokenWing(X) \Rightarrow \neg flies(X)$$

which contradict one another, no conclusive decision can be made about whether a bird with a broken wing can fly. But if we introduce a superiority relation $>$ with $r' > r$, then we can indeed conclude that the bird cannot fly. We assume that $>$ is acyclic.

It is not possible, in this paper, to give a complete formal description of the logic. However, we hope to give enough information about the logic to make the discussion of the denotational semantics intelligible.

A *rule* r consists of its *antecedent* (or *body*) $A(r)$ which is a finite set of literals, an arrow, and its *head*, which is a literal. Given a set R of rules, we denote the set of all strict rules in R by R_s, the set of strict and defeasible rules in R by R_{sd}, the set of defeasible rules in R by R_d, and the set of defeaters in R by R_{dft}. $R[q]$ denotes the set of rules in R with head q. If q is a literal, $\sim q$ denotes the complementary literal (if q is a positive literal p then $\sim q$ is $\neg p$; and if q is $\neg p$, then $\sim q$ is p).

A *defeasible theory* $\mathcal{T}$ is a triple $(F, R, >)$ where F is a finite set of literals (called *facts*), R a finite set of rules, and $>$ a superiority relation on the labels of R.

A *conclusion* of $\mathcal{T}$ is a tagged literal and can have one of the following four forms:

$+\Delta q$, which is intended to mean that q is definitely provable in $\mathcal{T}$ (i.e., using only facts and strict rules).

$-\Delta q$, which is intended to mean that we have proved that q is not definitely provable in $\mathcal{T}$.

$+\partial q$, which is intended to mean that q is defeasibly provable in $\mathcal{T}$.

$-\partial q$ which is intended to mean that we have proved that q is not defeasibly provable in $\mathcal{T}$.

Provability is based on the concept of a *derivation* (or proof) in $\mathcal{T} = (F, R, >)$. A derivation is a finite sequence $P = (P(1), \ldots P(n))$ of tagged literals constructed by inference rules. There are four inference rules (corresponding to the four kinds of conclusion) that specify how a derivation can be extended. ($P(1..i)$ denotes the initial part of the sequence P of length i):

> $+\Delta$: We may append $P(i+1) = +\Delta q$ if either
> $\quad q \in F$ or
> $\quad \exists r \in R_s[q] \ \forall a \in A(r) : +\Delta a \in P(1..i)$

This means, to prove $+\Delta q$ we need to establish a proof for q using facts and strict rules only. This is a deduction in the classical sense. To prove $-\Delta q$ it is required to show that every attempt to prove $+\Delta q$ fails in a finite time. Thus the inference rule for $-\Delta$ is the constructive complement of the inference rule for $+\Delta$ [16].

> $-\Delta$: We may append $P(i+1) = -\Delta q$ if
> $\quad q \notin F$ and
> $\quad \forall r \in R_s[q] \ \exists a \in A(r) : -\Delta a \in P(1..i)$

The inference rule for defeasible conclusions is complicated by the defeasible nature of DL: opposing chains of reasoning must be taken into account.

> $+\partial$: We may append $P(i+1) = +\partial q$ if either
> $\quad$(1) $+\Delta q \in P(1..i)$ or
> $\quad$(2) (2.1) $\exists r \in R_{sd}[q] \forall a \in A(r) : +\partial a \in P(1..i)$ and
> $\quad\quad\quad$(2.2) $-\Delta \sim q \in P(1..i)$ and
> $\quad\quad\quad$(2.3) $\forall s \in R[\sim q]$ either
> $\quad\quad\quad\quad$(2.3.1) $\exists a \in A(s) : -\partial a \in P(1..i)$ or
> $\quad\quad\quad\quad$(2.3.2) $\exists t \in R_{sd}[q]$ such that
> $\quad\quad\quad\quad\quad\quad \forall a \in A(t) : +\partial a \in P(1..i)$ and $t > s$

Let us work through this inference rule. To show that q is provable defeasibly we have two choices: (1) We show that q is already definitely provable; or (2) we need to argue using the defeasible part of $\mathcal{T}$ as well. In particular, we require that there must be a strict or defeasible rule with head q which can be applied (2.1). But now we need to consider possible "attacks", that is, reasoning chains in support of $\sim q$. To be more specific: to prove q defeasibly we must show that $\sim q$ is not definitely provable (2.2). Also (2.3) we must consider the set of all rules which are not known to be inapplicable and which have head $\sim q$ (note that here we consider defeaters, too, whereas they could not be used to support the conclusion q; this is in line with the motivation of defeaters given earlier). Essentially each such rule s attacks the conclusion q. For q to be provable, each such rule s must be counterattacked by a rule t with head q with the following properties: (i) t must be applicable at this point, and (ii) t must be stronger than s. Thus each attack on the conclusion q must be counterattacked by a stronger rule.

As with $-\Delta$, the inference rule for $-\partial$ is the constructive complement of the inference rule for $+\partial$.

$-\partial$: We may append $P(i+1) = -\partial q$ if
    (1) $-\Delta q \in P(1..i)$ and
    (2)   (2.1) $\forall r \in R_{sd}[q] \; \exists a \in A(r) : -\partial a \in P(1..i)$ or
          (2.2) $+\Delta \sim q \in P(1..i)$ or
          (2.3) $\exists s \in R[\sim q]$ such that
                  (2.3.1) $\forall a \in A(s) : +\partial a \in P(1..i)$ and
                  (2.3.2) $\forall t \in R_{sd}[q]$ either
                          $\exists a \in A(t) : -\partial a \in P(1..i)$ or $t \not> s$

3   A Denotational Semantics

The approach of denotational semantics is to map, using a function μ, every syntactic construct to its meaning, that is, the abstract thing that it denotes. The meaning of a compound syntactic object is defined in terms of the meaning of its components. Generally these definitions are recursive, and the meaning of each construct is then given by a fixedpoint of the corresponding equations.

In comparison to the denotational semantics of programming languages, the denotational semantics of DL appears simple since there are few syntactic constructs and there is no need to represent sequentiality or state. The meanings of all but one of the syntactic categories are defined non-recursively, in terms of the meaning of components. Only the semantics of an entire defeasible theory is defined recursively, that is, in terms of itself.

We first introduce some notation and then discuss our assumptions about DL. $\wp X$ denotes the powerset of X. $f + g$ denotes the function $(f + g)(X) = f(X) \cup g(X)$. When x is a tuple, we write $\pi_i x$ to denote the i'th element of x.

We assume a given language consisting of a set of function symbols Σ and a set of predicate symbols Π, all with fixed arities, an infinite set $Vars$ of variables, and an infinite set Lab of labels. We extend Lab to $Labels$ by the addition of a new element $\langle null \rangle$, which will be used as a placeholder for rules without a label. Thus Lab contains the labels that can be used in defining a theory, but $Labels$ is the set of labels used in the semantics.

Let $\mathcal{T} = (F, R, >)$ and let $\mathcal{L}$ be the set of literals generated by the language of $\mathcal{T}$. We assume that F, R, and $>$ are finite.

In all the functions to be presented, there is an implicit domain of interpretation $\mathcal{D}$. $\mathcal{D}$ consists of a set of values D and the interpretation of each function symbol f of arity n by a function $\hat{f} : D^n \to D$. Equality is interpreted by identity in D. In this paper we will consider only the Herbrand domain generated by an infinite set of constants, but we address later the issues in extending our results more generally. The set of evaluated literals is $EL = \{p(d_1, \ldots, d_n) \mid p \in \Pi, d_1, \ldots, d_n \in D\}$. We represent the conclusions of DL by a 4-tuple of sets of evaluated literals. Let $\mathbf{Conc} = (\wp EL)^4$. $\mathbf{Conc}$ contains elements such as $(\{emu(tweety), bird(tweety)\}, \{heavy(tweety), \neg heavy(tweety)\}, \{flies(tweety)\}, \{heavy(tweety)\})$.

We define a function μ from defeasible theories to $\mathbf{Conc}$, that is $\mu : \mathcal{T} \mapsto (+\Delta, -\Delta, +\partial, -\partial)$, which maps the defeasible theory $\mathcal{T}$ to the four sets of conclusions that can be derived from a theory [15].

The functions presented below act on elements of $\mathbf{Conc}$. Given an element X of $\mathbf{Conc}$, or any 4-tuple, we use a subscript $(+\Delta, -\Delta, +\partial,$ or $-\partial)$ to refer to the projection of X onto the corresponding field. For example, if $X = (A, B, C, D)$ then $X_{+\Delta}$ is A and $X_{-\partial}$ is D. We define the following order on $\mathbf{Conc}$: $(A_1, B_1, C_1, D_1) \leq (A_2, B_2, C_2, D_2)$ iff $A_1 \subseteq A_2$, $B_1 \subseteq B_2$, $C_1 \subseteq C_2$, and $D_1 \subseteq D_2$. Union is also defined pointwise, $(A_1, B_1, C_1, D_1) \cup (A_2, B_2, C_2, D_2) = (A_1 \cup A_2, B_1 \cup B_2, C_1 \cup C_2, D_1 \cup D_2)$, and extends in the obvious way to infinite unions.

A valuation is a function from variables to values in the domain. Thus $Valn$, the set of valuations is defined to be $Vars \to D$.

The meaning of a literal, given a single conclusion, is the collection of valuations that, when applied to the literal, produce the given conclusion. Since a conclusion may have one of four tags, when we generalize this statement to a set of conclusions, we use 4-tuples for both the concluded literals and the valuations.

For a literal in the body of a rule, we intend that $\mu[\![literal]\!]$ maps collections of conclusions to collections of the corresponding valuations that map $literal$ to one of the conclusions. That is, the meaning of a literal, given some conclusions, is the collections of valuations (one for each tag) that, when applied to the literal, produce one of the given conclusions.

However, we also need to use the meaning of a literal to define the appropriate instance of the literal by a valuation. This aspect of the literal is used when the literal appears in the head of a rule. Thus the type is:

$$\mu[\![literal]\!] : \mathbf{Conc} \to ((\wp Valn)^4 \times (Valn \to EL))$$

The second aspect of the meaning of a literal appears in the codomain of this expression purely to simplify the notation; it is not dependent on the input value from $\mathbf{Conc}$. We will use expressions such as $v(Head)$ as shorthand for $\pi_2(\mu[\![Head]\!](X))(v)$. Thus the meaning of a literal is defined as

$$\mu[\![literal]\!](X) = ((V_{+\Delta}, V_{-\Delta}, V_{+\partial}, V_{-\partial}), apply)$$

where $V_t = \{v \mid v(literal) \in X_t\}$ for each tag t, and $apply(v) = v(literal)$.

Define a function $\otimes$ by $(A, B, C, D) \otimes (E, F, G, H) = (A \cap E, B \cup F, C \cap G, D \cup H)$. This function is clearly commutative and associative, with identity

$(\mathcal{L}, \emptyset, \mathcal{L}, \emptyset)$, and so extends straightforwardly to a set of tuples. Note that $\otimes$ is monotonic wrt the pointwise extension of the containment ordering on $\wp \, Valn$.

The meaning of a rule body is simply the combination, by $\otimes$, of the (first part of the) meanings of its constituent literals.

$$\mu[\![Body]\!] : \mathbf{Conc} \to (\wp \, Valn)^4$$

$$\mu[\![Body]\!](X) = \bigotimes_{b \in Body} \pi_1 \mu[\![b]\!](X)$$

Before we define the meaning of a rule, we introduce some more types. $LATE = (Labels \times Arrows \times Tags \times EL)$. $Labels$ is the set of labels of rules, $Arrows = \{\to, \Rightarrow, \leadsto\}$, $Tags = \{+\Delta, \overline{-\Delta}, +\partial, \overline{-\partial}\}$, EL is the set of evaluated literals. $\overline{-\Delta}$ (respectively $\overline{-\partial}$) is intended to represent the complement of $-\Delta$ (respectively $-\partial$). Elements of $LATE$ are tentative conclusions (i.e. potential conclusions that might yet be defeated) including information on the rule used to produce the tentative conclusion (its label and its arrow). An example element of $LATE$ is $(\mathtt{rule1}, \Rightarrow, +\partial, flies(tweety))$.

The meaning of a rule is the function which maps a set of conclusions to further tentative conclusions which can be drawn using the rule. The tentative conclusions are only positive, in the sense that they are about inferences that could be made, rather than those that cannot be made. We represent a rule by $label : Body \hookrightarrow Head$, where $label$, $Body$, $\hookrightarrow$ and $Head$ are syntactic variables.

$$\mu[\![label : Body \hookrightarrow Head]\!] : \mathbf{Conc} \to \wp LATE$$

$$
\begin{aligned}
\mu[\![label : Body \ &\hookrightarrow \ Head]\!](X) = \\
&\{(label, \hookrightarrow, +\Delta, v(Head))| \quad \hookrightarrow \text{ is } \to \text{ and} \\
&\qquad\qquad\qquad\qquad\qquad\quad v \in \mu[\![Body]\!](X)_{+\Delta}\} \\
\cup \ &\{(label, \hookrightarrow, \overline{-\Delta}, v(Head))| \ \hookrightarrow \text{ is } \to \text{ and} \\
&\qquad\qquad\qquad\qquad\qquad\quad v \notin \mu[\![Body]\!](X)_{-\Delta}\} \\
\cup \ &\{(label, \hookrightarrow, +\partial, v(Head))| \ \hookrightarrow \in Arrows \text{ and} \\
&\qquad\qquad\qquad\qquad\qquad\quad v \in \mu[\![Body]\!](X)_{+\partial}\} \\
\cup \ &\{(label, \hookrightarrow, \overline{-\partial}, v(Head))| \ \hookrightarrow \in Arrows \text{ and} \\
&\qquad\qquad\qquad\qquad\qquad\quad v \notin \mu[\![Body]\!](X)_{-\partial}\}
\end{aligned}
$$

We consider rules without a label to be rules where the label is $\langle null \rangle$.

$$\mu[\![Body \hookrightarrow Head]\!](X) = \mu[\![\langle null \rangle : Body \hookrightarrow Head]\!](X)$$

The meaning of a fact is a constant function of the same type as rules: $\mathbf{Conc} \to \wp LATE$. Essentially, facts are treated as unlabelled, strict rules with empty bodies. This possibility was already pointed out in [2].

$$
\begin{aligned}
\mu[\![f]\!] = \lambda x. \quad &\{(\langle null \rangle, \to, +\Delta, v(f)) \mid v \in Valn\} \\
\cup \ &\{(\langle null \rangle, \to, \overline{-\Delta}, v(f)) \mid v \in Valn\}
\end{aligned}
$$

The meaning of a set of facts (or rules) is simply the sum of the meaning of every fact (or rule)

$$\mu[\![F]\!] = \sum_{f \in F} \mu[\![f]\!]$$

$$\mu[\![R]\!] = \sum_{r \in R} \mu[\![r]\!]$$

The meaning of an individual superiority statement is simply a binary relation expressed as a function, and has type $Bin\,Reln$, where $Bin\,Reln = Labels \times Labels \to Boolean$.

$$\mu[\![n_1 > n_2]\!](x, y) = \text{ if } (x = n_1 \wedge y = n_2) \text{ then } true \text{ else } false$$

The meaning of the superiority relation as a whole is simply the combination of the meaning of the individual statements in the obvious way.

$$\mu[\![>]\!](x, y) = \bigvee_{s \in >} \mu[\![s]\!]$$

The meaning of the theory $\mathcal{T}$ is defined as the least fixedpoint of a function $\mu_{\mathcal{T}}$ determined by the three components of $\mathcal{T}$: the facts F, the rules R and the superiority relation $>$.

$$\mu[\![\mathcal{T}]\!] : \textbf{Conc}$$

$$\mu[\![\mathcal{T}]\!] = lfp(\mu_{\mathcal{T}})$$

$\mu_{\mathcal{T}}$ is an auxiliary function, used for clarity, which maps a collection of conclusions to a new, larger collection of conclusions that can be drawn on the basis of the rules and the superiority relation. The requirement that $\mu[\![\mathcal{T}]\!]$ be a fixedpoint of $\mu_{\mathcal{T}}$ (i.e. a solution of $Z = \mu_{\mathcal{T}}(Z)$) is thus a requirement that $\mu[\![\mathcal{T}]\!]$ be deductively closed.

$$\mu_{\mathcal{T}} : \textbf{Conc} \to \textbf{Conc}$$

$$\mu_{\mathcal{T}}(X) = X \cup combine(\mu[\![>]\!], \mu[\![R]\!] + \mu[\![F]\!])(X)$$

combine performs the mediation, using the superiority relation, among the tentative conclusions produced by the rules and facts. It embodies most of the information that is part of the inference rules of DL and has been structured similarly to make the correspondence clear. For many variants of defeasible logic, only this function needs to be altered to produce a denotational semantics of the variant.

$$combine : (Bin\,Reln \times (\textbf{Conc} \to \wp LATE)) \to (\textbf{Conc} \to \textbf{Conc})$$

$$combine(\succ, f)(X) = (+\Delta, -\Delta, +\partial, -\partial)$$

where

$$+\Delta = \{p | \exists(n, \to, +\Delta, p) \in f(X)\}$$

$$-\varDelta = \{p|\ \not\exists(n,\to,\overline{-\varDelta},p) \in f(X)\}$$

$$+\partial = +\varDelta \cup \{p|$$
$$\not\exists(n,\to,\overline{-\varDelta},\sim p) \in f(X) \text{ and}$$
$$\exists(n_1,\hookrightarrow_1,+\partial,p) \in f(X) \text{ such that } \hookrightarrow_1 \text{ is } \to \text{ or } \Rightarrow, \text{ and}$$
$$\forall(n_2,\hookrightarrow_2,\overline{-\partial},\sim p) \in f(X)$$
$$\exists(n_3,\hookrightarrow_3,+\partial,p) \in f(X),$$
$$\hookrightarrow_3 \text{ is } \to \text{ or } \Rightarrow, \text{ and } n_3 \succ n_2$$
$$\}$$

$$-\partial = -\varDelta \cap \{p|$$
$$\exists(n,\to,+\varDelta,\sim p) \in f(X) \text{ or}$$
$$\forall(n_1,\hookrightarrow_1,\overline{-\partial},p) \in f(X) \text{ such that } \hookrightarrow_1 \text{ is } \to \text{ or } \Rightarrow,$$
$$\exists(n_2,\hookrightarrow_2,+\partial,\sim p) \in f(X)$$
$$\forall(n_3,\hookrightarrow_3,\overline{-\partial},p) \in f(X)$$
$$\hookrightarrow_3 \text{ is } \leadsto \text{ or } n_3 \not\succ n_2$$
$$\}$$

This ends the definition of the denotational semantics of DL.

4   Correctness

To show that this semantics is well-defined, we need to establish that a least fixedpoint of μ_T exists. Usually, in denotational semantics, all functions are chosen to be monotonic[1] over a complete lattice, and the existence of the least fixedpoint then follows by Tarski's result [23]. However, since we are dealing with a non-monotonic logic that option is not readily available. Specifically, the function μ_T is not monotonic. For example, consider the theory $(\emptyset, R, \emptyset)$ where $R = \{b \Rightarrow a\}$. Let $Y = \mu_T(\{b\}, \emptyset, \emptyset, \emptyset)$ and $Z = \mu_T(\{\neg a, b\}, \emptyset, \emptyset, \emptyset)$. Then $a \in Y_{+\partial}$ but $a \notin Z_{+\partial}$.

Nevertheless, we are able to establish that the least fixedpoint of μ_T exists and thus the semantics is well-defined.

Define
$$\mu_T \uparrow 0 = \emptyset$$
$$\mu_T \uparrow (\alpha + 1) = \mu_T(\mu_T \uparrow \alpha)$$
$$\mu_T \uparrow \alpha = \bigcup_{\beta < \alpha} \mu_T \uparrow \beta$$

where, in the last case, α is a limit ordinal. The semantics can be constructed using this definition.

Theorem 1.

$$lfp(\mu_T) = \mu_T \uparrow \omega$$

---

[1] A function f from a partially ordered set $(A, <_A)$ to a partially ordered set $(B, <_B)$ is *monotonic* if, for every $x, y \in A$, if $x <_A y$ then $f(x) <_B f(y)$.

The proof proceeds by showing, by induction, that $(\mu_T \uparrow \alpha) \leq X$ for every α and every X that is a fixedpoint of μ_T. Key to the proof are the containment relations holding as a result of $\mu_T \uparrow \alpha \leq X$, in particular, $\mu[\![R]\!](\mu_T \uparrow \alpha)_{+\partial} \subseteq \mu[\![R]\!](X)_{+\partial}$ and $\mu[\![R]\!](X)_{\overline{-\partial}} \subseteq \mu[\![R]\!](\mu_T \uparrow \alpha)_{\overline{-\partial}}$, where U_s denotes the set of all tuples u in U such that $\pi_3 u = s$. Thus, for example, $Y_{+\partial}$ denotes the subset of Y containing all tuples of the form $(\ldots, \ldots, +\partial, \ldots)$.

Furthermore, by the assumptions that the theory is finite and that the domain has only constants, $\mu_T \uparrow \omega$ is a fixedpoint of μ_T. The result follows immediately.

Since the semantics is well-defined, we can now address its correctness. Rather than determine its correctness with respect to the original proof theory, we will use the bottom-up formulation of the proof theory presented in [16]. That formulation is, in fact, an extension of the proof theory that permits non-propositional languages and infinite domains. The original proof-theoretic definitions [5, 19] implicitly assume that there are only finitely many ground instances of rules, and are inappropriate when the domain is infinite. If the domain consists of finitely many constants then [16] and [5, 19] are essentially equivalent.

The semantics is correct in the sense that it characterizes the conclusions that can be proved in the bottom-up formulation of the proof theory of DL. That is, the proof system is sound and complete with respect to this semantics.

Theorem 2. *Let T be a defeasible theory and μ as defined above.*

- $\mu[\![T]\!]_{+\Delta} = \{p \mid T \vdash +\Delta p\}$
- $\mu[\![T]\!]_{-\Delta} = \{p \mid T \vdash -\Delta p\}$
- $\mu[\![T]\!]_{+\partial} = \{p \mid T \vdash +\partial p\}$
- $\mu[\![T]\!]_{-\partial} = \{p \mid T \vdash -\partial p\}$

The proof is by induction on the level of iteration α. The use of the bottom-up formulation greatly simplifies the proof.

The denotational semantics has deliberately not addressed compositionality at the level of defeasible theories, so that the semantics reflects the proof theory exactly. The most reasonable operation on defeasible theories is union, defined by $T_1 \cup T_2 = (F_1 \cup F_2, R_1 \cup R_2, >_1 \cup >_2)$, where $T_i = (F_i, R_i, >_i)$. Although the denotational semantics is not compositional in the sense that the meaning of $T_1 \cup T_2$ can be determined from the meanings of T_1 and T_2, it can easily reflect the above definition through compositionality at the level of F, R and $>$.

5   Full Abstraction

A semantics is *fully abstract* if whenever the semantics of two things (of the same syntactic type) differ there is a context in which the two things produce different operational (in this case, proof-theoretic) results. By context we mean a theory with a "hole" such that once the hole is filled the resulting theory is syntactically correct.

If a semantics is fully abstract (and correct) then we can tell whether two syntactic items will behave equivalently or not by checking whether the semantics assigns the same meaning to both items. Thus a fully abstract correct semantics expresses exactly the same distinctions that would be observable from the proof theory, and no more.

For defeasible logic, we say a semantics is *fully abstract* if, for every syntactic category and every S_1 and S_2 in that category, $\mu[\![S_1]\!] \neq \mu[\![S_2]\!]$ implies there is a context $C[\ ]$ such that $\mathcal{P}[\![C[S_1]]\!] \neq \mathcal{P}[\![C[S_2]]\!]$ where $\mathcal{P}$ denotes the proof-theoretic semantics.

We start by characterizing, for some syntactic categories, when two syntactic objects have the same meaning. Two rules $Body_i \rightarrow Head_i$, for $i = 1, 2$, are subsumption-equivalent if there exists a variable renaming ρ such that $Head_1 = Head_2\rho$ and $Body_2\rho \subseteq Body_1$ and $Body_1\rho^{-1} \subseteq Body_2$.

Lemma 3. *Let $Literal_i$, $Body_i$, $label_i$ and $Head_i$ be syntactic variables ranging over literals, bodies, labels and literals respectively, for $i = 1, 2$.*

- *$\mu[\![Literal_1]\!] = \mu[\![Literal_2]\!]$ iff $Literal_1$ and $Literal_2$ are identical*
- *$\mu[\![Body_1]\!] = \mu[\![Body_2]\!]$ iff $Body_1 = Body_2$ as sets*
- *$\mu[\![label_1 : Body_1 \hookrightarrow_1 Head_1]\!] = \mu[\![label_2 : Body_2 \hookrightarrow_2 Head_2]\!]$ iff $label_1 = label_2$, $\hookrightarrow_1 = \hookrightarrow_2$, and $Body_1 \rightarrow Head_1$ is subsumption-equivalent to $Body_2 \rightarrow Head_2$*

The proof is straightforward, and very similar to a corresponding result for definite logic programs [14]. The possible presence of a literal and its negation in a body has no effect since the input X to the function is permitted to satisfy $\{p, \neg p\} \subseteq X_{+\Delta}$.

We can now show that the semantics is fully abstract in all syntactic categories except one. Specifically, the semantics is fully abstract for literals, bodies, rules, superiority statements, and the sets F of facts and the superiority relation $>$. It is only for the set of rules R that the semantics is not fully abstract.

Theorem 4. *The denotational semantics is fully abstract for every syntactic category, except the set of rules R.*

Proof. For bodies: If $\mu[\![B_1]\!] \neq \mu[\![B_2]\!]$, then $B_1 \neq B_2$ as sets, by the above lemma. Hence either $B_1 \not\subseteq B_2$ or $B_2 \not\subseteq B_1$ (or both). We consider only the first case, since the second is symmetrical. Let θ map all variables in B_1 to distinct constants. Then $B_1\theta$ is not an instance of B_2. Let $C[\ ] = (F, R, \emptyset)$, where $F = \{b\theta \mid b \in B_1\}$ and $R = \{[\ ] \Rightarrow h\}$, for an atom h not occurring in $B_1 \cup B_2$. Then $C[B_1] \vdash +\partial h$ but $C[B_2] \vdash -\partial h$. A similar argument applies to individual literals.

For rules: If $\mu[\![r_1]\!] \neq \mu[\![r_2]\!]$, then there are three cases by the above lemma: the difference is caused by labels, arrows, or the rules proper. Let r_i be $label_i : B_i \hookrightarrow_i h_i$ for $i = 1, 2$.

If r_1 and r_2 have different labels, we can assume, by symmetry, that $label_1 \neq \langle null \rangle$. Suppose this is the only difference between $\mu[\![r_1]\!]$ and $\mu[\![r_2]\!]$. Let $C[\ ] = (\emptyset, R, >)$, where $R = \{[\ ]\} \cup \{true \Rightarrow b\theta \mid b \in B_1\} \cup \{r : true \Rightarrow \sim h_1\theta\}$, $>$ contains only $r > label_1$, and r is a (non-null) label different from $label_1$ and $label_2$. Then $C[r_1] \vdash +\partial \sim h_1\theta$ but $C[r_2] \vdash -\partial \sim h_1\theta$.

Suppose r_1 and r_2 have different arrows but are otherwise subsumption-equal. Let $C[\ ] = (F, R, \emptyset)$, where $F = \{b\theta \mid b \in B_1\}$ and $R = \{[\ ]\}$. Then

- $\hookrightarrow_i$ is $\to$ iff $C[r_i] \vdash +\partial h_1 \theta$ and $C[r_i] \vdash +\Delta h_1 \theta$
- $\hookrightarrow_i$ is $\Rightarrow$ iff $C[r_i] \vdash +\partial h_1 \theta$ and $C[r_i] \vdash -\Delta h_1 \theta$
- $\hookrightarrow_i$ is $\rightsquigarrow$ iff $C[r_i] \vdash -\partial h_1 \theta$ and $C[r_i] \vdash -\Delta h_1 \theta$

Thus this context can distinguish r_1 and r_2.

Suppose r_1 and r_2 are not subsumption-equal. Then one rule, say r_1, does not subsume the other rule. Consequently, r_1 does not subsume $r_2 \theta$. Let $C[\ ] = (F, R, \emptyset)$, where $F = \{b\theta \mid b \in B_2\}$ and $R = \{[\ ]\} \cup \{true \Rightarrow \sim h_2 \theta\}$. Then $C[r_1] \vdash +\partial \sim h_2 \theta$ but $C[r_2] \vdash -\partial \sim h_2 \theta$.

For the set of facts: If $\mu[\![F_1]\!] \neq \mu[\![F_2]\!]$ then there is a tuple $(n, \hookrightarrow, t, f) \in \mu[\![F_1]\!] \backslash \mu[\![F_2]\!]$ (or vice versa). Let $C[\ ] = ([\ ], \emptyset, \emptyset)$. Then $C[F_1] \vdash +\Delta f$ but $C[F_2] \vdash -\Delta f$.

For superiority statements, full abstraction is trivial. For the superiority relation: If $\mu[\![>_1]\!] \neq \mu[\![>_2]\!]$ then there are labels a and b such that $a >_1 b$ but not $a >_2 b$ (or vice versa). Let $C[\ ] = (\emptyset, R, [\ ])$ where $R = \{a : true \Rightarrow p, b : true \Rightarrow \neg p\}$. Then $C[>_1] \vdash +\partial p$ but $C[>_2] \vdash -\partial p$.

To see that the semantics is not fully abstract for R consider the rule sets $R_1 = \{p \to q, q \to r\}$ and $R_2 = \{p \to q, q \to r, p \to r\}$. Clearly $\mu[\![R_1]\!] \neq \mu[\![R_2]\!]$ but in any context the proof-theoretic semantics are the same.

In a conventional logic programming setting we might overcome this problem by defining $\mu[\![R]\!]$ in terms of all unfoldings of rules of R. (See, for example, [6].) However, this approach is not immediately transferable to defeasible logics since tentative conclusions must be mediated by the superiority relation. It is perhaps possible to apply techniques used in giving compositional denotational semantics to concurrent languages (for example, something similar to failure sets) to solve this problem. Indeed, the result might be similar to the semantic kernel of [8]. This is certainly a topic for further investigation.

6 Further Work

Extending these results to other domains, – for example, the Herbrand domain with function symbols, or linear real arithmetic – faces two hurdles.

Firstly, the fixedpoint characterization is no longer valid. Consider the following example in a Herbrand domain.

$$p(X) \Rightarrow q(a)$$
$$p(X) \Rightarrow p(f(X))$$

In this case the fixedpoint characterization will produce the conclusion $-\partial q(a)$, which is not a valid conclusion in defeasible logic. The problem is essentially the same as the problem of representing finite failure in logic programs by fixedpoint techniques, although the function μ_T is considerably more complicated. Thus, in more powerful domains the semantics should be defined in terms of $\mu_T \uparrow \omega$, rather than $lfp(\mu_T)$.

This fact, and the relationship between Kunen's semantics of logic programs and defeasible logic [16] suggests that a model theory based on three-valued logic might be able to characterize $\mu_T \uparrow \omega$ in the same way that Kunen showed [13] that logical consequence in a three-valued logic characterizes $\Phi_P \uparrow \omega$, where Φ_P is a function introduced by Fitting [9]. However, the greater complexity of μ_T in comparison with Φ_P suggests that the required logic would be cumbersome. Nevertheless, this is a promising approach to achieving model-based semantics.

Secondly, in general, other domains require built-in relations - constraints [12]. The denotational semantics is easily adapted to handle constraints in rule bodies by defining

$$\mu[\![constraint]\!](X) = ((V, \overline{V}, V, \overline{V}), f)$$

where V is the set of valuations under which the constraint is true, $\overline{V}$ is the complement of V in $Valn$, and f is a dummy value that is never used. However, the full abstraction results will require further extension since, for example, the definition of subsumption-equal is inadequate when constraints are admitted.

7 Conclusion

The problem of finding a model theory for defeasible logic has been a longstanding one. This paper has defined a denotational semantics for the defeasible logic DL. This is a notable achievement since non-monotonicity is a difficult hurdle to overcome. The semantics is a step towards a model theory, but is not completely satisfactory since it is not fully abstract. Nevertheless, this work provides a sturdy basis for obtaining a satisfactory model theory.

Acknowledgements

Thanks to D. Billington, who introduced me to the problem of defining a model theory for defeasible logic, and gave me access to his extensive library of papers on defeasible logic, and to G. Antoniou and G. Governatori for discussions on defeasible logic. Thanks also to IC-Parc for the use of their facilities in preparing the camera-ready copy of this paper. This research was supported by the Australian Research Council under grant A49803544.

References

1. G. Antoniou, D. Billington, M.J. Maher, A. Rock, A Flexible Framework for Defeasible Logics, *Proc. American National Conference on Artificial Intelligence*, 2000, to appear.
2. G. Antoniou, D. Billington and M.J. Maher. Normal Forms for Defeasible Logic. In *Proc. Joint International Conference and Symposium on Logic Programming*, J. Jaffar (Ed.), 160–174. MIT Press, 1998.
3. G. Antoniou, D. Billington and M.J. Maher. On the analysis of regulations using defeasible rules. In *Proc. of the 32nd Annual Hawaii International Conference on System Sciences*. IEEE Press, 1999.

4. G. Antoniou, D. Billington, M.J. Maher, A. Rock, Efficient Defeasible Reasoning Systems. *Proc. Australian Workshop on Computational Logic*, 2000.

5. D. Billington. Defeasible Logic is Stable. *Journal of Logic and Computation* 3 : 370–400, 1993.

6. A. Bossi, M. Gabbrielli, G. Levi, M.C. Meo. A Compositional Semantics for Logic Programs. *Theoretical Computer Science* 122(1&2): 3–47, 1994.

7. S.N. Donnelly. Semantics, Soundness and Incompleteness for a Defeasible Logic. M.S. thesis, University of Georgia, 1999.

8. P.M. Dung and K. Kanchanasut. A Fixpoint Approach to Declarative Semantics of Logic Programs. *Proc. North American Conf. on Logic Programming*, 604–625, 1989.

9. M. Fitting, A Kripke-Kleene Semantics for Logic Programs, *Journal of Logic Programming*, 4, 295-312, 1985.

10. G. Governatori and M. Maher, An Argumentation-Theoretic Characterization of Defeasible Logic, *Proc. European Conf. on Artificial Intelligence*, 2000, to appear.

11. B.N. Grosof, Y. Labrou, and H.Y. Chan. A Declarative Approach to Business Rules in Contracts: Courteous Logic Programs in XML, *Proceedings of the 1st ACM Conference on Electronic Commerce (EC-99)*, ACM Press, 1999.

12. J. Jaffar and M.J. Maher, Constraint Logic Programming: A Survey, *Journal of Logic Programming 19 & 20*, 503–581, 1994.

13. K. Kunen, Negation in Logic Programming, *Journal of Logic Programming*, 4, 289–308, 1987.

14. M.J. Maher, Equivalences of Logic Programs, in: *Foundations of Deductive Databases and Logic Programming*, J. Minker (Ed), Morgan Kaufmann, 627–658, 1988.

15. M. Maher, G. Antoniou and D. Billington. A Study of Provability in Defeasible Logic. In *Proc. Australian Joint Conference on Artificial Intelligence*, 215–226, LNAI 1502, Springer, 1998.

16. M. Maher and G. Governatori. A Semantic Decomposition of Defeasible Logics. *Proc. American National Conference on Artificial Intelligence*, 299–305, 1999.

17. D. Makinson and K. Schlechta. Floating conclusions and zombie paths: two deep difficulties in the "directly skeptical" approach to defeasible inheritance nets. *Artificial Intelligence* 48(1991): 199–209.

18. V. Marek and M. Truszczynski. *Nonmonotonic Logic*, Springer 1993.

19. D. Nute. Defeasible Reasoning and Decision Support Systems. *Decision Support Systems* 4, 97–110, 1988.

20. D. Nute. Defeasible Logic. In D.M. Gabbay, C.J. Hogger and J.A. Robinson (eds.): *Handbook of Logic in Artificial Intelligence and Logic Programming Vol. 3*, Oxford University Press 1994, 353-395.

21. D.M. Reeves, B.N. Grosof, M.P. Wellman, and H.Y. Chan. Towards a Declarative Language for Negotiating Executable Contracts, *Proc. AAAI-99 Workshop on Artificial Intelligence in Electronic Commerce*, AAAI Press / MIT Press, 1999.

22. D.S. Scott. Logic and Programming Languages. *C.ACM* 20, 634–641, 1977.

23. A. Tarski. A Lattice-theoretical Fixpoint Theorem and its Applications. *Pacific Journal of Mathematics*, 5, 1955, 285–309.

Isoinitial Semantics for Logic Programs

Kung-Kiu Lau[1] and Mario Ornaghi[2]

[1] Dept. of Computer Science, University of Manchester, United Kingdom
kung-kiu@cs.man.ac.uk
[2] Dip. di Scienze dell'Informazione, Universita' degli studi di Milano, Italy
ornaghi@dsi.unimi.it

Abstract. The Herbrand model H of a definite logic program P is an initial model among the class of all the models of P, interpreting P as an initial theory. Such a theory (program) proves (computes) only positive literals (atoms) in P, so it does not deal with negation. In this paper, we introduce *isoinitial* semantics for logic programs and show that it can provide a rich semantics for logic programs, which can deal with not just negation, but also incomplete information, parametricity and compositionality.

We dedicate this paper to the memory of the originator of isoinitial semantics:
Pierangelo Miglioli (1946–1999).

1 Introduction

The intended model of a definite logic program P is its Herbrand model H. It interprets P under the Closed World Assumption [16]. Among the class of all the models of P, H interprets P as an *initial* theory [9]. A distinguishing feature of an initial theory P is that, in general, it proves (computes) only positive literals in P, so it does not deal with negation. One way to handle negation is to consider program *closures* (e.g. program completion). In this paper, we introduce *isoinitial* semantics [2] for (definite) logic programs, and we show that isoinitial closures are better able to handle negation than initial closures, and are, in general, richer than initial closures from the point of view of *incomplete information*, *parametricity* and *compositionality*.

We will discuss full first-order theories in general, and consider definite programs as a particular case, with its own peculiarities. Since it admits any kind of axioms, our treatment also applies to *normal* and *disjunctive* programs (which for lack of space we will only briefly mention in the Conclusion). Finally, we shall assume familiarity with the general terminology for logic programming, and refer readers to standard works such as [12] for this terminology.

The results of Sections 2 and 3 adapt the general results of [2, 14] to logic programs (for the first time), while the other results are mainly new.

J. Lloyd et al. (Eds.): CL 2000, LNAI 1861, pp. 223–238, 2000.

2 Initial and Isoinitial Models

In this section, we formally define, and exhibit examples of, theories with initial and isoinitial models. We show how we can characterise such models, and for isoinitial models, we state useful conditions for proving isoinitiality.

A Σ-theory is a set of Σ-sentences, where $\Sigma \equiv \langle F, R \rangle$ is a signature Σ with function symbols F and relation symbols R, where each symbol has an associated arity. For example, Peano Arithmetic is a *Nat*-theory, where *Nat* $\equiv \langle \{0^0, s^1, +^2, *^2\}, \{=^2\} \rangle$.[1]

We shall work in first-order logic with identity, i.e. identity $=$ and the usual identity axioms will always be understood. For example, we can introduce *Nat* as the signature $Nat \equiv \langle \{0^0, s^1, +^2, *^2\}, \{\} \rangle$, with $=$ being understood.

Let $\Sigma \equiv \langle F, R \rangle$ be a signature. As usual, a Σ-*structure* is a triple $\mathcal{M} \equiv \langle D, F^{\mathcal{M}}, R^{\mathcal{M}} \rangle$, where $F^{\mathcal{M}}$ is a F-indexed set of functions interpreting F, and $R^{\mathcal{M}}$ is an R-indexed set of relations interpreting R. Of course, the interpretation of a function symbol f^n is an n-ary function $f^{n\mathcal{M}} : D^n \to D$, and the interpretation of a relation symbol $r^m \in R$ is an m-ary relation $r^{m\mathcal{M}} \subseteq D^m$. When no confusion can arise, we may omit the arity, i.e. we write $f^{\mathcal{M}}$ instead of $f^{n\mathcal{M}}$ and $r^{\mathcal{M}}$ instead of $r^{m\mathcal{M}}$.

In a structure $\mathcal{M}$, terms and formulas are interpreted in the usual way. $t^{\mathcal{M}}$ will denote the value of a ground term t in $\mathcal{M}$, and $\mathcal{M} \models A$ will indicate that the sentence (sentences) A is (are) true in $\mathcal{M}$. A theory T is a set of sentences, and a *model* of T is a structure $\mathcal{M}$ such that $\mathcal{M} \models T$.

Finally, *homomorphisms*, *isomorphisms* and *isomorphic embeddings* are defined in the usual way. Since the latter are less popularly used in the literature than homomorphisms and isomorphisms, we briefly recall them here.

Definition 1. (Isomorphic Embeddings). An *isomorphic embedding* $i : \mathcal{J} \to \mathcal{M}$ is a homomorphism between the structures $\mathcal{J}$ and $\mathcal{M}$ that preserves the complements of relations, i.e.: $(\alpha_1, \ldots, \alpha_n) \notin r^{\mathcal{J}}$ entails $(i(\alpha_1), \ldots, i(\alpha_n)) \notin r^{\mathcal{M}}$.

Therefore, $\alpha \neq \beta$ entails $i(\alpha) \neq i(\beta)$, i.e. isomorphic embeddings are *injective*. Moreover, $\mathcal{J}$ is isomorphic to a substructure of $\mathcal{M}$ (viz. the i-image of $\mathcal{J}$), i.e. $\mathcal{J}$ is 'isomorphically embedded' in $\mathcal{M}$.

Now we can define initial and isoinitial models of Σ-theories.

Definition 2. (Initial Models). Let T be a first-order Σ-theory, and $\mathcal{I}$ be a model of T. $\mathcal{I}$ is an *initial model* of T iff, for every model $\mathcal{M}$ of T, there is a unique homomorphism $h : \mathcal{I} \to \mathcal{M}$.

Definition 3. (Isoinitial Models). Let T be a first-order Σ-theory, and $\mathcal{J}$ be a model of T. $\mathcal{J}$ is an *isoinitial model* of T iff, for every model $\mathcal{M}$ of T, there is a unique isomorphic embedding $i : \mathcal{J} \to \mathcal{M}$.

Example 1. Consider the simple signature $K \equiv \langle \{a^0, b^0\}, \{\} \rangle$, containing just two constant symbols a and b. The corresponding Herbrand interpretation H is defined by $D = \{a, b\}$, $a^H = a$ and $b^H = b$.[2]

---

[1] σ^n denotes a symbol σ with arity n.

[2] The standard interpretation of $=$ is understood.

H is an initial model of the empty theory $\emptyset$. Indeed, for every other model $\mathcal{M}$, the map h defined by $(h(a) = a^{\mathcal{M}}, h(b) = b^{\mathcal{M}})$ is the unique homomorphism from H into $\mathcal{M}$. The empty theory does not prevent interpretations where $a = b$.

H is not an isoinitial model of $\emptyset$ however. Indeed, there is no isomorphic embedding from H into models $\mathcal{M}$ such that $a^{\mathcal{M}} = b^{\mathcal{M}}$, since isomorphic embeddings have to preserve inequality.

In contrast, H is an isoinitial model of the theory $\{\neg a = b\}$. Indeed, for every model $\mathcal{M}$ of $\{\neg a = b\}$, we have $a^{\mathcal{M}} \neq b^{\mathcal{M}}$, and the map i such that $(i(a) = a^{\mathcal{M}}, i(b) = b^{\mathcal{M}})$ is the unique isomorphic embedding of H into $\mathcal{M}$.

In fact H is also an initial model of $\{\neg a = b\}$.

In the rest of the paper, we will consider *only* the particular case of *reachable* initial and isoinitial models. The treatment of non-reachable models requires concrete data [2] that are omitted for lack of space; isoinitiality entails initiality in the reachable case, whereas in the general case the two notions are independent.

Definition 4. (Reachable Models). A structure (model) $\mathcal{M} \equiv \langle D, F^{\mathcal{M}}, R^{\mathcal{M}} \rangle$ is *reachable* if, for every $\alpha \in D$, there is a ground term t such that $t^{\mathcal{M}} = \alpha$.

We can characterise reachable initial and isoinitial models as follows:

Theorem 1. *Let $\mathcal{J}$ be a reachable model of a Σ-theory T. Then $\mathcal{J}$ is an* initial *model of T if and only if the following* initiality condition *holds:*
for every ground atom A, $\mathcal{J} \models A$ iff ($\mathcal{M} \models A$, for every model $\mathcal{M}$ of T) (INI)
while it is an isoinitial *model of T if an only if the following* isoinitiality condition *holds:*
for every ground literal L, $\mathcal{J} \models L$ iff ($\mathcal{M} \models L$, for every model $\mathcal{M}$ of T). (ISO)

(The proof follows from the reachability hypothesis. We omit it for conciseness.)

Thus initial models represent *truth* of atomic formulas in every model, while isoinitial models represent both *truth* and *falsity* of atomic formulas in every model.

Now by the completeness theorem for first-order theories, we can prove:

Corollary 1. *In Theorem 1, we can replace* (INI) *and* (ISO) *by* (INI') *and* (ISO'):
for every ground atom A, $\mathcal{J} \models A$ iff $T \vdash A$. (INI')
for every ground literal L, $\mathcal{J} \models L$ iff $T \vdash L$. (ISO')

That is, initial models represent provability of *atomic formulas*, while isoinitial models represent provability of *literals*, i.e. they behave properly with respect to negation of atomic formulas.

Of course, in general, a first-order theory may have no initial or isoinitial models. To state the existence of such models, we could apply the above theoretical (characterisation) results. However, for isoinitial models, we can state a condition that is more useful in practice for proving isoinitiality:

Corollary 2. *In Theorem 1, we can replace* (ISO) *by the following* atomic completeness *condition: for every ground atom A, $T \vdash A$ or $T \vdash \neg A$.* (ATC)

In condition (ATC) models disappear altogether,[3] i.e., we have a purely proof-theoretic condition. This allows us to prove some interesting and useful results, that link classical and constructive proof theoretical properties with isoinitial models [14]. For example, we can prove the following theorem:

Theorem 2. *Let $K \equiv \langle F, \{\} \rangle$ be a signature containing a non-empty set F of function and constant symbols, with at least one constant symbol. Let H_F be the corresponding Herbrand structure, and let $CET(F)$ be Clark's Equality Theory for F. Then H_F is an isoinitial model of $CET(F)$.*

Proof. H_F is a model of $CET(F)$, and, being a term-model, it is trivially reachable. Atomic completeness follows from the fact that, for every ground atomic formula $t = t'$, $\emptyset \vdash t = t'$ if t and t' coincide, and $CET(F) \vdash \neg t = t'$, if t and t' are different.

3   Initial and Isoinitial Semantics for Closed Theories

In this section, we consider closed theories and their initial and isoinitial models. For conciseness, we will use the abbreviations *ini* for *initial semantics* (i.e. semantics based on initial models), *iso* for *isoinitial semantics* (i.e. semantics based on isoinitial models) and *sem* for a parameter standing for either *ini* or *iso*.

We will show that, for closed theories, *iso* is better able than *ini* to deal with *negation*. In the next section, we will show that for the special case of closed definite logic programs, *iso* also allows us to reason about *termination*.

Closed first-order Σ-theories are defined as follows:

Definition 5. (*Sem-Closed Σ-Theories*). A Σ-theory T is *sem-closed* if and only if it has a (reachable) *sem*-model.

Example 2. Consider the signature $K \equiv \langle F, \{\} \rangle$ (in Theorem 2) containing a non-empty set F of function and constant symbols, with at least one constant symbol. Let H_F be the corresponding Herbrand structure.

The empty theory $\emptyset$ is *ini*-closed, and H_F is an initial model of $\emptyset$. By contrast, $\emptyset$ is not *iso*-closed (it is not atomically complete). However, $CET(F)$ is an *iso*-closed theory, with isoinitial model H_F (see Theorem 2).

In general, *iso* is better equipped than *ini* to deal with *negation*: in Example 2, *iso* shows that $\emptyset$ lacks information with regard to negation, whereas *ini* does not show this. *ini* and *iso* correspond to two different ways of looking at negation, and, more generally, at the role of axioms. Indeed, as a corollary of (INI') and (ISO'), we get the following properties:

If $\mathcal{I}$ is an initial model, then for every ground atom A,

$$\mathcal{I} \models \neg A \text{ iff } T \nvdash A. \qquad \text{(INI'')}$$

If it is isoinitial, then for every ground atom A,

$$\mathcal{J} \models \neg A \text{ iff } T \vdash \neg A. \qquad \text{(ISO'')}$$

---

[3] However, models do not disappear completely from Theorem 1, because the existence of at least one reachable model $\mathcal{J}$ is always assumed.

(INI") generalises the Closed World Assumption (CWA) [16] to general first-order theories: a fact is *false* (in the intended reachable initial model) if and only if it cannot be proved.

(ISO") corresponds to Constructive Negation (CN) [6]: a fact is *false* (in the intended model) if and only if its *negation* can be proved.

Thus *ini* and *iso* subscribe to different views. *Ini* corresponds to a principle of *economy*: we look for the smallest set of axioms that allows us to derive the *positive* facts. In contrast, *iso* semantics corresponds to a principle of *richness*: we look for rich theories, that allow us, at least, to treat *negation* constructively.

Another remarkable difference is shown by the following corollary of (INI') and (ISO'):

Corollary 3. *Let T be sem-closed, and let $\exists x Q(x)$ be an existential sentence such that $T \vdash \exists x Q(x)$.*

If sem is ini and $Q(x)$ is a positive quantifier-free formula, then $T \vdash Q(t)$, for at least one ground t.

If sem is iso and $Q(x)$ is any quantifier-free formula, then $T \vdash Q(t)$, for at least one ground t.

That is, an *iso*-closed theory T is rich enough to prove the answers $\neg A(t)$ of negative existential queries $\exists x \neg A(x)$ that hold in the isoinitial model, whereas this is not guaranteed, in general, for *ini*-closed theories: the latter are guaranteed to answer only *positive* existential queries. Moreover, as is well known, with CWA the set of false ground atoms may not be recursively enumerable, whereas reachable isoinitial models are guaranteed to be computable [2]. Negation and computability are not the only reasons that induced us to consider isoinitial semantics, however. As we will show in forthcoming sections, we will also use isoinitial semantics to deal with *incomplete information, parametrisation and modularity.*

4 Closed Logic Programs

Now, we consider closed logic programs as closed theories. For lack of space we will focus on *definite* programs. Consequently we do not discuss normal programs, but we will show that even for definite programs, *iso* has another advantage of being able to reason about *termination*.

For a signature $\Sigma = \langle F, R \rangle$ with at least one constant symbol, interpretations over the term-domain H_F will be called *Herbrand Σ-structures* (or Σ-interpretations). As usual, a Herbrand Σ-interpretation can be uniquely represented as a set of ground atoms. Thus we will consider Herbrand Σ-structures as term models or as sets of ground atoms, interchangeably.

Let P be a logic program, with signature $\Sigma_P \equiv \langle F_P, R_P \rangle$. We will use $Cdef(p)$ to denote the completed definition of p in P (see, e.g., [12]). We will also use $Cdef(P)$ to denote the set of $Cdef(p)$, for $p \in R_P$.

The completion of P, $Comp(P)$, is then the union $CET(F_P) \cup Cdef(P)$.

Example 3. Consider the usual program P_{sum}:

$$sum(x, 0, x) \leftarrow$$
$$sum(x, s(i), s(v)) \leftarrow sum(x, i, v) \qquad (P_{sum})$$

for the sum of natural numbers (s is *successor*), with signature $\Sigma_{P_{sum}} \equiv \langle \{0^0, s^1\}, \{sum^3\} \rangle$. In this case, $CET(0^0, s^1)$ contains the axioms[4]

$$\{\forall x . \neg 0 = s(x), \quad \forall x, y . s(x) = s(y) \rightarrow x = y\} \cup \{\forall x . \neg s^{(n)}(x) = x | n > 0\}.$$

The completed definition of sum, $Cdef(sum)$, is (after some obvious simplifications): $\forall x, y, z . sum(x, y, z) \leftrightarrow (y = 0 \wedge z = x) \vee (\exists i, v . y = s(i) \wedge z = s(v) \wedge sum(x, i, v)))$.

The completion of P_{sum} is $Comp(P_{sum}) = CET(0^0, s^1) \cup Cdef(sum)$.

The minimum Herbrand model $\mathcal{M}(P)$ is defined in the usual way. We have the following theorem:

Theorem 3. *For a (definite) logic program P, $\mathcal{M}(P)$ is an initial model of P and of $Comp(P)$, but it is not an isoinitial model of P.*
Proof. The initiality of $\mathcal{M}(P)$ is well-known [9]. $\mathcal{M}(P)$ cannot be an isoinitial model of P, because P cannot be atomically complete (no negated formula is provable from it).

We might expect $\mathcal{M}(P)$ to be an isoinitial model of $Comp(P)$, but this is not necessarily so, as shown by the following example:

Example 4. Consider the program P_1 : $p(a) \leftarrow q(a)$ (P_1)
$\qquad\qquad\qquad\qquad\qquad\qquad\qquad\qquad q(a) \leftarrow p(a)$
with signature $\Sigma_1 \equiv \langle \{a^0\}, \{p^1, q^1\} \rangle$. $CET(a)$ is empty. $Cdef(p)$ is $\forall x . p(x) \leftrightarrow (x = a \wedge q(a))$, and $Cdef(q)$ is $\forall x . q(x) \leftrightarrow (x = a \wedge p(a))$.

For $Comp(P_1)$ to have a reachable isoinitial model, atomic completeness requires that $Comp(P_1) \vdash p(a)$ or $Comp(P_1) \vdash \neg p(a)$, and $Comp(P_1) \vdash q(a)$ or $Comp(P_1) \vdash \neg q(a)$. However these requirements are not met and, therefore, no reachable isoinitial model can exist for $Comp(P_1)$.

On the other hand, $\mathcal{M}(P_1)$ (where $p(a)$ and $q(a)$ are false) is an initial model of $Comp(P_1)$. Therefore P_1 and $Comp(P_1)$ are *ini*-closed, but not *iso*-closed.

Now consider the program P_2: $p(a) \leftarrow q(a)$ (P_2)
$Comp(P_2)$ is both *ini*- and *iso*-closed. Indeed, now $Cdef(q)$ is $\forall x . \neg q(x)$, and we can prove $\neg q(a)$ and $\neg p(a)$. $\mathcal{M}(P_2)$ is the same as $\mathcal{M}(P_1)$, but it is both initial and isoinitial for $Comp(P_2)$.

Finally, it is worth noting that while P_1 does not terminate with respect to the goals $\leftarrow p(a)$ and $\leftarrow q(a)$, P_2 finitely fails for both.

4.1 Termination

Example 4 suggests that termination (see [7] for a survey) and *iso*-closure are related. Indeed, we can prove the following result:

Definition 6. (Existential Ground-Termination). *Let P be a definite program. P existentially ground-terminates if and only if its Herbrand universe is not empty and, for every ground goal $\leftarrow A$, either there is a refutation of $\leftarrow A$, or $\leftarrow A$ finitely fails.*

---

[4] Here $s^{(n)}$ denotes the iteration of s for n times.

Theorem 4. *Let P be a definite program with a non-empty Herbrand universe. Comp(P) is iso-closed if and only if P existentially ground-terminates.*

Proof. If $Comp(P)$ is *iso*-closed, then it is atomically complete. By completeness of *SLDNF*-resolution for definite programs, P existentially ground-terminates. If P existentially ground-terminates, then $Comp(P)$ is atomically complete.

It follows that we can use termination analysis for stating isoinitiality.

Example 5. Consider the program P_{sum} in Example 3. We can prove that P_{sum} existentially ground-terminates. Therefore, we can conclude that its minimum Herbrand model is an isoinitial model of $Comp(P_{sum})$.

Moreover, the converse also holds, i.e. we can study existential ground-termination by studying isoinitiality, as the following example shows.

Example 6. Consider the following program P_{path}:
$$path(x, y) \leftarrow arc(x, y)$$
$$path(x, y) \leftarrow arc(x, z), path(z, y) \qquad\qquad (P_{path})$$
$$arc(1, 1) \leftarrow$$
$$arc(2, 2) \leftarrow$$
Its completion contains the axioms:
$$\neg 1 = 2$$
$$\forall x, y \,.\, path(x, y) \leftrightarrow arc(x, y) \vee \exists z \,.\, arc(x, z) \wedge path(z, y)$$
$$\forall x, y \,.\, arc(x, y) \leftrightarrow (x = 1 \wedge y = 1) \vee (x = 2 \wedge y = 2).$$
Instead of considering termination, we apply directly a model theoretic argument. We consider two term models $\mathcal{M}_1$ and $\mathcal{M}_2$. Both interpret *arc* in the same way, according to the axioms. In $\mathcal{M}_1$, the meaning of $path(x, y)$ is: "there is a finite path connecting x to y". In $\mathcal{M}_2$, the meaning of $path(x, y)$ is: "there is a finite path connecting x to y, or there is an infinite path starting from x". As we can see, both satisfy the axiom for *path*. In the first one, $path(1, 2)$ is false, while in the second one it is true. Therefore, we cannot have an isoinitial model. This entails that P_{path} does not existentially terminate for the goal $\leftarrow path(1, 2)$.

This model-theoretic argument applies to any graph, that is, we can define $\mathcal{M}_1$ and $\mathcal{M}_2$ that satisfy the axiom for *path* and interpret $path(a, b)$ in two different ways, if there is a cycle starting from a, but no finite path from a to b. In contrast, if the graph is finite and acyclic, or if it is infinite but *arc* is well founded, then both these interpretations interpret $path(a, b)$ in the same way for every a and b. On the other hand, for acyclic finite graphs, or infinite graphs with a well founded *arc*, the recursive clause for *path* existentially terminates.

5   Initial and Isoinitial Semantics for Open Theories

In this section we consider *sem*-open theories, namely theories without *sem*-models, and we will compare initial and isoinitial semantics from the point of view of *incomplete information*, *parametricity* and *compositionality*. We will show that *iso*-closures provide a rich semantics for these.

5.1   Incomplete Information

Definition 7. (*sem*-Open Σ-Theories). A Σ-theory T is *sem-open* if and only if it is consistent but has no *sem*-model.

We consider a *sem*-open Σ-theory as an incomplete axiomatisation of a *sem*-model, to be completed by adding new axioms and, possibly, new symbols to the signature Σ.

Here we will consider the simpler case where Σ is fixed, i.e., no new symbol is added. In this case, it is interesting to consider the *sem*-closures of a *sem*-open theory T, i.e., the theories T' that contain T,[5] and are *sem*-closed. The minimal *ini*-closures give rise to a poorer semantics compared to *iso*-closures, as we show in the following example.

Example 7. The theory $T_{disj} = \{p(a) \vee p(b)\}$ with signature $\langle \{a^0, b^0\}, \{p^1\} \rangle$ is both *ini*- and *iso*-open. In general, positive occurrences of $\vee$ and $\exists$ in the axioms give rise to theories that are both *ini* and *iso*-open.

T_{disj} has two minimal *ini*-closures, namely $T_{disj} \cup \{p(a)\}$ and $T_{disj} \cup \{p(b)\}$, and four minimal *iso*-closures, namely $T_{disj} \cup \{a = b\}$, $T_{disj} \cup \{\neg a = b, p(a), \neg p(b)\}$, $T_{disj} \cup \{\neg a = b, \neg p(a), p(b)\}$, $T_{disj} \cup \{\neg a = b, p(a), p(b)\}$.

This example shows that initial semantics allows more compact closures. However, (as we will see later in Example 8 in Section 6) isoinitial semantics is better at showing up missing or incomplete information. Dealing with incomplete information is an important issue for databases [8].

5.2   Parametricity

In this section, we introduce parametrised theories as a particular case of open theories.

A *parametrised* Σ-theory $T(\Pi)$ is a theory with signature $\Sigma = \langle F, R \rangle$ and a set $\Pi \subseteq F \cup R$ of parameters. We denote by $\Sigma_\Pi = \langle F \cap \Pi, R \cap \Pi \rangle$ the subsignature of the parameters.

A Σ_Π-structure $\mathcal{P}$ can be seen as a kind of parameter passing. To do so, we have to consider interpretations over different signatures. A signature $\Sigma \equiv \langle F, R \rangle$ is a *subsignature* of $\Sigma' \equiv \langle F', R' \rangle$, written $\Sigma \subseteq \Sigma'$, if and only if $F \subseteq F'$ and $R \subseteq R'$.

For $\Sigma \subseteq \Sigma'$, we have the well-known notions of *reduct* and *expansion*. The Σ-*reduct* of a Σ'-structure $\mathcal{N}$ is the Σ-structure $\mathcal{N}|\Sigma$ that has the same domain as $\mathcal{N}$ and interprets each symbol s of Σ in the same way as $\mathcal{N}$, i.e., $s^{\mathcal{N}|\Sigma} = s^{\mathcal{N}}$. Conversely, if $\mathcal{M} = \mathcal{N}|\Sigma$, $\mathcal{N}$ is said to be a Σ'-*expansion* of $\mathcal{M}$.

A well known property of reducts is that, for every Σ-formula G, $\mathcal{N} \models G$ iff $\mathcal{N}|\Sigma \models G$.

Now we can define the semantics of a parametrised theory $T(\Pi)$ by considering its $\mathcal{P}$-models:

---

[5] In the sense that $Theorems(T') \supseteq Theorems(T)$.

Definition 8. ($\mathcal{P}$-Models). Let $T(\Pi)$ be a Σ-theory, and $\mathcal{P}$ be a Σ_{Π}-interpretation. A $\mathcal{P}$-*model* of $T(\Pi)$ (if one exists) is a model $\mathcal{M}$ of T such that $\mathcal{M} \,|\, \Sigma_{\Pi} = \mathcal{P}$.

That is, $\mathcal{P}$-models are models that agree with the parameter passing $\mathcal{P}$. We can define $\mathcal{P}$-initial models and $\mathcal{P}$-isoinitial models in a similar manner to initial and isoinitial models. The difference is that here we use $\mathcal{P}$-homomorphisms and $\mathcal{P}$-isomorphisms.

Definition 9. ($\mathcal{P}$-Homomorphism and $\mathcal{P}$-(Isomorphic Embedding)). Let $\Pi \subseteq \Sigma$ be two signatures, $\mathcal{P}$ be a Π-structure, and $\mathcal{N}$ and $\mathcal{M}$ be two Σ-expansions of $\mathcal{P}$. A $\mathcal{P}$-*homomorphism* $h : \mathcal{M} \to \mathcal{N}$ is a homomorphism such that $h(s^{\mathcal{M}}) = s^{\mathcal{M}} = s^{\mathcal{P}}$, for every symbol s of Π. A $\mathcal{P}$-(*isomorphic embedding*) is a $\mathcal{P}$-*homomorphism* that preserves the complements of the relations.

Thus $\mathcal{P}$-homomorphisms and isomorphisms completely preserve the parameter passing $\mathcal{P}$, i.e., they work as identity over the parameters.

Now we can define parametric theories:

Definition 10. Let $\Sigma = \langle F, R \rangle$ be a signature and $T(\Pi)$ be a parametric Σ-theory. $T(\Pi)$ is *ini-parametric* if and only if, for every Σ_{Π}-interpretation $\mathcal{P}$, the class $MOD_{\mathcal{P}}(T(\Pi))$ of the $\mathcal{P}$-models of $T(\Pi)$ contains a $\mathcal{P}$-initial model $\mathcal{I}_{\mathcal{P}}$. If $\mathcal{I}_{\mathcal{P}}$ is $\mathcal{P}$-isoinitial in $MOD_{\mathcal{P}}(T(\Pi))$, then T is *iso-parametric*.

All the model-theoretic results that we have shown for initial and isoinitial models extend to $\mathcal{P}$-initial and $\mathcal{P}$-isoinitial models, considering the class of $\mathcal{P}$-models of a theory. Here reachability is not required, since the domain of the $\mathcal{P}$-models is completely left to $\mathcal{P}$.

With respect to provability, an open theory in general does not prove any ground atomic formula, since relation symbols are left open. We have to complete the theory, by adding a set Ax of new axioms, that characterises a parameter passing $\mathcal{P}$. Here we have the following *sufficient completeness problem*: how much of $\mathcal{P}$ has to be codified by Ax, in order to obtain a *sem*-complete theory $T(\Pi) \cup Ax$? It turns out that the use of constructive systems allows us to develop a proof theory for stating *iso*-parametricity (see [15]).

Another possibility is to characterise the minimal *iso*-closures, as we will see in Section 6.

5.3 Compositionality

Parametrised theories can be used for composing small well-defined theories into new larger theories [10]. Similarly, parametrised programs[6] can be used (and composed) as modules [4,5]. In this section, we study only the consequences of initial and isoinitial semantics for composition.

In general, a parametrised theory O_1 leaves open the intended meaning of its parameters and, possibly, the intended domain. O_1 can be used to produce a larger, composite theory, by composing it successively with other (closed or

---

[6] Usually called open programs.

parametrised) theories O_2, O_3, ... We can make sure that the final composite theory $O_1O_2O_3 \ldots$ is closed if we choose suitable closed sub-theories for the composition.

If composition is associative, i.e. $(O_1O_2)O_3 = O_1(O_2O_3)$, then each sequence $O_1O_2 \cdots O_n$ is equivalent to a two-step sequence O_1T, with $T = O_2 \cdots O_n$. For example, composition of logic programs is associative. Moreover, in many interesting cases, if O_1T is closed, then so is T. This is the case, for example, for program composition without mutual recursion. In the sequel we shall consider cases where T is assumed to be *sem*-closed.

So we start from a *sem*-closed theory T, with *sem*-model $\mathcal{I}$, and consider adding new constant, function or relation symbols to T. In general, the new symbols are *open symbols*, since, in the new language, T is no longer *sem*-closed. In our previous discussion, these symbols can be closed by the axioms of some O_1, but the question is: what is preserved of the *sem*-model $\mathcal{I}$ of T, by the *sem*-model $\mathcal{I}'$ of O_1T?

The following theorem provides a first answer:

Theorem 5. *Let $\Sigma \equiv \langle F, R \rangle$ be a signature, and T be a sem-closed Σ-theory, with sem-model $\mathcal{I} \equiv \langle D, F^{\mathcal{I}}, R^{\mathcal{I}} \rangle$. Let $\Sigma' \equiv \langle F', R' \rangle$ be a larger signature, and T' be a sem-closed theory containing T, with sem-model $\mathcal{I}'$. Then there is a unique sem-morphism $h : \mathcal{I} \to \mathcal{I}'|\Sigma$.*

The proof follows easily from the fact that $T \subseteq T'$ and, hence, $\mathcal{I}'|\Sigma \models T$.

The consequences of this theorem are the following:

Corollary 4. *Let T, T', $\mathcal{I}$, $\mathcal{I}'$ be as in Theorem 5. If sem is ini, then for every positive existential Σ-sentence $\exists(W)$, $\mathcal{I} \models \exists(W)$ entails $\mathcal{I}' \models \exists(W)$. If sem is iso, then for every existential Σ-sentence $\exists(Q)$, $\mathcal{I} \models \exists(Q)$ entails $\mathcal{I}' \models \exists(Q)$. Moreover, for a quantifier-free Σ-sentence, $\mathcal{I} \models Q$ iff $\mathcal{I}' \models Q$.*

The proof follows from Theorem 5, $\mathcal{I}'|\Sigma$ being a model of T.

This means that *iso*-closed theories preserve truth and falsity of quantifier-free formulas. This corresponds to the fact that $\mathcal{I}$ is isomorphically embedded into $\mathcal{I}'|\Sigma$. In initial semantics, $\mathcal{I}$ is only guaranteed to be homomorphic.

When the domain is preserved, *iso*-closure has a strong consequence:

Corollary 5. *Let T, T', $\mathcal{I}$, $\mathcal{I}'$, h be as in Theorem 5. If sem is iso and h is surjective, then, for every Σ-sentence S, $\mathcal{I} \models S$ iff $\mathcal{I}' \models S$.*

The proof follows from the fact that a surjective isomorphic embedding is an isomorphism.

Corollary 5 does not hold for initial semantics, because surjective homomorphisms are not necessarily isomorphisms.

Corollary 4 applies when we add new constant or function symbols, while Corollary 5 applies when we add only new predicates. This suggests that it is useful to start from a large signature, that contains all the possible function and constant symbols. Another, more reasonable alternative is to introduce many-sorted theories. In general, we can show that Corollary 5 can be extended to the many-sorted case, and it holds whenever the domains interpreting the old sorts are preserved, even if the larger signature contains new sorts, interpreted as new domains.

6 Open Logic Programs

Now, we consider open logic programs as *sem*-open theories. In general, the domain and/or some predicates are open. Predicates may be open because they are incompletely axiomatised, or because they are used as parameters.

6.1 Incomplete Information

In a program with incomplete information, open predicates are incompletely axiomatised.

Example 8. Consider the following informal specification:
   Every bird flies, if it is normal; tweety and pingu are birds.
   We do not know the entire domain of birds, and we do not say whether or not *tweety* and *pingu* are normal, that is, we have incomplete information. We could codify this situation by the open program P_{bird}:

$$flies(x) \leftarrow bird(x), normal(x)$$
$$bird(tweety) \leftarrow \qquad\qquad\qquad\qquad (P_{bird})$$
$$bird(pingu) \leftarrow$$

We leave *normal* as an open symbol, without any clause for it, because we do not have any information on it. *bird* is only partially axiomatised, i.e., its clauses are intended to fix it only in the known universe. Nevertheless, in contrast, the first clause is intended to *completely* define *flies*, since this happens in our informal problem.

P_{bird} is *ini*-closed. On the other hand, P_{bird} is *iso*-open, but there are minimal *iso*-closures that are at variance with our intention that *flies* is completely defined by the program. That is, initial semantics does not directly expose the presence of open symbols, while isoinitial semantics shows both that there is incomplete information and that the axiomatisation is too weak (in *iso*) to axiomatise our informal open problem. On the other hand, pure Horn clauses are not sufficiently expressive with respect to *iso*.

To get a more expressive language, we introduce the *open completion*, denoted by $Ocomp(P)$. Based on the idea that non-open predicates are completely defined by P, $Ocomp(P)$ contains the completed definition $Cdef(p)$ for every non-open predicate p, the clauses for open predicates q in P, and $CET(F_P)$ for the function and constant symbols of P.

Let P be a program with at least one open predicate, and with a non-empty Herbrand Universe. We can easily prove that $Ocomp(P)$ is *ini*-closed, but it is not *iso*-closed. That is, even using the open completion, initial semantics does not expose the fact that some information is missing, while isoinitial semantics does.

We consider the isoinitial models of the minimal *iso*-closures of $Ocomp(P)$ in a (possibly partial) domain as the *intended models* of the open program P in that domain. In this sense, $Ocomp(P)$ represents the interpretation of an open program P in the isoinitial semantics.

Example 9. In the informal problem, *bird* and *normal* are open. Thus, the open completion $Ocomp(P_{bird})$ of P_{bird} is: $\{\neg tweety = pingu, \forall x . flies(x) \leftrightarrow bird(x) \wedge normal(x), bird(tweety), bird(pingu)\}$. $Ocomp(P_{bird})$ is *ini*-closed, and in its initial model *tweety* and *pingu* do not fly. In contrast, $Ocomp(P_{bird})$ is *iso*-open. There are four minimal *iso*-closures, that is, four different ways of completing the information within the known domain $\{tweety, pingu\}$. One is:
$$Ocomp(P_{bird}) \cup \{normal(tweety), \neg normal(pingu)\}.$$
In its isoinitial model $\mathcal{I}_{bird}$, *tweety* flies, but *pingu* does not. By isoinitiality, if we add further individuals and further closed information on them, we get larger models, that contain (an isomorphic copy of) $\mathcal{I}_{bird}$ as a substructure.

6.2   Parametricity

In a parametric program P, *open* predicates occur in the body of clauses and act as parameters. P can be 'closed' by composition with different (closed, non-parametric) Q's, that compute the open predicates in different ways.

We assume that P completely specifies all its defined predicates, and parameters are *exactly* the predicates that are *not* defined by P. Moreover, the domain may be open, (i.e. we also consider the constant and function symbols (if any) as parameters), to be completed into a larger signature.

Let P be a parametric program with signature $\Sigma_P = \langle F_P, R_P \cup O \rangle$, where F_P are the constant and function symbols (if any) of P, and R_P are its defined predicates. We will use $\Pi_P = \langle F_P, O \rangle$ to denote the *parameter signature* of P.

Theorem 6. *A program P with parameter signature Π_P is ini-parametric.*

That is, for every Π_P-interpretation $\mathcal{P}$, there is a $\mathcal{P}$-initial model of P. It is easy to show that such a $\mathcal{P}$-initial model is the minimum $\mathcal{P}$-model[7] of P. This result holds for every interpretation $\mathcal{P}$, i.e., we do not necessarily require that $\mathcal{P}$ is reachable in the signature of program P.

Example 10. Consider the open program P_{times}:
$$times(x, 0, z) \leftarrow u(z) \qquad\qquad (P_{times})$$
$$times(x, s(y), z) \leftarrow times(x, y, w), q(x, w, z)$$
The parameters are $\Pi_{times} = \langle \{0^0, s^1\}, \{u^1, q^3\} \rangle$. If $\mathcal{P}_{sum}$ interprets $u(z)$ as $z = 0$ and $q(a, b, c)$ as $c = a + b$, then the $\mathcal{P}_{sum}$-initial model interprets $times(x, y, z)$ as $z = x * y$. If $\mathcal{P}_{prod}$ interprets $u(z)$ as $z = s(0)$ and $q(a, b, c)$ as $c = a * b$, then the $\mathcal{P}_{prod}$-initial model interprets $times(x, y, z)$ as $z = x^y$.

To introduce isoinitial semantics for parametric programs, we have to consider their open completion $Ocomp(P)$, as defined in the previous section. Here the open symbols are the parameters.

---

[7] It always exists, as shown in [11].

Example 11. The open completion $Ocomp(P_{times})$ contains $Cdef(times)$, i.e.
$$\forall x, v, z \,.\, times(x, v, z) \leftrightarrow (v = 0 \wedge u(z)) \vee$$
$$(\exists y, w \,.\, v = s(y) \wedge times(x, y, w) \wedge q(x, w, z))$$
and $CET(0, s)$.

While P and $Ocomp(P)$ are *ini*-parametric for every program P, this is no longer true for isoinitial semantics. As for closed programs, *iso*-parametricity of $Ocomp(P)$ depends on the termination properties of P. More precisely, we need to consider ground existential termination in a Π_P-interpretation $\mathcal{P}$ (formally defined in [11]). Informally, ground existential termination in $\mathcal{P}$ is defined in terms of the SLD-derivations and trees computed by an idealised $\mathcal{P}$-interpreter, that can solve the goals involving the parameters according to their interpretation in $\mathcal{P}$.

Theorem 7. *Let P be a program with parameter signature Π_P and open completion $Ocomp(P)$. $Ocomp(P)$ is iso-parametric in a class of Π_P-interpretations if and only if P ground existentially terminates in every interpretation of the class.*

That is, P ground existentially terminates in a Π_P-interpretation $\mathcal{P}$ if and only if there is a $\mathcal{P}$-isoinitial model of $Ocomp(P)$. The proof requires the results of [11] and the properties of $\mathcal{P}$-isoinitial models. We omit it for conciseness.

Example 12. Consider the open program P_{times}. $Ocomp(P_{times})$ is *iso*-parametric in the class of interpretations over the Herbrand structure corresponding to $CET(0, s)$. Indeed, in this class ground existential termination can be proved by the fact that $times(x, s(y), z)$ activates a recursive call with $y < s(y)$.

For an example where *iso*-parametricity fails, consider the following simple program P_p: $\qquad p(a) \leftarrow q(a) \qquad p(b) \leftarrow p(b) \qquad\qquad\qquad (P_p)$
Its parameters are $\Pi_p = \langle \{a^0, b^0\}, \{q^1\} \rangle$. Its open completion $Ocomp(P_p)$ contains the axioms: $\neg a = b, \ \forall x \,.\, p(x) \leftrightarrow (x = a \wedge q(a)) \vee (x = b \wedge p(b))$.
A possible Π_p interpretation is the term interpretation $\mathcal{P}$ with domain $\{a, b\}$ and q true in a and false in b. Every $\mathcal{P}$-model has to interpret $p(a)$ as true, but $p(b)$ can be interpreted as true by some $\mathcal{P}$-models and as false by others. Thus, a $\mathcal{P}$-isoinitial model cannot exist. This is a consequence of the presence of the cyclic clause $p(b) \leftarrow p(b)$.

6.3 Compositionality

Let P be a *sem*-parametric program with parameter signature Π_P, and let $\mathcal{P}$ be a Π_P-interpretation. Let Q be a *sem*-closed program that computes the parameters of P correctly with respect to $\mathcal{P}$, and let us consider the composite program $P \cup Q$. As remarked in Section 5, there is a sufficient completeness problem here. For $P \cup Q$, this problem can be stated as follows: which kind of goals have to be solved by Q, in order that it can replace the idealised $\mathcal{P}$-interpreter considered in the previous section?

For initial semantics the answer is easy, and is given by Theorem 8, while isoinitial semantics can expose *termination* problems in program composition and requires a more complex analysis (see Theorem 9).

Theorem 8. *Let P be a program with signature $\Sigma_P = \langle F_P, R_P \cup O \rangle$ and parameters $\Pi_P = \langle F_P, O \rangle$. Let $\Delta = \langle F, O \rangle$ be a signature such that $F \supseteq F_P$, and $\mathcal{J}$ be a reachable Δ-interpretation. Let $\mathcal{H}_{\mathcal{J}}$ be the set of ground atoms true in $\mathcal{J}$. Then $P \cup \mathcal{H}_{\mathcal{J}}$ is an ini-closed expansion of P with a reachable initial model $\mathcal{I}$. Moreover, $\mathcal{I}$ is isomorphic to the $(\mathcal{J} \mid \Pi_P)$-initial model of P.*

Proof. Since P is *ini*-parametric, it has a $\mathcal{J} \mid \Pi_P$-initial model, that we will indicate by $\mathcal{J}_P$. Since every model of $P \cup \mathcal{H}_{\mathcal{J}}$ is a model of P, there is a unique homomorphism $h : \mathcal{J}_P \to \mathcal{I}$. By the initiality of $\mathcal{I}$, there is a unique homomorphism $h' : \mathcal{I} \to \mathcal{J}_P$. Since $F_P \subseteq F$, $\mathcal{I}$ and $\mathcal{J}_P$ are F-reachable. This allows us to show that h' is the inverse map of h, i.e., h is an isomorphism.

Let P, Π_P, Δ, $\mathcal{J}$, $\mathcal{H}_{\mathcal{J}}$ and $\mathcal{J}_P$ as in Theorem 8. As an easy corollary, we can prove that, for a program Q with signature Δ, if the success set of Q coincides with $\mathcal{H}_{\mathcal{J}}$, then $\mathcal{M}(P \cup Q)$ is isomorphic to $\mathcal{J}_P$.

Informally, this means that, to get a program Q such that $P \cup Q$ correctly computes the $(\mathcal{J} \mid \Pi_P)$-initial model $\mathcal{J}_P$ of P, it suffices that the success set of Q coincides with the set of ground atoms true in $\mathcal{J}$. This result easily extends to the case where the signature Δ of Q contains the open predicates O of P and other auxiliary predicates not in the signature of P.

For isoinitial semantics of open programs, we have to consider the open completion $Ocomp(P)$. In this case, the answer to the sufficient completeness problem is more complex and involves termination, as we now explain.

Let us consider P, Π_P, Δ, $\mathcal{J}$, $\mathcal{H}_{\mathcal{J}}$ and $\mathcal{J}_P$ as in Theorem 8. As explained in the previous section, there is a $\mathcal{J} \mid \Pi_P$-isoinitial model of $Ocomp(P)$ if and only if P ground existentially terminates in $\mathcal{J}$. We can show that this model is also $\mathcal{J} \mid \Pi_P$-initial, i.e., it is $\mathcal{J}_P$.

Now, let Q be an *iso*-closed program with success set $\mathcal{H}_{\mathcal{J}}$. By Theorem 8, $\mathcal{M}(P \cup Q)$ is isomorphic to $\mathcal{J}_P$. However, $\mathcal{M}(P \cup Q)$ is an isoinitial model of $Comp(P \cup Q)$ if and only if $P \cup Q$ ground existentially terminates. The ground existential termination of $P \cup Q$ is not guaranteed by the *iso*-closure of Q. This is due to the fact that, in general, Q must terminate also for suitable non-ground goals, to get existential termination of $P \cup Q$. We can link this termination problem to the sufficient completeness problem by Theorem 9 below.

An *goal axiom* is a closed formula of the form $\exists x \,.\, G$ or $\neg \exists x \,.\, G$, where G is a conjunction of atoms and $\exists x$ is a possibly empty sequence of existential quantifiers. If it is empty, we will simply write G. A *goal theory* is a (possibly infinite) set of goal axioms.

We say that a closed program Q *computes* a goal theory T if and only if, for every $\exists x G \in T$, the goal $\leftarrow G$ is successful in Q, and for every $\neg \exists x G \in T$, $\leftarrow G$ is finitely failed in Q. We have the following theorem.

Theorem 9. *Let P be a program with parameter signature $\Pi_P = \langle F_P, O \rangle$, such that $Ocomp(P)$ is iso-parametric. Let $\mathcal{J}$ be a reachable Δ-interpretation, where $\Delta = \langle F, O \rangle$, with $F \subseteq F_P$, and let $\mathcal{J}_P$ be the $\mathcal{J} \mid \Pi_P$-isoinitial model of $Ocomp(P)$. Let Q be a closed program with signature Δ. If there is a goal theory T such that $\mathcal{J} \models T$, Q computes T and $Ocomp(P) \cup T$ is iso-closed, then $Comp(P \cup Q)$ is iso-closed and $\mathcal{J}_P$ is an isoinitial model of it.*

Proof. Since $Ocomp(P) \cup T$ is *iso*-closed and $\mathcal{J}_P$ is reachable, then one can show that $\mathcal{J}_P$ is an isoinitial model of $Ocomp(P) \cup T$. $Comp(Q) \vdash H$ for every $H \in T$, because Q computes T, and $Ocomp(P) \cup Comp(Q) = Comp(P \cup Q)$, because Q is a closed Δ-program. Therefore, the models of $Comp(P \cup Q)$ are a subset of those of $Ocomp(P) \cup T$ and $\mathcal{J}_P$ is an isoinitial model of $Comp(P \cup Q)$.

This theorem shows that there is a link between termination properties of program composition and the minimal *iso*-closures of $Ocomp(P)$. This justifies our choice of *iso*-closures as an interesting semantics for open programs.

Example 13. Consider the open program P_{times} and the axiom $Cdef(times)$ of $Ocomp(P_{times})$ of Example 11. We can prove, for example:
$$times(s0, s0, s0) \qquad \leftrightarrow$$
$$\exists w_1 \, . \, times(s0, 0, w_1) \wedge q(s0, w_1, s0) \leftrightarrow$$
$$\exists w_1 \, . \, u(w_1) \wedge q(s0, w_1, s0)$$
Thus, if a goal theory T proves $\exists w_1 \, . \, u(w_1) \wedge q(s0, w_1, s0)$, then $Ocomp(P_{times}) \cup T \vdash times(s0, s0, s0)$. If $T \vdash \neg \exists w_1 \, . \, u(w_1) \wedge q(s0, w_1, s0)$, then $Ocomp(P_{times}) \cup T \vdash \neg times(s0, s0, s0)$.

In general, T has to decide existential formulas of the form $\exists w_1, \ldots, w_n \, . \, u(w_1) \wedge q(a, w_1, w_2) \wedge \ldots \wedge q(a, w_n, c)$, in order that $Ocomp(P_{times}) \cup T$ be *iso*-closed.

This means that, for a closed program Q with predicates u and q, $P \cup Q$ existentially ground terminates, if and only if Q computes a goal theory T of the above kind.

7 Conclusion

The traditional view of a definite logic program (e.g., [9]) treats it as an initial theory. This in our opinion is too restrictive because it basically takes the Closed World view and does not provide a uniform semantics for negation and open programs, parametricity or compositionality. This view is therefore very much one of *programming-in-the-small*.

Our motivation is to search for a suitable uniform semantics for both *programming-in-the-large* and *programming-in-the-small*. We believe that isoinitial semantics fits the bill, for logic programs. It handles not only negation but also parametricity and compositionality in a uniform manner with respect to both closed and open programs. Moreover, constructive formal systems can help to formally prove isoinitiality and treat composition of *iso*-parametric theories [15]. Future work here will include a comparison with other semantics for modularity (e.g. [4,5]) and compositionality (e.g. [3,13]). Clearly such a uniform semantics is important if logic programming is to be used for large-scale software development. We have already used isoinitial semantics in our work in formal program development (e.g. [10]).

Finally, a brief comment on definite and normal programs. Under initial semantics, for every definite program D, both D and $Comp(D)$ are *ini-closed*, whereas for some normal programs N, both N and $Comp(N)$ are *ini-open*. Under isoinitial semantics, this asymmetry disappears if we consider $Comp(D)$ and

Comp(N) only: both definite and normal programs may be *iso*-open (and non-termination is one of the causes of *iso*-openness). For normal programs, other kinds of semantics have been proposed (for a survey see e.g. [1]). A comparison with these semantics is also one of our next steps. For example, we can link *iso*-closures and stable models by using open completion in a suitable way.

References

1. K.R. Apt and R. Bol. Logic programming and negation: a survey. *JLP* 19,20:9-71, 1994.
2. A. Bertoni, G. Mauri and P. Miglioli. On the power of model theory in specifying abstract data types and in capturing their recursiveness. *Fundamenta Informaticae* VI(2):127–170, 1983.
3. A. Bossi, M. Gabbrielli, G. Levi and M.C. Meo. A compositional semantics for logic programs. *TCS* 122:3-47, 1994.
4. A. Brogi, P. Mancarella, D. Pedreschi and F. Turini. Modular logic programming. *ACM TOPLAS* 16(4):1361–1398, 1994.
5. M. Bugliesi, E. Lamma and P. Mello. Modularity in logic programming. *JLP* 19,20:443–502, 1994.
6. D. Chan. Constructive negation based on the completed database. In *Proc. JIC-SLP'88*, pages 111-125, MIT Press, 1988.
7. D. De Schreye and S. Decorte. Termination of logic programs: The never-ending story. *JLP* 19,20:199-260, 1994.
8. M. Gelfond and V. Lifschitz. Classical negation in logic programs and disjunctive databases. *New Generation Computing* 9:365–385, 1991.
9. W. Hodges. Logical features of horn clauses. In D.M. Gabbay, C.J. Hogger, and J.A. Robinson. editors, *Handbook of Logic in Artificial Intelligence and Logic Programming, Volume 1*:449–503, Oxford University Press, 1993.
10. J. Küster Filipe, K.-K. Lau, M. Ornaghi, and H. Yatsu. On dynamic aspects of OOD frameworks in component-based software development in computational logic. In *Proc. LOPSTR'99, LNCS* 1817:43-62, Springer-Verlag, 2000.
11. K.-K. Lau, M. Ornaghi, and S.-Å. Tärnlund. Steadfast logic programs. *JLP* 38(3):259-294, 1999.
12. J.W. Lloyd. *Foundations of Logic Programming*. Springer-Verlag, 2nd edition, 1987.
13. P. Lucio, F. Orejas, and E. Pino. An algebraic framework for the definition of compositional semantics of normal logic programs. *JLP* 40:89-123, 1999.
14. P. Miglioli, U. Moscato and M. Ornaghi. Constructive theories with abstract data types for program synthesis. In D.G. Skordev, editor, *Mathematical Logic and its Applications*, pages 293–302, Plenum Press, 1986.
15. P. Miglioli, U. Moscato and M. Ornaghi. Abstract parametric classes and abstract data types defined by classical and constructive logical methods. *J. Symb. Comp.* 18:41–81, 1994.
16. R. Reiter. On closed world data bases. In H. Gallaire and J. Minker, editors, *Logic and Data Bases*, pages 293–322, Plenum Press, 1978.

Abstract Syntax for Variable Binders:
An Overview

Dale Miller

Department of Computer Science and Engineering
220 Pond Laboratory, The Pennsylvania State University
University Park, PA 16802-6106, USA
dale@cse.psu.edu

Abstract. A large variety of computing systems, such as compilers, interpreters, static analyzers, and theorem provers, need to manipulate syntactic objects like programs, types, formulas, and proofs. A common characteristic of these syntactic objects is that they contain variable binders, such as quantifiers, formal parameters, and blocks. It is a common observation that representing such binders using only first-order expressions is problematic since the notions of bound variable names, free and bound occurrences, equality up to alpha-conversion, substitution, etc., are not addressed naturally by the structure of first-order terms (labeled trees). This overview describes a higher-level and more declarative approach to representing syntax within such computational systems. In particular, we shall focus on a representation of syntax called *higher-order abstract syntax* and on a more primitive version of that representation called *λ-tree syntax*.

1   How Abstract Is Your Syntax?

Consider writing programs in which the data objects to be computed are syntactic structures, such as programs, formulas, types, and proofs, all of which generally involve notions of abstractions, scope, bound and free variables, substitution instances, and equality up to renaming of bound variables. Although the data types available in most computer programming languages are rich enough to represent all these kinds of structures, such data types do not have direct support for these common characteristics. Instead, "packages" need to be implemented to support such data structures. For example, although it is trivial to represent first-order formulas in Lisp, it is a more complex matter to write Lisp code to test for the equality of formulas up to renaming of variables, to determine if a certain variable's occurrence is free or bound, and to correctly substitute a term into a formula (being careful not to capture bound variables). This situation is the same when structures like programs or (natural deduction) proofs are to be manipulated and if other programming languages, such as Pascal, Prolog, and ML, replace Lisp.

Generally, syntax is classified into *concrete* and *abstract* syntax. The first is the textual form of syntax that is readable and typable by a human. This representation of syntax is implemented using strings (arrays or lists of characters).

J. Lloyd et al. (Eds.): CL 2000, LNAI 1861, pp. 239–253, 2000.

The advantages of this kind of syntax representation are that it can be easily read by humans and involves a simple computational model based on strings. The disadvantages of this style of representation are, however, numerous and serious. Concrete syntax contains too much information not important for many manipulations, such as white space, infix/prefix notation, and keywords; and important computational information is not represented explicitly, such as recursive structure, function–argument relationship, and the term–subterm relationship.

The costs of computing on concrete syntax can be overcome by parsing concrete syntax into *parse trees* (often also called *abstract syntax*). This representation of syntax is implemented using first-order terms, labeled trees, or linked lists, and it is processed using constructors and destructors (such as car/cdr/cons in Lisp) or using first-order unification (Prolog) or matching (ML). The advantages to this representation are clear: the recursive structure of syntax is immediate, recursion over syntax is easily accommodated by recursion in most programming languages, and the term-subterm relationship is identified with the tree-subtree relationship. Also, there are various semantics approaches, such as algebra, that provide mathematical models for many operations on syntax. One should realize, however, that there are costs associated with using this more abstract representation. For example, when moving to greater abstraction, some information is lost: for example, spacing and indenting of the concrete syntax is (generally) discarded in the parse tree syntax. Also, implementation support is needed to provide recursion and linked lists. These costs associated with using parse tree syntax are generally accepted since one generally does not mind the loss of pagination in the original syntax and since a few decades of programming language research has yielded workable and effective runtime environments that support the required dynamic memory demands required to process parse trees.

When representing syntax containing bound variables, there are, however, significant costs involved in not using a representation that is even more abstract than parse trees since otherwise the constellation of concepts surrounding bindings needs to be implemented by the programmer. There are generally two approaches to providing such implementations. The first approach treats bound variables as global objects and programs are then written to determine which of these global objects are to be considered free (global) and which are to be considered scoped. This approach is quite natural and seems the simplest to deploy. It requires no special meta-level support (all support must be provided explicitly by the programmer) and is the approach commonly used in text books on logic. A second approach uses the nameless dummies of de Bruijn [2]. Here, first-order terms containing natural numbers are used to describe alpha-equivalence classes of λ-terms: syntax is abstracted by removing bound variable names entirely. There has been a lot of success in using nameless dummies in low-level compilation of automated deduction systems and type systems. Consider, for instance, the work on explicit substitutions of Nadathur [25, 28] and Abadi, Cardelli, Curien, and Lévy [1]. Nadathur, for example, has recently built a compiler and abstract machine that exploits this representation of syntax [27].

While successful at implementing bound variables in syntax, nameless dummies, however do not provide a high-level and declarative treatment of binding.

We will trace the development of the ideas behind a third, more abstract form of syntactic representation, called λ-*tree syntax* [23] and the closely related notion of *higher-order abstract syntax* [36].

Logic embraces and explains elegantly the nature of bound variables and substitution. These are part of the very fabric of logic. So it is not surprising that our story starts and mostly stays within the area of logic.

2   Church's Use of λ-Terms within Logic

In [3], Church presented a higher-order logic, called the *Simple Theory of Types* (STT), as a foundation for mathematics. In STT, the syntax of formulas and terms is built on simply typed λ-terms. The axioms for STT include those governing the logical connectives and quantifiers as well as the more mathematical axioms for infinity, choice, and extensionality. The λ-terms of STT are also equated using the following equations of α, β, and η-conversion.

$$(\alpha) \qquad \lambda x.M = \lambda y.M[y/x], \qquad \text{provided } y \text{ is not free in } M$$
$$(\beta) \qquad (\lambda x.M)\, N = M\,[N/x]$$
$$(\eta) \qquad \lambda x.(M\ x) = M, \qquad \text{provided } x \text{ is not free in } M$$

Here, the expression $M[t/x]$ denotes the substitution of t for the variable x in M in which bound variables are systematically changed to avoid variable capture.

Church made use of the single binding operation of λ-abstraction to encode all of the other binding operators present in STT: universal and existential quantification as well as the definite description and choice operators. This reuse of the λ-binder in these other situations allows the notions of bound and free variables occurrences and of substitution to be solved once with respect to λ-binding and then be used to solve the associated problems with these other binding operations. In recent years, this same economy has been employed in a number of logical and computational systems.

Church used the λ-binder to introduce a new syntactic type, that of an *abstraction* of one syntactic type over another. For example, Church encoded the universal quantifier using a constant Π that instead of taking two augments, say, the name of a bound variable and the body of the quantifier, took one argument, namely, the abstraction of the variable over the body. That is, instead of representing universal quantification as, say, $\Pi(x, B)$ where Π has the type $\tau * o \rightarrow o$ (here, o is the type of formulas and τ is a type variable), it is represented as $\Pi(\lambda x.B)$, where Π has the type $(\tau \rightarrow o) \rightarrow o$. (This latter expression can be abbreviated using more familiar syntax as $\forall x.B$.) The λ-binder is used to construct the arrow ($\rightarrow$) type. Similarly, the existential quantifier used a constant Σ of type $(\tau \rightarrow o) \rightarrow o$ and the choice operator ι had type $(\tau \rightarrow o) \rightarrow \tau$: both take an abstraction as their argument.

Since Church was seeking to use this logic as a foundations for mathematics, λ-terms were intended to encode rich collections of mathematical functions that could be defined recursively and which were extensional. By adding higher-order quantification and axioms for infinity, extensionality, and choice, the equality of λ-term was governed by much more than simply the equations for α, β, and η-conversion. Hence, λ-abstractions could no longer be taken for expressions denoting abstractions of one syntactic types over another. For example, the formula $\Pi(\lambda x.(p\ x) \wedge q)$ would be equivalent and equal to the formula $\Pi(\lambda x.q \wedge (p\ x))$: there is no way in STT to separate these two formulas. Thus, the domain o became associated to the *denotation* or *extension* of formulas and not with their *intension*.

3 Equality Modulo $\alpha\beta\eta$-Conversion

One way to maintain λ-abstraction as the builder of a syntactic type is to weaken the theory of STT significantly, so that λ-terms no longer represent general functional expressions. The resulting system may no longer be a general foundations for mathematics but it may be useful for specifying computational processes. The most common approach to doing this weakening is to drop the axioms of infinity, extensionality, and choice. In the remaining theory, λ-terms are governed only by the rules of α, β, and η-conversion. The simply typed λ-calculus with an equality theory of α, β, η is no longer a general framework for functional computation although its is still rather rich [39].

The presence of β-conversion in the equality theory means that object-level substitution can be specified simply by using the meta-level equality theory. For example, consider the problem of instantiating the universal quantifier $\forall x.B$ with the term t to get $B[t/x]$. Using Church's representation for universal quantification, this operation can be represented simply as taking the expression (ΠR) and the term t and returning the term $(R\ t)$. Here, R denotes the abstraction $\lambda x.B$, so $(R\ t)$ is a meta-level β-redex that is equal to $B[t/x]$. Thus, β-reduction can encode object-level substitution elegantly and simply. For example, consider the following signature for encoding terms and formulas in a small object-logic:

$$\forall, \exists : (term \rightarrow formula) \rightarrow formula \qquad a, b : term$$
$$\supset : formula \rightarrow formula \rightarrow formula \qquad f : term \rightarrow term \rightarrow term$$
$$r, s : term \rightarrow formula \qquad\qquad t : formula.$$

The λ-term $\forall \lambda x.\exists \lambda y.\ r\ (f\ x\ y) \supset s\ (f\ y\ x)$ is of type *formula* and is built by applying the constant $\forall$ to the a λ-term of type *term* $\rightarrow$ *formula*, the syntactic type of a term abstracted over a formula. This universally quantified object-level formula can be instantiated with the term $(f\ a\ b)$ by first matching it with the expression $(\forall\ R)$ and then considering the term $(R\ (f\ a\ b))$. Since R will be bound to a λ-expression, this latter term will be a meta-level β-redex. If β is part of our equality theory, then this term is equal to

$$\exists \lambda y.r\ (f\ (f\ a\ b)\ y) \supset s\ (f\ y\ (f\ a\ b)),$$

which is the result of instantiating the universal quantifier.

Huet and Lang [13] were probably the first people to use a simply typed λ-calculus modulo α, β, η to express program analysis and program transformation steps. They used second-order variables to range over program abstractions and used second-order matching to bind such variables to such abstractions. The reliance on β-conversion also meant that the matching procedure was accounting for object-level substitution as well as abstractions. Second-order matching is NP-complete, in part, because reversing object-level substitution is complicated. There was no use of logic in this particular work, so its relationship to Church's system was rather minor.

In the mid-to-late 80's, two computational systems, Isabelle [32] and λProlog [26], were developed that both exploited the intuitionistic theory of implications, conjunctions, and universal quantification at all non-predicate types. In Isabelle, this logic was implemented in ML and search for proofs was governed by an ML implementation of tactics and tacticals. This system was intended to provide support for interactive and automatic theorem proving. λProlog implemented this logic (actually a extension of it called *higher-order hereditary Harrop formulas* [22]) by using a generalization of Prolog's depth-first search mechanism. Both systems implemented versions of unification for simply typed λ-terms modulo α, β, η conversion (often called *higher-order unification*). The general structuring of those unification procedures was fashioned on the unification search processes described by Huet in [12]. In λProlog, it was possible to generalize the work of Huet and Lang from simple template matching to more general analysis of program analysis and transformation [19–21].

The dependent typed λ-calculus LF [10] was developed to provide a high-level specification language for logics. This system contained quantification at higher-types and was based on an equality theory that incorporated α, β, and η-conversion (of dependent typed λ-calculus). Pfenning implemented LF as the Elf system [33] using a λProlog-style operational semantics. The earliest version of Elf implemented unification modulo α, β, η.

It was clear that these computer systems provided new ways to compute on the syntax of expressions with bound variables. The availability of unification and substitution in implementations of these meta-logics immediately allowed bound variable names to be ignored and substitutions for all data structures that contain bound variables to be provided directly.

Pfenning and Elliott in [36] coined the term *higher-order abstract syntax* for this new style of programming and specification. They also analyzed this style of syntactic specification and concluded that it should be based on an enrichment of the simply typed λ-calculus containing products and polymorphism, since they found that these two extensions were essential features for practical applications. To date, no computational system has been built to implement this particular notion of higher-order abstract syntax. It appears that in general, most practical applications can be accommodated in a type system without polymorphism or products. In practice, higher-order abstract syntax has generally come to refer to the encoding and manipulating of syntax using either simply or dependently typed λ-calculus modulo α, β, and η-conversion.

4   A Weaker Form of β-Conversion

Unification modulo α, β, and η conversion of λ-terms, either simply typed or dependently typed, is undecidable, even when restricted to second-order. Complexity results for matching are not fully know, although restricting to second-order matching is known to be NP-complete. Thus, the equalities implemented by these computer systems (Isabelle, λProlog, and Elf) are quite complex. This complexity suggests that we should find a simpler approach to using the λ-binder as a constructor for a syntactic type of abstraction. The presence of bound variables in syntax is a complication, but it should not make computations on syntax overly costly. We had some progress towards this goal when we weaken Church's STT so that λ-abstractions are not general functions. But since the equality and unification remains complex, it seems that we have not weakened that theory enough.

We can consider, for example, getting rid of β-conversion entirely and only consider equality modulo α, η-conversion. However, this seems to leave the equality system too weak. To illustrate that weakness, consider solving the following match, where capital letters denote the match variables:

$$\forall \lambda x (P \wedge Q) = \forall \lambda y ((ry \supset sy) \wedge t).$$

There is no substitution for P and Q that will make these two expressions equal modulo α and η-conversion: recall that we intend our meta-level to be a logic and that the proper logical reading of substitution does not permit variable capturing substitutions. Hence, the substitution

$$\{P \mapsto (rx \supset sx), Q \mapsto t\}$$

does not equate these two expressions: substituting into the first of these two terms produces a term equal to $\forall \lambda z ((rx \supset sx) \wedge t)$ and not equal to the intended term $\forall \lambda y ((ry \supset sy) \wedge t)$. If we leave things here, it seems impossible to do interesting pattern matching that can explore structure underneath a λ-abstraction.

If we change this match problem, however, by raising the type of P from *formula* to *term* $\to$ *formula* and consider the following matching problem instead,

$$\forall \lambda x (Px \wedge Q) = \forall \lambda y ((ry \supset sy) \wedge t)$$

then this match problem does, in fact, have one unifier, namely,

$$\{P \mapsto \lambda w (rw \supset sw), Q \mapsto t\}.$$

For this to be a unifier, however, the equality theory we use must allow $((\lambda w.rw \supset sw)\, x)$ to be rewritten to $(rx \supset sx)$. Clearly β will allow this, but we have really only motivated a much weaker version of β-conversion, in particular, the case when a λ-abstraction is applied to a bound variable that is not free in the abstraction. The restriction of β to the rule $(\lambda x.B)y = B[y/x]$, provided y is not free in $(\lambda x.B)$, is called β_0-conversion [15]. In the presence of α-conversion, this rule can be written more simply and without a proviso as $(\lambda x.B)x = B$. Our example can now be completed by allowing the equality theory to be based on α, β_0, and η-conversion. In such a theory, we have

$$\forall \lambda x((\lambda w(rw \supset sw)x) \wedge t) = \forall \lambda y((ry \supset sy) \wedge t).$$

If the λ-binder can be viewed as introducing a syntactic domain representing the abstraction of a bound variable from a term, then we can view β_0 as the rule that allows destructing a λ-binder by replacing it with a bound variable.

It is easy to imagine generalizing the example above to cases where match variables have occurrences in the scope of more than one abstraction, where different syntax is being represented, and where unification and not matching is considered. In fact, when examining typical λProlog programs, it is clear that most instances of β-conversion performed by the interpreter are, in fact, instances of β_0-conversion. Consider, for example, a term with a free occurrence of M of the form

$$\lambda x \ldots \lambda y \ldots (M \ y \ x) \ldots$$

Any substitution for M applied to such a term introduces β_0 redexes only. For example, if M above is instantiated with a λ-term, say $\lambda u \lambda v.t$, then the only new β-redex formed is $((\lambda u \lambda v.t) \ y \ x)$. This term is reduced to normal form by simply renaming in t the variables u and v to y and x — a very simple computation. Notice that replacing a β_0-redex $(\lambda x.B)y$ with $B[y/x]$ makes the term strictly smaller, which stands in striking contrast to β-reduction, where the size of terms can grow explosively.

5 L_λ-Unification

In [15], Miller introduced a subset of hereditary Harrop formulas, called L_λ, such that the equality theory of α, β, η only involved α, β_0, η rewritings. In that setting, Miller showed that unification of λ-terms is decidable and unary (most general unifiers exist when unifiers exist).

When L_λ is restricted to simply comparing two atomic formula or two terms, it is generally referred to as L_λ-unification or as higher-order pattern unification. More precisely, in this setting a unification problem a set of ordered pairs

$$\{(t_1, s_1), \ldots, (t_n, s_n)\},$$

where for $i = 1, \ldots, n$ and where t_i and s_i are simply typed λ-terms of the same type. Such a unification problem is an L_λ-unification problem if every free variable occurrence in that problem is applied to at most distinct bound variables. This severe restriction on the applications of variables of higher-type is the key restriction of L_λ.

This kind of unification can be seen both as a generalization of first-order unification and as a simplification of the unification process of Huet [12]. Any β-normal λ-term has the top-level structure $\lambda x_1 \ldots \lambda x_p(h \ t_1 \ldots t_q)$ where $p, q \geq 0$, the binder $x_1, \ldots, x_p$ is a list of distinct bound variables, the arguments $t_1, \ldots, t_q$ are β-normal terms, and the head h is either a constant, a bound variable (i.e., a member of $\{x_1, \ldots, x_p\}$), or a free variable. (We shall sometimes write $\bar{x}$ to denote a list of variables $x_1, \ldots, x_n$, for some n.) If the head is a free variable, the term is called *flexible*; otherwise, it is called *rigid*. Notice that if a term in L_λ is flexible, then it is of the form $\lambda x_1 \ldots \lambda x_n . V\ y_1\ \cdots\ y_p$ where each lists $x_1, \ldots, x_n$ and $y_1, \ldots, y_p$ contain distinct occurrences of variables and where the the set $\{y_1, \ldots, y_p\}$ is a subset of $\{x_1, \ldots, x_n\}$. Pairs in unification problems will be classified as either rigid-rigid, rigid-flexible, flexible-rigid, or flexible-flexible depending on the status of the two terms forming that pair. We can always assume that the two terms in a pair have the same binders: if not, use η to make the shorter binder longer and α to get them to have the same names.

We present the main steps of the unification algorithm (see for [15] for a fuller description). Select a pair in the given unification and choose the appropriate steps from the following steps.

Rigid-Rigid Step. If the pair is rigid-rigid and both terms have the same head symbol, say, $\langle \lambda \bar{x}.h t_1 \ldots t_n, \lambda \bar{x}.h s_1 \ldots s_n \rangle$, then replace that pair with the pairs $\langle \lambda \bar{x}.t_1, \lambda \bar{x}.s_1 \rangle, \ldots, \langle \lambda \bar{x}.t_n, \lambda \bar{x}.s_n \rangle$ and continue processing pairs. If the pair has different heads, then there is no unifier for this unification problem.

Flexible-Flexible Step. If the pair is flexible-flexible, then it is of the form $\langle \lambda \bar{x}.V y_1 \ldots y_n, \lambda \bar{x}.U z_1 \ldots z_p \rangle$ where $n, p \geq 0$ and where the lists $y_1, \ldots, y_n$ and $z_1 \ldots z_p$ are both lists of distinct variables and are both subsets of the binder $\bar{x}$. There are two cases to consider.

Case 1. If V and U are different, then this pair is solved by the substitution $[V \mapsto \lambda \bar{y}.W\bar{w}, U \mapsto \lambda \bar{z}.W\bar{w}]$, where W is a new free variable and $\bar{w}$ is a list enumerating the variables that are in both the list $\bar{y}$ and the list $\bar{z}$.

Case 2. If V and U are equal, then, given the typing of λ-terms, p and n must also be equal. Let $\bar{w}$ be an enumeration of the set $\{y_i \mid y_i = z_i, i \in \{1, \ldots, n\}\}$. We solve this pair with the substitution $[V \mapsto \lambda \bar{y}.W\bar{w}]$ (notice that this is the same via α-conversion to $[V \mapsto \lambda \bar{z}.W\bar{w}]$), where W is a new free variable.

Flexible-Rigid Step. If the pair is flexible-rigid, then that pair is of the form $\langle \lambda \bar{x}.V y_1 \ldots y_n, r \rangle$. If V has a free occurrence in r then this unification has no solution. Otherwise, this pair is solved using the substitution $[V \mapsto \lambda y_1 \ldots \lambda y_n.r]$.

Rigid-Flexible Step. If the pair is rigid-flexible, then switch the order of the pair and do the flexible-rigid step.

Huet's process [12], when applied to such unification problems, produces the same reduction except for the flexible-flexible steps. Huet's procedure actually does pre-unification, leaving flexible-flexible pairs as constraints for future unifications since general (non-L_λ) flexible-flexible pairs have too many solutions to actually enumerate effectively. Given the restrictions in L_λ, flexible-flexible pairs can be solved simply and do not need to be suspended.

Qian has shown that L_λ-unification can be done in linear time and space [38] (using a much more sophisticated algorithm than the one hinted at above). Nipkow has written a simple functional implementation of L_λ-unification [30] and has also showed that results concerning first-order critical pairs lift naturally to the L_λ setting [29].

It was also shown in [15] that L_λ-unification can be modified to work with untyped λ-terms. This observation means, for example, that the results about L_λ can be lifted to other type systems, not just the simple theory of types. Pfenning has done such a generalization to a dependent typed system [34]. Pfenning has also modified Elf so that pre-unification essentially corresponds to L_λ-unification: unification constraints that do not satisfy the L_λ restriction on free variables are delayed. The equality theory of Elf, however, is still based on full β-conversion.

Notice that unification in L_λ is unification modulo α, β_0, and η but unification modulo α, β_0, and η on unrestricted terms is a more general problem. For example, if g is a constant of type $i \to i$ and F is a variable of type $i \to i \to i$, the equation $\lambda x.F\ x\ x\ =\ \lambda y.g\ y$ has two solutions modulo α, β_0, η, namely, $F \mapsto \lambda u \lambda v.g\ u$ and $F \mapsto \lambda u \lambda v.g\ v$. Notice that this unification problem is not in L_λ since the variable F is applied to the bound variable x twice. As this example shows, unification modulo α, β_0, η is not necessarily unary.

6   Logic Programming in L_λ

Successful manipulation of syntax containing bound variables is not completely achieved by picking a suitable unification and equality theory for terms. In order to compute with λ-trees, it must be possible to define recursion over them. This requires understanding how one "descends" into a λ-abstraction $\lambda x.t$ in a way that is independent from the choice of the name x. A key observation made with respect to the design of such systems as Isabelle, λProlog, and Elf is that such a declarative treatment of bound variables requires the *generic* and *hypothetical* judgments that are found in intuitionistic logic (via implication and universal quantification) and associated dependent typed λ-calculi. The need to support universal quantification explicitly forces one to consider unification with both free (existentially quantified) variables and universally quantified variables. To handle unification with both kinds of variables present, Paulson developed $\forall$-*lifting* [31] and Miller developed *raising* [18] ($\forall$-lifting can be seen as backchaining followed by raising).

The name L_λ is actually the name of a subset of the hereditary Harrop formula used as a logical foundation for λProlog, except for restrictions on quantified variables made to ensure that only L_λ-unification occurs in interpreting the language. (L_λ is generally also restricted so as not to have the predicate quantification that is allowed in λProlog.) While we do not have adequate space here to present the full definition of the L_λ logic programming language (for that, see [15]) we shall illustrate the logic via a couple of examples.

We shall use inference figures to denote logic programming clauses in such a way that the conclusion and the premise of a rule corresponds to the head and body of the clause, respectively. For example, if A_0, A_1, and A_2 are syntactic variables for atomic formulas, then the two inference figures

$$\frac{A_1 \qquad A_2}{A_0} \qquad \frac{\forall x(A_1 \supset A_2)}{A_0},$$

denote the two formulas

$$\forall \bar{y}(A_1 \wedge A_2 \supset A_0) \quad \text{and} \quad \forall \bar{y}(\forall x(A_1 \supset A_2) \supset A_0)$$

The list of variables $\bar{y}$ is generally determined by collecting together the free variables of the premise and conclusion. In the inference figures, the corresponding free variables will be denoted by capital letters. The first of these inference rules denotes a simple Horn clause while the second inference rule is an example of a hereditary Harrop formula. The theory of higher-order hereditary Harrop formulas [22] provides an adequate operational and proof theoretical semantics for these kinds of clauses. The central restriction taken from L_λ-unification must be generalized to this setting. Note that in our examples this restriction implies that a variable in the list $\bar{y}$ can be applied to at most distinct variables that are either λ-bound or universally bound in the body of the clause.

Consider, for example, representing untyped λ-terms and simple types. Let tm and ty be two types for these two domains, respectively. The following four constants can be used to build objects in these two domains.

$$app : tm \to tm \to tm \qquad arr : ty \to ty \to ty$$
$$abs : (tm \to tm) \to tm \qquad i : ty$$

The constants app and abs are constructors for applications and abstractions, while the constants arr and i are used to denote functional (arrow) types and a primitive type.

To capture the judgment that an untyped λ-term has a certain simple type, we introduce the atomic judgment (predicate) $typeof$ that asserts that its first argument (a term of type tm) has its second argument (a term of type ty) as a simple type. The following two inference rules specify the $typeof$ judgment.

$$\frac{typeof\ M\ (arr\ A\ B) \qquad typeof\ N\ A}{typeof\ (app\ M\ N)\ B} \qquad \frac{\forall x(typeof\ x\ A \supset typeof\ (R\ x)\ B)}{typeof\ (abs\ R)\ (arr\ A\ B)}$$

Notice that the variable R is used in a higher-order fashion since it has an occurrence where it is an argument and an occurrence where it has an argument.

The conventional approach to specifying such a typing judgment would involve an explicit context of typing assumptions and an explicit treatment of bound variables names, either as names or as de Bruijn numbers. In this specification of the $typeof$ judgment, the hypothetical judgment (the intuitionistic implication) implicitly handles the typing context, and the generic judgment (the universal quantifier) implicitly handles the bound variable names via the use of eigenvariables.

Since the application of variables is restricted greatly in L_λ, object-level substitution cannot be handled simply by the equality theory of L_λ. For example, the clause

$$\frac{}{bredex\ (app\ (abs\ R)\ N)\ (R\ N)}$$

defines a predicate that relates the encoding of an untyped λ-term that represents a top-level β-redex to the result of reducing that redex. The formula that encodes this inference rule does not satisfy the L_λ restriction since the variable R is not applied to a λ-bound variable: notice that instances of $(R\ N)$ might produce (meta-level) β-redexes that are not β_0-redexes. Instead, object-level substitution can be implemented as a simple logic program. To illustrate this, consider the following two classes for specifying equality for untyped λ-terms.

$$\frac{copy\ M\ M' \qquad copy\ N\ N'}{copy\ (app\ M\ N)\ (app\ M'\ N')} \qquad \frac{\forall x\ \forall y\ (copy\ x\ y \supset copy\ (R\ x)\ (S\ y))}{copy\ (abs\ R)\ (abs\ S)}$$

Clearly, the atom $copy\ t\ t'$ is provable from these two clauses if and only if t and t' denote the same untyped λ-term. Given this specification of equality, we can now specify object-level substitution with the following simple clause:

$$\frac{\forall x\ (copy\ x\ N \supset copy\ (R\ x)\ M)}{subst\ R\ N\ M}$$

which axiomatizes a three place relation, where the type of the first argument is $i \to i$ and the type of the other two arguments is i. We can now finally re-implement $bredex$ so that it is now an L_λ program:

$$\frac{subst\ R\ N\ M}{bredex\ (app\ (abs\ R)\ N)\ M}$$

The entire specification $bredex$ is now an L_λ logic program. For a general approach to accounting for object-level substitution in L_λ, see [16].

For a specific illustration that classical logic does not support the notion of syntax when higher-orders are involved, consider the following signature.

$$p, q, r : term \to o \qquad g : (term \to term) \to term \qquad f : term \to term$$

and the two clauses

$$\frac{p\ X}{r\ (f\ X)} \qquad \frac{\forall x\ (p\ x \supset q\ (U\ x))}{r\ (g\ U)}$$

Using the familiar "propositions-as-types" paradigm, the three atomic formulas $p\ t_1, q\ t_2$, and $r\ t_3$ can be seen as specifying subtypes of the type $term$, that is, they can be read as $t_1 : p, t_2 : q$, and $t_3 : r$. Using this analogy, these two clauses would then read as the type declarations $f : p \to r$ and $g : (p \to q) \to r$. Now consider the question of whether or not there is a term of type r. Simple inspection reveals that there is no term of type r built from these two constants. Similarly, there is no intuitionistic proof of $\exists X.r\ X$ from the two displayed clauses. On the contrary, there is a classical logic proof of $\exists X.r\ X$ from these formulas. We leave it to the reader to ponder how classical logic can be so liberal to allow such a conclusion. (Hint: consider the classical logic theorem $(\exists w.p\ w) \vee (\forall w.\neg p\ w)$.)

7 λ-Tree Syntax

In contrast to *concrete syntax* and *parse tree syntax*, a third level of syntax representation, named λ-*tree syntax* was introduced in [23]. This approach to syntactic representation uses λ-terms to encode data and L_λ-unification and equality modulo α, β_0, and η to construct and deconstruct syntax. There is no commitment to any particular type discipline for terms nor is typing necessary.

As we have observed, a programming language or specification language that incorporates λ-tree syntax must also provide an abstraction mechanism that can be used to support recursion under term level abstractions. In logic or typed languages, this is achieved using eigenvariables (a notion of bound variable within a proof). Such a mechanism can be described in a logic programming setting, like λProlog, as one where new, scoped constants are introduced to play the role of bound variables.

While supporting λ-tree syntax is more demanding on the languages that implements it, there has been a lot of work in making such implementations feasible. Consider for example the work on explicit substitutions [1, 7, 25, 28] and the abstract machine and compiler Teyjus [27] for λProlog. The Isabelle theorem prover [32] implements L_λ and the Elf system [33] provides an effective implementation of L_λ within a dependently typed λ-calculus.

Support for λ-term syntax does not necessarily need to reside only in logic programming-like systems. In [14] Miller proposed an extension to ML in which pattern matching supported L_λ matching and where data types allowed for the scoped introduction of new constants (locally bound variables). A second type, written a' => b', was introduced to represent the type of syntactically abstracted variables: the usual function type, written a' -> b', was not used for that purpose. It is possible, following the techniques we described for L_λ, to implement in the resulting ML extension, a function **subst** that maps the first domain into the second, that is, **subst** has type (a' => b') -> (a' -> b'). To our knowledge, this language has not been implemented.

The need for the new term λ-*tree syntax* instead of the more common term *higher-order abstract syntax* can be justified for a couple of reasons. First, since types are not necessary in this style of representation, the adjective "higher-order", which refers to the order of types for variables and constants, seems inappropriate. Second, higher-order abstract syntax generally denotes the stronger notion of equality and unification that is based on full β-conversion. For example, Pfenning in [35] states that "higher-order abstract syntax supports substitution through λ-reduction in the meta-language". Thus, the term higher-order abstract syntax would not be appropriate for describing projects, such as L_λ and the proposal mentioned above for extending ML, in which β-reduction is not part of the meta-language.

8 Related Work

As we have mentioned, Church intended the function space constructor to be strong enough to model mathematical functions and not to support the weaker notion of representing an abstraction over syntactic types. As a result, we argued that Church's system should be weakened by removing not only the axioms of infinity, choice, and extensionality but also full β-conversion. On the other hand, there has been work in trying to recover higher-order abstract syntax from rich function spaces such as those found in Coq: the main issue there is to restrict the function space constructor to exclude "exotic" terms, like those inhabiting function spaces but which do not denote syntactic abstractions [4–6].

For conventional specifications using parse trees syntax, well understood semantic tools are available, such as those of initial algebras and models for equality. Similar tools have not yet been developed to handle λ-tree syntax. Since the logic that surrounds λ-tree syntax is that of intuitionistic logic, Kripke models might be useful: a simple step in this direction was taken in [17] by recasting the cut-elimination theorem for intuitionistic logic as a kind of initial model. Similarly, the notion of Kripke λ-models due to Mitchell and Moggi [24] could also be quite useful. The LICS 1999 proceedings contained three papers [9, 8, 11] that proposed semantics for abstract syntax containing bound variables that were based (roughly) on using initial models based on certain categories of sheaves. Pitts and Gabbay have used their semantics to develop an extension to ML that supports a notion of syntax somewhat similar to λ-tree syntax [37].

9   Conclusions

One might have some impatience with the idea of introducing a more high-level form of abstract syntax: just implement substitution and the associated support for bound variables and move on! But what we are discussing here is the foundations of syntax. The choices made here can impact much of what is built on top.

There is also the simple observation that with, say, the parse tree representation of syntax, it is natural to use meta-level application to encode object-level application. But application and abstraction are not two features that accidentally appear in the same logic: they are two sides of the same phenomenon, just as introduction and elimination rules in proof theory are two sides of a connective, and they need to be treated together. It should be just as natural to use meta-level abstractions to encode object-level abstractions, and indeed, this is what λ-tree syntax attempts to make possible.

Acknowledgments

I would like to thank Catuscia Palamidessi and the reviewers of this paper for their many useful comments that helped to improve this paper's presentation. This work was supported in part by NSF Grants INT-9815645 and CCR-9803971.

References

1. Martin Abadi, Luca Cardelli, Pierre-Louis Curien, and Jean-Jacques Lévy. Explicit substitutions. *Journal of Functional Programming*, 1(4):375–416, October 1991.
2. N. de Bruijn. Lambda calculus notation with nameless dummies, a tool for automatic formula manipulation, with application to the Church-Rosser Theorem. *Indag. Math.*, 34(5):381–392, 1972.
3. Alonzo Church. A formulation of the simple theory of types. *Journal of Symbolic Logic*, 5:56–68, 1940.
4. Joelle Despeyroux, Amy Felty, and Andre Hirschowitz. Higher-order abstract syntax in Coq. In *Second International Conference on Typed Lambda Calculi and Applications*, pages 124–138, April 1995.
5. Joelle Despeyroux and Andre Hirschowitz. Higher-order abstract syntax with induction in Coq. In *Fifth International Conference on Logic Programming and Automated Reasoning*, pages 159–173, June 1994.
6. Joelle Despeyroux, Frank Pfenning, and Carsten Schürmann. Primitive recursion for higher-order abstract syntax. In *Third International Conference on Typed Lambda Calculi and Applications*, April 1997.
7. G. Dowek, T. Hardin, and C. Kirchner. Higher-order unification via explicit substitutions. In D. Kozen, editor, *Logic in Computer Science*, pages 366–374, 1995.
8. M. P. Fiore, G. D. Plotkin, and D. Turi. Abstract syntax and variable binding. In *Logic in Computer Science*, pages 193–202. IEEE Computer Society Press, 1999.
9. M. J. Gabbay and A. M. Pitts. A new approach to abstract syntax involving binders. In *Logic in Computer Science*, pages 214–224. IEEE Computer Society Press, 1999.
10. Robert Harper, Furio Honsell, and Gordon Plotkin. A framework for defining logics. *Journal of the ACM*, 40(1):143–184, 1993.
11. M. Hofmann. Semantical analysis of higher-order abstract syntax. In *Logic in Computer Science*, pages 204–213. IEEE Computer Society Press, 1999.
12. Gérard Huet. A unification algorithm for typed λ-calculus. *Theoretical Computer Science*, 1:27–57, 1975.
13. Gérard Huet and Bernard Lang. Proving and applying program transformations expressed with second-order patterns. *Acta Informatica*, 11:31–55, 1978.
14. Dale Miller. An extension to ML to handle bound variables in data structures: Preliminary report. In *Informal Proceedings of the Logical Frameworks BRA Workshop*, June 1990. Available as UPenn CIS technical report MS-CIS-90-59.
15. Dale Miller. A logic programming language with lambda-abstraction, function variables, and simple unification. *J. of Logic and Computation*, 1(4):497–536, 1991.
16. Dale Miller. Unification of simply typed lambda-terms as logic programming. In *Eighth International Logic Programming Conference*, pages 255–269, Paris, France, June 1991. MIT Press.
17. Dale Miller. Abstract syntax and logic programming. In *Logic Programming: Proceedings of the First and Second Russian Conferences on Logic Programming*, number 592 in LNAI, pages 322–337. Springer-Verlag, 1992.
18. Dale Miller. Unification under a mixed prefix. *Journal of Symbolic Computation*, pages 321–358, 1992.
19. Dale Miller and Gopalan Nadathur. Higher-order logic programming. In Ehud Shapiro, editor, *Proceedings of the Third International Logic Programming Conference*, pages 448–462, London, June 1986.
20. Dale Miller and Gopalan Nadathur. Some uses of higher-order logic in computational linguistics. In *Proceedings of the 24th Annual Meeting of the Association for Computational Linguistics*, pages 247–255, 1986.

21. Dale Miller and Gopalan Nadathur. A logic programming approach to manipulating formulas and programs. In Seif Haridi, editor, *IEEE Symposium on Logic Programming*, pages 379–388, San Francisco, September 1987.

22. Dale Miller, Gopalan Nadathur, Frank Pfenning, and Andre Scedrov. Uniform proofs as a foundation for logic programming. *Annals of Pure and Applied Logic*, 51:125–157, 1991.

23. Dale Miller and Catuscia Palamidessi. Foundational aspects of syntax. In Pierpaolo Degano, Roberto Gorrieri, Alberto Marchetti-Spaccamela, and Peter Wegner, editors, *ACM Computing Surveys Symposium on Theoretical Computer Science: A Perspective*, volume 31. ACM, Sep 1999. Article number 10.

24. John C. Mitchell and Eugenio Moggi. Kripke-style models for typed lambda calculus. *Annals of Pure and Applied Logic*, 51, 1991.

25. Gopalan Nadathur. A fine-grained notation for lambda terms and its use in intensional operations. *Journal of Functional and Logic Programming*, 1999(2), March 1999.

26. Gopalan Nadathur and Dale Miller. An Overview of λProlog. In *Fifth International Logic Programming Conference*, pages 810–827, Seattle, Washington, August 1988. MIT Press.

27. Gopalan Nadathur and Dustin J. Mitchell. System description: Teyjus—a compiler and abstract machine based implementation of λProlog. In H. Ganzinger, editor, CADE-16, pages 287–291, Trento, Italy, July 1999. Springer LNCS.

28. Gopalan Nadathur and Debra Sue Wilson. A notation for lambda terms: A generalization of environments. *Theoretical Computer Science*, 198(1-2):49–98, 1998.

29. Tobias Nipkow. Higher-order critical pairs. In G. Kahn, editor, *Sixth Annual Sym. on Logic in Computer Science*, pages 342–349. IEEE, July 1991.

30. Tobias Nipkow. Functional unification of higher-order patterns. In M. Vardi, editor, *Eighth Annual Sym. on Logic in Computer Science*, pages 64–74. IEEE, June 1993.

31. Lawrence C. Paulson. The foundation of a generic theorem prover. *Journal of Automated Reasoning*, 5:363–397, September 1989.

32. Lawrence C. Paulson. Isabelle: The next 700 theorem provers. In Piergiorgio Odifreddi, editor, *Logic and Computer Science*, pages 361–386. Academic Press, 1990.

33. Frank Pfenning. Elf: A language for logic definition and verified metaprogramming. In *Fourth Annual Symposium on Logic in Computer Science*, pages 313–321, Monterey, CA, June 1989.

34. Frank Pfenning. Unification and anti-unification in the Calculus of Constructions. In G. Kahn, editor, *Sixth Annual Symposium on Logic in Computer Science*, pages 74–85. IEEE, July 1991.

35. Frank Pfenning. The practice of logical frameworks. In Hélène Kirchner, editor, *Proceedings of the Colloquium on Trees in Algebra and Programming*, volume LNCS 1059, pages 119–134. Springer-Verlag, 1996.

36. Frank Pfenning and Conal Elliot. Higher-order abstract syntax. In *Proceedings of the ACM-SIGPLAN Conference on Programming Language Design and Implementation*, pages 199–208. ACM Press, June 1988.

37. Andrew M. Pitts and Murdoch J. Gabbay. A meta language for programming with bound names modulo renaming (preliminary report). Draft January 2000.

38. Zhenyu Qian. Unification of higher-order patterns in linear time and space. *J. Logic and Computation*, 6(3):315–341, 1996.

39. Richard Statman. The typed λ calculus is not elementary recursive. *Theoretical Computer Science*, 9:73–81, 1979.

Goal-Directed Proof Search in Multiple-Conclusioned Intuitionistic Logic

James Harland, Tatjana Lutovac, and Michael Winikoff

Department of Computer Science
Royal Melbourne Institute of Technology
GPO Box 2476V, Melbourne, 3001, Australia
{jah,tanja,winikoff}@cs.rmit.edu.au
http://www.cs.rmit.edu.au/~{jah,tanja,winikoff}

Abstract. A key property in the definition of logic programming languages is the completeness of goal-directed proofs. This concept originated in the study of logic programming languages for intuitionistic logic in the (single-conclusioned) sequent calculus LJ, but has subsequently been adapted to multiple-conclusioned systems such as those for linear logic. Given these developments, it seems interesting to investigate the notion of goal-directed proofs for a multiple-conclusioned sequent calculus for intuitionistic logic, in that this is a logic for which there are both single-conclusioned and multiple-conclusioned systems (although the latter are less well known). In this paper we show that the language obtained for the multiple-conclusioned system differs from that for the single-conclusioned case, show how hereditary Harrop formulae can be recovered, and investigate contraction-free fragments of the logic.

1 Introduction

Logic programming is based upon the observation that if certain restrictions are placed on the class of formulae that can be used, then statements of mathematical logic can be interpreted as computer programs. In particular, computation consists of searching for a proof of a goal from a program, and the restrictions placed on both the program and the goal ensure that this proof search is sufficiently deterministic. The best known such restriction is to allow programs to consist of *Horn clauses* and goals to consist of existentially quantified conjunctions of atoms, which form the basis of the language *Prolog*.

When looking to extend such results to other logical systems, we proceed by starting from a logic $\mathcal{L}$ (or indeed a set of inference rules for $\mathcal{L}$) a proof search strategy $\mathcal{S}$, and then determining a set of goal formulae $\mathcal{G}$ and a set of program formulae $\mathcal{P}$ such that $\mathcal{S}$ is *complete* with respect to $\mathcal{L}$. This process amounts to a systematic method for designing logic programming languages, and has two important properties. Firstly, such a systematic process can uncover a richer, more expressive programming language. For example, analysis in intuitionistic logic has uncovered extensions to Horn clauses such as allowing implications, universal quantifiers, and negations in the bodies of clauses [3, 16], incorporation of higher-order facilities [16], and negations and disjunctions in the heads of clauses [17]. Secondly, this process can be applied to logics other than classical

J. Lloyd et al. (Eds.): CL 2000, LNAI 1861, pp. 254–268, 2000.

(or intuitionistic) logic. For example, a number of logic programming languages have been derived from linear logic including Lygon[11], Forum[15], LinLog [1], LO [2], Lolli [12], ACL [13], and $\mathcal{LC}$ [21].

A popular proof search strategy is the notion of *goal-directed proof* [16], which, roughly speaking, requires that the goal be decomposed before the program, and hence the computation uses the program as a context, and the goal as the controlling sequence of instructions. The original presentation of goal-directed proof (and its formalisation – *uniformity*) were derived for the *single-conclusioned* sequent calculus LJ. However, this notion has been generalised to multiple-conclusioned sequent calculi in much of the work on linear logic[1]. As pointed out in [23, section 3.1], there are some weaknesses in this approach, but it remains the best-known way to derive logic programming languages from inference rules.

In this paper we focus on the generalisation of uniformity to multiple-conclusioned logics. We investigate this question in the familiar territory of intuitionistic logic. The standard sequent calculus for intuitionistic logic is LJ, which is single-conclusioned. It is known that *hereditary Harrop formulae* are a logic programming language in intuitionistic logic, using goal-directed proof search in LJ. Further, there is evidence that this class of formulae is, in some sense, maximal [9] (at least for the first-order case).

Thus it would seem that the identification of logic programming languages in intuitionistic logic is a solved problem. However, it is less widely known that there are multiple-conclusioned sequent calculi for intuitionistic logic [22]. Whilst these are not as well known as LJ, they have been of some interest for the relationship between intuitionistic and classical inference [20]. Given such inference systems, the question naturally arises as to what logic programming languages would look like in such systems, and what the results of the previous analysis would be. This is a particularly interesting question given that there has been a significant amount of investigation of notions of goal-directed provability for multiple-conclusioned systems such as linear logic [1, 15, 19, 21] and classical logic [10, 18]. Thus it seems appropriate to investigate the design of logic programming languages via goal-directed provability for a multiple-conclusioned system for intuitionistic logic, and to compare the results with the single-conclusioned case.

2   Preliminaries

2.1   Sequent Calculi

Sequent calculi are due originally to Gentzen [7] and are often used in the analysis of proof systems. This is because sequent calculus rules are local (and hence conceptually straightforward to implement) and there is a natural distinction between programs and goals.

A sequent $\Gamma \vdash \Delta$ may be thought of as stating that if *all* the formulae in Γ are true, then *at least one* of the formulae in Δ is true. Γ is referred to as the *antecedent* and Δ as the *succedent*. The sequent calculus for classical logic, LK, is the best known (and arguably the simplest). Below we give a few of the rules for this calculus.

---

[1] Actually, there appear to be at least two distinct such generalisations.

$$\frac{}{F \vdash F} \text{ Axiom} \quad \frac{\Gamma \vdash F, \Delta \quad \Gamma, F \vdash \Delta}{\Gamma \vdash \Delta} \text{ Cut} \quad \frac{\Gamma \vdash F_1, F_2, \Delta}{\Gamma \vdash F_1 \vee F_2, \Delta} \vee R \quad \frac{\Gamma \vdash F, \Delta}{\Gamma, \neg F \vdash \Delta} L^{\perp}$$

$$\frac{\Gamma \vdash F_1, \Delta \quad \Gamma, F_2 \vdash \Delta}{\Gamma, F_1 \to F_2 \vdash \Delta} \to L \quad \frac{\Gamma, F_1 \vdash F_2, \Delta}{\Gamma \vdash F_1 \to F_2, \Delta} \to R \quad \frac{\Gamma, F_1 \vdash \Delta \quad \Gamma, F_2 \vdash \Delta}{\Gamma, F_1 \wedge F_2 \vdash \Delta} \wedge L$$

LK has the cut-elimination property [7], i.e. that any proof containing occurrences of the Cut rule can be replaced with a (potentially much larger) proof in which there are no occurrences of the Cut rule. Both of the other sequent calculus systems used in this paper (LJ and LM) also have the cut-elimination property.

2.2   Permutabilities

It is well known that the sequent calculus contains redundancies, in that there may be several trivially different proofs of the same sequent. In particular, the order of the rules can often be permuted, in that given a sequence of inference rules, we can change the order of the rules to obtain an equivalent sequence (i.e. one which has the same root and leaves as the original).

In order to study such properties, we require some further terminology [6]. The *active formulae* of an inference are the formulae which are present in the premise(s), but not in the conclusion. The *principal* formula of an inference is the formula which is present in the conclusion, but not in the premise(s). Intuitively, the inference converts the active formulae into the principal formula (but as discussed in [14], this is sometimes too simplistic).

When looking to permute the order of two inferences, it is necessary to check that the principal formula of the upper inference is not an active formula of the lower one; otherwise, no permutation is possible. When this property occurs, the two inferences are said to be in *permutation position* [6, 14].

For example, consider the two inferences below.

$$\frac{\dfrac{q \vdash p, q, r}{q \vdash p, q \vee r} \vee R}{\dfrac{\neg p, q \vdash q \vee r}{\neg p \wedge q \vdash q \vee r} \wedge L} \neg L \qquad \frac{\dfrac{q \vdash p, q, r}{\neg p, q \vdash q, r} \neg L}{\dfrac{\neg p, q \vdash q \vee r}{\neg p \wedge q \vdash q \vee r} \wedge L} \vee R$$

In either inference, we have the following:

Rule	Principal Formula	Active Formulae
$\wedge L$	$\neg p \wedge q$	$\neg p, q$
$\neg L$	$\neg p$	p
$\vee R$	$q \vee r$	q, r

Note that in the left-hand inference, as $\neg p$ is both the principal formula of $\neg L$ and an active formula of $\wedge L$, $\neg L$ and $\wedge L$ are not in permutation position. On the other hand, as the active formula of $\neg L$ is p, this is distinct from the principal formula of $\vee R$, which is $q \vee r$, and hence $\neg L$ and $\vee R$ are in permutation position. In particular, we can permute $\vee R$ below $\neg L$ (or alternatively $\neg L$ above $\vee R$) resulting in the right-hand inference above.

2.3   Intuitionistic Logic and LJ

The standard sequent calculus for intuitionistic logic, LJ, can be obtained from LK by requiring that in every sequent $\Gamma \vdash \Delta$ the succedent Δ contains at most one formula. Amongst other changes, this means that the conclusion of the $\neg$L rule must have an empty succedent. Other rules which are significantly affected are the $\rightarrow$L and $\vee$R rules, which have the following form in LJ:

$$\frac{\Gamma \vdash F_1 \quad \Gamma, F_2 \vdash F}{\Gamma, F_1 \rightarrow F_2 \vdash F} \rightarrow L \qquad \frac{\Gamma \vdash F_i}{\Gamma \vdash F_1 \vee F_2} \vee R$$

The $\rightarrow$L rule thus omits the duplication of F in the left-hand premise and the $\vee$R rule must choose which of F_1 and F_2 is to appear in the premise. As we shall see, this is a crucial difference between LJ and the multiple-conclusioned version.

2.4   Multiple-Conclusioned Systems for Intuitionistic Logic

Below is the multiple-conclusioned system taken from [22].

$$\frac{}{F \vdash F} \text{ Axiom} \qquad \frac{\Gamma \vdash F, \Delta \quad \Gamma, F \vdash \Delta}{\Gamma \vdash \Delta} \text{ Cut} \qquad \frac{\Gamma \vdash \Delta}{\Gamma, F \vdash \Delta} \text{ WL} \qquad \frac{\Gamma \vdash \Delta}{\Gamma \vdash F, \Delta} \text{ WR}$$

$$\frac{\Gamma, F, F \vdash \Delta}{\Gamma, F \vdash \Delta} \text{ CL} \qquad \frac{\Gamma \vdash F, F, \Delta}{\Gamma \vdash F, \Delta} \text{ CR} \qquad \frac{\Gamma, F_1, F_2 \vdash \Delta}{\Gamma, F_1 \wedge F_2 \vdash \Delta} \wedge L \qquad \frac{\Gamma \vdash F_1, \Delta \quad \Gamma \vdash F_2, \Delta}{\Gamma \vdash F_1 \wedge F_2, \Delta} \wedge R$$

$$\frac{\Gamma, F_1 \vdash \Delta \quad \Gamma, F_2 \vdash \Delta}{\Gamma, F_1 \vee F_2 \vdash \Delta} \vee L \qquad \frac{\Gamma \vdash F_1, F_2, \Delta}{\Gamma \vdash F_1 \vee F_2, \Delta} \vee R$$

$$\frac{\Gamma, F[y/x] \vdash \Delta}{\Gamma, \exists x F \vdash \Delta} \exists L \qquad \frac{\Gamma \vdash F[t/x], \Delta}{\Gamma \vdash \exists x F, \Delta} \exists R \qquad \frac{\Gamma, F[t/x] \vdash \Delta}{\Gamma, \forall x F \vdash \Delta} \forall L \qquad \frac{\Gamma \vdash F[y/x]}{\Gamma \vdash \forall x F, \Delta} \forall R$$

$$\frac{\Gamma \vdash F_1, \Delta \quad \Gamma, F_2 \vdash \Delta}{\Gamma, F_1 \rightarrow F_2 \vdash \Delta} \rightarrow L \qquad \frac{\Gamma, F_1 \vdash F_2}{\Gamma \vdash F_1 \rightarrow F_2, \Delta} \rightarrow R \qquad \frac{\Gamma \vdash F, \Delta}{\Gamma, \neg F \vdash \Delta} \neg L \qquad \frac{\Gamma, F \vdash}{\Gamma \vdash \neg F, \Delta} \neg R$$

The rules $\exists$L and $\forall$R have the usual side condition that y is not free in Γ, Δ or F.

Following [20], we refer to this system as **LM**. Unlike LJ, contraction on the right may be used arbitrarily here. Note that this is effectively negated by the form of the rules for $\forall$R, $\rightarrow$R and $\neg$R. Note also that the $\vee$R rule is classical (ie the LK rule), and the rules $\forall$R, $\rightarrow$R and $\neg$R are different from both LK and LJ. Following Wallen [22], let us call these latter rules *special* rules.

As an illustration of the differences between LK, LJ and LM, consider Peirce's formula $((p \rightarrow q) \rightarrow p) \rightarrow p$, which is provable classically, but not intuitionistically. The LK proof is below, as are the corresponding failed attempts in LJ and LM respectively (in left to right order).

$$\frac{\dfrac{\dfrac{\dfrac{p \vdash q, p}{\vdash p \rightarrow q, p} \rightarrow R \quad \dfrac{}{p \vdash p} \text{Ax}}{(p \rightarrow q) \vdash p \vdash p} \rightarrow L}{\vdash ((p \rightarrow q) \rightarrow p) \rightarrow p} \rightarrow R}$$

$$\frac{\dfrac{\overset{\textbf{\textit{X}}}{\dfrac{\dfrac{p \vdash q}{\vdash p \rightarrow q} \rightarrow R \quad \dfrac{}{p \vdash p} \text{Ax}}{(p \rightarrow q) \rightarrow p \vdash p}} \rightarrow L}{\vdash ((p \rightarrow q) \rightarrow p) \rightarrow p} \rightarrow R}$$

$$\frac{\dfrac{\overset{\textbf{\textit{X}}}{\dfrac{\dfrac{p \vdash q}{\vdash p \rightarrow q, p} \rightarrow R \quad \dfrac{}{p \vdash p} \text{Ax}}{(p \rightarrow q) \rightarrow p \vdash p}} \rightarrow L}{\vdash ((p \rightarrow q) \rightarrow p) \rightarrow p} \rightarrow R}$$

Note that in LK, the $\to$L rule does not make a choice between $p \to q$ and p, whereas in LJ it chooses p. In LM, the $\to$L does not make a choice between $p \to q$ and p, but the $\to$R rule does.

2.5 Goal-Directed Proofs

The logic programming interpretation of a sequent $\Gamma \vdash \Delta$ is that the antecedent Γ represents the program, and the succedent Δ the goal. Hence when searching for a proof of $\Gamma \vdash \Delta$ (i.e. performing computation), the search should be "driven" by Δ (and thus be goal-directed). The proof-theoretic characterisation of this property is the notion of *uniform proof* [16].

Definition 1. *An LJ proof is* uniform *if for every sequent $\Gamma \vdash \Delta$ in which Δ is a non-atomic formula, the inference rule used to derive $\Gamma \vdash \Delta$ is the right rule for the principal connective of Δ.*

Thus the search process must reduce a non-atomic succedent before it looks at the program. We also need a proof-theoretic account of resolution, which is given by the notion of a *simple proof* [16].

Definition 2. *An LJ proof is* simple *if for every occurrence of $\to$L the right hand premise is an axiom.*

Clearly it is possible for an LJ proof to be neither uniform nor simple. Hence the question is to identify a class of formulae for which simple uniform proofs are complete (i.e. do not "miss" any consequences). The fragment known as *hereditary Harrop formulae* (HHF) has these properties and is defined as follows, where A ranges over atomic formulae.

> *Definite formulae* $D ::= A \mid D \wedge D \mid G \to A \mid \forall x . D$
> *Goal formulae* $G ::= A \mid G \vee G \mid G \wedge G \mid D \to G \mid \forall x . G \mid \exists x . G$

A program, then, is a set of definite formulae, and a goal is a goal formula. We then have the following theorem.

Theorem 1 (Miller et. al [16]).
    Let $P \vdash G$ be a hereditary Harrop sequent. Then $P \vdash G$ iff $P \vdash G$ has a simple uniform proof in LJ.

3   Deriving a Logic Programming Language in LM

We now turn to the problem of identifying logic programming languages in LM. Following the above pattern, we need to find an appropriate conception of goal-directed proof in LM. Having done so, a class of formulae is then a logic programming language if for any P and G in the appropriate class, $P \vdash G$ is provable iff $P \vdash G$ has a goal-directed proof in LM. We can establish such a result by considering *permutabilities* of rules and showing that a given proof of $P \vdash G$ can always be transformed using permutabilities into a goal-directed proof. We are particularly interested in permuting right rules downwards (i.e. towards the root of the proof). A non-permuting right rule indicates a situation that needs to be avoided; this implies a constraint on the class of formulae considered to be a logic programming language.

3.1 Permutation Properties of LM

Since the only rules in LM which differ from LK are $\forall$R, $\rightarrow$R and $\neg$R these are the only ones whose permutation behaviour will differ from LK. Note that in LK all of the propositional logical rules permute with each other. The following table summarises when we can permute a right rule above a left to a left above a right.

	$\forall$R	$\neg$R	$\rightarrow$R	$\exists$R	$\wedge$R	$\vee$R
$\vee$L	✗	✗	✗	✓	✓	✓
$\rightarrow$L (right)	✗	✗	✗	✓	✓	✓
$\rightarrow$L (left)	*can be*	*eliminated*	*using W*	✓	✓	✓
$\wedge$L	✓	✓	✓	✓	✓	✓
$\forall$L	✓	✓	✓	✓	✓	✓
$\exists$L	✓	✓	✓	✗	✓	✓
$\neg$L	✓	✓	✓	✓	✓	✓

Note that we distinguish between the right rule appearing in permutation position above the left premise of $\rightarrow$L and above the right premise. We do not do this for $\vee$L as the two are symmetric. For the $\rightarrow$L (left) case the row marked "can be eliminated ... " corresponds to the transformation which replaces the left inference below with the right one, thus eliminating altogether the occurrence of the $\rightarrow$L rule.

$$\cfrac{\cfrac{\Gamma, F_3 \vdash F_4}{\Gamma \vdash F_1, F_3 \rightarrow F_4, \Delta} \rightarrow R \quad \Gamma, F_2 \vdash F_3 \rightarrow F_4, \Delta}{\Gamma, F_1 \rightarrow F_2 \vdash F_3 \rightarrow F_4, \Delta} \rightarrow L \qquad \cfrac{\cfrac{\Gamma, F_3 \vdash F_4}{\Gamma \vdash F_3 \rightarrow F_4, \Delta} \rightarrow R}{\Gamma, F_1 \rightarrow F_2 \vdash F_3 \rightarrow F_4, \Delta} WL$$

A point to note is that in LM, the $\vee$R rule can be permuted below the $\vee$L rule, which is not the case in LJ (but is the case in LK). As a result, it is possible to use disjunctions positively in programs in LM. This gives a proof-theoretic characterisation of the notion of *disjunctive logic programs* [17], which have been used to model certain types of uncertain information. This may be thought of as a particular instance of the general observation that there is a trade-off between the expressiveness of the language and the strength of the properties of the search strategy. In this case, no choice has to be made when the $\vee$R rule is applied, and hence a larger fragment of the logic may be used; *quid pro quo*, the resulting proofs no longer have the disjunctive property (i.e. that if $F_1 \vee F_2$ is provable, then so is F_i for some $i = 1, 2$). Note, though, that the $\exists$R rule cannot be permuted below the $\exists$L rule (just as in LK), and hence there is no corresponding property for $\exists$.

Hence the main observation is that the special rules do not permute downwards past $\vee$L or $\rightarrow$L on the right. Below is a proof in which $\rightarrow$R occurs above the right premise of $\rightarrow$L, but cannot be permuted downwards.

$$\cfrac{\cfrac{p \vdash p, q \rightarrow r, q \quad q \vdash p, q \rightarrow r, q}{p \vee q \vdash p, q \rightarrow r, q} \vee L \quad \cfrac{\cfrac{p \vee q, q, r \vdash r}{p \vee q, r \vdash q \rightarrow r, q} \rightarrow R}{}}{p \vee q, p \rightarrow r \vdash q \rightarrow r, q} \rightarrow L$$

Attempting to prove this sequent with $\rightarrow$R results in an unprovable premise:

$$\cfrac{\cfrac{p,q \vdash r,p \quad \cfrac{\text{✗}}{q,q \vdash r,p}}{p \vee q, q \vdash r, p} \vee L \quad \cfrac{}{p \vee q, r, q \vdash r}}{\cfrac{p \vee q, p \rightarrow r, q \vdash r}{p \vee q, p \rightarrow r \vdash q \rightarrow r, q} \rightarrow R} \rightarrow L$$

3.2 Identifying a Subset of the Logic

In order for a class of formulae to be a logic programming language (using a goal-directed proof search) we need to ensure that the no ("✗") cases in the above table cannot occur. We do this by ensuring that one of the non-permuting rules cannot occur by constraining the class of formulae to limit occurrences of the relevant connective. We have two orthogonal choices: (1) $\exists$L versus $\exists$R; and (2) The special rules ($\forall$R, $\neg$R and $\rightarrow$R) versus $\vee$L and $\rightarrow$L.

Note that the rules $\forall$L, $\wedge$L, $\neg$L, $\vee$R and $\wedge$R can be freely used. This yields the following four combinations:

	Right rules	Left rules
1.	$\wedge, \vee, \forall, \neg, \rightarrow$	$\forall, \wedge, \neg, \exists$
2.	$\wedge, \vee, \forall, \neg, \rightarrow, \exists$	$\forall, \wedge, \neg$
3.	$\wedge, \vee$	$\forall, \exists, \wedge, \vee, \neg, \rightarrow$
4.	$\wedge, \vee, \exists$	$\forall, \wedge, \vee, \neg, \rightarrow$

The first three possibilities don't appear to be very useful since they do not include Horn clauses: the first two possibilities do not allow implication on the left (and hence do not allow rules in programs) and the third possibility does not allow existential quantification in goals.

Hence the most useful language is the last one, which, when compared to hereditary Harrop formulae, allows disjunctions and negations on the left, but disallows universal quantifiers and implications on the right.

One question that quickly arises in any discussion of goal-directedness in a multiple-conclusioned setting is that there is a choice to be made between applicable right rules (whereas in the single-conclusioned case there is only one). Clearly there are only two possibilities: either the choice is arbitrary (and hence any choice will suffice) or it is not (and so more care must be taken to maintain completeness). The former is what is assumed in Forum, and hence all right rules must permute over each other. The latter is what is assumed in Lygon, and hence the possible execution strategies must be derived from an analysis of the permutation properties of the right rules, which in the case of Lygon, is based around Andreoli's analysis of such rules [1].

The following table summarises permutability properties among the right rules. A "✓" indicates that the right rule of the column can be permuted below the right rule of the row. A "-" indicates that it is not possible for the pair of rules to occur in permutation position and a "(✗)" indicates that although a normal permutation is not possible, a sub-proof with the same premises and conclusion is possible which only applies the special rule. For example consider the transformation below:

$$\dfrac{\dfrac{\Gamma, G \vdash H}{\Gamma \vdash F_1, F_2, G \to H} \to R}{\Gamma \vdash F_1 \vee F_2, G \to H} \vee R \quad \Longrightarrow \quad \dfrac{\Gamma, G \vdash H}{\Gamma \vdash F_1 \vee F_2, G \to H} \to R$$

This is similar to the case involving a special rule above the left premise of $\to$L.

	∀-R	¬-R	→-R	∃-R	∧-R	∨-R
∀-R	-	-	-	-	-	-
¬-R	-	-	-	-	-	-
→-R	-	-	-	-	-	-
∃-R	(✗)	(✗)	(✗)	✓	✓	✓
∧-R	(✗)	(✗)	(✗)	✓	✓	✓
∨-R	(✗)	(✗)	(✗)	✓	✓	✓

Thus, for LM, all right rules effectively permute over each other and so proof search can arbitrarily choose an applicable right rule without any loss of completeness.

3.3   Formal Results

Hence we arrive at the following notion of goal-directness and class of formulae.

Definition 3. *An LM proof is* uniform *if every sequent which contains a non-atomic formula in the succedent is the conclusion of a right rule.*

Definition 4. *LM-definite formulae and LM-goal formulae are given by the grammar:*

$$LM\text{-}definite\ formulae\ D ::= A \mid D \wedge D \mid D \vee D \mid \neg G \mid G \to D \mid \forall x \,.\, D$$
$$LM\text{-}goal\ formulae \quad\ G ::= A \mid G \vee G \mid G \wedge G \mid \exists x \,.\, G$$

Note that although negations occurring positively in programs are permitted according to uniformity, they are in some sense not goal directed in that it is possible to have programs which are provable regardless of the goal given. For example, $p, \neg p \vdash G$ is provable for any goal formula G.

Theorem 2 (Uniformity). *Let $\mathcal{P}$ be a set of LM-definite formulae and $\mathcal{G}$ be a set of LM-goal formulae. Then $\mathcal{P} \vdash \mathcal{G}$ has an LM-proof iff $\mathcal{P} \vdash \mathcal{G}$ has a uniform proof.*

Proof. (sketch) The basic idea is that since all of the possible right rules permute down over all of the possible left rules we can eliminate non-uniform inferences by permuting right rules down so they are beneath left rules. The details are more subtle and are omitted due to space limitations.   □

As for simple proofs, we need to restrict the formulae in the programs to be *clausal*, i.e. of the form $G \to A$ rather than $G \to D$. This is done so that when permuting other left rules down below $\to$L on the right, we can be sure that the two rules are always in permutation position (as an atom can never be the principal formula). Hence we arrive at the following definition.

Definition 5. *Clausal LM-definite formulae are given by the grammar:*

$$D ::= A \mid D \wedge D \mid D \vee D \mid G \to A \mid \forall x \,.\, D$$

Then it is straightforward to show the following result from the permutation properties by a simple inductive argument.

Theorem 3. *Let $\mathcal{P}$ be a set of clausal LM-definite formulae and $\mathcal{G}$ be a set of LM-goal formulae. Then $\mathcal{P} \vdash \mathcal{G}$ has an LM-proof iff $\mathcal{P} \vdash \mathcal{G}$ has a simple uniform proof.*

Proof. By theorem 2, there is a uniform proof of $\mathcal{P} \vdash \mathcal{G}$. From the permutation properties we know that any occurrences of $\exists$R, $\vee$R or $\wedge$R can be permuted down past $\to$L on the right. By a similar argument, it can be shown that any occurrences of $\wedge$L, $\neg$L, $\vee$L and $\forall$L can be permuted downwards. Hence the right premise of an occurrence of $\to$L must be the conclusion of either an axiom, or another $\to$L. The following permutation can be applied to the highest non-simple occurrence of $\to$L in a chain of $\to$L to make it simple. We repeat this until all occurrences of $\to$L in the chain are simple.

$$
\cfrac{
\Gamma, G_2 \to A_2 \vdash G_1, \Delta
\qquad
\cfrac{
\Gamma, A_1 \vdash G_2, \Delta \quad \Gamma, A_1, A_2 \vdash \Delta
}{
\Gamma, G_2 \to A_2, A_1 \vdash \Delta
} \; {\to}\,\mathrm{L}
}{
\Gamma, G_1 \to A_1, G_2 \to A_2 \vdash \Delta
} \; {\to}\,\mathrm{L}
$$

$$\Downarrow$$

$$
\cfrac{
\cfrac{
\cfrac{
\cfrac{\Gamma, G_2 \to A_2 \vdash G_1, \Delta}{\Gamma, G_2 \to A_2 \vdash G_1, G_2, \Delta}\;\mathrm{WR}
\quad
\cfrac{\Gamma, A_1 \vdash G_2, \Delta}{\Gamma, G_2 \to A_2, A_1 \vdash G_2, \Delta}\;\mathrm{WL}
}{
\Gamma, G_2 \to A_2, G_1 \to A_1 \vdash G_2, \Delta
}\; {\to}\,\mathrm{L}
\qquad
\Gamma, G_1 \to A_1, G_2 \to A_2, A_2 \vdash \Delta
}{
\Gamma, G_2 \to A_2, G_1 \to A_1, G_2 \to A_2 \vdash \Delta
}\; {\to}\,\mathrm{L}
}{
\Gamma, G_1 \to A_1, G_2 \to A_2 \vdash \Delta
}\;\mathrm{CL}
$$

Consider the sequent $\Gamma, A_1, A_2 \vdash \Delta$ in the first inference. Since it is the conclusion of an axiom rule (modulo structural rules) we have that either $A_2 \vdash \Delta$, or $A_1 \vdash \Delta$, or $F \vdash \Delta$ for some $F \in \Delta$. In the last two cases we can simply delete the top occurrence of $\to$L altogether thus making the remaining $\to$L simple. In the remaining case we have that $\Gamma, G_1 \to A_1, G_2 \to A_2, A_2 \vdash \Delta$ and hence the permutation has produced a simple occurrence of $\to$L as desired. $\qquad\qquad\square$

Theorem 4. *LM-definite and LM-goal formulae are not a logic programming language in LJ.*

Proof. LM-definite and LM-goal formulae allow disjunction as a top-level connective. The sequent $p \vee q \vdash p \vee q$ is provable, but does not have a uniform (in the sense of definition 1) proof. $\qquad\qquad\square$

Hence the analyses for LM and LJ lead to different logic programming languages. However, whilst HHF do not qualify "directly" as a logic programming language in LM, it is possible to recover HHF as a logic programming language in LM by a simple analysis of the role of disjunctions in programs.

4   Definite Formulae in LM

One interpretation of the results of the previous sections is that whilst it is possible to use disjunctions positively in programs in an intuitionistic setting by using LM rather than LJ, the cost is that the richer language of HHF cannot be used. On the other hand, it is well-known that in LJ, HHF can be used, but at the cost of not allowing disjunctions in programs. However, we can recover HHF without changing inference rules by omitting disjunctions in programs (and hence not using the ∨L in proofs). We explore this issue in this section.

It is not hard to show that in LM, WL can always be permuted upwards, and WR can either be permuted upwards or "absorbed" by the special rules. For the latter case, note the transformation below.

$$\cfrac{\cfrac{\Gamma \vdash F[y/x]}{\Gamma \vdash \forall x F, \Delta} \forall R}{\Gamma \vdash \forall x F, F', \Delta} WR \quad \Longrightarrow \quad \cfrac{\Gamma \vdash F[y/x]}{\Gamma \vdash \forall x F, F', \Delta} \forall R$$

Hence we can use the form of the axiom rule below, and omit the WL and WR rules.

$$\overline{\Gamma, F \vdash F, \Delta} \; Axiom'$$

This means that we can show the following result.

Theorem 5. *Let* $\Gamma \vdash \Delta$ *be a provable sequent in LM in which* ∨L *does not occur. Then either* $\Gamma \vdash$ *is provable in LM or* $\Gamma \vdash F$ *for some* $F \in \Delta$ *is provable in LM.*

Note the strength of the contrapositive of this result; if a proof requires multiple conclusions, then it must include an occurrence of ∨L.

Proof. We proceed by induction on the size of the proof. In the base case, $\Gamma \vdash \Delta$ is just an axiom, and clearly the result is trivially true. Hence we assume the result is true for all proofs of no more than a given size. The cases for CL, ∧L, ∧R, ∃L, ∃R, ∀L, ¬L and the special rules are all trivial. That leaves CR, ∨R, and →L.

CR: The previous sequent is $\Gamma \vdash F, F, \Delta$, and so by the hypothesis we have that either $\Gamma \vdash F'$ for some $F' \in \Delta$, in which case we are done, or $\Gamma \vdash F$ in which case we are done.

∨R: The previous sequent is $\Gamma \vdash F_1, F_2, \Delta$, and so by the hypothesis we have that either $\Gamma \vdash F$ for some $F \in \Delta$, in which case we are done, or $\Gamma \vdash F_i$, in which case we can derive $\Gamma \vdash F_1 \vee F_2$ via WR and ∨R.

→L: The previous sequents are $\Gamma \vdash F_1, \Delta$ and $\Gamma, F_2 \vdash \Delta$, and so by the hypothesis, we have that $\Gamma, F_2 \vdash F'$ for some $F' \in \Delta$ and either $\Gamma \vdash F$ for some $F \in \Delta$, in which case we can derive $\Gamma, F_1 \to F_2 \vdash F$ by WL, or we have $\Gamma \vdash F_1$. In the latter case we have $\Gamma \vdash F_1$ and $\Gamma, F_2 \vdash F'$, and hence we have $\Gamma, F_1 \to F_2 \vdash F'$.   □

Thus once (positive) disjunctions are removed from programs (i.e. antecedents), we essentially recover LJ.

In particular, this shows that we can use the following versions of $\to$L and $\lor$R:

$$\frac{\Gamma \vdash F_1 \quad \Gamma, F_2 \vdash F}{\Gamma, F_1 \to F_2 \vdash F} \qquad \frac{\Gamma \vdash F_i}{\Gamma \vdash F_1 \lor F_2}$$

These are clearly just the LJ rules. This means that by using this form of $\to$L, we can recover the downwards permutability of the special rules over $\to$L. For example, consider the $\to$R rule and the transformation below:

$$\frac{\dfrac{\Gamma, F_2, F_3 \vdash F_4}{\Gamma \vdash F_1 \quad \Gamma, F_2 \vdash F_3 \to F_4, \Delta} \to R}{\Gamma, F_1 \to F_2 \vdash F_3 \to F_4, \Delta} \to L \quad\Longrightarrow\quad \frac{\dfrac{\dfrac{\Gamma \vdash F_1}{\Gamma, F_3 \vdash F_1} \, WL \quad \Gamma, F_2, F_3 \vdash F_4}{\Gamma, F_1 \to F_2, F_3 \vdash F_4} \to L}{\Gamma, F_1 \to F_2 \vdash F_3 \to F_4, \Delta} \to R$$

Thus we can recover the completeness of uniform and simple (LJ) proofs by using particular properties of LM. This, together with the earlier arguments about disjunctions in LM, may be seen as evidence that the approach using LM is more general than using LJ.

5   Contraction-Free Fragments

One issue which becomes relevant in the analysis involving LM is the role of contraction in succedents. In LJ, such contraction is forbidden; in LM, a naive interpretation would require that each formula be copied before being used as the principal formula of a rule application. However, it is not hard to show that the CR rule is only necessary when such a rule application is $\exists$R — in all other cases the CR rule can either be permuted upwards or can be eliminated.

That such contractions are necessary is shown by the following proof.

$$\frac{\dfrac{\dfrac{p(a) \vdash p(a), p(b) \quad p(b) \vdash p(a), p(b)}{p(a) \lor p(b) \vdash p(a), p(b)} \lor L}{\dfrac{p(a) \lor p(b) \vdash p(a), \exists x p(x)}{\dfrac{p(a) \lor p(b) \vdash \exists x p(x), \exists x p(x)}{p(a) \lor p(b) \vdash \exists x p(x)} CR} \exists R}}{} \exists R$$

Hence an implementation will require existentially quantified goals to be copied. However, Theorem 5 shows that such copying will not be necessary in the absence of disjunctions in programs, or for any fragment which does not contain existentially quantified goals. In particular, this argument shows that the propositional fragment does not require contraction on the right.

It is then interesting to pursue the question of whether contraction on the left is required in the propositional case. Dyckhoff [4] has shown that it is possible to use a more intricate proof system in which contraction is not needed at all for any propositional fragment. In our case, we are interested in determining whether the standard rules of LM are contraction-free for various propositional fragments.

An intriguing result is that propositional Horn clauses are contraction-free, but propositional hereditary Harrop formulae are not. That the latter are not may be shown by the following proof:

$$
\cfrac{
  \cfrac{
    \cfrac{
      \cfrac{
        \cfrac{
          \cfrac{
            \cfrac{\overline{p \vdash p}}{p \vdash p \vee (p \to q)} \vee R
          }{(p \vee (p \to q)) \to q, p \vdash q} \to L
        }{(p \vee (p \to q)) \to q \vdash p \to q} \to R
      }{(p \vee (p \to q)) \to q \vdash p \vee (p \to q)} \vee R
    }{(p \vee (p \to q)) \to q, (p \vee (p \to q)) \to q \vdash q} \to L
  }{(p \vee (p \to q)) \to q \vdash q} CL
}{}
$$

However, if we try to omit the contraction, we quickly arrive at an unprovable sequent:

$$
\cfrac{
  \cfrac{\textcolor{red}{\pmb{X}}}{\vdash p \vee (p \to q)}
}{(p \vee (p \to q)) \to q \vdash q} \to L
$$

It is interesting to note that Dyckhoff shows in [4] that the formula $\neg\neg(p \vee \neg p)$ requires contraction in LJ; this formula is essentially the same as the above formula under the transformation of $\neg F$ to $F \to \bot$.

We now proceed to show that propositional Horn clauses do not require contraction. We denote by $\mathcal{D}_{\wedge,\vee,\to,\neg}\mathcal{G}_{\wedge,\vee,\to,\neg}$ the fragment defined by the following rules:

$$D ::= A \mid D \wedge D \mid D \vee D \mid \neg G \mid G \to A$$
$$G ::= A \mid G \wedge G \mid G \vee G \mid \neg D \mid D \to G$$

We use similar notation for smaller fragments such as $\mathcal{D}_{\wedge,\to}\mathcal{G}_{\wedge,\vee,\to}$.

Definition 6. *Given an occurrence $\Gamma, F \vdash F, \Delta$ of the Axiom' rule, we refer to Γ as the* context.

In a proof Φ of a propositional sequent $\Gamma \vdash \Delta$, a formula F in Γ is passive *if is not the principal formula of any rule occurrence in Φ, and F is in the context of every occurrence of the Axiom' rule.*

Now in order to show that a given fragment is contraction-free, we proceed by showing that if a contraction is used, then the formula that is copied by the rule is passive (i.e. plays no active part in the proof).

It is not hard to show that CL permutes up past all propositional rules except $\to$L.

Hence, we need only consider occurrences of CL which are immediately below $\to$L, and for which the principal formula of $\to$L is an active formula of CL, i.e.

$$
\cfrac{
  \cfrac{\Gamma, F_1 \to F_2 \vdash F_1 \qquad }{\Gamma, F_1 \to F_2, F_1 \to F_2 \vdash F_2} \to L
}{\Gamma, F_1 \to F_2 \vdash F_2} CL
$$

Theorem 6. *Let Φ be a proof of a $\mathcal{D}_{\wedge,\to}\mathcal{G}_{\wedge,\vee}$ sequent $P \vdash G$. Then for every occurrence*

$$\dfrac{\dfrac{\dfrac{\Psi}{\Gamma, F_1 \to F_2 \vdash F_1}}{\Gamma, F_1 \to F_2, F_1 \to F_2 \vdash F_2} \to L}{\Gamma, F_1 \to F_2 \vdash F_2}\, CL$$

of CL and $\to L$ in Φ, $F_1 \to F_2$ is passive in Ψ.

Proof. We proceed by induction on the number of occurrences of $\to L$ in Φ. Consider an occurrence of $\to L$ closest to the leaves. As there are no occurrences of $\to L$ in Ψ, $F_1 \to F_2$ is clearly passive.

Hence we assume that the result holds for proofs which contain no more than a given number of occurrences of $\to L$.

Consider an occurrence of $\to L$ as above. If $F_1 \to F_2$ is not passive in Ψ, then there must be an occurrence of $\to L$ in Ψ in which $F_1 \to F_2$ is the principal formula. It is not hard to see that as the goals consist only of conjunctions and disjunctions (and hence the antecedents in the proof can never be changed), this must be of the form

$$\dfrac{\dfrac{\dfrac{\dfrac{\dfrac{\Xi}{\Gamma, F_1 \to F_2 \vdash F_1}}{\Gamma, F_1 \to F_2, F_1 \to F_2 \vdash F_2} \to L}{\Gamma, F_1 \to F_2 \vdash F_2}\, CL}{\dfrac{\dfrac{\dfrac{\Psi}{\Gamma, F_1 \to F_2 \vdash F_1}}{\Gamma, F_1 \to F_2, F_1 \to F_2 \vdash F_2} \to L}{\Gamma, F_1 \to F_2 \vdash F_2}}}{}\, CL$$

By the hypothesis we know that $F_1 \to F_2$ is passive in Ξ.

Now as there is a sequent identical to one closer to the leaves, we can eliminate the part of the proof between these two occurrences, and in particular we can remove the copy of the identical sequent closer to the root. □

In a similar manner, it is not hard to show that the $\mathcal{D}_{\wedge,\to}\mathcal{G}_{\wedge,\to,\neg}$ fragment is also contraction-free.

Theorem 7. *Let Φ be a proof of a $\mathcal{D}_{\wedge,\to}\mathcal{G}_{\wedge,\to,\neg}$ sequent $P \vdash G$. Then for every occurrence*

$$\dfrac{\dfrac{\dfrac{\Psi}{\Gamma, F_1 \to F_2 \vdash F_1}}{\Gamma, F_1 \to F_2, F_1 \to F_2 \vdash F_2} \to L}{\Gamma, F_1 \to F_2 \vdash F_2}\, CL$$

of CL and $\to L$ in Φ, $F_1 \to F_2$ is passive in Ψ.

Proof. Similar to the above argument. □

Hence we arrive at the following classification:

- $\mathcal{D}_{\wedge,\to}\mathcal{G}_{\wedge,\vee}$ (Horn clauses) is contraction-free.
- $\mathcal{D}_{\wedge,\to}\mathcal{G}_{\wedge,\to,\neg}$ is contraction-free.

- $\mathcal{D}_{\wedge,\to}\mathcal{G}_{\vee,\to}$ is not contraction-free (see above).
- $\mathcal{D}_{\wedge,\to}\mathcal{G}_{\vee,\neg}$ is not contraction-free (Dyckhoff [4]).

Note that the third case implies that propositional hereditary Harrop formulae are not contraction-free. Note also that these cases cover all the fragments of $\mathcal{D}_{\wedge,\to}\mathcal{G}_{\wedge,\vee,\to,\neg}$.

6 Conclusions and Further Work

We have seen that the permutation properties of LM mean that the straightforward application of the notion of goal-directed proof from the single-conclusioned case results in a different class of formulae than hereditary Harrop formulae, and in particular that disjunctions may be used in programs. We have also seen that it is possible to recover hereditary Harrop formulae by not using such disjunctions. This suggests that LM is a potentially more general framework for logic programming languages based on intuitionistic logic than LJ.

Another topic of interest is the relationship between search in LM and search in LJ. In particular, the search properties of LM may be thought of as allowing "delayed" choices when compared with LJ, particularly for the $\vee R$ and $\to L$ rules as mentioned above. This means that an attempt at a proof in LM may correspond to more than one such attempt in LJ; a correspondence of this sort seems worthy of further investigation.

Another property of interest is the precise notion of equivalence used. It is known that for hereditary Harrop formulae in LJ, there is no increase in power by allowing clauses of the form $G \to D$, due to the following intuitionistic equivalences[2]:

$$G \to (D_1 \wedge D_2) \equiv (G \to D_1) \wedge (G \to D_2)$$
$$G \to (G' \to D) \equiv (G \wedge G') \to D$$
$$G \to (\forall x D) \equiv \forall x (G \to D) \text{ where } x \text{ is not free in } G.$$

In the LM case, this is no longer true, due to the presence of clauses of the form $D_1 \vee D_2$, and that $G \to (D_1 \vee D_2)$ is not intuitionistically equivalent to $(G \to D_1) \vee (G \to D_2)$. However, it should be noted that this equivalence does hold in a slightly stronger logic (called Gödel-Dummett logic in [5]), in which this is one of the *Independence of Premise* rules. This logic is also relevant to issues of program equivalence [8], and so an investigation of the proof theory of such a logic and its relation to LM would be particularly interesting.

Acknowledgements

The authors are grateful to Pablo Armelin, Roy Dyckhoff and David Pym for stimulating discussions. The first author is grateful for the hospitality of the Department of Computer Science of Queen Mary and Westfield College, University of London during a period of sabbatical leave.

---

[2] One consequence of the first equivalence is that there is no benefit to considering multi-headed clauses for hereditary Harrop formulae as in Lygon, Forum, or LO.

References

1. J.-M. Andreoli. Logic Programming with Focusing Proofs in Linear Logic. *Journal of Logic and Computation*, 2(3), 1992.
2. J.-M. Andreoli and R. Pareschi. Linear Objects: Logical Processes with Built-in Inheritance. In David H. D. Warren and Péter Szeredi, editors, *Proceedings of the Seventh International Conference on Logic Programming*, pages 496–510, Jerusalem, 1990. The MIT Press.
3. K. Clark. Negation as Failure. In H. Gallaie and J. Minker, editors, *Logic and Databases*, pages 293–323. Plenum Press, 1978.
4. R. Dyckhoff. Contraction-free Sequent Calculi for Intuitionistic Logic. *Journal of Symbolic Logic*, 57:795–807, 1992.
5. R. Dyckhoff. A Deterministic Terminating Sequent Calculus for Gödel-Dummett logic. *Logic Journal of the IGPL*, 7:319–326, 1999.
6. D. Galmiche and G.Perrier. On Proof Normalisation in Linear Logic. *Theoretical Computer Science*, 135:67–110, 1994.
7. G. Gentzen. Untersuchungen über das logische Schliessen. *Math. Zeit.*, 39:176–210,405–431, 1934.
8. J. Harland. On Normal Forms and Equivalence for Logic Programs. In Krzysztof Apt, editor, *Proceedings of the Joint International Conference and Symposium on Logic Programming*, pages 146–160, Washington, DC, 1992. ALP, MIT Press.
9. J. Harland. A Proof-Theoretic Analysis of Goal-Directed Provability. *Journal of Logic and Computation*, 4(1):69–88, January 1994.
10. J. Harland. On Goal-Directed Provability in Classical Logic. *Computer Languages*, 23:161–178, 1997.
11. J. Harland, D. Pym, and M. Winikoff. Programming in Lygon: An Overview. In M. Wirsing, editor, *Lecture Notes in Computer Science*, pages 391–405. Springer, July 1996.
12. J. Hodas and D. Miller. Logic Programming in a Fragment of Intuitionistic Linear Logic. *Information and Computation*, 110(2):327–365, 1994.
13. N. Kobayash and A. Yonezawa. ACL - A Concurrent Linear Logic Programming Paradigm. In Dale Miller, editor, *Logic Programming - Proceedings of the 1993 International Symposium*, pages 279–294, Vancouver, Canada, 1993. The MIT Press.
14. T. Lutovac and J. Harland. Towards the Automation of the Design of Logic Programming Languages. Technical Report 97-30, Department of Computer Science, RMIT, 1997.
15. D. Miller. Forum: A Multiple-Conclusion Specification Logic. *Theoretical Computer Science*, 165(1):201–232, 1996.
16. D. Miller, G. Nadathur, F. Pfenning, and A. Ščedrov. Uniform Proofs as a Foundation for Logic Programming. *Annals of Pure and Applied Logic*, 51:125–157, 1991.
17. J. Minker and A. Rajasekar. A Fixpoint Semantics for Disjunctive Logic Programs. *Journal of Logic Programming*, 9(1):45–74, July 1990.
18. G. Nadathur. Uniform Provability in Classical Logic. *Journal of Logic and Computation*, 8(2):209–230, 1998.
19. D. Pym and J. Harland. A Uniform Proof-theoretic Investigation of Linear Logic Programming. *Journal of Logic and Computation*, 4(2):175–207, April 1994.
20. E. Ritter, D. Pym, and L. Wallen. On the Intuitionistic Force of Classical Search. to appear in *Theoretical Computer Science*, 1999.
21. P. Volpe. Concurrent Logic Programming as Uniform Linear Proofs. In G. Levi and M. Rodríguez-Artalejo, editors, *Proceedings of the Conference on Algebraic and Logic Programming*, pages 133–149. Springer, 1994.
22. Lincoln Wallen. *Automated Deduction in Nonclassical Logics*. MIT Press, 1990.
23. M. Winikoff. *Logic Programming with Linear Logic*. PhD thesis, University of Melbourne, 1997.

Efficient EM Learning with Tabulation for Parameterized Logic Programs

Yoshitaka Kameya and Taisuke Sato

Dept. of Computer Science, Graduate School of Information Science and Engineering
Tokyo Institute of Technology
Ookayama 2-12-1, Meguro-ku, Tokyo, Japan, 152-8552
kame@mi.cs.titech.ac.jp, sato@cs.titech.ac.jp

Abstract. We have been developing a general symbolic-statistical modeling language [6, 19, 20] based on the logic programming framework that semantically unifies (and extends) major symbolic-statistical frameworks such as hidden Markov models (HMMs) [18], probabilistic context-free grammars (PCFGs) [23] and Bayesian networks [16]. The language, PRISM, is intended to model complex symbolic phenomena governed by rules and probabilities based on the *distributional semantics*[19]. Programs contain statistical parameters and they are automatically learned from randomly sampled data by a specially derived EM algorithm, the graphical EM algorithm. It works on support graphs representing the shared structure of explanations for an observed goal. In this paper, we propose the use of tabulation technique to build support graphs, and show that as a result, the graphical EM algorithm attains the same time complexity as specilized EM algorithms for HMMs (the Baum-Welch algorithm [18]) and PCFGs (the Inside-Outside algorithm [1]).

1 Introduction

We have been developing a general symbolic-statistical modeling language [19, 20, 6] based on the logic programming framework that semantically unifies (and extends) major symbolic-statistical frameworks such as hidden Markov models (HMMs) [18], probabilistic context-free grammars (PCFGs) [23] and Bayesian networks [16]. The language, PRISM (*programming in statistical modeling*), is intended to model complex symbolic phenomena governed by rules and probabilities using the *distributional semantics*[19]. Programs contain statistical parameters and they are automatically learned from randomly sampled data by a specially derived EM algorithm, the *graphical EM algorithm*. It works on *support graphs* representing the shared structure of explanations for an observed goal. In this paper, we propose the use of tabulation technique to build support graphs, and show that as a result, the graphical EM algorithm attains the same time complexity as specilized EM algorithms for HMMs (the Baum-Welch algorithm [18]) and PCFGs (the Inside-Outside algorithm[1]). Our subject in this paper is inter-deciplinary, concerning logic programming, probability theory, statistics and formal languages, and the reader is assumed to be familiar with basics of these deciplines [5, 11, 18, 22, 23].

J. Lloyd et al. (Eds.): CL 2000, LNAI 1861, pp. 269–284, 2000.

The rest of this paper is as follows. After having a look at background in the next section, and preparing basic materials of PRISM in Sec 3, we present an efficient learning algorithm for PRISM (Sec. 4). We evaluate the time complexity of our algorithm in Sec. 5. Sec. 6 contains a conclusion. Throughout the paper, we use Prolog conventions for logic programs.

2   Background

2.1   Constraint Approach and Distribution Approach

Since our work is at the crossroads of logic programming and probability, it might help to first review various attempts made to integrate probability with logic, or logic programming (though we do not claim exhaustiveness of the list at all). In reviewing, one can immediately notice there are two different basic attitudes towards the use of probability in logic or logic programming. One type, *constraint approach*, emphasizes the role of probabilities as constraints and does not necessarily seek for a unique probability distribution over logical formulas. The other type, *distribution approach*, explicitly defines a unique distribution by model theoretical means or proof theoretical means, to compute various probabilities of propositions.

A typical constraint approach is seen in the early work of probabilistic logic by Nilsson [15]. He considered probabilities assigned to formulas in a knowledge base as constraints on the possible range of probability of a formula of interest. He used linear programming techniques to solve constraints that necessarily delimits the applicability of his approach to finite domains. Turining to logic programming, probabilistic logic programming formalized by Ng and Subrahmanian used clauses of the form $A : \mu \leftarrow F_1 : \mu_1, \ldots, F_n : \mu_n$ annotated by probability intervals μ_is [13]. Lakshmanan and Sadri also used annotated clauses $A \xleftarrow{c} B_1, \ldots, B_n$ where $c = \langle I_b, I_d \rangle$ in the formalization of their probabilistic logic programming. Here I_b represents an expert's belief interval, I_d a doubt interval respectively [10]. Both formalizations only allowed for a finite number of constant and predicate symbols, but no function symbols[10, 13].

Some of the early works of the distribution approach to combining probability with logic programs came out of the Bayesian network community[1]. Breese made a first attempt to use logic programs to automatically build a Bayesian network from a query [2]. After identifying atoms relevant to the query, a local Baysian network for them is constructed to compute posterior probabilities. Logical variables can appear in atoms but no function symbol was allowed [2] (see also [14] for recent development of the use of logic programs to build Bayesian networks). Poole proposed "probabilistic Horn abduction" [17]. His program consists of definite clauses and *disjoint declarations* of the form disjoint([$h_1:p_1, \ldots, h_n:p_n$]) which specifies a probability distribution over the hypotheses (abducibles) $\{h_1, \ldots, h_n\}$. He assigned unique probabilities to all

---

[1] A Bayesian network is a finite directed acyclic graph representing probabilistic dependences between (continuous or discrete) random variables [16]

ground atoms with the help of the theory of logic programming, and furthermore proved that Bayesian networks are representable in his framework [17]. He however imposed various conditions (the covering property, the acyclicity property, etc [17]) on the class of applicable programs.

In a more linguistic vein, Muggleton formulated SLP (Stochastic Logic Programming) procedurally, as an extension of logic programming to PCFGs [12]. So, a clause C, which must be range-restricted[2], is annotated with a probability p like $p : C$. The probability of a goal G is the products of such ps appearing in its derivation, but with a modification such that if a subgoal g can invoke n clauses, $p_i : C_i$ $(1 \leq i \leq n)$ at some derivation step, the probability of choosing k-th clause is normalized, that is $p_k / \sum_{i=1}^{n} p_i$. SLP was further extended by Cussens by introducing the notion of loglinear models for SLD refutation proofs and defining probabilities of ground atoms in terms of their SLD-trees and "features"[3].

2.2   Limitations and Problems

Approaches described so far have more or less similar limitations and problems. Descriptive power confined to finite domains is the most common limitation, which is due to the use of linear programming techniques [15], or due to the syntactic restrictions not allowing for infinitely many constant, function or predicate symbols [10, 13]. Bayesian networks have the same limitation as well (only a finite number of random variables are representable). Also there are various semantic/syntactic restrictions on logic programs. For instance the acyclicity condition [14, 17] prevents the use of clauses with local variables unconditionally, and the range-restrictedness [3, 12] excludes programs such as the usual membership Prolog program. These restrictions would cause problems when we model the distribution of infinitely many objects such as natural language sentences [11].

There is another type of problem, the inconsistent assignment of probabilities. Think of extensions of PCFGs to logic programs [3, 12]. Since they define the probability $\mathbf{Pr}(A)$ of an atom A in terms of syntactic features of the proof trees for A, it is quite possible for $\mathbf{Pr}(A)$ and $\mathbf{Pr}(A \wedge A)$ to differ as their proof trees are different, though logically, they are one and the same.

Last but not least, there is a big problem common to any approach using probabilities: *where do the numbers come from?* Generally speaking, if we use n binary random variables, we need to get 2^n probabilities to completely specify their joint distribution, and this kind of attempt quickly becomes impossible as n grows. Also if there are "hidden variables" in the model such as true causes of a disease, we need lots of work to get reliable probabilities of those variables. Despite these difficulties, all approaches in subsection 2.1 assume *their numbers are given a priori*, and none of them address the problem of how to find probabilities, excepts attempts to use learning techniques for Bayesian networks [8].

---

[2] A syntactic property that variables appearing in the head also appear in the body of a clause. So, a unit clause must be ground.

2.3   The Idea of PRISM

We have been developing a general symbolic-statistical modeling language called PRISM since 1995 along the line of the distribution approach that is free of limitations mentioned above [19, 20]. It is a probabilistic logic programming language equipped with a new semantic framework termed the *distributional semantics* [19], an extension of the least Herbrand model semantics to possible world semantics with a distribution. Theoretically, a PRISM program $DB = F \cup R$ is comprised of a denumerable[3] number of ground facts (hypotheses, abducibles) F and a denumerable number of rules (definite clauses) R in a first-order language with a denumerable number of constant symbols, function symbols and predicate symbols. F is supposed to come with a *basic distribution* P_F that is a completely additive probability measure. So every ground atom in F is considered a random variable taking on 1 (true) or 0 (false). A sampling of P_F determines a set F' of true atoms, which in turn determines the set of true atoms as $M_{DB}(F' \cup R)$ where M_{DB} denotes the least Herbrand model of $F' \cup R$. Hence, every ground atom in DB is a random variable. Their joint distribution P_{DB}, a completely additive probability measure as an extension of P_F, is defined to be the denotation (declarative semantics) of DB (the *distributional semantics*) [19].

Thanks to a general semantic framework, we need none of restrictions such as no function symbols and a finite number of constant and predicate symbols [2, 4, 8, 10, 13], the acyclicity [14, 17] and the covering assumption [17], the range-restrictedness of clauses [3, 12], or the finiteness of domains [2, 4, 15]. A user can write whatever program he/her likes at their own risk without a fear of inconsistent probabilities. Also we succeeded in deriving a new EM learning algorithm for learning statistical parameters in PRISM programs (BS programs) [19], and hence every program can learn from positive examples. So far, we have confirmed the descriptive/learning power of PRISM by tackling various domains including three major symbolic-statistical models, HMMs, PCFGs and Bayesian networks [20].[4]

2.4   Problem of Computational Complexity

The major problem with the current implementation of PRISM is the slow speed of learning. After determining the scope of symbolic-statistical phenomena we model such as stochastic language generation, we write a parameterized model DB ($= F \cup R$) that can explain conceivable observations (sentences for instance). If independent observations $G_1, \ldots, G_T$ are given, we let our EM algorithm to learn statistical parameters in DB by (locally) maximizing $\prod_t P_{DB}(G_t = 1)$. The learning process starts with collecting all such $S \subseteq F$ that $S \cup R \models G$ for each observation G_t. This all solution search usually contains a lot of redundancy,

---

[3] We hereafter use a term "denumerable" as a synonym of "countably infinite." The finite case is similarly treated.

[4] Koller has proposed a probabilistic functional language [9] which can represent HMMs, PCFGs and Bayesian networks, but left the problem of declarative semantics and learning untouched.

and in case of HMMs, we end up in the time complexity exponential in the length of an input string. The reason is obvious: in the stochastic automata such as HMMs, the number of transition paths is exponential, but the Baum-Welch algorithm [18], the specialized EM algorithm for HMMs, achieves linear time complexity by taking advantage of structure-sharing of transition paths represented as a trellis diagram, which corresponds to the reuse of solved subgoals in logic programming. We therefore introduced a reuse mechanism of solved goals such as OLDT search [21] in PRISM, and thus rederived the whole EM algorithm to combine with the OLDT search. Owing to this entire reconstruction, our EM algorithm, though applicable to even type-0 stochastic grammars, has achieved the same time complexity as specialized EM algorithms as far as HMMs and PCFGs are concerned, as described in the sequel.

3   PRISM Programs

In this section, we define PRISM programs and the related concepts. See also the basic idea of the distributional semantics in Sec. 2.3.

Definition 1. *A PRISM program is a definite clause program $DB = F \cup R$ which satisfies the following conditions on facts F, their distribution P_F and rules R.*

1. *F is a set of ground atoms of the form $\mathtt{msw}(i,n,v)$. The arguments i and n are called group-id (or switch name) and trial-id, respectively. We assume that a finite set V_i of ground terms is associated with each i, and $v \in V_i$ holds.[5] V_i corresponds to a set of possible values of switch i.*
2. *Let V_i be $\{v_1, v_2, \ldots, v_{|V_i|}\}$. Then, one of the ground atoms $\mathtt{msw}(i,n,v_1)$, $\mathtt{msw}(i,n,v_2)$, $\ldots$, $\mathtt{msw}(i,n,v_{|V_i|})$ becomes exclusively true (takes the value 1) on each trial. For each i, $\theta_{i,v} \in [0,1]$ is a parameter of the (marginal) probability of $\mathtt{msw}(i,\cdot,v)$ being true ($v \in V_i$), and $\sum_{v \in V_i} \theta_{i,v} = 1$ holds.*
3. *For each ground terms i, i', n, n', $v \in V_i$ and $v' \in V_{i'}$, random variable $\mathtt{msw}(i,n,v)$ is independent of $\mathtt{msw}(i',n',v')$ if $n \neq n'$ or $i \neq i'$.*
4. *Define $head(R)$ as a set of atoms appearing in the head of R. Then, $F \cap head(R) = \emptyset$.*

In the first condition, we introduce a predicate $\mathtt{msw}/3$ to represent a basic probabilistic choice such as coin-tossing ($\mathtt{msw}$ stands for *multi-valued switch*). A ground atom $\mathtt{msw}(i,n,v)$ represents an event "a switch named i takes on v as a sample value on the trial n." We combine these switches to build a probability distribution of complex phenomena. The second and the third condition say that a logical variable $\mathtt{V}$ in $\mathtt{msw}(i,n,\mathtt{V})$ behaves like a random variable which is realized to v_k with probability θ_{i,v_k} ($k = 1\ldots|V_i|$).[6] Moreover, from the third condition, the logical variables $\mathtt{V1}$ and $\mathtt{V2}$ in $\mathtt{msw}(i,n_1,\mathtt{V1})$ and $\mathtt{msw}(i,n_2,\mathtt{V2})$ can

---

[5] As described before, we consider DB as a denumerable set of ground clauses, i and n are arbitrary ground terms in the Herbrand universe.

[6] These probabilities are either learned or given by the user.

be seen as *independent and identically distributed* (i.i.d.) random variables if n_1 and n_2 are different ground terms. The fourth condition says that no $\text{msw}(\cdot, \cdot, \cdot)$ appears in the head of R.

3.1   A Program Example

We here pick up a PRISM program which represents an HMM, also known as a probabilistic regular grammar. HMMs define a probability distribution over the strings of given alphabets, and can be considered as probabilistic string generators [18], in which an output string is a sample from the defined distribution. The HMM represented below[7] has two states $\{\text{s0}, \text{s1}\}$ and outputs a symbol a or b in each state. For simplicity, the length of output strings is fixed to three.

```
(1)  target(hmm/1).              (4)  values(init,[s0,s1]).
(2)  data('hmm.dat').            (5)  values(out(_),[a,b]).
(3)  table([hmm/1,hmm/3]).       (6)  values(tr(_),[s0,s1]).
(7)  hmm(Cs):-                    % To generate a string (chars) Cs...
         msw(init,null,Si),      %      Set initial state to Si, and then
         hmm(1,Si,Cs).           %      Enter the loop with clock = 1.
(8)  hmm(T,S,[C|Cs]):- T=<3,     % Loop:
         msw(out(S),T,C),        %      Output C in state S.
         msw(tr(S),T,NextS),     %      Transit from S to NextS.
         T1 is T+1,              %      Put the clock ahead.
         hmm(T1,NextS,Cs).       %      Continue the loop (recursion).
(9)  hmm(T,_,[]):- T>3.          % Finish the loop if clock > 3.
```

Procedurally, the above HMM program simulates the generation process of strings (see the comments in the program). Clauses $(7)\sim(9)$ represent the probabilistic behavior of the HMM. In clause (8), to output a symbol C, we use different switches $\text{out}(\text{S})$ conditional on the state S.[8] Note that T in $\text{msw}(\text{out}(\text{S}),\text{T},\text{C})$ is used to guarantee the independency among the choices at each time step. Recursive clauses like (8) are allowed in the distributional semantics, and so are in PRISM. Clauses $(1)\sim(6)$ contain additional information about the program. Clause (1) declares only the ground atoms containing $\text{hmm}/1$ are observable. $\text{hmm}([\text{a},\text{b},\text{a}])$ being true means this HMM generates the string aba. Clause (2) specifies a file storing learning data. Clause (3) specifies the table predicates (described later) are $\text{hmm}/1$ and $\text{hmm}/3$. We can read that $V_{\text{init}} = \{\text{s0}, \text{s1}\}$, $V_{\text{out}(\cdot)} = \{\text{a}, \text{b}\}$, $V_{\text{tr}(\cdot)} = \{\text{s0}, \text{s1}\}$ from clauses $(4)\sim(6)$.

---

[7] The clause numbers are not written in the actual program.

[8] Generally speaking, a conditional probability table (CPT) of a random variable X can be represented by the switch $\text{msw}(f(c_1, c_2, \ldots, c_n), \cdot, x)$, where n is the number of conditional variables, f is the id of X, c_i ($i = 1 \ldots n$) is the value of each conditional variable C_i, and x is one of X's possible values $x_1, x_2, \ldots, x_k$. Of course, $V_{f(c_1, c_2, \ldots, c_n)} = \{x_1, x_2, \ldots, x_k\}$ should be declared in advance.

3.2   Further Definitions and Assumptions

For the learning algorithm for PRISM, we need some definitions and assumptions. For the moment, we assume the set I of group-ids coincides with the Herbrand universe of DB. Based on I, a(-n infinite-dimension) *parameter space* Θ is defined as follows:

$$\Theta \stackrel{\text{def}}{=} \prod_{i \in I} \{\langle \theta_{i,v_1}, \ldots, \theta_{i,v_{|V_i|}} \rangle \mid V_i = \{v_1, \ldots, v_{|V_i|}\}, \sum_{v \in V_i} \theta_{i,v} = 1\}. \quad (1)$$

We next define the probabilistic inconsistency (consistency), probabilistic exclusiveness, and independency w.r.t. facts and goals.

Definition 2. *Consider a PRISM program $DB = F \cup R$ and a set S of facts in F ($S \subseteq F$). S is said to be* p-inconsistent *if $P_F(\boldsymbol{S}=\boldsymbol{1}|\boldsymbol{\theta}) = 0$ for any parameters $\boldsymbol{\theta} \in \Theta$.[9] Otherwise, S is said to be* p-consistent. *Consider two sets S_1 and S_2 of facts in F, which are p-consistent. Then S_1 is said to be* p-exclusive *to S_2 if $S_1 \cup S_2$ is p-inconsistent. Furthermore, let B_1 and B_2 be arbitrary two atoms in $head(R)$. Then, B_1 is said to be* p-exclusive *to B_2 if and only if $P_{DB}(B_1 = 1, B_2=1|\boldsymbol{\theta}) = 0$ for any $\boldsymbol{\theta} \in \Theta$.*

Definition 3. *For each B in $head(R)$, let $S^{(1)}, \ldots, S^{(m)}$ be minimal subsets of F such that*

$$comp(R) \models B \leftrightarrow S^{(1)} \vee \cdots \vee S^{(m)}, \quad (2)$$

where $0 \leq m$ and $comp(R)$ is the completion [5] *of R.[10] Then, each of $S^{(1)}, \ldots, S^{(m)}$ is referred to as a* minimal support set *or an* explanation *for B. We put $\psi_{DB}(B) = \{S^{(1)}, \ldots, S^{(m)}\}$.*

Together with a PRISM program $DB = F \cup R$, we always consider a (denumerable) subset $obs(DB)$ of $head(R)$, which is referred to as a set of observable atoms. Each $G \in obs(DB)$ is called a *goal*. Note that the following assumptions are made only for *practical* reasons (e.g. program termination and efficiency), and that the distributional semantics itself does not require these assumptions.

Assumption 1. *Consider a PRISM program DB. In Eq. 2, m is finite ($m < \infty$), and each of $S^{(1)}, \ldots, S^{(m)}$ is a finite set* (finite support condition). *For any $G \in obs(DB)$, explanations in $\psi_{DB}(G)$ are p-consistent and p-exclusive* (exclusiveness condition). *Goals in $obs(DB)$ are p-exclusive to each another, and $\sum_{G \in obs(DB)} P_{DB}(G=1|\boldsymbol{\theta}) = 1$ holds for some parameter $\boldsymbol{\theta} \in \Theta$* (uniqueness condition).

From the uniqueness condition, we know that just one atom in $obs(DB)$ becomes true at each observation. Suppose we make T ($< \infty$) independent observations, and G_t is the atom obtained at the t-th observation ($G_t \in obs(DB)$, $t = 1 \ldots T$). *Observed data* $\mathcal{G}$ is a finite sequence $\langle G_1, G_2, \ldots, G_T \rangle$. Then, I is redefined here as a set of the group-ids of relevant switches to $\mathcal{G}$, i.e. $I \stackrel{\text{def}}{=} \bigcup_{t=1}^{T} \bigcup_{S \in \psi_{DB}(G_t)} \{i \mid \exists n, v(\texttt{msw}(i, n, v) \in S)\}$. Also, we redefine Θ as the (finite-dimension) parameter space by Eq. 1.

---

[9] $\boldsymbol{S}$ is a random vector whose elements are in S. $\boldsymbol{1}$ (resp. $\boldsymbol{0}$) is a vector consisting of all 1s (resp. 0s). $\boldsymbol{S}=\boldsymbol{1}$ means all atoms in S are true.

[10] We sometimes consider a conjunction of atoms $A_1, A_2, \ldots$ as a set $\{A_1, A_2, \ldots\}$.

4 Learning PRISM Programs

Learning a PRISM program means *maximum likelihood estimation* (MLE) of the parameters in the program. That is, given observations $\mathcal{G} = \langle G_1, \ldots, G_T \rangle$, we find the parameter $\boldsymbol{\theta} \in \Theta$ which (locally) maximizes the *likelihood* $\Lambda(\mathcal{G}|\boldsymbol{\theta}) \stackrel{\text{def}}{=} \prod_{t=1}^{T} P_{DB}(G_t = 1|\boldsymbol{\theta})$.[11] Although the PRISM program is affected by the behavior, hence by the parameters $\boldsymbol{\theta}$ of switches $\mathrm{msw}(\cdot, \cdot, \cdot)$ it contains, we cannot directly observe their behavior (i.e. these switches are "hidden"). Hence we apply the EM algorithm [22]. The learning procedure comprises two phases:

- *Find* all explanations $\psi_{DB}(G_t)$ for each goal G_t $(t = 1 \ldots T)$.
- *Run* the EM algorithm based on the statistics from $\psi_{DB}(G_t)$ $(t = 1 \ldots T)$.

In the rest of this section, we first quickly derive a naive version of the EM algorithm,[12] assuming ψ_{DB}. We then introduce *support graphs*, a compact datastructure for ψ_{DB}. After the introduction of support graphs, the *graphical EM algorithm*, an efficient EM algorithm working on support graphs, is described.

4.1 Naive Approach

To derive an EM algorithm for PRISM, we must define a Q *function*. First, from the exclusiveness and the uniqueness condition, it is easily shown that explanations in $\Delta_{DB} \stackrel{\text{def}}{=} \bigcup_{G \in obs(DB)} \psi_{DB}(G)$ are all p-exclusive each other. Besides, also from the uniqueness condition,

$$\sum_{G \in obs(DB)} P_{DB}(G = 1|\boldsymbol{\theta}) = \sum_{G \in obs(DB)} \sum_{S \in \psi_{DB}(G)} P_{DB}(\boldsymbol{S} = 1|\boldsymbol{\theta})$$
$$= \sum_{S \in \Delta_{DB}} P_{DB}(\boldsymbol{S} = 1|\boldsymbol{\theta}) = 1$$

holds for any $\boldsymbol{\theta} \in \Theta$. Hence, exactly one of the explanations in Δ_{DB} is true. Since Δ_{DB} is denumerable, we can consider an isomorphic map $f : \Delta_{DB} \to \boldsymbol{N}^+$, where $\boldsymbol{N}^+$ is a set of positive integers, and temporarily introduce a new random variable E on Ω_F such that $E = f(S)$ if $S \in \Delta_{DB}$ is exclusively true ($\boldsymbol{S} = 1$), or $E = 0$ otherwise. Now we are in a position to define the Q function:

$$Q(\boldsymbol{\theta}', \boldsymbol{\theta}) \stackrel{\text{def}}{=} \sum_{t=1}^{T} \sum_{e \in \boldsymbol{N}} P_{DB}(E = e|G_t = 1, \boldsymbol{\theta}) \log P_{DB}(E = e, G_t = 1|\boldsymbol{\theta}'), \quad (3)$$

where $\boldsymbol{N}$ is a set of non-negative integers. It is easy to show $Q(\boldsymbol{\theta}', \boldsymbol{\theta}) \geq Q(\boldsymbol{\theta}, \boldsymbol{\theta}) \Rightarrow P_{DB}(G_t = 1|\boldsymbol{\theta}') \geq P_{DB}(G_t = 1|\boldsymbol{\theta})$. Therefore, for MLE, starting with some parameters $\boldsymbol{\theta}^{(0)}$, we iteratively update parameters by $\boldsymbol{\theta}^{(m+1)} := \mathrm{argmax}_{\boldsymbol{\theta}} Q(\boldsymbol{\theta}, \boldsymbol{\theta}^{(m)})$

---

[11] Under the exclusiveness condition, each marginal probability of G_t being true is calculated as below. $\sigma_{i,v}(S)$ is defined as $\sigma_{i,v}(S) \stackrel{\text{def}}{=} \left| \left\{ n \mid \mathrm{msw}(i, n, v) \in S \right\} \right|$.

$$P_{DB}(G_t = 1|\boldsymbol{\theta}) = \sum_{S \in \psi_{DB}(G_t)} P_F(\boldsymbol{S} = 1|\boldsymbol{\theta}) = \sum_{S \in \psi_{DB}(G_t)} \prod_{i \in I, v \in V_i} \theta_{i,v}^{\sigma_{i,v}(S)},$$

[12] In [6], PRISM* programs are introduced to remove computationally intractable terms. We here present an alternative way to remove them.

until the *log-likelihood* $\log \Lambda(\mathcal{G}|\boldsymbol{\theta})$ converges. Transforming Eq. 3, the following formula is obtained:

$$Q(\boldsymbol{\theta}',\boldsymbol{\theta}) = \sum_{i\in I, v\in V_i} \eta(i,v,\boldsymbol{\theta}) \log \theta'_{i,v} \leq \sum_{i,v} \left(\eta(i,v,\boldsymbol{\theta}) \log \frac{\eta(i,v,\boldsymbol{\theta})}{\sum_{v'\in V_i} \eta(i,v',\boldsymbol{\theta})} \right),$$

where $\eta(i,v,\boldsymbol{\theta}) \stackrel{\text{def}}{=} \sum_{t=1}^{T} \frac{1}{P_{DB}(G_t=1|\boldsymbol{\theta})} \sum_{S\in\psi_{DB}(G_t)} P_F(\boldsymbol{S}=1|\boldsymbol{\theta})\sigma_{i,v}(S)$. Hence, we reach the procedure *learn-naive* in Fig. 1 that finds the MLE of the parameters. The array variable $\eta[i,v]$ contains $\eta(i,v,\boldsymbol{\theta})$ under the current $\boldsymbol{\theta}$. In this procedure, the calculations for $P_{DB}(G_t=1|\boldsymbol{\theta})$ and $\eta[i,v]$ (Line 2, 5 and 9) are computationally intractable when $|\psi_{DB}(G_t)|$ is exponential (though finite) in the complexity of the model.[13]

4.2 Tabulation Approach

For efficient computation of $P_{DB}(G_t=1|\boldsymbol{\theta})$ and $\eta[i,v]$, we introduce structure-sharing of explanations by tabulation, which requires more assumptions on DB. We assume that a set of table predicates $table(DB)$ is declared in advance (like the HMM program in Sec. 3.1). Let τ_{DB}^* be a set of ground atoms containing the table predicate in $table(DB)$. We use $comp(R)$, the completion of rules R, again in the following assumption.

Assumption 2. *Let DB be a PRISM program which satisfies the finite support condition, the exclusiveness condition, and the uniqueness condition. Assume that, for each $t = 1 \ldots T$, the following condition holds for some finite ordered subset $\tau_{DB}^t = \{\tau_1^t, \ldots, \tau_{K_t}^t\}$ of τ_{DB}^*:*[14]

$$comp(R) \models \left(G_t \leftrightarrow \tilde{S}_{0,1}^t \vee \cdots \vee \tilde{S}_{0,m_0}^t \right) \tag{4}$$

$$\wedge \left(\tau_1^t \leftrightarrow \tilde{S}_{1,1}^t \vee \cdots \vee \tilde{S}_{1,m_1}^t \right) \wedge \cdots \wedge \left(\tau_{K_t}^t \leftrightarrow \tilde{S}_{K_t,1}^t \vee \cdots \vee \tilde{S}_{K_t,m_{K_t}}^t \right),$$

where

- *Letting G_t be τ_0^t, each of $\tilde{S}_{k,1}^t, \ldots, \tilde{S}_{k,m_k}^t$ is a subset of $F \cup \{\tau_{k+1}^t, \ldots, \tau_{K_t}^t\}$, and is also called a t-explanation*[15] *for τ_k^t (for $k = 0 \ldots K_t$). We here put $\tilde{\psi}_{DB}(\tau_k^t) \stackrel{\text{def}}{=} \{\tilde{S}_{k,1}, \ldots, \tilde{S}_{k_{m_k}}\}$ (for $k = 0 \ldots K_t$).*
- *Each of $\tilde{S}_{k,1}^t, \ldots, \tilde{S}_{k,m_k}^t$ ($k = 0 \ldots K_t$) is a set of independent atoms.*[16]

Each τ_k^t ($k = 1 \ldots K_t$) is referred to as a table atom. *We call the former condition* acyclic support condition, *and the latter* independent support condition.

---

[13] For example, the complexity of the HMM depends on the number of states, the length of input/output string or the number of output alphabets.

[14] From the finite support condition, for $k = 0 \ldots K_t$, m_k is finite and each of $\tilde{S}_{k,1}^t, \ldots, \tilde{S}_{k,m_k}^t$ is finite. Also, from the exclusive condition, $\tilde{S}_{k,1}^t, \ldots, \tilde{S}_{k,m_k}^t$ are p-consistent and p-exclusive ($k = 0 \ldots K_t$). Besides, from the uniqueness condition, $G_{t'} \notin \tau_{DB}^t$ holds for any $t, t' = 1 \ldots T$.

[15] Prefix "t-" is an abbreviation of "tabled-".

[16] For $B_1, B_2 \in head(R)$, B_1 is independent of B_2 if $P_{DB}(B_1 = y_1, B_2 = y_2|\boldsymbol{\theta}) = P_{DB}(B_1 = y_1|\boldsymbol{\theta}) \cdot P_{DB}(B_2 = y_2|\boldsymbol{\theta})$ for any $y_1, y_2 \in \{0,1\}$ and any $\boldsymbol{\theta} \in \Theta$.

1: **procedure** *learn-naive* $(DB, \mathcal{G})$ **begin**

2:     Select some $\boldsymbol{\theta}$ from Θ; $\lambda^{(0)} := \sum_{t=1}^{T} \log P_{DB}(G_t = 1 | \boldsymbol{\theta})$;

3:     **repeat**

4:         **foreach** $i \in I, v \in V_i$ **do**

5:             $\eta[i, v] := \sum_{t=1}^{T} \frac{1}{P_{DB}(G_t = 1 | \theta)} \sum_{S \in \psi_{DB}(G_t)} P_F(\boldsymbol{S} = 1 | \boldsymbol{\theta}) \sigma_{i,v}(S)$;

6:         **foreach** $i \in I, v \in V_i$ **do**

7:             $\theta_{i,v} := \eta[i, v] / \sum_{v' \in V_i} \eta[i, v']$;

8:         $m := m + 1$;

9:         $\lambda^{(m)} := \sum_{t=1}^{T} \log P_{DB}(G_t = 1 | \boldsymbol{\theta})$

10:     **until** $\lambda^{(m)} - \lambda^{(m-1)} < \varepsilon$

11: **end.**

Fig. 1. A procedure for naive approach.

The task here is to construct such $\tilde{\psi}_{DB}$ and τ_{DB}^t from the source PRISM program. One way is to use OLDT (*OLD with tabulation*) [21], a complete search technique for logic programs. In OLDT, a (sub-)goal g containing a table predicate is registered into a *solution table*, whereas the instance of g is registered in a *lookup table*. The latter reuses solutions in the solution table. In what follows, we illustrate our tabulation approach by using the HMM program in Sec. 3.1.

First, we translate the PRISM program to another logic program. Similarly to the translation of *definite clause grammars* (DCGs) in Prolog, we add two arguments (which forms *D-list*) to each predicate for collecting t-explanations. In the case of the HMM program, the translation results in:

```
(T1)   top_hmm(Cs,X):- tab_hmm(Cs,X,[]).
(T3)   tab_hmm(Cs,[hmm(Cs)|X],X):- hmm(Cs,_,[]).
(T3')  tab_hmm(T,S,Cs,[hmm(T,S,Cs)|X],X):- hmm(T,S,Cs,_,[]).
(T4)   e_msw(init,T,s0,[msw(init,T,s0)|X],X).
(T4')  e_msw(init,T,s1,[msw(init,T,s1)|X],X).
  :
(T7)   hmm(Cs,X0,X1):- e_msw(init,null,Si,X0,X2), tab_hmm(1,Si,Cs,X2,X1).
(T8)   hmm(T,S,[C|Cs],X0,X1):-
           T=<3, e_msw(out(S),T,C,X0,X2), e_msw(tr(S),T,NextS,X2,X3),
           T1 is T+1, tab_hmm(T1,NextS,Cs,X3,X1).
(T9)   hmm(T,S,[],X,X):- T>3.
```

Clauses (Tj) and (Tj') correspond to the original clause (j), respectively. In the translated program, $p/(n + 2)$ is a table predicate if p/n is a table predicate in the original program. We use the predicate `tab_p`$/(n + 2)$ to keep the t-explanations (in Eq. 4). Note that `tab_p`$/(n + 2)$ is called instead of the table predicate $p/(n + 2)$. We then apply OLDT search while noting (i) added D-list does not influence the original OLDT procedure, and (ii) we associate a list of t-explanations with each solution. For example, running OLDT for the above translated program gives the solution table in Fig. 2. Finally, we extract $\tilde{\psi}_{DB}$, the set of all t-explanations, from this table. The remaining task is to get totally

```
hmm([a,b,a]): [hmm([a,b,a]):[[m(init,null,s0),hmm(1,s0,[a,b,a])],
                             [m(init,null,s1),hmm(1,s1,[a,b,a])]]]
hmm(1,s0,[a,b,a]):
  [hmm(1,s0,[a,b,a]):[[m(out(s0),1,a),m(tr(s0),1,s0),hmm(2,s0,[b,a])],
                      [m(out(s0),1,a),m(tr(s0),1,s1),hmm(2,s1,[b,a])]]]
hmm(1,s1,[a,b,a]):
  [hmm(1,s1,[a,b,a]):[[m(out(s1),1,a),m(tr(s1),1,s0),hmm(2,s0,[b,a])],
  :                   [m(out(s1),1,a),m(tr(s1),1,s1),hmm(2,s1,[b,a])]]]
```

Fig. 2. Solution table (m is an abbreviation of msw).

ordered table atoms, i.e. the ordered set τ_{DB}^t, respecting the acyclicity in Eq. 4. Obviously, it can be done by topological sorting.

To help visualizing our learning algorithm, we introduce a data-structure called *support graphs*, though the algorithm itself is defined using only $\tilde{\psi}_{DB}$ and the ordered set τ_{DB}^t. As illustrated in Fig 3 (a), the support graph for G_t ($t = 1 \ldots T$), a graphical representation of Eq. 4, consists of disconnected subgraphs, each of which is labeled with the corresponding table atom τ_k^t in τ_{DB}^t ($k = 1 \ldots K_t$). Each subgraph labeled τ_k^t comprises two special nodes, the *start node* and the *end node*, and *explanation graphs*, each of which corresponds to a t-explanation $\tilde{S}_{k,j}^t$ in $\tilde{\psi}_{DB}(\tau_k^t)$ ($j = 1 \ldots m_k$). An explanation graph of $\tilde{S}_{k,j}^t$ is cascaded nodes, where each node is labeled with a table atom τ or a switch $\mathsf{msw}(\cdot,\cdot,\cdot)$ in $\tilde{S}_{k,j}^t$. It is called a *table node* or a *switch node*. Support graphs have a similar structure to *recursive transition networks* (RTNs). Fig 3 (b) is the support graph for hmm([a,b,a]) obtained from the solution table in Fig 2. Each table node labeled τ refers to the subgraph labeled τ, so data-sharing is achieved by the distinct table nodes referring to the same subgraph.

4.3 Graphical EM Algorithm

We describe here a new learning algorithm, the *graphical EM algorithm*, that works on support graphs (more specifically, on $\tilde{\psi}_{DB}$ and τ_{DB}^t). We prepare four

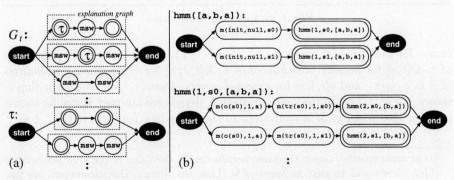

Fig. 3. A support graph (a) in general form, (b) for the HMM program with $G_t = $ hmm([a,b,a]). A double-circled node refers to a table node.

1: **procedure** *learn-gEM* $(DB, \mathcal{G})$
2: **begin**
3:   Select some θ from Θ;
4:   *get-inside-probs*$(DB, \mathcal{G})$;
5:   $\lambda^{(0)} := \sum_{t=1}^{T} \log \mathcal{P}[t, G_t]$;
6:   **repeat**
7:     *get-expectations*$(DB, \mathcal{G})$;
8:     **foreach** $i \in I, v \in V_i$ **do**
9:       $\eta[i, v] :=$
10:        $\sum_{t=1}^{T} \eta[t, i, v] / \mathcal{P}[t, G_t]$;
11:    **foreach** $i \in I, v \in V_i$ **do**
12:      $\theta_{i,v} := \eta[i, v] / \sum_{v' \in V_i} \eta[i, v']$;
13:    *get-inside-probs*$(DB, \mathcal{G})$;
14:    $\lambda^{(m)} := \sum_{t=1}^{T} \log \mathcal{P}[t, G_t]$
15: **until** $\lambda^{(m)} - \lambda^{(m-1)} < \varepsilon$
16: **end.**

1: **procedure** *get-inside-probs* $(DB, \mathcal{G})$
2: **begin**
3:   **for** $t := 1$ **to** T **do begin**
4:     Put $G_t = \tau_0^t$;
5:     **for** $k := K_t$ **downto** 0 **do begin**
6:       $\mathcal{P}[t, \tau_k^t] := 0$;
7:       **foreach** $\tilde{S} \in \tilde{\psi}_{DB}(\tau_k^t)$ **do begin**
8:         Put $\tilde{S} = \{A_1, A_2, \ldots, A_{|\tilde{S}|}\}$;
9:         $\mathcal{R}[t, \tau_k^t, \tilde{S}] := 1$;
10:        **for** $\ell := 1$ **to** $|\tilde{S}|$ **do**
11:          **if** $A_\ell = \mathtt{msw}(i, \cdot, v)$ **then**
12:            $\mathcal{R}[t, \tau_k^t, \tilde{S}] \mathrel{*}= \theta_{i,v}$
13:            **else** $\mathcal{R}[t, \tau_k^t, \tilde{S}] \mathrel{*}= \mathcal{P}[t, A_\ell]$;
14:          $\mathcal{P}[t, \tau_k^t] \mathrel{+}= \mathcal{R}[t, \tau_k^t, \tilde{S}]$
15:      **end** /* **foreach** $\tilde{S}$ */
16:    **end** /* **for** k */
17: **end** /* **for** t */
18: **end.**

1: **procedure** *get-expectations* $(DB, \mathcal{G})$ **begin**
2:   **for** $t := 1$ **to** T **do begin**
3:     Put $G_t = \tau_0^t$; $\mathcal{Q}[t, \tau_0^t] := 1$; **for** $k := 1$ **to** K_t **do** $\mathcal{Q}[t, \tau_k^t] := 0$;
4:     **for** $k := 0$ **to** K_t **do**
5:       **foreach** $\tilde{S} \in \tilde{\psi}_{DB}(\tau_k^t)$ **do begin**
6:         Put $\tilde{S} = \{A_1, A_2, \ldots, A_{|\tilde{S}|}\}$;
7:         **for** $\ell := 1$ **to** $|\tilde{S}|$ **do**
8:           **if** $A_\ell = \mathtt{msw}(i, \cdot, v)$ **then** $\eta[t, i, v] \mathrel{+}= \mathcal{Q}[t, \tau_k^t] \cdot \mathcal{R}[t, \tau_k^t, \tilde{S}]$
9:           **else** $\mathcal{Q}[t, A_\ell] \mathrel{+}= \mathcal{Q}[t, \tau_k^t] \cdot \mathcal{R}[t, \tau_k^t, \tilde{S}] / \mathcal{P}[t, A_\ell]$
10:      **end** /* **foreach** $\tilde{S}$ */
11: **end** /* **for** t */
12: **end.**

Fig. 4. Graphical EM algorithm.

arrays for each support graph for G_t $(t = 1 \ldots T)$: $\mathcal{P}[t, \tau]$ for *inside probabilities* of τ, $\mathcal{Q}[t, \tau]$ for *outside probabilities* of τ, $\mathcal{R}[t, \tau, \tilde{S}]$ for *explanation probabilities* of $\tilde{S}$ in $\tilde{\psi}_{DB}(\tau)$, and $\eta[t, i, v]$ for *expected counts* of $\mathtt{msw}(i, \cdot, v)$. The algorithm is shown in Fig. 4. Due to the space limitation, details are omitted. It can be shown however that *learn-gEM* is equivalent to the procedure *learn-naive* (Sec. 4.1).[17]

---

[17] To be more specific, under the same parameters θ, the value of $\eta[i, v]$ in *learn-naive* (Line 5) is equal to that in *learn-gEM* (Line 10). Hence, the parameters are updated to the same value. Furthermore, starting with the same initial parameters, the converged parameters are also the same.

As shown in Sec. 4.1, *learn-naive* is the MLE procedure, hence the following theorem holds.

Theorem 1. *Let DB be a PRISM program, and $\mathcal{G}$ be the observed data. Then learn-gEM finds $\theta^* \in \Theta$ which (locally) maximizes the likelihood $\Lambda(\mathcal{G}|\theta)$.*

5 Complexity

In this section, we estimate the time complexity of our learning method in case of PRISM programs for PCFGs, and compare with the Inside-Outside algorithm. Since our method comprises two phases (OLDT and the graphical EM), we estimate the computation time in each phase.

In the Inside-Outside algorithm, time complexity is measured by N, the number of non-terminals, and L, the number of terminals in the input/output sentence. Assuming that the target grammar is in *Chomsky normal form*, the worst-case time complexity is the computation time for the largest grammar, i.e. a set of all combinations of terminals and non-terminals. Hence, we may start with a logic program (not a PRISMprogram) representing the largest grammar:

$$\left\{ q(i,d,d') \text{:- } q(j,d,d''), q(k,d'',d') \mid i,j,k = 1\dots N,\ 0 \le d < d'' < d' \le L \right\}$$
$$\cup \left\{ q(i,d,d') \mid i = 1\dots N,\ 0 \le d \le L-1,\ d' = d+1 \right\}. \tag{5}$$

$q(i,d,d')$ says that the i-th non-terminal spans from $(d+1)$-th word to d'-th word. The textual order over the clauses "$q(i,d,d')$:- $q(j,d,d''), q(k,d'',d')$" is the lexicographic order over the tuples (i,j,k,d,d',d''). We then make an exhaustive search for the query by OLDT. Assuming that the solution table is accessible in $O(1)$ time, the time complexity of OLDT is measured by the number of nodes in OLDT tree (the search tree for OLDT). We fix the search strategy to *multi-stage depth-first strategy* [21]. Let T_d be an OLDT tree for the query ?-$q(1,d,L)$. Fig. 5 illustrates the case of $0 \le d \le L-3$. As can be seen, even for this simple grammar, the tree has many similar subtrees, so we put them together (see [**Note**] in Fig. 5). Then, due to the depth-first strategy, T_d has a recursive structure, i.e. T_{d+1} is a part of T_d. We enumerate h_d, the number of the nodes in T_d but not in T_{d+1}. The node with an underlined leftmost atom is a lookup node, which only *consumes* the solution obtained in other place. From Fig. 5, $h_d = O(N^3(L-d)^2)$.[18] Total time for OLDT search is the number of nodes in the OLDT tree for ?-$q(1,0,L)$ (the whole sentence), that is, $\sum_{d=0}^{L-3} h_d = O(N^3 L^3)$.[19] In the case of a DCG program below, it can be proved similarly that the time complexity is $O(N^3 L^3)$.

$$\left\{ q(i,\text{L0},\text{L1})\text{:- } q(j,\text{L0},\text{L2}), q(k,\text{L2},\text{L1}) \mid i,j,k = 1\dots N \right\}$$
$$\cup \left\{ q(i,\text{L0},\text{L1})\text{:- } \text{L0=}[w|\text{L1}] \mid i = 1\dots N,\ w \text{ is a terminal symbol} \right\}$$

---

[18] We here focus on the subtree T_d'. Each of j, i', j' ranges from 1 to N, and $\left| \{(e,e') \mid d+2 \le e' < e \le L-1\} \right| = O((L-d)^2)$. Hence, the number of nodes in T_d' is $O(N^3(L-d)^2)$. The number of nodes in T_d but neither in T_{d+1} nor in T_d' is negligible, therefore $h_d = O(N^3(L-d)^2)$.

[19] The number of nodes of T_{L-1} and T_{L-2} is negligible.

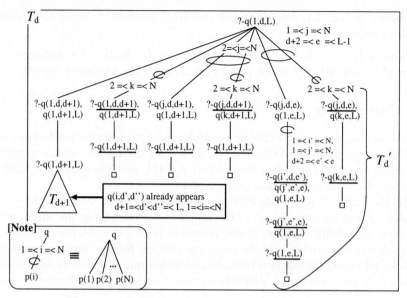

Fig. 5. an OLDT tree T_d for the query ?-q(1,d,L).

Since our method respects the original OLDT procedure, the search time for the corresponding PRISM program given T observed goals is $O(N^3 L^3 T)$.

On the other hand, the learning time of the graphical EM algorithm is propotional to the size of the support graphs used, i.e. the number of nodes in the graphs. It is easily shown, from the description of *learn-gEM*, that the size of the graphs is $O(\xi_{num} \xi_{maxsize} T)$, where $\xi_{num} \stackrel{\text{def}}{=} \max_{1 \le t \le T} |\tilde{\Delta}_{DB}^t|$, $\xi_{maxsize} \stackrel{\text{def}}{=} \max_{1 \le t \le T, \tilde{S} \in \tilde{\Delta}_{DB}^t} |\tilde{S}|$, and $\tilde{\Delta}_{DB}^t \stackrel{\text{def}}{=} \bigcup_{\tau \in \tau_{DB}^t} \tilde{\psi}_{DB}(\tau)$. In the case of the PCFG program, $\xi_{num} = O(N^3 L^3)$ and $\xi_{maxsize} = O(1)$. Hence, the computation time per update of the graphical EM algorithm is $O(N^3 L^3 T)$. We therefore have:

Proposition 1. *Let DB be a PRISM program representing a PCFG, and $\mathcal{G} = \langle G_1, G_2, \ldots, G_T \rangle$ be the observed data. We assume each table operation in OLDT search is done in time $O(1)$. Then OLDT search for the goal G_t and each iteration in learn-gEM is done in time $O(N^3 L^3 T)$.*

$O(N^3 L^3 T)$ is also the time complexity of the Inside-Outside algorithm, hence our algorithm is as efficient as the Inside-Outside algorithm.[20] Similarly, we can show that, for HMM programs like ones in Sec. 3.1, the search and the learning time is $O(\hat{N}^2 LT)$, the same order as that of the Baum-Welch algorithm ($\hat{N}$ is the number of states).

---

[20] Ours can be better than the Inside-Outside algorithm as only relevant grammar rules are involved in the EM learning phase as is observed experimentally.

6   Conclusion

We have proposed an efficient EM learning algorithm for the parameterized logic programs which seamlessly unifies logical semantics and probabilistic semantics. It is shown our general algorithm works as efficiently as the specialized EM algorithms such as the Baum-Welch algorithm and the Inside-Outside algorithm. Furthermore, due to the generality of the language and the learning algorithm, our framework can be applied to the stochastic grammars with context dependencies such as the bigram model of production rules [7], in which case the time complexity of the EM learning is polynomial (details are omitted). The omitted details in this paper will be included in the full paper we are preparing.

References

1. Baker, J. K., Trainable grammars for speech recognition, *Proc. of Spring Conf. of the Acoustical Society of America*, pp.547–550, 1979.
2. Breese, J. S., Construction of belief and decision networks, *Computational Intelligence*, Vol.8, No.4, pp.624–647, 1992.
3. Cussens, J., Loglinear models for first-order probabilistic reasoning, *Proc. of UAI'99*, pp.126–133, 1999.
4. Dekhtyar, A. and Subrahmanian, V. S., Hybrid probabilistic programs, *Proc. of ICLP'97*, pp.391–405, 1997.
5. Doets, K., *From Logic to Logic Programming*, The MIT Press, 1994.
6. Kameya, Y., Ueda, N. and Sato, T., A graphical method for parameter learning of symbolic-statistical models, *Proc. of DS'99*, LNAI 1721, pp.264–276, 1999.
7. Kita, K., Morimoto, T., Ohkura, K., Sagayama, S. and Yano, Y., Spoken sentence recognition based on HMM-LR with hybrid language modeling, *IEICE Trans. on Information & Systems*, Vol.E77-D, No.2, 1994.
8. Koller, D. and Pfeffer, A., Learning probabilities for noisy first-order rules, *Proc. of IJCAI'97*, pp.1316–1321, 1997.
9. Koller, D., McAllester, D. and Pfeffer, A., Effective Bayesian Inference for Stochastic Programs, *Proc. of AAAI'97*, pp.740–747, 1997.
10. Lakshmanan, L. V. S. and Sadri, F., Probabilistic deductive databases, *Proc. of ILPS'94*, pp.254–268, 1994.
11. Manning, C. D. and Schütze, H., *Foundations of Statistical Natural Language Processing*, The MIT Press, 1999.
12. Muggleton, S., Stochastic logic programs, In *Advances in Inductive Logic Programming* (Raedt,L.De ed.), OSP Press, pp.254–264, 1996.
13. Ng, R. and Subrahmanian, V. S., Probabilistic logic programming, *Information and Computation*, Vol.101, pp.150–201, 1992.
14. Ngo, L. and Haddawy, P., Answering queries from context-sensitive probabilistic knowledge bases, *Theoretical Computer Science*, Vol.171, pp.147–177, 1997.
15. Nilsson, N. J., Probabilistic logic, *Artificial Intelligence*, Vol.28, pp.71–87, 1986.
16. Pearl, J., *Probabilistic Reasoning in Intelligent Systems*, Morgan Kaufmann, 1988.
17. Poole, D., Probabilistic Horn abduction and Bayesian networks, *Artificial Intelligence*, Vol.64, pp.81–129, 1993.
18. Rabiner, L. and Juang, B., *Foundations of Speech Recognition*, Prentice-Hall, 1993.
19. Sato, T., A statistical learning method for logic programs with distribution semantics, *Proc. of ICLP'95*, pp.715–729, 1995.

20. Sato, T. and Kameya, Y., PRISM: a language for symbolic-statistical modeling, *Proc. of IJCAI'97*, pp.1330–1335, 1997.
21. Tamaki, H. and Sato, T., OLD resolution with tabulation, *Proc. of ICLP'86*, LNCS 225, pp.84–98, 1986.
22. Tanner, M., *Tools for Statistical Inference* (2nd ed.), Springer-Verlag, 1986.
23. Wetherell, C.S., Probabilistic languages: a review and some open questions, *Computing Surveys*, Vol.12, No.4, pp.361–379, 1980.

Model Generation Theorem Proving with Finite Interval Constraints

Reiner Hähnle[1], Ryuzo Hasegawa[2], and Yasuyuki Shirai[3]

[1] Department of Computing Science, Chalmers Technical University
41296 Gothenburg, Sweden
reiner@cs.chalmers.se
[2] Department of Intelligent Systems, Kyushu University
Kasuga Kouen 6-1, Kasuga-shi, Fukuoka 816, Japan
hasegawa@ar.is.kyushu-u.ac.jp
[3] Information Technologies Development Department
Mitsubishi Research Institute, Inc., Tokyo 100-8141, Japan
shirai@mri.co.jp

Abstract. Model generation theorem proving (MGTP) is a class of deduction procedures for first-order logic that were successfully used to solve hard combinatorial problems. For some applications the representation of models in MGTP and its extension CMGTP is too redundant. Here we suggest to extend members of model candidates in such a way that a predicate p can have not only terms as arguments, but at certain places also subsets of totally ordered finite domains. The ensuing language and deduction system relies on constraints based on finite intervals in totally ordered sets and is called IV-MGTP. It is related to constraint programming and many-valued logic, but differs significantly from either. We show soundness and completeness of IV-MGTP. First results with our implementation show considerable potential of the method.

1 Introduction

Model generation theorem proving (MGTP) is a class of deduction procedures for first-order logic in conjunctive normal form (CNF) that have been successfully used to solve hard combinatorial problems [9]. The procedural semantics of first-order CNF formulas as defined by MGTP is based on bottom-up evaluation. MGTP operates on range-restricted non-Horn rules over positive literals, and it is proof confluent. Together, this ensures completeness even without backtracking. MGTP is closely related [6] to hypertableaux [2]. CMGTP [14] is an extension of MGTP that allows negated atoms in rules and approximates their declarative semantics with an additional inference rule. Very efficient implementations of (C)MGTP were realized [8].

In MGTP (CMGTP), interpretations (called *model candidates*) are represented as finite sets of ground atoms (literals). In many situations this turns out being too redundant: take, for example, variables I, J ranging over the domain $\text{dom} = \{1, \ldots, 4\}$, and interpret $\leq$, $+$ naturally. A rule like "$p(I), \text{dom}(J), I + J \leq 4 \to q(J)$" splits into three model extensions: $q(1)$, $q(2)$, $q(3)$, if $p(1)$ is

J. Lloyd et al. (Eds.): CL 2000, LNAI 1861, pp. 285–299, 2000.
© Springer-Verlag Berlin Heidelberg 2000

present in the current model candidate. Now assume we have the rule "$q(I)$, $q(J)$, $I \neq J \to \perp$" saying that q is functional in its argument and, say, $q(4)$ is derived. Then all three branches must be refuted separately. Note that the rules above do not take advantage of pattern matching (the arguments of the predicates are flat).

Totally ordered, finite domains occur naturally in many problems. In such problems, situations like the one just sketched are common. Here[1] we set out to enhance MGTP with mechanisms to deal with them efficiently. Informally, we suggest two extensions of MGTP: first, the arguments of predicates can contain certain finite domain constructors based on intervals. The first rule on the previous page could be rephrased as "$p([I, I]) \to q([1, 4 - I])$", where $[i, j]$ denotes the set $\{k \in \text{dom} \mid i \leq k \leq j\}$. Second, to make full use of this extended language, elements of model candidates M are generalised as well. In the example, if $p(1) \in M$, then the rule is triggered with $\{I \leftarrow 1\}$ and results in the single extension of M with $q(\{1, 2, 3\})$, rather than in three extensions as before. The functionality of selected arguments will be built in, so the second rule above is not needed. One could even write a more general rule like "$p([1, I]) \to q([1, 4 - I])$", which has two advantages: it is still useful, if p is undetermined in the current model candidate, and (a suitably extended version of) pattern matching can be used on the term $[1, I]$. Because intervals play a central role, we gave the name IV-MGTP to the present extension of MGTP.

The paper is organised as follows: in Section 2 some standard definitions are collected, while in Section 3 the formal syntax and semantics of IV-MGTP is defined. A deduction procedure for IV-MGTP programs is given in Section 4. Like other extensions of model generation and logic programming, such as CMGTP [14], general logic programs, or signed logic programs [12], the IV-MGTP procedure is not complete with respect to the standard semantics, but it turns out to be characterisable by extended interpretations [12], which are suitably adapted to the present purpose, see Section 5. Section 6 summarises first results obtained with IV-MGTP, and Section 7 discusses related work and gives a brief outlook to future research. The full version of this paper is available at ftp://ftp.cs.chalmers.se/pub/users/reiner/iv-paper.ps.gz

2   Standard Definitions

Terms and Literals. Terms and atoms are defined as usual over a **signature** Σ consisting of **constant symbols** C_Σ, **function symbols** F_Σ, **predicate symbols** P_Σ. Variables from a set $TVar$ occurring in terms are called **term variables** to distinguish them from variables occurring in constraints. The set of variable free or **ground terms** is denoted $Term^0_\Sigma$, the set of variable free or **ground atoms** with $Atom^0_\Sigma$. A **literal** is either an atom or an expression $\neg L$, where L is an atom.

---

[1] A preliminary version of the present paper appeared in unpublished proceedings [7].

Rules and Programs. **Clauses** are written in **rule notation** and are expressions of the form $C \to D$, where C and D are finite sequences of atoms or literals. The expression $L \in C$ denotes that L occurs in the sequence C. C is called the **antecedent** of $C \to D$ and D its **succedent**. Using explicitly named atoms such a rule is written $L_1, \ldots, L_k \to M_1; \ldots; M_l$. Write $\top$ for the empty antecedent and $\bot$ for the empty succedent. Sometimes it is convenient to refer to the **clause representation** of a rule $C \to D$, which is $\neg L_1 \vee \cdots \vee \neg L_k \vee M_1 \vee \cdots \vee M_l$. In that case the antecedent literals can be selected with $\overline{C} = \neg L_1 \vee \cdots \vee \neg L_k$ and the succedent literals with $\overline{D} = M_1 \vee \cdots \vee M_l$.

As usual, **ground literals, rules, clauses** etc., are variable free expressions. A rule is **range-restricted**, if all variables occurring in its succedent occur already in its antecedent. Therefore, a range-restricted rule with empty antecedent must be ground. The first occurrence (reading from left to right) of a variable in a rule is called **free**, all other occurrences are **bound**. In a range-restricted rule only bound variables occur in the succedent.

An **MGTP program** P is a finite set of range-restricted rules, where only atoms occur in antecedents and succedents. If the restriction to atoms is lifted to literals, one obtains the language of **CMGTP**. To avoid technical complications, we assume that the signature Σ of the terms occurring in a program P contains at least one constant symbol, so that $Term_\Sigma^0$ and $Atom_\Sigma^0$ are non-empty. If a program P contains no constant symbol, we add artificially the constant t_0.

Domains. A **domain** is a finite, totally ordered set N, which is represented by a set of natural numbers of the form $\{1, \ldots, n\}$. This implies that domains are *homogeneous*, that is, initial segments with identical length from different domains are indistinguishable. **Constraint variables** $I, J, \ldots$ from a set $CVar$ hold elements from a domain N, while **domain variables** $U, V, \ldots$ from a set $DVar$ hold subsets of a domain N.

Rules will contain constraint and domain variables in a way made precise later. We note for now that the notions of range-restrictedness and free/bound variable are defined exactly as for term variables.

3   Syntax and Semantics of IV-MGTP

3.1   Motivation

We set out to enhance MGTP with finite domain constraints. First, we motivate our central definition from the point of view of signed formula logic (SFL) [12] and constraint logic programming (CLP) over finite domains [13].

In SFL rules are defined over signed atoms, where a signed atom is of the form $S{:}L$, and where in turn S is a non-empty subset of a domain N and L is an atom. Atoms L are interpreted N-valued and a signed atom $S{:}L$ is satisfied iff the interpretation of L takes on a value in S.

If $L = p(t_1, \ldots, t_r)$, then $S{:}L$ is equivalent to the MGTP atom $p(t_1, \ldots, t_r, x)$, where: (i) x is constrained to values from $S \subseteq N$; (ii) p is **functional** at the $r + 1$-st argument, that is, $p(t_1, \ldots, t_r, i)$ and $p(t_1, \ldots, t_r, j)$ have the same value iff $i = j$; (iii) p is **total** at the $r+1$-st argument, that is, $p(t_1, \ldots, t_r, x)$ is satisfied for at least one value of x.

A different notation for $S{:}p(t_1, \ldots, t_r)$ inspired by finite domain CLP is to write "$p(t_1, \ldots, t_r, x)$, $x :: S$". Lifting the restriction that constraints can only occur in one argument of an atom yields

$$p(t_1, \ldots, t_r, x_1, \ldots, x_m), \ x_1 :: S_1, \ldots, x_m :: S_m \ , \tag{1}$$

where $S_1 \subseteq N_1, \ldots, S_m \subseteq N_m$. The actual order of constrained and unconstrained arguments is irrelevant. We chose to group them in order to simplify notation. The intended meaning of (1) is as in CLP: it is satisfiable iff $p(t_1, \ldots, t_r, c_1, \ldots, c_m)$ is satisfied by some interpretation $\mathbf{I}$ with $\mathbf{I}(c_j) \in S_j$, $1 \leq j \leq m$. In contrast to CLP we do not allow the x_i to occur in the S_j, so we can just as well replace each x_i with S_i in $p(t_1, \ldots, t_r, x_1, \ldots, x_m)$. This gives the more compact and readable notation

$$p(t_1, \ldots, t_r, S_1, \ldots, S_m) \ , \tag{2}$$

for what we call from now a **constrained atom**. Further differences between IV-MGTP and CLP are discussed in Section 7.1.

3.2   The Language of IV-MGTP

Constrained atoms (2) explicitly stipulate subsets of domains and thus are in **solved** or **canonical form**. The language of IV-MGTP needs to admit other forms of atoms, in order to be practically useful.

For a start, an IV-MGTP atom $p(\ldots)$ may contain domain variables from $DVar$ at the constraint places of p. Our domains are totally ordered; we take advantage from this by admitting **interval** and **extraval** notation to specify subsets of domains. In addition, the boundary values of intervals and extravals can be constraint variables from $CVar$. To summarise, an **IV-MGTP atom** is an expression $p(t_1, \ldots, t_r, \kappa_1, \ldots, \kappa_m)$, where the κ_i have one of the following forms:

1. $\{i_1, \ldots, i_r\}$, where $i_j \in N$ for $1 \leq j \leq r$ (κ_i is in **solved form**);
2. $]\iota_1, \iota_2[$, where ι_j for $j = 1, 2$ are from $N \cup CVar$; the intended meaning is $]\iota_1, \iota_2[= \{i \in N \mid i < \iota_1 \text{ or } i > \iota_2\}$;
3. $[\iota_1, \iota_2]$, where ι_j for $j = 1, 2$ are from $N \cup CVar$; the intended meaning is $[\iota_1, \iota_2] = \{i \in N \mid \iota_1 \leq i \leq \iota_2\}$;
4. $U \in DVar$.

It is legal to write empty set constraints, such as "$\{\}$". Note that an IV-MGTP atom whose constraints are all in solved form is a constrained atom.

Further forms of constraints might be useful, but are not considered for now. One has to find a trade-off between implementability and usability. Our current applications only justify the forms defined so far.

IV-MGTP rules are defined like MGTP rules, but are based on IV-MGTP atoms. Not only the term variables, but also constraint and domain variables of an IV-MGTP rule must be **range-restricted**, i.e., all constraint/domain variables occurring in the succedent of the rule must occur in the antecedent already.

By way of extension of the corresponding mechanism in MGTP [9], we allow an arbitrary ground decidable *guard* or *condition* cond over term and *constraint* variables to occur in the antecedent of an IV-MGTP rule. The term and constraint variables occurring in cond must be bound. For example, a rule with antecedent $p([I, J])$ and condition cond $= J - I \leq 1$ is intended to be applicable to all constrained atoms of the form $p(S)$ which constrain the value of p to contain at most two model elements.

A finite set of IV-MGTP rules satisfying the conditions above is called an **IV-MGTP program**. Different arguments of constrained atoms can be associated with different domains, so predicate symbols must be declared. For each $p \in P_\Sigma$ with constrained arguments, an IV-MGTP program contains a **declaration** line of the form "declare $p(t, \ldots, t, j_1, \ldots, j_m)$".

If the i-th place of p is t, then the i-th argument of p is a standard term; if the i-th place of p is a positive integer j, then the i-th argument of p is a constraint over the domain $\{1, \ldots, j\}$. If a constraint declaration is "1", then one should consider to omit it altogether, as "declare $p(1)$" is equivalent to "declare". The free, that is, first occurrence of a constraint or domain variable in an expression determines also its domain.

Each IV-MGTP atom $p(t_1, \ldots, t_r, \kappa_1, \ldots, \kappa_m)$ consists of two parts, the standard **term part** $p(t_1, \ldots, t_r)$ and the **constraint part** $\langle \kappa_1, \ldots, \kappa_m \rangle$. Each of r and m can be 0. The latter, $m = 0$, is in particular the case for a predicate that has no declaration. Such a predicate is assumed to be implicitly declared as "declare $p(t, \ldots, t)$". By this convention, every MGTP program is also an IV-MGTP program.

3.3 Formal Semantics of IV-MGTP

Substitutions. Recall that there are three kinds of variables that occur in IV-MGTP programs: term variables $TVar$, constraint variables $CVar$, domain variables $DVar$. An **(IV-MGTP) ground substitution** σ maps term variables to ground terms, constraint variables over a domain N to N, and domain variables over a domain N to $2^N - \{\emptyset\}$.

Interpretations. Let $\mathbb{N}^+$ denote the positive integers. Then any domain is contained in $\mathbb{N}^+$. To simplify things we assume in the following $\mathbb{N}^+ \subseteq C_\Sigma$. With this in mind, assume "declare $p(t, \ldots, t, j_1, \ldots, j_m)$", then any subset of $(Term_\Sigma^0)^r \times \{1, \ldots, j_1\} \times \cdots \times \{1, \ldots, j_m\}$ is a **IV-MGTP pre-interpretation** of p. In other words, any standard Herbrand interpretation (restricted to suitable domains for the constraint part) is also an IV-MGTP pre-interpretation. In an **IV-MGTP interpretation I**, only the constraint part is handled in a slightly non-standard way: the constrained arguments of p are **functional**, so the same must be true for $\mathbf{I}(p)$. If p is declared as above, then for all $\langle t_1, \ldots, t_r \rangle \in (Term_\Sigma^0)^r$

there is at most one $\langle i_1, \ldots, i_m \rangle \in \{1, \ldots, j_1\} \times \cdots \times \{1, \ldots, j_m\}$ such that $\langle t_1, \ldots, t_r, i_1, \ldots, i_m \rangle \in \mathbf{I}(p)$.

The constraint part of an IV-MGTP ground atom can without loss of generality be assumed in solved form, because variable free intervals and extravals can be trivially converted to sets of domain values. *In the following we assume that all ground constraints are automatically converted into solved form.*

Satisfaction. A IV-MGTP ground atom $L = p(t_1, \ldots, t_r, S_1, \ldots, S_m)$ is **satisfied** by an IV-MGTP interpretation $\mathbf{I}$ (in symbols $\mathbf{I} \models L$) iff there are $i_1 \in S_1, \ldots, i_m \in S_m$ such that $\langle t_1, \ldots, t_r, i_1, \ldots, i_m \rangle \in \mathbf{I}(p)$. A set of IV-MGTP ground atoms M is satisfied iff $\mathbf{I} \models L$ for each $L \in M$. Note that an atom of the form $p(\ldots, \{\}, \ldots)$ is unsatisfiable.

A ground IV-MGTP rule is satisfied by $\mathbf{I}$ iff at least one of the atoms in its antecedent or **cond** is not satisfied by $\mathbf{I}$ or at least one of the atoms in its succedent is satisfied by $\mathbf{I}$. Obviously, $C \to D$ is satisfied iff $\overline{C}$ is satisfied or **cond** is not satisfied or $\overline{D}$ is satisfied. An IV-MGTP rule r is satisfied by $\mathbf{I}$ iff $\mathbf{I} \models r\sigma$ for every ground substitution σ. Finally, an IV-MGTP program P is satisfied by $\mathbf{I}$ iff $\mathbf{I} \models r$ for all $r \in P$.

The sets S_i in the constrained part of an IV-MGTP literal are independent of each other, that is, an IV-MGTP literal can only represent rectangles in domain spaces. We stress that in IV-MGTP we did not essentially change the notion of an Herbrand interpretation (we stipulated functionality and domain restrictions for constrained arguments). What we did change (in fact: generalise) is the notion of an atom. While in classical logic a maximal, consistent set of ground literals specifies exactly one interpretation, this particular relationship becomes one-many in the case of IV-MGTP.

4   The IV-MGTP Deduction Process

4.1   Model Candidates

In the MGTP deduction process, a list of current model candidates is kept that represent Herbrand interpretations. In MGTP model candidates are identified with sets of ground atoms. The same holds in IV-MGTP, only that certain places of a predicate contain a ground constraint in solved form (that is: a subset of a domain) instead of a ground term. While in MGTP a model candidate containing ground atoms $\{L_1, \ldots, L_r\}$ represents exactly one possible interpretation of the set of atoms $\{L_1, \ldots, L_r\}$, in IV-MGTP one single model candidate represents many IV-MGTP interpretations which differ in the constraint parts.

Thus, in the following high-level description of the IV-MGTP deduction process, model candidates can be conceived as sets of constrained atoms of the form (2), where the S_i are subsets of the appropriate domain. If M is a model candidate, $p(t_1, \ldots, t_r)$ the ground term part, and $\langle S_1, \ldots, S_m \rangle$ the constraint part of a constrained atom in M, then define $M(p(t_1, \ldots, t_r)) = \langle S_1, \ldots, S_m \rangle$.

Formally, a **model candidate** M is a *partial* function that maps ground instances of the term part of constrained atoms "declare $p(t, \ldots, t, j_1, \ldots, j_m)$"

into $(2^{\{1,\ldots,j_1\}} - \{\emptyset\}) \times \cdots \times (2^{\{1,\ldots,j_m\}} - \{\emptyset\})$. Note that $M(p(t_1, \ldots, t_r))$ can be undefined.

4.2   Conjunctive Matching

Let $r = C \to D \in P$ be an IV-MGTP rule, M a model candidate. We say that **conjunctive matching (CJM) can be applied to (the antecedent) of r and M** if there is a ground substitution σ such that for each atom of the form $p(t_1, \ldots, t_r, \kappa_1, \ldots, \kappa_m) \in C$: (i) $M(p(t_1, \ldots, t_r)\sigma) = \langle S_1, \ldots, S_m \rangle$; (ii) For all $1 \leq i \leq m$: $S_i = \kappa_i\sigma$ if κ_i is a domain variable and $S_i \subseteq \kappa_i\sigma$ otherwise; (iii) $\mathsf{cond}\sigma$ in the antecedent of $r\sigma$ is satisfied.

4.3   Inconsistency

A model candidate M **is inconsistent with** a constrained ground atom of the form $p(t_1, \ldots, t_r, S_1, \ldots, S_m)$ iff $M(p(t_1, \ldots, t_r)) = \langle S_1', \ldots, S_m' \rangle$ and $S_i \cap S_i' = \emptyset$ for some $i \in \{1, \ldots, m\}$. For example, $p(a, [1,2], [3,4])$ is inconsistent with $M(p(a)) = \langle \{2\}, \{2\} \rangle$.

4.4   Subsumption

The task of the subsumption check is to avoid deriving atoms that would not further constrain the current model candidate. Formally, we say that a constrained ground atom $p(t_1, \ldots, t_r, S_1', \ldots, S_m')$ **is implied** by model candidate M iff $M(p(t_1, \ldots, t_r)) = \langle S_1, \ldots, S_m \rangle$ and $S_i \subseteq S_i'$ for $1 \leq i \leq m$. (Obviously, this is a special case of conjunctive matching.)

Let D be the succedent of an IV-MGTP rule to which conjunctive matching can be applied in M with substitution σ, then $D\sigma$ is said to be **subsumed** by M iff there is a constrained atom L in $D\sigma$ such that L is implied by M.

4.5   Model Candidate Update

Besides rejection, subsumption, and extension of a model candidate, in IV-MGTP there is a fourth possibility not present in MGTP.

Example 1. Let $D = p(\{1, 2\})$ and assume $M(p) = \langle \{2, 3\} \rangle$. Neither is the single atom in D inconsistent with M nor is it subsumed by M. Yet the information contained in D is not identical to the information contained in M and it can be used to refine M to $M(p) = \langle \{2\} \rangle$.

Another possibility is that M holds no restriction on p so far: $M(p) = N$, where N is the domain of the single argument of p. Again, M can be refined, here to $M(p) = \langle \{1, 2\} \rangle$.

In general we define model candidate update or the addition of information to model candidates as follows: let $L = p(t_1, \ldots, t_r, S_1, \ldots, S_m)$ be a constrained ground atom consistent with model candidate M; $p' = p(t_1, \ldots, t_r)$ is the ground term part of L. Then the **update** $M + L$ of M with L is:

$$(M + L)(q) = \begin{cases} \langle S_1, \ldots, S_m \rangle & q = p' \text{ and } M(p') \text{ undefined} \\ \langle S_1 \cap S_1', \ldots, S_m \cap S_m' \rangle & q = p' \text{ and } M(p') = \langle S_1', \ldots, S_m' \rangle \\ M(q) & \text{otherwise} \end{cases} .$$

Example 2. To gain further insight into the process of model candidate update let us redo Example 1 in plain MGTP. The constrained atom $D = p(\{1, 2\})$ corresponds to the disjunction $D' = p(1); p(2)$ of classical atoms, while $M = \{p(\{2, 3\})\}$ corresponds to *two* MGTP model candidates: $M' = \{p(2)\}$, $M'' = \{p(3)\}$. Moreover, the functionality axiom "$p(I), p(J), I \neq J \to \bot$" is added. D' is subsumed by M', so M' is unchanged. On the other hand, M'' is rejected (in the MGTP sense) by D' and functionality, so we are left with M' only. But M' contains exactly the information of $M + p(\{1, 2\}) = p(\{2\})$.

We see that, in MGTP terms, model candidate update is really a combination of subsumption and rejection.

4.6   IV-MGTP Procedure

The following definition gives the procedural semantics of IV-MGTP programs. It is modeled after the high-level description of the standard MGTP procedure [4]. Let $M_\emptyset$ be the **undefined model candidate**, where $M_\emptyset(p(t_1, \ldots, t_r))$ is undefined for all $t_1, \ldots, t_r \in Term_\Sigma^0$ and "declare $p(t, \ldots, t, j_1, \ldots, j_m)$".

For a given IV-MGTP program P, let $\mathcal{M}$ be a set of IV-MGTP model candidates, inductively defined as follows:

Initialisation $M_\emptyset \in \mathcal{M}$.

Update $M \in \mathcal{M}$ is not rejected, CJM can be applied to the antecedent of $C \to D \in P$ and M with substitution σ, $D\sigma$ is not subsumed by M, and not all constrained atoms in $D\sigma$ are inconsistent with M. Let $D'\sigma \neq \bot$ consist of the atoms in $D\sigma$ consistent with M.

Then M is **extendible (with $D'\sigma$)**, the elements of $\mathcal{M}' = \bigcup_{L \in D'\sigma}(M + L)$ are called **immediate successor of** M, and $\mathcal{M}$ becomes $(\mathcal{M} - \{M\}) \cup \mathcal{M}'$.

Rejection CJM can be applied to the antecedent of $r = C \to D \in P$ and M with substitution σ and all constrained atoms in $D\sigma$ are inconsistent with M.[2] Then M is **rejected** (by r).

Those elements of a set $\mathcal{M}$ that are neither rejected nor extendible are the **IV-MGTP models** of P.

Example 3. Consider the program consisting of rules $R_1 = \top \to p(\{1\}); p(\{2\})$, $R_2 = \top \to p([1, 2])$, $R_3 = \top \to p([2, 3])$. Any of the rules can be trivially applied to the undefined model candidate, because the antecedents are empty. Update of $M_\emptyset$ with R_1 results in two new model candidates with $M_1(p) = \langle \{1\} \rangle$ and $M_2(p) = \langle \{2\} \rangle$. R_2 can be applied to neither of them, because its succedent is subsumed. If we apply first R_2 to $M_\emptyset$ instead, then the result is $M_3(p) = \langle \{1, 2\} \rangle$ and extension with R_1 is possible. It yields again M_1 and M_2. R_3 is rejected in M_1, and subsumed in M_2, however, it can be used to update M_3 to M_2.

---

[2] This is in particular the case when $D = \bot$.

5   Soundness and Completeness

Theorem 1 (Soundness). *If P is a satisfiable IV-MGTP program, then P has an IV-MGTP model.*

IV-MGTP cannot be complete with respect to the semantics that has been used up to now. The reason is essentially the same as for incompleteness of resolution and hypertableaux with unrestricted selection function [6].[3] It can be demonstrated with the simple example $P = \{\top \to p, \neg q \to \neg p, q \to \bot\}$. The program P is unsatisfiable, yet deduction procedures based on selection of only antecedent (or only succedent) literals cannot detect this. Likewise, the incomplete treatment of negation in CMGTP comes up with the incorrect model $\{p\}$ for P. This incompleteness also occurs in IV-MGTP. Assume p and q are defined "declare $p(2)$" and "declare $q(2)$". The idea is to represent a positive literal p with $p(2)$ and a negative literal $\neg p$ with $p(1)$. Consider

$$P' \quad = \quad \{\top \to p(\{2\}),\ q(\{1\}) \to p(\{1\}),\ q(\{2\}) \to \bot\} \tag{3}$$

which is unsatisfiable (recall that p and q are functional), but has an IV-MGTP model, where $M(p) = \langle\{2\}\rangle$, and $M(q)$ is undefined.

The example shows that already the ground Horn case with one constrained argument causes problems. Exactly this case is handled in so-called *signed formula logic programming* (SFLP), where Lu [12] suggested a possible solution: he conceived a non-standard semantics called *extended interpretations* for SFLP that characterises a certain procedural semantics. This procedural semantics, defined for the one-argument Horn case, happens to be quite similar to that of IV-MGTP (see Section 7.2 for a more detailed account of the relation between SFLP and IV-MGTP).

There are more IV-MGTP models than satisfying interpretations as is exemplified by (3). So our solution is to admit additional interpretations that account for the remaining IV-MGTP models.

The basic idea underlying extended interpretations (briefly: e-interpretations) is to introduce the disjunctive information inherent to constraints into the interpretations themselves. Recall that IV-MGTP interpretations essentially are normal Herbrand interpretations (with some arguments functional and over a suitable domain). In contrast to this, model candidates contain IV-MGTP ground atoms with constraints. **Extended interpretations** are defined exactly as model candidates, i.e., partial functions $\mathbf{I}$ mapping ground instances of the term part of IV-MGTP atoms with predicate symbol p into $(2^{\{1,\ldots,j_1\}} - \{\emptyset\}) \times \cdots \times (2^{\{1,\ldots,j_m\}} - \{\emptyset\})$, if p is defined "declare $p(t,\ldots,t,j_1,\ldots,j_m)$". In the following we normally use M, M' as meta variables for model candidates and $\mathbf{I}$, $\mathbf{I}'$ for e-interpretations, but it is sometimes convenient to use the same letter for both which we do without an explicit (but trivial) conversion function.

An extended interpretation $\mathbf{I}$ does **e-satisfy** an IV-MGTP ground atom $L = p(t_1,\ldots,t_r,S_1,\ldots,S_m)$ iff $\mathbf{I}(p(t_1,\ldots,t_r))$ is defined, has the value $\langle S'_1,\ldots,S'_m\rangle$,

---

[3] As in the ground case positive hypertableaux [2] and MGTP are virtually indistinguishable [6], this finding is not surprising.

and $S_i' \subseteq S_i$ for all $1 \leq i \leq m$.[4] Equivalently, using the terminology of model candidates we could have expressed e-satisfaction as "CJM can be applied to L and $\mathbf{I}$". E-satisfaction of rules and programs is defined exactly as before, only relative to e-interpretations.

Our previous notation for updates (Section 4.5) can be generalised to cover extended interpretations: $\mathbf{I} + \mathbf{I}' = \mathbf{I} + \Sigma_{p \in Atom_{\Sigma}^{0}} \mathbf{I}'(p)$.

Example 4. The program P' in (3) is unsatisfiable, but it is e-satisfiable by $\mathbf{I}(p) = \langle\{2\}\rangle$, $\mathbf{I}(q) = \langle\{1,2\}\rangle$, because $\mathbf{I}(q)$ neither satisfies $q(\{1\})$ nor $q(\{2\})$, hence both the second and third rule are satisfied as q occurs in the antecedent.

Consider the single-rule programs P_1 containing $\top \to p(\{1\}); p(\{2\})$ and P_2 containing $\top \to p([1,2])$. They cannot be distinguished with IV-MGTP interpretations: both are satisfied exactly by $\mathbf{I}_1 = \{p(1)\}$ and $\mathbf{I}_2 = \{p(2)\}$. The e-interpretations $\mathbf{I}_1'(p) = \langle\{1\}\rangle$ and $\mathbf{I}_2'(p) = \langle\{2\}\rangle$ corresponding to $\mathbf{I}_1$ and $\mathbf{I}_2$ satisfy P_1 and P_2 as well, but there is a further e-interpretation $\mathbf{I}'(p) = \langle\{1,2\}\rangle$ satisfying P_2, but not P_1.

The relationship between interpretations and e-interpretations of IV-MGTP programs is stated in the next lemma. We say an e-interpretation (or a model candidate) $\mathbf{I}$ is **definite** iff $\mathbf{I}(p(t_1, \ldots, t_r)) = \langle S_1, \ldots, S_m \rangle$ implies $|S_1| = \cdots = |S_m| = 1$.

Lemma 1. *Let $\mathbf{I}$ be an IV-MGTP interpretation that satisfies the IV-MGTP program P. Then the e-interpretation $\mathbf{I}'$ defined as*

$$\mathbf{I}'(p(t_1, \ldots, t_r)) = \begin{cases} \langle\{i_1\}, \ldots, \{i_m\}\rangle & \langle t_1, \ldots, t_r, i_1, \ldots, i_m \rangle \in \mathbf{I}(p) \\ undefined & otherwise \end{cases}$$

e-satisfies P. If $\mathbf{I}'$ is a definite e-interpretation that e-satisfies P, then the interpretation $\mathbf{I}$ defined as follows satisfies P:

$$\langle t_1, \ldots, t_r, i_1, \ldots, i_m \rangle \in \mathbf{I}(p) \quad iff \quad \mathbf{I}'(p(t_1, \ldots, t_r)) = \langle\{i_1\}, \ldots, \{i_m\}\rangle$$

Theorem 2 (Completeness). *An IV-MGTP program P having an IV-MGTP model M is e-satisfiable by M (viewed as an e-interpretation).*

Corollary 1. *If an IV-MGTP program P has a definite IV-MGTP model M' then P is satisfied by the IV-MGTP interpretation M (using the terminology of Lemma 1).*

Theorem 3 (E-Soundness). *If an IV-MGTP program P is e-satisfiable then P has an IV-MGTP model.*

---

[4] The concept of e-interpretation and e-satisfaction occurs already in [5], where it was used to simplify some definitions. Its relevancy for SFLP was first noticed in [12].

6   Results

We developed an IV-MGTP prototype system in Java and made experiments on a Sun Ultra 5 under JDK 1.2. The results are compared with those on the same problems formulated and run with CMGTP [14], also written in Java [8]. We consider two types of finite domain constraint satisfaction problems: cryptarithmetic and channel routing. For these problems, many specialised solvers employing heuristics were developed. Our experiments are not primarily intended to compare IV-MGTP with such solvers, but to show the effectiveness of the representation and its domain calculation in the IV-MGTP procedure.

6.1   Cryptarithmetic

We demonstrate the effect of IV-MGTP with the well-known cryptarithmetic problem $SEND + MORE = MONEY$. The problem is to find instances of the variables $\{ D, E, M, N, O, R, S, Y \}$ satisfying the computation displayed on the right-hand side.

$$
\begin{array}{r}
S\ E\ N\ D \\
+\quad M\ O\ R\ E \\
\hline
M\ O\ N\ E\ Y
\end{array}
$$

To solve this problem we need, among others, the rule $D + E = 10 \times Z + Y$, where Z ranges over $\{0,1\}$, while D, E, and Y range over $\{0,1,\ldots,9\}$. The domain of Y can be narrowed by the minimum and maximum values of the variables D, E, Z. IV-MGTP can implement such domain calculation using intervals/extravals, which enables to prune redundant branches by refutation of domains.

CMGTP (or MGTP), however, lack the notion of a variable domain, so one has to represent possible values a variable may take with multiple literals. Thus, in CMGTP, constraint propagation cannot be implemented with domain calculation. Table 1 compares IV-MGTP and CMGTP for the cryptarithmetic problem.

Table 1. Experimental results for cryptarithmetic problem.

	IV-MGTP	CMGTP
models	1	1
total branches	12	3308
runtime(msec)	391	4793

Both systems found the unique model, but differed in the numbers of failed branches. The comparison of total branches generated by CMGTP and IV-MGTP exhibits that IV-MGTP has a considerable pruning effect, and thus creates a much smaller proof tree than CMGTP.

6.2   Channel Routing

Channel routing problems in VLSI design can be represented as constraint satisfaction problems, in which connection requirements (what we call *nets*) between terminals must be solved under the condition that each net has a disjoint path from all others. For these problems, many specialised solvers employing heuristics were developed. Our experiments are not primarily intended to compare IV-MGTP with such solvers, but to show the effectiveness of the interval/extraval representation and its domain calculation in the IV-MGTP procedure.

Here we consider a multi-layer channel which consists of multiple layers, each of which has multiple tracks. We assume in addition, to simplify the problem, that each routing path contains no dog-legs and contains only one track. By this assumption, the problem can be formalised to determine the layer and the track numbers for each net with the help of constraints that express the two binary relations: *not equal* and *above*; *not equal(N_1,N_2)* means that the net N_1 and N_2 do not share the same track. *above(N_1,N_2)* means that if N_1 and N_2 share the same layer, the track number of N_1 must be larger than that of N_2 (trivially, the *not equal* relation includes the *above* relation). For example, *not equal* constraints for nets N_1 and N_2 are represented in IV-MGTP as follows:

$$p(N_1, [L, L], [T_1, T_1]), \ p(N_2, [L, L], [T_{21}, T_{22}]), \ N_1 \neq N_2 \rightarrow p(N_2, [L, L],]T_1, T_1[)$$

where the predicate p has two constraint domains: layer number L and track number T_i. We experimented with problems consisting of 6, 8, 10, and 12 net patterns on the 2 layers channel each of which has 3 tracks. The results are shown in Table 2.

Table 2. Experimental results for channel routing problems.

Number of Nets = 6

	IV-MGTP	CMGTP
models	250	840
branches	286	882
runtime(msec)	168	95

Number of Nets = 10

	IV-MGTP	CMGTP
models	4998	51922
branches	6238	52000
runtime(msec)	2311	3882

Number of Nets = 8

	IV-MGTP	CMGTP
models	1560	10296
branches	1808	10302
runtime(msec)	706	470

Number of Nets = 12

	IV-MGTP	CMGTP
models	13482	538056
branches	20092	539982
runtime(msec)	7498	31681

IV-MGTP reduces the number of models considerably. For example, we found the following model in a 6-net problem:

$$\{p(1, [1, 1], [3, 3]), p(2, [1, 1], [1, 1]), p(3, [1, 1], [2, 2]),$$
$$p(4, [2, 2], [2, 3]), p(5, [2, 2], [1, 2]), p(6, [1, 1], [2, 3])\} \ ,$$

which contains 8 $(= 1 \times 1 \times 1 \times 2 \times 2 \times 2)$ CMGTP models. The advantage of using IV-MGTP representation and interpretation is that the different feasible track numbers can be represented as interval constraints. In CMGTP the above IV-MGTP model is split into 8 different models. Obviously, as the number of nets increases, the reduction ratio of the number of models becomes larger.

We conclude that IV-MGTP can effectively suppress unnecessary case splitting by using interval constraints, and hence, reduce the total size of proofs.

7   Related and Future Work

7.1   Constraint Logic Programming

IV-MGTP is reminiscent of finite domain CLP [13], but there are a number of fundamental differences. In contrast to MGTP, (C)LP systems proceed by top-down reasoning, they do not enforce range-restrictedness (which is pointless, as they are not proof confluent), and are defined on Horn clauses; the MGTP procedure is proof confluent and strongly complete, if rules are selected fairly and thus requires no backtracking. Thus we have "committed choice" computation without sacrificing completeness. The philosophy of IV-MGTP is to provide a theorem prover with a certain capability to deal with totally ordered finite domain constraints; it has few operators to manipulate them and no optimisation component. A complete constraint solver is not implemented. In CLP, on the other hand, the constraint solver often carries the bulk of computation, and logical inference is less efficient.

There is some similarity between IV-MGTP and Interval CLP [3]. The latter is more general in that it can be used to approximate real-valued relations and to narrow real-valued intervals, whereas IV-MGTP is optimized to work with finite domains. Bottum-up computation in IV-MGTP allows natural propagation of inconsistent constraints, while CLP needs other mechanisms to avoid redundant search such as dependency-directed backtracking. In addition, IV-MGTP gives the user explicit control over case-splitting in succedents of rules.

The committed choice constraint language $CHR^\vee$ [1] accommodates bottom-up reasoning and non-Horn rules. It would be possible to write a meta-interpreter for IV-MGTP in $CHR^\vee$. There are no experimental data in [1], so it is difficult to evaluate, however, $CHR^\vee$ is implemented on top of Prolog-based implementations of CHR, and pattern matching on constraint constructors is not available. Moreover, there is no completeness result like Theorem 2.

From a language design point of view, in CLP *variables* are declared, rather than predicates. A central feature of MGTP-like procedures, needed for strong completeness [6] as well as efficiency, is that only ground atoms are stored in model candidates. The variable-centred view of CLP is not an option. In IV-MGTP constraints are attached to predicates (not to variables which occur in predicates), so predicate arguments fulfil the task of variables. The semantics of CLP does *not* impose functionality on constrained arguments in interpretations, for example, in CLP a query of the form "$? - p(S), S::1..1, p(T), T::2..2$" succeeds, because variables as opposed to predicates are declared.

7.2   Signed Formula Logic (Programming)

The principal differences between (C)LP and MGTP deduction sketched in the previous subsection apply to the comparison with SFLP as well. It was pointed out in Section 3.1 that IV-MGTP atoms can be seen as a generalisation of signed atoms in SFL. While partially or totally ordered domains are often considered in SFL, the syntax of signs/constraints is usually limited to forms $\{i_1, \ldots, i_r\}$ (the solved form in our setting) and $\uparrow i$ (the order filter on N generated by i). Constraint variables are sometimes admitted [11], but usually missing in concrete implementations. On the semantic side, in SFLP e-interpretations are *total* functions, that is, $\mathbf{I}(p)$ is defined for all ground atoms p. In SFLP, for example, the query "$?- \{1, \ldots, n\}{:}p$" succeeds (if $N = \{1, \ldots, n\}$ is the domain, see Section 3.1 for SFL notation). The equivalent IV-MGTP program consisting of the single rule $p(\{1, \ldots, n\}) \to \bot$ (where p is assumed "declare $p(n)$") has the IV-MGTP model $M_\emptyset$, that is, $\mathbf{I}(p)$ is undefined.

7.3   IV-MGTP and CMGTP

CMGTP [14] is a special case of IV-MGTP: for each r-ary predicate p in CMGTP let p' be a corresponding $r + 1$-ary IV-MGTP predicate declared "$p(t, \ldots, t, 2)$".

Now replace each CMGTP literal of the form $p(t_1, \ldots, t_r)$ with the IV-MGTP atom $p(t_1, \ldots, t_r, \{2\})$ and each literal of the form $\neg p(t_1, \ldots, t_r)$ with $p(t_1, \ldots, t_r, \{1\})$. CMGTP contains an additional rule $p(\ldots), \neg p(\ldots) \to \bot$. This is not necessary in IV-MGTP, because of functionality.

7.4   Paraconsistent Reasoning

There is a close relationship between the functionality requirement for constraints in IV-MGTP interpretations, the non-emptiness of e-interpretations, and paraconsistent reasoning: the functionality requirement for constraints in IV-MGTP interpretations $\mathbf{I}$ corresponds to the restriction to non-empty constraints in e-interpretations $\mathbf{I}'$: assume "declare $p(2)$" for p. Then $\mathbf{I}(p)$ is functional iff not both $\mathbf{I} \models p(\{i\})$ and $\mathbf{I} \models p(\{j\})$ for $i \neq j$ iff $p(\{i\}) + p(\{j\}) \neq p(\emptyset)$ iff $\mathbf{I}'(p) \neq \langle \emptyset \rangle$. Consider the IV-MGTP program $P = \{\top \to p(\{1\}),\ \top \to p(\{2\})\}$. It is neither satisfiable nor e-satisfiable. In *paraconsistent reasoning* [10], however, one infers from it the atom $p(\emptyset)$ indicating that inconsistent information is entailed about p. Lifting the non-emptiness restriction on e-interpretations still gives a well-defined, non-trivial semantics and captures paraconsistent reasoning [12].

It is possible to generalise the IV-MGTP deduction procedure for paraconsistent reasoning by a minor modification. See the full paper for details.

7.5   Future Work

CMGTP programs are complete even with respect to standard interpretations provided that antecedents of rules are **consistent** [6]: for all literals L, L' occurring in the antecedent of any ground instance of a rule, $\{L, L'\}$ is a consistent set. The straightforward generalisation to domains of size greater than two fails to guarantee completeness, but the matter should be investigated more thoroughly.

The language of IV-MGTP constraints can be made richer, but the more complicated constraints are, the more computational burden is shifted to constraint solving and the specific advantages of MGTP might vanish; in any case, the trade-offs must be better understood. The speed of our implementation should be improved. The reduction of generated models (see Section 6) shows the IV-MGTP paradigm to be quite effective, but it needs to be more efficient to play out its full strength. Experience with implementation of (C)MGTP shows that careful coding makes a difference in the order of several magnitudes [8].

References

1. S. Abdennadher and H. Schütz. CHR$^\vee$: A flexible query language. In T. Andreasen, H. Christansen, and H. L. Larsen, eds., *Proc. Int. Conf. on Flexible Query Answering Systems FQAS, Roskilde, Denmark*, vol. 1495 of *LNCS*, pp. 1–15. Springer-Verlag, 1998.
2. P. Baumgartner, U. Furbach, and I. Niemelä. Hyper tableaux. In J. J. Alferes, L. M. Pereira, and E. Orłowska, eds., *Proc. European Workshop: Logics in Artificial Intelligence*, vol. 1126 of *LNCS*, pp. 1–17. Springer-Verlag, 1996.
3. F. Benhamou. Interval constraint logic programming. In A. Podelski, editor, *Constraint programming: basics and trends, Chatillon Spring School, Chatillon-sur-Seine, France, 1994*, vol. 910 of *LNCS*, pp. 1–21. Springer-Verlag, 1995.
4. H. Fujita and R. Hasegawa. A model generation theorem prover in KL1 using a ramified-stack algorithm. In K. Furukawa, editor, *Proc. 8th Int. Conf. on Logic Programming, Paris/France*, pp. 535–548. MIT Press, 1991.
5. R. Hähnle. *Automated Deduction in Multiple-Valued Logics.* OUP, 1994.
6. R. Hähnle. Tableaux and related methods. In A. Robinson and A. Voronkov, eds., *Handbook of Automated Reasoning.* Elsevier Science Publishers, to appear, 2000.
7. R. Hähnle, R. Hasegawa, and Y. Shirai. Model generation theorem proving with interval constraints. In F. Benhamou, W. J. Older, M. van Emden, and P. van Hentenryck, eds., *Proc. of ILPS Post-Conf. Workshop on Interval Constraints, Portland/OR, USA*, Dec. 1995.
8. R. Hasegawa and H. Fujita. A new implementation technique for a Model-Generation Theorem Prover to solve constraint satisfaction problems. Research Reports on Inf. Sci. and El. Eng. Vol. 4, No. 1, pp. 57–62, Kyushu Univ., 1999.
9. R. Hasegawa, H. Fujita, and M. Koshimura. MGTP: a model generation theorem prover—its advanced features and applications. In D. Galmiche, editor, *Proc. Int. Conf. on Automated Reasoning with Analytic Tableaux and Related Methods, Pont-à-Mousson, France*, vol. 1227 of *LNCS*, pp. 1–15. Springer-Verlag, 1997.
10. M. Kifer and E. L. Lozinskii. A logic for reasoning with inconsistency. *Journal of Automated Reasoning*, 9(2):179–215, Oct. 1992.
11. M. Kifer and V. S. Subrahmanian. Theory of generalized annotated logic programming and its applications. *Journal of Logic Programming*, 12:335–367, 1992.
12. J. J. Lu. Logic programming with signs and annotations. *Journal of Logic and Computation*, 6(6):755–778, 1996.
13. U. Montanari and F. Rossi. Finite Domain Constraint Solving and Constraint Logic Programming. In F. Benhamou and A. Colmerauer, eds., *Constraint Logic Programming: Selected Research*, pp. 201–221. The MIT press, 1993.
14. Y. Shirai and R. Hasegawa. Two approaches for finite-domain constraint satisfaction problem: CP and MGTP. In L. Stirling, editor, *Proc. 12th Int. Conf. on Logic Programming*, pp. 249–263. MIT Press, 1995.

Combining Mobile Processes and Declarative Programming

Rachid Echahed and Wendelin Serwe

Laboratoire LEIBNIZ – Institut IMAG, CNRS
46, avenue Felix Viallet, F-38031 Grenoble, FRANCE
Tel: (+33) 4 76 57 48 91; Fax: (+33) 4 76 57 46 02
Rachid.Echahed@imag.fr, Wendelin.Serwe@imag.fr

Abstract. We propose a general framework for combining mobile processes and declarative programming languages, e.g., functional, logic or functional-logic languages. In contrast to existing concurrent extensions of declarative languages, we distinguish clearly between the notion of processes and that of functions or predicates. Thus, our framework is generic and may be applied to extend several kinds of declarative languages. It also extends PA process algebra in order to deal with parameter passing, mobile processes and interactive declarative programming. In our setting, declarative programs are dynamic and may be modified thanks to the actions performed by processes.

1 Introduction

Classical declarative languages, i.e., functional, logic and functional-logic languages, aim to provide high-level descriptions of applications or systems. These languages have well-known nice features (e.g., abstraction, readability, compilation techniques, proof methods etc.) since functions and predicates are well mastered mathematical concepts which have been successfully used in describing algorithms even before the invention of computers. However, these concepts, which constitute the basis of classical functional-logic languages, are not sufficient to capture the whole complexity of real-world applications [30] where interactivity, concurrency and distributivity are needed.

On the other hand, processes have been used as a means for the description of interactive applications. Informally, a process can be described as the set of its possible runs, i.e., the set of possible action-sequences which can be performed by the process. Thus, it is immediate that processes are different from functions or predicates.

Most existing concurrent extensions of declarative languages do not distinguish clearly between processes and the concepts underlying the declarative language, but rather try to *encode* processes in terms of the latter [4, 5, 8–11, 13, 16, 17, 21, 23–28]. Thus each of these approaches seems to be tailored for a specific language rendering the extension to a general framework not straightforward.

Classically, declarative languages allow one to describe functions by means of equations (rewrite rules) or lambda abstractions and predicates by Horn clauses

J. Lloyd et al. (Eds.): CL 2000, LNAI 1861, pp. 300–314, 2000.
© Springer-Verlag Berlin Heidelberg 2000

(with constraints). As for processes, there are as many ways to define them as there are different programming styles (including temporal logic programming). Nevertheless, process algebras have been well investigated, see e.g., [3], and provide a clean framework for the description of concurrent processes. An extension, that allows the communication structure to vary, is the π-calculus [20]. It provides a basis for modelling mobile computations.

But similar to concurrent extensions of declarative languages, programming languages uniquely based on process calculi *encode* the notions of functions and predicates via processes, e.g., [22].

This paper aims at a new combination of mobile processes and declarative languages where we distinguish clearly between, on the one hand, concepts which are definable in classical declarative languages, such as functions, predicates or constraints and (mobile) processes on the other hand. Thus the merit of our contribution is to propose a new framework where each part of a mobile, concurrent, functional and/or logic application can be described by the most appropriate known theoretical concept, instead of encoding all these different concepts in a sole framework. Our resulting proposal extends both, declarative programming with mobile processes, and PA process algebra in order to deal with parameter passing, mobile processes and interactive declarative programming.

Theoretically, our framework can be characterised as a new (modal) theory whose models are Kripke-structures. Practically, we provide a new full and rigorous combination of programming paradigms, providing the respective advantages of functional, logic, functional-logic, concurrent and mobile programming in addition to the advantages proper to the combination, in the same way as it was already the case for the integration of functional and logic programming.

The rest of the paper is organised as follows: The next section gives a broad outline of our framework. Section 3 discusses the definitions of actions. The definition of processes is given in Sect. 4 and some examples are presented in Sects. 5 and 6. In Sect. 7 we give the operational semantics. A comparison with some related work is subject of Sect. 8. Finally, Sect. 9 concludes.

2 Overview of Our Proposal

In our framework, an application is modelled via several components. Due to space limitations, we focus in this paper on applications with a single component; but the framework presented here can be extended easily to several components. Roughly speaking, a program or a component in our framework will consist of two parts $C = (\mathcal{F}, \mathcal{P})$. $\mathcal{P}$ is a set of process definitions and $\mathcal{F}$ is a set of formulæ describing a traditional declarative program, called a *store* in the sequel. The execution model of a component can be schematised as in Fig. 1. Processes (p_i) communicate by modifying the common store $\mathcal{F}$, i.e., by altering, in a non-monotonic way, the current theory described by the store, for example by simply redefining constants (e.g., adding a message in a queue) or by adding or deleting formulæ in $\mathcal{F}$. Hence, the execution of processes will cause the transformation of the store $\mathcal{F}$. Every change of the store is the result of the execution of an *action*. Thus actions constitute the basic entities for building processes. In general, processes are also able to modify the stores of other components and thus interact with the environment of their component. Orthogonally, the store can be used as usual for a functional-logic program, i.e., for goal solving or the evaluation of expressions.

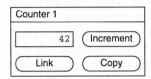

Fig. 1. execution model   **Fig. 2.** a counter window

A real-world instance of a system as depicted in Fig. 1 is for example the file-system on a UNIX-workstation: while there are processes running which may modify the store, i.e., the file-system, it is always possible to investigate the current state by commands as `ls` or `find`. Following the same idea, there are some processes keeping the list of currently logged users up-to-date; this list can be consulted via the command `who`. This investigation may be done "on-line", that is to say, the set of possible questions a user might ask is not known in advance; in fact, the user might ask *any* well-formed question.

Another example is an application emitting flight tickets. Obviously, declarative languages are well-suited to describe the function calculating the price of a ticket. However, if we want to allow the modification of this function without stopping the entire application, then we need to extend classical declarative languages.

To illustrate our extension further, we consider a (simplistic) application inspired from [15], a system of multiple counters. The application starts by creating a window (as shown in Fig. 2) representing a counter which can be incremented manually. In the window of the counter, a copy-button and a link-button allow one to create new counter windows: the former creates an independent counter (with an associated new window) and initialises it with the current value of the counter being copied; the latter creates a new view (i.e., a new window) of the same counter. All links (or views) of a same counter should behave identically, e.g., they increase the counter at the same time. Additionally we may want to use the current value of the counters for some calculations, in the same way as we would like to use any other constant in a classical declarative language. A sample of our solution for this problem is subject of Sect. 5.

This example illustrates some of the difficulties when modelling concurrent processes, such as dynamic creation of new constants (e.g., counters, windows and the corresponding channels) or resources shared by several processes. Obviously, we need to extend a pure declarative language to cope with this *interactive* application. This has also been noted in the literature on declarative programming: "Some interactions appear most straightforward to express in an imperative style, and we should not hesitate to do so" [29].

3 Actions

In our framework, an application may be composed of several components, each consisting of a store and a set of processes. These processes execute actions modifying the stores of different components. Classical examples of actions are for instance tell of ccp (see Sect. 8) which adds a constraint to a constraint store, or setq of Scheme which updates destructively the value of a constant. Other examples of actions concern interaction with the environment, as for instance the commands controlling external physical machines, e.g., opening a door or starting an engine.

Actions are composed of a guard and a sequence of elementary actions. Informally, an elementary action is a function(al), that when supplied with its arguments, returns a total recursive function from stores to stores.

Definition 1. *An* action α *is a pair consisting of a guard g and a sequence of pairs of a storename (expression) s_i and an (parameterised) elementary action a_i, written: $[g \Rightarrow \langle s_1, a_1 \rangle; \ldots ; \langle s_n, a_n \rangle]$. A guard is a formula whose validity (in the (current) store) is decidable. An elementary action a is a total recursive mapping whose type is of the following shape: $types\_of\_arguments \to (store \to store)$.*

Roughly speaking, executing an action means to test the validity of the guard in the (local) store, and, upon the validity of the guard, to execute (atomically) the sequence of the elementary actions, $\langle s_i, a_i \rangle$, that is to say replace the store denoted by the storename (expression) s, say $\mathcal{F}$, by the result of the application of the elementary action a to it, i.e., $a(\mathcal{F})$. Informally, a storename can be seen as a symbolic identifier for a store in the same way as the symbolic host-names stand for (numeric) IP-addresses. In the sequel, we will note a sequence $\gamma_1; \ldots ; \gamma_n$ as γ_i. Thus, an action $[g \Rightarrow \langle s_1, a_1 \rangle; \ldots ; \langle s_n, a_n \rangle]$ will be represented by $[g \Rightarrow \langle s_i, a_i \rangle_i]$.

Due to space limitations, we suppose in this paper that the set of elementary actions is given, and thus restrain ourselves to give below just some examples of useful elementary actions. In our full framework [12], actions are definable by the programmer.

We call skip the elementary action which does not modify the store. Certainly the most common elementary action is assignment $(:=)$. $:=$ takes two parameters: the name c of a constant (traditionally considered as a variable) and a (new) value v. Thus we introduce a new parameterised type $\mathtt{Name}(t)$ to denote the type of the name of a symbol of type t. If c is of type $\mathtt{Name}(t)$, we denote by $c\uparrow$ the associated symbol of type t. Hence, $:=(c, v)(\mathcal{F})$ represents the store obtained from $\mathcal{F}$ by erasing all equations of the form $c\uparrow == term$ and adding the new equation $c\uparrow == v$. In the sequel, and by abuse of notation, we write c in place of $c\uparrow$ whenever there is no ambiguity.

The elementary action tell (respectively, del) adds (respectively, removes) clauses to (respectively, from) the store.

As all processes of a component share the store, broadcasting messages between processes is realised naturally via the common store by executing appropriate elementary actions. To simulate message passing, we can use elementary actions handling queues representing the buffers for (incoming) messages. To send a message, e.g., m, to a process, we need to know the name, e.g., q, of its queue for incoming messages (q is a constant of type $\text{Name}(List(messages))$). Executing the elementary action $\text{enq}(q, m)$ will put our message in the queue of our (communication-) partner. To read a message from a queue, we access the queue, i.e., q, just as we usually access a constant. In order to erase a message from the queue (after having read it), we introduce the elementary action $\text{deq}(q)$.

Another important elementary action handles the creation of new symbols: $\text{new}(s, t)$ introduces two new symbols in the store, namely s of type $\text{Name}(t)$ and $s\uparrow$ of type t. s stands for the name of (or a reference to) the symbol $s\uparrow$. In the multiple counters example, new allows the creation of new counters and the associated communication channels with the window-system.

Example 1. The following is an example of an action, inspired from the program of the "Dining Philosophers" given in Sect. 6:

$$\left[\begin{array}{ccc} \begin{array}{l} \text{stick}(x) \\ \text{stick}(x{+}1 \bmod n) \end{array} \;\wedge\; & \Rightarrow & \begin{array}{l} \langle F, \text{del}(\text{stick}(x))\rangle; \\ \langle F, \text{del}(\text{stick}(x{+}1 \bmod n))\rangle; \\ \langle F, \text{tell}(\text{is\_eating}(x))\rangle \end{array} \end{array} \right]$$

This action says that whenever the sticks number x and $x{+}1 \bmod n$ are available on the table (i.e., $(\text{stick}(x) \wedge \text{stick}(x{+}1 \bmod n))$ holds in the store F), then the philosopher number x can get these sticks (i.e., remove them from the table by deleting the corresponding predicates via the elementary actions $\text{del}(\text{stick}(x))$ and $\text{del}(\text{stick}(x + 1 \bmod n))$ from the store F) and start eating (i.e., add the predicate $\text{is\_eating}(x)$ to F by using the elementary action $\text{tell}(\text{is\_eating}(x))$).

4   Processes

Before giving the formulæ defining processes, we introduce first the notion of process-terms. Such terms are constructed by means of basic processes as well as operators which combine processes into new ones.

Basic processes are success, i.e., the process which terminates successfully, (guarded) actions α, or process calls $p(t_1, \ldots, t_n)$. As usual in process algebra (see, e.g., [3]), we provide some operators for combining processes: parallel ($\|$) and sequential (;) composition, nondeterministic choice (+) and choice with priority ($\oplus$). The last operator is not very common, but we found it necessary to model critical applications where nondeterminism is not acceptable [1]. The intended meaning of the process term $p_1 \oplus p_2$ is: "execute the process p_2 only if the process p_1 cannot be executed", i.e., the process p_1 has a higher priority than the process p_2.

Definition 2. *A process term p is a well-typed expression defined by the following grammar:*

$$p ::= \text{success} \mid \left[g \Rightarrow \langle s_i, a_i \rangle_i\right] \mid p(t_1, \ldots, t_n) \mid p;p \mid p \parallel p \mid p+p \mid p \oplus p$$

Process abstractions are intended to give a description of the behaviour of processes. Some restrictions are required on the (recursive) definitions of process abstractions in order to avoid pathologic cases, especially processes with an infinite branching degree. A common solution to avoid such problems consists in requiring process abstractions to be *guarded*.

Definition 3. *A process abstraction p is defined by a sentence of the form*

$$p(x_1, \ldots, x_n) \Leftarrow \bigoplus_{i=1}^{m} \alpha_i; \ p_i$$

where (for each i) α_i is an action and p_i is a process term. For a readable presentation, we omit here some formal technical conditions on the use of variables.

According to definition 3 a process abstraction is defined by a set (ordered by priority) of "formulæ", which consist of a (guarded) action and a process term.

Example 2. inc-dec is a process on a store C receiving via a queue named q messages for incrementation (*inc*) or decrementation (*dec*) of the value of a counter named *val*.

$$\begin{aligned}
\text{inc-dec} \Leftarrow & \ [head(q) == inc \Rightarrow \langle C, val{:=}val{+}1 \rangle; \ \langle C, deq(q) \rangle]; \ \text{inc-dec} \\
\oplus & \ [head(q) == dec \Rightarrow \langle C, val{:=}val{-}1 \rangle; \ \langle C, deq(q) \rangle]; \ \text{inc-dec}
\end{aligned}$$

The elementary action new presented in the previous section allows to extend the signature of the store with new symbols for functions or predicates. As these symbols are created dynamically and can be passed, we can model mobile processes in the same way as in the π-calculus [20], namely by passing the *names* of communication channels.

As an example, consider a process, p_1, which creates a new channel, q, of type t and communicates it to a process p_2 in order to receive messages from p_2 via channel q. The creation of q is performed by the action $\text{new}(q, List(t))$. There are several ways for p_1 to communicate the channel q to p_2 (e.g., by sending q through a channel or by using parameter passing). Since channels in our setting are modelled as changing constants, passing q to p_2 requires some caution. Indeed, passing the channel q to p_2 does not mean passing the *value* of q but rather its name (or a reference to it) in order to enable p_2 to send messages to p_1 via q.

5   Example of the Multiple Counters

Our solution for the problem of the multiple counters presented in Sect. 2 separates the counters from the window system. This is similar to real window systems, where applications may run on a machine connected via the network to the machine controlling the monitor. Thus we have two stores: one for the processes modelling the counters, say C, and one for the window system, say X. In this paper, we focus on the component with store C.

The store C describes a theory for counters. We model a counter c as a constant of type Cnt, i.e., a pair $\langle val, wins \rangle$, where $c.val$ indicates the current value of the counter c and $c.wins$ is a list of the window identifiers of the windows associated with c, i.e., the windows displaying the value of c. The only (high-level) events (occurring in a counter window) we consider are clicks on the different buttons. Thus we define the type $Evts$ to be the set $\{inc, copy, link\}$. In this paper, we assume that the translation of the low-level events, e.g., "click at position (x, y)" is handled by another process. For a counter c, the function bmp returns the bitmap to display for c.

The store X of the window system is a description of a theory for windows and contains in the (changing) constant $winlist$ descriptions for all the windows currently displayed on the screen. Each descriptor contains at least the identifier of the window, its position, the bitmap to be displayed and the event-queue where the events occurring in the window should be sent to. To simplify, we do not precise the data-structure of $winlist$ further.

Figure 3 shows the process abstractions for the processes located on the store C. The process abstraction controlling a counter-window is cnt_ctrl. It has three parameters: the name c of the associated counter, the identifier w of the window and the name e of the event-queue to which the window system sends all the events occurring in the window w. cnt_ctrl takes the (high-level) events (occurring in the window w) one by one from the queue e and reacts accordingly. For instance an event representing a click on the copy-button will create a new counter, named c', and a new event-queue, named e', send a request for creating a new window to the queue $newwins$ on the store X and launch a concurrent process for handling the new window for the counter named c'. An event corresponding to a click on the increment-button will increment the counter c and trigger the redrawing of all windows associated to c by executing the elementary action refresh_wins on the store X. refresh_wins has two parameters: a list of window identifiers l and a bitmap b. For each window identifier w in l, it updates the bitmap associated to w in the constant $winlist$.

The creation of a new window proceeds in two steps: requests sent to the store X are eventually acknowledged by the attribution of a new window identifier. These requests are pairs of a bitmap for the window and the name of the event-queue where events occurring in the window should be sent to. Hence, before starting a process controlling a new window, we have to wait for this acknowledgement. For this, we use another process abstraction, namely create_win.

6   Example of the Dining Philosophers

Coping with mutual exclusion is simple in our framework, since the execution of actions is (locally) atomic, see Sect. 7. Thus, we can easily program the problem

$$\begin{aligned}
&\text{cnt\_ctrl}(c\colon \textbf{Name}(\mathit{Cnt});\ e\colon \textbf{Name}(\mathit{List}(\mathit{Evts}));\ w\colon \mathit{Wid}) \Leftarrow \\
&\quad \left[head(e) == inc \Rightarrow \begin{array}{l} \langle C,\ c.val{:=}c.val{+}1\rangle;\ \langle C,\ \text{deq}(e)\rangle; \\ \langle X,\ \text{refresh\_wins}(c.wins, bmp(c))\rangle \end{array} \right];\ \text{cnt\_ctrl}(c, e, w) \\
&\oplus \left[head(e) == copy \Rightarrow \begin{array}{l} \langle C,\ \text{new}(c', \mathit{Cnt})\rangle;\ \langle C,\ c'.wins{:=}nil\rangle;\ \langle C,\ c'.val{:=}c.val\rangle; \\ \langle C,\ \text{new}(e', \mathit{List}(\mathit{Evts}))\rangle;\ \langle C,\ e'{:=}nil\rangle; \\ \langle X,\ \text{enq}(newwins, \langle bmp(c), e'\rangle)\rangle;\ \langle C,\ \text{deq}(e)\rangle \end{array} \right]; \\
&\qquad \text{create\_win}(c', e') \parallel \text{cnt\_ctrl}(c, e, w) \\
&\oplus \left[head(e) == link \Rightarrow \begin{array}{l} \langle C,\ \text{new}(e', \mathit{List}(\mathit{Evts}))\rangle;\ \langle C,\ e'{:=}nil\rangle; \\ \langle C,\ \text{deq}(e)\rangle;\ \langle X,\ \text{enq}(newwins, \langle bmp(c), e'\rangle)\rangle \end{array} \right]; \\
&\qquad \text{create\_win}(c, e') \parallel \text{cnt\_ctrl}(c, e, w) \\[4pt]
&\text{create\_win}(c\colon \textbf{Name}(\mathit{Cnt});\ e\colon \textbf{Name}(\mathit{List}(\mathit{Evts}))) \Leftarrow \\
&\quad \left[head(newwids).evt == e \Rightarrow \begin{array}{l} \langle C,\ c.wins{:=}cons(head(newwids).wid, c.wins)\rangle; \\ \langle C,\ \text{deq}(newwids)\rangle \end{array} \right]; \\
&\qquad \text{cnt\_ctrl}(c, e, head(c.wins))
\end{aligned}$$

Fig. 3. Process abstractions for processes located on the store C

of the "Dining Philosophers" by using an action which atomically tests for the presence of the two sticks (or forks) and gets them, if they are present.

We model the situation with two predicates: $stick(x)$ and $is\_eating(y)$. The former represents the fact that stick x is lying on the table, and the latter holds whenever philosopher y is eating. We can model the behaviour of a philosopher by the process abstractions of Fig. 4.

$$\begin{aligned}
&\text{thinks}(x, n\colon \mathit{Nat}) \Leftarrow \left[\begin{array}{l} stick(x) \quad \wedge \\ stick(x{+}1 \bmod n) \end{array} \Rightarrow \begin{array}{l} \langle F,\ \text{del}(stick(x))\rangle; \\ \langle F,\ \text{del}(stick(x{+}1 \bmod n))\rangle; \\ \langle F,\ \text{tell}(is\_eating(x))\rangle \end{array} \right];\ \text{eats}(x, n) \\[6pt]
&\text{eats}(x, n\colon \mathit{Nat}) \Leftarrow \left[true \Rightarrow \begin{array}{l} \langle F,\ \text{del}(is\_eating(x))\rangle \\ \langle F,\ \text{tell}(stick(x))\rangle \\ \langle F,\ \text{tell}(stick(x{+}1 \bmod n))\rangle \end{array} \right];\ \text{thinks}(x, n)
\end{aligned}$$

Fig. 4. Process abstractions for the Dining Philosophers (located on store F)

Note that we need neither low-level synchronisation (like semaphores), nor auxiliary constructions (as placing the table in a separate room or asymmetric philosophers) nor any special assumptions about the underlying logic program.

7   Operational Semantics

To simplify the presentation, we consider in this paper only the operational semantics of a single component, since the semantics presented here can be easily extended to several components. Informally, a component in our framework is a pair $C = \langle \mathcal{F}, \mathcal{P} \rangle$ where $\mathcal{F}$ stands for the store (with storename s) and $\mathcal{P}$ for the set of process abstractions.

The operational semantics of a component has to take into account two different aspects, namely the execution of processes and actions, and interactive goal-solving or expression evaluation. Thus, we present the operational semantics in two steps. First, we describe the execution of processes by a transition system T. Then we combine these rules in an "orthogonal" way with rules describing the interactive use of the store, leading to a second transition system $\mathcal{T}$ which defines the operational semantics of a component.

The operational semantics of a process is the set of sequences of actions that can be observed when executing a process. The execution of a process is described by the transition system $T = \langle Q, \longrightarrow, \langle \mathcal{F}^i, p^i, nil \rangle \rangle$. The states of T, i.e., Q, are triples, e.g., $\langle \mathcal{F}, p, m \rangle$, consisting of a store $\mathcal{F}$, a process term p and a mail-box m, acting as a fifo-channel on which the component receives (sequences of) elementary actions to execute (emanating from other components). In the sequel, we represent the mail-boxes as lists, and write $[e]$ for the (singleton) list $cons(e, nil)$ and $l_1 :: l_2$ for the concatenation of the lists l_1 and l_2. The initial state of T is built from the initial store $\mathcal{F}^i$ and the initial process term p^i, which are both specified by the programmer. The transition relation $\longrightarrow$ is defined by a set of inference rules shown in Fig. 5.

According to Rule (R1), execution of the process success is always possible and yields the special symbol ss. The latter witnesses successful termination.

The execution of a closed action, i.e., an action without free variables, is described by Rule (R2), under the premise of the validity of the guard in the current store $(\mathcal{F} \vdash g)$. Since an action may contain elementary actions on several stores, we have to distinguish between elementary actions meant for the local store (denoted by the (storename) constant self) and all the others. In the first case, we update the local store, in the second we send a message containing the sequence of elementary actions (together with their arguments) to the remote component which has to ensure the execution.

Hence, Rule (R2) uses two auxiliary functions, namely $exec$ and sel. sel filters the elementary actions for a given storename from a sequence of pairs of storenames and elementary actions, and $exec$ describes the execution of a sequence of elementary actions. Their definitions are as follows:

$$sel(s, l) = \begin{cases} l & \text{if } l \text{ is empty, i.e., } l = nil, \\ cons\big(\mathsf{a}, sel(s, tail(l))\big) & \text{if } head(l) = \langle s', \mathsf{a} \rangle \text{ and } s = s', \\ sel(s, tail(l)) & \text{otherwise.} \end{cases}$$

$$exec(\mathsf{a}_1; \ldots; \mathsf{a}_n, \mathcal{F}) = \mathsf{a}_n \underbrace{(\cdots(}_{n-2} \mathsf{a}_2(\mathsf{a}_1(\mathcal{F}))\underbrace{)\cdots)}_{n-2}$$

$$(R1) \frac{}{\langle \mathcal{F}, \text{success}, m \rangle \longrightarrow \langle \mathcal{F}, \text{ss}, m' \rangle}$$

$$(R2) \frac{\mathcal{F} \vdash g}{\langle \mathcal{F}, [g \Rightarrow \langle s_i, a_i \rangle_i], m \rangle \longrightarrow \langle exec(sel(\text{self}, \langle s_i, a_i \rangle_i), \mathcal{F}), \text{ss}, m' \rangle}$$

$$(R3) \frac{(p(x_1, \ldots, x_n) \Leftarrow \bigoplus_{i=1}^{m} \alpha_i; \; p_i) \in \mathcal{P}}{\langle \mathcal{F}, (\bigoplus_{i=1}^{m} rename(\alpha_i; \; p_i))[v_i/x_i], m \rangle \longrightarrow \langle \mathcal{F}', p', m' \rangle}{\langle \mathcal{F}, p(v_1, \ldots, v_n), m \rangle \longrightarrow \langle \mathcal{F}', p', m' \rangle}$$

$$(R4) \frac{\langle \mathcal{F}, p_1, m \rangle \longrightarrow \langle \mathcal{F}', p_1', m' \rangle}{\langle \mathcal{F}, p_1; p_2, m \rangle \longrightarrow \langle \mathcal{F}', p_1'; p_2, m' \rangle} p_1' \neq \text{ss} \qquad (R4') \frac{\langle \mathcal{F}, p_1, m \rangle \longrightarrow \langle \mathcal{F}', \text{ss}, m' \rangle}{\langle \mathcal{F}, p_1; p_2, m \rangle \longrightarrow \langle \mathcal{F}', p_2, m' \rangle}$$

$$(R5) \frac{\langle \mathcal{F}, p_1, m \rangle \longrightarrow \langle \mathcal{F}', p_1', m' \rangle}{\langle \mathcal{F}, p_1 \parallel p_2, m \rangle \longrightarrow \langle \mathcal{F}', p_1' \parallel p_2, m' \rangle} p_1' \neq \text{ss} \qquad (R5') \frac{\langle \mathcal{F}, p_1, m \rangle \longrightarrow \langle \mathcal{F}', \text{ss}, m' \rangle}{\langle \mathcal{F}, p_1 \parallel p_2, m \rangle \longrightarrow \langle \mathcal{F}', p_2, m' \rangle}$$

$$(R6) \frac{\langle \mathcal{F}, p_1, m \rangle \longrightarrow \langle \mathcal{F}', p_1', m' \rangle}{\langle \mathcal{F}, p_1 + p_2, m \rangle \longrightarrow \langle \mathcal{F}', p_1', m' \rangle}$$

$$(R7) \frac{\langle \mathcal{F}, p_1, m \rangle \longrightarrow \langle \mathcal{F}', p_1', m' \rangle}{\langle \mathcal{F}, p_1 \oplus p_2, m \rangle \longrightarrow \langle \mathcal{F}', p_1', m' \rangle} \qquad (R7') \frac{\langle \mathcal{F}, p_2, m \rangle \longrightarrow \langle \mathcal{F}', p_2', m' \rangle}{\langle \mathcal{F}, p_1 \oplus p_2, m \rangle \longrightarrow \langle \mathcal{F}', p_2', m' \rangle} \\ \text{if } \nexists p_1'(\neq p_1), \nexists \mathcal{F}'' \text{ s.t. } \langle \mathcal{F}, p_1 \rangle \longrightarrow \langle \mathcal{F}'', p_1' \rangle$$

Fig. 5. Inference rules defining the transition relation $\longrightarrow$ of T
We omitted the symmetric versions of the rules (R5), (R5′) and (R6).
The side-condition $\exists m'' \colon m' = m \colon\colon m''$ applies to all rules.

Note that the execution of an action is (locally) atomic, i.e., all the elementary actions (for a same store) of an action are executed in a single step. An example for the usefulness of the atomic execution of actions is the program for the dining philosophers (see Sect. 6) where a philosopher may take the two needed sticks in a single atomic step.

According to Rule (R3), a call to a process abstraction corresponds to execute an (instantiated) *variant* of the definition of the process abstraction. Such a variant is obtained by renaming in the defining "formulæ" of the process abstraction the symbols defined in elementary actions **new** by fresh ones. We denote this renaming by the operation *rename*. This is similar to the application of clauses in logic programming, where implicitly each variable is renamed by a fresh one, i.e., a new and unused variable.

Rules (R4) to (R6) describe the standard semantics of the operators ;, $\parallel$ and +. In the process-term $p_1 \oplus p_2$, the process p_2 will only be executed when (in the current store) an execution of p_1 is impossible (see Rule (R7′)). In contrary, p_1 can be executed independently from the executability of p_2 (see Rule (R7)).

Intuitively, the modifications of the channel m model the reception of (sequences of) elementary actions emanating from other components of the system. Due to space limitations we do not detail these communications between components further. However, the execution of elementary actions from the channel m is described by the rule (R8):

$$\text{(R8)}\frac{}{\langle \mathcal{F}, p, [(a_i)_i] :: m\rangle \longrightarrow \langle exec((a_i)_i, \mathcal{F}), p, m'\rangle}\exists m'' : m' = m :: m''$$

Besides the execution of the processes modifying the store, described by the transitions system T, the operational semantics of a component C has another, orthogonal aspect, namely the classical operational semantics of the underlying declarative program used for interactive goal-solving. We suppose that the latter is described by a relation $\twoheadrightarrow$.

Therefore we can describe the operational semantics of a component C via a new transition system, $\mathcal{T} = \langle \mathcal{Q}, \longmapsto, \langle \mathcal{F}^i, p^i, nil, g^i\rangle\rangle$, where g^i denotes the (possibly empty) initial goal the user wants to solve. The states of $\mathcal{T}$ are *configurations*, i.e., tuples $\langle \mathcal{F}, p, m, g\rangle$, where $\mathcal{F}$ is the current store, p is the current process term, m is the mailbox and g is the current expression to evaluate (according to the operational semantics of the underlying declarative language).

Classically, configurations of a concurrent language are described only by the first two parts, say $\langle \mathcal{F}, p\rangle$, which are enough to express the execution of processes. As for declarative languages, a configuration classically uses the first and the fourth parts $\langle \mathcal{F}, g\rangle$ which allow to express the rules of the operational semantics $\twoheadrightarrow$ of the declarative language. Combining these two operational semantics adds the possibility to run concurrent applications without loosing the characteristics of declarative languages. For instance, goals can be solved while the processes keep on running.

The transition relation of $\mathcal{T}$, i.e., $\longmapsto$, is defined by the two inference rules:

$$\text{(G)}\frac{\langle \mathcal{F}, g\rangle \twoheadrightarrow \langle \mathcal{F}, g'\rangle}{\langle \mathcal{F}, p, m, g\rangle \longmapsto \langle \mathcal{F}, p, m', g'\rangle}\exists m'' : m' = m :: m'' \qquad \text{(P)}\frac{\langle \mathcal{F}, p, m\rangle \longrightarrow \langle \mathcal{F}', p', m'\rangle}{\langle \mathcal{F}, p, m, g\rangle \longmapsto \langle \mathcal{F}', p', m', g^i\rangle}$$

Rule (G) concerns interactive goal-solving, i.e., the use of the operational semantics of the declarative language, as for instance goal solving (in logic languages) or evaluation of expressions (in functional languages). In the example of the dining philosophers, we might ask for the eating philosophers by solving the goal is_eating(x). Rule (P) describes the modifications of the store by the processes via the transition system T. When a process modifies the store, we have to restart the goal-solving at the initial goal (g^i), as the modification may invalidate the already achieved derivation. Obviously, rule (P) has to be refined. For instance, if the execution of a process does not alter the definitions used so far in the evaluation of the goal, restarting the goal-solving is unnecessary.

8   Related Work

Due to lack of space we do not survey all the propositions in the area in depth, but focus on some of those which are close to our suggested framework.

One of the main advantages of logic programming is its semantics (least Herbrand model). However, if we consider a Horn clause such as $p(x) \Leftarrow q, p(x)$, the denotation of p is empty according to the classical semantics of logic programs (i.e., for any x, $p(x)$ does not hold). But seen as a process, the semantics of p is the infinite sequence q^ω. Hence, we preferred to distinguish processes and predicates, which is not the case for most concurrent extensions of logic programming.

Besides this fundamental difference, there are several similarities. In concurrent constraint programming (ccp, [24]), agents communicate also via a common (constraint) store. However, the only actions on this store are telling a new constraint and asking if the current store entails a constraint. While the original model is limited to a monotonic evolution of the store, there have been several suggestions for non-monotonic extensions, e.g., [4, 9, 10, 13, 25–27]. These extension either provide new built-in actions [9, 10, 27] or use non-monotonic logics, as logic with defaults [25] or linear logic [4, 13, 26].

The logic programming language Prolog provides two "predicates" that allow one to modify the logic program by adding and deleting clauses, namely assert and retract [11]. Since these "extra-logical operators" have no declarative reading, they have been interpreted in [5, 8] as send and receive operations on a multiset of atoms, called "blackboard". Our approach is more general, as our stores allow the modification of more than only a multiset of atoms.

The notion of *ports* as a many-to-one communication medium has been introduced in AKL [17]. It is argued that the introduced port primitives have a "logical reading" and preserve the monotonicity of the constraint store. In our non-monotonic setting, we can provide the behaviour of ports via appropriate (elementary) actions, e.g., enq and deq. Recently, the idea of ports, has been extended and integrated into the functional-logic language Curry in order to cope with distributed applications [16].

Pure functional programs can also be easily parallelised: as the evaluation of expressions has no side-effects, the function-arguments can be evaluated in parallel. But this *implicit* parallelism is to be distinguished from (by the programmer) *explicitly* specified concurrency. Several concurrent extensions have been suggested for functional languages, most of them do not distinguish between processes and functions [21, 23].

Concurrent Haskell (CH) [21] introduces new primitives starting processes (e.g., forkIO) which can communicate and synchronise via mutable variables (of a new built-in type MVar). These primitives are meant as "raw iron from which more friendly abstractions can be built" [21]. This is different from our philosophy: we want to exhibit the high-level abstractions needed for easy programming and not the minimal set of low-level primitives. Also, our actions together with, e.g., "changing constants", are a more flexible support for communication. CML [23] also provides new primitives, supporting a synchronisation mechanism based on "events", a new abstract type representing "potential communication". To effectively communicate, a process has to synchronise on an event.

Facile [28] extends the functional language ML with "behaviour-expressions" and (synchronous communication) "channels". As behaviour-expressions can be transformed into a value, called a process "script", programming with processes in a functional style is supported. A script s can be executed by evaluating

spawn s which has the side-effect of spawning a new process. Thus, Facile allows functions and processes to use each other mutually. In our framework, the use of processes for the definition of functions or predicates is not necessary. However, the communication between processes in Facile is restricted to message passing through channels, which is a special case of the communication via stores.

Our framework extends classical process algebras, e.g., CCS [19], CSP [6] or ACP [3] in several aspects. First, our processes (and actions) are parameterised. Second, our actions have a precise semantics as transformations of a global store. Last but not least, our framework provides the possibility of (interactive) declarative programming, i.e., evaluation of expression and goal solving, along with concurrent execution of processes.

Our elementary action **new** together with the parameterised type $\mathtt{Name}(t)$ allows to model mobility in the same way as the π-calculus [20]. However, the communication mechanism of the π-calculus is synchronous and exclusively based on message passing (thus one-to-one), whereas our framework is based on asynchronous, broadcasting communication via a shared store. Thus, our proposal is more related to the asynchronous trend of the π-calculus. Our guards allow the atomic reception on several channels, whereas in the π-calculus processes can only wait on a single channel. Extensions of the (asynchronous) π-calculus without this restriction are the join-calculus [14] and $\mathcal{L}_\pi$ [7].

In the join-calculus [14] processes can be seen as communicating via a multiset of messages: sending a message corresponds to place it in the multiset, and the "joint reception" of several messages is blocking and removes the received messages from the multiset. Thus broadcast is not provided directly and has to be encoded as in any π-calculus-based language.

Last but not least, promising approaches using linear logic as a basis to define frameworks for the description of the semantics of higher-level languages which integrate declarative programming with object-oriented or concurrent features have been proposed in the literature, see e.g., [2, 7, 18]. These approaches can be adapted to our framework in order to give an alternative semantics based on proof search in linear logic.

9   Conclusion

We have presented a generic framework for the combination of mobile processes and declarative programming languages. Our proposition differs from most related frameworks in that it distinguishes syntactically and semantically between the notion of processes and that of functions or predicates. Thus our framework does not force programmers to encode some concepts by means of others, but allows to express everything by the most appropriate concept.

Processes are parameterised and communicate asynchronously via the modification of stores. Classical communication media, namely channels, are modelled as (changing) constants. This view of channels has both, a functional reading and a (constraint) logical reading. New channels (as well as new functions) can be created thanks to the (built-in) action **new**. This action, combined with the parameterised type Name(t), allows one to model mobility and thus generalises the notions introduced in the π-calculus to declarative languages.

The complete formal definitions of this framework together with the extension to several components can be found in [12]. The implementation of a prototype is under progress.

Acknowledgements.

We are grateful to Bernd Braßel, Michael Hanus, and Frank Steiner for fruitful discussions on a preliminary version of this paper.

References

1. J.-R. Abrial. *Formal Methods for Industrial Applications*, volume 1165 of *LNCS*, chapter Steam-Boiler Control Specification Problem, pages 500–510. Springer, 1996.
2. J.-M. Andreoli and R. Pareschi. Linear objects: Logical processes with built-in inheritance. *New Generation Computing*, 9(3–4):445–473, 1991. selected papers from the 7th Int. Conf. on Logic Programming, 1990.
3. J. C. M. Baeten and W. P. Weijland. *Process Algebra*. Number 18 in Cambridge Tracts in Theoretical Computer Science. Cambridge University Press, 1990.
4. E. Best, F. de Boer, and C. Palamidessi. Partial order and SOS semantics for linear constraint programs. In D. Garlan and D. L. Métayer, editors, *Proc. of the 2nd Int. Conf. on Coordination: Languages and Models (Coordination '97)*, volume 1282 of *LNCS*, pages 256–273, Berlin, September 1997. Springer.
5. A. Brogi and P. Ciancarini. The concurrent language, Shared Prolog. *ACM TOPLAS*, 13(1):99–123, January 1991.
6. S. D. Brookes, C. A. R. Hoare, and A. W. Roscoe. A theory of communicating sequential processes. *Journal of the ACM*, 31(3):560–599, July 1984.
7. L. Caires and L. Monteiro. Verifiable and executable logic specifications of concurrent objects in $\mathcal{L}_\pi$. In C. Hankin, editor, *Proc. of the 7th European Symp. on Programming (ESOP '98)*, volume 1381 of *LNCS*, pages 42–56, Lisbon, March–April 1998. Springer.
8. M. Carro and M. Hermenegildo. Concurrency in prolog using threads and a shared database. In *Proc. of the 16th Int. Conf. on Logic Programming (ICLP '99)*, Las Cruces, November 1999. MIT Press.
9. P. Codognet and F. Rossi. Nmcc programming: Constraint enforcement and retraction in cc programming. In *Proc. of ICLP '95*. MIT Press, 1995.
10. F. S. de Boer, J. N. Kok, C. Palamidessi, and J. J. M. M. Rutten. Non-monotonic concurrent constraint programming. In *Proc. of the Int. Symp. on Logic Programming (ILPS '93)*, pages 315–334. The MIT Press, 1993.
11. P. Deransart, A. Ed-Dbali, and L. Cervoni. *Prolog: The Standard, Reference Manual*. Springer, 1996.
12. R. Echahed and W. Serwe. A multiparadigm programming scheme. Technical Report, forthcoming.
13. F. Fages, P. Ruet, and S. Soliman. Phase semantics and verification of concurrent constraint programs. In *Proc. of the 13th Annual IEEE Symp. on Logic in Computer Science (LICS '98)*, 1998.

14. C. Fournet and G. Gonthier. The reflexive chemical abstract machine and the join-calculus. In *Proc. of the 23rd Symp. on Principles of Programming Languages (POPL '96)*, pages 372–385, St. Petersburg Beach, Florida, January 1996.

15. GUI Fest '95 Post-Challenge: multiple counters. available at http://www.cs.chalmers.se/~magnus/GuiFest-95/, July 24–July 28 1995. organized by Simon Peyton Jones and Phil Gray as a part of the Glasgow Research Festival.

16. M. Hanus. Distributed programming in a multi-paradigm declarative language. In G. Nadathur, editor, *Proc. of the Int. Conf. on Principles and Practice of Declarative Programming (PPDP '99)*, volume 1702 of *LNCS*, pages 188–205, Paris, 1999. Springer.

17. S. Janson, J. Montelius, and S. Haridi. Ports for objects in concurrent logic programs. In Agha, Wegner, and Yonezawa, editors, *Research Directions in Concurrent Object-Oriented Programming*. The MIT Press, 1993.

18. D. Miller. Forum: A multiple-conclusion specification logic. *Theoretical Computer Science*, 165(1):201–232, September 1996.

19. R. Milner. *A calculus of communicating systems*, volume 92 of *LNCS*. Springer, 1980.

20. R. Milner, J. G. Parrow, and D. J. Walker. A calculus of mobile processes. *Information and Computation*, 100(1):1–77, September 1992.

21. S. L. Peyton Jones, A. D. Gorden, and S. Finne. Concurrent Haskell. In *Proc. of the 23rd Symp. on Principles of Programming Languages (POPL '96)*, pages 295–308, St Petersburg Beach, Florida, January 1996.

22. B. C. Pierce and D. N. Turner. Pict: A programming language based on the pi-calculus. In G. Plotkin, C. Stirling, and M. Tofte, editors, *Proof, Language and Interaction: Essays in Honour of Robin Milner*. MIT Press, 1998.

23. J. H. Reppy. *Concurrent Programming in ML*. Cambridge University Press, 1999.

24. V. A. Saraswat. *Concurrent Constraint Programming*. ACM Doctoral Dissertation Awards. MIT Press, 1993.

25. V. A. Saraswat, R. Jagadeesan, and V. Gupta. Timed default concurrent constraint programming. *Journal of Symbolic Computation*, 22(5–6):475–520, November–December 1996.

26. V. A. Saraswat and P. Lincoln. Higher-order, linear, concurrent constraint programming. Technical report, Xerox PARC, 1992.

27. G. Smolka. *Computer Science Today: Recent Trends and Developments*, volume 1000 of *LNCS*, chapter The Oz Programming Model, pages 324–343. Springer, 1995. Jan van Leeuwen (Ed.).

28. B. Thomsen, L. Leth, and T.-M. Kuo. FACILE — from toy to tool. In F. Nielson, editor, *ML with Concurrency: Design, Analysis, Implementation and Application*, Monographs in Computer Science, chapter 5, pages 97–144. Springer, 1996.

29. P. Wadler. How to declare an imperative. *ACM Computing Surveys*, 29(3):240–263, September 1997.

30. P. Wegner. Interactive foundations of computing. *Theoretical Computer Science*, 192(2):315–351, February 1998.

Representing Trees with Constraints

Ben Curry[1]*, Geraint A. Wiggins[2], and Gillian Hayes[1]

[1] Institute of Perception, Action and Behaviour, Division of Informatics
University of Edinburgh, Edinburgh EH1 1HN
[2] Department of Computing, School of Informatics
City University, Northampton Square, London EC1V 0HB

Abstract. This paper presents a method for representing trees using constraint logic programming over finite domains. We describe a class of trees that is of particular interest to us and how we can represent the set of trees belonging to that class using constraints. The method enables the specification of a set of trees without having to generate all of the members of the set. This allows us to reason about sets of trees that would normally be too large to use. We present this research in the context of a system to generate expressive musical performances and, in particular, how this method can be used to represent musical structure.

1 Introduction

This paper describes how constraints can be used to represent a specific class of trees that have the following properties:

Rooted - each tree has a node distinguished as the root node.
Ordered - the children of each node are distinct and cannot be re-ordered without changing what the tree represents.
Constant Depth - the leaf nodes of each tree are all the same distance from the root.
Strict - at each depth, one of the nodes has at least two successors.

The number of distinct trees in this class is large for each n, where n is the number of leaf nodes. If $n \geq 10$ the set of trees described can not easily be manipulated or used within a computer system. We present here an efficient way of representing this large set of trees, using constraint logic programming, that enables us to use this class of trees in our research.

The structure of the paper is as follows. The next section explains why we are interested in representing sets of trees in the context of music. We then present some implementation details including our representation and the constraints used to specify the trees of interest. Some results are presented that illustrate the effectiveness of this method. Finally, we end with our conclusions.

---

* Ben Curry is supported by UK EPSRC postgraduate studentship 97305827

J. Lloyd et al. (Eds.): CL 2000, LNAI 1861, pp. 315–325, 2000.

2   Motivation: Grouping Structure

This work forms part of our research into creating an expressive musical performer that is capable of performing a piece of music alongside a human musician in an expressive manner.

An expressive performance is one in which the performer introduces variations in the timing and dynamics of the piece in order to emphasise certain aspects of it. Our hypothesis is that there is a direct correlation between these expressive gestures and the musical structure of the piece and we can use this link to generate expressive performances.

The theory of musical structure we are using is the Generative Theory of Tonal Music (GTTM) by Lerdahl and Jackendoff (1983). The theory is divided into four sections that deal with different aspects of the piece's musical structure. We are particularly interested in the *grouping structure* which corresponds with how we segment a piece of music, as we are listening to it, into a hierarchy of groups. It is this hierarchy of groups that we seek to represent with our trees.

The rules are divided into two types: *well-formedness* rules that specify what structures are possible; and *preference* rules that select, from the set of all possible structures, those that correspond most closely to the score.

The rules defining grouping structures are based on principles of change and difference. Figure 1 shows four places where a grouping boundary may be detected (denoted by a '*'). The first case is due to a relatively large leap in pitch between the third and fourth notes in comparison to the pitch leaps between the other notes. The second boundary occurs because there is a change in dynamics from piano to forte. The third and fourth boundaries are due to changes in articulation and duration respectively.

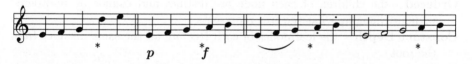

Fig. 1. Points in the score where grouping rules may apply

Figure 2 shows an example of a grouping structure for a small excerpt of music. We can see that the music has been segmented into five different groups, one for each collection of three notes. The musical rest between the third and fourth groups causes a higher level grouping boundary that makes two higher level groups which contain the five groups. These groups are then contained within one large group at the highest level.

The grouping structure can be represented with a tree. Figure 3 shows a tree representation (inverted, to aid comparison) for the grouping structure shown in Fig. 2. The leaf nodes at the top of the tree correspond to the notes in the score, and the branches convey how the notes are grouped together. This is an example of the class of tree we are trying to represent. From this point onwards the trees will be presented in the more traditional manner, i.e. the leaf nodes at the bottom and the root node at the top.

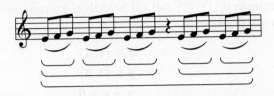

Fig. 2. An example grouping structure

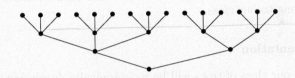

Fig. 3. Tree representing the grouping structure shown in Fig. 2

Although the GTTM grouping rules are presented formally, the preference rules introduce a large amount of ambiguity. For a particular piece of music, there are many possible grouping structures which would satisfy the preference rules. The purpose of the present research is to devise a way to represent this large set of possible structures in an efficient way so that they can be used by a computer system.

Using our hypothesis of the link between musical structure and expressive performance, one of the core ideas of our research is to use rehearsal performances by the human musician to disambiguate the large set of possible grouping trees. The expressive timing used by the musician in these rehearsals provides clues as to how the musician views the structure of the piece. A consistent pattern of timing deviations across a number of performances will enable us to high-light points in the score where the musician agrees with the possible grouping boundaries.

3   Using Constraints

This section of the paper explains how we use constraint logic programming (Van Hentenryck, 1989) to represent sets of trees. Although constraints have been used in the areas of music composition (e.g. Henz 1996) and tree drawing (e.g. Tsuchida 1997), this research is concerned with an efficient representation of large numbers of tree structures, which is a problem distinct from these.

Constraint logic programming over finite domains enables the specification of a problem in terms of variables with a range of possible values (known as the *domain* of the variable) and equations that specify the relationships between the variables. For example if (1), (2) and (3) hold then we can narrow the domains of x and y as shown in (4):

$$x \in \{1..4\} \tag{1}$$
$$y \in \{3..6\} \tag{2}$$
$$x + y \geq 9 \tag{3}$$
$$x \in \{3..4\} \wedge y \in \{5..6\} \tag{4}$$

The following sections outline the representation and the constraints we use to specify the class of trees. We begin by discussing the representation of the nodes and then present the five types of constraints used to ensure that the trees generated belong to our class.

3.1   Representation

We know that our class of trees will be monotonically decreasing in width from the leaf nodes up to the root and, therefore, we can represent the set of trees by a triangular point lattice of nodes[1]. Figure 4 shows the point lattices for trees of width $n = 3$ and $n = 4$.

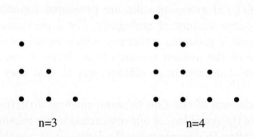

n=3   n=4

Fig. 4. Point lattices for trees of width 3 and 4

Each node has the following variables (illustrated in Fig. 5):

1. *id*: a unique identifier;
2. *uplink*: a connection to the level above;

---

[1] An implementation detail means that there is always a path from the highest node of the point lattice to the leaf nodes, but this highest node should not be considered the root node. The root node may occur at any height in the point lattice and is identified as the highest node with more than one child.

3. Downlink values which represent all the nodes on the level below that are connected to this one.

The *id* is specified as an (x,y) coordinate to simplify the implementation details. The *uplink* variable contains an integer that represents the x-coordinate of the node on the level above to which this node is connected i.e. node *(uplink,* $y + 1$*)*. The downlink values, specified by a lower *(dl)* and upper *(du)* bound, refer to a continuous range of nodes on the level below that may be connected to this one i.e. nodes *(dl, y − 1)*...*(du, y − 1)*.

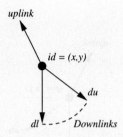

Fig. 5. A typical node

The next sections present the constraints that are applied to the nodes in order to create the specific set of trees in which we are interested. They begin by specifying the domains of the variables and then constraining the nodes so that only those trees that belong to our class can be generated.

3.2   Node Constraints

The first task is to define the domains of the variables for each node. Due to the triangular shape of the point lattice, the uplink for each node is constrained to point either upwards, or up and to the left of the current node. We constrain the downlink for each node to span the nodes directly below, and below and to the right of the current node.

The constraints (given in (5)-(8)) define the domains of the *uplink* and downlink range (i.e. *dl* and *du*) for each node[2]. The *uplink* lies in the range $\{0..x\}$ where x is the x-coordinate of the current node. The zero in the range is used when the node is not connected to the level above.

$$domain([uplink]) = \{0..x\} \tag{5}$$
$$domain([dl, du]) = \{0..n\} \tag{6}$$
$$(dl = 0) \oplus (dl \geq x) \tag{7}$$
$$du \geq dl \tag{8}$$

---

[2] The $\oplus$ in (7) denotes exclusive-or.

The downlink specifiers dl and du are constrained in a similar way to lie in a range from $\{0..n\}$ with the added constraints that du has to be greater than or equal to dl and that dl either equals zero or is greater than or equal to x. Figure 6 shows how these constraints relate to the direction of the connections to and from each node.

Constraint (9) handles the situation of a node which is not used in a tree. If the *uplink* of the node is zero then the downlinks of the node must also be zero.

$$((dl = 0) \Leftrightarrow (du = 0)) \wedge ((dl = 0) \Leftrightarrow (uplink = 0)) \tag{9}$$

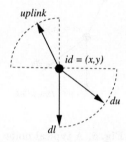

Fig. 6. Constraining the Uplinks and Downlinks

3.3 Level Constraints

To ensure that the connections between two levels do not cross, constraints (10) and (11) are applied to each pair of adjacent nodes. For a pair of nodes A and B, with A directly to the left of B, the $uplink_B$ must either point to the same node as the $uplink_A$ or to the node to the right of it or, if it is unused, be equal to zero (10).

$$(uplink_B = uplink_A) \vee (uplink_B = uplink_A + 1) \vee (uplink_B = 0) \tag{10}$$

Once one of the uplinks on a particular level becomes equal to zero, all the uplinks to the right of it must also be zero (11). This prevents the situation of an unconnected node in the midst of connected ones.

$$(uplink_A = 0) \Rightarrow (uplink_B = 0) \tag{11}$$

Figure 7 shows examples of correct and incorrect mid-sections of a tree under these new constraints. The bottom example is incorrect because it violates constraints (10) and (11).

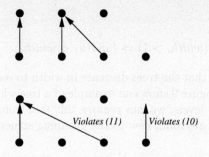

Fig. 7. A correct (*top*) and incorrect (*bottom*) mid-section of a tree

3.4 Consistency Constraints

If the current node refers to a node in the level above, the *x*-coordinate of this node must appear within its downlink range. Constraint (12) ensures that if this node points to a node on the level above, the downlink range of that node must include this one. Figure 8 shows how this constraint affects two nodes where the lower one is connected to the upper one.

$$(x_{above} = uplink_{this}) \Leftrightarrow ((x_{this} \geq dl_{above}) \wedge (x_{this} \leq du_{above})) \tag{12}$$

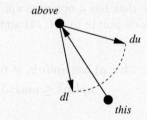

Fig. 8. Ensuring connectivity between nodes

3.5 Width Constraints

We now constrain the trees to decrease in width as we travel from the leaf nodes to the root node. The width of a level is defined as the number of nodes that have a non-zero uplink on that level. Constraint (13) deals with this situation with the precondition that the width of the current level is greater than 1. This precondition is necessary to allow situations such as the first four trees in Fig. 10 where we consider the root node to be at the point where branching begins.

$$(width_i > 1) \Rightarrow (width_j < width_i) \tag{13}$$

We want to ensure that the trees decrease in width to reduce the search space as much as possible. Figure 9 shows an example of a tree which does not decrease in width between two levels, we can remove this tree from our search space as it does not contribute anything new to the grouping structure as we move from level i to level j.

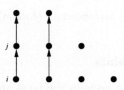

Fig. 9. A section of a tree that does not decrease in width

3.6   Edge Constraints

The last step is to ensure that the uplink of the rightmost[3] node on a level points inwards (the rightmost node in Fig. 7 is an example of this). We find the maximum x of the level above that has a non-zero *uplink* and then ensure that the *uplink* of the rightmost node points to it ((14) and (15)).

$$\mathcal{S} = \{x : id(x, y) \text{ has } uplink_x \neq 0\} \tag{14}$$

$$uplink \leq max(\mathcal{S}) \tag{15}$$

3.7   Valid Trees

The constraints given in §3.2 to §3.6 define the set of trees which belong to our class. Figure 10 shows an example set of width $n = 4$. The white nodes are ones that appear in the generated solutions but are not considered to be part of the tree since the root of the tree is the highest node with more than one child.

3.8   Using the Constraint Representation

The constraints which have been defined in the sections above describe a general class of trees. The next step is to introduce aspects of the grouping structure to

---

[3] By 'rightmost' we mean the node on the current level with the maximum x-coordinate that has a non-zero uplink.

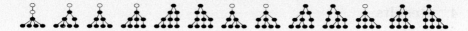

Fig. 10. All the trees of width four ($n = 4$)

reduce this large set of trees to only those trees that correspond to the piece of music being analysed.

Every point in the musical score where a grouping boundary could occur is identified, for each of these points we then measure the relative strength of this boundary against the surrounding ones. Every boundary point can then be used to determine the shape of the tree by ensuring that every pair of notes intersected by a boundary corresponds to a pair of nodes separated in the tree set.

To separate the nodes in a tree, we need to ensure that the parents of the nodes are not the same, and if we have a measure of relative strength between boundaries, we can specify how far towards the root the nodes need to be separated. The algorithm below shows how this is implemented:

> $Repel(id_A, id_B, strength)$
>   **if** $(strength \geq 1)$ **then**
> $parent(id_A) \neq parent(id_B)$
> $Repel(parent(id_A), parent(id_B), strength - 1)$
>   **endif**

This recursive predicate takes two nodes and a strength argument and recursively ensures that the nodes are separated up to a height *strength*. Figure 11 shows an example tree where the tree is divided into two subtrees by a *Repel* constraint that is applied with *strength* = 1 between the second and third leaf nodes.

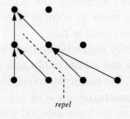

Fig. 11. How *Repel* affects the tree

4 Results

We generated all the trees up to width $n = 7$ and found a similarity with an entry in the Online Encyclopedia of Integer Sequences (Sloane, 2000). It matched a sequence discovered by the mathematician Arthur Cayley (1891) based upon this particular class of trees which has the recurrence shown in (16) and (17)[4]

This recurrence defines the number of trees that belong to our class that are of width n.

$$a(0) = 1 \tag{16}$$

$$a(n) = \sum_{k=1}^{n} \binom{n}{k} a(n-k) \tag{17}$$

Using our representation, the approximate formula, derived experimentally, for the number of constraints to represent the set of all the trees of width n is given in (18).

$$Constraints \approx \frac{2}{3}n^3 + 11n^2 - \frac{2}{3}n - 24 \tag{18}$$

The number of trees of width n grows rapidly (e.g. the number of trees of width 50 is 1.995×10^{72}). By contrast, the number of constraints it takes to represent the same number of trees is 1.1×10^5.

Figure 12 shows how the number of trees grows in comparison to the number of constraints as we increase the width of the tree. The number of trees increases at a greater than exponential rate whereas the number of constraints increases at a low-order polynomial rate.

5 Conclusions

This paper presents our research on representing a specific class of trees with constraint logic programming. Although the number of constraints needed to represent these large sets of trees is comparatively small, the computational time needed to solve the constraints is not.

The representation currently restricts the trees to have leaf nodes at the same depth; however, it does allow the addition of quite simple constraints to change the class of trees represented. For example, to restrict the trees to strictly binary trees we need only add the constraint $du = dl + 1$.

With the use of constraints we have delayed the generation of trees until we have added all the possible restrictions, this offers a great reduction in complexity and allows us to manipulate trees of greater width than would normally be possible.

---

[4] Where $\binom{n}{k}$ is the standard n choose k formula given by: $\frac{n!}{k!(n-k)!}$

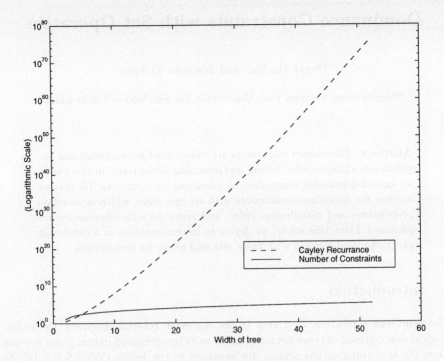

Fig. 12. A graph showing how the number of trees and number of constraints grows with the width of the tree

References

Cayley A.: On the Analytical Forms Called Trees. Coll. Math. Papers, Vol. 4. Cambridge University Press (1891)

Henz M., Lauer S. and Zimmermann D.: COMPOzE – Intention-based Music Composition through Constraint Programming. Proceedings of the 8th IEEE International Conference on Tools with Artificial Intelligence, IEEE Computer Society Press (1996)

Lerdahl F. and Jackendoff R.: A Generative Theory of Tonal Music. MIT Press (1983)

Sloane N. J. A.: The On-Line Encyclopedia of Integer Sequences. Published electronically at http://www.research.att.com/~njas/sequences/ (2000)

Tsuchida K., Adachi Y., Imaki T. and Yaku T.: Tree Drawing Using Constraint Logic Programming. Proceedings of the 14th International Conference of Logic Programming, MIT Press (1997)

Van Hentenryck P.: Constraint Satisfaction in Logic Programming. Logic Programming Series, MIT Press (1989)

Dominance Constraints with Set Operators

Denys Duchier and Joachim Niehren

Programming Systems Lab, Universität des Saarlandes Saarbrücken

Abstract. Dominance constraints are widely used in computational linguistics as a language for talking and reasoning about trees. In this paper, we extend dominance constraints by admitting set operators. We present a solver for dominance constraints with set operators, which is based on propagation and distribution rules, and prove its soundness and completeness. From this solver, we derive an implementation in a constraint programming language with finite sets and prove its faithfullness.

1 Introduction

The dominance relation of a tree is the ancestor relation between its nodes. Logical descriptions of trees via dominance were investigated in computer science since the beginning of the sixties, for instance in the logics (W)SkS [15, 16]. In computational linguistics, the importance of dominance based tree descriptions for deterministic parsing was discovered at the beginning of the eighties [9]. Since then, tree descriptions based on dominance constraints have become increasingly popular [14, 1]. Meanwhile, they are used for tree-adjoining and D-tree grammars [17, 13, 3], for underspecified representation of scope ambiguities in semantics [12, 4] and for underspecified descriptions of discourse structure [5].

A dominance constraint describes a finite tree by conjunctions of literals with variables for nodes. A dominance literal $x \triangleleft^* y$ requires x to denote one of the ancestors of the denotation of y. A labeling literal $x{:}f(x_1, \ldots, x_n)$ expresses that the node denoted by x is labeled with symbol f and has the sequence of children referred to by $x_1, \ldots, x_n$. Solving dominance constraints is an essential service required by applications in e.g. semantics and discourse. Even though satisfiability of dominance constraints is NP-complete [8], it appears that dominance constraints occurring in these applications can be solved rather efficiently [2, 7].

For a typical application of dominance constraints in semantic underspecification of scope we consider the sentence: *every yogi has a guru*. This sentence is semantically ambiguous, even though its syntactic structure is uniquely determined. The trees in Figure 1 specify both meanings: either there exists a common guru for every yogi, or every yogi has his own guru. Both trees (and thus meanings) can be represented in an underspecified manner through the dominance constraint in Figure 2.

In this paper, we propose to extend dominance constraints by admitting set operators: union, intersection, and complementation can be applied to the relations of dominance $\triangleleft^*$ and inverse dominance $\triangleright^*$. Set operators contribute

J. Lloyd et al. (Eds.): CL 2000, LNAI 1861, pp. 326–341, 2000.
© Springer-Verlag Berlin Heidelberg 2000

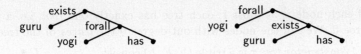

Fig. 1. Sets of trees represent sets of meanings.

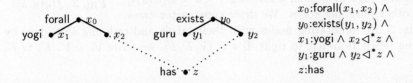

x_0:forall(x_1, x_2) $\wedge$
y_0:exists(y_1, y_2) $\wedge$
x_1:yogi $\wedge$ $x_2 \lhd^* z$ $\wedge$
y_1:guru $\wedge$ $y_2 \lhd^* z$ $\wedge$
z:has

Fig. 2. A single tree description as underspecified representation of all meanings.

a controlled form of disjunction and negation that is eminently well-suited for constraint propagation while less expressive than general Boolean connectives. Set operators allow to express proper dominance, disjointness, nondisjointness, nondominance, and unions thereof. Such a rich set of relations is important for specifying powerful constraint propagation rules for dominance constraints as we will argue in the paper.

We first present a system of abstract saturation rules for propagation and distribution, which solve dominance constraints with set operators. We illustrate the power of the propagation rules and prove soundness, completeness, and termination in nondeterministic polynomial time. We then derive a concrete implementation in a constraint programming language with finite sets [11, 6] and prove its faithfulness to the abstract saturation rules. The resulting solver is not only well suited for formal reasoning but also improves in expressiveness on the saturation based solver for pure dominance constraints of [8] and produces smaller search trees than the earlier set based implementation of [2] because it requires less explicit solved forms. For omitted proofs, we globally refer to the extended version of this paper available from http://www.ps.uni-sb.de/Papers/.

2 Dominance Constraints

We first define tree structures and then dominance constraints with set operators which are interpreted in the class of tree structures. We assume a signature Σ of function symbols ranged over by $f, g, \ldots$, each of which is equipped with an arity $\mathsf{ar}(f) \geq 0$. Constants – function symbols of arity 0 – are ranged over by a, b. We assume that Σ contains at least one constant and one symbol of arity at least 2. We are interested in finite constructor trees that can be seen as ground terms over Σ such as $f(g(a, b))$ in Fig. 3.

We define an *(unlabeled) tree* to be a finite directed graph (V, E). V is a finite sets of *nodes* ranged over by u, v, w, and $E \subseteq V \times V$ is a finite set of *edges*. The in-degree of each node is at most 1; each tree has exactly one *root*, i.e. a node with in-degree 0. We call the nodes with out-degree 0 the *leaves* of the tree.

A *(finite) constructor tree* τ is a triple (V, E, L) consisting of a tree (V, E), and *labelings* $L : V \to \Sigma$ for nodes and
$L : E \to N$ for edges, such that any node $u \in V$ has exactly
one outgoing edge with label k for each $1 \leq k \leq \mathsf{ar}(\sigma(\pi))$,
and no other outgoing edges. We draw constructor trees

Fig. 3. $f(g(a, b))$

as in Fig. 3, by annotating nodes with their labels and ordering the edges by increasing labels from left to right. If $\tau = (V, E, L)$, we write $V_\tau = V$, $E_\tau = E$, $L_\tau = L$.

Definition 1. *The* tree structure $\mathcal{M}^\tau$ *of a finite constructor tree τ over Σ is the first-order structure with domain V_τ which provides the* dominance relation $\lhd^{*\tau}$ *and a* labeling relation *of arity* $\mathsf{ar}(f) + 1$ *for each function symbol $f \in \Sigma$. These relations are defined such that for all $u, v, u_1, \ldots, u_n \in V_\tau$:*

$$u \lhd^{*\tau} v \qquad \text{iff there is a path from } u \text{ to } v \text{ with egdes in } E_\tau;$$
$$u{:}f^\tau(v_1, \ldots, v_n) \text{ iff } L_\tau(u) = f, \mathsf{ar}(f) = n, \text{ and } L(u, v_i) = i \text{ for all } 1 \leq i \leq n$$

We consider the following *set operators* on binary relations: inversion $^{-1}$, union $\cup$, intersection $\cap$, and complementation $\neg$. We write $\rhd^{*\tau}$ for the inverse of dominance $\lhd^{*\tau}$, equality $=^\tau$ for the intersection $\lhd^{*\tau} \cap \rhd^{*\tau}$, inequality $\neq^\tau$ for the complement of equality, proper dominance $\lhd^{+\tau}$ as dominance but not equality, $\rhd^{+\tau}$ for the inverse of proper dominance, and disjointness $\perp^\tau$ for $\neg\lhd^{*\tau} \cap \neg\rhd^{*\tau}$. Most importantly, the following partition holds in all tree structures $\mathcal{M}^\tau$.

$$V_\tau \times V_\tau \quad = \quad \uplus\{=^\tau, \lhd^{+\tau}, \rhd^{+\tau}, \perp^\tau\}$$

Thus, all relations that set operators can generate from dominance $\lhd^{*\tau}$ have the form $\cup\{r^\tau \mid r \in R\}$ for some set of relation symbols $R \subseteq \{=, \lhd^+, \rhd^+, \perp\}$.

For defining the constraint language, we let x, y, z range over an infinite set of node variables. A *dominance constraints with set operators* φ has the following abstract syntax (that leaves set operators implicit).

$$\varphi ::= x\,R\,y \mid x{:}f(x_1, \ldots, x_n) \mid \varphi \wedge \varphi' \mid \mathsf{false}$$

where $R \subseteq \{=, \lhd^+, \rhd^+, \perp\}$ is a set of relation symbols and $n = \mathsf{ar}(f)$. Constraints are interpreted in the class of tree structures over Σ. For instance, a constraint $x\,\{=, \perp\}\,y$ expresses that the nodes denoted by x and y are either equal or lie in disjoint subtrees. In general, a set R of relation symbols is interpreted in $\mathcal{M}^\tau$ as the union $\cup\{r^\tau \mid r \in R\}$.

We write $\mathsf{Vars}(\varphi)$ for the set of variables occurring in φ. A *solution* of a constraint φ consists of a tree structure $\mathcal{M}^\tau$ and a variable assignment $\alpha :$ $\mathsf{Vars}(\varphi) \to V_\tau$. We write $(\mathcal{M}^\tau, \alpha) \models \varphi$ if all constraints of φ are satisfied by $(\mathcal{M}^\tau, \alpha)$ in the usual Tarskian sense. For convenience we admit syntactic sugar and allow to write constraints of the form $x\,S\,y$ where S is a set expression:

$$S ::= R \mid = \mid \lhd^* \mid \rhd^* \mid = \mid \neq \mid \lhd^+ \mid \rhd^+ \mid \perp \mid \neg S \mid S_1 \cup S_2 \mid S_1 \cap S_2 \mid S^{-1}$$

Propagation Rules:

(Clash)	$x \emptyset y \;\rightarrow\;$ **false**	
(Dom.Refl)	$\varphi \;\rightarrow\; x \vartriangleleft^* x$	(x occurs in φ)
(Dom.Trans)	$x \vartriangleleft^* y \wedge y \vartriangleleft^* z \;\rightarrow\; x \vartriangleleft^* z$	
(Eq.Decom)	$x{:}f(x_1, \dots, x_n) \wedge y{:}f(y_1, \dots, y_n) \wedge x{=}y \;\rightarrow\; \bigwedge_{i=1}^{n} x_i{=}y_i$	

(Lab.Ineq)	$x{:}f(\dots) \wedge y{:}g(\dots) \;\rightarrow\; x{\neq}y$	if $f \neq g$
(Lab.Disj)	$x{:}f(\dots, x_i, \dots, x_j, \dots) \;\rightarrow\; x_i \bot x_j$	where $1 \leq i < j \leq n$
(Lab.Dom)	$x{:}f(\dots, y, \dots) \;\rightarrow\; x \vartriangleleft^+ y$	

(Inter)	$x R_1 y \wedge x R_2 y \;\rightarrow\; x R y$	if $R_1 \cap R_2 \subseteq R$
(Inv)	$x R y \;\rightarrow\; y R^{-1} x$	
(Disj)	$x \bot y \wedge y \vartriangleleft^* z \;\rightarrow\; x \bot z$	
(NegDisj)	$x \vartriangleleft^* z \wedge y \vartriangleleft^* z \;\rightarrow\; x \neg \bot y$	
(Child.up)	$x \vartriangleleft^* y \wedge x{:}f(x_1, \dots, x_n) \wedge \bigwedge_{i=1}^{n} x_i \neg \vartriangleleft^* y \;\rightarrow\; y{=}x$	

Distribution Rules:

(Distr.Child)	$x \vartriangleleft^* y \wedge x{:}f(x_1, \dots, x_n) \;\rightarrow\; x_i \vartriangleleft^* y \vee x_i \neg \vartriangleleft^* y$	$(1 \leq i \leq n)$
(Distr.NegDisj)	$x \neg \bot y \;\rightarrow\; x \vartriangleleft^* y \vee x \neg \vartriangleleft^* y$	

Fig. 4. Saturation rules D of the Base Solver

Clearly, every set expression S can be translated to a set R of relation symbols denoting the same relation. In all tree structures, $x \neg S y$ is equivalent to $\neg\, x S y$ and $x S_1 \cup S_2 y$ to $x S_1 y \vee x S_2 y$. Thus our formalism allows a controlled form of negation and disjunction without admitting full Boolean connectives.

3 A Saturation Algorithm

We now present a solver for dominance constraints with set operators. First, we give a base solver which saturates a constraint with respect to a set of propagation and distribution rules, and prove soundness, completeness, and termination of saturation in nondeterministic polynomial time. Second, we add optional propagation rules, which enhance the propagation power of the base solver.

The base solver is specified by the rule schemes in Figure 4. Let D be the (infinite) set of rules instantiating these schemes. Each rule is an implication between a constraint and a disjunction of constraints. We distinguish *propagation* rules $\varphi_1 \rightarrow \varphi_2$ which are deterministic and *distribution* rules $\varphi_1 \rightarrow \varphi_2 \vee \varphi_3$ which are nondeterministic.

Proposition 1 (Soundness). *The rules of D are valid in all tree structures.*

The inference system D can be interpreted as a saturation algorithm which decides the satisfiability of a constraint. A propagation rule $\varphi_1 \rightarrow \varphi_2$ applies to a constraint φ if all atomic constraints in φ_1 belong to φ but at least one of the atomic constraints in φ_2 does not. In this case, saturation proceeds with $\varphi \wedge \varphi_2$. A distribution rule $\varphi_1 \rightarrow \varphi_2 \vee \varphi_3$ applies to a constraint φ if both rules $\varphi_1 \rightarrow \varphi_2$ and $\varphi_1 \rightarrow \varphi_3$ could be applied to φ. In this case, one of these two rules is non-deterministically chosen and applied. A constraint is called D-saturated if none of the rules in D can be applied to it.

Proposition 2 (Termination). *The maximal number of iterated D-saturation steps on a constraint is polynomially bounded in the number of its variables.*

Proof. Let φ be a constraint with m variables. Each D-saturation step adds at least one new literal to φ. Only a $O(m^2)$ literals can be added since all of them have the form xRy where $x, y \in \mathsf{Vars}(\varphi)$ and R has 16 possible values.

Next, we illustrate prototypical inconsistencies and how D-saturation detects them. We start with the constraint $x{:}f(x_1, x_2) \wedge x_1 \triangleleft^* z \wedge x_2 \triangleleft^* z$ in Fig. 5 which is unsatisfiable since siblings cannot have a common descendant. Indeed, the disjointness of the siblings $x_1 \perp x_2$ can be

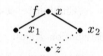

Fig. 5. (Neg.Disj)

derived from (Lab.Disj) whereas $x_1 \neg \perp x_2$ follows from (NegDisj) since x_1 and x_2 have the common descendant z.

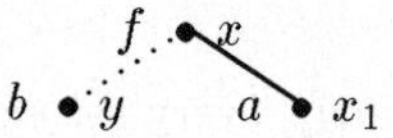

To illustrate the first distribution rule, we consider the unsatisfiable constraint $x{:}f(x_1) \wedge x \triangleleft^* y \wedge x_1{:}a \wedge y{:}b$ in Fig. 6 where $a \neq b$. We can decide the position of y with respect to x by applying rule (Distr.Child)

Fig. 6. (Distr.Child)

which either adds $x_1 \triangleleft^* y$ or $x_1 \neg \triangleleft^* y$. (1) If $x_1 \neg \triangleleft^* y$ is added, propagation with (Child.up) yields $x=y$. As x and y carry distinct labels, rule (Lab.Ineq) adds $x \neq y$. Now, we can deduce $x \emptyset y$ by intersecting equality and inequality (Inter). Thus, the (Clash) rule applies. (2) If $x_1 \triangleleft^* y$ is added then (Child.up) yields $x_1 = y$ which again clashes because of distinct labels.

The second distribution rules helps detect the inconsistency of $x{:}f(z) \wedge y{:}g(z)$ in Fig 7 where $f \neq g$. In a first step one can infer from (Lab.Dom) that $x \triangleleft^+ z$ and $y \triangleleft^+ z$. As the (Inter) rule allows to weaken relations, we

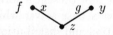

Fig. 7. (Distr.NegDisj)

also have $x \triangleleft^* z$ and $y \triangleleft^* z$, i.e. $x \neg \perp y$ by (NegDisj), so that (Distr.NegDisj) can deduce either $x \triangleleft^* y$ or $x \neg \triangleleft^* y$. Consider the case $x \triangleleft^* y$, from $y \triangleleft^+ z$ derive $z \neg \triangleleft^* y$ by (Inv, Inter), and (Child.up) infers $y=x$ resulting in a clash due to the distinct labels. Similarly for the other case.

Definition 2. *A D-solved form is a D-saturated constraint without* false.

The intuition is that a D-solved form has a back-bone which is a *dominance forest*, i.e. a forest with child and dominance edges. For instance, Fig 8 shows the dominance forest underlying $x_1{:}f(x_4) \land x_4 \lhd^* x_5 \land x_4 \lhd^* x_6 \land x_2 \lhd^* x_3 \land x_5 \perp x_6$ which becomes D-solved when D-propagation.

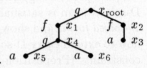

Fig. 8. D-solved form

We would like to note that the set based solver for dominance constraints of [2] insists on more explicit solved forms: for each two variables, one of the relations $\{=, \lhd^+, \rhd^+, \perp\}$ must be selected. For the dominance forest in Fig. 8, this leads to 63 explicit solutions instead of a single D-solved form. The situation is even worse for the formula $x_1 \lhd^* x_2 \land x_2 \lhd^* x_3 \land \ldots \land x_{n-1} \lhd^* x_n$. This constraint can be deterministically D-solved by D-propagation whereas the implementation of [2] computes a search tree of size 2^n.

Proposition 3 (Completeness). *Every D-solved form has a solution.*

The proof is given in the Section 4. The idea for constructing a solution of a D-solved form is to turn its underlying dominance forest into a tree, by adding labels such that dominance children are placed at disjoint positions whenever possible. For instance, a solution of the dominance forest in Fig. 8 is drawn in Fig. 9. Note that this solution does also satisfy $x_5 \perp x_6$ which be-

Fig. 9. A solution.

longs to the above constraint but not to its dominance forest. This solution is obtained from the dominance forest in Fig. 8 by adding a root node and node labels by which all dominance edges are turned into child edges.

Theorem 1. *Saturation by the inference rules in D decides the satisfiability of a dominance constraint with set operators in non-deterministic polynomial time.*

Proof. Let φ be a dominance constraint with set operators. Since all rules in D are sound (Proposition 1) and terminate (Proposition 2), φ is equivalent to the disjunction of all D-solved forms reachable from φ by non-deterministic D-saturation. Completeness (Proposition 3) yields that φ is satisfiable iff there exists a D-solved reachable from φ.

We can reduce the search space of D-saturation by adding optional propagation rules O. Taking advantage of set operators, we can define rather powerful propagation rules. The schemes in Fig 10, for instance, exploit the complementation set operators, and are indeed supported by the set based implementation of Section 6. For lack of space, we omit further optional rules that can be expressed by set operators and are also implemented by our solver. Instead, we illustrate O in the situation below which arises naturally when resolving scope ambiguities as in Figure 2.

$x{:}f(x_1, x_2) \land y{:}g(y_1, y_2) \land x_2 \lhd^* z \land y_1 \lhd^* z \land x \lhd^* y$

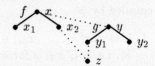

(Child.down) $x \lhd^+ y \wedge x{:}f(x_1, \ldots, x_n) \wedge \bigwedge_{i=1, i \neq j}^{n} x_i \neg \lhd^* y \quad \rightarrow \quad x_j \lhd^* y$

(NegDom) $x \perp y \wedge y \neg \perp z \quad \rightarrow \quad x \neg \lhd^* z$

Fig. 10. Some Optional Propagation Rules O

We derive $x \lhd^+ y$ by (Lab.Ineq,Inter), $x_1 \perp x_2$ by (Lab.Disj), and $x_2 \neg \perp y$ by (Dom. Trans,NegDisj). We combine the latter two using optional rule (NegDom) into $x_1 \neg \lhd^* y$. Finally, optional rule (Child.down) yields $x_2 \lhd^* y$ whereby the situation is resolved.

4   Completeness Proof

We now prove Proposition 3 which states completeness in the sense that every D-solved form is satisfiable. We proceed in two steps. First, we identify *simple D-solved forms* and show that they are satisfiable (Proposition 4). Then we show how to extend every D-solved form into a simple D-solved form by adding further constraints (Proposition 5).

Definition 3. *A variable x is* labeled *in φ if $x{=}y$ in φ and $y{:}f(y_1, \ldots, y_n)$ in φ for some variable y and term $f(y_1, \ldots, y_n)$. A variable y is a* root variable *for φ if $y \lhd^* z$ in φ for all $z \in \mathsf{Vars}(\varphi)$. We call a constraint φ* simple *if all its variables are labeled, and if there is a root variable for φ.*

Proposition 4. *A simple D-solved form is satisfiable.*

Proof. By induction on the number of literals in a simple D-solved form φ. φ has a root variable z. Since all variables in φ are labeled there is a variable z' and a term $f(z_1, \ldots, z_n)$ such that $z{=}z' \wedge z'{:}f(z_1, \ldots, z_n) \in \varphi$. We pose:

$$V = \{x \in \mathsf{Vars}(\varphi) \mid x{=}z \in \varphi\} \text{ and } V_i = \{x \in \mathsf{Vars}(\varphi) \mid z_i \lhd^* x \in \varphi\}$$

for all $1 \leq i \leq n$. To see that $\mathsf{Vars}(\varphi)$ is covered by $V \cup V_1 \cup \ldots \cup V_n$, let $x \in \mathsf{Vars}(\varphi)$ such that $z_i \lhd^* x \notin \varphi$ for all $1 \leq i \leq n$. Saturation with (Distr.Child) derives either $z_i \lhd^* x$ or $z_i \neg \lhd^* x$; but $z_i \lhd^* x \notin \varphi$ by assumption, therefore $z_i \neg \lhd^* x \in \varphi$ for all $1 \leq i \leq n$. (Child.up) infers $z{=}x \in \varphi$, i.e. $x \in V$. For a set $W \subseteq \mathsf{Vars}(\varphi)$ we define $\varphi_{|W}$ to be the conjunction of all literals $\psi \in \varphi$ with $\mathsf{Vars}(\psi) \subseteq W$.

$$\varphi \models\mid \varphi' \quad \text{holds where} \quad \varphi' =_{\text{def}} \varphi_{|V} \wedge z{:}f(z_1, \ldots, z_n) \wedge \varphi_{|V_1} \wedge \ldots \wedge \varphi_{|V_n}$$

$\varphi \models \varphi'$ follows from $\varphi' \subseteq \varphi$. To show $\varphi' \models \varphi$ we prove that each literal in φ is entailed by φ'

1. Case $x{:}g(x_1, \ldots, x_m) \in \varphi$ for some variable x and term $g(x_1, \ldots, x_m)$: If $x \in V_i$, i.e. $z_i \lhd^* x \in \varphi$ for some $1 \leq i \leq n$ then $x{:}g(x_1, \ldots, x_m) \in \varphi_{|V_i}$ since φ is

saturated under (Lab.Dom, Dom.Trans). Otherwise $x \in V$, i.e. $z=x \in \varphi$, and thus $z=x \in \varphi_{|V}$. Since φ is clash free and saturated under (Lab.Ineq,Clash), $f=g$ and $n=m$ must hold. Saturation with respect to (Eq.Decom) implies $z_i=x_i \in \varphi$ for all $1 \le i \le n$ and hence $z_i=x_i \in \varphi_{|V_i}$. All together, the right hand side φ' contains $z=x \wedge z{:}f(z_1, \ldots, z_n) \wedge \bigwedge_{i=1}^n z_i=x_i$ which entails $x{:}g(x_1, \ldots, x_m)$ as required.

2. Case $xRy \in \varphi$ for some variables x, y and relation set $R \subseteq \{=, \lhd^+, \rhd^+, \perp\}$. Since $x, y \in V \cup V_1 \cup \ldots \cup V_n$ we distinguish 4 possibilities:

   (a) $x \in V_i$, $y \in V_j$, where $1 \le i \ne j \le n$. Here, $x \perp y \in \varphi$ by saturation under (Lab.Disj, Inv, Disj). Clash-freeness and saturation under (Inter, Clash) yield $\perp \in R$. Finally, φ' entails $z_i \perp z_j$ and thus $x \perp y$ which in turn entails xRy.

   (b) When $x, y \in V$ (resp. V_i), by definition $xRy \in \varphi_{|V}$ (resp. $\varphi_{|V_i}$)

   (c) $x \in V$ and $y \in V_i$. Here, $x \lhd^+ y \in \varphi$ by saturation under (Lab.Dom, Dom.Trans). Thus $\lhd^+ \in R$ by saturation under (Inter, Clash) and clash-freeness of φ. But φ' entails $z \lhd^+ z_i$ and thus $x \lhd^+ y$ which in turn entails xRy.

   (d) The case $x \in V$ and $y \in V_i$ is symmetric to the previous one.

Next note that all $\varphi_{|V_i}$ are simple D-solved forms. By induction hypothesis there exist solutions $(\mathcal{M}^{\tau_i}, \alpha_i) \models \varphi_{|V_i}$ for all $1 \le i \le n$. Thus $(\mathcal{M}^{f(\tau_1, \ldots, \tau_n)}, \alpha)$ is a solution of φ if $\alpha_{|V_i} = \alpha_i$ and $\alpha(x) = \alpha(z)$ is the root node of $f(\tau_1, \ldots, \tau_n)$ for all $x \in V$. □

An *extension of a constraint* φ is a constraint of the form $\varphi \wedge \varphi'$ for some φ'. Given a constraint φ we define a partial ordering $\prec_\varphi$ on its variables such that $x \prec_\varphi y$ holds if and only if $x \lhd^* y$ in φ but not $y \lhd^* x$ in φ. If x is unlabeled then we define the set $\mathsf{con}_\varphi(x)$ of variables *connected to* x *in* φ as follows:

$$\mathsf{con}_\varphi(x) = \{y \mid y \text{ is } \prec_\varphi \text{ minimal with } x \prec_\varphi y\}$$

Intuitively, a variable y is connected to x if it is a "direct dominance child" of x. So for example, $\mathsf{con}_{\varphi_1}(x) = \{y\}$ and $\mathsf{con}_{\varphi_1}(y) = \{z\}$ for:

$$\varphi_1 := x \lhd^* x \wedge x \lhd^* y \wedge x \lhd^* z \wedge y \lhd^* z,$$

Definition 4. *We call* $V \subseteq \mathsf{Vars}(\varphi)$ *a* φ-disjointness *set if for any two distinct variables* $y_1, y_2 \in V$, $y_1 \neg\perp y_2$ *not in* φ.

The idea is that all variables in a φ-disjointness set can safely be placed at disjoint positions in at least one of the trees solving φ.

Lemma 1. *Let* φ *be D-saturated,* $x \in \mathsf{Vars}(\varphi)$. *If* V *is a maximal* φ-disjointness *set in* $\mathsf{con}_\varphi(x)$ *then for all* $y \in \mathsf{con}_\varphi(x)$ *there exists* $z \in V$ *such that* $y=z$ *in* φ.

Proof. If $y\neg\perp z$ *not in* φ for all $z \in V$ then $\{y\} \cup V$ is a disjointness set; thus $y \in V$ by maximality of V. Otherwise, there exists $z \in V$ such that $y\neg\perp z$ *in* φ. Saturation of φ with respect to rules (Distr.NegDisj, Inter) yields $y\lhd^* z$ *in* φ or $z\lhd^* y$ *in* φ. In both cases, it follows that $z=y$ *in* φ since z and y are both $\prec_\varphi$ minimal elements in the set $\mathsf{con}_\varphi(x)$.

Lemma 2 (Extension by Labeling). *Every D-solved form φ with an unlabeled variable x can be extended to a D-solved form with strictly fewer unlabeled variables, and in which x is labeled.*

Proof. Let $\{x_1, \ldots, x_n\}$ be a maximal φ-disjointness set included in $\mathsf{con}_\varphi(x)$. Let f be a function symbol of arity n in Σ, which exists w.l.o.g. Otherwise, f can be encoded from a constant and a symbol of arity ≥ 2 whose existence in Σ we assumed. We define the following extension $\mathsf{ext}(\varphi)$ of φ:

$$\mathsf{ext}(\varphi) =_{\mathrm{def}} \varphi \wedge x{:}f(x_1, \ldots, x_n) \wedge$$

$$\bigwedge \{xRz \wedge zR^{-1}x \mid \lhd^+ \in R,\ x_i\lhd^* z \text{ in } \varphi,\ 1 \leq i \leq n\} \wedge \qquad (1)$$

$$\bigwedge \{yRz \mid \perp \in R,\ x_i\lhd^* y \text{ in } \varphi,\ x_j\lhd^* z \text{ in } \varphi,\ 1 \leq i{\neq}j \leq n\} \qquad (2)$$

Note that x is labeled in $\mathsf{ext}(\varphi)$ since $x=x \in \varphi$ by saturation under (Dom.Refl). We have to verify that $\mathsf{ext}(\varphi)$ is D-solved, i.e. that none of the D-rules can be applied to $\mathsf{ext}(\varphi)$. We give the proof only for two of the more complex cases.

1. (Distr.Child) cannot be applied to $x{:}f(x_1, \ldots, x_n)$: suppose $x\lhd^* y$ *in* φ and consider the case $y\lhd^* x$ *not in* φ. Thus $x \prec_\varphi y$ and there exists $z \in \mathsf{con}_\varphi(x)$ with $z\lhd^* y$ *in* φ. Lemma 1 and the maximality of the φ-disjointness set $\{x_1, \ldots, x_n\}$ yield $x_j=z$ *in* φ for some $1 \leq j \leq n$. Thus, $x_j\lhd^* y$ *in* φ by (Dom.Trans) and (Distr.Child) cannot be applied with x_j. For all such $1 \leq i \neq j \leq n$ we can derive $x_i\perp y$ by (Lab.Dom, Disj, Inv), thus $x_i\neg\lhd^* y$ by (Inter) and (Distr.Child) cannot be applied with x_i either.

2. (Inter) applies when $R_1 \cap R_2 \subseteq R$, yR_1z *in* $\mathsf{ext}(\varphi)$, and yR_2z *in* $\mathsf{ext}(\varphi)$. We prove yRz *in* $\mathsf{ext}(\varphi)$ for the case where yR_1z *in* φ and yR_2z is contributed to $\mathsf{ext}(\varphi)$ by (2). Thus, $\perp \in R_2$ and there exists $1 \leq i{\neq}j \leq n$ such that $x_i\lhd^* y$ *in* φ and $x_j\lhd^* z$ *in* φ. It is sufficient to prove $\perp \in R_1$ since then $\perp \in R_1 \cap R_2 \subseteq R$ which implies yRz *in* φ. We assume $\perp \notin R_1$ and derive a contradiction. If $\perp \notin R_1$ then $R_1 \subseteq \{=, \lhd^+, \rhd^+\}$. Thus, weakening yR_1z *in* φ with (Inter) yields $y\neg\perp z$ *in* φ. Next, we can apply (Distr.NegDisj) which proves either $y\lhd^* z$ *in* φ or $y\neg\lhd^* z$ *in* φ.

    (a) If $y\lhd^* z$ *in* φ then $x_i\lhd^* z$ *in* φ follows from (Dom.Trans) and $x_i\neg\perp x_j$ *in* φ from (NegDisj). This contradicts our assumption that $\{x_1, \ldots, x_n\}$ is a φ-disjointness set.

    (b) If $y\neg\lhd^* z$ *in* φ then we have $y\neg\lhd^* z$ *in* φ and $y\neg\perp z$ *in* φ from which on can derive $y\rhd^* z$ *in* φ with (Inter) and $z\lhd^* y$ *in* φ with (Inv). From (Dom.Trans) we derive $x_j\lhd^* y$ *in* φ. Since we already know $x_j\lhd^* y$ *in* φ

$$\mathcal{B} ::= \mathsf{false} \mid X_1{=}X_2 \mid I \in D \mid i \in S \mid i \notin S \qquad (D \subseteq \Delta)$$
$$\mathcal{C} ::= \mathcal{B} \mid S_1 \cap S_2{=}\emptyset \mid S_3 \subseteq S_1 \cup S_2 \mid \mathcal{C}_1 \wedge \mathcal{C}_2 \mid \mathcal{C}_1 \text{ or } \mathcal{C}_2$$

Fig. 11. Finite Domain and Finite Set Constraints

we can apply (NegDisj) which shows $x_i \neg \perp x_j$ in φ. But again, this contradicts that $\{x_1, \ldots, x_n\}$ is a φ-disjointness set. $\qquad \square$

Proposition 5. *Every D-solved form can be extended to a simple D-solved form.*

Proof. Let φ be D-solved. W.l.o.g., φ has a root variable, else we choose a fresh variable x and consider instead the D-solved extension $\varphi \wedge \bigwedge \{xRy \wedge yR^{-1}x \mid \vartriangleleft^+ \in R, \, y \in \mathsf{Vars}(\varphi)\}$. By Lemma 2, we can successively label all its variables. $\qquad \square$

5   Constraint Programming with Finite Sets

Current constraint programming technology provides no support for our D-saturation algorithm. Instead, improving on [2], we reformulate the task of finding solutions of a tree description as a constraint satisfaction problem solvable by constraint programming [11,6]. In this section, we define our target language. Its propagation rules are given in Fig 12 and are used in proving correctness of implementation. Distribution rules, however, are typically problem dependent and we assume that they can be programmatically stipulated by the application. Thus, the concrete solver of Section 6 specifies its distribution rules in Figure 13.

Let $\Delta = \{1 \ \ldots \ \mu\}$ be a finite set of integers for some large practical limit μ such as 134217726. We assume a set of *integer variables* with values in Δ and ranged over by I and a set of *set variables* with values in 2^Δ and ranged over by S. Integer and finite set variables are also both denoted by X.

The abstract syntax of our language is given in Fig 11. We distinguish between *basic constraints* $\mathcal{B}$, directly representable in the constraint store, and *non-basic constraints* $\mathcal{C}$ acting as propagators and amplifying the store. The declarative semantics of these constraints is obvious (given that $\mathcal{C}_1 \text{ or } \mathcal{C}_2$ is interpreted as disjunction). We write $\beta \models \mathcal{C}$ if β is an assignment of integer variables to integers and set variables to sets which renders $\mathcal{C}$ true (where set operators and Boolean connectives have the usual meaning).

We use the following abbreviations: we write $I{\neq}i$ for $I \in \Delta \setminus \{i\}$, $S_1 \parallel S_2$ for $S_1 \cap S_2{=}\emptyset$, $S{=}D$ for $\bigwedge\{i \in S \mid i \in D\} \wedge \{i \notin S \mid i \in \Delta \setminus D\}$, $S_1 \subseteq S_2$ for $S_1 \subseteq S_2 \cup S_3 \wedge S_3{=}\emptyset$, and $S = S_1 \uplus S_2$ for $S_1 \parallel S_2 \wedge S \subseteq S_1 \cup S_2 \wedge S_1 \subseteq S \wedge S_2 \subseteq S$

The propagation rules $\leadsto_P$ for inference in this language are summarized in Fig 12. The expression $\mathcal{C}_1 \text{ or } \mathcal{C}_2$ operates as a *disjunctive propagator* which does not invoke any case distinction. The propagation rules for disjunctive propagators use the saturation relation $\leadsto_P^{\circledast}$ induced by $\leadsto_P$ which in turn is defined by

Equality: $X_1 {=} X_2 \wedge \mathcal{B}[X_j] \leadsto_P \mathcal{B}[X_k] \quad \{j,k\} = \{1,2\}$ (eq.subst)

Finite domain integer constraints:

$$I \in D_1 \wedge I \in D_2 \leadsto_P I \in D_1 \cap D_2 \qquad\qquad\text{(fd.conj)}$$
$$I \in \emptyset \leadsto_P \text{false} \qquad\qquad\text{(fd.clash)}$$

Finite sets constraints:

$$i \in S \wedge i \notin S \leadsto_P \text{false} \qquad\qquad\text{(fs.clash)}$$
$$S_1 \cap S_2 {=} \emptyset \wedge i \in S_j \leadsto_P i \notin S_k \quad \{j,k\} = \{1,2\} \qquad\text{(fs.disjoint)}$$
$$S_3 \subseteq S_1 \cup S_2 \wedge i \notin S_1 \wedge i \notin S_2 \leadsto_P i \notin S_3 \qquad\text{(fs.subset.neg)}$$
$$S_3 \subseteq S_1 \cup S_2 \wedge i \in S_3 \wedge i \notin S_j \leadsto_P i \in S_k \quad \{j,k\} = \{1,2\} \qquad\text{(fs.subset.pos)}$$

Disjunctive propagators:

$$\frac{\mathcal{B} \wedge \mathcal{C} \leadsto_P^{\oplus} \text{false}}{\mathcal{B} \wedge (\mathcal{C} \text{ or } \mathcal{C}') \leadsto_P \mathcal{C}'} \qquad \frac{\mathcal{B} \wedge \mathcal{C}' \leadsto_P^{\oplus} \text{false}}{\mathcal{B} \wedge (\mathcal{C} \text{ or } \mathcal{C}') \leadsto_P \mathcal{C}} \qquad \text{(commit)}$$

Fig. 12. Propagation Rules

recursion through $\leadsto_P^{\oplus}$. Clearly, all propagation rules are valid formulas when seen as implications or as implications between implications in case of (commit).

6   Reduction to Finite Set Constraints

We now reduce dominance constraints with set operators to finite set constraints of the language introduced above. This reduction yields a concrete implementation of the abstract dominance constraint solver when realized in a constraint programming system such as [11, 6].

The underlying idea is to represent a literal $x\,R\,y$ by a membership expression $y {\in} R(x)$ where $R(x)$ is a set variable denoting a finite set of nodes in a tree. This idea is fairly general in that it does not depend on the particular relations interpreting the relation symbols. Our encoding consists of 3 parts:

$$\llbracket \varphi \rrbracket = \bigwedge_{x \in \mathsf{Vars}(\varphi)} \mathsf{A}_1(x) \bigwedge_{x,y \in \mathsf{Vars}(\varphi)} \mathsf{A}_2(x,y) \wedge \mathsf{B}\llbracket \varphi \rrbracket$$

$\mathsf{A}_1(\,\cdot\,)$ introduces a node representation per variable, $\mathsf{A}_2(\,\cdot\,)$ axiomatizes the treeness of the relations between these nodes, and $\mathsf{B}\llbracket \varphi \rrbracket$ encodes the specific restrictions imposed by φ.

Representation. When observed from a specific node Up_x x, the nodes of a solution tree (hence the variables $Side_x$ that they interpret) are partitioned into 4 regions: x itself, all nodes above, all nodes below, and all nodes to the side. The main idea is to introduce corresponding set variables.

Let MAX be the maximum constructor arity used in φ. For each formal variable x in φ we choose a distinct integer ι_x to represent it, and introduce $7 +$ MAX constraint set variables written Eq_x, Up_x, $Down_x$, $Side_x$, $Equp_x$, $Eqdown_x$,

$Parent_x$, $Down_x^i$ for $1 \leq i \leq$ MAX, and one constraint integer variable $Label_x$. First we state that $x = x$:

$$\iota_x \in Eq_x \tag{3}$$

Eq_x, Up_x, $Down_x$, $Side_x$ encode the set of variables that are respectively equal, above, below, and to the side (i.e. disjoint) of x. Thus, posing $\mathcal{I} = \{\iota_x \mid x \in \mathsf{Vars}(\varphi)\}$ for the set of integers encoding $\mathsf{Vars}(\varphi)$, we have:

$$\mathcal{I} = Eq_x \uplus Down_x \uplus Up_x \uplus Side_x$$

We can improve propagation by introducing $Eqdown_x$ and $Equp_x$ as intermediate results. This improvement is required by (Dom.Trans):

$$\mathcal{I} = Eqdown_x \uplus Up_x \uplus Side_x \quad (4) \qquad\qquad Eqdown_x = Eq_x \uplus Down_x \qquad (6)$$
$$\mathcal{I} = Equp_x \uplus Down_x \uplus Side_x \quad (5) \qquad\qquad Equp_x = Eq_x \uplus Up_x \qquad\qquad (7)$$

$Down_x^i$ encodes the set of variables in the subtree rooted at x's ith child (empty if there is no such child):

$$Down_x = \uplus\{Down_x^i \mid 1 \leq i \leq \text{MAX}\} \tag{8}$$

We define $A_1(x)$ as the conjunction of the constraints introduced above:

$$A_1(x) = (3) \wedge (4) \wedge (5) \wedge (6) \wedge (7)$$

Wellformedness. Posing $\mathbf{Rel} = \{=, \lhd^+, \rhd^+, \perp\}$. In a tree, the relationship that obtains between the nodes denoted by x and y must be one in $\mathbf{Rel}$. We introduce an integer variable C_{xy}, called a choice variable, to explicitly represent it and contribute a well-formedness clause $A_3[\![x \, r \, y]\!]$ for each $r \in \mathbf{Rel}$. Freely indentifying the symbols in $\mathbf{Rel}$ with the integers 1,2,3,4, we write:

$$A_2(x, y) \quad = \quad C_{xy} \in \mathbf{Rel} \wedge \bigwedge\{A_3[\![x \, r \, y]\!] \mid r \in \mathbf{Rel}\} \tag{9}$$
$$A_3[\![x \, r \, y]\!] \quad \equiv \quad D[\![x \, r \, y]\!] \wedge C_{xy} = r \text{ or } C_{xy} \neq r \wedge D[\![x \, \neg r \, y]\!] \tag{10}$$

For all $r \in \mathbf{Rel}$, it remains to define $D[\![x \, r \, y]\!]$ and $D[\![x \, \neg r \, y]\!]$ encoding the relations $x \, r \, y$ and $x \, \neg r \, y$ resp. by set constraints on the representations of x and y.

$$
\begin{aligned}
D[\![x = y]\!] \quad &= \quad Eq_x = Eq_y \wedge Up_x = Up_y \wedge Down_x = Down_y \wedge Side_x = Side_y \\
&\qquad \wedge Eqdown_x = Eqdown_y \wedge Equp_x = Equp_y \\
&\qquad \wedge Parent_x = Parent_y \wedge Label_x = Label_y \wedge_i Down_x^i = Down_y^i \\
D[\![x \, \neg= y]\!] \quad &= \quad Eq_x \parallel Eq_y \\
D[\![x \lhd^+ y]\!] \quad &= \quad Eqdown_y \subseteq Down_x \wedge Equp_x \subseteq Up_y \wedge Side_x \subseteq Side_y \\
D[\![x \, \neg\lhd^+ y]\!] \quad &= \quad Eq_x \parallel Up_y \wedge Down_x \parallel Eq_y \\
D[\![x \perp y]\!] \quad &= \quad Eqdown_x \subseteq Side_y \wedge Eqdown_y \subseteq Side_x \\
D[\![x \, \neg\perp y]\!] \quad &= \quad Eq_x \parallel Side_y \wedge Side_x \parallel Eq_y
\end{aligned}
$$

$$C_{xy} \in \{=, \lhd^+\} \quad \leadsto_\mathrm{D} \quad C_{x_i y} \in \{=, \lhd^+\} \vee C_{x_i y} \notin \{=, \lhd^+\} \quad \text{for } x{:}f(x_1, \dots, x_n) \text{ in } \varphi$$

$$C_{xy} \neq \bot \quad \leadsto_\mathrm{D} \quad C_{xy} \in \{=, \lhd^+\} \vee \ C_{xy} \notin \{=, \lhd^+\}$$

Fig. 13. Problem specific distribution rules

Problem Specific Constraints. The third part $\mathsf{B}[\![\varphi]\!]$ of the translation forms the additional problem-specific constraints that further restrict the admissibility of wellformed solutions and only accept those that are models of φ. The translation is given by clauses (11,12,13).

$$\mathsf{B}[\![\varphi \wedge \varphi']\!] \quad = \quad \mathsf{B}[\![\varphi]\!] \wedge \mathsf{B}[\![\varphi']\!] \tag{11}$$

A pleasant consequence of the introduction of choice variables C_{xy} is that any dominance constraint $x \, R \, y$ can be translated as a restriction on the possible values of C_{xy}. For example, $x \lhd^* y$ can be encoded as $C_{xy} \in \{1, 2\}$. More generally:

$$\mathsf{B}[\![x \, R \, y]\!] \quad = \quad C_{xy} \in R \tag{12}$$

Finally the labelling constraint $x : f(y_1 \ \dots \ y_n)$ requires a more complex treatment. For each constructor f we choose a distinct integer ι_f to encode it.

$$\mathsf{B}[\![x : f(y_1 \ \dots \ y_n)]\!] \quad = \quad Label_x = \iota_f \wedge^{j=\mathrm{MAX}}_{j=n+1} Down^j_x = \emptyset$$

$$\wedge^{j=n}_{j=1} Parent_{y_j} = Eq_x \wedge Down^j_x = Eqdown_{y_j} \wedge Up_{y_j} = Equp_x \tag{13}$$

Definition of the Concrete Solver. For each problem φ we define a search strategy specified by the distribution rules of Figure 13. These rules correspond precisely to (Distr.Child, Distr.NegDisj) of algorithm-D and are to be applied in the same non-deterministic fashion. Posing $\leadsto \ = \ \leadsto_\mathrm{P} \cup \leadsto_\mathrm{D}$, we define our concrete solver as the non-deterministic saturation $\leadsto^\circledast$ induced by $\leadsto$ and write $\varphi_1 \leadsto^\circledast \varphi_2$ to mean that φ_2 is in a $\leadsto^\circledast$ saturation of φ_1. While the abstract solver left this point open, in order to avoid unnecessary choices, we further require that a $\leadsto_\mathrm{D}$ step be taken only if no $\leadsto_\mathrm{P}$ step is possible.

7   Proving Correctness of Implementation

We now prove that $[\![\varphi]\!]$ combined with the search strategy defined above yields a sound and complete solver for φ. Completeness is demonstrated by showing that the concrete solver obtained by $[\![\varphi]\!]$ provides at least as much propagation as specified by the rules of algorithm D, i.e. whenever $x \, R \, y$ is in a $\rightarrow^\circledast$ saturation of φ then $C_{xy} \in R$ is in a $\leadsto^\circledast$ saturation of $[\![\varphi]\!]$.

Theorem 2. $[\![\varphi]\!]$ *is satisfiable iff* φ *is satisfiable.*

This follows from Propositions 6 and 7 below.

Proposition 6. *If φ is satisfiable then $\llbracket \varphi \rrbracket$ is satisfiable.*

We show how to construct a model β of $\llbracket \varphi \rrbracket$ from a model $(\mathcal{M}^\tau, \alpha)$ of φ. We define the variable assignment β as follows: $\beta(Up_x) = \{\iota_y \mid \alpha(y) \lhd^+ \alpha(x)\}$ and similarly for $Eq_x, Down_x, Side_x, Eqdown_x, Equp_x$, $\beta(Parent_x) = \{\iota_y \mid \exists k \; \alpha(y)k = \alpha(x)\}$, $\beta(Down_x^k) = \{\iota_y \mid \alpha(y) \rhd^* \alpha(x)k\}$, $\beta(Label_x) = \iota_{L_r(\alpha(x))}$ and $\beta(C_{xy}) = R$ if $\alpha(x) \, R \, \alpha(y)$ in $\mathcal{M}^\tau$. We have that if $(\mathcal{M}^\tau, \alpha) \models \varphi$ then $\beta \models \llbracket \varphi \rrbracket$.

Proposition 7. *If $\llbracket \varphi \rrbracket$ is satisfiable, then φ is satisfiable.*

We prove this by reading a D-solved form off a model β of $\llbracket \varphi \rrbracket$.

$$\varphi' \quad \equiv \quad \varphi \wedge \bigwedge_{x,y} \bigwedge_{R' \supseteq R} x \, R' \, y \qquad \text{where } R = \beta(C_{xy})$$

φ' is a D-solved form containing φ: all relationships between variables are fully resolved and all their generalizations have been added. The only possibility is that D-rules might derive a contradiction. However, if $\varphi' \to_P^\circledast$ false then $\llbracket \varphi' \rrbracket \rightsquigarrow_P^\circledast$ false (Lemma 4) which would contradict the existence of a solution β. Therefore φ' is a O-solved form and φ is satisfiable.

We distinguish propagation and distribution rules; in algorithm D they are written $\to_P$ and $\to_D$, and in our concrete solver $\rightsquigarrow_P$ and $\rightsquigarrow_D$. We write $\varphi'' \preccurlyeq \varphi'$ for φ'' *is stronger than* φ' and define it as the smallest relation that holds of atomic constraints and such that false $\preccurlyeq$ false and $x \, R \, y \preccurlyeq x \, R' \, y$ iff $R \subseteq R'$.

Proposition 8 (Stronger Propagation). *For each rule $\varphi \to_P \varphi'$ of algorithm D, there exists $\varphi'' \preccurlyeq \varphi'$ such that $\llbracket \varphi \rrbracket \rightsquigarrow_P^\circledast \llbracket \varphi'' \rrbracket$.*

The proof technique follows this pattern: each φ' is of the form $x \, R \, y$ and we choose $\varphi'' = x R' y$ where $R' \subseteq R$. Assume $\llbracket \varphi \rrbracket$ as a premise. Show that $\llbracket \varphi \rrbracket \wedge \mathcal{C} \rightsquigarrow_P^\circledast$ false. Notice that a clause $\mathcal{C}$ or $\mathcal{C}'$ is introduced by $\llbracket \varphi \rrbracket$ as required by (10). Thus $\mathcal{C}'$ follows by (commit). Then show that $\llbracket \varphi \rrbracket \wedge \mathcal{C}' \rightsquigarrow_P^\circledast \llbracket \varphi'' \rrbracket$. For want of space, we include here only the proof for rule (NegDisj).

Lemma 3. $\llbracket x \lhd^* y \rrbracket \rightsquigarrow_P^\circledast \iota_y \in Eqdown_x$ *(proof omitted)*

Proposition 9. $\llbracket x \lhd^* z \wedge y \lhd^* z \rrbracket \rightsquigarrow_P^\circledast \llbracket x \neg\!\perp y \rrbracket$

Proof. From the premises $\llbracket x \lhd^* z \rrbracket$ and $\llbracket y \lhd^* z \rrbracket$, i.e. $C_{xz} \in \{=, \lhd^+\}$ and $C_{yz} \in \{=, \lhd^+\}$, we must show $\llbracket x \neg\!\perp y \rrbracket$ i.e. $C_{xy} \neq \perp$. By Lemma 3 we obtain $\iota_z \in Eqdown_x$ and $\iota_z \in Eqdown_y$. Since $\mathcal{I} = Eqdown_y \uplus Up_y \uplus Side_y$, we have $\iota_z \notin Side_y$. Now consider the non-basic constraint $Eqdown_x \subseteq Side_y$ which occurs in $D\llbracket x \perp y \rrbracket$: from $\iota_z \in Eqdown_x$ it infers $\iota_z \in Side_y$ which contradicts $\iota_z \notin Side_y$. Therefore, the well-formedness clause $D\llbracket x \perp y \rrbracket \wedge C_{xy} = \perp$ or $C_{xy} \neq \perp \wedge D\llbracket x \neg\!\perp y \rrbracket$ infers its right alternative by rule (commit). Hence $C_{xy} \neq \perp$. $\square$

Lemma 4. *(1) if $\varphi \to_P^\circledast \varphi'$, then there exists $\varphi'' \preccurlyeq \varphi'$ such that $\llbracket \varphi \rrbracket \rightsquigarrow_P^\circledast \llbracket \varphi'' \rrbracket$. (2) if $\varphi \to_P^\circledast \varphi_1$ and $\varphi_1 \to_D \varphi_2$, then there exists $\varphi_1' \preccurlyeq \varphi_1$ such that $\llbracket \varphi \rrbracket \rightsquigarrow_P^\circledast \llbracket \varphi_1' \rrbracket$ and $\llbracket \varphi_1' \rrbracket \rightsquigarrow_D \llbracket \varphi_2 \rrbracket$.*

(1) follows from Proposition 8, and (2) from (1) and the fact that the concrete distribution rules precisely correspond to those of algorithm D.

Proposition 10 (Simulation). *The concrete solver simulates the abstract solver: if $\varphi \to^{\circledast} \varphi'$ then there exists $\varphi'' \preccurlyeq \varphi'$ such that $[\![\varphi]\!] \rightsquigarrow^{\circledast} [\![\varphi'']\!]$.*

Follows from Lemma 4.

Theorem 3. *(1) every $\rightsquigarrow^{\circledast}$ saturation of $[\![\varphi]\!]$ corresponds to a D-solved form of φ and (2) for every D-solved form of φ there is a corresponding $\rightsquigarrow^{\circledast}$ saturation of $[\![\varphi]\!]$.*

(1) from Proposition 10. (2) Consider a $\rightsquigarrow^{\circledast}$ saturation of $[\![\varphi]\!]$. As in Proposition 7, we can construct a D-solved form φ' of φ by reading off the current domains of the choice variables C_{xy}. If φ' was not D-solved, then $\to^{\circledast}$ could infer a new fact, but then by Proposition 10 so could $\rightsquigarrow^{\circledast}$ and it would not be a saturation.

8   Conclusion

In this paper, we extended dominance constraints by admitting set operators. Set operators introduce a controlled form of disjunction and negation that is less expressive than general Boolean connectives and remains especially well-suited for constraint propagation. On the basis of this extension we presented two solvers: one abstract, one concrete.

The design of the abstract solver is carefully informed by the needs of practical applications: it stipulates inference rules required for efficiently solving dominance constraints occurring in these applications. The rules take full advantage of the extra expressivity afforded by set operators. We proved the abstract solver sound and complete and that its distribution strategy improves over [2] and may avoid an exponential number of choice points. This improvement accrues from admitting less explicit solved forms while preserving soundness.

Elaborating on the technique first presented in [2], the concrete solver realizes the desired constraint propagation by reduction to constraint programming using set constraints. We proved that the concrete solver faithfully simulates the abstract one, and thereby shed new light on the source of its observed practical effectiveness. The concrete solver has been implemented in the concurrent constraint programming language Oz [10], performs efficiently in practical applications to semantic underspecification, and produces smaller search trees than the solver of [2].

References

1. R. Backofen, J. Rogers, and K. Vijay-Shanker. A first-order axiomatization of the theory of finite trees. *Journal of Logic, Language, and Information*, 4:5–39, 1995.
2. D. Duchier and C. Gardent. A constraint-based treatment of descriptions. In *Int. Workshop on Computational Semantics*, Tilburg, 1999.
3. D. Duchier and S. Thater. Parsing with tree descriptions: a constraint-based approach. In *Int. Workshop on Natural Language Understanding and Logic Programming*, Las Cruces, New Mexico, 1999.
4. M. Egg, J. Niehren, P. Ruhrberg, and F. Xu. Constraints over lambda-structures in semantic underspecification. In *Joint Conf. COLING/ACL*, pages 353–359, 1998.
5. C. Gardent and B. Webber. Describing discourse semantics. In *Proceedings of the 4th TAG+ Workshop*, Philadelphia, 1998.
6. C. Gervet. Interval propagation to reason about sets: Definition and implementation of a practical language. *Constraints*, 1(3):191–244, 1997.
7. A. Koller, K. Mehlhorn, and J. Niehren. A polynomial-time fragment of dominance constraints. Technical report, Programming Systems Lab, Universität des Saarlandes, Apr. 2000. Submitted.
8. A. Koller, J. Niehren, and R. Treinen. Dominance constraints: Algorithms and complexity. In *Logical Aspects of Comp. Linguistics 98*, 2000. To appear in LNCS.
9. M. P. Marcus, D. Hindle, and M. M. Fleck. D-theory: Talking about talking about trees. In *21st ACL*, pages 129–136, 1983.
10. Mozart. The mozart programming system. http://www.mozart-oz.org/.
11. T. Müller and M. Müller. Finite set constraints in Oz. In F. Bry, B. Freitag, and D. Seipel, editors, *13. Workshop Logische Programmierung*, pages 104–115, Technische Universität München, 1997.
12. R. Muskens. Order-Independence and Underspecification. In J. Groenendijk, editor, *Ellipsis, Underspecification, Events and More in Dynamic Semantics.* DYANA Deliverable R.2.2.C, 1995.
13. O. Rambow, K. Vijay-Shanker, and D. Weir. D-tree grammars. In *Proceedings of ACL'95*, pages 151–158, MIT, Cambridge, 1995.
14. J. Rogers and K. Vijay-Shanker. Reasoning with descriptions of trees. In *Annual Meeting of the Association for Comp. Linguistics (ACL)*, 1992.
15. J. W. Thatcher and J. B. Wright. Generalized finite automata theory with an application to a decision problem of second-order logic. *Mathematical Systems Theory*, 2(1):57–81, August 1967.
16. W. Thomas. Automata on Infinite Objects. In J. v. Leeuwen, editor, *Handbook of Theoretical Computer Science, Formal Models and Semantics*, volume B, chapter 4, pages 133–191. The MIT Press, 1990.
17. K. Vijay-Shanker. Using descriptions of trees in a tree adjoining grammar. *Computational Linguistics*, 18:481–518, 1992.

Better Communication for Tighter Cooperation

Petra Hofstedt

Department of Computer Science, Berlin University of Technology

Abstract. We propose a general scheme for the cooperation of different constraint solvers. A uniform interface for constraint solvers allows to formally specify information exchange between them and it enables the development of an open and very flexible combination mechanism. This mechanism allows the definition of a wide range of different cooperation strategies according to the current requirements such that our overall system forms a general framework for cooperating constraint solvers.

1 Introduction

Often it is desirable and advantageous to combine several constraint solving techniques because this combination makes it possible to solve problems that none of the single solvers can handle alone.

Example 1. Let an electric circuit be given with a resistor R_1 of $0.1M\Omega$ connected in parallel with a variable resistor R_2 of between $0.1M\Omega$ and $0.4M\Omega$, a capacitor K is in series connection with the two resistors. Also, there is a kit of electrical components in which capacitors of $1\mu F, 2.5\mu F, 5\mu F, 10\mu F, 20\mu F$, and $50\mu F$ are available.

We want to know which capacitor to use in our circuit such that the time until the voltage of the capacitor reaches 99% of the final voltage is between 0.5s and 1s, i.e. the duration until the capacitor is loaded is between 0.5s and 1s. Thus, the input constraint conjunction is $R_1 = 10^5 \wedge R_2 = [10^5, 4 \cdot 10^5] \wedge (1/R) = (1/R_1) + (1/R_2) \wedge V_K = V \times (1 - exp(-t/(R \times K))) \wedge V_K = 0.99 \times V \wedge t = [0.5, 1] \wedge K \in \{10^{-6}, 2.5 \cdot 10^{-6}, 5 \cdot 10^{-6}, 10^{-5}, 2 \cdot 10^{-5}, 5 \cdot 10^{-5}\}$.

This constraint conjunction can be solved using different cooperating constraint solvers. A solver for rational interval arithmetic infers from the constraint conjunction $R_1 = 10^5 \wedge R_2 = [10^5, 4 \cdot 10^5] \wedge (1/R) = (1/R_1) + (1/R_2)$ the new constraint $R = [5 \cdot 10^4, 8 \cdot 10^4]$. Let's assume that, since the interval solver is able to handle constraints of rational arithmetic, it also computes from $V_K = V \times (1 - E) \wedge V_K = 0.99 \times V$, where $E = exp(-t/(R \times K))$, the new constraint $E = 0.01$. This constraint is given to a constraint solver which is able to handle functions, like exp, ln, sin, and cos, to infer from the constraint conjunction $E = 0.01 \wedge E = exp(F)$, where $F = -t/(R \times K)$, the constraint $F = ln(0.01)$. Now, the interval solver is able to compute the constraint $1.3572 \cdot 10^{-6} \leq K \leq 4.3429 \cdot 10^{-6}$ from the constraints $F = ln(0.01), F = -t/(R \times K), R = [5 \cdot 10^4, 8 \cdot 10^4]$, and $t = [0.5, 1]$. The last step is done by a finite domain constraint solver which uses the constraints $K \in \{10^{-6}, 2.5 \cdot 10^{-6}, 5 \cdot 10^{-6}, 10^{-5}, 2 \cdot 10^{-5}, 5 \cdot 10^{-5}\}$ and

J. Lloyd et al. (Eds.): CL 2000, LNAI 1861, pp. 342–357, 2000.

$1.3572 \cdot 10^{-6} \leq \text{K} \leq 4.3429 \cdot 10^{-6}$ to choose the capacitor which we are searching for from the kit: $\text{K} = 2.5 \cdot 10^{-6}$ holds. □

In this paper, we define a combination mechanism for constraint solvers that supports openness and flexibility. Both properties result from the definition of a uniform interface for the solvers. The combination is open in the sense that whenever a new constraint system with associated constraint solver is developed, it can be easily incorporated into the whole system independently of its constraint domain and the language in which the constraint solver is implemented. It is flexible because the definition of different strategies for the cooperation of the single solvers is possible in a simple way.

We start with basic definitions concerning constraint systems and constraint solvers in Sect. 2. Section 3 is dedicated to the description of the mechanism for the combination of different constraint solvers. Section 3.1 shows the overall architecture. The syntax of a language which enables the specification of mixed constraints of different constraint systems is described in Sect. 3.2. Section 3.3 defines our uniform interface for constraint solvers. In Sect. 3.4, we show the general way of defining cooperation strategies for constraint solvers in our framework. In Sect. 4, we discuss our approach and we compare it with other related work.

2   Constraint Systems and Constraint Solvers

Let S be a set of sorts. X^s denotes the set of variables of sort $s \in S$. $X = \dot{\bigcup}_{s \in S} X^s$ is a many sorted set of variables ($\bigcup$ denotes the disjoint union).

A (many sorted) *signature* $\Sigma = (S, F, R; ar)$ is defined by a set S of sorts, a set F of function symbols, and a set R of predicate symbols. S, F, and R are mutually disjoint. The function $ar : F \cup R \to S^*$ is called arity function of the signature Σ. For every $f \in F$, $ar(f) \neq \epsilon$ holds. In the following, we will also denote S, F, R, and ar by S_Σ, F_Σ, R_Σ, and ar_Σ, respectively. We write $f : s_1 \times \ldots \times s_n \to s$ (and $r : s_1 \times \ldots \times s_m$) to denote that $f \in F$ with $ar(f) = s_1 \ldots s_n s$ (and $r \in R$ with $ar(r) = s_1 \ldots s_m$, resp.). The *set* $\mathcal{T}(F, X)^s$ *of terms over* F *of sort* $s \in S$ with variables from X is defined as usual.

A Σ-*structure* $\mathcal{D} = (\{\mathcal{D}^s \mid s \in S\}, \{f^{\mathcal{D}} \mid f \in F\}, \{r^{\mathcal{D}} \mid r \in R\})$ consists of 1. an S-sorted family of nonempty carrier sets $\mathcal{D}^s$, 2. a family of functions $f^{\mathcal{D}}$, and 3. a family of predicates $r^{\mathcal{D}}$. Given $f \in F$ with $ar(f) = s_1 \ldots s_n s$, $f^{\mathcal{D}}$ is an n-ary function such that $f^{\mathcal{D}} : \mathcal{D}^{s_1} \times \ldots \times \mathcal{D}^{s_n} \to \mathcal{D}^s$. Given $r \in R$ with $ar(r) = s_1 \ldots s_m$, $r^{\mathcal{D}}$ is an m-ary predicate such that $r^{\mathcal{D}} \subseteq \mathcal{D}^{s_1} \times \ldots \times \mathcal{D}^{s_m}$.

Definition 1 (Constraint System, Constraint, Constraint Domain). *A constraint system   is a tuple* $\zeta = \langle \Sigma, \mathcal{D} \rangle$, *where* $\Sigma = (S_\Sigma, F_\Sigma, R_\Sigma; ar_\Sigma)$ *is a signature and* $\mathcal{D}$ *is a* Σ-*structure. For every* $s \in S_\Sigma$, R_Σ *contains at least a predicate symbol* $=_{s, \Sigma}$ *with the usual equality predicate* $=_s^{\mathcal{D}}$.

A constraint over Σ *is a string of the form* $r\, t_1 \ldots t_m$ *where* $r \in R_\Sigma^{s_1 \times \ldots \times s_m}$ *and* $t_i \in \mathcal{T}(F_\Sigma, X)^{s_i}$. *The set of constraints over* Σ *is denoted by* $Cons(\Sigma)$. $(\mathcal{D}, Cons(\Sigma))$ *is called a* constraint domain. □

The terms over F_Σ and the constraints in $Cons(\Sigma)$ can be considered as particular expressions of a first order language. In the following, constraints are typically denoted by c and c_i.

For every finite set $Y \subseteq X$, let $\tilde{Y}$ denote an arbitrary enumeration, i.e. a sequence, of the variables of Y. Let ψ be a formula of first order predicate logic, and let $\{x_1, \ldots, x_n\}$ be the set of free variables of ψ. The *universal closure* $\forall\psi$ and the *existential closure* $\exists\psi$ of formula ψ are defined as follows: $\forall\psi = \forall x_1 \ldots \forall x_n : \psi$ and $\exists\psi = \exists x_1 \ldots \exists x_n : \psi$, resp. $\exists_{-\tilde{Y}}\psi$ denotes the existential closure of formula ψ except for the variables of $\tilde{Y}$.

A conjunction $C = \bigwedge_{i \in \{1,\ldots,n\}} c_i$ of constraints $c_1, \ldots, c_n$ is called *satisfiable* in $\mathcal{D}$ if $\mathcal{D} \models \exists C$ holds. It is called *valid* in $\mathcal{D}$ if $\mathcal{D} \models \forall C$ holds, *unsatisfiable* in $\mathcal{D}$ if $\mathcal{D} \not\models \exists C$ holds, and *invalid* in $\mathcal{D}$ if $\mathcal{D} \not\models \forall C$ holds, respectively.

Let $\mathcal{D} = (\{\mathcal{D}^s \mid s \in S\}, \{f^\mathcal{D} \mid f \in F\}, \{r^\mathcal{D} \mid r \in R\})$ be a Σ-structure, and let $C = \bigwedge_{i \in \{1,\ldots,n\}} c_i$ be a conjunction of constraints $c_1, \ldots, c_n$ over Σ. Let $var(C)$ denote the set of variables which occur in C. A *solution* of C in $\mathcal{D}$ is a valuation $\sigma : V \to \bigcup_{s \in S} \mathcal{D}^s$ of a finite set V of variables, $var(C) \subseteq V$, such that $(\mathcal{D}, \sigma) \models \forall C$ holds. Solving a conjunction C of constraints means finding out whether there is a solution for C or not.

A *constraint solver* consists of a collection of tests and operations, e.g. constraint satisfaction, constraint entailment, constraint projection, and simplification (see [5]), which can be used to solve and to transform constraints of a constraint system. A solver works on a constraint store. A constraint store $C \in CStore$ consists of a disjunction of constraint conjunctions; in particular, C has the property that it is satisfiable in the corresponding domain $\mathcal{D}$.

3   Combination of Constraint Solvers

3.1   The Architecture

Figure 1 shows the architecture of our overall system for cooperating constraint solvers. It consists of two levels: At *object level* different constraint solvers CS_ν, $\nu \in L$, $L = \{1, \ldots, l\}$, infer about objects of their constraint domains. To every individual solver CS_ν a constraint store C^ν is assigned. A constraint store C^ν contains the already propagated constraints of constraint system ζ_ν. Propagating a constraint $c \in Cons(\Sigma_\nu)$ means to add c to the constraint store C^ν if the conjunction of c and C^ν is satisfiable. In this case the propagation is successful, otherwise it fails. At *meta level* the *meta constraint solver* handles both the constraint solvers and constraints as objects. It coordinates the work of the different object level solvers, i.e. it realizes the cooperation between the solvers under a certain strategy (see Sect. 3.4.3). The meta solver manages the *constraint pool* which contains the constraints which have not been propagated so far.

Initially, the constraint pool contains the constraints which we want to solve. The meta constraint solver takes constraints from the constraint pool and passes them to the constraint solvers of the corresponding constraint domains (step 1). Each of the individual constraint solvers is able to handle a subset of the given

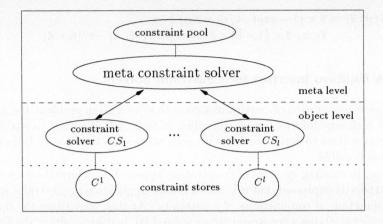

Fig. 1. Architecture of the overall system

set of constraints of the constraint pool independently of the other solvers, the individual solvers propagate the received constraints to their stores (step 2). The meta constraint solver manages the exchange of information between the individual solvers. It forces them to extract information from their constraint stores. This information which has again the form of constraints is added by the meta constraint solver to the constraint pool (step 3). The procedure of steps 1-3 is repeated until the pool contains either the constraint *false* or the constraint *true* only, i.e. the given constraints are solved. If the constraint pool contains *false* only, then the initially given conjunction of constraints is unsatisfiable. If the pool contains *true* only, then the system could not find a contradiction. Solutions can be retrieved from the current constraint stores. Using the described mechanisms, each individual solver deals with more information than only that of its associated constraints of the initially given constraint conjunction.

3.2 Syntax

Assume that for every $\nu \in L, L = \{1, \ldots, l\}$, a constraint system $\zeta_\nu = \langle \Sigma_\nu, \mathcal{D}_\nu \rangle$ with associated constraint solver CS_ν is given. We want to solve a conjunction $(c_1 \wedge \ldots \wedge c_n)$ of constraints $c_i, i \in \{1, \ldots, n\}$, where every c_i may contain function symbols and predicate symbols of different constraint systems. It is necessary to detect overloaded symbols by analysis and to convert every conjunction of constraints into a conjunction such that every constraint is defined by function symbols and predicate symbols of exactly one constraint system. This is done by a function *Simplify* which is provided by the meta constraint solver.

Example 2. Given two constraint systems $\zeta_i = \langle \Sigma_i, \mathcal{D}_i \rangle$ with $\Sigma_i = (S_i, F_i, R_i; ar_i)$, $i \in \{1, 2\}$, where $=_1 \in R_1$, $\{\times, -, /\} \subseteq F_1$, and $=_2 \in R_2$, $exp \in F_2$, the following transformation is performed:

$$Simplify(\ V_K = V \times (1 - exp(-t/(R \times K))) \ ) \ =$$
$$V_K =_1 V \times (1 - E) \wedge E =_2 exp(F) \wedge F =_1 -t/(R \times K). \qquad \Box$$

3.3   A Uniform Interface for Constraint Solvers.

To enable a cooperation of constraint solvers to solve a given problem, the solvers need to exchange information as described in Sect. 3.1. We want to enable the constraint solvers to communicate with each other such that a very tight cooperation is possible.

Often, in existing systems of cooperation approaches, information exchange is not explicitly expressed, but it is talked about 'application of constraint solvers to a disjunction of conjunctions of constraints'. At this, sometimes the form of the result of applying a constraint solver is fixed [8], in others neither the form of the results nor the involved variables or the constraint systems which can work with these results are described [3, 6]. Thus, to provide a general framework for cooperating solvers, we split the handling of constraints into two parts and define *our uniform interface* for a constraint solver CS_ν by the following functions, $\nu, \mu \in L$ (the set of constraint stores of a constraint system ζ_ν is denoted by $CStore_\nu$):

1. $tell: Cons(\Sigma_\nu) \times CStore_\nu \rightarrow \{true_{changed}, true_{redundant}, false\} \times CStore_\nu$
2.(a) $proj: \mathcal{P}(X) \times CStore_\nu \rightarrow CStore_\nu$
2.(b) $proj^{\nu \rightarrow \mu}: \mathcal{P}(X) \times CStore_\nu \rightarrow CStore_\mu$

1. The function *tell* is due to constraint satisfaction, i.e. an operation which is usually offered by constraint solvers. Function *tell* adds a constraint $c \in Cons(\Sigma_\nu)$ to a constraint store $C \in CStore_\nu$ if the conjunction of c and C is satisfiable. If c can be inferred by C, i.e. if $\mathcal{D}_\nu \models \forall(C \longrightarrow c)$ holds, then the result is $true_{redundant}$, and C does not change. If c cannot be inferred by C but the conjunction of c and C is satisfiable, i.e. if $(\mathcal{D}_\nu \not\models \forall(C \longrightarrow c)) \wedge (\mathcal{D}_\nu \models \exists(C \wedge c))$ holds, then we get $true_{changed}$, and the constraint store becomes $C \wedge c$. If the conjunction of C and c is unsatisfiable, i.e. $\mathcal{D}_\nu \not\models \exists(C \wedge c)$ holds, then the result is $false$, and C does not change. To enable the use of incomplete constraint solvers we allow to define *tell* in such a way that $tell(c, C) = (true_{changed}, C \wedge c)$ holds if the satisfaction algorithm cannot find out whether $\mathcal{D}_\nu \models \exists(C \wedge c)$ holds or not. (A more appropriate definition of *tell* for incomplete solvers which, for example, allows to delay particular constraints is left out because of space limitations.)

2.(a) The function *proj* is due to the operation constraint projection of constraint solvers. Usually, the aim of projecting a constraint store $C \in CStore_\nu$ wrt a sequence $\tilde{Y}$ (with $Y \in \mathcal{P}(X)$) of variables which occur in C is to find a disjunction C' of conjunctions of constraints which is equivalent to $\exists_{-\tilde{Y}} C$ and where the variables which do occur in C but not in $\tilde{Y}$ are eliminated: $\mathcal{D}_\nu \models \forall(\exists_{-\tilde{Y}} C \longleftrightarrow C')$. However, since sometimes it is not possible to compute C' or it is not possible to compute it efficiently, we define our interface function *proj* as follows: A constraint store C is projected wrt a set $Y \subseteq X$ of variables.

The result is a disjunction C' of conjunctions of constraints induced by $\exists_{-\tilde{Y}} C$: $\mathcal{D}_\nu \vDash \forall (\exists_{-\tilde{Y}} C \longrightarrow C')$.

2.(b) The projection of a constraint store C^ν, $\nu \in L$, generates a disjunction of conjunctions of constraints of $Cons(\Sigma_\nu)$. Since we want to use projections for information exchange between the different constraint solvers, we need a projection of a constraint store C^ν wrt a constraint system ζ_μ, $\mu \in L$. Thus, we use the function $proj \colon \mathcal{P}(X) \times CStore_\nu \to CStore_\nu$ of a constraint solver CS_ν and a conversion function $conv^{\nu \to \mu} \colon CStore_\nu \to CStore_\mu$ to define the function $proj^{\nu \to \mu} \colon \mathcal{P}(X) \times CStore_\nu \to CStore_\mu$ which projects a constraint store C^ν wrt a constraint system ζ_μ and a subset of the set of common variables of the sorts of S_{Σ_ν} and S_{Σ_μ}. The result of the projection of C^ν wrt ζ_μ is a disjunction of conjunction of constraints of $Cons(\Sigma_\mu)$:

$$
\begin{array}{|l|}
\hline
proj^{\nu \to \mu}(Y, C^\nu) = conv^{\nu \to \mu}(proj(Y, C^\nu)), \text{ where} \\
\mu, \nu \in L, C^\nu \in CStore_\nu, Y \subseteq X^s, s \in S_{\Sigma_\nu} \cap S_{\Sigma_\mu}. \\
proj^{\nu \to \mu}(Y, C^\nu) = \bigvee_{\gamma \in \{1,\ldots,u\}} (\bigwedge_{\delta \in \{1,\ldots,t_\gamma\}} c_{\gamma,\delta}), \text{ where for every} \\
\gamma \in \{1,\ldots,u\}, \delta \in \{1,\ldots,t_\gamma\} \text{ holds: } c_{\gamma,\delta} \in \{true, false\} \cup Cons(\Sigma_\mu). \\
\hline
\end{array}
$$

Thus, each single constraint solver can be regarded as black box constraint solver equipped with a projection function which allows the projection of the constraint store wrt a set of variables. These black box solvers are extended by functions for converting a projection wrt another constraint system.

Example 3. The simplest case is the projection of valuations. Consider the finite domain constraint solver CS_3 of our example. Let $X_{Ex} = \{R, R_1, R_2, V, V_K, K, E, F, t\}$ hold, i.e. X_{Ex} is the set of variables of our example. The projection functions $proj^{3 \to \mu}$, $\mu \in \{1, 2\}$, are defined as follows:

$proj^{3 \to \mu}(Y, C) = conv^{3 \to \mu}(proj(Y, C))$, where

$$
proj(Y, C) = \begin{cases} \bigvee_{i \in \{1,\ldots,n\}} (x =_3 val_i) & \text{if } Y = \{x\},\ x \in X_{Ex}, \text{ and } val_i \in \mathbb{R},\ i \in \\ & \{1,\ldots,n\}, \text{ are the possible values that } x \\ & \text{can take such that } \mathcal{D}_3 \vDash \exists(\sigma_i(C)) \text{ holds,} \\ & \text{where } \sigma_i(x) = val_i, \\ true & \text{otherwise.} \end{cases}
$$

$$
conv^{3 \to \mu}(C) = \begin{cases} \bigvee_{i \in \{1,\ldots,n\}} (x =_\mu val_i) & \text{if } C = \bigvee_{i \in \{1,\ldots,n\}} (x =_3 val_i),\ x \in X_{Ex}, \\ true & \text{otherwise.} \end{cases} \qquad \square
$$

To prevent a loss of information at the communication of the solvers, the operation projection must be monotonous, i.e. in the following, for every $\nu, \mu \in L$, Property 1 is required:

Property 1 (Monotonicity of the Operation Projection).

> If C is the projection of the constraint store C^ν wrt a constraint system ζ_μ and a set of variables Y, i.e. $proj^{\nu \to \mu}(Y, C^\nu) = C$, and
>
> C'^ν is the new constraint store after the successful propagation of some constraint $c \in Cons(\Sigma_\nu)$ to the store C^ν, i.e. $tell(c, C^\nu) = (result, C'^\nu)$ and
>
> if C' is the projection of C'^ν wrt ζ_μ and Y, i.e. $proj^{\nu \to \mu}(Y, C'^\nu) = C'$,
>
> then C is redundant wrt C', i.e. $\mathcal{D}_\mu \vDash \forall(C' \longrightarrow C)$.
>
> At this, $result \in \{true_{changed}, true_{redundant}\}$, $Y \subseteq X^s$, $s \in S_{\Sigma_\nu} \cap S_{\Sigma_\mu}$.

Note 1. To avoid a possible increase of the computation cost because of a high number of projected constraints in the pool, the projection functions and the conversion functions must be defined cautiously.

In the following, we require the functions *tell*, *proj*, and $proj^{\nu \to \mu}$, $\nu, \mu \in L$, to be computable.

3.4   Operational Semantics

We define the notion of an overall configuration in a bottom-up manner. Two basic relations which lift the application of the functions *tell* and *proj* to the level of overall configurations provide the basis for a stepwise definition of the operational semantics in the following sections.

3.4.1   Preliminaries.

In the following, we mark each constraint store C^ν, $\nu \in L$, by a tag t_ν, $t_\nu \in \{0, 1, 2, 3\}$, i.e. we write $C^\nu[t_\nu]$. This tag indicates various changes of a constraint store after its last projection (to be explained later).

The conjunction $\bigwedge_{\nu \in L} C^\nu[t_\nu]$ of all constraint stores $C^\nu[t_\nu]$, $\nu \in L$, corresponds to the block of constraint stores of the individual solvers in Fig.1. A constraint store contains the already propagated constraints. If $c_1, \ldots, c_n$ have been successfully propagated to store C^ν of the solver CS_ν and the associated constraint system $\zeta_\nu = \langle \Sigma_\nu, \mathcal{D}_\nu \rangle$, then $\mathcal{D}_\nu \vDash \forall(C^\nu \longrightarrow \bigwedge_{i \in \{1, \ldots, n\}} c_i)$ holds.

A *configuration* $\mathcal{G} = \mathcal{P} \odot (\bigwedge_{\nu \in L} C^\nu[t_\nu])$ corresponds to the architecture of the overall system (Fig.1). It consists of the constraint pool $\mathcal{P}$ which is a set of constraints which we want to solve and the conjunction $\bigwedge_{\nu \in L} C^\nu[t_\nu]$ of constraint stores. An *overall configuration* $\mathcal{H}$ consists of a *formal disjunction* $\dot{\bigvee}_{j \in \{1, \ldots, m\}} \mathcal{G}_j = \mathcal{G}_1 \dot{\vee} \ldots \dot{\vee} \mathcal{G}_m$ of configurations $\mathcal{G}_1, \ldots, \mathcal{G}_m$, $m > 0$. Ξ is the set *of overall configurations*. In this work, formulas of the form $\mathcal{H} = \mathcal{G} \dot{\vee} \mathcal{H}'$, with $\mathcal{H}' = \mathcal{G}_1 \dot{\vee} \ldots \dot{\vee} \mathcal{G}_m$, $m \geq 0$, appear, where $m = 0$ means that $\mathcal{H} = \mathcal{G}$ holds, i.e. $\mathcal{H}'$ is an empty formal disjunction. Formal disjunction $\dot{\vee}$ is commutative.

The *initial overall configuration* $\mathcal{H}_0$ consists of one configuration $\mathcal{H}_0 = \mathcal{G}_0 = \mathcal{P} \odot (\bigwedge_{\nu \in L} C_0^\nu[t_\nu])$, where for every $\nu \in L$, $t_\nu = 0$, and $\mathcal{P} = \{c_1, \ldots, c_n\}$ is the constraint pool (if $(c_1 \wedge \ldots \wedge c_n)$ is the constraint conjunction which we want to solve), and the constraint stores $C_0^\nu[0]$ are empty: $C_0^\nu[0] = (true)$.

If $\mathcal{H} = \{false\} \odot (\bigwedge_{\nu \in L} C_0^\nu[0])$ or $\mathcal{H} = \bigvee_{\kappa \in \{1,\ldots,\lambda\}} (\{true\} \odot (\bigwedge_{\nu \in L} C^\nu \kappa[0]))$, $\lambda \in I\!N$, then the overall configuration $\mathcal{H}$ is in *normal form*.

Example 4. Consider the input constraint conjunction of Example 1. Given the constraint systems $\zeta_\nu = \langle \Sigma_\nu, \mathcal{D}_\nu \rangle$ with $\Sigma_\nu = (S_\nu, F_\nu, R_\nu; ar_\nu)$, $\nu \in \{1, 2, 3\}$, where $=_\nu \in R_\nu$, $\{+, -, \times, /, [\,]\} \subseteq F_1$, $exp \in F_2$, and $\{\in, \leq\} \subseteq R_3$, after applying the function $Simplify$ the following conjunction is to be handled:
$R_1 =_1 10^5 \wedge R_2 =_1 [10^5, 4 \cdot 10^5] \wedge (1/R) =_1 (1/R_1) + (1/R_2) \wedge V_K =_1 V \times (1 - E) \wedge$
$E =_2 exp(F) \quad \wedge \quad F =_1 -t/(R \times K) \quad \wedge \quad V_K =_1 0.99 \times V \quad \wedge \quad t =_1 [0.5, 1] \quad \wedge$
$K \in \{10^{-6}, 2.5 \cdot 10^{-6}, 5 \cdot 10^{-6}, 10^{-5}, 2 \cdot 10^{-5}, 5 \cdot 10^{-5}\}$.

We assign the names $c_1, \ldots, c_9$ to the constraints in the above given order. $\mathcal{G}_0 = \{c_1, \ldots, c_9\} \odot (C_0^1[0] \wedge C_0^2[0] \wedge C_0^3[0])$ is the initial overall configuration, where $\forall \nu \in \{1, 2, 3\}: C_0^\nu[0] = (true)$.   □

3.4.2 Basic Relations.

In the following, we define two basic relations for the formal description of the communication between the solvers. As we will see in the following sections, these relations allow a fine grain description of the cooperation of the solvers according to the current requirements, i.e. a tight cooperation of constraint solvers.

1. The relation $prop \subseteq \bigcup_{\nu \in L} Cons(\Sigma_\nu) \times \Xi \times \Xi$ lifts the application of the function $tell$ to the level of overall configurations. $prop(c, \mathcal{G}, \mathcal{H})$ holds, if the propagation of a constraint c of the constraint pool of the configuration $\mathcal{G}$ to the appropriate constraint store of $\mathcal{G}$ yields the overall configuration $\mathcal{H}$.

$prop(c, \mathcal{G}, \mathcal{H})$ holds, where $\mathcal{G} = \mathcal{P} \odot (\bigwedge_{\mu \in L} C^\mu[t_\mu])$,
if $c \in \mathcal{P}$, $c \in Cons(\Sigma_\nu) \backslash \{true, false\}$, $\nu \in L$, $t_\nu \in \{0, 1, 2, 3\}$, and one of the following cases holds:

1. $\mathcal{H} = (\mathcal{P} \backslash \{c\}) \odot ((\bigwedge_{\mu \in L \backslash \{\nu\}} C^\mu[t_\mu]) \wedge C'^\nu[1])$ if
   $tell(c, C^\nu) = (true_{changed}, C'^\nu)$, $t_\nu \in \{0, 1, 2\}$,
2. $\mathcal{H} = (\mathcal{P} \backslash \{c\}) \cup \{true\} \odot ((\bigwedge_{\mu \in L \backslash \{\nu\}} C^\mu[t_\mu]) \wedge C^\nu[t'_\nu])$ if
   $tell(c, C^\nu) = (true_{redundant}, C^\nu)$,
   $t'_\nu = 2$ if $t_\nu \in \{0, 2\}$, and $t'_\nu = 1$ if $t_\nu = 1$,
3. $\mathcal{H} = (\mathcal{P} \backslash \{c\}) \cup \{false\} \odot ((\bigwedge_{\mu \in L \backslash \{\nu\}} C^\mu[t_\mu]) \wedge C^\nu[3])$ if
   $tell(c, C^\nu) = (false, C^\nu)$, $t_\nu \in \{0, 1, 2\}$,
4. $\mathcal{H} = (\mathcal{P} \backslash \{c\}) \odot (\bigwedge_{\mu \in L} C^\mu[t_\mu])$ if $t_\nu = 3$.

According to the definition of the operation $tell$ we distinguish the cases (1)-(3). The tag t_ν, $\nu \in L$, of the constraint store $C^\nu[t_\nu]$ indicates changes of the store after its last projection: $t_\nu = 0$ denotes that no propagation of constraints to C^ν was done, $t_\nu = 1$ reports that a nonredundant constraint was successfully propagated, $t_\nu = 2$ notices that only redundant constraints have been propagated, and $t_\nu = 3$ indicates a failing propagation. If the propagation of a constraint failed, i.e. $t_\nu = 3$, then the constraint pool contains $false$ and further constraint propagations are irrelevant (case (4)). Figure 2.1. shows the changes of a tag t_ν in dependence of the relation $prop$.

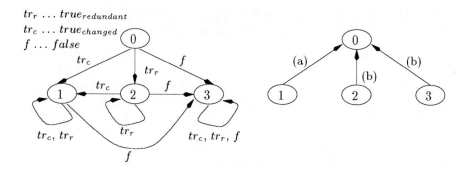

$tr_r \ldots true_{redundant}$
$tr_c \ldots true_{changed}$
$f \ldots false$

Fig.2.1. Changes of tag t_ν by *prop*   **Fig.2.2.** Changes of tag t_ν by *put_proj*

$prop(c, \mathcal{H}, \mathcal{H}')$ holds, where $\mathcal{H} = \dot{\bigvee}_{j\in\{1,\ldots,m\}} \mathcal{G}_j$, $\mathcal{H}' = \dot{\bigvee}_{j\in\{1,\ldots,m\}} \mathcal{H}'_j$,
if $\forall j \in \{1, \ldots, m\}$: $prop(c, \mathcal{G}_j, \mathcal{H}'_j)$.

The validity of the relation *prop* for some constraint c and two overall configurations $\mathcal{H} = \dot{\bigvee}_{j\in\{1,\ldots,m\}} \mathcal{G}_j$ and $\mathcal{H}' = \dot{\bigvee}_{j\in\{1,\ldots,m\}} \mathcal{H}'_j$ is due to the validity of *prop* for every $j \in \{1, \ldots, m\}$ for c and the configurations $\mathcal{G}_j$ and $\mathcal{H}'_j$.

2. The relation $put\_proj \subseteq L \times \mathcal{P}(L \times \mathcal{P}(\mathcal{P}(X))) \times \varXi \times \varXi$ lifts the application of the function *proj* to the level of overall configurations. $put\_proj(\nu, ProjSet, \mathcal{G}, \mathcal{H})$ holds (case (a)), if the overall configuration $\mathcal{H}$ is reached from the configuration $\mathcal{G}$ by projection of the constraint store C^ν ($t_\nu = 1$) of $\mathcal{G}$ wrt every ζ_μ and every set of $XSet_{\mu,\nu}$, where $ProjSet = \bigcup_{\mu\in L\setminus\{\nu\}} \{(\mu, XSet_{\mu,\nu})\}$, and adding these projections to the constraint pool of $\mathcal{G}$. ($XSet_{\mu,\nu}$, $\mu \in L\setminus\{\nu\}$, contains sets of variables of the common sorts of $\varSigma_\mu$ and $\varSigma_\nu$. The constraint store C^ν is projected wrt each of these sets and ζ_μ.) For better understanding see Example 5.

If C^ν of $\mathcal{G}$ has not changed by a constraint propagation before ($t_\nu \in \{0, 2\}$), or the change of C^ν is not relevant for further derivation ($t_\nu = 3$) (case (b)), then ν, $ProjSet$ and $\mathcal{G}$ are in relation to $\mathcal{H}$ (according to put_proj), where no projection is added to the pool of $\mathcal{G}$. This use of the tags t_ν, $\nu \in L$, (see Fig.s 2.1. and 2.2.) prevents unnecessary projections.

$put\_proj(\nu, \bigcup_{\mu\in L\setminus\{\nu\}}\{(\mu, XSet_{\mu,\nu})\}, \mathcal{G}, \mathcal{H})$, with $\nu, \mu \in L$,
$XSet_{\mu,\nu} \in \mathcal{P}(\mathcal{P}(X^s))$, $s \in S_{\varSigma_\nu} \cap S_{\varSigma_\mu}$, and

(a) $\mathcal{G} = \mathcal{P} \odot ((\bigwedge_{r\in L\setminus\{\nu\}} C^r[t_r]) \wedge C^\nu[1])$,
  $\mathcal{H} = \dot{\bigvee}_{\alpha\in\{1,\ldots,m\}}(\mathcal{P} \cup \bigcup_{\theta\in\{1,\ldots,n_\alpha\}}\{c_{\alpha,\theta}\} \odot ((\bigwedge_{r\in L\setminus\{\nu\}} C^r[t_r]) \wedge C^\nu[0]))$,
  where $\bigwedge_{\mu\in L\setminus\{\nu\}}(\bigwedge_{Z\in XSet_{\mu,\nu}}(proj^{\nu\to\mu}(Z, C^\nu))) =$
$$\dot{\bigvee}_{\alpha\in\{1,\ldots,m\}}(\bigwedge_{\theta\in\{1,\ldots,n_\alpha\}} c_{\alpha,\theta}), \text{ or}$$
(b) $\mathcal{G} = \mathcal{P} \odot ((\bigwedge_{r\in L\setminus\{\nu\}} C^r[t_r]) \wedge C^\nu[t_\nu])$, $t_\nu \in \{0, 2, 3\}$, and
  $\mathcal{H} = \mathcal{P} \odot ((\bigwedge_{r\in L\setminus\{\nu\}} C^r[t_r]) \wedge C^\nu[0])$.

As for the relation *prop* the validity of *put_proj* for two overall configurations $\mathcal{H}$ and $\mathcal{H}'$ is due to the validity of *put_proj* for their configurations.

$$put\_proj(\nu, ProjSet, \mathcal{H}, \mathcal{H}'), \text{ where } \mathcal{H} = \bigvee_{j \in \{1,\ldots,m\}} \mathcal{G}_j, \mathcal{H}' = \bigvee_{j \in \{1,\ldots,m\}} \mathcal{H}'_j,$$
$$\text{if } \forall j \in \{1,\ldots,m\}: put\_proj(\nu, ProjSet, \mathcal{G}_j, \mathcal{H}'_j).$$

Example 5. Consider our example, when in the last step CS_3 produces the constraint $\mathtt{K} =_3 2.5 \cdot 10^{-6}$, i.e. the constraint store C''^3 of CS_3 'contains' the valuation $\sigma(\mathtt{K}) = 2.5 \cdot 10^{-6}$. We want to project C''^3 wrt ζ_1 and ζ_2 for information exchange. Let $\mathcal{G} = \mathcal{P} \odot (C^1[0] \wedge C^2[0] \wedge C''^3[1])$ be the current configuration. The relation $put\_proj(3, ProjSet, \mathcal{G}, \mathcal{H})$ with $ProjSet = \{(1, \{\{\mathtt{K}\}, \{\mathtt{t}\}\}), (2, \{\{\mathtt{K}\}, \{\mathtt{R}\}\})\}$ describes that the overall configuration $\mathcal{H}$ is reached from configuration $\mathcal{G}$ by projecting the constraint store C''^3 wrt constraint system ζ_1 and each of the sets $\{\mathtt{K}\}$ and $\{\mathtt{t}\}$ and wrt system ζ_2 and each of the sets $\{\mathtt{K}\}$ and $\{\mathtt{R}\}$ and adding the projections to the pool. The set $ProjSet$ fixes pairs of a constraint system and a set of sets of variables for a directed projection.

$$put\_proj(3, ProjSet, \mathcal{G}, \mathcal{H}), \text{ where } ProjSet = \{(1, \{\{\mathtt{K}\}, \{\mathtt{t}\}\}), (2, \{\{\mathtt{K}\}, \{\mathtt{R}\}\})\},$$
$$\bigwedge_{\mu \in \{1,2\}} (\bigwedge_{Z \in XSet_{\mu,3}} (proj^{3 \to \mu}(Z, C''^3)))$$
$$= (\bigwedge_{Z \in \{\{\mathtt{K}\}, \{\mathtt{t}\}\}} (proj^{3 \to 1}(Z, C''^3))) \wedge (\bigwedge_{Z \in \{\{\mathtt{K}\}, \{\mathtt{R}\}\}} (proj^{3 \to 2}(Z, C''^3)))$$
$$= proj^{3 \to 1}(\{\mathtt{K}\}, C''^3) \wedge proj^{3 \to 1}(\{\mathtt{t}\}, C''^3) \wedge (\bigwedge_{Z \in \{\{\mathtt{K}\}, \{\mathtt{R}\}\}} (proj^{3 \to 2}(Z, C''^3)))$$
$$= \mathtt{K} =_1 2.5 \cdot 10^{-6} \wedge true \wedge \mathtt{K} =_2 2.5 \cdot 10^{-6} \wedge true$$
$$\mathcal{H} = \mathcal{P} \cup \{\mathtt{K} =_1 2.5 \cdot 10^{-6}, \mathtt{K} =_2 2.5 \cdot 10^{-6}, true\} \odot (C^1[0] \wedge C^2[0] \wedge C''^3[0]). \quad \square$$

3.4.3 Defining Strategies for Cooperating Constraint Solvers.

Now, we want to use the above defined basic relations for a stepwise definition of the operational semantics. The coordination of the individual constraint solvers which is specified by the operational semantics is controlled by the meta constraint solver. To enable a tight cooperation of the different solvers to reach an efficient computation behaviour, we need to take into account various influences on such a combined system.

Example 6. Consider the input constraint conjunction of Example 4. Constraint $c_5 = (\mathtt{E} =_2 exp(\mathtt{F}))$ is handled by the constraint solver CS_2 which is able to infer about functions, like exp, ln, sin, and cos; constraint $c_9 = (\mathtt{K} \in \{10^{-6}, 2.5 \cdot 10^{-6}, 5 \cdot 10^{-6}, 10^{-5}, 2 \cdot 10^{-5}, 5 \cdot 10^{-5}\})$ is handled by the finite domain constraint solver CS_3, all other constraints are constraints for which the constraint solver CS_1 for rational interval arithmetic is responsible. Figure 3 shows the information exchange between the constraint solvers during the process of solving the constraint conjunction as done in Example 1. Constraints which label arrows between constraint solvers express that they are projections from one solver which are propagated to the other solver.

Figure 3 shows one possible order of application of the constraint solvers on the given constraint conjunction. The computation effort depends on the order of application of the solvers. An arbitrary order of solver application does not need to yield the constraint $\mathtt{K} =_3 2.5 \cdot 10^{-6}$ as fast. For example, using CS_2 to find a

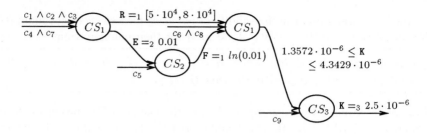

Fig. 3. Information exchange of cooperating solvers according to Example 1

valuation for **F** requires a computation of a valuation for **E** by CS_1 before. This leads to the question of how to describe an appropriate coordination strategy. □

There are many influences, like properties of the particular constraint solvers as well as properties of the underlying hardware architecture, for instance, parallel processors, on the choice of an appropriate cooperation strategy to optimize the computation effort. This yields the necessity to define different coordination strategies for cooperating solvers. If the single solvers for the cooperation are chosen, the interfaces of the solvers are fixed, and the external influences are known, then we can start to design a cooperation strategy. In the following, we illustrate the way of defining strategies in general, we do not go into detail wrt particular influences.

In general, in one derivation step one or more configurations $\mathcal{G}_j$, $j \in \{1, \ldots, m\}$, are rewritten by a formal disjunction $\mathcal{HG}_j$ of configurations (for $i \in \{1, \ldots, m+1\}$, $\mathcal{H}_i$ denotes a (possibly empty) formal disjunction):

$$\mathcal{H}_1 \dot{\vee} \mathcal{G}_1 \quad \dot{\vee} \ldots \dot{\vee} \mathcal{H}_j \dot{\vee} \mathcal{G}_j \quad \dot{\vee} \ldots \dot{\vee} \mathcal{H}_m \dot{\vee} \mathcal{G}_m \quad \dot{\vee} \mathcal{H}_{m+1} \implies$$
$$\mathcal{H}_1 \dot{\vee} \mathcal{HG}_1 \dot{\vee} \ldots \dot{\vee} \mathcal{H}_j \dot{\vee} \mathcal{HG}_j \dot{\vee} \ldots \dot{\vee} \mathcal{H}_m \dot{\vee} \mathcal{HG}_m \dot{\vee} \mathcal{H}_{m+1}$$

Thus, first, we define a derivation relation for configurations and, based on this, we define a derivation relation for overall configurations. The following three steps build a general frame for the definition of strategies for cooperating solvers:

1. Definition of a derivation relation for configurations (*production level*).
2. Defining a derivation relation for overall configurations (*application level*).
3. Definition of a reduction system for the derivation of overall configurations.

In the following, showing four examples of strategy definitions, we instantiate the general frame by specifying the steps 1, 2, and 3.

1. Definition of a derivation relation for configurations: For simplification, in our example strategies constraint stores are projected wrt all other constraint systems and wrt each of the variables of the common sorts of the two concerned constraint systems. To summarize this we define the relation *project*:

$project(\nu, \mathcal{H}, \mathcal{H}')$ holds if $put\_proj(\nu, ProjSet, \mathcal{H}, \mathcal{H}')$ holds, where
$ProjSet = \bigcup_{\mu \in L \setminus \{\nu\}} \{(\mu, XSet_{\mu,\nu})\}$ with $XSet_{\mu,\nu} = \bigcup_{x \in X^s, s \in S_{\Sigma_\nu} \cap S_{\Sigma_\mu}} \{\{x\}\}$.

Let us consider the simplest possibility to define a derivation step for a configuration $\mathcal{G} = \mathcal{P} \odot (\bigwedge_{r \in L} C^r[t_r])$: Exactly one constraint $c \in Cons(\Sigma_\nu)$ is chosen (nondeterministically) from the constraint pool $\mathcal{P}$ of $\mathcal{G}$ and it is propagated to C^ν building C'^ν and the new configuration $\mathcal{H}$. This is followed by a projection of C'^ν by means of *project* (i.e. a projection wrt all other constraint systems ζ_μ and every variable of the common sorts of ζ_ν and ζ_μ).

$\mathcal{G} \overset{sub}{\longrightarrow}^\nu \mathcal{H}$ holds if $\mathcal{G} = \mathcal{P} \odot (\bigwedge_{r \in L} C^r[0])$ is not in normal form,
$\exists \mathcal{H}' \in \Xi$: $prop(c, \mathcal{G}, \mathcal{H}') \wedge project(\nu, \mathcal{H}', \mathcal{H})$,
where $c \in \mathcal{P}$, $c \in Cons(\Sigma_\nu) \backslash \{true, false\}$, $\nu \in L$.

If, in a number of such steps, constraints $c_1, \ldots, c_n$ from the pool are propagated one after the other, such that they are all constraints of exactly one constraint system, then each projection is redundant wrt the following projections because of Property 1. Avoiding such redundant projections leads to the definition of the relation $\overset{sub}{\longrightarrow}_+^\nu$, $\nu \in L$:

$\mathcal{G} \overset{sub}{\longrightarrow}_+^\nu \mathcal{H}$ holds if $\mathcal{G} = \mathcal{H}_1 = \mathcal{P} \odot (\bigwedge_{r \in L} C^r[0])$ is not in normal form and
$\exists \mathcal{H}_2, \ldots, \mathcal{H}_{n+1} \in \Xi$: $\bigwedge_{i \in \{1, \ldots, n\}} prop(c_i, \mathcal{H}_i, \mathcal{H}_{i+1}) \wedge project(\nu, \mathcal{H}_{n+1}, \mathcal{H})$,
where $\nu \in L$, $c_1, \ldots, c_n \in \mathcal{P}$, $c_1, \ldots, c_n \in Cons(\Sigma_\nu) \backslash \{true, false\}$, $n \geq 1$.

Example 7. Recall our example to see the difference between $\overset{sub}{\longrightarrow}^\nu$ and $\overset{sub}{\longrightarrow}_+^\nu$. Consider the situation, when CS_3 gets the constraint $c_9 = (\text{K} \in \{10^{-6}, 2.5 \cdot 10^{-6}, 5 \cdot 10^{-6}, 10^{-5}, 2 \cdot 10^{-5}, 5 \cdot 10^{-5}\})$ from the input constraint conjunction and afterwards the constraint $c_{10} = (1.3572 \cdot 10^{-6} \leq \text{K} \leq 4.3429 \cdot 10^{-6})$ from CS_1, both to be propagated to the current constraint store C^3 of CS_3.

Using $\overset{sub}{\longrightarrow}^\nu$, in the first step c_9 is added to C^3 which yields C'^3, which is projected. The second $\overset{sub}{\longrightarrow}^\nu$ step adds c_{10} to C'^3 which yields C''^3. Using $\overset{sub}{\longrightarrow}_+^\nu$ we avoid the projections of C'^3 which are redundant wrt the later following projections of C''^3 because of Property 1. Thus, moreover, the handling of the redundant projections of C'^3 by CS_1 and CS_2 is avoided.   □

If we want to fix the order of the constraint systems constraints of which are propagated next, then we simply give an order $<$ on constraint systems and we use the relation $\overset{sub}{\longrightarrow}_+^<$ which is defined as follows:

$\mathcal{G} \overset{sub}{\longrightarrow}_+^< \mathcal{H}$ holds if $\mathcal{G} \overset{sub}{\longrightarrow}_+^\nu \mathcal{H}$, $\nu \in L$, and
there is no $\mu \in L$, $\mu \neq \nu$, $\mu < \nu$, s.t. $\exists \mathcal{H}' \in \Xi$: $\mathcal{G} \overset{sub}{\longrightarrow}_+^\mu \mathcal{H}'$.

Similarly, we can define an order of constraints to be propagated which enables to regard choice heuristics, for example to delay particular constraints, as for naive solving nonlinear constraints [1].

Hitherto, constraints of exactly one constraint system ζ_ν, $\nu \in L$, are propagated and afterwards the associated constraint store C^ν is projected while all other individual constraint solvers than CS_ν are idle. However, since each of the

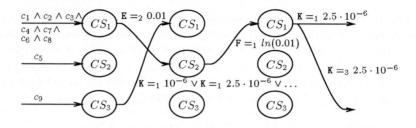

Fig. 4. Information exchange handling the input constraint conjunction using $\xrightarrow{sub}_{par}$

individual constraint solvers is able to handle a subset of the constraint pool independently of the other constraint solvers, the solvers may work in parallel:

$G \xrightarrow{sub}_{par} \mathcal{H}$ holds if $G = \mathcal{H}_1 = \mathcal{P} \odot (\bigwedge_{r \in L} C^r[0])$ is not in normal form and $\exists \mathcal{H}_2, \ldots, \mathcal{H}_{n+m+1} \in \Xi: (\mathcal{H}_{n+m+1} = \mathcal{H}) \wedge$
$\bigwedge_{i \in \{1, \ldots, n\}} prop(c_i, \mathcal{H}_i, \mathcal{H}_{i+1}) \wedge \bigwedge_{l_\nu \in L} project(l_\nu, \mathcal{H}_{n+\nu}, \mathcal{H}_{n+\nu+1})$, where $\mathcal{P} \backslash \{true, false\} = \bigcup_{i \in \{1, \ldots, n\}} \{c_i\}$, $n \geq 1$, and $L = \{l_1, \ldots l_m\}$.

This definition describes the sequential execution of propagations followed by projections. However, propagations of constraints of different constraint systems are independent as well as projections of constraint stores of different constraint systems do. Thus, they can be performed in arbitrary order, in special in parallel and the behaviour defined by the relation $\xrightarrow{sub}_{par}$ can be regarded (and if we have a parallel computer system it can as well be performed) as follows: The constraint pool $\mathcal{P}$ of the configuration $G = \mathcal{P} \odot (\bigwedge_{\nu \in L} C^\nu[0])$ is split into subsets $\mathcal{P}_\nu$ of constraints, $\nu \in L$, with $\forall c \in \mathcal{P}_\nu: c \in Cons(\Sigma_\nu)$. These subsets are passed to their associated solvers which, in parallel, propagate all constraints of their received subsets. Afterwards they project their constraint stores. The resulting overall configuration is built by composition of the results of the single solvers.

The advantages of the derivation relation $\xrightarrow{sub}_{par}$ are, first, that the individual constraint solvers can work in parallel, and second, that redundant projections are avoided as well as by relation $\xrightarrow{sub}_{+}^{\nu}$.

Example 8. Parallel work of all constraint solvers of our example handling the input constraint conjunction yields the trace and the information exchange of Fig.4. To allow a comparison to the trace in Example 6 only the incoming constraints which are propagated to the associated stores of the solvers by *tell* and the outgoing constraints, i.e. projections of the constraint stores are given. Only the relevant projections are shown and changes of constraint stores are left out.

The cooperating solvers find the capacitor which we are searching for in parallel after 3 $\xrightarrow{sub}_{par}$ steps while Example 6 suggested to need at least 4 steps. □

Our framework allows to define many other possible strategies for the derivation of configurations by varying the use of the basic relations. Moreover, in our four example strategies a constraint store is projected wrt each other constraint system and wrt each single variable of the common sorts of two constraint systems (fixed by the auxiliary predicate *project*). This causes overhead; designing specialized systems of cooperating solvers, this overhead can be avoided by a more appropriate application of *put_proj* in the definition of the strategy.

2. Defining a derivation relation of overall configurations: The most simple case is to define a derivation step for overall configurations on the base of the derivation of exactly one (nondeterministically chosen) configuration:

$\mathcal{G}\dot{\vee}\mathcal{H} \leadsto_1 \mathcal{H}'\dot{\vee}\mathcal{H}$ holds, where $\mathcal{H} = \mathcal{G}_1\dot{\vee}\ldots\dot{\vee}\mathcal{G}_m$, $m \geq 0$, if $\mathcal{G} \leadsto_2 \mathcal{H}'$, and

if $\leadsto_2 = \bigcup_{\nu \in L} \xrightarrow{sub}_\nu$ then $\leadsto_1 = \longrightarrow_{seq}$,   if $\leadsto_2 = \xrightarrow{sub}_+^<$ then $\leadsto_1 = \longrightarrow_{seq+}^<$,

if $\leadsto_2 = \bigcup_{\nu \in L} \xrightarrow{sub}_+^\nu$ then $\leadsto_1 = \longrightarrow_{seq+}$,   if $\leadsto_2 = \xrightarrow{sub}_{par}$ then $\leadsto_1 = \longrightarrow_{par}$.

Other possibilities are, for example, to allow a derivation step for several configurations in parallel or concurrently.

We add further, specific rules at application level, i.e. simplification rules $\longrightarrow_0$ for overall configurations:

1. $\mathcal{P} \odot (\bigwedge_{\nu \in L} C^\nu[t_\nu])\dot{\vee}\mathcal{H} \longrightarrow_0 \mathcal{H}$, $t_\nu \in \{0,1,2,3\}$,
   if $false \in \mathcal{P}$ and $\mathcal{H} = \mathcal{G}_1\dot{\vee}\ldots\dot{\vee}\mathcal{G}_m$, $m > 0$,
2. $\mathcal{P} \odot (\bigwedge_{\nu \in L} C^\nu[t_\nu]) \longrightarrow_0 \{false\} \odot (\bigwedge_{\nu \in L} C^\nu[t_\nu])$, $t_\nu \in \{0,1,2,3\}$,
   if $false \in \mathcal{P}$ and $\exists c \in \mathcal{P} : c \neq false$,
3. $\{false\} \odot (\bigwedge_{\nu \in L} C^\nu[t_\nu]) \longrightarrow_0 \{false\} \odot (\bigwedge_{\nu \in L} C_0^\nu[0])$, $t_\nu \in \{0,1,2,3\}$,
   if $\exists \mu \in L: C^\mu[t_\mu] \neq C_0^\mu[0]$, $t_\mu \in \{0,1,2,3\}$.

3. Definition of a reduction system for the derivation of overall configurations:

Definition 2. *We define the reduction systems* $(\Xi, \Longrightarrow_{seq})$, $(\Xi, \Longrightarrow_{seq+})$, $(\Xi, \Longrightarrow_{seq+}^<)$, *and* $(\Xi, \Longrightarrow_{par})$, *where* Ξ *is the set of overall configurations and* $(\Longrightarrow_{seq} = \longrightarrow_{seq} \cup \longrightarrow_0)$, $(\Longrightarrow_{seq+} = \longrightarrow_{seq+} \cup \longrightarrow_0)$, $(\Longrightarrow_{seq+}^< = \longrightarrow_{seq+}^< \cup \longrightarrow_0)$, *and* $(\Longrightarrow_{par} = \longrightarrow_{par} \cup \longrightarrow_0)$. □

The defined reduction systems are used for the derivation of an initial overall configuration to normal form. For example, using the reduction system $(\Xi, \Longrightarrow_{seq})$, in every derivation step, one constraint of the constraint pool of a configuration is propagated to its associated constraint store, followed by a projection of the newly built constraint store wrt all other constraint systems.

The λ conjunctions $\bigwedge_{\nu \in L} C^\nu \kappa[0]$, $\kappa \in \{1, \ldots, \lambda\}$, of the current constraint stores of a normal form $\bigvee_{\kappa \in \{1,\ldots,\lambda\}} \{true\} \odot (\bigwedge_{\nu \in L} C^\nu \kappa[0])$ contain constraints which describe the set of solutions. The initially given constraint conjunction has no solution if the derivation yields the normal form $\{false\} \odot (\bigwedge_{\nu \in L} C_0^\nu[0])$.

Solving constraint conjunctions using cooperating constraint solvers according to our framework no solutions are lost wrt the intersection of the solution sets of a computation of the single constraint solvers if $\forall \nu, \mu \in L: proj^{\nu \to \mu}$ is sound, i.e. a projection of a constraint store C^ν wrt to a constraint system ζ_μ and a set of variables V, is valid in $\mathcal{D}_\mu$ under all assignments $\sigma : V_\mu \cap V_\nu \to \bigcup_{s \in S_\nu \cap S_\mu} \mathcal{D}^s$, where σ is obtained by restricting a solution $\sigma_\nu : V_\nu \to \bigcup_{s \in S_\nu} \mathcal{D}^s$ of C^ν (wrt $\mathcal{D}_\nu$) to the variables of the common sorts of ζ_μ and ζ_ν; $V_\nu, V_\mu, V \subseteq X$. Because of the information exchange between the cooperating solvers they are able to solve constraint conjunctions which single constraint solvers are not able to handle.

4 Conclusion and Related Work

We have presented a general scheme for cooperating constraint solvers. A uniform interface for the solvers allows to formally specify the information exchange between them. Because of the modularity of our definitions of the basic relations and of the derivation relations at production level as well as at application level, we are able to define a wide range of derivation strategies for cooperating solvers. To analyse the particular influences of the choice of a strategy on the computation effort is one task of future research. Since our approach allows the integration of constraint solvers of very different constraint systems, it is possible to integrate different host languages into the system by treating them as constraint solvers. In [2] we have shown the integration of the functional logic language Curry. This new point of view on the host language of such a system and the possibility to define tight cooperation strategies according to the current requirements allow to specify a wide range of systems of cooperating solvers such that our overall system forms a general framework for cooperating solvers.

Cooperating solvers have been investigated from different points of view. Hong [3] addresses the issue of confluence for a system of cooperating solvers. The strategy of this system can be described using our sequential strategy $\Longrightarrow_{seq}$. The cooperative schemes for solving systems of constraints over real numbers [7, 8] introduced by Rueher resp. Rueher and Solnon describe concurrent work of the individual solvers. Such concurrent strategies can be described in our framework by strategies similar to $\Longrightarrow_{seq+}$. The environment for executing constraint solver combinations of Monfroy [6] provides three fixed cooperation primitives, where two of them correspond to our strategies $\Longrightarrow_{seq+}^{<}$ and $\Longrightarrow_{par}$. However, our approach allows a finer grained definition of strategies according to the current requirements. As far as for these approaches the form of constraints exchanged between the solvers is given, we are able to express that as well by means of our interface function *proj*. The main idea behind the combination approach in [9], which is an extension of the CLP scheme of Jaffar and Lassez [4], is a mechanism which controls variable equality sharing. We think that our approach is more general wrt information exchange, because in our system this is done by projections, where variable equality sharing is only one instance of it. The investigation of different cooperation strategies is left out in [9].

Acknowledgement

The author would like to thank Wolfgang Grieskamp and Heiko Vogler for discussions, careful reading, and helpful comments.

References

1. A. Colmerauer. Naive solving of non-linear constraints. In F. Benhamou and A. Colmerauer, editors, *Constraint Logic Programming. Selected Research*, pages 89–112. MIT Press, 1993.
2. P. Hofstedt. A functional logic language as hostlanguage for a system of combined constraint solvers. In R. Echahed, editor, *8th International Workshop on Functional and Logic Programming*, pages 119–132. Grenoble, France, 1999.
3. H. Hong. Confluency of cooperative constraint solvers. Technical Report 94-08, Research Institute for Symbolic Computation, Linz, Austria, 1994.
4. J. Jaffar and J.-L. Lassez. Constraint logic programming. Technical Report 74, Monash University, Melbourne, Australia, 1986.
5. J. Jaffar and M.J. Maher. Constraint logic programming: A survey. *Journal of Logic Programming*, 19&20:501–581, 1994.
6. E. Monfroy. *Solver Collaboration for Constraint Logic Programming*. PhD thesis, Centre de Recherche en Informatique de Nancy. INRIA-Lorraine, 1996.
7. M. Rueher. An architecture for cooperating constraint solvers on reals. In A. Podelski, editor, *Constraint Programming*, volume 910 of *LNCS*. Springer-Verlag, 1995.
8. M. Rueher and C. Solnon. Concurrent cooperating solvers over reals. *Reliable Computing*, 3:3:325–333, 1997.
9. C. Tinelli and M.T. Harandi. Constraint logic programming over unions of constraint theories. *The Journal of Functional and Logic Programming*, Article 6, 1998.

Arc Consistency Algorithms
via Iterations of Subsumed Functions

Rosella Gennari

Institute of Logic, Language and Computation, ILLC
Department of Philosophy, University of Amsterdam, N. Doelenstraat 15
1012 CP Amsterdam, The Netherlands
gennari@hum.uva.nl

Abstract. We provide here an extension of a general framework introduced in [Apt99b,Apt99c] that allows to explain several local consistency algorithms in a systematic way. In this framework we proceed in two steps. First, we introduce a generic iteration algorithm on partial orderings and prove its correctness. Then we instantiate this algorithm with specific partial orderings and functions to obtain specific local consistency algorithms. In particular, using the notion of subsumption, we show that the algorithms AC4, HAC-4, AC-5 and our extension HAC-5 of AC-5 are instances of a single generic algorithm.

1 Introduction

Constraint programming consists of formulating and solving constraint satisfaction problems. One of the most important techniques developed in this area is local consistency that aims at pruning the search space while maintaining equivalence. Our work stems from the framework devised in [Apt99b,Apt99c]; there the author introduces an algorithm, the Generic Iteration algorithm (GI), able to explain most of the usual local consistency algorithms in term of fixpoints of functions. In this paper, we develop the GI algorithm into a new one, the Generic Iteration Algorithm with Subsumed Functions, briefly GISF; our new algorithm can account for more local consistency algorithms than GI does, namely arc and hyper arc consistency ones. In fact the (hyper) arc consistency algorithms that we study in this paper all share a common feature: they are split in two parts; a first pruning takes place, then a new program - not interleaved with the previous one - performs a "local" action of pruning. Since the two programs are not interleaved, the GI algorithm cannot account for those kinds of (hyper) arc consistency algorithms; while our GISF algorithm can do it. Moreover the GI algorithm is an instance of our GISF algorithm. This article is organized as follows: we introduce our GISF algorithm and the general framework in Section 2. We show how constraint satisfaction problems can be encoded in that framework in Section 3. Afterwards, we show how GISF can account for some arc and hyper arc consistency algorithms; namely HAC-4 and AC-4, cf. Subsection 4.1 and 4.2; AC-5 and our generalization of it HAC-5, cf. Subsection 4.4 and 4.3.

J. Lloyd et al. (Eds.): CL 2000, LNAI 1861, pp. 358–372, 2000.
© Springer-Verlag Berlin Heidelberg 2000

2   The Generic Iteration Algorithm with Subsumed Functions

The GI algorithm of [Apt99b,Apt99c] can only iterate functions that belong to a unique set F. Now, our algorithm GISF feeds the set G of functions to iterate with functions from two possibly different sets, F and H; both sets H and F contain functions defined on the same set D. Further, we initialize G with the set H while the operator *update* can only select functions to iterate from the other set F.

GENERIC ITERATION ALGORITHM WITH SUBSUMED FUNCTIONS (GISF)

1. $d := \bot$;
2. $G := H$;
3. **while** $G \neq \emptyset$ **do**
4.   choose $g \in G$;
5. $G := G - \{g\}$;
6. $G := G \cup update(G, F, g, d)$;
7. $d := g(d)$
8. **od**

Our *update* operator has to satisfy the following three conditions:

A. if $g(d) \neq d$, then the following functions have to be in $update(G, F, g, d)$: all $f \in F - G$ such that $f(d) = d$ and $f(g(d)) \neq g(d)$;
B. $g(d) = d$ implies $update(G, F, g, d) = \emptyset$;
C. if $g(g(d)) \neq g(d)$, then g is in $update(G, F, g, d)$.

Remark 1. Suppose that g is *idempotent*; that is, for every $d \in D$, $g(g(d)) = g(d)$. In this case, g does not need to be added to $update(G, F, g, d)$ according to the third condition **C**.

The sets F and H are not arbitrary but related as in the following definition.

Definition 1. *Let f and g two functions on a set D; g subsumes f iff $g(d) = d$ implies $f(d) = d$. Let F and H be two sets of functions defined on the same set D; we say that the set H subsumes the set F iff each function of F is subsumed by a function of H; thus we write $subs(F, H)$.*

Remark 2. Observe that $subs(H, H)$ is always valid; this means that $subs$ is a reflexive relation. In general, it might not be trivial to check whether the subsumption relation holds between two functions f and g defined on the same set. However, suppose that $\langle D, \sqsubseteq \rangle$ is a partial ordering with bottom and that f is an inflationary function. If $f(d) \sqsubseteq g(d)$ for every $d \in D$, then indeed g subsumes f.

Now it is clear that our algorithm generalizes the GI one: in fact, it is enough to set $F = H$ in GISF and exploit the fact that $subs$ is a reflexive relation, cf. Remark 2.

Proposition 1. *The* GI *algorithm is an instance of the* GISF *algorithm.*

The following result was already in [Apt99b,Apt99c]; we shall use it to prove the correctness of GISF.

Lemma 1 (Stabilization, [Apt99b,Apt99c]). *Consider a partial ordering $\langle D, \sqsubseteq \rangle$ with bottom $\perp$ and a set K of monotonic functions on D; suppose that an iteration of the functions from K starting from $\perp$ eventually stabilizes at a common fixpoint d of the functions from K. Then d is the least common fixpoint of all functions from K.*

Theorem 1. (GISF) *Let $\langle D, \sqsubseteq \rangle$ be a partial ordering with the least element $\perp$; suppose that H and F are two sets of functions on D; if $subs(F, H)$ holds and K is $H \cup F$, then the following statements are valid.*

i. *Every terminating execution of the* GISF *algorithm computes in d a common fixpoint of the functions in K.*

ii. *Suppose that all functions of K are monotonic. Then every terminating execution of the* GISF *algorithm computes in d the least common fixpoint of all the functions of K.*

iii. *Suppose that K is finite and all of its functions are inflationary; further suppose that the strict partial order on D satisfies the ascending chain condition (ACC), namely that there are not infinite ascending chains. Then every execution of the* GISF *algorithm terminates.*

Proof. First we prove claim *i* by showing that the predicate $I := \forall f \in H - G \; f(d) = d$ is an invariant of the **while** loop. Suppose that the predicate I is true before we enter the **while** loop (observe that, when we enter the loop for the first time, the predicate is trivially true because $H - G$ is the empty set). After the execution of the loop, we have to inspect the functions which could be deleted from G; that is the function g. If $g(d) = d$, then $g(g(d)) = g(d)$ and so we could safely add g to $H - G$. Suppose now that $g(d) \neq d$; because of condition **C**, g could be added to $H - G$ only if $g(g(d)) = g(d)$. Our argument shows that the predicate I is trivially true after an execution of the **while** loop; therefore it is an invariant of the loop. This means that, upon the termination of the algorithm, the following condition holds: $(G = \emptyset) \wedge I$. Hence, for every g in H, $g(d) = d$; since all functions from F are subsumed by functions from H, then d is a fixpoint of all functions of $H \cup F = K$.

Claim *ii* follows from *i* and the Stabilization Lemma 1 applied to K.

Finally we prove *iii*. Let us consider the strict orderings $\langle D, \sqsupset \rangle$ and $\langle \mathbb{N}, < \rangle$, where $\sqsupset$ is the reverse of $\sqsubseteq$ and $\mathbb{N}$ is the set of natural numbers. We can define the following lexicographic order $<_{lex}$ on the set $D \times \mathbb{N}$:

$$(d, n) <_{lex} (d', n') \text{ iff } d \sqsupset d' \text{ or } n < n'.$$

By hypothesis, all functions in K are inflationary, so at each iteration of the **while** loop the cardinality of K strictly decreases with respect to $<$. By assumption, the strict order $\sqsubseteq$ satisfies the ACC, hence the are not infinite descending chains in the lexicographic order $<_{lex}$; the latter fact implies that the algorithm terminates. □

Note 1. If the set D is finite, then any relation of (strict) partial order on D is finite; further there is a finite number of different functions on D. Hence, if the set D is finite, the conditions in the last point of the previous theorem respectively on the order and on the set of functions K are trivially satisfied.

3 GISF for Constraint Satisfaction Problems

Our aim is to apply the GISF algorithm to solve constraint satisfaction problems; therefore we need to relate the last ones to the notions so far introduced. In the following, first we provide the definitions of constraints and constraint satisfaction problems that we shall need; then we make explicit the connections with the results from the previous section.

Consider a finite sequence X of $n > 0$ different variables, say $x_1, \ldots, x_n$, with associated domains $D_1, \ldots, D_n$; from now onwards, we shall always denote the Cartesian product $D_1 \times \cdots \times D_n$ with D.

Definition 2. *A scheme s on $n > 0$ is a strictly growing sequence of different integers from $1, \ldots, n$.*

Let s be the scheme $\langle i_1, \ldots, i_m \rangle$ on n; we denote the Cartesian product $D_{i_1} \times \cdots \times D_{i_n}$ with $D[s]$. For instance, if $D_1 = \{0\}$, $D_2 = \{2, 6\}$, $D_3 = \{4\}$ and s is the scheme $\langle 1, 3 \rangle$, then $D[s]$ is the set $\{(0, 4)\}$. Further, we shall denote the elements of $D[s]$ with $d[s]$, where d is a tuple of $D_1 \times \cdots \times D_n$.

Definition 3. *Let X be a sequence of $n > 0$ different variables with domains $D_1, \ldots, D_n$, the set D the Cartesian product $D_1 \times \cdots \times D_n$ and s a scheme on n; a constraint on s is a subset of $D[s]$; we shall write $C(s)$ or simply C when no confusion can arise. A constraint satisfaction problem on X, briefly CSP, is a triple $\langle X, D, C \rangle$ where C is a set of constraints (on schemes on n) and D is $D_1 \times \cdots \times D_n$.*

Yet we have not introduced any orderings; the following definition will fill our gap.

Definition 4. *Given a CSP, the domain order relation[1] $\sqsubseteq$ associated with it is the reverse of the set inclusion relation on the power set of D; namely, for every subset $A := A_1 \times \cdots \times A_n$ and $B := B_1 \times \cdots \times B_n$ of $D := D_1 \times \cdots \times D_n$, we write $A \sqsubseteq B$ iff $A \supseteq B$.*

---

[1] We could have given a more general notion of domain order, allowing it to be any relation of partial order on $\wp(D)$ with D as bottom; but the definition we give is sufficient for our purposes. Even a broader generalization can be found in [Apt99a], where the author replaces $\wp(D)$ with a family of subsets based on D closed with respect to $\cap$.

Observe that, by definition of $\sqsubseteq$, we have the following equivalence:

$$A \sqsubseteq B \text{ iff, for every } i = 1, \ldots, n, \text{ we have that } A_i \supseteq B_i.$$

Notice also that D is the top of $\langle \wp(D), \subseteq \rangle$; therefore it is the bottom of $\langle \wp(D), \sqsubseteq \rangle$.

Remark 3. From now onwards we shall always be dealing with functions f such that $f : \wp(D) \longrightarrow \wp(D)$; the order $\sqsubseteq$ on $\wp(D)$ is specified as above. Notice that a function $f : \wp(D) \longrightarrow \wp(D)$ is inflationary with respect to $\sqsubseteq$ iff, for every subset B of D, we have that $f(B) \subseteq B$.

We can now specialize GISF to the case in which the ordering is $\langle \wp(D), \sqsubseteq \rangle$; we call this instantiation of the GISF algorithm GISF *on compound domains*, briefly CGISF. The *update* operator has still to satisfy the conditions **A**, **B** and **C** given for GISF. Hence the previous results and remarks are applicable to CGISF as well; we get immediately the following result for free as a corollary of Theorem 1.

Corollary 1. (CGISF) *Consider a CSP $\langle X, D, \mathcal{C} \rangle$ with the associated domain order and two sets of functions H and F on D such that $subs(F, H)$ holds. Moreover, suppose that all functions in $K := H \cup F$ are monotonic. Then the following statements are valid.*

  i. *Every terminating execution of the CGISF algorithm computes the least common fixpoint of all the functions from K.*
 iii. *Suppose that K is finite and all of its functions are inflationary; further, suppose that the strict domain order satisfies the ACC. Then every execution of the CGISF algorithm terminates, computing the least common fixpoint of all the functions from K.*

Finally we introduce the notion of local consistency that we shall study in the rest of the paper, cf. also [MS99].

Definition 5. *Consider a constraint satisfaction problem $CSP := \langle X, D, \mathcal{C} \rangle$. The problem CSP is hyper arc consistent iff, for all of its constraints $C(s)$, the following condition is satisfied: for all $i \in s$ and $a \in D_i$, there exists $d \in D[s]$ such that $d \in C(s)$ and $a = d[i]$.*

If a CSP has only binary constraints $C(i, j)$, instead of hyper arc consistency we simply speak of *arc consistency*.

4   Arc and Hyper Arc Consistency Algorithms

In the next subsections, we shall instantiate the CGISF algorithm with ad hoc designed functions in order to enforce arc and hyper arc consistency on constraint satisfaction problems. First we consider the algorithms HAC-4 for hyper arc consistency and AC-4 for binary arc consistency and prove that CGISF can be instantiated to them, cf. Subsection 4.2 and 4.1 respectively; then we do the same with the algorithms AC-5 and HAC-5 in Subsection 4.4 and 4.3.

4.1   The Algorithm HAC-4 for Hyper Arc Consistency

We show here that the HAC-4 algorithm of [MM88] is an instance of the CGISF algorithm. The HAC-4 algorithm enforces hyper arc consistency by constructing the greatest hyper arc consistent problem included in the input constraint satisfaction problem. First we describe the original algorithm HAC-4; afterwards we devise some functions and show how CGISF can be instantiated to HAC-4 by means of those functions.

Table 1. Algorithm HAC-4 for hyper arc consistency

```
1. input: List;
2. while List ≠ ∅ do
3.   choose (i, a) ∈ List;
4.   List := List − {(i, a)}
5.   for C(s) and i ∈ s do
6.     for d ∈ S(C, a, i) do
7.       for j ∈ s, b = d[j] do
8.         S(C, b, j) := S(C, b, j) − {d};
9.         if S(C, b, j) = ∅ then
10.          List := List ∪ {(j, b)};
11.          D[j] := D[j] − {b}
12.        fi
13.      od
14.    od
15.  od
16. od
17. od
```

Before HAC-4 starts, an initial pruning and a construction of structures take place: the pairs (i, a) of elements $a \in D_i$ that do not have any supports in some constraints of the problem are removed from their domain D_i and stored in the set of deleted elements called *List*. The HAC-4 algorithm starts by choosing an element (i, a) from *List*; chosen a tuple d that belongs to a constraint of the problem and that supports a, HAC-4 removes d and propagates the effects of its elimination on its components different from a. Since we want to instantiate CGISF to HAC-4, we need to introduce the necessary functions on $\wp(D)$. In the following, we devise two classes of such functions. Let B any subset of D.

a. For every D_i, $a \in D_i$ and constraint $C(s)$ such that $i \in s$, we define a function $\pi(i, a, C)(B) := B'$ where $B' := B'_1 \times \ldots \times B'_n$ and, for every $k = 1, \ldots, n$, we have

$$
B'_k := \begin{cases} B_i - \{a\} & \text{if } k = i \text{ and we have that} \\ & \forall d \, (d \in B[s] \text{ and } d[i] = a \Rightarrow d \notin C(s)), \\ \\ B_k & \text{otherwise.} \end{cases}
$$

Basically, $\pi(i, a, s)$ removes the element a from the domain B_i iff a has no supports in $C(s)$.

b. For all constraints $C(s)$ of the problem and $d \in C(s)$, we define a function $\pi(i, d, C)(B) := B'$ where $B' := B'_1 \times \ldots \times B'_n$ and, for every $k = 1, \ldots, n$, we have

$$
B'_k := \begin{cases} B_i - \{d\,[i]\} & \text{if } k = i \text{ and } \forall\, d'\,(d' \in B\,[s] \text{ and } d'\,[i] = d\,[i] \Rightarrow d' \notin C), \\[2mm] B_k & \text{otherwise.} \end{cases}
$$

Intuitively, the function $\pi(i, d, C)$ removes the element $a := d\,[i]$ from its domain B_i iff d, the unique support for a, has been removed from $B\,[s]$.

Remark 4. Observe that, for every constraint $C(s)$ of the problem and $i \in s$, the function $\pi(i, d, C(s))$ is subsumed by $\pi(i, d\,[i], C(s))$; in fact

$$
\pi(i, d\,[i], C(s)) \subseteq \pi(i, d, C(s)).
$$

We shall initialize G with the functions $\pi(i, a, C)$ and F with the functions $\pi(i, d, C)$.

Note 2. The functions $\pi(i, a, C(s))$ and $\pi(i, d, C(s^*))$ are idempotent, inflationary and monotonic with respect to the domain order $\sqsubseteq$.

Hence, due to Remark 1 and Note 2, our *update* operator needs only to satisfy conditions **A** and **B** given in Section 2. We define it as follows.

- If $\pi(i, a, C(s))(B) = B$, then $update(G, F, \pi(i, a, C(s)), B)$ is the empty set. Otherwise $update(G, F, \pi(i, a, C(s), B))$ is the set of functions $\pi(j, d, C(s^*))$ from $F - G$ that satisfy the following conditions:
  i1. $d\,[i] = a$, $j \in s$ and $j \neq i$;
  ii1. for all $d' \in B\,[s^*]$ such that $a = d'\,[i]$ we have that $d' \notin C(s^*)$.
- Similarly, if $\pi(i, d, C(s))(B) = B$, then $update(G, F, \pi(i, d, C(s)), B)$ is the empty set. If it is not the case, then the set $update(G, F, \pi(i, d, C(s))$ only contains the functions $\pi(j, d^*, C(s^*))$ of $F - G$ that satisfy the following conditions:
  i2. $i \in s^*$, $j \neq i$ and $d^*\,[i] = d\,[i]$;
  ii2. for all $d' \in B\,[s^*]$ such that $d\,[i] = d'\,[i]$ we have that $d' \notin C(s^*)$.

It is immediate to check that that *update* operator fulfills conditions **A** and **B**. Moreover, after executing CGISF with all the functions of H, the set G only contains functions of F.

Theorem 2. *Consider a CSP $\langle X, D, \mathcal{C} \rangle$ with the associated domain order and the sets of functions H and F defined above; then we have the following results.*
(Partial correctness) Every terminating execution of the CGISF algorithm computes the greatest arc consistent problem contained in the given one.
(Total correctness) Suppose that D is finite; then every execution of the CGISF algorithm terminates.

Proof. Indeed a fixpoint of the functions from H is a hyper arc consistent problem contained in the given one; as $subs(F, H)$ holds, a fixpoint of the functions from $H \cup F$ is a hyper arc consistent problem $\langle X, D', \mathcal{C} \rangle$ such that D' is a subset of D. Now it is enough to observe that if D is finite so is $H \cup F$ and the strict partial order on D satisfies the ACC, cf. Note 1. Our statements immediately follow from Proposition 2 and Corollary 1. □

In the next theorem, we prove that the CGISF algorithm can be instantiated to the HAC-4 algorithm by means of the functions $\pi(j, d, C)$.

Theorem 3. (CGISF for HAC-4) *Each iteration of the HAC-4 algorithm is equivalent to one or more iterations of the CGISF algorithm.*

Proof. First we execute the CGISF algorithm with the functions $\pi(i, a, C(s))$ of H; this way we prune the search space and propagate the effects of the removal of each a that has no supports from its domain D_i by means of the *update* operator. In parallel, for each D_i and a removed from D_i, the pairs (i, a) are stored in *List* before starting the HAC-4 algorithm. The structures $S(C(s^*), a, i)$, where $C(s^*)$ is a constraint of the problem, contain all the tuples d such that $d \in C(s^*)$ and $d[i] = a$. Let (i, a) be the pair that we pick out from *List* (line 3. of HAC-4), $C(s^*)$ a constraint of the problem on s^* with $i \in s^*$ (line 5. of HAC-4) and d a tuple of $C(s^*)$ that supports a (line 6. of HAC-4). For each $j \neq i$ and $j \in s^*$, for each $b = d[j]$ (line 7. of HAC-4), the HAC-4 algorithm deletes d from $S(C(s^*), b, j)$ (line 8. of HAC-4) because a does not belong to D_i any more. In parallel we choose the function $\pi(j, d, C(s^*))$ in CGISF; the CGISF algorithm removes $\pi(j, d, C(s^*))$ from the set G of functions to inspect. Observe that the function that we select is available in $F - G$, because of our choice of the *update* operator. In the **if-then** sub-program HAC-4 eliminates b from D_j and adds (j, b) to *List* iff b does not have any more support in $C(s^*)$ after the removal of d; so does the function $\pi(j, d, C(s^*))$, which removes b from D_j iff it has no more supports in $C(s^*)$ and propagates the effects of the removal of b by means of the *update* operator. □

4.2 AC-4 for Binary Constraint Satisfaction Problems

In case of normalized binary CSP's, the AC-4 algorithm of [MH86] becomes an instance of CGISF. In order to obtain a compact notation, we shall also assume to have at our disposal the *transposed constraint* $C^T := C(j, i)$ of each constraint $C = C(i, j)$ of the given problem, where $(b, a) \in C^T$ iff $(a, b) \in C$. First we describe the original algorithm AC-4. In order to execute the AC-4 algorithm a series of structures need to be created. The algorithm in Table 2 initializes those structures, performing two different actions:

1. it stores in *List* the pairs (i, a) such that $a \in D_i$ has no support in D_j, deletes a from its domain D_i and, by means of the condition $M[i, a] = 1$, records that a has been deleted;
2. it adds (j, b) to $S[i, a]$ if $(a, b) \in C(i, j)$ so that, if a happens to be deleted, then we know that we have to check whether b has still supports in D_j.

Table 2. Algorithm to initialize data structures

$List := \emptyset$;
for $C(i,j)$ constraint of the problem **do**
    for $a \in D_i$ **do**
        $S[i,a] := \emptyset$;
        $M[i,a] := 0$;
        $Total := 0$;
            for $b \in D_j$ **do**
                if $(a,b) \in C(i,j)$ **then**
                    $Total := Total + 1$;
                    $S[j,b] := S[j,b] \cup \{(i,a)\}$
                fi
        od
        if $Total = 0$ **then**
            $D_i := D_i - \{a\}$;
            $List := List \cup \{(i,a)\}$;
            $M[i,a] := 1$;
        fi
        $Counter[(i,j),a] := Total$
    od
od

Table 3. Elimination of inconsistencies from the domains in AC-4

while $List \neq \emptyset$ **do**
    choose and remove (i,a) from $List$;
    for $(j,b) \in S[i,a]$ **do**
        $Counter[(j,i),b] := Counter[(j,i),b] - 1$;
        if $Counter[(j,i),b] = 0$ **and** $M[j,b] = 0$ **then**
            $D_j := D_j - \{b\}$;
            $List := List \cup \{(j,b)\}$;
            $M[j,b] := 1$
        fi
    od
do

The algorithm in Table 3 inspects each b that supports a which has been removed; if a happens to have been the unique support of b and b has not been deleted yet, then b is removed from its domain D_j and (j,b) is added to $List$.

We show how CGISF can be instantiated to AC-4 in the following. Notice that the functions that we are about to use are the ones devised in Subsection 4.1; however we prefer to rewrite them for normalized binary CSP's in order to make explicit the link with AC-4.

a. For every D_i, $a \in D_i$ and constraint $C(i,j)$, we define a new function $\pi(a,i,j)$ such that $\pi(a,i,j)(B) := B'$, where B' is defined as the set $B'_1 \times \ldots \times B'_n$ and, for every $k = 1, \ldots, n$, we have

$$B'_k := \begin{cases} B_i - \{a\} & \text{if } k = i \text{ and we have that} \\ & \forall b \, (b \in B_j \Rightarrow (a,b) \notin C(i,j)), \\ \\ B_k & \text{otherwise,} \end{cases}$$

Basically, $\pi(a,i,j)$ removes the element a from the domain B_i iff a has no support in B_j, where $j \neq i$.

b. For every $(a,b) \in C(i,j)$, we define a function $\pi(a,i,b,j)(B) := B'$ where $B' := B'_1 \times \ldots \times B'_n$ and, for every $k = 1, \ldots, n$, we have

$$B'_k := \begin{cases} B_i - \{a\} & \text{if } k = i, \, a_i \in B_i, b \notin B_j \text{ and we have that} \\ & \forall c \, (c \in B_j \Rightarrow (a,c) \notin C(i,j)), \\ \\ B_k & \text{otherwise,} \end{cases}$$

Intuitively, the function $\pi(a,i,b,j)$ removes the element a from its domain B_i iff $a \in B_i$ and b, which is the unique support of a in $B_j \cup \{b\}$, does not belong to B_j.

Remark 5. Observe that, again, for every $i = 1, \ldots, n$ and $a \in D_i$, the functions $\pi(a,i,b,j)$ are all subsumed by $\pi(a,i,j)$. Hence the set H contains all functions $\pi(a,i,j)$; while F is the set of functions $\pi(a,i,b,j)$.

If $\pi(a,i,j)(B) = B$, then $update(G,F,\pi(a,i,j),B)$ is the empty set. Otherwise the set $update(G,F,\pi(a,i,j),B)$ is given by the functions $\pi(b,k,a,i)$ from $F - G$ that satisfy the following conditions:

i. $k \neq i$ and $(a,b) \in C(i,k)$,
ii. if $a' \in B_i$ then $(a',c) \notin C(i,k)$.

Similarly, if $\pi(a,i,c,j)(B) = B$, the set $update(G,F,\pi(a,i,c,j),b)$ is the emtpy set; otherwise it is given by the functions $\pi(b,k,a,i)$ from $F - G$ that satisfy the previous conditions i and ii. The *update* operator above defined satisfies conditions **A** and **B**; **C** is satisfied because those functions are idempotent, cf. Remark 1. We claim that the CGISF algorithm can be instantiated to the AC-4 algorithm. In order to prove our claim we just need to prove the following proposition and then exploit the result in Theorem 2.

Proposition 2. *Given a CSP, consider an iteration of the CGISF algorithm in which only functions from H are chosen. Then the output CSP is the same as the one generated by means of the algorithm in Table 2.*

Proof. The algorithm in Table 2 initializes data structures: for each D_i, $a \in D_i$ and constraint $C(i,j)$, the algorithm checks whether a has a support in D_j. If and only if a has no supports in D_j, then a is removed from D_i and D_i is set to $D_i - \{a\}$. In parallel, we execute CGISF with the functions of H; the function $\pi(a, i, j)$ removes a from D_i iff a has no support in D_j; again D_i is set to $D_i - \{a\}$. The algorithm in Table 2 propagates the effects of the elimination of a on the elements $b \in D_k$ of which a was a support by adding (i, a) to $S[k, b]$ and *List*. The CGISF algorithm removes the function $\pi(a, i, j)$ from G; moreover it adds to G all the functions $\pi(b, k, a, i)$ that are indexed by b such that $(a, b) \in C(i, k)$. After we execute CGISF with all the functions of H, we leave only functions from F in G, and never introduce the functions of H again.   □

We get our claim as a corollary of Theorem 3 and Proposition 2.

Corollary 2. *Each iteration of the* AC-4 *algorithm is equivalent to one or more iterations of the* CGISF *algorithm.*

4.3   The Algorithm HAC-5 for Hyper Arc Consistency

The AC-5 algorithm for enforcing arc consistency on binary constraint problems was presented in [HDT92]. However the procedure that the authors proposed there can be slightly modified in order to enforce hyper arc consistency. In this subsection, first we define two kinds of functions, namely $\pi(s, i)$ and $\pi(s, i, j, b)$; then we explain how they can account for the two-step behaviour of the AC-5 algorithm but to achieve hyper arc consistency. All those functions are defined on subsets B of $D := D_1 \times \cdots \times D_n$; given a constraint $C(s)$ of the problem, $i, j \in s$, and an element $b \in D_j$, we define the following two classes of functions.

1. $\pi(s, i)(B) := B'$, where $B'_i = B_i - \Delta_1(i)$ if $\Delta_1(i)$ is the set

$$\{a \in B_i : \forall d \, (d \in B[s] \land d[i] = a \Rightarrow d \notin C(s))\}$$

   while $B'_k = B_k$ whenever $k \neq i$. Basically $\pi(s, i)$ removes the elements of B_i that do not have supports in the constraint $C(s)$ of the problem.
2. $\pi(s, i, j, b)(B) := B'$, where, if $b \notin B_j$, $B'_i = B_i - \Delta_2(i)$ and $\Delta_2(i)$ is the subset of B_i of elements a that satisfy the following condition:

$$\exists d \in C(s) \text{ s.t. } d[i] = a, \, d[j] = b \land \forall d' \, (d' \in B[s] \land d'[i] = a \Rightarrow d' \notin C(s)),$$

   while $B'_k = B_k$ if $b \in B_j$ or $B_k \neq B_i$. Intuitively, $\pi(s, i, j, b)$ removes the elements of B_i that do not have more supports in $C(s)$ after the removal of b from D_j, for $i, j \in s$.

The set H contains the functions $\pi(s, i)$, while F only contains the functions $\pi(s, i, j, b)$. Moreover every function $\pi(s, i)$ subsumes all functions $\pi(s, i, j, b)$ such that $b \in D_j$; in fact we have the following relation:

$$\pi(s, i) \subseteq \bigcap_{j \in s, \, b \in D_j} \pi(s, i, j, b).$$

When we execute CGISF, we can first select and delete all functions $\pi(s, i)$; when each $\pi(s, i)$ is processed, the operator *update* adds the suitable functions $\pi(s, i, j, b)$ to G. When there are no more functions of H to inspect, we execute CGISF with the functions $\pi(s, i, j, b)$.

Note 3. The functions $\pi(s, i)$ and $\pi(s, i, j, b)$ are idempotent, inflationary and monotone with respect to the domain order $\sqsubseteq$.

Because of the previous note and Remark 1, our *update* operator needs to satisfy only conditions **A** and **B**. Hence we define *update* as follows:

- if $\pi(s, i)(B) \neq B$, then $update(G, F, \pi(s, i), B)$ is the subset of $F - G$ of functions $\pi(t, k, i, a)$ such that $a \in \Delta_1(i)$, where $\Delta_1(i)$ is defined as above; otherwise it is the empty set;
- if $\pi(s, j, i, a)(B) \neq B$, then $update(G, F, \pi(s, j, i, a), D)$ is the subset of $F - G$ of functions $\pi(t, k, j, b)$ such that $b \in \Delta_2(j)$, where $\Delta_2(j)$ is defined as above; otherwise it is the empty set.

Theorem 4. *Consider a CSP $\langle X, D, \mathcal{C} \rangle$ with the associated domain order and the set of functions H and F defined above; then we have the following.*
(Partial correctness) Every terminating execution of the CGISF *algorithm computes the greatest arc consistent problem contained in the given one.*
(Total correctness) Suppose that D is finite; then every execution of the CGISF *algorithm terminates.*

Proof. Indeed a fixpoint of the functions from H is a hyper arc consistent problem contained in the given one; as $subs(F, H)$ holds, a fixpoint of the functions from $H \cup F$ is a hyper arc consistent problem that is also a subset of the input CSP. Now it is enough to observe that if D is finite then so is $H \cup F$ and the strict partial order on D satisfies the ACC, cf. Note 1. Our statements follow immediately from Proposition 3 and Corollary 1. $\square$

Remark 6. Observe that, as in the case of HAC-4, after CGISF inspects all the functions $\pi(s, i)$ of H, G contains only functions $\pi(s, i, j, b)$ of F.

4.4   AC-5 for Binary Constraint Satisfaction Problems

As in the case of AC-4, we claim that the AC-5 algorithm of [HDT92] can be seen as an instance of our CGISF algorithm when we work with normalized binary CSP's. In order to avoid a cumbersome notation, we shall also assume to have at our disposal the *transposed constraint* $C^T := C(j, i)$ of each constraint $C = C(i, j)$ of the given problem, where $(b, a) \in C^T$ iff $(a, b) \in C$. In this subsection, first we describe the original algorithm AC-5. Then we prove our claim by showing how CGISF can be instantiated to AC-5.

The algorithm by [HDT92] is reproduced in Table 4; it is split into two steps, as we explain in the following.

1. For any constraint $C(i,j)$ of the given CSP, the procedure *arc-cons* creates the subset $\Delta(i)$ of D_i of elements a that are not supported by any element of D_j in $C(i,j)$; then, for each $a \in \Delta(i)$, all triples $\langle (k,i), a \rangle$ such that $C(k,i)$ is a constraint of the problem are added to Q and the elements of the set $\Delta(i)$ are deleted from D_i.
2. In the second step, a triple $\langle (i,j), b \rangle$ is selected and deleted from Q; if D_i and D_j are not empty and b has been removed from D_j, then the procedure *loc-arc-cons* updates the set $\Delta(i) \subseteq D_i$ adding all elements a that are no (more) supported in $C(i,j)$ by any element of D_j (after b has been removed from D_j); then, for each $a \in \Delta(i)$, all triples $\langle (k,i), a \rangle$ such that $C(k,i)$ is a constraint of the problem are added to Q and the elements of $\Delta(i)$ are removed from D_i.

Table 4. The arc-consistency algorithm `AC-5`

```
Q := [ ]
for (i, j) ∈ arc(G) do
        arc-cons(i, j, Δ(i));
        for k ≠ i, and a ∈ Δ(i) do Q := Q ∪ {⟨(k, i), a⟩} od;
        Dᵢ := Dᵢ − Δ(i)
od
while Q ≠ [ ] do
        choose ⟨(i, j), b⟩ ∈ (Q, i, j, b);
        local-arc-cons(i, j, b, Δ(i));
        for k ≠ i, and a ∈ Δ(i) do Q := Q ∪ {⟨(k, i), a⟩} od;
        Dᵢ := Dᵢ − Δ(i)
od
```

As pointed out in [HDT92], `AC-5` is a generic algorithm which can be instantiated to `AC-4` by slightly changing the definition of the sets $\Delta(i)$; in the latter case, the functions that we use for `AC-4` are adopted. In case the definition of $\Delta(i)$ is chosen as stated above, we need new functions to express `AC-5`. Basically, we use the functions of the previous subsection and refine them for normalized binary CSP's. We shall call those functions $\pi(i,j)$ and $\pi(i,j,b)$, because s is either i,j or j,i; we shall use them to account for the two-step behaviour of the algorithm in Table 4. For each constraint $C(i,j)$ and element $b \in D_j$ we define the functions as follows:

1. $\pi(i,j)(B) := B'$, where $B'_i = B_i - \Delta_1(i)$ if $\Delta_1(i)$ is the set
$$\{a \in B_i : \forall b\,(b \in B_j \Rightarrow (a,b) \notin C(i,j))\}$$
while $B'_k = B_k$ whenever $k \neq i$;
2. $\pi(i,j,b)(B) := B'$, where $B'_i = B_i - \Delta_2(i)$ if $b \notin B_j$ and $\Delta_2(i)$ is
$$\{a \in B_i : (a,b) \in C(i,j) \land \forall c\,(c \in B_j \Rightarrow (a,c) \notin C(i,j))\}$$
while $B'_k = B_k$ otherwise.

The set H contains the functions $\pi(i,j)$, while F only contains the functions $\pi(i,j,b)$. Moreover every function $\pi(i,j)$ subsumes all functions $\pi(i,j,b)$ such that $b \in D_j$.

The first part of the AC-5 algorithm is encoded in the actions of inspecting and deleting all functions $\pi(i,j)$ from G in our algorithm; when each $\pi(i,j)$ is processed, the operator *update* propagates the effects of the (possible) reduction of D_i by adding the suitable functions $\pi(i,j,b)$ to G. Besides we want to instantiate CGISF to the second part of the AC-5 algorithm by means of the functions $\pi(i,j,b)$ of F. Therefore we define *update* as follows:

- if $\pi(i,j)(B) \neq B$, then $update(G,F,\pi(i,j),B)$ is the subset of $F-G$ of functions $\pi(k,i,a)$ such that $a \in \Delta_1(i)$; otherwise it is the empty set;
- if $\pi(j,i,a)(B) \neq B$, then $update(G,F,\pi(j,i,a),D)$ is the subset of $F-G$ of functions $\pi(k,j,b)$ of $F-G$ such that $b \in \Delta_2(j)$; otherwise it is the empty set.

It is immediate to check that the *update* operator satisfies conditions **A** and **B**; the third condition **C** trivially holds because the considered functions are idempotent and what we observe in Remark 1. Now we can show that CGISF can be instantiated to AC-5.

Theorem 5. *Each iteration of the* CGISF *algorithm is equivalent to one or more iterations of the* CGISF *algorithm.*

Proof. After one execution of the first **for** loop of AC-5, all the elements a of D_i that have no supports in a domain D_j are removed from D_i; then the triples $\langle (k,i),a \rangle$ are added to the set Q of elements to inspect in the second **for** loop; namely all $\langle (k,i),a \rangle$ such that a has been removed from D_i and $C(k,i)$ is a constraint of the problem. In parallel, CGISF selects $\pi(i,j)$ and removes from D_i the elements that are not supported in $C(i,j)$ by any element of D_j; afterwards, the effect of that removal are propagated by *update* which adds G all the functions $\pi(k,i,a)$ such that a has been removed from D_i and $C(k,i)$ is a constraint of the given CSP. Let us analyze the second part of AC-5 and see how CGISF can be instantiated to it by means of the functions $\pi(j,i,a)$. If the triple $\langle (j,i),a \rangle$ is chosen from Q, then we execute CGISF with $\pi(a,i,j)$. The procedure *local-arc-cons* removes from D_i all the elements a that have lost their unique support in D_j after the removal of b; by executing CGISF with $\pi(i,j,b)$ we perform the same action. When the AC-5 algorithm adds all the triples $\langle (k,i),a \rangle$ indexed by a removed from D_i to Q, the *update* operator performs the same action with the associated functions. □

5   Conclusions

In this article we refined the general framework for local consistency introduced in [Apt99b,Apt99c] that explains various local consistency algorithms in a uniform way. In our algorithm GISF, we used two sets of functions instead of only one; the relation of subsumption between those two sets was introduced and proved to be sufficient to guarantee the (partial) correctness of the algorithm itself. Thanks to `GISF`, we could clarify the two-step behaviour of the algorithms `AC-4` of [MH86], `HAC-5` of [MM88] and `AC-5` of [HDT92]: the functions of one set perform a "global" action, loosely speaking; instead the functions of the other set work more "locally", precisely as it happens in those algorithms. The use of a more general yet unique framework helped also to make explicit the underlying differences between the algorithms `AC-4` and `AC-5`; in fact the sets of functions needed to express them by means of the `GISF` algorithm are different. Moreover we extended the `AC-5` algorithm to a hyper consistency algorithm.

Lately, we demonstrated that the `PC-4` algorithm is an instance of `GISF`, too; in fact the `PC-4` algorithm is split in two parts like the arc consistency algorithms that we discussed in this paper. In the future, we would like to investigate further properties of functions, like subsumption or commutativity in [Apt99c], in order to derive new constraint propagation algorithms or optimize some of the existing ones. Finally a richer structure than a partial ordering could also be studied in order to guarantee the termination of `GISF`; which is not a meaningless task, because the termination of `GISF` is not ensured if the variable domains are infinite and the order does not satisfy the ACC, as it happens in fuzzy and probabilistic constraint satisfaction problems.

References

[Apt99a] K.R. Apt, *The Essence of Constraint Propagation*, Theoretical Computer Science, 221(1-2), pp. 179–210, 1999.

[Apt99b] K.R. Apt, *The Rough Guide to Constraint Propagation*, Proc. of the 5th International Conference on Principles and Practice of Constraint Programming (CP'99), (invited lecture), Springer-Verlag Lecture Notes in Computer Science 1713, pp. 1–23.

[Apt99c] K.R. Apt, *The Role of Commutativity in Constraint Propagation Algorithms*, submitted for publication.

[HDT92] P. van Hentenryck, Y. Deville and C. Teng, *A generic arc-consistency algorithm and its specializations*, Artificial Intelligence, 57, pp. 291–321, 1992.

[MS99] K. Marriott and P. Stuckey, *Programming with Constraints*, MIT Press, 1998.

[MH86] R. Mohr and T. Henderson, *Arc and Path Consistency Revisited*, Artificial Intelligence, 28, pp. 225–233, 1986.

[MM88] R. Mohr and G. Masini, *Good old discrete relaxation*, Proc. of the 8th European Conference on Artificial Intelligence (ECAI), pp. 651–656, Pitman Publisher, 1988.

AVAL: An Enumerative Method for SAT

Gilles Audemard, Belaid Benhamou, and Pierre Siegel

Laboratoire d'Informatique de Marseille
Centre de Mathématiques et d'Informatique
39, Rue Joliot Curie - 13453 Marseille cedex 13 - France
Tel : 04 91 11 36 25 - Fax : 04 91 11 36 02
{audemard,benhamou,siegel}@lim.univ-mrs.fr

Abstract. We study an algorithm for the SAT problem which is based on the Davis and Putnam procedure. The main idea is to increase the application of the unit clause rule during the search. When there is no unit clause in the set of clauses, our method tries to produce one occuring in the current subset of binary clauses. A literal deduction algorithm is implemented and applied at each branching node of the search tree. This method AVAL is a combination of the Davis and Putnam principle and of the mono-literal[1] deduction procedure. Its efficiency comes from the average complexity of the literal deduction procedure which is linear in the number of variables. The method is called "AVAL" (avalanch) because of its behaviour on hard random SAT problems. When solving these instances, an avalanche of mono-literals is deduced after the first success of literal production and from that point, the search effort is reduced to unit propagations, thus completing the remaining part of enumeration in polynomial time.

Keywords: Satisfiability, deduction, enumeration...

1 Introduction

Some progresses have been realized in solving SAT problem. In particular, application of local search methods [13] to hard satisfiable SAT instances gives satisfying results. However, they can not deal with unsatisfiable instances.

To solve such instances, one usually uses systematic methods based on the Davis and Putnam procedure [3] (DP). DP efficiency comes from the property of unit clause propagation. This method, and its well known improvements (SATO [14], C-SAT [4], POSIT [6] [7], SATZ [10]...) find their limits when applied to SAT random instances located in the transition phase.

This paper introduces the method AVAL based on DP procedure to improve search efficiency and uses it as a base method to study the behaviour of enumeration methods on hard SAT instances. The improvement consists in maximizing the use of unit clause propagation during the search. To do that, a literal production algorithm (LP) is implemented. This procedure is called when there is no explicit mono-literal in the set of clauses, to produce new ones from the subset of binary clauses and to use them as new propagations. Such propagations are not done by the classical method of Davis and Putnam. The AVAL method is a

---

[1] A mono-literal means a unit clause.

J. Lloyd et al. (Eds.): CL 2000, LNAI 1861, pp. 373–383, 2000.

combination of DP and of the literal production procedure. Its efficiency comes from the average complexity of the literal production process which is linear in the number of variables.

The literal production procedure deduces literals occuring in the subset of binary clauses. Such literals are more likely to be logical consequence of the current set of clauses than any others. The LP procedure is called at each branching node when the classic unit clause rule of DP does not apply. This minimizes the number of branching nodes (choice nodes) and provides a robust algorithm which is less sensitive to heuristics. This algorithm can be used in practice to analyze the limits of systematic methods in solving hard SAT instances.

The paper is organized as following: In section 2, we study the literal production algorithm. Section 3 describes the avalanche method (AVAL), the heuristics and the pre-processing used. Section 4 shows experimental results on a large variety of problems: hard random instances and problems of both challenges DIMACS and Beijing. A comparison of AVAL with other algorithms among the most powerful ones like POSIT [6] and SATZ [11] is done. section 5 concludes.

2   Literal Production

Let's give some definitions we shall use. Let $V = \{x_1...x_n\}$ be a set of boolean variables, a literal l is a variable x_i or its negation $\overline{x_i}$. A monotone literal is a literal occuring exclusively either in its positive or negative form. A clause is a disjunction of literals $c_i = l_1 \vee l_2... \vee l_{n_i}$. A unit clause (a mono-literal) is a clause of one literal. The conjunctive normal form of a propositional formula C is a conjunction of clauses $C = c_1 \wedge c_2... \wedge c_m$. We can consider C as a set of clauses $C = \{c_1..., c_m\}$. The SAT decision problem is defined as follows: is there an assignment of the variables so that the formula C is satisfied, i.e all the clauses of the set C are satisfied?

If l is logically implied by the set of clauses C, then we write $C \models l$. When a system of clauses C is unsatisfiable, we note it by $C \models \square$, where $\square$ denotes the empty clause. The k-SAT problem is the problem SAT where all clauses have exactly k literals. 3-SAT is known to be the simplest form of k-SAT which remains NP-Complete.

The Davis and Putnam procedure is a real improvement of the Quine method [12] thanks to both unit clause and monotone literal rules (cf proposition 1). Methods like C-SAT [4] and SATZ [10] do more unit propagations. In the same spirit, our work consist in revealing, at lower cost, unit clauses that DP does not consider in exploiting them in order to reduce the size of the search tree. The main property used in DP is the following.

Proposition 1. *Let S be a SAT problem and x be a mono-literal or a monotone literal then S is satisfiable if and only if $S \wedge \{x\}$ is satisfiable.*

If there is no mono-literal in the current set of clauses at a given node of the search tree, our algorithm tries to produce one. For efficiency reasons we restrict the production process to literals occuring in binary clauses. These literals are more likely to be produced.

Let I be the current instantiation and C_I be the set of the clauses C simplified by the instantiation I. If l is a literal occuring in a binary clause of C_I, then producing l from C_I ($C_I \models l$) is equivalent to proving the unsatisfiability of $C_I \wedge \{\neg l\}$. Two cases are possible:

1. If $C_I \wedge \{\neg l\} \models \square$ then l is produced by C_I and considered as a mono-literal. Thus, $I = I \cup \{l\}$
2. If $C_I \wedge \{\neg l\} \not\models \square$ then l is not produced by C_I, and this failure deduction highlights several literals which can not be deduced by C_I. It will be useless to consider them as candidates for production.

The efficiency of the literal production is due to this elimination of useless variables. Formally:

Proposition 2. *Let B_I be the set of binary clauses of C_I and V_{B_I} be its set of literals. Let $l \in V_{B_I}$, if $C_I \cup \{\neg l\} \models a_{i \in \{1..n\}}$ such that $C_I \cup \{\neg l\} \not\models \square$ then $\forall a_{i \in \{1..n\}} \in V_{B_I}$, $C_I \cup \{a_i\} \not\models \square$.*

Proof. Let $l \in V_{B_I}$, suppose that $C_I \cup \{\neg l\} \models a_{i \in \{1..n\}}$ and $C_I \cup \{\neg l\} \not\models \square$. If there exists $a_{j \in \{1..n\}}$ such that $C_I \cup \{a_j\} \models \square$, then, $C_I \cup \{\neg l\} \cup \{a_j\} \models \square$. But $C_I \cup \{\neg l\} \cup \{\neg a_j\} \models \square$, hence $C_I \cup \{\neg l\} \models \square$. This make a contradiction with the hypothesis. $\square$

The literals $\{\neg a_1, .., \neg a_n\}$ can not be logical consequences of C_I. Thus, considering them for production is irrelevant. The previous proposition gives the literal production algorithm (LP) described in figure 1. In the following, we show the mechanism algorithm.

Example 1. Let the set of clauses $C = \{x_1 \vee \neg x_2 \vee \neg x_3, x_1 \vee x_2, \neg x_2 \vee x_3\}$. The literals $V_{B_I} = \{x_1, x_2, \neg x_2, x_3\}$ appears in the binary clauses.

We try to produce x_3. $C \wedge \{\neg x_3\} \models \neg x_2, x_1$. So, $C \wedge \{\neg x_2\} \not\models \square$ then x_2 can't be deduced by C and $Candidate[x_2] = False$. Now, literals candidate to production are $\{x_1, \neg x_2\}$.

We try to produce x_1. $C \wedge \{\neg x_1\} \models x_2, x_3, \square$. So, $C \models x_1$. x_1 is produced by C.

Remark 1. In the algorithm of figure 1, $Candidate[x] = True$ expresses the fact that x is a candidate to production.

The LP algorithm deduces literals among those appearing in binary clauses. Its termination, correctness, completeness and complexity are studied in the following propositions.

Proposition 3. *Let C be the current set of clauses, and l a literal occuring in a binary clause. If LP produces l ($LP(C) \models l$) then $C \equiv C \cup \{l\}$.*

Proof. Let l be a literal produced by LP. Then, $(C \cup \{\neg l\}) \models \square$.

But $C \equiv (C \wedge l) \vee (C \wedge \{\neg l\}$. Thus, $C \equiv C \cup \{l\}$ and LP correctness is proved. $\square$

```
Procedure LP(C : set of clauses ; I : instantiation)
Return : a literal l if C ⊨ l
         0 if ∄l ∈ V_{B_I} such that C ⊨ l

Begin
For All l ∈ V_{B_I} do Candidate[l] = True
For All l ∈ V_{B_I} such that Candidate[l] = True Do Begin
        Candidate[l] = False
        I' = I ∪ {¬l}
        While C_{I'} ≠ ∅ and ∃x ∈ V_{C_{I'}}, x is a unit clause and □ ∉ C_{I'} Do
                Begin
                I' = I' ∪ {x}
                Candidate[¬x]=False
                End
        If □ ∈ C_{I'} Then Return l
        End
Return 0
End
```

Algorithm 1: Literal Production Algorithm (LP)

Proposition 4. *If C_I is the current set of clauses, and B_I the subset of binary clauses, then the algorithm terminates and its complexity in worst case is in $O(|V_{B_I}| \times |V_{C_I}|)$.*

Proof. When, LP tries to deduce l ($C_I \models l$?), it propagates in the worst case V_{C_I} unit clauses. If l is not deductible ($C_I \not\models l$), the LP procedure tries to deduce an other literal among those of V_{B_I}. The worst case is when all the propagated literals occuring in the failure of producing l ($C_I \models l$?) are not in V_{B_I}. In this case LP tries V_{B_I} literals. Thus its complexity in the worst case is in order of $O(|V_{B_I}| \times |V_{C_I}|)$. □

The C-SAT method [4] does some local deduction on selected variables, but does not take advantage of the literals that are not potential candidates for production (see proposition 2) despite Boufkhad remarked these irrelevant literals in his thesis [1]. In [7] (POSIT) Freeman uses a kind of literal production on selected variables but does not suppress the irrelevant literals. Elimination of these useless literals allows to obtain a literal production algorithm whose average time complexity is linear in practice (see algorithm 1).

3 The Avalanch Method (AVAL)

The combination of the literal production algorithm (LP) and the DP procedure yields the enumeration method AVAL.

The difference between DP and AVAL is that AVAL calls the procedure LP to produce a mono-literal when no explicit unit clause exists in the current set of clauses. This prevents for visiting some nodes that DP visits. When LP succeeds, the returned literal is considered as a mono-literal. In case of failure we choose via heuristics the next literal, thus creating a new choice point in the search tree. Exploiting the literals produced by LP, leads to minimizing the number of choice points in the search tree (for a given heuristic). The algorithm 2 sketches the AVAL method. The first call to AVAL is made with the parameter values : $I = \emptyset$ and $C = C_\emptyset$.

```
Procedure AVAL(C : Set of Clause ; I : Instantiation)
Return : True if C is satisfiable by I
         False otherwise

Begin
If  C = ∅ Then Return True
If  C contains an empty clause Then Return False
If  C contains an unit clause l Then Return AVAL(C_{l}, I ∪ {l})
q=LP()
If  q ≠ 0 Then Return AVAL(C_{q}, I ∪ {q})
Choose by heuristic a literal p ∈ C
If  AVAL(C_{p}, I ∪ {p})
    Then Return True
    Else Return AVAL(C_{¬p}, I ∪ {¬p})
End
```

Algorithm 2: AVAL Method

3.1 Heuristics

Heuristics are used when there is no mono-literal in the current set of clauses and when LP does not produce one. We use the MOM heuristic (Maximum Occurrence in minimum size clauses) (Freeman [6]) which chooses the variable with the greatest number of occurrences in the minimum size clauses and the UP (Unit Propagation) heuristic which takes advantage of unit propagation. These heuristics allow to produce new binary clauses which favor the production of mono-literals when calling LP. Let us summarize them.

Mom Heuristic: If l is a literal then $w(l) = \sum_{\neg l \in C_i} 5^{-|C_i|}$ is its weight. MOM heuristic chooses the variable which maximizes the function used by Freeman in [6]: $H(x) = 1024.w(x).w(\neg x) + w(x) + w(\neg x)$.

UP Heuristic: UP heuristic (see [6] and [10]) exploits unit propagation more than MOM heuristic does and gives more binary clauses which help LP to produce literals as soon as possible during the search. Let C_I be the current set of clauses, x a variable of C_I, $C_I' = C_I \wedge x$ and $C_I'' = C_I \wedge \neg x$. After unit propagation on both C_I' and C_I'', UP chooses the variable which shortens a maximum number of clauses in C_I' and C_I''. We use this heuristic to select the variables for the first choice points of the search tree where the procedure LP usually fails to produce literals.

3.2 Pre-processing

Before starting the search, we do some pre-processings which consists in adding resolvants to the set of clauses. This usually reduces the search space. We use the same technique as the one of Chu Min Lee in [10]. Only resolvants of size less than 3 are considered and can to be used to produce other resolvants. The resolvants technique consists in the following rules: Two binary clauses can create only unary one. A binary and a ternary clauses can create only a binary one. Two ternary clauses produce a resolvant of size less or equal to 3. The process is maintained until saturation. This pre-processing allows a gain of nearly 10% for the hard random problems.

4 Experiments

We first compare our method AVAL with the classic Davis and Putnam Method. We study the behaviour of AVAL during search and compare it with two known algorithms (SATZ [10] and POSIT [6]) on different problems: instances of both challenges DIMACS and Beijing, and random 3-SAT instances. Random problems are generated as follows: Let c be the number of clauses and v be the number of variables, we generate randomly c clauses among the $2^3\binom{v}{3}$ possible ones. Many research works showed that there is transition phase for the random k-SAT problems : there is a critical value of the ratio $\frac{c}{v}$ before which problems are few constrained (have many models) and after which problems are very constrained (have no models). The hard problems are in the neighborhood of this critical value. The existence of the threshold for 3-SAT was proven by Friedgut [8] but the critical value is still not known. We only know bounds ($3.03 \leq \frac{c}{v} \leq 4.64$), (Dubois and al [5]). For 2-SAT, the value is equal to one (Chvatal [2], Goerdt [9]).

The results are measured on a PC Pentium 200 with 64 Mo of RAM. The code of the program is written in C and includes 1300 lines. All CPU times are given in seconds.

4.1 Comparison between DP and AVAL

We compared the AVAL and DP methods augmented by the MOM and UP heuristics on hard random SAT instances. The samples of each test are 50 randomly generated instances with a ratio ($\frac{c}{v} = 4.25$). Tables 1 and 2 show the results obtained.

We can see that AVAL surpasses DP in both the number of search nodes and the CPU time. This confirms the efficiency of the LP procedure in producing literals and the advantage in combining it with DP. The gain increases as the number of variable grows giving a promising way to solve large scale problems. We can also see the benefit of using UP heuristic to define the variable assignment order. For this reason we use it in AVAL to compare the method with both SATZ and POSIT methods which out perform C-SAT [4].

Using the LP procedure in an enumerative method leads to minimizing the number of branchings. Indeed, LP efficiently produces literals, thus avoiding some choice points in the search tree. This optimizes in some way, the number of branching for the enumerative method with respect to the heuristic used for the variable ordering.

Table 1. Comparison between DP and AVAL (Nodes)

Number of Variables	140	160	180	200	220	240
DP + MOM	756	1165	3193	6736	18997	51733
AVAL + MOM	69	98	245	474	1212	2672
DP + UP + MOM	654	1047	2709	5271	15373	33000
AVAL + UP + MOM	58	82	189	335	923	2072

Table 2. Comparison between DP and AVAL (Time)

Number of variables	140	160	180	200	220	240
DP + MOM	0.219	0.355	1.01	2.269	7.055	19.8
AVAL + MOM	0.176	0.273	0.717	1.554	4.508	12.1
DP + UP + MOM	0.261	0.409	1.039	2.131	6.15	14.8
AVAL + UP + MOM	0.228	0.339	0.79	1.535	4.50	10.5

4.2   Success Rate of the Literal Production

Table 3. Success rate of literal production

Nb of variables	100	140	180	220	260
Nb of tests	170	860	3795	14136	62672
Nb of success	152	784	3494	13105	58372
%	89	91	92	92	93

Results of table 3 confirm that about 90% of calls to LP succeed to produce a literal. This is a promising result and explains the gain in number of nodes when comparing AVAL to DP. Experiments on random instances show that after the depth $\frac{v}{21}$ in the search tree, AVAL search efforts only consist in unit propagations. Indeed, all the calls to LP succeed to produce literals. Literal production failures (about 10%) correspond to calls to LP in the top part of the search tree. In practice, an avalanch of mono-literals is observed after the first literal production. Such phenomenon occurs after nearly the depth $\frac{v}{21}$ and the search process is achieved in linear time complexity. This phenomenon is observed for the classical method DP too, but later, after a depth of $\frac{v}{13}$ in the search tree. This explains the difference between the efficiency of AVAL and DP. The more early the avalanch, the more efficient the algorithm. Thus, one can think that a minimal bound of the number of nodes that an enumerative method (w.r.t a given heuristic) has to explore is reached with the method AVAL.

4.3   Efficiency of Our Method

Theoretical complexity in the worst case of the LP algorithm is in $O(|V_{B_I}||V_{C_I}|)$. But in practice the average complexity is linear in the number of variables. This is confirmed by the experimental results of table 4. The ratio $\frac{b}{a}$ gives the average number of unit propagations for one call to the literal production procedure LP. Its variation is linear with respect to the number of variables. This allows to perform LP at each node of the search tree which explains the efficiency of AVAL.

Table 4. Complexity of the LP algorithm

Nb of variables	100	140	180	220	260
$a=nb$ call of LP	170	860	3795	14136	62672
$b=nb$ Unit Prop	9919	73303	420363	1930100	10216322
ratio $\frac{b}{a}$	58	85	110	136	163

4.4   Threshold of Unit Clauses Production

The number of binary clauses in the current set of clauses has a great impact on literal production. The more the number of binary clauses, the more the chance to succeed in producing a literal. As AVAL performances depend on the efficiency of literal production, it is important to know in practice how many binary clauses are necessary to produce a literal. In theory, the threshold of the satisfiability problem for 2-SAT random instances is reached when the ratio number of clauses to the number of variable is equal to one. This means that literal production shall succeed when the number of binary clauses is equal to the number of variables. But in practice literal production is guaranteed with a fewer number of binary clauses. Table 5 reports experiments on random 3-SAT instances which show that for a ratio $\frac{c}{v} \geq 0.7$ the procedure LP always succeeds in producing a literal. This means that $0.7 \times v$ binary clauses always produce a literal. This number of binary clauses is maintained at each node of the search tree after a depth of $\frac{v}{21}$ and make an avalanch of unit clauses. It will be interesting to study the existence of a theorical threshold for literal production.

Table 5. Ratio nb binary / nb prop

Nb of Variables	100	140	180	220	260	300
$\frac{c}{v}$		0.702	0.708	0.747	0.748	0.744	0.757

4.5   Comparison with SATZ and POSIT

We compared both SATZ and POSIT methods to our method AVAL on hard random SAT instances, on the basis of the CPU times and the number of nodes. The number of variables stands from 100 to 400 (by a step of 50) and the samples of each test are 100 random instances when the number of variables is greater than 300, 200 otherwise. The instances are generated in the transition phase ($\frac{c}{v} = 4.25$). Table 6 shows the results. We can see that AVAL solves problems with 400 variables in the hard region in less than 2 hours in average. AVAL is better than both SATZ and POSIT in the number of nodes. Because of sophisticated heuristics (application of UP to selected variables) SATZ gives the best CPU times. AVAL and POSIT CPU times are comparable.

Table 6. Random Problems.

Nb of variables		100	150	200	250	300	350	400
AVAL	Time (sec)	0.069	0.268	1.681	12,1	100	610	5278
	Nodes	14	72	382	2182	13 946	70 405	502 803
SATZ	Time (sec)	0.068	0.205	0.856	4,399	30.6	189	1096
	Nodes	18	111	590	3089	18 371	100 014	521 349
POSIT	Time (sec)	0.016	0.148	1.074	8.605	65.7	407	3698
	Nodes	39	264	1502	10094	65 505	334 847	2 898 510

4.6   Challenges Beijing and DIMACS

We also compared the three methods on problems of the DIMACS and Beijing challenges. The maximum time that an algorithm can spend in solving an instance is limited to two hours (7200 seconds). Problems of the challenge Beijing are listed individually and those of DIMACS are gathered into classes. *Time* denotes the total time spent in solving all the problems of a class. When a problem is not solved in two hours, its CPU time is considered as 2 hours. The symbol $\#M$ indicates the number of problems in a class and $\#S$ the number of solved problems. Tables 7 and 8 show the results.

Problems of the challenge Beijing, listed in table 7, are mostly planning and scheduling problems. We resolve one more instance than SATZ and four more instances than POSIT. Except the problem 2_bit_add_12, AVAL CPU times are comparable to those of both SATZ and POSIT.

For the DIMACS challenge, AVAL solved less instances than SATZ for the classes: dubois, ii16 and ssa, and less instances than POSIT for the class ii16. But only AVAL is able to solve the whole problems in class ii32. POSIT solved half of the class aim200. These results show the advantage of combining literal deduction algorithm LP with DP.

Table 7. Challenge Beijing.

Problem	AVAL		SATZ		POSIT	
	Time	*Nodes*	*Time*	*Nodes*	*Time*	*Nodes*
2bitadd_10	3706	2 116 944	>7200	-	>7200	-
2bitadd_11	6.4	4 838	113	120 982	>7200	-
2bitadd_12	35.2	28 843	0.265	99	0.04	35
2bitcomp_5	0.02	11	0.01	6	0.01	34
2bitmax_6	0.06	14	0.05	7	0.05	12
3bitadd_31	>7200	-	>7200	-	>7200	-
3bitadd_32	>7200	-	3101	297 652	>7200	-
3blocks	2.2	16	1.6	7	2.38	669
4blocks	1184	18 823	930	228 040	>7200	-
4blocksb	11.5	97	8	8	70	8424
e0ddr2-10-by-5-1	2657	705	86	35	>7200	-
e0ddr2-10-by-5-4	617	661	86	32	2726	34759
enddr2-10-by-5-1	38	10	>7200	-	>7200	-
enddr2-10-by-5-8	66	15	81	30	>7200	-
ewddr2-10-by-5-1	41	15	124	40	143	250
ewddr2-10-by-5-8	861	238	92	39	>7200	-

Table 8. Challenge DIMACS

Pb Class	#M	AVAL		SATZ		POSIT	
		#S	Time	#S	Time	#S	Time
aim-50	24	24	14	24	14	24	0.3
aim-100	24	24	3.55	24	3.4	24	320
aim-200	24	24	4.2	24	3.85	12	86400
dubois	13	8	43274	12	38665	8	45500
hole	5	5	180	5	213	5	444
ii8	14	14	15.4	14	5	14	0.77
ii16	10	8	14967	10	104	9	7268
ii32	17	17	2060	16	7638	15	14410
jnh	50	50	12.84	50	11	50	0.25
par8	10	10	0.7	10	0.66	10	0.05
par1	10	10	288	10	403	10	33
ssa	8	7	10500	8	826	7	7231

5   Conclusion

Systematic search methods based on the Davis and Putnam procedure use unit propagation. But, only the explicit mono-literals occuring in the set of clauses are considered. AVAL does more propagation than these methods. Indeed, when there is no explicit mono-literal in the current set of clauses, AVAL calls the procedure LP to produce one before branching. Produced literals are propagated as mono-literals, thus minimizing the number of branching nodes. The LP algorithm produces literals appearing in binary clauses with a linear time complexity ($O(v)$ in practice). This allows to use LP at each branching node of the search tree, thus increasing the efficiency of the AVAL method.

We studied the behaviour of AVAL on hard random SAT instances generated in the neighbourhood of the threshold area and we observed two different parts in the search tree when solving such instances by AVAL.The hard part is the one formed by the first levels of the search tree. AVAL shows that enumerative methods have to spend a lot of time in this part of the search tree which contains all the branching nodes. Future work will consist to aim at finding variable ordering heuristics and techniques in order to reduce the search space of this part.

References

1. Y. Boufkhad. *Aspects probabilistes et algorithmiques du problème de satisfaisabilité.* PhD thesis, Univertsité de Jussieu, 1996.
2. V. Chvátal and B. Reed. Mick Gets Some (the odds are on this side). In *33rd IEEE Symposium on Foundation of Computers Science,* 1992.
3. M. Davis and H. Putnam. A computing procedure for quantification theory. *JACM,* 1960.
4. O. Dubois, P. André, Y. Boufkhad, and J. Carlier. Sat versus unsat. *AMS, DI-MACS Series in Discrete Mathematics and Theoretical Computer Science,* 26, 1996.
5. O. Dubois and Y. Boufkhad. A General Upper Bound for the Satisfiability Threshold of random r-sat formulae. *Journal of Algorithms,* 1996.
6. J.W. Freeman. *Improvements to Propositionnal Satisfiability Search Algorithms.* PhD thesis, Univ. of Pennsylvania, Philadelphia, 1995.
7. J.W. Freeman. Hard random 3-SAT problems and the Davis-Putnam procedure. *Artificial Intelligence,* 81(2):183–198, 1996.
8. E. Friegut. Necessary and sufficient conditions for sharp threolds of graphs properties and the k-sat problem. Technical report, Institute of Mathematics, The Hebrew University of Jerusalem, 1997.
9. A. Goerdt. A threshold for unsatisfiability. In *Mathematical Foundations of Computer Science,* volume 629, pages 264–274. Springer, 1992.
10. Chu Min Li and Anbulagan. Heuristics based on unit propagation for satisfiability problem. In *proceedings of IJCAI 97,* 1997.
11. Chu Min Li and Anbulagan. Look-Ahead Versus Look-Back for Satisfiability Problems. In *proceedings of CP97,* pages 341–355, 1997.
12. W.V. Quine. Methods of logics. *Henry Holt, New York,* 1950.
13. B. Selman, H. Levesque, and D. Mitchell. A New Method for Solving Hard Satisfiability Problems. In *Proceedings of the 10th National Conference on Artificial Intelligence AAAI'94,* 1994.
14. H. Zhang. SATO: An efficient propositional prover. In *Proceedings of the 14th International Conference on Automated deduction,* 1997.

Constraint Logic Programming for Local and Symbolic Model-Checking

Ulf Nilsson and Johan Lübcke

Dept of Computer and Information Science
Linköping University, 581 83 Linköping, Sweden
{ulfni,johlu}@ida.liu.se

Abstract. We propose a model checking scheme for a *semantically complete* fragment of CTL by combining techniques from constraint logic programming, a restricted form of constructive negation and tabled resolution. Our approach is *symbolic* in that it encodes and manipulates sets of states using constraints; it supports *local* model checking using goal-directed computation enhanced by tabulation. The framework is parameterized by the constraint domain and supports any finite constraint domain closed under disjunction, projection and complementation. We show how to encode our fragment of CTL in constraint logic programming; we outline an abstract execution model for the resulting type of programs and provide a preliminary evaluation of the approach.

1 Introduction

Model checking [5], is a technique for automatic verification of safety and liveness properties in finite, reactive systems. Given a model of the system and a property – often expressed in some temporal logic [10] such as CTL (computation tree logic) or the mu-calculus – model checking amounts to checking if a given initial state of the system satisfies the desired property. The early approaches relied on fixed point techniques where all states satisfying the given property were explicitly enumerated. Since even small (finite) systems tend to have very large state spaces early attempts were quite restrictive.

More recently it was observed that sets of states could be represented implicitly e.g. by logic formulas – so called *symbolic model checking* [15]. In combination with very efficient representations of such formulas, e.g. *BDDs*, it is often possible to verify considerably larger – but still finite – systems. There are now several model checking systems around and model checking has been successfully applied both to hardware verification problems [2] and verification of computer protocols [11]. There is on-going work to extend model checking also to infinite systems.

A complementary approach to reduce the search space is to try to avoid generating as much as possible of it. As pointed out above, the aim of model checking is to verify if a property holds in the initial state(s). By checking the formula and its sub-formulas only in those states that are reachable from the

J. Lloyd et al. (Eds.): CL 2000, LNAI 1861, pp. 384–398, 2000.

initial state(s) it is often possible to substantially reduce the state space. This is known as *local* (or *on-the-fly*) model checking (e.g. [19]).

Model checking has many characteristics in common with logic programming; a logic program is a symbolic description of a model (the so-called least Herbrand model in case of definite programs or the standard model in the case of stratified logic programs) and by means of resolution it is possible to verify certain properties (expressed by means of *queries*) of that model. This process is demand-driven in the sense that only the part of the model necessary to verify the property/query is produced. That is, the model is described symbolically and generated on-the-fly (locally) when needed for the verification of a specific property/query.

Recently there have been several attempts to formalize and host model checking inside the logic programming paradigm. One of the first attempts were reported by the logic programming group at Stony Brook [16]. They describe an implementation of a model checking system called XMC [9] in the logic programming system XSB (a logic programming system based on tabulation [4]). In XMC the system model is described in a CCS-like language and properties are described in the alternation free fragment of the modal mu-calculus. While providing a "symbolic" description of states (CCS formulas), the approach does not offer an implicit representation of *sets* of states in the true sense of symbolic model checking. However, XMC relies on local checking and the results reported in [16] show that the approach can compete with state-of-the-art model checkers, although implemented in a general purpose logic programming system.

Independently Charatonik and Podelski [3], and Delzanno and Podelski [7, 8] described an alternative approach to model checking in which the transition relation between states is encoded as a (constraint) logic program; the temporal properties to be checked can also be encoded as a (constraint) logic program, and by use of the immediate consequence operator, they were able to characterize the meaning of the temporal operators of CTL in terms of least and greatest fixed points of compositions of the two programs. By means of the well-established magic templates transformation Delzanno and Podelski also introduced a way of achieving local model checking for some of the temporal operators of CTL. A novel feature of [3, 7, 8] is that the approach facilitates approximation of properties of infinite state systems.

We should also mention the early work of Rauzy, who developed the constraint language Toupie (e.g. [17]). This is a equational constraint language with support for computing least and greatest solutions of sets of mutually recursive equations. Toupie is symbolic and, in a restricted sense, local; the actual checking of a property is preceded by a reachability analysis which eliminates some (but not all) states where the property does not need to be checked.

In this paper we propose an encoding of a *semantically complete* fragment of the temporal specification language CTL using techniques from constraint logic programming (CLP) [13], constructive negation [20] and tabulation [22]. Our approach is fully symbolic in that it encodes and manipulates sets of states using constraints; it also fully supports local model checking of all temporal operators using goal-directed search in combination with tabulation techniques similar to those in [16]. The approach is parameterized by the constraint domain, which means that any finite constraint language equipped with disjunctive constraints, projection and complementation can be used together with the scheme.

In the next section we give preliminary notions from constraint logic programming and present the temporal specification language CTL. In Section 3 we describe a (schematic) constraint logic program that encodes the semantic equations of CTL and discuss its correctness in Section 4. In Section 5 we give an abstract execution model specialized for the program schema. The execution model is embodied in a prototype implementation whose preliminary evaluation is presented in Section 6.

2   Preliminaries

We survey basic concepts and terminology from the field of constraint logic programming and provide a short summary of model checking – in particular the temporal specification language CTL (Computation Tree Logic).

2.1   Constraint Logic Programming

Constraint logic programs are defined in the usual way, see e.g. [13, 12]. A program is a set of clauses where each clause is an implicitly universally quantified expression of the form

$$A_0 \leftarrow C, L_1, \ldots, L_n. \qquad (n \geq 0)$$

where A_0 is an atomic formula, $L_1, \ldots, L_n$ are literals, and C is a constraint. (In what follows we use A and B to denote atomic formulas, L to denote literals, and C to denote constraints.) A *goal* is an expression

$$\leftarrow C, L_1, \ldots, L_n. \qquad (n \geq 0)$$

In what follows we frequently consider clauses where $n = 0$ and goals where $n = 1$. A clause of the form $A \leftarrow C$ is called an *answer* while a goal of the form $\leftarrow C, A$ is referred to as a *call*. (As usual, a call denotes the logic formula $\forall \neg (C \wedge A)$; that is, $\neg \exists (C \wedge A)$.)

We assume the existence of a sufficiently large set of variables VAR ranging over the constraint domain. By a *valuation* over a domain D we mean a mapping $\theta : \text{VAR} \to D$. The set of all valuations is denoted VAL. A valuation θ is called a *solution* of a constraint C iff $D \models C\theta$. By $sol(C)$ we denote the set of all solutions of C. A constraint is said to be *satisfiable* iff $sol(C) \neq \emptyset$.

An answer $A \leftarrow C$ represents the set of all atomic formulas $A\theta$ such that $\theta \in sol(C)$. We use the notation $[\![A \leftarrow C]\!]$ to denote this set. Similarly, a call $\leftarrow C, A$ represents the set of all $A\theta$ such that $\theta \in sol(C)$. We introduce the following order $\sqsubseteq$ on answers and calls:

$$(A \leftarrow C_1) \sqsubseteq (A \leftarrow C_2) \text{ iff } [\![A \leftarrow C_1]\!] \subseteq [\![A \leftarrow C_2]\!]$$
$$(\leftarrow C_1, A) \sqsubseteq (\leftarrow C_2, A) \text{ iff } [\![\leftarrow C_1, A]\!] \subseteq [\![\leftarrow C_2, A]\!]$$

Answers of the form $A \leftarrow$ *false* are minimal, and answers of the form $A \leftarrow$ *true* are maximal in the $\sqsubseteq$-ordering. Two answers $A \leftarrow C_1$ and $A \leftarrow C_2$ are said to be equivalent (denoted $A \leftarrow C_1 \simeq A \leftarrow C_2$) iff $A \leftarrow C_1 \sqsubseteq A \leftarrow C_2 \sqsubseteq A \leftarrow C_1$; similarly with calls.

We do not assume a specific constraint domain, but we assume that the language CON of constraints is closed under four operations $\otimes:$ CON $\times$ CON $\rightarrow$ CON, $\oplus:$ CON $\times$ CON $\rightarrow$ CON, $\pi:$ VAR$^* \times$ CON $\rightarrow$ CON, $\neg:$ CON $\rightarrow$ CON, satisfying the following:[1]

- $sol(C_1 \otimes C_2) = sol(C_1) \cap sol(C_2)$
- $sol(C_1 \oplus C_2) = sol(C_1) \cup sol(C_2)$
- $\theta \in sol(\pi_{\overline{x}} C)$ iff $(\exists \theta') \in sol(C)$ such that $\theta(x_i) = \theta'(x_i)$ for every $(x_i \in \overline{x})$
- $sol(\neg C) = $ VAL $\setminus sol(C)$

That is, we require that the language contains *conjunctive* and *disjunctive* constrains, as well as *projection* and *complementation*. This is not a limitation of our approach as such, but rather a requirement of any approach to represent sets of states symbolically and exactly. We introduce $C_1 \setminus C_2$ as a short-hand for $C_1 \otimes \neg C_2$. Conjunctive constraints are available in most constraint domains, but the other operations are not always available; CLP(B) (boolean constraints) and CLP(FD) (finite domain constraints) usually support all four operations (although some operations may be computationally expensive).

Note that $[\![A \leftarrow C_1]\!] \cup [\![A \leftarrow C_2]\!] = [\![A \leftarrow C_1 \oplus C_2]\!]$ (provided that $C_1 \oplus C_2$ exists and satisfies the requirement above). We refer to $A \leftarrow C_1 \oplus C_2$ as the *join* of $A \leftarrow C_1$ and $A \leftarrow C_2$. A goal $\leftarrow C, A$ represents the formula $\neg \exists (C \wedge A)$ so the join of two goals $\leftarrow C_1, A$ and $\leftarrow C_2, A$ equals $\leftarrow C_1 \oplus C_2, A$.

Note that answers are really universally quantified formulas, so we can, and will, take the join also of answers $A_1 \leftarrow C_1$ and $A_2 \leftarrow C_2$ when A_1 and A_2 are equal modulo renaming of variables provided that the answers are appropriately renamed first. We will do similarly with calls.

A logic formula or a term is said to be *ground* if it contains no variables.

2.2   Model Checking and CTL

We briefly survey the temporal logic CTL (Computation Tree Logic); or rather a semantically complete subset of CTL. For an extensive survey of CTL and temporal logics, see e.g. [15, 10]. CTL is a branching time specification language for discrete dynamic systems. Formulas in CTL are used to specify properties of states and state transitions. In this context a state is characterized by a finite set of *state variables* and a *state* is a *valuation* of the variables – i.e. an assignment of values to the state variables. States are here denoted by σ. It is often assumed that the state variables are boolean, but it is also possible to

---

[1] We do not require the constraint language to be equipped with these operations; only that a new semantically equivalent constraints can be obtained. For instance $\exists x F(x) \equiv F(0) \vee F(1)$ in the case of projection.

have finite domain variables or even variables with infinite domains (in which case checking properties is generally undecidable).

Let c be a set of primitive constraints – for instance, boolean variables or simple equations involving finite domain variables. The abstract syntax of the CTL fragment that we consider here is defined as follows:

$$F ::= c \mid F_1 \wedge F_2 \mid F_1 \vee F_2 \mid \neg F \mid ex(F) \mid eg(F) \mid eu(F_1, F_2)$$

It should be noted that the fragment is semantically complete. That is, temporal operators not discussed here (e.g. ag and ef) can be expressed by means of the operators above (cf. [5]).

A *model* M is a (transition-) relation between states, written $\sigma_1 M \sigma_2$. It is assumed that there is at least one transition from every state (possibly to itself). The model M defines a set of infinite computation paths of states $\sigma_0 \sigma_1 \ldots$, written $\sigma_0 \sigma_1 \ldots \in M$. *Model checking* in CTL is the problem of deciding whether a given system model M and a given initial state σ (or a set of states) satisfies a CTL specification F, written $M, \sigma \models F$. The semantics of the satisfaction relation is defined as follows:

$$
\begin{array}{ll}
M, \sigma_0 \models c & \text{iff } \sigma_0(c) = 1 \\
M, \sigma_0 \models F_1 \wedge F_2 & \text{iff } M, \sigma_0 \models F_1 \text{ and } M, \sigma_0 \models F_2 \\
M, \sigma_0 \models F_1 \vee F_2 & \text{iff } M, \sigma_0 \models F_1 \text{ or } M, \sigma_0 \models F_2 \text{ or both} \\
M, \sigma_0 \models \neg F & \text{iff } M, \sigma_0 \not\models F \\
M, \sigma_0 \models ex(F) & \text{iff there is a path } \sigma_0 \sigma_1 \ldots \in M \text{ such that } M, \sigma_1 \models F \\
M, \sigma_0 \models eg(F) & \text{iff there is a path } \sigma_0 \sigma_1 \ldots \in M \text{ such that } M, \sigma_i \models F \\
& \quad \text{for every } i \geq 0 \\
M, \sigma_0 \models eu(F_1, F_2) & \text{iff there is a path } \sigma_0 \sigma_1 \ldots \in M \text{ and an } i \geq 0 \text{ such that} \\
& \quad M, \sigma_i \models F_2 \text{ and } M, \sigma_j \models F_1 \text{ for every } 0 \leq j < i
\end{array}
$$

Since the model M is static it is common to write simply $s \models F$ when the transition relation is clear from the context.

Figure 1 depicts a model involving a single state variable S with the domain $S \in 0\,..\,3$. In this model the property $eg(S < 2)$ holds in the initial state $S = 0$, since there is an infinite path where S is always less than 2. Also the property $eu(S \neq 1, S = 3)$ holds in the same model and the same initial state, since there is a path where $S \neq 1$ until S becomes 3.

The semantic equations given above can be extended to sets of states: $M, S \models F$ iff $M, \sigma \models F$ for each $\sigma \in S$.

3   A CLP Formalization of CTL

In this section we show that the semantic equations of CTL can be naturally defined using (constraint) logic programming. We introduce two binary predicates – *holds*/2 and *step*/2; the atomic formula $holds(F, S)$ expresses that a CTL formula F holds in the state(s) S. The predicate $step(S_1, S_2)$ expresses that there are transitions from all states in S_1 to some state in S_2. We will encode CTL formulas – even CTL state variables – as ground terms, while sets of states will

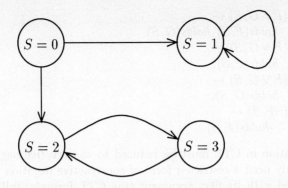

Fig. 1. State machine with a finite domain state variable

be represented as a *constraint* between CLP variables; later we show how to couple CTL variables (encoded as constants) and CLP variables.

Note that the satisfaction relation *holds*/2 does not explicitly involve the actual model; the transition relation is rather encoded in the relation *step*/2. To describe the system model (or the transition relation) we need two copies of the state variables – say S_1 and S_2.[2] The set of all transitions can then be defined in the following schematic way:

$$step(S_1, S_2) \leftarrow C(S_1, S_2).$$

where $C(S_1, S_2)$ is a constraint which is (equivalent to) a disjunction of all possible transitions. For instance, the system in Figure 1 (with only a single state variable) can be described as follows using a finite domain constraint:

$$step(S_1, S_2) \leftarrow$$
$$(S_1 = 0 \wedge S_2 = 1) \vee (S_1 = 0 \wedge S_2 = 2) \vee \cdots \vee (S_1 = 3 \wedge S_2 = 2).$$

Note that it is perfectly possible to give an intensional definition of the transition relation; for example, it is possible to express composition of models in a natural way. If we have sub-systems encoded by the relations $step_1, \ldots, step_n$, then the parallel composition can be defined schematically as follows:

$$step(S_1, S_2) \leftarrow$$
$$step_1(S_1, S_2), \ldots, step_n(S_1, S_2).$$

In what follows we assume nothing about *how* the transition relation is defined; only that it is correct: that is, $\sigma_1 M \sigma_2$ iff $step(\sigma_1, \sigma_2)$ is a consequence of the program.[3]

The meaning of the standard boolean connectives can be defined straightforwardly:

---

[2] To simplify the notation we consider only a single state variable, but S_1 and S_2 can be also tuples of state variables.

[3] By abuse of notation we sometimes view a state (which is defined as a function from state variables to values) also as a tuple of values.

(C_1) $holds(F \wedge G, S) \leftarrow$
  $holds(F, S), holds(G, S).$
(C_2) $holds(F \vee G, S) \leftarrow$
  $holds(F, S).$
(C_3) $holds(F \vee G, S) \leftarrow$
  $holds(G, S).$
(C_4) $holds(\neg F, S) \leftarrow$
  $\sim holds(F, S).$

Note that negation in CTL must be reduced to *constructive* negation in CLP. Actually we only need a restricted form of constructive negation – $holds/2$ will always be called with its first argument (the CTL formula) fully instantiated so there will be no need to construct (and then complement) any Herbrand constraints. For this to work we require that a goal $\leftarrow holds(F, S)$ has only a finite number of answers, and that the constraint (representing these answers) can be complemented (see e.g. [20] for details on negation in constraint logic programming).

The temporal operators ex and eu can be defined similarly:

(C_5) $holds(ex(F), S_1) \leftarrow$
  $step(S_1, S_2), holds(F, S_2).$
(C_6) $holds(eu(F, G), S) \leftarrow$
  $holds(G, S).$
(C_7) $holds(eu(F, G), S_1) \leftarrow$
  $holds(F, S_1), step(S_1, S_2), holds(eu(F, G), S_2).$

The only problem is caused by the CTL formula $eg(F)$: it is typically defined as a greatest fixed point; namely the largest set of states (1) where F holds and (2) where every state has at least one transition back to some state in the set. In a previous paper we extended CLP with a mechanism for computing greatest fixed points [14]. It is also possible to solve the problem by use of several nested negations, but negation means complementation which is often an expensive operation.

On the other hand, if we assume that the state space is finite it is possible to formulate the semantics of $eg(F)$ as a least fixed point, using the following trivial observation.

Proposition 1. Let M be a finite transition system, then $M, \sigma_0 \models eg(F)$ iff there exists a finite path $\sigma_0 \dots \sigma_i$ such that $M, \sigma_j \models F$ for all $0 \leq j \leq i$ and $\sigma_i = \sigma_k$ for some $0 \leq k < i$. ∎

By an F-path we mean a finite non-empty path where F holds in every state (except possibly the last one). F-paths can be characterized as follows.

(C_8) $path(F, S_1, S_2) \leftarrow$
  $holds(F, S_1), step(S_1, S_2).$
(C_9) $path(F, S_1, S_3) \leftarrow$
  $path(F, S_1, S_2), holds(F, S_2), step(S_2, S_3).$

Now the property $eg(F)$ obviously holds in a state σ if there is an F-path $\sigma_0 \ldots \sigma_i$ such that $\sigma_0 = \sigma_i = \sigma$. Moreover, $eg(F)$ must hold in a *set* S of states, if for every $\sigma \in S$ there is an F-path $\sigma \ldots \sigma_i$ such that $\sigma_i \in S$. Consequently:

(C_{10}) $holds(eg(F), S) \leftarrow$
    $path(F, S, S)$.

In addition, $eg(F)$ must hold in every state where F holds and where there is a transition to a state where $eg(F)$ holds.

(C_{11}) $holds(eg(F), S_1) \leftarrow$
    $holds(F, S_1), step(S_1, S_2), holds(eg(F), S_2)$.

These eleven clauses are sufficient for defining the semantics of CTL.

Finally we have to encode the primitive constraints of CTL. We illustrate the principle by example only, since this depends very much on the particular constraint domain, and what primitive constraints that are being used. As pointed out, CTL formulas (including state variables) are encoded as ground terms, but for each state variable we also need a constraint variable. Each primitive CTL constraint is then lifted to the meta level. In case of a boolean domain we may for instance introduce one clause (using the syntax of SICStus Prolog) for each boolean state variable c_i of our CTL formula:

$holds(c_i, [X_1, \ldots, X_i, \ldots, X_n]) \leftarrow sat(X_i)$.

That is, the boolean state variable c_i is satisfied in a state $[X_1, \ldots, X_i, \ldots, X_n]$ if the constraint $sat(X_i)$ is satisfied.

The system model in Figure 1 involves a single state variable S with the finite domain 0..3. The following clauses illustrate how some primitive constraints can be encoded using CLP(fd):

$holds(s = N, S) \leftarrow S = N$.
$holds(s < N, S) \leftarrow S \in 0..(N-1)$.

4   Correctness

We now have to show that the relation $holds/2$, as defined by the CLP program P above, is equivalent to the satisfaction relation in Section 2.2, provided that P contains correct definitions of $step$ and the primitive constraints.

The program P is a general constraint logic program. There are a number of different semantic frameworks for logic programs with negation (see e.g. [1]). Fortunately it can be shown that the program described in the previous section is (locally) stratified, and for such programs there is a well-established *standard model*[4] (usually denoted M_P) which coincides with most other semantic frameworks.

---

[4] This standard model should not be confused with the model in model checking.

In order to prove equivalence we have to assume that $step/2$ is equivalent to the transition relation; that is

$$M_P \models step(\sigma_1, \sigma_2) \text{ iff } \sigma_1 M \sigma_2.$$

We also have to assume that P contains an equivalent definition of the primitive constraints:

$$M_P \models holds(c, \sigma) \text{ iff } M, \sigma \models c.$$

Theorem 2. Let F be a CTL formula, σ a state and P a constraint logic program as described above. If $step/2$ is a correct realization of the transition relation M, and if the primitive constraints are correct then:

$$M, \sigma \models F \text{ iff } M_P \models holds(F, \sigma)$$

∎

The theorem can be shown by rule induction using the fact that the size of the CTL formula in the head of each clause is never smaller than the size of CTL formulas in the body of the same clause.

5 An Abstract Model of Computation

In this section we describe an abstract model of execution for the restricted type of constraint logic programs considered here. The model is goal-directed, uses tabulation and a restricted form of constructive negation. It should be noted that while the model has been used as a basis for a prototype implementation (see Section 6), and may serve as a basis for a real implementation, there are many design decisions (intentionally) left open.

There are two reasons why we need a new model (rather than using an existing CLP system):

- no CLP system known to us has support for constructive negation (see [20]) which is necessary in order to deal with negation in CTL;
- the program in Section 3 is highly recursive; in fact, the rules for $eg(F)$ and $eu(F_1, F_2)$ would, in most cases, result in infinite computations in existing CLP systems.

However, both problems can be repaired; at least in the presence of CLP programs with a finite number of solutions. Constructive negation fits very well with constraint logic programming. The main difficulty being that we have to be able to compute the complement of a constraint (which was one of our initial assumptions). When it comes to infinite (and repeated) computations it is possible to use *tabulation*, or memoization, (e.g. [22,6,4]). Efficient systems based on tabulation (and similar techniques) exist for logic programming, most notably XSB [18]. There are frameworks for extending tabulation also to constraints [21], but general and efficient implementations are not yet available.

Our execution model relies on the notion of a *table*. The table is used to record all procedure invocations and all answers to each procedure invocation. Informally a table is a set of answers and calls modulo the equivalence $\simeq$. Moreover the table will be kept in a standardized form, obtained by joining answers (and calls); for instance, the answers, $A \leftarrow C_1$ and $A \leftarrow C_2$ will be combined into $A \leftarrow C_1 \oplus C_2$. As a result the table will contain at most one answer per atomic formula (modulo $\simeq$), and similarly for calls.[5]

The ordering $\sqsubseteq$ on answers and calls extends to tables. Hence, $T_1 \sqsubseteq T_2$ iff whenever $A \leftarrow C_1 \in T_1$, then there is an answer $A \leftarrow C_2 \in T_2$ such that $A \leftarrow C_1 \sqsubseteq A \leftarrow C_2$, and similarly with calls.

Given an initial table T_0, a computation is a sequence of tables

$$T_0 \rhd T_1 \rhd \ldots \rhd T_n \text{ such that } T_i \sqsubseteq T_{i+1} \text{ for } 0 \leq i \leq n-1$$

and where each table T_{i+1} is obtained from T_i by application of a so-called *extension* ($\rhd$) to be defined below. Each extension adds a new answer or call to the current table, and this process proceeds until no further extensions are possible (or more precisely until nothing new can be added to the table). The initial table T_0 typically contains a single call $\{\leftarrow C, A\}$ – in our case the goal is typically on the form $\leftarrow C(S), holds(f, S)$ where f is a CTL formula, and $C(S)$ a constraint on S encoding the set of states where we want to check f. However, it is also possible to start from other initial tables; both standard (global) model checking and Rauzy's approach can be simulated by alternative initial tables as discussed in the next section.

Before defining the actual extensions we first introduce two auxiliary transition relations $\overset{c}{\Rightarrow}$ (call) and $\overset{a}{\Rightarrow}$ (answer) between clauses. The relation $\overset{c}{\Rightarrow}$ describes partial instantiation and constraining of clauses, and the relation $\overset{a}{\Rightarrow}$ corresponds to resolution with answers (both positive and negative subgoals can be resolved). Let T be a table, then:

Call: If $(\leftarrow C', B) \in T$, $C \otimes C'$ is satisfiable and $\theta = \text{mgu}(A, B)$, then[6]

$$(A \leftarrow C, L_1, \ldots, L_n) \overset{c}{\Rightarrow} (A \leftarrow C \otimes C', L_1, \ldots, L_n)\theta.$$

Answer I: If $(B \leftarrow C') \in T$, $C \otimes C'$ is satisfiable and $\theta = \text{mgu}(A_1, B)$, then

$$(A \leftarrow C, A_1, L_2, \ldots, L_n) \overset{a}{\Rightarrow} (A \leftarrow C \otimes C', L_2, \ldots, L_n)\theta.$$

Answer II: If $(B \leftarrow C') \in T$, $C \setminus C'$ is satisfiable and $\theta = \text{mgu}(A_1, B)$, then

$$(A \leftarrow C, \sim A_1, L_2, \ldots, L_n) \overset{a}{\Rightarrow} (A \leftarrow C \setminus C', L_2, \ldots, L_n)\theta$$

---

[5] On the other hand, our model is an abstract one, and in an actual implementation we may decide to keep table entries separate.

[6] Here, and in the following transitions, we implicitly assume that the expressions are first appropriately renamed apart.

We then define $\overset{ca^{\bullet}}{\Rightarrow}$ as the relational composition of $\overset{c}{\Rightarrow}$ with the transitive and reflexive closure of $\overset{a}{\Rightarrow}$. That is, $\overset{ca^{\bullet}}{\Rightarrow} \equiv \overset{c}{\Rightarrow}(\overset{a}{\Rightarrow})^{*}$.

The (three) extensions can now be defined as follows:

1. $T \triangleright T \cup \{A' \leftarrow \pi_{A'}C'\}$ if there is a program clause $A \leftarrow C, L_1, \ldots, L_n$ such that
$$A \leftarrow C, L_1, \ldots, L_n \overset{ca^{\bullet}}{\Rightarrow} A' \leftarrow C'$$

2. $T \triangleright T \cup \{\leftarrow \pi_{A_i'}C', A_i'\}$ if there is a program clause $A \leftarrow C, L_1, \ldots, L_n$ and formulas $A', L'_{i+1}, \ldots, L'_n$ such that
$$A \leftarrow C, L_1, \ldots, L_n \overset{ca^{\bullet}}{\Rightarrow} A' \leftarrow C', A_i', L'_{i+1}, \ldots, L'_n$$

3. $T \triangleright T \cup \{\leftarrow \pi_{A_i'}C', A_i'\}$ if there is a program clause $A \leftarrow C, L_1, \ldots, L_n$ and formulas $A', L'_{i+1}, \ldots, L'_n$ such that
$$A \leftarrow C, L_1, \ldots, L_n \overset{ca^{\bullet}}{\Rightarrow} A' \leftarrow C', \sim A_i', L'_{i+1}, \ldots, L'_n$$

A computation is a saturation process where the extensions above are applied until no further extensions are possible. The extensions can be applied non-deterministically with one restriction; extensions relying on the transition Answer II (answer resolution with a negative subgoal) should not be applied until the answer for the corresponding positive subgoal is completed. In our particular case it means that we must not generate answers on the form $holds(\neg f, S) \leftarrow C(S)$ until we have exhausted all possibilities to extend $holds(f, S) \leftarrow C(S)$. (See [6, 4] for details on how to deal with negation in tabled resolution.)

6   A Preliminary Experimental Evaluation

Since there is presently no CLP system that supports constructive negation and tabulation, we had to implement a prototype system in order to evaluate the approach outlined above. Instead of building a general purpose system we have hard-coded the CLP program in Section 3 and the extensions described above. The prototype supports boolean constraints and uses Jørn Lind-Nielsen's BDD library BuDDy[7] to represent boolean constraints.

One of the main benefits of local model checking, is that it reduces the state space in which we have to check a property; it should be noted that this is not always productive in combination with symbolic model checking – there is not always a direct correspondence between the size of a BDD and the set of states that it represents. For example, the set of *all* states is represented by the boolean expression *true* which is a one-node BDD. Hence, for evaluation purposes it would probably have been better to pick another domain (or another representation of boolean expressions). However, even for BDDs we can report improvement in some cases, as illustrated below.

Since there are relatively few clauses in our program the various extensions were hard-coded. As an example, consider for the clause defining $\wedge$:

---

[7] http://www.itu.dk/research/buddy/

(C_1) $holds(F \wedge G, S) \leftarrow$
         $holds(F, S), holds(G, S).$

The clause represents two possible uses of extension by call (the two body literals), and one use of extension by answer. Figure 2 shows the dependencies between the different entries in the table. The arrows describe dependencies between table entries. The labels on edges refer to the three different types of extensions. The fact that entries for the answers of sub-formulas depend on the corresponding calls are visualized by dashed edges. Each time a table entry is updated, all entries depending on that entry are scheduled for execution.

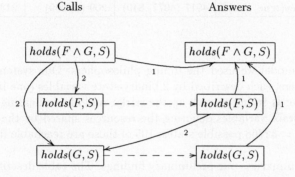

Fig. 2. Dependencies between table entries due to (C_1).

Because of the prototype nature of our system it is not meaningful to compare the run-time of our system with others. On the other hand, the framework described in Section 5 is general enough to simulate both local model checking and global model checking (the standard approach to symbolic model checking) as well as the restricted type of local checking used by Rauzy [17] (where we first compute all reachable states and then apply a global algorithm).

Local: In this approach the initial table is loaded with a single call as described in Section 5. This amounts to a top-down traversal of the CTL formula making use of all of the three extensions.

Global: Here the initial table is loaded with calls of the form $\leftarrow true, holds(f, S)$ for each sub-formula f of the CTL formula that we want to check. This results in a bottom-up traversal of the CTL formula; i.e. we first compute the set of states where the inner-most formulas hold, followed by larger and larger sub-formulas. Only extension (1) is needed for this.

Filtered Global: Here we first compute the set of all states $C(S)$ reachable from the initial state; then the initial table is loaded with calls of the form $\leftarrow C(S), holds(f, S)$ for each sub-formula f of the CTL formula that we want to check. We use only extension (1) but each answer is filtered with the states $C(S)$.

Table 1. The size of BDDs for local checking, global checking and filtered global checking. The numbers are (1) the total number of nodes in the BDDs, and (in parentheses) the total number of BDD nodes in all (2) call and all (3) answer entries.)

CTL formula	Local	Global	Filtered global
$eat1 \land eat2$	32 (30, 2)	4 (0, 4)	128 (0, 128)
$ex(ex(eat1 \land eat2))$	267 (265, 2)	525 (0, 525)	109 (0, 109)
$\neg eu(true, \neg ex(true))$	897 (681, 216)	3831 (0, 3831)	786 (0, 786)
$eu(stick1, eat1 \land eat2)$	63 (60, 3)	61 (0, 61)	249 (0, 249)
$ex(eat1)$	65 (64, 1)	302 (0, 302)	130 (0, 130)
$ex(ex(ex(eat1)))$	377 (291, 86)	1385 (0, 1385)	376 (0, 376)
$\neg eu(true, \neg eu(true, init))$	4917 (4077, 840)	209 (0, 209)	2137 (0, 2137)

As a sample model we used the dining philosophers. Our system consisted of five philosophers, each described by 2 binary state variables (one indicating that the philosopher is trying to pick up the sticks, and one indicating success), and 5 additional state variables denoting the resources shared by the philosophers. This gives $2^{15} = 32768$ possible states; 105 of those are reachable from the initial state.

Table 1 summarizes our preliminary findings. The table describes the size of all final BDDs in the three different approaches. In addition we show how the total number of BDD nodes is divided between call and answer entries. The size of the BDDs is probably a better measure than run-time since operations are generally polynomial in the size of BDDs, but the size of a BDDs may in the worst case grow exponentially in the number of boolean parameters. We would like to point out that boolean constraints and BDDs is not the best domain and representation to demonstrate the usefulness of local, symbolic model checking, since large sets of states may have very compact representations as BDDs. Moreover, the dining philosophers is not the best example, since there are relatively few synchronization points. In spite of this, there are several properties where local checking beats global checking. Most notably the property $\neg eu(true, \neg ex(true))$ which is saying that there is "no deadlock". On the other hand there are other properties where global checking beats local checking; in particular the property $\neg eu(true, \neg eu(true, init))$ which states that it is always possible to return to the initial state from any reachable state. It should be observed that the figures in the last column are somewhat misleading since they do not include the size of the BDD that represents the set of all reachable states.

7   Conclusions

We have encoded a *semantically complete* fragment of CTL in a constraint logic programming framework extended with constructive negation and tabulation. We have also described an abstract model of execution which encompasses both local and global model checking as well as filtered global checking. In this framework we can combine symbolic model checking with different degrees of local model checking. Our framework is parameterized by the constraint domain, which means that any constraint language over a finite domain and equipped with disjunctive constraints, projection and complementation can be used. The program is very succinct and basically corresponds to the semantic equations of CTL.

As far as we know this is the first formalization of a semantically complete fragment of CTL which supports both *symbolic* model checking, and *on-the-fly* generation of the state space; i.e. local model checking. Other approaches such as XMC [16] supports local model checking, but not symbolic model checking, while the approach of Delzanno and Podelski ([7] and [8]) allows for symbolic checking, but not for a semantically complete fragment of CTL, and there is only limited support for local checking. Rauzy's constraint language Toupie [17] combines symbolic checking with a reachability analysis but the two are not intertwined, as in our approach.

Acknowledgements

We are grateful to the comments from the anonymous referees. The work has been supported by the Swedish Research Council for Engineering Sciences (TFR) and by CENIIT.

References

1. K. Apt and R. Bol. Logic Programming and Negation: A Survey. *J. Logic Programming*, 19/20:9–71, 1994.
2. J. R. Burch, E. M. Clarke, D. E. Long, K. I. McMillan, and D. L. Dill. Symbolic Model Checking for Sequential Circuit Verification. *IEEE Trans on Computer-Aided Design of Integrated Circuits*, 13(4):401–424, 1994.
3. W. Charatonik and A. Podelski. Set-Based Analysis of Reactive Infinite-State Systems. In *Proc. of TACAS'98*, Lecture Notes in Computer Science 1384, pages 358–375. Springer-Verlag, 1998.
4. W. Chen and D. S. Warren. Tabled Evaluation With Delaying for General Logic Programs. *J. ACM*, 43(1):20–74, 1996.
5. E. Clarke, O. Grumberg, and D. Peled. *Model Checking*. MIT Press, 2000.
6. L. Degerstedt. *Tabulation-based Logic Programming*. PhD thesis, Linköping studies in Science and Technology, dissertation no 462, 1996.
7. G. Delzanno and A. Podelski. Model Checking Infinite-State Systems using CLP. Technical report MPI-I-98-2-012, Max-Planck-Institut für Informatik, 1998.
8. G. Delzanno and A. Podelski. Model Checking in CLP. In *Proc of TACAS'99, Amsterdam*, Lecture Notes in Computer Science 1579. Springer Verlag, 1999.
9. Y. Dong, X. Du, Y.Ramakrishna, I. Ramakrishnan, S. Smolka, O. Sokolsky, E. Stark, and D. Warren. Fighting Livelock in the i-Protocol: A Comparative Study of Verification Tools. In *Proc of TACAS'99, Amsterdam*, Lecture Notes in Computer Science 1579. Springer Verlag, 1999.

398   Ulf Nilsson and Johan Lübcke

10. E. A. Emerson. Temporal and Modal Logics. In Jan van Leeuwen, editor, *Handbook on Theoretical Computer Science*, volume B, pages 995–1072. Elsevier Science, 1990.
11. G. Holzmann. *Design and Validation of Computer Protocols*. Prentice-Hall, 1991.
12. J. Jaffar and J-L. Lassez. Constraint Logic Programming. In *Conf. Record of 14th Annual ACM Symp. on POPL*, pages 111–119, 1987.
13. J. Jaffar and M. Maher. Constraint Logic Programming: A Survey. *J. Logic Programming*, 19/20:503–581, 1994.
14. J. Lübcke and U. Nilsson. On-the-fly CTL Model-checking using Constraint Logic Programming. In *Intl Workshop on Constraint Programming for Time-Critical Applications, COTIC99*, 1999.
15. K. McMillan. *Symbolic Model Checking*. Kluwer Academic Publishers, 1993.
16. Y. S. Ramakrishna, C. R. Ramakrishnan, I. V. Ramakrishnan, S. Smolka, T. Swift, and D. S. Warren. Efficient Model Checking using Tabled Resolution. In *Proc of Computer Aided Verification (CAV)*, Lecture Notes in Computer Science 1254. Springer Verlag, 1997.
17. A. Rauzy. Toupie = Mu-calculus + Constraints. In *Proc. of Computer Aided Verification 1995*, Lecture Notes in Computer Science 939, pages 114–126. Springer Verlag, 1995.
18. K. Sagonas et al. *The XSB Programmer's Manual Version 2.0*, 1999.
19. C. Stirling and D. Walker. Local Model Checking in the Modal Mu-calculus. *Theoretical Computer Science*, 89(1):161–177, 1991.
20. P. Stuckey. Constructive Negation for Constraint Logic Programming. In *Proc of Logic in Computer Science (LICS'91)*, 1991.
21. D. Toman. Memoing Evaluation for Constraint Extensions of Datalog. *J. Constraints*, 2:337–359, 1997.
22. D. S. Warren. Memoing for Logic Programs. *CACM*, 35(3):93–111, 1992.

A CLP Framework for Computing Structural Test Data

Arnaud Gotlieb[1], Bernard Botella[1], and Michel Rueher[2]

[1] Thomson-CSF Detexis, Centre Charles Nungesser 2, av. Gay-Lussac
78851 Elancourt Cedex, France
{Arnaud.Gotlieb,Bernard.Botella}@detexis.thomson-csf.com
[2] Université de Nice–Sophia-Antipolis, I3S
ESSI, 930, route des Colles - B.P. 145
06903 Sophia-Antipolis, France
rueher@essi.fr, http://www.essi.fr/~rueher

Abstract. Structural testing techniques are widely used in the unit testing process of softwares. A major challenge of this process consists in
generating automatically test data, i.e., in finding input values for which
a selected point in a procedure is executed. We introduce here an original framework where the later problem is transformed into a CLP(FD)
problem. Specific operators have been introduced to tackle this kind of
application. The resolution of the constraint system is based upon entailment techniques. A prototype system — named INKA— which allows
to handle a non-trivial subset of programs written in C has been developed. First experimental results show that INKA is competitive with
traditional ad–hoc methods. Moreover, INKA has been used successfully
to generate test data for programs extracted from a real application.

1 Introduction

Structural testing techniques are widely used in the unit or module testing process. Structural testing requires:

1. Identifying a set of statements in the procedure under test, the covering
   of which implies the coverage of some criteria (e.g., statement or branch
   coverage);
2. Computing test data so that each statement of the set is reached.

The second point —called ATDG[1] problem in the following— is the corner
stone of structural testing since it arises for a wide range of structural criteria.
The ATDG problem is undecidable in the general case since it can be reduced
to the halting problem. Classical ad-hoc methods fall into three categories:

– Random test data generation techniques which blindly try values [Nta98]
  until the selected point is reached;

---

[1] Automatic Test Data Generation

J. Lloyd et al. (Eds.): CL 2000, LNAI 1861, pp. 399–413, 2000.

- Symbolic-execution techniques [Kin76,DO93] which replace input parameters by symbolic values and which statically evaluate the statements along the paths reaching the selected point;
- Dynamic methods [Kor90,FK96] which are based on actual execution of procedure and which use heuristics to select values, e.g. numerical direct search methods.

The limit of these techniques mainly comes from the fact that they "follow one path" in the program and thus fail to reach numerous points in a procedure. A statement in a program may be associated with the set of paths reaching it, whereas a test datum on which the statement is executed follows a single path. However, there are numerous non-feasible paths, i.e., there is no input data for which such paths can be executed. Furthermore, if the procedure under test contains loops, it may contain an infinite number of paths.

We introduce here an original framework where the ATDG problem is transformed into a CLP problem over finite domains. Roughly speaking, this framework can be defined by the following three steps:

1. Transformation of the initial program into a CLP(FD) program with some specific operators which have been introduced to tackle this kind of application ;
2. Transformation of the selected point into a goal to solve in the CLP(FD) system ;
3. Solving the resulting constraint system to check whether at least one feasible control flow path going through the selected point exists, and to generate automatically test data that correspond to one of these paths.

The two first steps are based on the use of the "Static Single Assignment" form [CFR+91] and control-dependencies [FOW87]. They have been carefully detailed in [GBR98].

In this paper, we mainly analyze the third step: the constraint solving process. The key-point of our approach is the use of constraint entailment techniques to drive this process efficiently. In the proposed CLP framework test data can be generated without following one path in the program.

To validate this framework, a prototype system — named INKA— has been developed over the CLP(FD) library of Sicstus Prolog. It allows to handle a nontrivial subset of programs written in C. The first experimental results show that INKA overcomes random generation techniques and is competitive with other methods. Moreover, INKA has been used successfully to generate test data for programs extracted from a real application.

Before going into the details, let us illustrate the advantage of our approach on a very simple example.

1.1 Motivating Example

Let us consider the small toy–program given in Fig. 1. The goal is to generate a test datum, i.e. a pair of values for (x, y), for which statement 10 is executed.

"Static Single Assignment" techniques and control-dependencies analysis yield the following constraint system[2]:

$\sigma_1 = (x, y, z, t_1, t_2, u \in (0..2^{32} - 1) \wedge$

$\quad (z = x * y) \wedge (t_1 = 2 * x) \wedge (z \leq 8) \wedge (u \leq x) \wedge (t_2 = t_1 - y) \wedge (t_2 \leq 20)$

Variables t_1 and t_2 denote the different renaming of variable t.

```
int foo(int x, int y)
      int z, t, u;
1.    { z = x * y;
2.      t = 2 * x;
3.      if (x < 4)
4.          u = 10;
        else
5.          u = 2;
6.      if (z ≤ 8)
7.          { if (u ≤ x)
8.              { t = t - y;
9.                if (t ≤ 20)
10.                   { ...
```

Fig. 1. Program foo

Local consistency techniques like *interval–consistency* [HSD98] cannot achieve any significant pruning: the domain of x will be reduced to $0..2^{16} - 1$ while no reduction can be achieved on the domain of y. So, the search space for (x, y) contains $(2^{16} - 1) \times (2^{32} - 1)$ possible test data. However, more information could be deduced from the program. For instance, the following relations could be derived from the first **if_then_else** statement (lines 3,4,5):

$\quad (x \geq 4 \wedge u = 2)$ holds if $\neg(x < 4 \wedge u = 10)$ holds

$\quad (x < 4 \wedge u = 10)$ holds if $\neg(x \geq 4 \wedge u = 2)$ holds

Entailment mechanisms allow to capture such information. Indeed, since $\neg(x < 4 \wedge u = 10)$ is entailed by $u \leq x$, we can add to the store the constraint $(x \geq 4 \wedge u = 2)$. Filtering $x \geq 4 \wedge u = 2 \wedge \sigma_1$ by *interval-consistency* reduces the domain of x to $4..11$ and the domain of y to $0..2$.

This example shows that entailment tests may help to drastically reduce the search space. Of course, the process becomes more tricky when several conditional statements and loop statements are inter-wound.

Outline of the Paper. The next section introduces the notation and some basic definitions. Section 3 details how the constraint system over CLP(FD) is generated. Section 4 details the constraint solving process. Section 5 reports

---

[2] In this context, an **int** variable has an unsigned long integer value, i.e. a value between 0 and $2^{32} - 1$.

the first experimental results obtained with INKA, while section 6 discusses the extensions of our framework.

2   Notations and Basic Definitions

A *domain* in FD is a non-empty finite set of integers. A variable which is associated to a domain in FD is called a FD_variable and will be denoted by an upper-case letter. *Primitive constraints* in CLP(FD) are built with variables, domains, the $\in$ operator, arithmetical operators in $\{+, -, \times$ div, mod $\}$ [3] and the relations $\{>, \geq, =, \neq, \leq, <\}$. Note that the negation of a primitive constraint is also a primitive constraint. In the following, c possibly subscripted denotes exclusively a primitive constraint. A *constraint-store* σ is a conjunction of primitive and non-primitive constraints.

Non-primitive constraints are composed of combinators and guarded–constraints. *Combinators* are boolean combination of constraints. For example, the constraint $\texttt{element}(I, L, V)$ which express that V is the Ith element in the list L is a combinator.

Guarded-constraints are built by using the blocking ask operator [HSD98] and are denoted $C_1 \longrightarrow C_2$, where C_1 and C_2 stand for constraints. C_1 is called the guard. The operational semantic of $C_1 \longrightarrow C_2$ is given by the following rules:

- The constraint $C_1 \longrightarrow C_2$ is removed and C_2 is added to σ when C_1 is entailed by σ;
- The constraint $C_1 \longrightarrow C_2$ is just removed when $\neg C_1$ is entailed by σ;
- The constraint $C_1 \longrightarrow C_2$ is suspended when neither C_1 nor $\neg C_1$ are entailed by σ;

Note that C_1 and C_2 are not restricted to be primitive and that checking whether $\neg C_1$ is entailed may require to compute the negation of a non-primitive constraint.

Entailment operations are based on partial consistencies. Two partial entailment tests have been introduced in [HSD98]: *domain-entailment* and *interval-entailment*. They are based upon *domain-consistency* and *interval-consistency*. Let $X_1, \ldots, X_n$ be FD_variables, let $D_1, \ldots, D_n$ be domains and let C be a constraint[4].

Definition 1 *(Domain-Consistency)*
A constraint C is domain-consistent if for each variable X_i and value $v_i \in D_i$ there exists values $v_1, \ldots, v_{i-1}, v_{i+1}, \ldots, v_n$ in $D_1, \ldots, D_{i-1}, D_{i+1}, \ldots, D_n$ such that $C(v_1, \ldots, v_n)$ holds. A store σ is domain-consistent if for every constraint C in σ, C is domain-consistent.

Interval consistency is based on an approximation of finite domains by finite sets of successive integers. More precisely, if D is a domain, D^* is defined by the set $\{\min(D), \ldots, \max(D)\}$ where $\min(D)$ and $\max(D)$ denote respectively the minimum and maximum values in D.

---

[3] div and mod represent the Euclidean division and remainder
[4] we assume that all the constraints are implicitly defined on $X_1, \ldots, X_n$

Definition 2 *(Interval-Consistency)*
A constraint C is interval-consistent if for each variable X_i and value $v_i \in \{min(D_i), max(D_i)\}$ there exist values $v_1, \dots, v_{i-1}, v_{i+1}, \dots, v_n$ in $D_1^*, \dots, D_{i-1}^*, D_{i+1}^*, \dots, D_n^*$ such that $C(v_1, \dots, v_n)$ holds. A store σ is interval-consistent if for every constraint C in σ, C is interval-consistent.

The following relaxations of entailment are introduced in [HSD98]:

Definition 3 *(Domain-Entailment)*
A constraint $C(X_1, \dots, X_n)$ is domain-entailed by $D_1, \dots, D_n$ iff, for all values $v_1, \dots, v_n$ in $D_1, \dots, D_n$, $C(v_1, \dots, v_n)$ holds.

Definition 4 *(Interval-Entailment)*
A constraint $C(X_1, \dots, X_n)$ is interval-entailed by $D_1, \dots, D_n$ iff, for all values $v_1, \dots, v_n$ in $D_1^*, \dots, D_n^*$, $C(v_1, \dots, v_n)$ holds.

We introduce here another partial entailment test which is based on refutation:

Definition 5 *(abs-Entailment)*
A constraint C is abs-entailed by a store σ iff, filtering $\sigma \wedge \neg C$ by domain-consistency or interval-consistency yields an empty domain.

3   Generation of the Constraint System

Let P be a single procedure written in an imperative language, let n be a point (either a statement or a branch) in P. Solving the ATDG problem requires to compute a vector of input[5] values of P such that n is executed.

For the sake of simplicity, we first introduce the constraint system generation technique for an `array_if_while` language over integers. Procedure calls are handled in our framework but we assume that there is only one mechanism for passing arguments: the call–by–value mechanism. Programs must be well-structured and must avoid floating-point variables. A procedure is assumed to have a single return statement.

Next subsection recalls the general principles of the "Static Single Assignment" form [CFR+91]. The following subsections detail the transformation process of a program under SSA form into a CLP program.

3.1   Static Single Assignment Form

The SSA form is a version of a procedure on which every variable has a unique definition and every use of a variable is reached by this definition. The SSA form of a basic block is obtained by a simple renaming ($i = i + 1$ yields $i_2 = i_1 + 1$). For the control structures, SSA form introduces special assignments, called ϕ-functions, to merge several definitions of the same variable. For example, the SSA form of the `if_then_else` statement is illustrated in the top of Fig. 2. The

---

[5] An input variable is either a formal parameter or a referenced global variable

if $(x < 4)$	**if** $(x < 4)$
$\quad u = 10;$	$\quad u_1 = 10;$
else	**else**
$\quad u = 2;$	$\quad u_2 = 2;$
	$\quad u_3 = \phi(u_1, u_2);$
$j = 1;$	$j_1 = 1;$
	/* Heading - while */
	$j_3 = \phi(j_1, j_2);$
while $(j * u \leq 16)$	**while** $(j_3 * u_3 \leq 16)$
$\quad j = j + 1$	$\quad j_2 = j_3 + 1;$

Fig. 2. SSA form of control statements

ϕ-function of the statement $u_3 = \phi(u_1, u_2)$ returns one of its argument: if the flow comes from the *then*- part then the ϕ-function returns u_1, otherwise it returns u_2.

For other structures such as loops, the ϕ-functions are introduced in a special heading which is executed at every iteration. The ϕ-functions work as usual: this explains the counter-intuitive renaming of variables (see Fig. 2).

For convenience, a list of ϕ-functions will be written with a single statement: $x_2 := \phi(x_1, x_0), \ldots, z_2 := \phi(z_1, z_0) \iff v_2 := \phi(v_1, v_0)$ where v_i stands for a vector of variables.

3.2   Generation of the CLP Program

The basic idea is to translate each statement of the SSA form into a primitive constraint or a combinator, in order to build a CLP program. A clause is generated for each procedure P of the program. The head of the clause has several arguments:

– A list of FD_variables associated with the parameters of P ;
– A list of FD_variables associated with the referenced globals of P ;
– A list of FD_variables associated with the local variables used inside the decisions of P ;
– A list of FD_variables associated with the globals defined inside P ;
– A single FD_variable associated with the expression returned by P.

Now, let us detail the transformation process.

Declaration. A type declaration of a variable x_i is translated into a primitive constraint of the form: $X_i \in Min_T..Max_T$ where Min_T (resp. Max_T) is the minimum (resp. maximum) value of the type T. Such a constraint prevents overflows of values, a condition which is required to generate a test datum on which a selected point is reached.

Array. SSA form provides special expressions to handle arrays: $access(a_0, k)$ which evaluates to the kth element of a_0, and $update(a_0, j, w)$ which evaluates to an array a_1 which has the same size and the same elements as a_0, except for j where value is w. *access* and *update* expressions are transformed into `element/3` constraints:

- $v = access(a_0, k)$ is translated into $\texttt{element}(K, A_0, V)$;
- a definition statement $a_1 = update(a_0, j, w)$ is translated into
  $\texttt{element}(J, A_1, W) \quad \bigwedge_{I \neq J}(\texttt{element}(I, A_0, V) \land \texttt{element}(I, A_1, V))$.

Conditional. The *if_then_else* statement is treated by using a combinator, called `ite/3`. For example, the *if_then_else* statement of Fig. 2 is translated into: $\texttt{ite}(X < 4, U_1 = 10 \land U_3 = U_1, U_2 = 2 \land U_3 = U_2)$. The conditional statement express an exclusive disjunction between two paths. So, $\texttt{ite}(c, C_1 \land \ldots \land C_n, C_1' \land \ldots \land C_m')$ holds iff $(c \land C_1 \land \ldots \land C_n)$ or $(\neg c \land C_1' \land \ldots \land C_m')$ holds, where c is a primitive constraint, and $C_1, \ldots, C_n, C_1', \ldots, C_m'$ are primitive or non-primitive constraints. The operational semantic of combinator `ite/3` is based on the following rules:

Definition 6 `ite/3` *(Operational Semantic)*
$\texttt{ite}(c, C_1 \land \ldots \land C_n, C_1' \land \ldots \land C_m')$ *is reduced to the four following guarded-constraints:*

- $c \longrightarrow C_1 \land \ldots \land C_n$
- $\neg c \longrightarrow C_1' \land \ldots \land C_m'$
- $\neg(c \land C_1 \land \ldots \land C_n) \longrightarrow (\neg c \land C_1' \land \ldots \land C_m')$
- $\neg(\neg c \land C_1' \land \ldots \land C_m') \longrightarrow (c \land C_1 \land \ldots \land C_n)$

The first two guarded-constraints result from the operational semantic of the *if_then_else* statement in an imperative language. The last two are introduced to allow a more effective pruning. c and $\neg c$ are included in the guards to facilitate the detection of inconsistencies by *abs-entailment* (see section 4).

Loop. Unlike the conditional, the *while* statement under SSA form cannot be translated directly. A *while* statement in SSA form is of the general form: $v_2 = \phi(v_0, v_1)$ *while* (c) $\{C_1; \ldots; C_p\}$ where v_0 is the vector of input variables of the *while*, v_1 is the vector of variables defined inside the body of the *while*, and v_2 is the vector of variables used inside and outside the *while*. This statement is transformed into a $\texttt{w}(c, V_0, V_1, V_2, C_1 \land \cdots \land C_p)$ combinator, which is a constraint generation program.
$\texttt{w}(c, V_0, V_1, V_2, C_1 \land \ldots \land C_p)$ holds iff $(\neg \dot{c} \land V_0 = V_2)$ or $(\dot{c} \land \dot{C_1} \land \ldots \land \dot{C_p} \land \texttt{w}(c, V_1, V_3, V_2, \ddot{C_1} \land \ldots \land \ddot{C_p}))$ holds, where c is a primitive constraint, $\dot{c} = subs(V_2 \leftarrow V_0, c)$; V_0, V_1 and V_2 are three vector of FD_variables, V_3 is a newly created vector of FD_variables, $\dot{C_1} = subs(V_2 \leftarrow V_0, C_1), \ldots, \dot{C_p} = subs(V_2 \leftarrow V_0, C_p)$, and $\ddot{C_1} = subs(V_1 \leftarrow V_3, C_1), \ldots, \ddot{C_p} = subs(V_1 \leftarrow V_3, C_p)$; *subs* being the substitution of variables over a term.

The operational semantic of w/5 is defined by the following rules:

Definition 7 w/5 *(Operational Semantic)*
$w(c, V_0, V_1, V_2, C_1 \wedge \ldots \wedge C_p)$ *is reduced to the four following guarded-constraints:*

- $\dot{c} \longrightarrow (\dot{C}_1 \wedge \ldots \dot{C}_p \wedge w(c, V_1, V_3, V_2, \ddot{C}_1 \wedge \ldots \wedge \ddot{C}_p))$
- $\neg \dot{c} \longrightarrow V_0 = V_2$
- $\neg(\dot{c} \wedge \dot{C}_1 \wedge \ldots C_p) \longrightarrow (\neg \dot{c} \wedge V_0 = V_2)$
- $\neg(\neg \dot{c} \wedge V_0 = V_2) \longrightarrow (\dot{c} \wedge \dot{C}_1 \wedge \ldots \dot{C}_p \wedge w(c, V_1, V_3, V_2, \ddot{C}_1 \wedge \ldots \wedge \ddot{C}_p))$

The first two guarded-constraints result from the behavior of the *while* statement. Whenever the decision of the statement $\dot{c}$ is verified, then the body is executed and another w/5 is stated. When the decision is refuted, the body is skipped and the input variables of the statement are equated to the vector of used variables.

The third guarded-constraint is based on the following observation: if the constraints of the body are inconsistent w.r.t the current information in the store, then the loop cannot be performed. The last guarded-constraint comes from the following observation: if the value of a variable is different before and after the *while* statement, then the body of the loop must be executed at least once. Note that the guards of both combinators are either primitive constraints or negations of conjunction of constraints, so the implementation of *abs-entailment* becomes straightforward (see section 4).

Let us illustrate how w/5 works on the example of Fig. 2. The *while_do* statement is translated into: $w(J_3 * U_3 \leq 16, [J_1], [J_2], [J_3], J_2 = J_3 + 1)$. If the store contains $J_1 = 1, J_3 = U_3$, then the fourth guarded-constraint is activated because $\neg(\neg(J_1 * U_3 \leq 16) \wedge J_1 = J_3)$ is entailed by the store. So, the following constraints are added to the store: $J_1 * U_3 \leq 16 \wedge J_2 = J_1 + 1 \wedge w(J_3 * U_3 \leq 16, [J_2], [J_\#], [J_3], J_\# = J_3 + 1)$ where $J_\#$ is a newly created variable.

Procedure Call. A procedure call is translated into a goal to solve. For example, a statement such as $v = foo(x, 29)$ is translated into
$foo([X, 29], [], Liste\_of\_locals, [], V)$, where foo is the name of the clause generated for the procedure foo and $Liste\_of\_locals$ is a the list of FD_variables associated to local variables and referenced in the decisions of the procedure. Such a mechanism allows the treatment of recursive procedure.

3.3   Generation of the CLP Goal

The decisions which must be verified to reach a given point in a procedure are called the *control-dependencies* [FOW87]. They are syntactically determined in well-structured procedures. For loop statements, these decisions are computed dynamically. Let $C(foo, 10)$ be the *control-dependencies* associated with point 10 in the procedure foo of Fig. 1. So, we have: $C(foo, 10) = (Z \leq 8) \wedge (U_3 \leq X) \wedge (T_2 \leq 20)$. The selected point determines a goal to solve with the clauses of the generated CLP(FD) program :

$$\longleftarrow C(foo, 10), foo([X, Y], [], [X, Z_1, U_3, T_2], [], RET)$$

The generated CLP program for program `foo` and the goal associated with point 10 are given in the Fig. 3.

$$\text{foo}([X,Y],[],[X,Z_1,U_3,T_2],[],RET) \longleftarrow$$
$$X,Y,Z,T_1,T_2,U_1,U_2,U_3,RET \in 0..2^{32} - 1,$$
$$Z = X * Y,$$
$$T_1 = 2 * X,$$
$$\text{ite}(X < 4, U_1 = 10 \wedge U_3 = U_1, U_2 = 2 \wedge U_3 = U_2),$$
$$\text{ite}(Z \leq 8,$$
$$\quad \text{ite}(U_3 \leq X, T_2 = T_1 - Y \wedge$$
$$\quad\quad \text{ite}(T_2 \leq 20,$$
$$\quad\quad\quad ...$$
$$RET = ...$$

$$\longleftarrow (Z \leq 8) \wedge (U_3 \leq X) \wedge (T_2 \leq 20), foo([X,Y],[],[X,Z_1,U_3,T_2],[],RET)$$

Fig. 3. CLP Program generated for the program foo

4   Solving the Goal

In our framework, the constraint solving process is based on:

1. A filtering process based on partial consistency techniques and entailment techniques ;
2. A search procedure which combines an enumeration process and a constraint propagation step.

In view of the operational semantics of combinators introduced in the previous section, there are several operations to be implemented. They include an entailment test, an algorithm for processing the guarded–constraints, and the implementation of the combinators themselves.

4.1   Entailment Test

Three levels of entailment relaxations may be used to achieve entailment tests: *domain–entailment*, *interval–entailment* and *abs–entailment*, defined in section 2.

Consider the following example: $\sigma = (X \in 1..100) \wedge (Y \in 9..11) \wedge (X \neq Y)$ and the question " is $(X * Y \neq 100)$ entailed by σ ?".

The constraint is neither interval-entailed, nor domain-entailed because $(X = 10, Y = 10)$ does not verify the constraint. Thus, in our framework, we have implemented *abs–entailment* which is more effective —at least on our problems—

than *domain-entailment* and *interval-entailment*. Practically, we add the negation of the considered constraint C to the store before starting a filtering step by interval–consistency. When the domain of one variable is reduced to an empty set, constraint C is entailed ; when all the constraints are interval–consistent, no deduction can be done and the previous store must be restored. For instance, filtering the store $\sigma \wedge \neg C = (x \in 1..100) \wedge (y \in 9..11) \wedge (x \neq y) \wedge (x * y = 100)$ by interval-consistency leads to an empty domain for both variables, and then proves that the constraint $x * y \neq 100$ is *abs-entailed*.

This relaxation of entailment can be seen as a proof by refutation. Technically, *abs-entailment* requires to compute the negation of the considered constraint C. Since we only test the entailment of primitive constraints or the negation of conjunctions of constraints in our framework, this computation becomes straightforward.

Note also that no suspension will remain in the constraint store at the end of the resolution, since the last step of the solving process is an enumeration step.

4.2   Processing Guarded–Constraints

The guarded–constraints are evaluated iteratively in the store. The algorithm for processing guarded–constraints is given in Fig. 4.

/* Let C_1, C_2 be two constraints and σ be the current store */
/* Process $C_1 \longrightarrow C_2$ in σ */

    if filtering $\sigma \wedge \neg C_1$ by interval–consistency yields an inconsistency
    then   /* C_1 is *abs-entailed* by σ */

$$\sigma \leftarrow (\sigma \cup \{C_2\}) \setminus \{C_1 \longrightarrow C_2\};$$

    if filtering $\sigma \wedge C_1$ by interval–consistency yields an inconsistency
    then   /* $\neg C_1$ is abs-entailed by σ */

$$\sigma \leftarrow \sigma \setminus \{C_1 \longrightarrow C_2\};$$

    if neither C_1 nor $\neg C_1$ are abs–entailed by σ
    then continue
        /* The guarded-constraint $C_1 \longrightarrow C_2$ is suspended in σ */

Fig. 4. Algorithm for processing guarded–constraints

Note that the second rule can be ignored until the end of the computation because it does not add any constraint to the store. Two kind of problems may occur with this algorithm:

- The store may contain other guarded–constraints which are activated as soon as a filtering is started ;
- The store may contain a non–terminating combinator. In fact, some w/5 combinator may introduce guarded–constraints which will recursively put other w/5 combinators in the store. This pitfall can be seen as a consequence of the halting problem.

A practical solution for both difficulties consists in ignoring any other guarded–constraint or combinator of the store during the filtering of $\sigma \wedge \neg C_1$. Other awakening policies exist[Got00] but are not discussed in this paper.

4.3   Search Process

Filtering by partial consistencies does not always yield a solution, thus a search step is necessary. Note that, up to this point, no choice point has been set up. In fact, the disjunctions introduced by the combinators are "captured" by the entailment tests. As usual, the search is interleaved with constraint propagation. Since the class of programs is unbound, experiments are the best way to determine a good heuristic for the ATDG problem. We have tested the *first-fail*, *first-fail constrained*, *domain-splitting* heuristics among others. Iterative domain–splitting yields the best results in average [Got00].

The search process stops in one of the following states:

- **Success: A solution of the constraint system was found.** In our framework, such a solution is a test datum on which the selected point n is reached in the procedure P, hence it is a solution to the ATDG problem.
- **Success: The inconsistency of the constraint system has been detected.** If an inconsistency of the store is detected during the initial filtering step or during the search process, we can state that n is unreachable in P, i.e. there is no test datum on which n is executed[6]; hence, the ATDG problem has no solution. This is an important information for the tester.
- **Failure: The search process did not reach a success state during the allowed amount of CPU time.** This can result from the non–termination problem of w/5. Consider a reachable point n in a procedure containing a loop which does not terminate for certain input values. If such an input is tried during the search process, the w/5 combinator will not terminate.
  Note that no information can be deduced when the process is stopped before the end. It is not possible to determine whether it is a consequence of an infinite loop or just a very long search. In both cases, we say that our technique fails to find a solution of the ATDG problem.

5   First Experimental Results

We compare our CLP framework with a random test data generation method and the dynamic approach of [Kor90,FK96]. We implemented the random method by

---

[6] sometimes called dead code

using the `drand48` C function, which generates pseudo-random numbers with the well-known linear congruential algorithm and 48-bit integer arithmetic. TEST-GEN is an implementation of the dynamic method for Pascal programs. The tool is not available, hence we base the comparison on the results published in [FK96]. The symbolic execution method has been implemented in a tool called GODZILLA [DO93] but the tool is dedicated to mutation analysis of Fortran programs making the experimental comparison very difficult.

5.1   Our Prototype System

INKA operates on a restricted subset of the C language. Unstructured statements such as *goto* statement are not handled in our framework. Pointer arithmetic, dynamic allocated structures, pointer functions, type casting, involve difficult problems to solve. Pointers are only partially supported by INKA (see section 6). Although, floating point numbers are finite in essence, they introduce problems[7] which cannot be solved within the framework introduced here. All the types of integer variables (char,short, long,...) and almost all the C operators (34 out of 42) are handled (by capturing their behavior into user–defined constraints).

INKA includes a C parser, a SSA form generator and a Constraint system producer over the `clp(fd)` library of Sicstus Prolog.

5.2   Experiments

We only present our experiments on three classical academic programs of the Software Testing Community and one real–world program but INKA has been used successfully on several other programs [Got00]. The academic programs[8] are 1) "bsearch" [DO93] which is a binary search in a sorted array; 2) a program published in [FK96] named "sample" which contains arrays, loops and a lot of dependencies; 3) the famous program "trityp" [DO93] which contains numerous non-feasible paths.

Finally, we introduce the results for a real–world program extracted from an avionic project, named "ardeta03". This program mainly contains complex C structures and bitwise operations but does not contain loops.

5.3   Test Procedure

For each program, a test datum for each basic block (sequence of statements without branching) is generated. Of course, this approach is not optimal to reach a complete block coverage since no coverage information is reused between two generations.

---

[7] The evaluation process of an arithmetical expression in a CLP system and the evaluation of the same expression in the operational software may yield different results

[8] The source code of these programs are available at
http://www.essi.fr/~rueher/trityp.htm

For each selected block, we have compared INKA to the random method, and to the published results of TESTGEN. We have performed our experiments on a 300Mhz Sun UltraSparc 5. A time-out of 10 seconds per block was set. In 10 seconds, the random method generated approximatively 10^5 test data, while INKA generated only one test datum. To limit the factor of "bad luck" which may occur with the random method, we repeated 10 times the generation with different initial values for the linear congruential algorithm, and we only considered the best results.

[FK96] introduces the results of TESTGEN on the three academic programs among others. The TESTGEN technique starts with a random generation of value which determines the success of the method. They performed their experiments on a PC with 60Mhz–Pentium processor. A time–out was set to 5 minutes and the same test procedure as ours was applied, except that they repeated 10 times their search for each block. Their "coverage represents the percentage of nodes for which at least one try was successful in finding input data" [FK96]. According to this definition, they found 100% for each program.

5.4   Results

The results are shown in Fig. 5. The number of lines of code and the number of statement blocks are reported in the first two columns; whereas an estimate of the search space is reported in the third column (number of possible test data). The last three columns contain the results of block coverage obtained with the three different approaches.

Programs	loc	blocks	test data	TESTGEN*	Random**	INKA**
bsearch	21	10	$> 10^{50}$	100%	100%	100%
sample	33	14	$> 10^{100}$	100%	93%	100%
trityp	40	22	$> 10^{10}$	100%	86%	100%
ardeta03	157	38	$> 10^{60}$	–	74%	100%

(*) 50 minutes on PC Pentium (60Mhz) for each block
(**) 10 seconds on Sun Sparc 5 (300Mhz) under Solaris 2.5 for each block

Fig. 5. Comparison on block coverage

5.5   Analysis

TESTGEN did allow 50 minutes per block whereas INKA did not spent more than 10 seconds on each block. The tests with TESTGEN have been done on a PC with 60Mhz-Pentium processor while INKA was run on 300Mhz Sun UltraSparc 5. If we assume that there is less than a factor 30 between these two computers, INKA is still 10 time faster than TESTGEN[9].

---

[9] Note that INKA is written in Prolog while TESTGEN is written in C

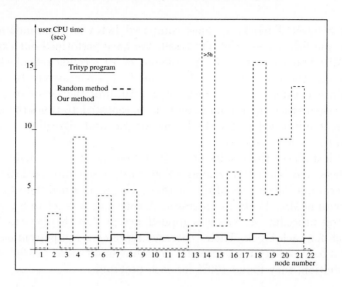

Fig. 6. Time required to generate a solution for each block

Let us see in more details what appends on one of the programs. We report in Fig. 6 the curve of times required to generate a solution for the program "trityp" by the last two methods. First, note that the time required by the random method is smaller on some blocks. In fact, INKA requires a nominal time to generate the constraint system and to solve it, even if it is very easy to solve. Second, note that the random method fails on some blocks. For instance, the block 14 which requires for the random method to generate a sequence of three equal integers. On the contrary, this block does not introduce a particular difficulty for INKA, because such a constraint is easily propagated.

6   Perspective

First experiments are promising but, of course, more experiments have to be performed on non-academic programs to validate the proposed approach. The main extension of our CLP framework concerns the handling of pointer variables. Unlike scalars, pointer variables cannot directly be transformed into logical variables because of the aliasing problem. In fact, an undirect reference and a variable may refer to the same memory location at some program point. In [Got00], we proposed to handle this problem for a restricted class of pointers: pointers to stack–allocated variables. Our approach, based on a pointer analysis, does not handle dynamically allocated structures. For some classes of applications, this restriction is not important. However, the treatment of all pointer variables is essential to extend our CLP framework to a wide spread of real–world applications.

Acknowledgements

Patrick Taillibert and Serge Varennes gave us invaluable help on the work presented in this paper. Thanks to François Delobel for its comments on an earlier draft of this paper. This research is part of the Systems and Software Tools Support department of THOMSON-CSF DETEXIS.

References

[CFR⁺91] Ron Cytron, Jeanne Ferrante, Barry K. Rosen, Mark N. Wegman, and F. Kenneth Zadeck. Efficently Computing Static Single Assignment Form and the Control Dependence Graph. *Transactions on Programming Languages and Systems*, 13(4):451–490, October 1991.

[DO93]   R. A. Demillo and A. J. Offut. Experimental Results from an Automatic Test Case Generator. *Transactions on Software Engineering Methodology*, 2(2):109–175, 1993.

[FK96]   Roger Ferguson and Bogdan Korel. The Chaining Approach for Software Test Data Generation". *ACM Transactions on Software Engineering and Methodology*, 5(1):63–86, January 1996.

[FOW87]   Jeanne Ferrante, Karl J. Ottenstein, and J. David Warren. The Program Dependence Graph and its use in optimization. *Transactions on Programming Languages and Systems*, 9-3:319–349, July 1987.

[GBR98]   Arnaud Gotlieb, Bernard Botella, and Michel Rueher. Automatic Test Data Generation Using Constraint Solving Techniques. In *Proc. of the Sigsoft International Symposium on Software Testing and Analysis*, Clearwater Beach, Florida, USA, March 2-5 1998. *Software Engineering Notes*,23(2):53-62. disponible at http://www.essi.fr/ rueher/.

[Got00]   A. Gotlieb. *Automatic Test Data Generation using Constraint Logic Programming*. PhD thesis, PHD Dissertation (in French), Université de Nice–Sophia Antipolis, January 2000.

[HSD98]   Pascal Van Hentenryck, Vijav Saraswat, and Yves Deville. Design, implementation, and evaluation of the constraint language cc(fd). *Journal of Logic Programming*, 37:139–164, 1998. Also in CS-93-02 Brown–University 1993.

[Kin76]   James C. King. Symbolic Execution and Program Testing. *Communications of the ACM*, 19(7):385–394, July 1976.

[Kor90]   Bogdan Korel. Automated Software Test Data Generation. *IEEE Transactions on Software Engineering*, 16(8):870–879, august 1990.

[Nta98]   S. Ntafos. On Random and Partition Testing. In *Proceedings of Sigsoft International Symposium on Software Testing and Analysis*, volume 23(2), pages 42–48, Clearwater Beach, FL, March,2-5 1998. ACM, SIGPLAN Notices on Software Engineering.

Modelling Digital Circuits Problems
with Set Constraints

Francisco Azevedo and Pedro Barahona
{fa,pb}@di.fct.unl.pt
Departamento de Informática, Universidade Nova de Lisboa
2825-114 Caparica — Portugal

Abstract. A number of diagnostic and optimisation problems in Electronics Computer Aided Design have usually been handled either by specific tools or by mapping them into a general problem solver (e.g. a propositional Boolean SAT tool). This approach, however, requires models with substantial duplication of digital circuits. In Constraint Logic Programming, the use of extra values in the digital signals (other than the usual 0/1) was proposed to reflect their dependency on some faulty gate. In this paper we present an extension of this modelling approach, using set variables to denote dependency of the signals on sets of faults, to model different circuits problems. We then show the importance of propagating constraints on sets cardinality, by comparing Cardinal, a set constraint solver that we implemented, with a simpler version that propagates these constraints similarly to Conjunto, a widely available set constraint solver. Results show speed ups of Cardinal of about two orders of magnitude, on a set of diagnostic problems.

1   Introduction

A number of problems in Electronics Computer Aided Design (ECAD) has been widely studied and they are still the subject of active research, with a variety of approaches. The evolution of the area, with new technologies and continuous new requirements and needs, makes it a suitable application field for CLP [12], whose usefulness was already exemplified and discussed [17].

One particular sub-area of ECAD that deserves plenty of attention is that of Automatic Test Pattern Generation (ATPG), which aims at checking whether a circuit is faulty or not. In this context, a digital circuit (e.g. a VLSI chip) is regarded as a black box, performing some function, and one has only access to its inputs and outputs. The basic problem consists of finding an input test pattern for a specific faulty gate, i.e. an input that makes the output dependent on whether the gate is faulty or not. In general, one is not interested in the basic problem but rather in some related and more complex problems.

One such problem is the generation of minimal sets of test patterns, i.e. in finding sets of test patterns with minimum cardinality that cover all the possible faults in a digital circuit. A related problem is finding maximal test patterns, i.e. those that maximise the number of faults they unveil. A third problem, diagnosis, aims at generating patterns for a circuit that would produce different outputs for different sets of faulty gates. The problem is not only interesting in itself, but has possible applications on the related optimisation problems.

J. Lloyd et al. (Eds.): CL 2000, LNAI 1861, pp. 414-428, 2000.

These problems have usually been handled either by specific tools or by modelling them in some appropriate form to be subsequently dealt with by a general problem solver (e.g. a Boolean SAT-based solver [15]). Current techniques to deal with the problem of diagnosis try to generate input vectors that cause different outputs in two circuits. In [9] one tries to detect one fault assuming the circuit has the other; in [8] one tries to detect one fault without detecting the other; finally, in [14] one tries to detect both, and after undetect one of them. The complexity of the diagnosis increases significantly with the extra circuitry involved, thoug, and modelling the above referred optimisation problems into a SAT solver poses a more challenging problem with respect to the multiplication of circuits [13], and the associated combinatorics.

As an alternative to Boolean satisfiability, a CLP system presented in [16] adds two extra values to the usual Boolean 0/1 values to code the dependency of a digital signal on the (faulty) state of a gate. With this extension, a test pattern is an input of the circuit that yields an output with one such extra value. In [2], this idea was adopted and extended further for diagnostic problems, by introducing a logic whose 8 values were used not only to represent dependency on a faulty gate, but also to discriminate the dependencies between two sets of faulty gates. Nevertheless, this 8-valued logic does not allow the modelling of ATPG related optimisation problems.

In this paper we discuss an alternative approach using CLP over sets as a unifying modelling framework for all these ATPG related problems, whereby the dependency on sets of faults is modelled by explicit consideration of these sets in the signals that are carried throughout the digital circuit.

Although avoiding the duplication of circuitry required by the Boolean approach, the domains of the variables in this new modelling become more complex, requiring the handling of set constraints, and their efficient constraint solving. Conjunto [6] was a first language to represent set variables by set intervals with a lower and an upper bound considering set inclusion as the partial ordering. Consistency techniques are then applied to set constraints by interval reasoning [3]. This language, implemented as an ECLiPSe [4] library, represented a great improvement over previous CLP languages with set data structures [6].

Conjunto makes a limited use of the information about the cardinality of set variables. The reason for this lies in the fact that it is in general too costly to derive all the inferences one might do over the cardinality information, in order to tackle the problems Conjunto had initially been designed for (i.e. large scale set packing and partitioning problems) [7]. Nonetheless, and given their nature, we anticipated that some use of this information could be quite useful and speed up the solving of ATPG related problems. We thus developed a new constraint solver over sets with two versions. The first fully uses constraint propagation on sets cardinality; the other uses a more limited amount of constraint propagation, similar to that used in Conjunto. In the following we will refer to these versions as Cardinal and „Conjunto", respectively.

In this paper we present a formal definition of Cardinal and show that, in a preliminary evaluation with diagnostic problems in digital circuits, it has a significant speed up (over 100 times, in average) over „Conjunto". The paper is organised as follows. Section 2 addresses the modelling of ATPG problems with set constraints. Section 3 describes Cardinal. Section 4 presents some implementation issues as well as preliminary results. Section 5 summarises conclusions and discusses further work.

2   Modelling

A digital circuit is composed of gates performing the usual Boolean logic operations (and, xor, not, …) on their input bits to determine the output bits. A digital signal has two possible values, 0 or 1, and the circuit gates (or their connections) might be faulty. We will only address the usual stuck-at-X faults (X= 0 or 1), whereby the output of a gate is X regardless of its input.

For some circuit under consideration, let n_i and n_o be the number of input and output bits, respectively, I is the set of all possible inputs ($\#I=2^{n_i}$), $out(b,i,F)$ the output value for bit number b ($b \in 1..n_o$) under input i ($i \in I$) when the circuit exhibits a set of faults F. With such notation, a number of ATPG related problems can be formulated:

1. **ATPG (Basic).** Find an input test pattern i for a set of faults F, i.e. an input for which some output bit of the circuit is different when the circuit has faults F or has no faults.

$$test(F,i) \Leftrightarrow \exists b \in 1..n_o, out(b,i,F) \neq out(b,i,\varnothing)$$

2. **Diagnosis.** Find an input test pattern i that differentiates two diagnostic sets F and G, i.e. an input i for which some output bit of the circuit is different when the circuit has faults F or G

$$diff(\{F,G\},i) \Leftrightarrow \exists b \in 1..n_o, out(b,i,F) \neq out(b,i,G)$$

Let D now denote a set of diagnostic sets (these can be a set of more common faults, but in the limit D may represent all possible sets of faults in the circuit). The next two related optimisation problems deal with sets with varying cardinality.

3. **Maximisation.** Find an input i which is a test pattern for a maximum number of diagnoses in D. Set $D_i \subseteq D$ now denotes the set of faulty gates for which input i is an input test pattern, i.e.

$$D_i = \{F : F \in D \wedge test(F,i)\}$$
$$max(D,i) \Leftrightarrow \forall j \in I, \#D_j \leq \#D_i\}$$

4. **Minimisation.** Find a minimal set S of input test patterns that cover all diagnoses in D (the definition of covering is given below, and $P(I)$ is the power-set of I).

$$cover(D,S) \Leftrightarrow \forall F \in D, \exists i \in S : test(F,i)$$
$$min(D,S) \Leftrightarrow cover(D,S) \wedge \forall S' \in P(I), \#S' \geq \#S \vee \neg cover(D,S')$$

Given these ATPG related problems, we now present two alternatives to model them, the first representing digital signals with sets and Booleans, the second adopting a pure set representation.

2.1   Modelling Digital Signals with Sets and Booleans

Since the faulty behaviour can be explained by several of the possible faults, we represent a signal not only by its normal value but also by the set of diagnoses it depends on. More specifically, a signal is denoted by a pair L-N, where N is a Boolean value (representing the Boolean value of the circuit if it had no faults) and L is a set of diagnostic sets, that might change the signal into the opposite value. For instance, $X=\{\{f/0,g/0\}, \{i/1\}\}$-$0$ means that signal X is normally 0 but if both gates f and g are stuck-at-0, or gate i is stuck-at-1, then its actual value is 1. Thus $\varnothing$-N represents a signal with constant value N, independent of any fault.

Any circuit gate either belongs or not to the universe D of possible faults. We next show how to model the different gate types to process signals in the form of pairs L-N.

2.1.1   Normal Gates

Normal gates (those with no faults included in D) fully respect the Boolean operation they represent. We discuss the behaviour of not- and and-gates as illustrative of these gates, the others can be modelled as combinations of these.

Given the above explanation of the encoding of digital signals, it is easy to see that, for a normal not-gate whose input is signal L-N, the output is simply L-$\overline{N}$, since the set of faults on which it depends is the same as the input signal.

As for the and-gate, three distinct situations may arise as illustrated below:

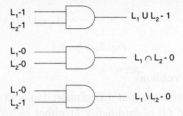

Fig. 1. And-gate

In the absence of faults the output is the conjunction of the normal inputs. However, the output may be different from this normal value due to faulty inputs. In the first case of Fig. 1, with two 1s as normal inputs, it is enough that a fault in either set $L1$ or $L2$ occurs for the output to change, thus justifying the disjunction of the sets in the output signal. In the second case (two 0s), it is necessary that faults occur in both $L1$ and $L2$ to invert the output signal, thus imposing an intersection of the input sets. In the last case, to obtain an output different from the normal 0 value, it is necessary to invert the normal 0 input (i.e. to have faults in set $L1$) but not the normal 1 input (i.e. no faults in set $L2$) which justifies the set difference in the output.

2.1.2   S-Buffers

The gates that participate in the universe of faults D (i.e. that can either be stuck-at-0 or stuck-at-1) may be modelled by means of a normal gate to which a special buffer, an S-buffer, is attached to the output. As such, all gates are considered normal, and only S-buffers can be stuck. An S-buffer for a gate g has associated to it a set L_S of diagnostic sets where g appears as stuck. Since g can appear either as stuck-at-0 or stuck-at-1, we split this set in two (L_{S0} and L_{S1}), one for each type of diagnoses:

$$L_{S0} = \{\text{diag} \in D: g/0 \in \text{diag}\}$$
$$L_{S1} = \{\text{diag} \in D: g/1 \in \text{diag}\}$$
$$L_S = L_{S0} \cup L_{S1}$$

Table 1. S-buffer output

In	Out
$\varnothing$-0	L_{S1}-0
$\varnothing$-1	L_{S0}-1
L_i-0	$L_{S1} \cup (L_i \setminus L_{S0})$ - 0
L_i-1	$L_{S0} \cup (L_i \setminus L_{S1})$ - 1

The modelling of S-buffers is shown in Table 1. When the input is 0 independently of any fault, the S-buffer output would normally be also 0, but if it is stuck-at-1 then it becomes 1, thus depending on set L_{S1}. More generally, if the normal input is 0 but dependent on L_i, the output depends not only on L_{S1} but also on input dependencies L_i (except if they include fault $g/0$). The same reasoning can be applied to the case where the normal input signal is 1, and the whole Table 1 is generalised as shown in Fig.2.

$$L_i\text{-}N \xrightarrow{\quad L_s \quad} L_{S\bar{N}} \cup (L_i \setminus L_{SN})\text{-}N$$

Fig. 2. S-buffer

2.1.3   Modelling the Problems

To model the diagnosis problem, and differentiate faults in set F from faults in set G, (the universe is thus $D=\{F,G\}$ of cardinality 2), either $\{F\}$-N or $\{G\}$-N must be present in a circuit output bit. In any case, a bit L-N must be present in the output where $\#L=1$.

The goal of the maximisation problem is to maximise the number of output dependencies, i.e. the number of diagnoses covered by the input test pattern. The goal is then *maximise* $\#(\cup_b L_b)$ where b ranges over all the output bits b with signals L_b-N_b.

The fourth problem (minimisation) is a typical set covering problem: the test patterns (i) are the resources, and the diagnoses (F) are the services we want to cover with the minimum of resources. Each diagnosis can be tested by a number of test patterns, and each test pattern can test a number of diagnoses. The relation between these services and resources is *test(F,i)*, which is not fully known a priori, though.

2.2   Modelling Digital Signals with Sets

With the previous representation, all digital signals are represented by a pair: a set of faults on which it depends plus a Boolean value that the signal takes if there were no faults at all. Both the set and the Boolean value can be variables, enforcing constraints on two domains to be expressed for each gate, and the modelling presented above implies an extensive use of disjunctive constraints, with the corresponding exponential complexity. For instance, to express the above and-gates, one needs to know the Boolean values of the signals to select the appropriate set constraint.

It would thus be very convenient to join the two domains into a single one. Intuitively, to incorporate the two domains, the new one should be richer than any of them. But there is also the possibility of using a simpler one if the loss of information is not important for the problem, or if it can be compensated by the introduction of extra constraints. This latter alternative is the one we follow here.

More specifically, we propose the use of a transformation *transf*, where signals *L-0* are simply represented as *L*, and *L-1* as $\overline{L}$ (the complement of *L*, w.r.t *D*):

$$transf(S) = \begin{cases} L, & S = L - 0 \\ \overline{L}, & S = L - 1 \end{cases}$$

Though *transf* is not a bijective function (both *L-0* and $\overline{L}$ *-1* are transformed into *L*), we argue that it is quite useful to model our problems. For example, with this representation, the and-gate and the S-buffer are simply stated as follows:

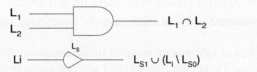

Fig. 3. And-gate and S-buffer over sets

The correctness of this new simplified representation can be checked by simple analysis of each case, shown in Tables 2 and 3.

Table 2. Application of *transf* function to the inputs and output of an and-gate

I1	transf(I1)	I2	transf(I2)	I1∧I2	tranf(I1∧I2)
L_1-1	$\overline{L_1}$	L_2-1	$\overline{L_2}$	$L_1 \cup L_2$-1	$\overline{L_1 \cup L_2} = \overline{L_1} \cap \overline{L_2}$
L_1-0	L_1	L_2-0	L_2	$L_1 \cap L_2$-0	$L_1 \cap L_2$
L_1-0	L_1	L_2-1	$\overline{L_2}$	$L_1 \backslash L_2$-0	$L_1 \backslash L_2 = L_1 \cap \overline{L_2}$

Table 3. Application of transf function to the input and output of an S-buffer

In	transf(In)	S-buffer output	transf(output)
L_i-0	L_i	$L_{S1} \cup (L_i \backslash L_{S0})$ - 0	$L_{S1} \cup (L_i \backslash L_{S0})$
L_i-1	$\overline{L_i}$	$L_{S0} \cup (L_i \backslash L_{S1})$ - 1	$\overline{L_{S0} \cup (L_i \backslash L_{S1})} = \overline{L_{S0}} \cap \overline{L_i \cap \overline{L_{S1}}} =$
			$\overline{L_{S0}} \cap (\overline{L_i} \cup L_{S1}) = (\overline{L_{S0}} \cap \overline{L_i}) \cup (\overline{L_{S0}} \cap L_{S1})$
			$= (\overline{L_i} \cap \overline{L_{S0}}) \cup L_{S1} = L_{S1} \cup (\overline{L_i} \backslash L_{S0})$

In Table 2, the transformed output set is always the intersection of the transformed input sets, i.e. *transf(I1)* ∧ *transf(I2)* = *transf(I1* ∧ *I2)*. Similarly, in Table 3, *s_buffer(L_S,transf(Input))* = *transf(s_buffer(L_S, Input))*.

For completion, it may be also noticed that the other gate operations can be expressed with the expected set operations:

L ▷∘— $\overline{L}$ $\begin{matrix} L_1 \\ L_2 \end{matrix}$ ⊐— $L_1 \cup L_2$ $\begin{matrix} L_1 \\ L_2 \end{matrix}$ ⊐— $(L_1 \cap \overline{L_2}) \cup (\overline{L_1} \cap L_2)$

Fig. 4. Other gates over sets

2.2.1   Modelling the Problems

To solve the diagnosis problem with this representation based exclusively on sets, it is still sufficient to ensure that a set L with cardinality 1 is present in an output bit of the circuit. Being $D=\{F,G\}$ the set of diagnoses F and G to differentiate, it is equivalent to have in an output bit an L (#L=1), in the sets representation, or to have an L-N (#L=1) in the mixed representation (pairs Set-Boolean).

Proof.

⇒   If L (#L=1) is present in an output bit, it represents either L-0 (#L=1) or $\overline{L}$-1 (#$\overline{L}$=1, since #D=2). In either case, it solves the problem.

⇐   If an L-N (#L=1) is present in an output bit, it is either L-0 (represented as L) or L-1 (represented as $\overline{L}$). In either case, the represented set has cardinality 1.

Therefore, the loss of information incurred by the transformation used has no effect in this problem, since it is not necessary to add any new constraints to solve it.

Modelling the maximisation problem in a circuit c, is not so straightforward. Since a digital signal coded as D does not necessarily mean a dependency on all diagnoses (it can represent D-0, as well as $\varnothing$-1), maximising the union of all the output bits is not adequate. In fact, it is necessary to know exactly whether an output signal depends on its set or on its complement. This can be done as shown in Fig. 5.

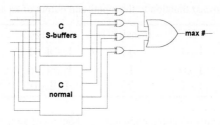

Fig. 5. Modelling the maximisation problem with sets

Circuit c with S-buffers is kept as before, but now the circuit with no S-buffers is added, sharing the input bits and with the corresponding output bits xor-ed. Values inside the normal circuit are necessarily independent of any faults, and can only be represented as $\varnothing$ (for $\varnothing$-0) and D (for $\varnothing$-1). The xor gates in the output bits receiving a set L from the faulty circuit and either $\varnothing$ or D (the universe) from the normal one, recover the correct dependency set of the signal as being either L or $\overline{L}$ (if the normal value were 0 or 1, respectively). A maximisation on the union of these real fault dependencies can be performed to obtain a desired solution of the problem.

The reduction of the problem size by eliminating the Boolean part of the domain is now compensated by the duplication of constraints. Still, what could naively be seen as an useless manipulation, allows an active use of constraints by a set constraint solver avoiding the choice-points that would otherwise be necessary.

Moreover, the exponential component of search, labelling, is only performed at the circuit with S-buffers (the other circuit simply checks this labelling). This is in contrast with Boolean SAT approaches, which consider one extra circuit for each diagnosis, which is unacceptable, in practice, for a large set of diagnoses [15].

The minimisation problem is a meta-problem: it involves sets of solutions to set problems. A set variable S could be used ranging from $\emptyset$ to $P(I)$, where set S of inputs is constrained to cover diagnoses D. The goal is then to minimise the cardinality of S.

To find a test pattern for a single diagnosis F using sets, we need to model a faulty and a normal circuit xor-ing the outputs and checking if at least one set value $\{F\}$ is obtained. This is equivalent to the SAT approach for obtaining test patterns.

The ideal is to consider all diagnoses D at the same time, with set constraints, and include or remove elements from S during the computation, updating the diagnoses covered until D is reached, and then start finding smaller sets for S in a branch-and-bound manner. This is still an open problem and perhaps the maximisation problem can be used to solve this minimisation one, by obtaining intermediate solutions.

3   Cardinal Set Solver

Clearly a constraint solver over sets is required to deal with these set problem models directly. Conjunto [6] represents set variables by set intervals with a lower and an upper bound considering set inclusion as the partial ordering. In Conjunto, a set domain variable S is specified by an interval $[a,b]$ where a and b are known sets, representing the greatest lower bound and the lowest upper bound of S, respectively. The cardinality of S is a finite domain variable C ($\#S{=}C$). This cardinality information, however, is largely disregarded until it is known to be equal to the cardinality of one of the set bounds, in which case an inference rule is triggered to instantiate the set.

Inferences using cardinalities can be very useful to more rapidly conclude the non-satisfiability of a set of constraints, thus improving efficiency of combinatorial search problem solving. As a simple example, if Z is known to be the set difference between Y and X, both contained in set $\{a,b,c,d\}$, and it is also known that X has exactly 2 elements, it should be inferred that the cardinality of Z can never exceed 2 elements (i.e. from $X,Y \subseteq \{a,b,c,d\}$, $\#X{=}2$, $Z{=}Y\backslash X$ it should be inferred that $\#Z \le 2$), and thus immediately detect a failure upon the posting of a constraint such as $\#Z{=}3$.

Inference capabilities such as these (and other more complex discussed below) are particularly important when solving set problems where cardinality plays a especial role, as is the case of the circuit problems seen above.

In this section we present a new constraint solver, Cardinal, that makes a number of such inferences. Cardinal is formally presented as a set of rewriting rules on a constraint store. This store maintains constraints over sets and over finite domains (the cardinality of the sets), but we only describe the rewriting rules of the set constraints (we assume that a finite domain constraint solver maintains bounded arc-consistency, or interval consistency, on these constraints).

3.1   A Set Constraint Solver: Cardinal

The universe notion is necessary not only for the set complement operation, but also for the especial cardinality inferences we propose. Hence we will use U to denote the set universe domain (for the proposed circuit problems, the universe is the set of diagnoses D), and u to denote the cardinality of U ($u = \#U$).

A set variable X is represented by $[a_x,b_x]_{Cx:Dx}$ (or simply as $[a_x,b_x]_{Cx}$) where a_x is its greatest lower bound (i.e. the elements known to belong to X), b_x its lowest upper bound (i.e. the elements not excluded from X), C_x its cardinality (a finite domain variable) with domain D_x. In the remainder, a_x, b_x, C_x and D_x will refer to these set X's attributes if no confusion arises. Given the transformation presented above, independent values such as the circuit inputs are represented by $[\varnothing, U]_{Cx:\{0,u\}}$.

Cardinal implements a number of set constraints such as inclusion, equality, difference, membership and disjointness, together with set operations (union, intersection, difference and complement), as built-in. We only describe here the operations of sets complement and binary intersection and the equality and inclusion constraints, since these are enough to model the circuit problems.

3.1.1   Set Variable

When a variable is declared as a set variable, it is simply included in the constraint store, ensuring the bounds of the variable and that its cardinality C is a finite domain variable with domain D:

$$\overline{\{tell(X \in [a,b]_{C:D})\} \mapsto \{X \in [a,b]_C, C::D\}} \tag{1}$$

A number of inferences are subsequently maintained. The cardinality must always remain inside the limits given by the set bounds (the triggers of these inferences are shown in parenthesis next to the rewriting rules, and may correspond to one or more variables becoming ground, changing bounds, or being bound in the Prolog sense):

(X: changed bounds) $$\frac{n = \#a_x, m = \#b_x}{\{\} \mapsto \{C_x \geq n, C_x \leq m\}} \tag{2}$$

As in Conjunto, a set variable becomes one of its bounds if their cardinality is the same (this rule is triggered only when C_x becomes a fixed value):

(Cx: ground) $$\frac{C_x = \#a_x}{\{\} \mapsto \{X = a_x\}} \qquad \frac{C_x = \#b_x}{\{\} \mapsto \{X = b_x\}} \tag{3}$$

When there are two domains declared for the same set variable, their intersection must be computed and the cardinalities made equal:

$$\frac{a = a_1 \cup a_2, b = b_1 \cap b_2}{\{X \in [a_1,b_1]_{C_1}, X \in [a_2,b_2]_{C_2}\} \mapsto \{X \in [a,b]_{C_1}, C_1 = C_2\}} \tag{4}$$

Eventually a failure may be detected, either because the lower bound of a set is not included in its upper bound, or the domain of the cardinal becomes empty:

(X: changed bounds) $$\frac{not(a_x \subseteq b_x)}{\{\} \mapsto fail} \qquad \frac{D_x = \varnothing}{\{\} \mapsto fail} \tag{5}$$

3.1.2   Set Complement

For the set complement constraint it is assumed the existence of an universe of cardinality u, that is used in a finite domain constraint, $C_y = u - C_x$, over the sets cardinalities. In general, the finite domains constraint solver maintains bounded arc consistency on this constraint. Nevertheless, we ensure full arc consistency when the constraint is posted:

$$\frac{}{\{tell(X = \overline{Y})\} \mapsto \{Cy = u - Cx, X = \overline{Y}\}} \tag{6}$$

Whenever there is an update of the bounds of one of the sets, the bounds of its complement must also be updated accordingly:

(X: changed bounds) $$\frac{a = \overline{bx}, b = \overline{ax}}{\{X = \overline{Y}\} \mapsto \{X = \overline{Y}, Y \in [a,b]\}} \tag{7}$$

(Y: changed bounds) $$\frac{a = \overline{by}, b = \overline{ay}}{\{X = \overline{Y}\} \mapsto \{X = \overline{Y}, X \in [a,b]\}} \tag{8}$$

Assuming that the universe is not empty, a set cannot be the same as its complement:

(X or Y: changed bounds) $$\frac{}{\{X = \overline{Y}, X = Y\} \mapsto fail} \tag{9}$$

When the two sets are ground, their complementary nature can be easily checked:

(X and Y: ground) $$\frac{ground(X), ground(Y), ax = \overline{ay}}{\{X = \overline{Y}\} \mapsto \{\}} \qquad \frac{ground(X), ground(Y), ax \neq \overline{ay}}{\{X = \overline{Y}\} \mapsto fail} \tag{10}$$

Of course, this rule could be checked even when X or Y are not ground. Nevertheless, such check would only add to the overhead without useful inferences being made.

3.1.3 Set Equality

When two sets are told to be equal, so does their cardinality:

$$\frac{}{\{tell(X = Y)\} \mapsto \{X = Y, Cx = Cy\}} \tag{11}$$

When one bound of the set is updated, so does the corresponding bound of any set equal to it (the situation is similar to that of two domains for the same set):

(X or Y: ch. bounds) $$\frac{a = ax \cup ay, b = bx \cap by}{\{X = Y, X \in [ax,bx], Y \in [ay,by]\} \mapsto \{X = Y, X \in [a,b], Y \in [a,b]\}} \tag{12}$$

Again, when sets are ground, the equality is easily tested:

(X and Y: ground) $$\frac{ground(X), ground(Y), ax = ay}{\{X = Y\} \mapsto \{\}} \qquad \frac{ground(X), ground(Y), ax \neq ay}{\{X = Y\} \mapsto fail} \tag{13}$$

Of course, if only one of the sets becomes ground, the previous rule enforces the other set either to become with the same bounds (and ground, in which case this rule eliminates the equality constraint) or with an empty domain, causing a failure.

3.1.4 Set Inclusion

If Y contains X, then C_y is greater (or equal) than C_x:

$$\frac{}{\{tell(X \subseteq Y)\} \mapsto \{X \subseteq Y, Cx \leq Cy\}} \tag{14}$$

When the lower bound (glb) of X increases, the lower bound of Y may also increase; and when the upper bound (lub) of Y decreases, so might happen to X:

(X: changed glb)
$$\frac{a = ax \cup ay}{\{X \subseteq Y\} \mapsto \{X \subseteq Y, Y \in [a, by]\}} \tag{15}$$

(Y: changed lub)
$$\frac{b = bx \cap by}{\{X \subseteq Y\} \mapsto \{X \subseteq Y, X \in [ax, b]\}} \tag{16}$$

If b_x is contained in a_y, or X is the same as Y, the constraint $X \subseteq Y$ is trivially satisfied, and can be eliminated from the store:

(X or Y: bound)
$$\frac{ground(X) \vee ground(Y), bx \subseteq ay}{\{X \subseteq Y\} \mapsto \{\}} \qquad \frac{}{\{X \subseteq Y, X = Y\} \mapsto \{X = Y\}} \tag{17}$$

3.1.5   Set Intersection

While for the set complement the universe must be given, for the intersection Z of sets X and Y, the universe can be considered as the union of the upper bounds ($U = b_x \cup b_y$), u being its cardinality.

The following rule states that the intersection of two sets must be contained in both sets, and posts a special constraint on the cardinality of the set intersection:

$$\frac{}{\{tell(Z = X \cap Y)\} \mapsto \{Z = X \cap Y, tell(Z \subseteq X), tell(Z \subseteq Y), tell(C_z = X \otimes Y)\}} \tag{18}$$

The special cardinality constraint over sets ($C_z = X \otimes Y$) ensures that each possible value for C_z has a supporting cardinality pair in domains D_x and D_y when the intersection is posted. Before formalising this operation, we first analyse what can be the domain of cardinality C_z be. If we take possible cardinality values cx of D_x and cy of D_y, and the sum of cx and cy exceeds u, there must be common elements to X and Y, and their intersection has at least $cx + cy - u$ elements.

To reason about the upper bound, C_z can never exceed cx nor cy since Z is the sets intersection. The elements in a_x not in b_y (i.e. $a_x \backslash b_y$) can safely be subtracted from cx since they are definitely not part of the intersection, but are counted in cx (so an upper bound can be $cx - \#a_x \backslash b_y$). A similar reasoning may be done for Y, yielding another upper bound. A final upper bound can thus be considered the minimum of the two (i.e. $min(cx - \#(a_x \backslash b_y), cy - \#(a_y \backslash b_x))$).

Thus for each pair cx and cy, an integer range for C_z is calculated, and the ranges for all such pairs are eventually merged. This can in fact be regarded as maintaining arc-consistency between the cardinalities of X, Y and Z, when $Z = X \cap Y$. In fact, this arc-consistency is enforced when the constraint is first told:

$$\tag{19}$$
$$\frac{}{\{tell(C_z = X \otimes Y)\} \mapsto \{C_z \in \{n : \exists i \in Dx, j \in Dy, i + j - u \leq n \leq min(i - \#(ax \backslash by), j - \#(ay \backslash bx))\}\}}$$

The usefulness of this rule for the problems we address, can be illustrated with the diagnosis problem. Let us take two sets X and Y which can both be $\varnothing$ or $D = \{f, g\}$, and have them intersected (this is a typical case when two input bits are connected through an and-gate). While their set domain is the convex closure of the two bounds, their cardinality can only be 0 or 2. To find the cardinality domain of their intersection we examine cardinality pairs $<cx, cy> = <0,0>$, $<0,2>$, $<2,0>$ and $<2,2>$. The three first pairs, yield only value 0 as a possible intersection cardinality, since one set has no elements. Pair $<2,2>$ yields single value 2, since u is also 2 ($cx + cy - u = 2 + 2 - 2 = 2$). Thus the final cardinality domain for the sets intersection is also $\{0,2\}$. If only interval reasoning were performed on cardinality, the result would be the full range $\{0,1,2\}$.

Instead of checking pairs of integers, it is equivalent and more efficient to check pairs of sub-ranges and their bounds when the constraint is posted. Nevertheless, this arc consistency is very costly to maintain, so it is only checked when the constraint is posted. Subsequently, only bounded arc consistency is maintained on the cardinality of the sets (by the underlying finite domains constraint solver):

$$\text{(X: changed glb or Y: changed lub)} \quad \frac{n = \#(ax \setminus by)}{\{Z = X \cap Y\} \mapsto \{Z = X \cap Y, Cz \leq Cx - n\}} \tag{20}$$

$$\text{(X: changed lub, Y: changed glb)} \quad \frac{n = \#(ay \setminus bx)}{\{Z = X \cap Y\} \mapsto \{Z = X \cap Y, Cz \leq Cy - n\}} \tag{21}$$

$$\text{(X or Y: changed lub)} \quad \frac{n = \#bx + \#by - \#bz}{\{Z = X \cap Y\} \mapsto \{Z = X \cap Y, Cz \geq Cx + Cy - n\}} \tag{22}$$

A number of other inferences are performed regarding intersection. The lower bound of the set intersection is kept as the intersection of the lower bounds of the arguments:

$$\text{(X or Y: changed glb)} \quad \frac{a = ax \cap ay}{\{Z = X \cap Y\} \mapsto \{Z = X \cap Y, Z \in [a, bz]\}} \tag{23}$$

If both arguments are the same set, their intersection is that set (idempotence):

$$\text{(X or Y: bound)} \quad \frac{}{\{Z = X \cap Y, X = Y\} \mapsto \{X = Y, tell(Z = X)\}} \tag{24}$$

If intersection Z is known to be the same set as one of its arguments, then the intersection constraint may be eliminated (as $Z \subseteq Y$ and $Z \subseteq X$):

$$\text{(X or Y: bound)} \quad \frac{}{\{Z = X \cap Y, X = Z\} \mapsto \{X = Z\}} \quad \frac{}{\{Z = X \cap Y, Y = Z\} \mapsto \{Y = Z\}} \tag{25}$$

Conversely, if an argument contains the other, the intersection is the included set:

$$\text{(X or Y: bound)} \quad \frac{ground(Y), bx \subseteq ay}{\{Z = X \cap Y\} \mapsto \{tell(Z = X)\}} \quad \frac{ground(X), bx \subseteq ax}{\{Z = X \cap Y\} \mapsto \{tell(Z = Y)\}} \tag{26}$$

Although inclusion could be inferred more generally, for efficiency reasons this rule is only triggered when either one of the arguments is ground. These four simplification/simpagation rules [5] exploit the fact that the universe is the neutral element of the intersection. Here, the universe is the set argument containing the other.

All common elements to X and Y must be in Z. That is, X and Y must have no common elements outside Z. This is a costly operation, so it is performed only once (when Z is ground):

$$\text{(Z: ground)} \quad \frac{bx' = bx \setminus (ay \setminus az), by' = by \setminus (ax \setminus az)}{\{Z = X \cap Y\} \mapsto \{Z = X \cap Y, X \in [ax, bx'], Y \in [ay, by']\}} \tag{27}$$

4   Implementation and Results

We used ECLiPSe with attributed variables to implement Cardinal, a set constraint solver with cardinality inferences based on the above rules. The attributes of a set variable are its domain and its cardinality together with lists of suspended goals, since we used the underlying predicate suspension handling mechanism. The cardinality is an integer variable to be handled by the ECLiPSe finite domain library. To represent the domain of set S as a set interval we need its bounds a_s and b_s. Since $a_s \subseteq b_s$, it is enough to store a_s as the definite elements of S, and the difference $b_s \backslash a_s$ as the possible extra elements of S. For efficiency reasons, the sizes of its two bounds are also stored.

Gate constraints are currently implemented based on just two basic set operations: complement (not-gate) and binary intersection (and-gate). Set complement constraints take as arguments the universe and the input and output set variables. In general, constraints perform all the possible inferences when posted (interval-consistency on the sets; arc-consistency on their cardinalities), while their subsequent maintenance only ensures arc-consistency on their bounds. The rationale for this is that it is worth spending more time trying to reduce domains, only if this effort is not done too often.

Our labelling strategy for circuit problems finds for the relevant output bits and S-buffers, the inputs they depend on. These are then labelled by assigning values (0 or u) to their cardinality. If successful, the rest of the circuit input is labelled.

To assess the advantages of cardinality inferences, we took off inferences from Cardinal that are not implemented in Conjunto (i.e. rewrite rules 6, 14, 18 to 22 and 24 to 27 presented in section 3). As mentioned before, this simpler version is referred to as „Conjunto". We then tried to solve the same problems for the standard ISCAS digital circuits benchmarks [10] using Cardinal and „Conjunto". From a set of diagnosis benchmarks created over these circuits [1], we randomly picked pairs of diagnoses to differentiate. The results are shown in Table 4 (times reported in seconds on a Pentium III, 500 Mhz).

Table 4. Experimental Results

circuit	Diag1	Diag2	Diff.	„Conjunto"	Cardinal	Speed-up
c432	380gat/0	415gat/1	X	8.1	0.4	20.3
c432	431gat/0	428gat/1	√	39.4	1.3	30.3
c432	431gat/0	419gat/0	√	37.9	1.4	27.1
c432	428gat/1	419gat/0	X	24.0	1.0	24.0
c1908	1541/1	1538/0	√	24.2	3.2	7.6
c1908	860/1	72/1	√	156.3	1.3	120.2
c1908	72/1	71/0	X	194.9	1.0	194.9
c3540	855/0	707/1	√	4.1	6.1	0.7
c3540	955/0	954/0	X	3482.8	2.4	1451.2
c3540	855/0	707/1	√	1.8	3.2	0.6
c3540	403/0	3544/1	√	352.1	2.9	121.4
c6288	5671gat/0	5537gat/1	√	> 86400	11.0	> 7854.5
c6288	6288gat/1	6285gat/0	√	> 3600	8.9	> 404.5
c6288	813gat/0	6123gat/0	√	> 3600	8.9	> 404.5

This table, with results for 4 ISCAS circuits, indicates the time that Cardinal and „Conjunto" needed to find a differentiating test pattern between *Diag1* and *Diag2* (marked as √) or to prove it is impossible (i.e. the faults are indistinguishable, shown as X). For example, the first line reports that the differentiation of gate 380gat stuck-at-0 from gate 415gat stuck-at-1, in circuit c432, took 8.1 seconds in Conjunto and 0.4 seconds in Cardinal.

Globally, it can be stated that Cardinal showed a speed-up of two orders of magnitude compared to „Conjunto" on this set of problems (and others we tried) although, as expected, the improvement was not uniform over all the tests.

While for circuit c432 Cardinal showed a consistent speed-up around 25, for larger circuits the variation can be quite large. In circuits c1908 and c3540, the speed-up ranges from 0.6 to 1451.2, Cardinal being more efficient in harder problems (specially those where there is no differentiating pattern between the two diagnoses). For the two instances in circuit c3540 where there was an easy solution for „Conjunto", Cardinal was slower due to the extra inferences performed, and the times thus reflect this overhead. The extra computing effort may be largely compensated, as tests in c6288 show, where Cardinal easily found a solution, whereas „Conjunto" had to be aborted in all three tests after one hour (one particular test was even kept running for one day of unsuccessful processing). Of course, the speed-up can be arbitrarily large as long as not enough propagation was achieved and we start labelling variables, since the execution time is exponential on the number of these variables.

Due to all the especial inferences and list processing, we expected Cardinal to experience problems with larger circuits or in problems with many diagnoses. Also, since the general feeling is that, in practice, it is very costly to perform all the desired inferences over sets and their cardinalities, we tried to create another version with n-ary gates but with less inferences, which produced results that were midway between „Conjunto" and Cardinal. The fact is that Cardinal still managed to efficiently solve problems for the largest of the benchmark circuits (c7552), so no improvements were obtained by reducing inferences.

5   Conclusions and Further Research

In this paper we showed how to model ATPG related problems in digital circuits with a constraint logic programming approach. We reckon our approach has great potential in this area, since competing alternatives, based on SAT, require substantial duplication of the circuits under consideration. In contrast, our technique uses set variables to denote dependency of faults and is able to model the problems without adding extra circuitry (more precisely, without imposing the labelling of more variables, the exponential part of search).

Since we deal with set variables and set constraints, we realise that existing set constraint solvers were not adequate to handle these problems as they were not using actively important information about the cardinality of the sets, a key feature in these problems. We therefore implemented an optimised set constraint solver, Cardinal, and compared it with a simplified version with propagation similar to that of the widely available solver, Conjunto. Preliminary experimental results show that Cardinal obtains a speed up of about two orders of magnitude over „Conjunto", in a set of diagnostic problems.

428 Francisco Azevedo and Pedro Barahona

We are now working on two directions. On the one hand we will compare our results with results obtained with specialised SAT based tools dealing with the same problems. On the other hand, we will implement a second version of Cardinal that deals with optimisation problems. We are now starting a project with colleagues using a SAT tool, and we expect to have soon available more substantial evaluation results and comparison of the approaches.

Acknowledgements: The first author was financially supported by „Sub-Programa Ciência e Tecnologia do 2° Quadro Comunitário de Apoio". We would also like to thank the anonymous referees and Carmen Gervet for their helpful comments.

References

1 F. Azevedo and P. Barahona. *Benchmarks for Differential Diagnosis*, at URL http://www-ssdi.di.fct.unl.pt/~fa/differential-diagnosis/benchmarks.html, 1998.

2 F. Azevedo and P. Barahona. *Constraints over an Eight-Valued Logic to Differentiate Diagnostic Theories*, to appear in Proceedings of the 14th European Conference on Artificial Intelligence (ECAI 2000), W. Horn (Ed.), IOS Press, Amsterdam, 2000.

3 F. Benhamou, *Interval Constraint Logic Programming, in Constraint Programming: Basics and Trends*, LNCS 910, A. Podelski (Ed.), Springer, March 1995.

4 ECRC, *ECLiPSe (a) user manual, (b) extensions of the user manual, Technical Report*, ECRC, 1994.

5 T. Frühwirth, *Constraint Handling Rules*, in Constraint Programming: Basics and Trends, LNCS 910, A. Podelski (Ed.), Springer, 1995.

6 C. Gervet, *Interval Propagation to Reason about Sets: Definition and Implementation of a Practical Language*, Constraints, vol. 1(3), Kluwer, pp.191-244, March 1997.

7 C. Gervet, personal communication

8 T. Gruning, U. Mahlstedt, H. Koopmeiners, DIATEST: *A Fast Diagnostic Test Pattern Generator for Combinational Circuits*, Proceedings of the IEEE International Conference on Computer-Aided Design (ICCAD91), pp. 194-197, 1991

9 I. Hartanto*1, V. Boppana, W.K. Fuchs, J.H. Patel, *Diagnostic Test Pattern Generation For Sequential Circuits*, Proc. 15th VLSI Test Symposium (VTS), Monterey, pp.196-202, 1997.

10 ISCAS. *Special Session on ATPG*, Proc. IEEE Symposium on Circuits and Systems, 1985.

11 J. Jaffar and J.-L. Lassez. *Constraint Logic Programming*, Proceedings of the 14th ACM Symposium on Principles of Programming Languages, pp. 111-119, 1987.

12 J. Jaffar and M. J. Maher. *Constraint Logic Programming: A Survey*, Journal of Logic Programming, 19(20):503-581, 1994.

13 V. Manquinho and J. Marques Silva, *On using satisfiability based pruning techniques in covering algorithms*, Proc. ACM/IEEE Design, Automation and Test in Europe Conf. 2000.

14 I. Pomeranz, S.M. Reddy, *A Diagnostic Test Generation Procedure for Synchronous Sequential Circuits based on Test Elimination*, International Test Conference (ITC98). Washington, D.C., USA, pp. 1074-1083, 1998.

15 L. G. Silva, L. M. Silveira and J. P. Marques-Silva, *Algorithms for Solving Boolean Satisfiability in Combinational Circuits*, in Proc. of the IEEE/ACM Design and Test in Europe Conference (DATE), 1999.

16 H. Simonis. *Test Generation using the Constraint Logic Programming Language CHIP*, in Proc. of the 6th International Conf. on Logic Programming, MIT Press, pp 101-112, 1989.

17 H. Simonis. *Constraint Logic Programming Language as a Digital Circuit Design Tool*, Thesis, 1992.

Promoting Constraints to First-Class Status

Tobias Müller

Programming System Lab, Universität des Saarlandes
Postfach 15 11 50, D-66041 Saarbrücken, Germany
tmueller@ps.uni-sb.de

Abstract. This paper proposes to promote constraints to first-class status. In contrast to constraint propagation, which performs inference on values of variables, first-class constraints allow reasoning about the constraints themselves. This lets the programmer access the current state of a constraint and control a constraint's behavior directly, thus making powerful new programming and inference techniques possible, as the combination of constraint propagation and rewriting constraints à la term rewriting. First-class constraints allow for *true* meta constraint programming. Promising applications in the field of combinatorial optimization include early unsatisfiability detection, constraint reformulation to improve propagation, garbage collection of redundant but not yet entailed constraints, and finding minimal inconsistent subsets of a given set of constraints for debugging immediately failing constraint programs.

We demonstrate the above-mentioned applications by means of examples. The experiments were done with Mozart Oz but can be easily ported to other constraint solvers.

Keywords: Constraint programming, first-class constraints, early failure detection, simplification and garbage collection of constraints, minimal sets of inconsistent constraints.

1 Introduction

This paper proposes to promote constraints to first-class status and presents three applications for combinatorial problems. In contrast to constraint propagation, which performs inference on values of variables, first-class constraints allow reasoning about the constraints themselves. This lets the programmer access the current state of a constraint and control a constraint's behavior directly, thus making powerful new programming and inference techniques possible, as the combination of constraint propagation and rewriting constraints à la term rewriting. Promising applications in the field of combinatorial optimization include early unsatisfiability detection, constraint reformulation to improve propagation, and garbage collection of redundant but not yet entailed constraints.

Commonly, a constraint that reflects its validity to a 0/1-variable is called a meta constraint. This notion is slightly misleading since this reflection does not allow for true meta programming in the sense of self-reasoning and self-modification. Hence Smolka coined the term *reified* constraints, which we use in this paper, instead of meta constraints (first used in [6]). First-class constraints are orthogonal to reified constraints and allow for *true* meta constraint programming. For example, one can obtain the name

J. Lloyd et al. (Eds.): CL 2000, LNAI 1861, pp. 429–447, 2000.
© Springer-Verlag Berlin Heidelberg 2000

and the parameters of a first-class constraint and learn whether it is already entailed or not. Furthermore, one can explicitly discard a first-class constraint and can turn its propagation on or off. We demonstrate these operations in the following application areas:

Early Failure Detection. Due to the limited view of a single constraint on the constraint store, reasoning and especially failure detection is limited too. Often recognizing a certain constraint pattern makes it possible to spot an inconsistency much earlier than constraint propagation can do and sometimes constraint propagation on its own is not able to detect the inconsistency at all. For example $x < y \land y < x$ is obviously inconsistent. But the time ordinary finite domain propagation takes to detect the inconsistency is proportional to the domain size of x and y, and hence, can be quite long. Reasoning about the constraints themselves can detect the unsatisfiability of this constraint immediately.

Constraint Simplification. Constraints fed into a constraint solver can often be improved regarding their propagation behavior. Common sub-constraints, for example, can be collapsed and constraints can be reformulated to provided for better domain pruning.

Garbage Collection. Usually constraints are garbage collected as soon as they are entailed by the constraint store. But typically that requires the parameter of the constraints to be determined. In many cases constraints could be discarded earlier. Consider the finite domain constraint $x + 1 = z \land x \leq z$. The constraint $x \leq z$ can be discarded since it is implied by $x + 1 = z$.

Minimal Sets of Inconsistent Constraints. Like every kind of programming, constraint programming is prone to error. A common programming error is to put up an incorrect model a given problem or to implement a constraint model incorrectly. This frequently results in inconsistent constraints which cause immediate failure. Debugging such symptoms is supported by finding sets of constraints that are responsible for the inconsistency.

First-class constraints are defined as an abstract data type, i. e., in terms of operations on them. They are true first-class citizens: they can occur at any position where primitive values can occur too, e. g., as parameters of applications, as return values of functions, or as parts of composite data structures. That makes the new powerful programming techniques possible and allows the programmer, for example, to combine constraint inference on variable values with rewriting techniques to implement hybrid constraint solvers. Furthermore first-class constraints can be used for prototyping sophisticated new constraints.

To our knowledge existing systems do not provide first-class constraints even though it is straightforward to add them to existing solvers (cf. Sect. 8). It is not sufficient to have access to a C++ object representing a constraint as in ILOG Solver [14, 7]. A first-class constraint is a value of an abstract data type defined by a set of operations (cf. Sect. 2).

First-class constraints have been implemented with Mozart Oz [9] and the extensions are orthogonal to the existing solver and do not impose any performance penalty when not using first-class constraints.

Plan of the Paper. Sect. 2 defines first-class constraints as abstract data types. The following sections investigate early failure detection, simplification, garbage collection of constraints, and finding minimal sets of consistent constraints. Sect. 7 contrasts the expressiveness of first-class constraints with reified constraints, Sect. 8 discusses implementation issues and Sect. 9 comments on related work. The paper closes with concluding remarks.

2 Constraints as First-Class Values

This section introduces a general model for constraint inference serving as a base for the promotion of constraints to first-class status. Then first-class constraints are introduced as values of an abstract data type.

A Model for Constraint Inference. Constraint inference involves a *constraint store*, holding so-called *basic* constraints. A basic constraint is of the form $x = v$ (x is bound to a value v), $x = y$ (x is equated to another variable y), or $x \in D$ (x takes its value in D). Attached to the constraint store are *non-basic* constraints.

Together with the constraint store they form a *computation space*. A computation space can be asked, among other things, if propagation has reached a fix-point [16].

Non-basic constraints, as for example "$x + y = z$", are more expressive than basic constraints and, hence, require more computational effort. In the following we call a non-basic constraint "constraint". A constraint is realized by a computational agent (a so-called *propagator*) observing the basic constraints of its *parameters* (which are variables in the constraint store; in the example x, y, and z). The purpose of a constraint is to infer new basic constraints for its parameters and add them to the store. A constraint terminates (fails) if it is inconsistent with the constraint store or if it is explicitly represented by the basic constraints in the store, i. e., it is entailed by the store. A computation space becomes entailed as soon as all constraints are entailed or it becomes failed as soon as at least one constraint fails.

First-Class Constraints. A first-class constraint is a value of an abstract data type and is hence defined in terms of its operations. It can be handled like any other primitive value, i.e, it can be part of composite data structures or can be used in applications or expressions.

Operations on first-class constraints are provided by the module `Constraint`. Access to operations is obtained by the ".-"operator and operations are applied by the "{}"-operator.

Note that reflective operations are typically *non-monotonic*, i. e., the produced result depends on the current state of the solver. Hence, these operations can be safely applied only if propagation has reached a fix-point. This has to be taken into account when adding new basic constraints to the constraint store while reasoning over first-class constraints. Adding new basic constraints typically requires the recomputation of the fix-point resulting in a changed set of first-class constraints to reason about.

First we define a minimal set of operations, i. e., this set does not contain operations which can be expressed by other operations of this set. Then we introduce operations that make more concise and elegant programming possible.

The following operations designate the minimal set of operations to be provided:

The first two operations are required to obtain access to a first-class constraint and to be able to identify a value as a first-class constraint.

- C <- { F } (for short <--operator) creates the constraint F, adds it to the current computation space, and binds C to an abstract value referring to F.
- C <-# { F } (for short <-#-operator) creates the constraint F, adds it inactive, i. e., the propagation is turned off, to the current computation space, and binds C to an abstract value referring to F. The <-#-operator is used in conjunction with the following abstraction:
- {Constraint.activate C} turns constraint propagation of constraint C on.
- {Constraint.is C B} binds B to **true** if C refers to a constraint and otherwise to **false**.

Obviously C <- { F } can be expressed by combining C <-# { F } and {Constraint.activate C} but it is added for convenience since it is the usual way to create a first-class propagator.

Programming with first-class constraints typically involves rewriting sets of constraints to operationally more efficient formulations (the most efficient one is of course **true**). That requires discarding the redundant constraint which is replaced. Furthermore, reasoning about constraints may take into account that a constraint has already become entailed by the constraint store, i. e., can be ignored.

- {Constraint.discard C} discards C explicitly, i. e., C is removed from the computation space. By discarding a constraint, its whole host space may become entailed.
- {Constraint.isEntailed C B} binds B to **true** if C is entailed, either explicitly by the operation discard or by entailment through the constraint store, and otherwise to **false**.

To be able to reason about constraints the programmer needs to identify what kind of constraint she is dealing with and what the parameters of the constraints are like. The question of which parameters are equal is especially interesting because it makes reformulations of constraints possible.

- {Constraint.getName C N} binds N to the name of C.
- {Constraint.getParameters C Ps} binds Ps to the parameters of C.
- {Constraint.identifyParameters Vs Ids} maps the list of variables Vs to a list of integer identifiers Ids by assigning to each element in Vs the index of its first occurrence in Vs. Thus equal variables can be detected easily.

Additionally, we propose operations that have turned out to be useful and convenient in the applications discussed in this paper.

- {Constraint.toString C S} binds S to a textual representation of C.
- {Constraint.reflectSpace Rs Cs} takes a list Rs of variables. It collects all propagators that have at least one variable of Rs as a parameter. Furthermore, it collects propagators which share parameters with collected propagators. Thus, the transistive closure of all propagators "reachable" from Rs is computed. The collected propagators are turned into some normal form and returned in the list Cs.

The application of Constraint.reflectSpace makes it possible to use first-class constraints in an orthogonal way since the original constraint program needs not be modified (cf. Sect. 3 and Sect. 4).

3   Early Failure Detection

One of the major goals of constraint programming is to avoid exploration of parts of the search tree that do not contain any solutions. But there are cases where propagation takes significant time to detect failure or is even unable to do so. An example for potential long lasting propagation are the finite domain constraints $x < y \land y < x$ and $2x = y \land 2u = v \land y + 1 = v$ assuming sufficiently large domains.[1] An example for an unsatisfiable constraint that cannot be spotted without any meta reasoning is $x, y, z \in \{0, 1\} \land x \neq y \land x \neq z \land y \neq z$.

This section demonstrates how meta constraint programming can be used to detect unsatisfiable constraints where ordinary constraint propagation fails to do so. Thus the search tree can be significantly pruned and bigger instances of the problem can be solved.

We use as example a modified Hamiltonian path problem, where the aim is to find a path through a given directed graph from an arbitrary starting node to an arbitrary ending node such that all nodes of the graph are visited once and the path is valid for the reverse direction too.

The Constraint Model and Its Implementation. The problem data is given as set $Arcs$ of 2-tuples $arc(f, T)$, where the set $T \subseteq \{1, \ldots, n\}$ contains all nodes $t \in T$ such that there is an arc from node f to t. Every of the n nodes of the graph is represented by a finite domain variable $x_i \in \{1, \ldots, n\}$ which represents the position of the ith node; the variables have to be pairwise distinct (constraint (1)). Constraint (2) expresses the path from the starting node to the ending node. Node x_i is the successor of x_f if $x_i = x_f + 1$ holds. Note the extra clause for the ending point. The constraint (3) is dual to constraint (2) and models the reverse path.

$$distinct(x_1, \ldots, x_n) \tag{1}$$

$$\forall \ arc(f, T) \in Arcs : \bigvee_{i \in T} (x_i = x_f + 1) \lor x_f = n \tag{2}$$

$$\forall \ arc(f, T) \in Arcs : \bigvee_{i \in T} (x_i + 1 = x_f) \lor x_f = 1 \tag{3}$$

---

[1] Due to the significant propagation time, we used these constraints in [13] to benchmark the propagation performance of our constraint solver.

We have implemented the constraint model one-to-one with Mozart Oz finite domain constraints and used disjunctive combinators producing choice-points to obtain the same behavior as the program used in [4]. The search strategy is naïve, i. e., it picks from the left-most finite domain variable x_l the minimum element m and creates a choice-point $x_l = m \lor x_l \neq m$.

Deriving an Early-Failure Criterion. Deriving a criterion is a creative process and it is hard to give any guidelines. But it is helpful to have a tool handy that displays the constraints in a node of the search tree. Mozart Oz [9] offers a combination of such tools, namely the Oz Explorer [15] and the Oz Propagator Viewer.[2]

The figure shows a part of the constraints of a node of the search tree without early failure detection. One may notice the constraints $distinct(\dots, x_3, \dots, x_{10}, \dots)$ $\land 1 - x_2 + x_3 = 0 \land 1 - x_2 + x_{10} = 0$ (last two lines). Substitution of the two equations yields $x_3 = x_{10}$, which contradicts the con-

straint $distinct(\dots, x_3, \dots, x_{10}, \dots)$ (top line). Generalization of this observation leads to an early failure detection criterion: the set D contains all indices of variables required to be pairwise distinct (derived from the parameters of the $distinct$-constraint). The criterion is: $\exists C_1, C_2 : C_1 \equiv 1 + a_i x_i + a_j x_j = 0 \land C_2 \equiv 1 + a_k x_k + a_l x_l = 0 \land a_{i,j,k,l} \neq 0 \land i = k \land j \neq l \land j, l \in D \land a_j = a_l \rightarrow$ failure.

Adding the Early Failure Detection Criterion. The early failure detection code is completely factored out. It is embedded in the procedure `DetectFailureEarly` which is applied as soon as constraint propagation reaches a fix-point, i. e., right before the creation of a new choice-point.[3] The procedure reflects the constraints to their first-class representation `Cs` according to a normal form. The variable `EqCs` refers to the equational constraints and the variable `DistinctCs` to the pairwise distinct constraints. Then for each $distinct$-constraint a set D is computed and stored in the list of sets values `DistinctSets` (see [12] for details on integer sets in Mozart Oz). Here the implementation is more general than required for this example.

```
proc {DetectFailureEarly RootVars}
    Cs          = {Constraint.reflectSpace RootVars}
    EqCs        = {FilterEqualityConstraints Cs}
    DistinctCs  = {FilterDistinctConstraints Cs}
    DistinctSets = {ComputeDistinctSets DistinctCs}
```

---

[2] The Propagator Viewer is still experimental and not yet official part of the Mozart Oz distribution. It can be obtained from the author.

[3] Mozart Oz provides means to synchronize on reaching a propagation fix-point: A unary procedure can be passed to the search engine and this procedure is applied to the solution variable of a search problem as soon as a fix-point is reached.

Then two nested loops (procedures ForAllTail[4] and ForAll[5] applying anonymous procedures $) try to match the appropriate equational constraints according to the early failure detection criterion. An equational constraint is represented by a tuple ´=:´(P LHS RHS) where P is a reference to the actual constraint and LHS (RHS) is the left hand-side (right hand-side) of the equation. The left resp. right hand-side is represented by a list of addend tuples addend(Sign Coeff Var) where Sign is the sign (-1 or 1), Coeff is the absolute value of the coefficient, and Var is a reference to the variable.

Constraints of form $1 + ax + by = 0$ are isolated by pattern matching and the pattern for such a constraint is ´=:´(_ [A1 A2 A3] 0)[6] as it can be found in the **case**-statements.

```
  in
    {ForAllTail EqCs
      proc {$ Tail}
         case Tail of   (´=:´(_ [A X1 X2] 0))  |  T then
             {ForAll T
               proc {$ TC}
                  case TC of ´=:´(_ [B Y1 Y2] 0) then
```

After isolating two matching equational constraints the constant addends are compared and it is checked if the variables are in a D-set. The predicate Some is true if at least one of the elements of the list passed (here DistinctSets) evaluates the 2nd argument function to **true**.

```
                      if A == B andthen
                         {Some DistinctSets
                          fun {$ Set}
                              {VarIsInSet X1 Set}
                              andthen {VarIsInSet X2 Set}
                              andthen {VarIsInSet Y1 Set}
                              andthen {VarIsInSet Y2 Set}
                          end}
                      then
```

Here the anonymous function $ checks if the variables of the addends are in one and the same D-set. It uses the predicate VarIsInSet which checks if a variable is in a given set. The connector **andthen** is a short-circuit conjunction.

```
                         if {IsEqAddend X1 Y1}
                                    andthen {IsNeqAddend X2 Y2}
                            orelse {IsEqAddend X1 Y2}
                                    andthen {IsNeqAddend X2 Y1}
                            orelse {IsEqAddend X2 Y1}
```

---

[4] The procedure {ForAllTail List Proc} applies the unary procedure Proc to all non-nil tails of list List.

[5] The procedure {ForAll List Proc} applies the unary procedure Proc to all elements of list List.

[6] Note that there is an order on the addends: the first one is constant, the next ones contain variables and the variables are subject to a certain order.

```
                       andthen {IsNeqAddend X1 Y2}
                orelse {IsEqAddend X2 Y2}
                       andthen {IsNeqAddend X1 Y1}
             then fail % raise failure
             end
          end
       end % case
    end}
  end % case
end}
end % DetectFailureEarly
```

Finally, the variables of the addends are tested to meet the early failure detection criterion and if so, failure is raised by the statement **fail**. The predicate IsEqAddend (IsNeqAddend) tests if two addends are equal (not equal). The individual applications of IsEqAddend are connected by the short-circuit disjunction orthen.

Evaluation. Table 1 shows the effectiveness of the presented technique impressively. Entries '-' indicate that after 100.000 nodes of the search tree no solution was found and search was aborted.

Table 1. Effectiveness of early failure detection.

# nodes	no early failure detection solution found after # choices/# failures	with early failure detection solution found after # choices/# failures	# detected failures
10	72/52	72/52	0
20	-	160/124	1
30	-	298/244	68
40	-	499/406	162
50	-	499/406	162

By accident the results for problems with 40 and 50 nodes are identical. The first solution was found on a 200MHz Pentium Pro in a range from a tenth of a second till less than a minute depending on the problem. But the benchmarks aim at demonstrating the effectiveness of the technique, and the early failure detection code has not been particularly optimized.

Early failure detection requires constraints to be first-class values in order to reflect the state of the constraint solver for making symbolic detection of inconsistent constraints possible.

4   Constraint Simplification

This section demonstrates another constraint programming technique made possible by first-class constraints. It is not unusual that a constraint model and consequently its implementation contains redundant constraints or constraints in a formulation that does not allow for the strongest possible propagation.

Consider the constraint $x + x = y \wedge x \in \{1, 2\} \wedge y \in \{3, 4\}$. Without exploiting the equality of the two variables on the left hand-side the constraint cannot deduce that the only valid instantiation is $x = 2 \wedge y = 4$. Hence the simplification $x + x = y \rightarrow 2x = y$ improves constraint propagation significantly.

This section reuses the Hamiltonian path problem defined in Sect. 3 but uses reified constraints instead of disjunctive combinators. A reified constraint connects a constraint C with a 0/1-variable B: $(C \leftrightarrow B) \wedge B \in \{0, 1\}$. Variable B is bound to $1(0)$ if C is entailed (disentailed). As long as B is unbound C does not add any constraints to the constraint store. In case B is bound to $1(0)$ the reified constraint is replaced by $C(\neg C)$. Reified constraints are used mainly for handling over-constrained problems, i.e., problems where not all constraints can be fulfilled at once, or for modeling disjunctive constraints as in the following case.

The Constraint Model and Its Implementation. The constraint model expresses the disjunctions by reified constraints. The parentheses "()" enclosing the equations indicate reification. Constraint (5) stands for the path from the starting to the ending node and constraint (6) for the same path in reverse direction.

$$distinct(x_1, \ldots, x_n) \qquad (4)$$

$$\forall\ arc(f, T) \in Arcs : \left((x_f = n) + \sum_{i \in T}(x_i = x_f + 1) \right) = 1 \qquad (5)$$

$$\forall\ arc(f, T) \in Arcs : \left((x_f = 1) + \sum_{i \in T}(x_i + 1 = x_f) \right) = 1 \qquad (6)$$

Deriving a Simplification Rule. In this case finding a suitable rule is easy. Regard the lines in the figure starting with the variables x_{16} and x_3. In both cases the corresponding constraints reify $1 + x_1 - x_2 = 0$. That makes it possible to equate x_{16} and x_3 and to discard a copy of $1 + x_1 - x_2 = 0$. In general $\exists (C_i \leftrightarrow B_i), (C_j \leftrightarrow B_j) :$ $C_i = C_j \rightarrow B_i = B_j \wedge discard(C_j)$.

```
— ⟶  Propagator Viewer: 93 propagators in space #1        · ⬚ ✕
Viewer
distinct( x1 x2 x17 x18 x19 x20 x21 x22 x23 x24 )
k29 <=> ( 1 + x2 - x24 = 0 )
x16 <=> ( 1 + x1 - x2 = 0 )
x37 <=> ( 1 - x2 + x24 = 0 )
x34 <=> ( 10 - x2 = 0 )
x32 <=> ( 1 + x2 - x22 = 0 )
x13 <=> ( 1 - x1 + x2 = 0 )
x10 <=> ( 1 - x1 = 0 )
x8 <=> ( 1 - x1 + x2 = 0 )
x5 <=> ( 10 - x1 = 0 )
x3 <=> ( 1 + x1 - x2 = 0 )
x73 <=> ( 1 + x23 - x24 = 0 )
x70 <=> ( 10 - x24 = 0 )
x68 <=> ( 1 - x22 + x24 = 0 )
```

The proposed simplification has two effects: it removes redundant propagation by discarding superfluous constraints, and it strengthens the constraint store by adding equality constraints.[7]

Adding Constraint Simplification. Constraint simplification is executed whenever propagation reaches its fix-point. It reflects the constraints of a computation space with `Constraint.reflectSpace` to obtain direct access to the constraints, and function `FilterReified` filters out all reified constraints $(C \leftrightarrow B)$ since the other constraints are

---

[7] In Mozart Oz equality is represented directly in the constraint store.

of no interest. The result is stored in `ReCs`. Furthermore, `FilterReified` generates a textual representation of C using `Constraint.toString` which is used as index for the dictionary `Dict` to easily identify reified constraints which are identical modulo the 0/1-variable B.

```
fun {SimplifyAndCollect RootVars}
   ReCs = {FilterReified {Constraint.reflectSpace RootVars}}
   Dict = {NewDictionary}
in
```

For each reified constraint the actual simplification is done in a `ForAll` loop which calls an anonymous procedure $. This procedure accesses the components of its argument by pattern matching: `I` is the textual representation index, `P` is a reference to the reified constraint itself, `C` the reified constraint, and `B` is a 0/1-variable. Note that `#` is the infix tuple constructor and hence `I#reified(P C B)` is a 2-tuple matched against the argument passed to the anonymous procedure.

```
   {ForAll ReCs
    proc {$ I#reified(P C B)}
       if {Dictionary.member Dict I} then
          reified(P1 C1 B1) = {Dictionary.get Dict I}
       in
          B1 = B
          {Constraint.discard P}
       else
          {Dictionary.put Dict I reified(P C B)}
       end
    end}
   % return 0/1-variables of the reified constraints
   {RetrieveBools Dict}
end % SimplifyAndCollect
```

Using `Dictionary.member` the procedure checks if a reified constraint is already stored under the textual representation index `I`. If so, the individual components of the entries are retrieved by pattern matching[8], the 0/1-variables are equated, and the constraint referred to by `P` is stated to be entailed by `Constraint.discard`. That is exactly what the simplification rule requires. In case the reified constraint is not yet stored in `Dict` a new entry is created by `Dictionary.put`. Finally, the 0/1-variables of the reified constraints are retrieved and returned by `RetrieveBools`.

The search strategy branches over the 0/1-variables of the reified constraints (5) and (6) returned by `SimplifyAndCollect` to stay as close as possible to the program used in Sect. 3.

Evaluation. The number of 0/1-variables coming from the reified constraints is significantly reduced by simplification. In combination with the additional equality constraints, this leads to an enormous reduction of choice points (see Table 2), even better than for early failure detection in Sect. 3.

---

[8] The return value of the function application `{Dictionary.get Dict I}` is matched against the tuple `reified(P1 C1 B1)` and the newly introduced variables `P1 C1 B1` are bound accordingly.

Table 2. Effectiveness of constraint simplification.

# nodes	no simplification solution found after # choices/# failures	with simplification solution found after # choices/# failures	# simplified constraints
10	292/288	4/2	26
20	-	19/0	60
30	-	19/94	118
40	-	2673/2632	158
50	-	122/73	199

Only for the graph with 40 nodes the number of choice points is much greater. This indicates that the search strategy used is not stable enough against variations of the problems, but this is not the focus of this paper.

Constraint simplification requires constraints to be first-class values in order to reflect the state of the constraint solver and thus making symbolic constraint simplifications possible.

5 Garbage Collection of Constraints

Usually constraint solvers collect redundant constraints as they become entailed by the constraints in the store. Even if their memory is not freed due the implementation of the solver, they are at least not rerun anymore if their parameters receive new basic constraints. For example, consider $x \leq y \wedge x \in \{0, \ldots, 3\} \wedge y \in \{3, \ldots, 6\}$, and suppose the $\leq$-constraint is entailed by the basic constraints $x \in \{0, \ldots, 3\} \wedge y \in \{3, \ldots, 6\}$ and is garbage collected. That is not always the case, as demonstrated for the no-overlap constraint in the tiling problem.

The Problem Description and the Constraint Model. A given number of square tiles has to be placed on a master plate (see figure). The tiles must not exceed the master plate along the x- and y-axis. This is enforced by the *capacity*-constraint which is not of interest here. Furthermore, the tiles must not overlap which is enforced by the *nonoverlap*-constraint. Consider the square tiles T_1 and T_2 with length l_1 and l_2. Their positions on the master plate are determined by their left lower corners (x_1, y_1) and (x_2, y_2) which results in the *nonoverlap*-constraint

$$x_1 + l_1 \leq x_2 \vee x_2 + l_2 \leq x_1 \vee y_1 + l_1 \leq y_2 \vee y_2 + l_2 \leq y_1. \tag{7}$$

The constraint (7) is encoded by the reified constraint

$$(x_1 + l_1 \leq x_2) + (x_2 + l_2 \leq x_1) + (y_1 + l_1 \leq y_2) + (y_2 + l_2 \leq y_1) \geq 1.$$

Note the $\geq$-constraint which is necessary since two tiles can be non-overlapping in both the x- and y-axis. This constraint causes the trouble regarding garbage collection since as soon as one of its reified constraints is valid the remaining three constraints could be discarded. But this is impossible without first-class constraints because a reified constraint cannot be discarded, it just reduces to its embedded positive or negative constraint.

Implementation Issues. The encoding of the *nonoverlap*-constraint by the procedure ImposeNonOverlap catches the references to the individual constraints involved, i. e., the reified ≤-constraints and the ≥-constraint. This is achieved by using the <--operator. The *nonoverlap*-constraint returns these references wrapped in the tuple nonoverlap(P0 [P1 P2 P3 P4]).

```
fun {ImposeNonOverlap X1 Y1 L1 X2 Y2 L2}
   B1 B2 B3 B4 P0 P1 P2 P3 P4
in
   P1 <- {(X1 + L1 =<: X2) = B1}
   P2 <- {(X2 + L2 =<: X1) = B2}
   P3 <- {(Y1 + L1 =<: Y2) = B3}
   P4 <- {(Y2 + L2 =<: Y1) = B4}
   P0 <- {B1 + B2 + B3 + B4 >=: 1}

   nonoverlap(P0 [P1 P2 P3 P4])
end
```

The procedure CollectNonOverlapConstraints is called when propagation has reached a fix-point. It receives as its argument a list of tuples produced by ImposeNonOverlap and checks for all tuples if the enclosed ≥-constraint is entailed by applying Constraint.isEntailed to P0. If so, the remaining reified constraints are determined to be entailed by Constraint.discard.

```
proc {CollectNonOverlapConstraints NonOverlapConstraints}
   {ForAll NonOverlapConstraints
    proc {$ nonoverlap(P0 Ps)}
       if {Constraint.isEntailed P0} then
          {ForAll Ps proc {$ P}
                        if not {Constraint.isEntailed P}
                        then {Constraint.discard P} end
                     end}
       end
    end}
end
```

Evaluation. Table 3 shows the number of reified ≤-constraints garbage collected for different instances of the tiling problem.

The third column shows the amount of memory saved which is in balance with the overhead imposed by the extra data structures used.

The proposed garbage collection scheme relies on first-class constraints for detecting redundant constraints and for explicitly discarding such constraints since they cannot be garbage collected yet by entailment.

Table 3. Effectiveness of constraint garbage collection.

# tiles	# collected constraints	saved memory
6	18	5K
9	44	11K
17	197	100K
21	1528	1.7M

6   Computing Minimal Sets of Inconsistent Constraints

Solving a combinatorial problem by constraint programming requires expressing the problem in terms of constraints, i.e., finding a constraint model, and implement the conceived constraint model as a constraint program for a concrete constraint solver. This process is prone to error. The first run of the constraint program frequently results in an immediate failure of the solver, caused by an inconsistent set of constraints. The set of constraints is usually large and only a subset is responsible for the failure. Hence, being able to find minimal inconsistent subsets of constraints of a given set of constraints may simplify debugging the above-described situation significantly. Note that there may be several minimal inconsistent sets of constraints since several errors may occur at once.

Idea. According to the model presented in Sect. 2, constraint propagation takes place in computation spaces. A failed space hosts an inconsistent set of constraints. Finding minimal sets of inconsistent constraints starts by reflecting the last consistent state of the failed computation space. Reflection comprises all basic constraints, i.e., constraints of the form $x \in D$ and $x = y$, and all propagators. Such a reflection makes it possible to restore the constraints of the last consistent state of the failed space in a fresh space. Since such a restoring would immediately result in a failure, the propagators are imposed as *inactive first-class propagators*, i.e., they are imposed with propagation turned off. A solution is a set of inconsistent propagators. Hence, the fresh space is appropriately wrapped to propagate its failure as solution. The starting point for searching a solution that all propagators are inactive. Search turns propagation successively on for every propagator and then checks whether the set of active propagators is inconsistent or not.

Implementation. The last consistent state of a failed computation space is reflected by `Constraint.reflectSpace` and equal variables are spotted by `Constraint.identifyParameters`. The reflected propagators are imposed as inactive first-class propagators using the `<-#`-operator in a fresh computation space to be able to catch failure. Furthermore, every propagator is assigned a unique integer identifier and is connected via its corresponding first-class value to a $0/1$-variable such, that constraining the $0/1$-variable to 1 (0) activates (discards) the propagator. That makes it possible to use the standard search library on finite domain variables. A possible solution is a set of integers denoting a set of inconsistent propagators.

We are interested in minimal sets of inconsistent constraints. Branch-and-bound search is used to ensure that new solutions are either a proper subset of an already found solution or a distinct set of inconsistent constraints. An appropriate order constraint, which ensures that new solutions meet the above condition, has to take into account two cases:

1. A new solution N is a proper subset of the current solution O, i. e., $N \subset O$ resp. $N \setminus C \neq \emptyset$ where $C = N \cap O$.
2. A new solution N is distinct to the set of inconsistent constraints O, i. e., $O \setminus C \neq \emptyset \wedge N \setminus C \neq \emptyset$ where $C = N \cap O$.

These two conditions can be collapsed to $O \setminus (N \cap O) \neq \emptyset$. The implementation of the order constraint uses Mozart Oz's finite set constraints [12].

A first minimal set of inconsistent constraints is found by starting with all propagator's propagation turned on and successively turning propagation off. As soon as turning a propagator inactive makes the set of active propagators not immediately inconsistent, this propagator is kept active. Thus, by processing all propagators once, a first minimal set of inconsistent constraints is found. Finding other possible sets requires backtracking to the first propagator turned inactive and turning this propagator active and continue search from there. The order constraint described above prunes the search space further by disallowing solutions subsuming already known ones.

Example. Consider the inconsistent set of constraints composed of the constraints $c_{1...5}$: $x <_{c1} y \wedge y <_{c2} z \wedge z <_{c3} x \wedge z <_{c4} u \wedge u <_{c5} x$. As one can easily see, there are two minimal sets of constraints that are not in a subset relation: $S1 = \{c1, c2, c3\}$ and $S2 = \{c1, c2, c4, c5\}$.

Expectedly, the search routine finds two solutions $S1$ and $S2$, as the corresponding search tree shows (see the rhombus-shaped nodes in the Mozart Explorer display [15] in Fig. 1).

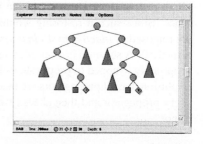

We use the Mozart Constraint Investigator [10] to present the solutions graphically. The first solution, corresponding to $S1$, is shown as a variable graph in Fig. 2(a), i. e., the nodes of the graph denote variables and edges represent propagators. Thick solid edges stand for propagators being part of the set of inconsistent constraints.

The propagator graph in Fig. 2(b) depicts propagators as nodes and variables shared be-

Fig. 1. Search tree of example.

tween propagators as edges between the respective propagators. Propagators being part of the inconsistent set of constraints are shaded. Having propagators, represented by their nodes, identified as being responsible for a failure, the Investigator allows to highlight their occurrence in the source code by simply clicking the respective propagator node.

The second solution, corresponding to $S2$, is shown as the variable graph in Fig. 3 and reveals a second reason for the example set constraints being inconsistent.

First-class constraints are the key to this application since they make it possible to reflect a failed computation space and to do search over constraints by explicitly turning propagation on and off.

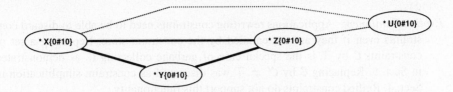

(a) Parameter graph where failed propagator edges are thick solid line.

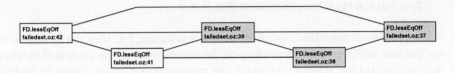

(b) Constraint graph where nodes of failed propagators are shaded.

Fig. 2. First solution (left-most solution (rhombus) node in Fig. 1).

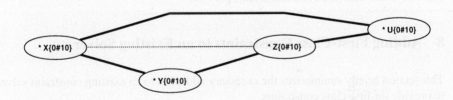

Fig. 3. Variable graph of second solution (right-most solution (rhombus) node in Fig. 1).

7   First-Class Constraints vs. Reified Constraints

This section summarizes the unique features of first-class constraints used in the presented applications and argues why the expressiveness of first-class constraints goes far beyond what can be expressed with reified constraints.

Reflection. First-class constraints make it possible to reflect the propagator's name and parameters to values. Reified constraints do not offer reflection.

Activation and Deactivation. Applications searching over sets of constraints (cf. Sect. 6) have to be able to impose propagators with propagation turned off and then to toggle propagation as computation proceeds. Initially, reified constraints ($C \leftrightarrow B \in \{0, 1\}$) are inactive w. r. t. propagation. Turning propagation on is done by constraining B to 1. But once turned on, propagation cannot be turned off due to monotonicity of reified constraints. [9] Although not mentioned so far, propagation of a first-class constraint C can be turned off by calling {Constraint.deactivate C}.

Explicit Entailment. Applications rewriting constraints need to be able to discard constraints even if they are not entailed by the constraint store. Replacing a set of constraints $\mathcal{C}$ by $\top$ is the special case of garbage collecting $\mathcal{C}$, as demonstrated in Sect. 5. Replacing $\mathcal{C}$ by $\mathcal{C}' \neq \top$ was discussed as constraint simplification in Sect. 4. Reified constraints do not support this functionality.

Checking for Entailment. It is frequently necessary to find out if a constraint is already entailed or not. First-class constraints provide the operation Constraint.isActive. Reified constraints can be used for entailment checking too, where $B = 1$ indicates entailment. The constraint $C \wedge (C \leftrightarrow B \in \{0,1\})$ does this test but it must be ensured that $B \neq 0$.

Operations on first-class constraints are non-monotonic, i. e., they can be undone or can produce different result depending on the current state of the computation space they are applied on. Reified constraints are monotonic, i. e., they *cannot* be undone and in conjunction with a certain set of other constraints they always reach the same fix-point. In fact, first-class constraints and reified constraints are *orthogonal concepts* and reified constraints can of course be first-class constraints too (cf. Sect. 5 where the *nonoverlap*-constraint uses reified first-class constraints). The use of the notion *meta* is somewhat misleading since true meta programming is only possible with the expressiveness that first-class constraints provide.

8   Adding First-Class Constraints to an Existing Solver

This section briefly summarizes the necessary additions to an existing constraint solver to provide for first-class constraints.

Promoting a constraint to first-class status means giving the programmer direct access to it and thus being able to inspect and control the constraint. This is straightforwardly done by introducing a data type referring to constraints.

Inspecting a constraint (cf. getName and getParameters in Sect. 2) requires being able to retrieve a constraint's parameters and name. Constraint solvers implemented in C++ typically represent a constraint as an object such that it is easy to add appropriate member functions and keep the changes local to the actual constraints.

Furthermore, first-class constraints need to have a unique identity to enable the check for equality of first-class constraints.[10] This can be done by deriving an identity from the memory address of the object representing a constraint. But care must be taken for garbage collection and all kinds of operations that change the location of a constraint in memory.

---

[9] Note that constraining B to 0 imposes the negative constraint $\neg C$.

[10] This paper ignores identity on first-class constraints. But if one has to implement reflect-Space just with the other operations, to guarantee termination one has to check equality of constraints.

Discarding a constraint and checking for entailment (cf. `discard` and `isEntailed` in Sect. 2) typically requires setting a flag in the constraint representation. The constraint solver has to check right before the execution of a constraint whether it was explicitly entailed in the mean-time, i. e., between wake-up and execution, or not.

The programming techniques presented in Sect. 3, Sect. 4, and Sect. 5 need to detect the fix-point of constraint propagation. Hence the constraint language has to provide a combinator that allows the programmer to do so. Implementation may simply check if the propagation queue, which maintains constraints to be executed next, is empty.

The experimental implementation of first-class constraints was straightforward since Mozart Oz provides so-called extensions. They are intended to allow the programmer to add new data types via a C++ interface [8]. There were no modifications necessary to the actual propagation engine such that there are no performance penalties.

9 Related Work

One approach at gaining more control and expressivity over constraints was the idea to exploit a constraint's truth value as proposed for the cardinality constraint in [18]. Applying arithmetic and boolean operations to constraint's truth values was explored in [1]. These constraints are usually called meta or reified constraints. They are available in nearly all current constraints solvers.

Meta-programming as known from Lisp or Prolog means manipulating a program by another program. Therefore, the program code is represented as a term of the respective programming language and then submitted to a meta-interpreter written in this language. Such a scheme for the constraint programming language CLP($\mathcal{R}$) is proposed in [5]. They use `quote` and `eval` functions which are analogous to the corresponding Lisp functions.

Solvers dedicated to a certain set of constraints as well as dedicated constraints can of course do the same analysis as discussed in this paper. In [4] early failure detection as described in Sect. 3 has been proposed as a by-product of analyzing the impact of simplifications for equational constraints on the propagation behavior.

ILOG Solver [7] is a C++ library for constraint programming in C++. It does not support first-class constraints as presented in this paper but ILOG Solver 4.4 allows the user to define a new constraint by defining a new class of constraints derived from the library class `IlcConstraintI`. It is straightforward to provide the required extra functionality according to Sect. 8 by adding appropriate member functions to the class definition of the new constraint.

Constraint Handling Rules (CHR) [3] are a committed-choice language for rewriting constraints towards a solved form which eventually denotes a solution. A CHR program is a set of guarded rules of the form $H \;\; op \;\; G \mid B$ where $op \in \{\texttt{<=>}, \texttt{==>}\}$, $H = H_1, \ldots, H_i$, $G = G_1, \ldots, G_j$, and $B = B_1, \ldots, B_k$. A multi-head H is a sequence of CHR, the guard G is a sequence of built-in constraints, and the body B is a sequence of CHR and built-in constraints. A rule fires as soon as a the CHR store implies H and the constraint store implies G. Then the CHR and constraint store are extended by B. A propagation rule ($op = \texttt{==>}$) extends the appropriate stores by redundant constraints B. A simplification rule ($op = \texttt{<=>}$) behaves like a propagation rule but additionally removes H from the CHR store. CHR can be used to implement the techniques proposed in Sect. 3 and Sect. 4 due to the multi-heads of the rules. For example, the inconsistent constraint $x < y \wedge y < x$ can be detected by the following CHR rule:

```
less(x,y),less(y,x) <=> true | false.
```

To the best of our knowledge none of the above-mentioned approaches, nor other existing systems, offer the same expressiveness or generality as the scheme proposed in this paper, to promote constraints to first-class status.

10   Conclusion and Future Work

We have introduced constraints as first-class citizens and investigated possible fields of application. Furthermore, we have demonstrated programming techniques using first-class constraints, have proved their effectiveness, and argued that first-class constraints and reified constraints are orthogonal concepts (cf. Sect. 7).

The experiments have shown that the programmer needs appropriate analysis tools to find powerful meta-constraint propagation rules especially for the techniques discussed in Sect. 3 and Sect. 4. Furthermore, the effects of simplification and garbage collection may overlap since simplified constraints become redundant and can be discarded.

The experiments were done with Mozart Oz using the Oz Explorer and the Oz Propagator Viewer. The experimental implementation of first-class constraint was straightforward since Mozart Oz provides adequate programming interfaces to extend the constraint solver's functionality easily from user level [8, 11].

Extending an existing constraint solver can be done with minimal effort and without performance penalties when first-class constraints are not used.

Acknowledgements. I am grateful to Warwick Harwey for discussing with me issues of early failure detection and pointing me to the Hamiltonian path problem as a suitable example. Katrin Erk, Leif Kornstaedt, Kevin Ng Ka Boon and Christian Schulte gave helpful comments on earlier versions of the paper. Furthermore, Christian brought the tiling example in Sect. 5 to my attention. Moreover, I am grateful to Ulrich Neumerkel for discussing ideas about inconsistent sets of constraints. The graphs in Sect. 6 were drawn with *daVinci* [17]. Last but not least I would like to thank the anonymous referees for their comments.

References

1. Frédéric Benhamou and William J. Older. Applying interval arithmetic to real, integer and boolean constraints. *Journal of Logic Programming*, 1997.
2. M. Dincbas, P. Van Hentenryck, H. Simonis, A. Aggoun, T. Graf, and F. Berthier. The constraint logic programming language CHIP. In *Proceedings of the International Conference on Fifth Generation Computer Systems FGCS-88*, pages 693–702, Tokyo, Japan, December 1988. Institute for New Generation Computer Technology (ICOT),Tokyo, Japan.

3. Thom Früwirth. Theory and practice of constraint handling rules. *Special Issue on Constraint Logic Programming, Journal of Logic Programming*, 37(1–3), October 1998.
4. Warwick Harvey and Peter J. Stuckey. Constraint representation for propagation. In M. Maher and J.-F. Puget, editors, *Proceedings of the Fourth International Conference on Principles and Practice of Constraint Programming (CP98)*, Lecture Notes in Computer Science, pages 235–249, Pisa, Italy, October 1998. Springer-Verlag.
5. Nevin Heintze, Spiro Michaylov, Peter J. Stuckey, and Roland H. C. Yap. Meta-programming in CLP($\mathcal{R}$). *Journal of Logic Programming*, 33(3):221–259, December 1997.
6. Martin Henz and Jörg Würtz. Using Oz for college timetabling. In E.K. Burke and P. Ross, editors, *Practice and Theory of Automated Timetabling, First International Conference, Selected Papers, Edinburgh 1995*, volume 1153 of *Lecture Notes in Computer Science, Springer*, pages 162–178. Springer-Verlag, Berlin-Heidelberg, 1996.
7. ILOG S. A., URL: http://www.ilog.com/. *ILOG Solver 4.4, User's Manual*, 1999.
8. Michael Mehl, Tobias Müller, Christian Schulte, and Ralf Scheidhauer. Interfacing to C and C++. Technical report, Mozart Consortium, 1999. Available at http://www.mozart-oz.org/documentation/foreign/index.html.
9. The Mozart Consortium. *The Mozart Programming System*. http://www.mozart-oz.org/.
10. Tobias Müller. Practical investigation of constraints with graph views. In Konstantinos Sagonas and Paul Tarau, editors, *Proceedings of the International Workshop on Implementation of Declarative Languages (IDL'99)*, September 1999.
11. Tobias Müller. The Mozart Constraint Extensions Reference. Technical report, Mozart Consortium, 1999. Available at http://www.mozart-oz.org/documentation/cpiref/index.html.
12. Tobias Müller and Martin Müller. Finite set constraints in Oz. In François Bry, Burkhard Freitag, and Dietmar Seipel, editors, *13. Workshop Logische Programmierung*, pages 104–115, Technische Universität München, 17–19 September 1997.
13. Tobias Müller and Jörg Würtz. Extending a concurrent constraint language by propagators. In Jan Małuszyński, editor, *Proceedings of the International Logic Programming Symposium*, pages 149–163. The MIT Press, Cambridge, 1997.
14. Jean-François Puget and Michel Leconte. Beyond the glass box: Constraints as objects. In John Lloyd, editor, *Logic Programming – Proceedings of the 1995 International Symposium*, pages 513–527. The MIT Press, Cambridge, December 1995.
15. Christian Schulte. Oz Explorer: A visual constraint programming tool. In Lee Naish, editor, *Proceedings of the Fourteenth International Conference on Logic Programming*, pages 286–300, Leuven, Belgium, 8-11 July 1997. The MIT Press, Cambridge.
16. Christian Schulte. Programming constraint inference engines. In Gert Smolka, editor, *Proceedings of the Third International Conference on Principles and Practice of Constraint Programming*, volume 1330 of *Lecture Notes in Computer Science*, Schloss Hagenberg, Linz, Austria, October 1997. Springer-Verlag, Berlin-Heidelberg.
17. Universität Bremen, Group of Prof. Dr. Bernd Krieg-Brückner. *The Graph Visualization System daVinci*. http://www.informatik.uni-bremen.de/~davinci/.
18. Pascal Van Hentenryck and Yves Deville. The Cardinality Operator: A new Logical Connective for Constraint Logic Programming. In Koichi Furukawa, editor, *Proceedings of the International Conference on Logic Programming*, pages 745–759, Paris, France, 1991. The MIT Press.
19. Pascal Van Hentenryck, Vijay Saraswat, and Yves Deville. Design, implementation and evaluation of the constraint language cc(FD). In Andreas Podelski, editor, *Constraints: Basics and Trends*, volume 910 of *Lecture Notes in Computer Science*. Springer Verlag, 1995.

Developing Finite Domain Constraints –
A Data Model Approach

Kit-ying Hui and Peter M. D. Gray

Department of Computing Science
King's College, University of Aberdeen
Aberdeen AB24 3UE, Scotland, United Kingdom
{khui|pgray}@csd.abdn.ac.uk

Abstract. We describe a technique for formulating a problem for solution by a finite domain constraint solver, where the finite domains can be modelled in correspondence with an Entity-Relationship diagram or UML Class diagram. This works particularly well where data for the problem is retrieved from database(s) over a network, but we believe the modelling discipline will be more generally useful. We show how relationships are conveniently represented using the *infers* operator of the *generalised constraint propagation* (*Propia*) library of ECLiPSe. Further, we can then express sets of quantified constraints over the data model in the declarative Colan language, and use this to generate equivalent ECLiPSe code directly. The user then has only to maintain the declarative version of the constraints, which are much easier to read. They can also be reused in many ways by fusing them with constraints from other sources, as in the KRAFT project. An important subclass of such constraints behave as conditional constraints which need delayed application, and we discuss experience in making such constraints more active in the solving process.

1 Introduction

Finite domain (FD) constraint solving is now a well established technique, and forms the basis of constraint logic programming (CLP) systems such as CHIP and ECLiPSe. However, even with the assistance of these packages, it is quite daunting for the average procedural programmer to use it. Thus, in the KRAFT project [8] we have been researching ways to generate CLP programs for FD solution from declarative constraint descriptions, that are much easier to read and understand. We also encourage the re-use of such descriptions by having them available over an extranet.

The unusual thing about our constraint descriptions is that they are expressed (and type-checked) against a data model that gives the semantics of the domain. Thus, many people think of an entity-relationship diagram (or UML class diagram) as being a useful diagrammatic guide and visualisation of the types of entities and relationships in a database (or an OO application), but they do not think of it as an operational basis for forming queries or specifications. However, in [7] we showed how quantified constraints can be expressed

J. Lloyd et al. (Eds.): CL 2000, LNAI 1861, pp. 448–462, 2000.

```
constrain each t in tutor
    such that astatus(t)="research"
no s in advises(t) has grade(s) =< 30;

constrain each r in residue to have
    distance(atom(r,"sg"),
      atom(disulphide(r),"sg")) < 3.7;
```

Fig. 1. The above examples demonstrate how Daplex/Colan [1] expresses a constraint on a university database containing student records. The same constraint language is applicable to the domain of protein structure modelling, as in the example restricting bond lengths.

in a very readable form of first order logic, including evaluable functions. An example is given in figure 1. Here a variable t ranges over an entity type **tutor**. which is populated with stored object instances. Each of these instances may be related to instances of student entities through the relationship **advises**. These entities can be restricted by the values of attributes such as **grade**. There are also other entity types such as **residue** (representing parts of protein chains) which have method functions for determining distances by computation [1]. The constraint then expresses a formula of logic which is true when applied to all the instances in a database, or even to instances in a solution database which is yet to be populated with constructed solutions. In this latter case it is behaving as a specification, rather than as an integrity constraint.

The great advantage of this approach when formulating combinatorial problems is that each **entity** type forms the natural basis for one or more finite domains. The values in the domains become tokens or object identifiers for the objects themselves. They thus naturally have a finite set of values. The **attributes** of the objects may have continuous values representing spatial or temporal values. These values are considered as components of objects and held in tuples as constants or Prolog variables. They can be accessed and tested in the normal way. We do not need to map them onto finite domains unless the problem requires it. The instances of **relationships**, as described below, can be represented by asserted facts, just like tuples in a relational database table, referencing the object identifier values of the related objects. In this form we can use the *infers* construct, for *generalised constraint propagation* in the ECLiPSe *Propia* library, to prune values from the finite domains.

2   Specifying a CSP by Database Integrity Constraints

A constraint is an excellent declarative way to specify domain-specific semantic features in a particular data model. It is an important abstraction which extends a data model in various ways so that it can address questions of importance today, in the era of the Internet. Recently, it has also been realised that constraints

---

[1] A fuller description is given in http://www.csd.abdn.ac.uk/~pfdm

are a highly suitable representation for knowledge in distributed agent-based applications [2], enabling novel approaches to the solution of design and configuration problems. When used as mobile knowledge which is exported and attached to data, constraints restrict the way in which the data can be used and form relationships with other objects. This mobility, together with its declarativeness, allows constraints to be transported, transformed, combined and manipulated in a distributed environment.

We have chosen to use the Colan language [1] developed for the P/FDM functional database system because it is based on Shipman's Daplex language [11], which is being used for its original purpose of integrating data expressed in different local databases using different local schemas. We have found this constraint language (figure 1) to be independent of the problem domain and able to represent the knowledge stored in a variety of local data models. It has the power of first order logic with safe expressions restricted by mixed quantifiers over finite domains of objects stored in databases or finite subranges of integers. It also has much of the power of a functional programming language for recursive computation.

To specify a CSP by database integrity constraints expressed in Colan, we visualise a *solution database* which is empty and yet to be populated by the solutions of a CSP, after it is solved. Figure 2 shows the ER diagram of our example *solution database* for configuring PC. We restrict the combination of values which can be stored and qualified as solutions to the CSP by imposing integrity constraints against the *solution database* schema, thus formalising the CSP specification. In practice, the *solution database* may simply provide a framework for CSP specification and does not physically exist or contain any data. Here are some example constraints imposed on the *solution database* and serve as CSP specifications:

```
constrain all p in pc
    to have cpu(p)="pentium2"

constrain all p in pc
    such that name(has_os(p))="winNT"
to have memory(p) >= 64
```

These example constraints expressed in Colan are quantified constraints with the last one being a *conditional constraint* which only applies when a certain condition is true. The implementation of *conditional constraints* and *quantified constraints*, which form the basic patterns of constraint specification in Colan, will be discussed in section 4. Note that, although we use a syntax originally devised for database integrity constraints, here we extend it to problems that need a CSP solver, not just a database engine.

To solve a CSP, we retrieve candidate data values from other populated databases, test them against the required constraints, and optionally store the qualified ones into the *solution database*. Candidate data in our example are usually provided by different vendors giving the available components for PC

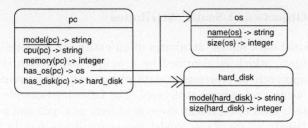

Fig. 2. In this ER diagram, we have three entities pc, hard_disk and os linked together by their attributes. The single-valued attribute has_os(pc) is represented by a single-arrow while the multi-valued attribute has_disk(pc) is denoted by a double-arrow. Attributes underlined are keys of their respective entity class.

configuration. For illustration purpose, we populate our single vendor database with the following values of partially configured PC, OS and hard-disk, although in real practice these candidate data may be stored in distributed databases:

pc object-id	model(pc)	cpu(pc)	memory(pc)	has_disk(pc)
pc1	"P5-120"	"pentium"	32	disk1, disk2
pc2	"P5-233"	"pentium"	32	disk2, disk3
pc3	"P2-333"	"pentium2"	64	disk3, disk4

os object-id	name(os)	size(os)
os1	"win95"	300
os2	"linux"	200
os3	"winNT"	500

hard_disk object-id	model(hard_disk)	size(hard_disk)
disk1	sg-256	256
disk2	wd-512	512
disk3	ib-1024	1024
disk4	ib-2048	2048

It is important to note that these values are originally stored in the vendor database instead of the *solution database*. Some attributes, like has_os, are not populated in the vendor databases as a configuration is not yet made. It is only when the CSP is solved that values for these attributes are determined and qualified values (as solutions) are copied into the *solution database*.

3   Compiling Data Objects into CLP Structures

A CLP program reasons over CLP data structures and therefore we have to compile constraints and data into their corresponding CLP program codes and data structures before the CLP system can utilise them.

3.1   Data Objects and Scalar Attributes

In the functional data model, attributes of an entity are modelled as functions on a data object, which is identified by a unique *object identifier*. A simple but flexible approach to represent a data object and its attributes in a CLP system is by using Prolog term structures. The following example shows how a pc/5 structure is used to represent three *pc* objects pc1, pc2 and pc3 with their respective attribute values of *cpu, model, memory* and *has_disk*. In this example, the *has_disk* attribute is multi-valued and contains the *object-id* of all related *harddisk* data objects as a list:

```
pc(pc1,'P5-120'pentium,32,[disk1,disk2]).
pc(pc2,'P5-233'pentium,32,[disk2,disk3]).
pc(pc3,'P2-333'pentium2,64,[disk3,disk4]).
```

Instead of using these facts as a passive test against instantiated values, ECLiPSe supports the use of a user-defined predicate (e.g. pc/5) as an active constraint by *generalised constraint propagation* [10]. The following ECLiPSe goal constrains the finite domain variables Pc, Model, Cpu, Memory and Disks to the value combination as specified by pc/5:

```
pc(Pc,Model,Cpu,Memory,Disks) infers most
```

An alternative representation is to model the relationship between an object and each of its attributes by a separate constraint. The following example shows how the object/2 and fnval/5 (meaning *'function value'*) term structures are used to represent data objects and the single-valued attributes model, cpu, memory, and the multi-valued attribute has_disk of the object pc1:

```
object(pc,pc1).
fnval(model,[pc],[pc1],string,'P5-120').
fnval(cpu,[pc],[pc1],string,pentium).
fnval(memory,[pc],[pc1],integer,32).
fnval(has_disk,[pc],[pc1],hard_disk,disk1).
fnval(has_disk,[pc],[pc1],hard_disk,disk2).
```

This approach offers a uniform representation across different entity classes and attributes by modelling the relationship between the input arguments and output value of a function. Type information is included to make it self-describing and to discriminate between overloaded functions. The single-tuple approach (e.g. pc/5), on the other hand, has to change its arity when the number of attribute changes in representing objects of different entity classes. As a result, we choose to use the fnval/5 structure to represent the attributes of a data object. Once these facts are established, we can use the following ECLiPSe goals to set up the constraints between the domain variables Pc, Model, Cpu, Memory and Disk:

```
object(pc,Pc) infers most,
fnval(model,[pc],[Pc],string,Model) infers most,
fnval(cpu,[pc],[Pc],string,Cpu) infers most,
fnval(memory,[pc],[Pc],integer,Memory) infers most,
fnval(has_disk,[pc],[Pc],hard_disk,Disk) infers most,
```

3.2   Relationships between Objects

In the functional data model, relationships between objects are modelled as attributes and thus are also represented as functions. Instead of returning scalar values, these functions return the *object identifiers* of the related data objects and we can use the same technique as described in section 3.1. The example in section 3.1 shows two *hard_disk* objects disk1 and disk2 are related to a single PC pc1:

```
fnval(has_disk,[pc],[pc1],hard_disk,disk1).
fnval(has_disk,[pc],[pc1],hard_disk,disk2).
```

Once again, the infers operator of *generalised constraint propagation* in ECLiPSe allows these facts to be used as an active constraint, like the following goal:

```
fnval(has_disk,[pc],[Pc],hard_disk,Disk) infers most
```

4   Constraint Compilation

4.1   Existentially Quantified Constraint

Quantified constraints in Colan [1] fall into two main categories. They are either *universally* quantified or *existentially* quantified. To facilitate the compilation of quantified constraints into CLP codes, we have implemented two meta-predicates forall/3 and exist/3. When supplied with the set of quantified variables and ECLiPSe code fragments compiled from the *generator* and *predicate* of a quantified constraint, these two meta-predicates behave as a *universal quantifier* and an *existential quantifier* respectively. They are defined in an ECLiPSe module to provide the required runtime support.

By default, a CSP implemented as a CLP program has an implicit *existential quantifier* over each involved variable. When we execute a CLP program and find the solutions to a CSP, we have found *"the existence of values in the value domains of the involved variables such that all required constraints are satisfied"*.

Assume that we want to restrict the existence of a PC in the *solution database* such that it has at least one installed hard-disk of a capacity greater than or equal to 1024 unit. This requirement can be written as a first-order logic expression:

$$(\exists p, d, s) \quad pc(p) \wedge harddisk(d) \wedge has\_disk(p, d) \wedge size(d, s) \wedge (s \geq 1024)$$

By searching for the existence of solution for variable Pc, Disk and Size, the following ECLiPSe program posts the same constraint:

```
post(Pc,Disk,Size) :-
    object(pc,Pc) infers most,
    object(harddisk,Disk) infers most,
    fnval(has_disk,[pc],[Pc],harddisk,Disk) infers most,
    fnval(size,[harddisk],[Disk],integer,Size) infers most,
    Size #>= 1024.
solve(Pc,Disk,Size) :-
    post(Pc,Disk,Size),
    indomain(Pc), indomain(Disk), indomain(Size).
```

Therefore, the `exist/3` meta-predicate can simply be implemented as:

```
exist(Variables,Generator_code,Predicate_code) :-
    call(Generator_code),
    call(Predicate_code).
```

where `Generator_code` defines the initial domains of the involved variables, and `Predicate_code` imposes the required constraint. `Variables` is the list of involved variables which are shared between `Generator_code` and `Predicate_code` and serve as a means to link the two program fragments.

Now our previous example can be expressed in term of the `exist/3` meta-predicate. Notice how the generator and predicate codes are linked by the shared variables `Pc`, `Disk` and `Size` and the use of the `infers` operator as discussed in section 3:

```
post(Vars) :-
    Vars=[Pc,Disk,Size],
    Gen_code=
        (object(pc,Pc) infers most,
         object(harddisk,Disk) infers most,
         fnval(has_disk,[pc],[Pc],harddisk,Disk) infers most,
         fnval(size,[harddisk],[Disk],integer,Size) infers most
        ),
    Pred_code=(Size #>= 1024),
    exist(Vars,Gen_code,Pred_code).
```

The following captured log shows how the domains of `Pc`, `Disk` and `Size` are reduced after the constraint is posted. `pc1` is removed as none of its `hard-disks` satisfies the requirement:

```
[eclipse 2]: post(V).
V = [_173{[pc2, pc3]}, _281{[disk3, disk4]}, _770{[1024, 2048]}]
```

4.2   Conditional Constraints

Conditional constraints are constraints which require their guarding conditions to be satisfied before the constraints are applied. A *conditional constraint* has the operational semantics of an *"if-then-else"* statement where we cannot decide which one of the two branches to take before the guarding condition is evaluated. The following example specifies that `"linux"` must be used when a `PC` has 64 units or more memory, otherwise the use of `"win95"` is enforced:

```
if memory(p) >= 64
    then name(has_os(p)) = "linux"
    else name(has_os(p)) = "win95"
```

We define a meta-predicate `if_then_else/4` on a set of variables with the testing condition and the two alternate branches of the decision. In general, there are two approaches to implementing a conditional constraint: passive or active. A passive approach delays evaluating the *guarding condition* until all variables are instantiated. This is similar to a generate-and-test strategy. An active one takes an aggressive approach to make its decision as soon as enough information is available, and if possible, without fully instantiating all the involved variables.

We use the technique of applying the *guarding condition* as a constraint and detect the change in the solution space, which is based on the fact that when there is a combination of variable values that fails the *guarding condition*, applying the *guarding condition* as a constraint either removes this combination of values, or creates a *delayed-goal* [2] . Applying the *guarding condition* as a constraint has three possible outcomes:

1. **The *guarding condition* fails to apply as a constraint**
   In this case, the *guarding condition* must fail as no value combination within the variable domains can satisfy it. Therefore, we execute the *else* branch of the conditional constraint.
2. **The *guarding condition* applies with delayed-goals**
   When the *guarding condition* applies with delayed-goals, it means some decisions cannot be made. In this case, we have to suspend our conditional constraint until more information is available.
3. **The *guarding condition* applies without any delayed-goal**
   When the *guarding condition* applies without any delayed-goal, we can proceed to detect any change in the solution space. If the solution space has changed, then the original variable domains must have some variable combinations violating the *guarding condition*. In this case, we have to suspend our decision until the variables are more constrained. However, if the solution space has not changed and there is no delayed-goal, then we are sure that no value combination in the variable domains will violate the guarding condition. In this case, we can safely execute the *then* branch.

Ideally, this approach allows us to evaluate the *guarding condition* as soon as possible without fully instantiating all domain variables. In actual implementation, however, we found that it is difficult to detect the potential change of the solution space without exploring all value combinations, which is not an efficient

---

[2] A delayed-goal in ECLiPSe is a goal waiting for a certain event to occur.

solution as we try to avoid instantiating any variable, if possible. Thus in real practice, we choose to suspend our decision even if there is no delayed goal in applying the *guarding condition* as a constraint. The *then* branch is only executed when all involved variables are ground and the condition gets evaluated. Even so, this will detect a failure of the condition earlier than a purely passive approach.

The evaluation of a conditional constraint is thus a loop of awakening and suspension until the *guarding condition* finally succeeds or fails (figure 3). To detect the presence of any delayed-goal in applying a constraint, we use the ECLiPSe predicate `subcall/2` which executes a constraint and gets the list of introduced delayed-goals. Now the need to check for the presence of any delayed-goal in each iteration of the loop creates a technical problem. When the constraint is awakened, applying the *predicate* for a second time does not give us any new information if the constraint is already applied in a previous iteration. That means we should not apply the *guarding condition* in any previous iteration but only compute the possible change in domains and detect the presence of any delayed-goal introduced. This is an interesting problem as we have to know what will happen when a constraint (i.e. the guarding condition) is imposed without really applying it, thus performing a trial application of a constraint.

The key to this problem is the Prolog predicate `findall/3`. As `findall/3` finds all solutions to its non-deterministic goal by backtracking, it executes the goal that contains `subcall/2`, collects information and undoes it. As a result, delayed-goals and domain change information are collected but the constraint is finally undone, with the results of all constraint application instances in a list.

Figure 3 describes the implementation of the `if_then_else/4` meta-predicate. This solution of `if_then_else/4` works well with a 'suspension-aware' implementation of a quantified constraint and we can have a conditional constraint nested in the predicate part of a quantified constraint. The aggressive evaluation of the *guarding condition* encourages an early but decisive application of constraints which helps cutting down variable domains.

In general, the presence of conditional constraints in a CSP shifts the behaviour of the constraint solver from *prune-and-search* towards *generate-and-test*, as some decisions cannot be made until more constraint information is available. In the worst case, all constraints may have to be delayed until all variables are instantiated. However, the constraint solver should be able to give us the best combination of active and passive constraint processing by wakening constraints as soon as they are applicable. The suspension mechanism of ECLiPSe allows constraints to be posted together but processed at different time, only when they are ready. This differs significantly from a LP system where the order of constraint processing (consistency test) is determined by the order of constraint posting.

The following example illustrates the behaviour of the `if_then_else/4` meta-predicate. Notice that the *guarding condition* is compiled into a constraint when we call `if_then_else/4`:

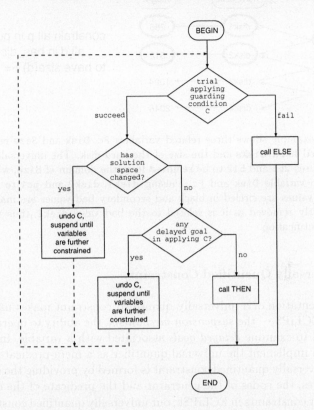

Fig. 3. The implementation of the meta-predicate if_then_else/4.

```
post_active([Pc,Os,Name,Memory]) :-
    object(pc,Pc) infers most,
    object(os,Os) infers most,
    fnval(has_memory,[pc],[Pc],integer,Memory) infers most,
    fnval(name,[os],[Os],string,Name) infers most,
    Vars=[Memory],
    If=(Memory #>=64),                %the 'active' test
    Then=(Name #= 'linux'),
    Else=(Name #= 'win95'),
    if_then_else(Vars,If,Then,Else). %call if_then_else/4
```

As soon as we post the extra constraint **Memory #< 64**, the correct OS is chosen:

```
[eclipse 2]: post_active(V), V=[Pc,Os,Name,Memory],Memory #< 64.

V = [Pc{[pc1, pc2]}, os1, win95, 32]
```

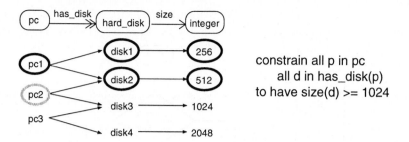

constrain all p in pc
all d in has_disk(p)
to have size(d) >= 1024

Fig. 4. This example shows three related variables Pc, Disk and Size representing a PC, its installed hard-disks and the size of the hard-disk. The universally quantified constraint causes 256 and 512 to be removed from the domain of Size, whose changes propagates to variable Disk and Pc, causing disk1, disk2 and pc1 to be removed. Primary bad values are circled in black and secondary bad values are marked in grey. pc2 is indirectly removed as it is related to the bad value disk2, thus violating the universal quantification.

4.3   Universally Quantified Constraint

Our implementation of a universally quantified constraint makes use of several facilities in ECLiPSe – the *suspension mechanism*, the ability to operate on *finite domains* and to examine *delayed goals* associated with a variable. In particular, we choose to implement the universal quantifier as a meta-predicate forall/3, so that a universally quantified constraint is formed by providing the set of quantified variables, the codes of the generator and the predicate of the constraint.

Like other constraints in ECLiPSe, our universally quantified constraint works by solution elimination, where values violating the constraint are removed from their respective domains. When the *predicate* part of the quantified constraint is imposed, some values are removed as a direct consequence. We call these values *primary bad values* as they are promptly removed by the constraint (figure 4). However, these *primary bad values* are not the only ones to be removed. If there are related variables which are also universally quantified, we also have to remove values that these variables will take which are associated with a *bad value*. These *secondary bad values* are indirectly removed by the universal quantification because of their relationship to the *primary bad values*. As the imposed constraint propagates through the related variables, this process of indirect value removal continues.

To achieve the desired behaviour of universal quantification, we have to collect information on the *bad values* that violate the required constraint, so that we can determine what values to remove, either directly or indirectly. We use the same technique as in the implementation of the *conditional constraint* (section 4.2), where we trial-apply a constraint and compute the difference of the involved variable domains before and after the constraint is imposed.

We have a loop of *suspension-and-awakening* until the *predicate* applies without any delayed-goal (see figure 5). This implementation encourages an early

utilisation of constraint information, which in turn allows an early triggering of
conditional constraints instead of waiting for variable instantiation. The overall
solving process is thus pushed towards a *prune-and-search* strategy rather than
generate-and-test. It also has the major advantage of being 'suspension-aware',
which allows the proper handling of nested *quantified constraints*.

Our example constraint requires all `hard_disk` installed in a `PC` to have a
size of `1024` units or more:

$$(\forall p, d, s)\, pc(p) \land harddisk(d) \land has\_disk(p, d) \land size(d, s) \longrightarrow s \geq 1024$$

The following ECLiPSe codes defines a predicate `post/1` which posts the
universally quantified constraint on variables `Pc`, `Disk` and `Size` with the meta-
predicate `forall/3`:

```
post(Vars) :-
    Vars=[Pc,Disk,Size],
    Gen_code=(
        object(pc,Pc) infers most,
        object(harddisk,Disk) infers most,
        fnval(pc,[pc],[Pc],harddisk,Disk) infers most,
        fnval(size,[harddisk],[Disk],integer,Size) infers most
        ),
    Pred_code=(Size #>= 1024),
    forall(Vars,Gen_code,Pred_code).
```

Here are the variable domains of the three variables `Pc`, `Disk` and `Size` after
calling `post/1`. Notice how `Pc` is instantiated by posting the constraint alone:

```
[eclipse 3]: post(V).
V = [pc3, _346{[disk3, disk4]}, _835{[1024, 2048]}]
```

5   Related Work

Early work in generation of CLP code from CoLan-style constraints is reported
in [3]. This shows how the classic eight queens problem can be described as constraints on sets of data values and then code-generated in CHIP. The emphasis
here is on how to deal with nested loops and other control issues. The data
model for this is very simple and does not include relationships, instead it just
compares numerical attributes:

```
constrain each q in queen to have row(q) in {1 to 8};
constrain each q in queen
  so that no q1 in queen has (q1 <> q and
  (col(q1)=col(q) or row(q1)=row(q) or
  abs(row(q1)-row(q)) = abs(col(q1)-col(q)) ));
```

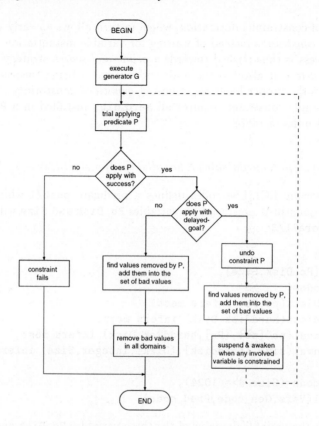

Fig. 5. The implementation of the meta-predicate `forall/3`.

The KRAFT project worked in a domain of configuration of telecommunication equipment, including various specialised subtypes of equipment and many complex relationships. Examples of various complex constraints that we have compiled are given in [5]. These may be more representative of real-life engineering problems than the commonly used examples of magic squares and eight queens. Another example of complex engineering assembly data that has been very neatly captured in an object-relational model [4] with a query language similar to ours is given in [9]. This is an area where scientists traditionally work directly in Fortran with large matrices passed to Finite Element packages; yet the data-model based representation interfaced to the FE package paid off in extra flexibility and scalability, and in clarity of problem formulation. By analogy, one should be able to use it with a constraint solver.

Recently Freuder, in an invited address [6], has identified modelling as "the transformation of the customer's statement of the problem into a form suitable for efficient processing by constraint algorithms or languages". He admits that it is largely a black art at present and calls for improved facilities, in order to get wider usage of CLP. This is echoed in a recent conference paper [12] including a simple declarative high-level language EaCL which is intended as a "solver-independent representation" for transmitting specifications across a net. Thus EaCL acts as a high level language in which to capture the problem, with aims similar to CoLan. Instead of using objects with attributes, as in our model, EaCL works directly in terms of named finite domain variables, possibly in an array. The ER model is, instead, naturally independent of the data storage representation. Thus there is a choice of whether to keep object attributes in one tuple or in several. There is also a choice of arrays or collections of tuples. This is a new field that is opening up, with many varieties of description yet to be explored.

6 Conclusions

The use of a Data Model is well established in the structured database world. Correspondingly Class Diagrams are a well established part of the UML modelling language used by object-oriented programmers. Thus people are increasingly used to relating data values to this formalism. Many combinatorial constraint problems that suit finite domains also have data in this form. We conjecture that many of these problems, especially in the area of configuration, are ripe for an automatic generation approach which would save the end user from maintaining CLP code.

We have described our own approach, as used in the KRAFT project, in the hope of encouraging others to follow suit. Once one has the idea of how to use a data model in this way, the details of how to generate the code are relatively straightforward. We have found the ECLiPSe system particularly suitable as a target, because of its use of generalised constraint propagation from stored data. Once one uses this framework, one can then see particular patterns in the generated code, which then call for improved performance. We believe that conditional constraints are one such pattern, and we have described a way to compile them into code that uses the constraint in a more active fashion. Certain kinds of universal constraint have similar considerations.

We believe that increased facilities for automatic generation of CLP are needed to make this technique more widely usable. As these get more widely used they will stimulate improved implementation of time-critical operations that are commonly generated. We look forward to future developments combining program transformation with improved algorithms to tackle the conditional constraint problem.

Acknowledgements

The work of Kit Hui was supported by grants from BT and EPSRC under the KRAFT project.

References

1. N. Bassiliades and P.M.D Gray. CoLan: a Functional Constraint Language and Its Implementation. *Data and Knowledge Engineering*, 14:203–249, 1994.
2. P.S. Eaton, E.C. Freuder, and R.J. Wallace. Constraints and agents: Confronting ignorance. *AI Magazine*, 19(2):51–65, 1998.
3. S.M. Embury and P.M.D. Gray. The Declarative Expression of Semantic Integrity in a Database of Protein Structure. In A. Illaramendi and O. Díaz, editors, *Data Management Systems: Proceedings of the Basque International Workshop on Information Technology (BIWIT 95)*, pages 216–224, San Sebastían, Spain, July 1995. IEEE Computer Society Press.
4. G. Fahl, T. Risch, and M. Sköld. AMOS — an Architecture for Active Mediators. In *Proc. Workshop on Next Generation Information Technologies and Systems (NGITS'93)*, Haifa, Israel, June 1993.
5. N. J. Fiddian, P. Marti, J-C. Pazzaglia, K. Hui, A. Preece, D. M. Jones, and Z. Cui. A knowledge processing system for data service network design. *BT Technical Journal*, 17(4):117–130, October 1999.
6. E.C. Freuder. Modeling: The final frontier. In *Proc. First Int'l Conf'ce on the Practical Application of Constraint Technologies and Logic Programming(PACLP99)*, 1999. London.
7. P. M. D. Gray, S. M. Embury, K. Hui, and G. J. K. Kemp. The evolving role of constraints in the functional data model. *Journal of Intelligent Information Systems*, 12:113–137, 1999.
8. P.M.D. Gray, A. Preece, N.J. Fiddian, W.A. Gray, T.J.M. Bench-Capon, M.J.R. Shave, N. Azarmi, M. Wiegand, M. Ashwell, M. Beer, Z. Cui, B. Diaz, S.M.Embury, K.Hui, A.C.Jones, D.M.Jones, G.J.L.Kemp, E.W.Lawson, K.Lunn, P.Marti, J.Shao, and P.R.S.Visser. KRAFT: Knowledge Fusion from Distributed Databases and Knowledge Bases. In R.R. Wagner, editor, *Proceedings of the Eighth International Workshop on Database and Expert Systems Applications*, pages 682–691, Toulouse, France, September 1997. IEEE Computer Society Press.
9. Kjell Orsborn. *On Extensible and Object-Relational Database Technology for Finite Element Analysis Applications*. PhD thesis, Linkoeping University, Sweden, 1996.
10. Thierry Le Provost and Mark Wallace. Generalised constraint propagation over the CLP scheme. Technical Report ECRC-91-1, ECRC, 1991. Also appears in *Journal of Logic Programming*, 16(3):319–359, 1993.
11. D.W. Shipman. The Functional Data Model and the Data Language DAPLEX. *ACM Transactions on Database Systems*, 6(1):140–173, March 1981.
12. E. Tsang, P. Mills, R. Williams, J. Ford, and J. Borrett. A computer aided constraint programming system. In *Proc. First Int'l Conf'ce on the Practical Application of Constraint Technologies and Logic Programming(PACLP99)*, 1999.

Concurrent Constraint Programming with Process Mobility

David Gilbert[1] and Catuscia Palamidessi[2]

[1] Department of Computing, City University
drg@soi.city.ac.uk

[2] Department of Computer Science and Engineering, Penn State University
catuscia@cse.psu.edu

Abstract. We propose an extension of concurrent constraint programming with primitives for process migration within a hierarchical network, and we study its semantics.

To this purpose, we first investigate a "pure" paradigm for process migration, namely a paradigm where the only actions are those dealing with transmissions of processes. Our goal is to give a structural definition of the semantics of migration; namely, we want to describe the behaviour of the system, during the transmission of a process, in terms of the behaviour of the components. We achieve this goal by using a labeled transition system where the effects of sending a process, and requesting a process, are modeled by symmetric rules (similar to handshaking-rules for synchronous communication) between the two partner nodes in the network.

Next, we extend our paradigm with the primitives of concurrent constraint programming, and we show how to enrich the semantics to cope with the notions of environment and constraint store.

Finally, we show how the operational semantics can be used to define an interpreter for the basic calculus.

1 Introduction

Concurrent constraint programming (ccp) [16] is a computational paradigm which combines the notions of concurrency and constraints. Classical ccp is based on a shared (constraint) store and, as such, it implies a centralized computational model.

In this work, we aim at enriching the ccp paradigm with the notion of localities, local stores and environments, and process migration. More precisely, we consider a distributed version of ccp where processes (or agents) run at specific sites, and have associated a local environment of procedure declarations, and a local store of constraints. The sites are organized hierarchically, and therefore an agent may contain sub-agents. The computation of a process only depends on its local code and data; however, a crucial characteristic that we wish to describe is the ability of an agent to *move* from site to site in the network, and bring along its environment and store.

J. Lloyd et al. (Eds.): CL 2000, LNAI 1861, pp. 463–477, 2000.

Our main goal is to provide a Structural Operational Semantics for such an extension of ccp, namely a semantics in which the behaviour of complex processes is defined in terms of the behaviour of their components. This results in the usual advantages for reasoning and for the definition of formal tools. In the long-term our motivation is to be able to describe and reason about the migration of *software agents* in a distributed system.

1.1   Process Migration versus Link Mobility

The term "mobility" has become associated with two meanings – firstly that of reconfiguring a network by changing the links or connections between nodes, and secondly the ability of a node within a network to migrate its position, thus also reconfiguring the topology of the network. In order to avoid confusion, we use *link mobility* to describe the former, and *process mobility*, or *migration*, for the latter. In this work, we are concerned with process mobility.

The classical work on link mobility is Milner's *π-calculus* [12]. Migration has been described by Cardelli [3,7], and formalized in work on *agent-passing* calculi, for example *Plain CHOCS*[17] and *Strictly-Higher-Order π-calculus* [14]. For a study of the correspondence between the two concepts, see Sangiorgi [15].

An important consideration in migration is that of locality, namely the explicit association between agents and specific sites. Several calculi supporting this notion have been presented recently; see for instance [5,6,10]. Of these, however, only Fournet et al's Distributed Join Calculus [10] treats locality in combination with migration. This is done in style of the Chemical Abstract Machine, by creating a flat model of local solutions with associated local names, and organising them as an implicit tree of nested locations. In contrast with [10], we describe migration in the SOS style, maintaining the network structure explicitly as it is done in [5]. Another difference with [10] is that we are able to describe migration to a sublocation, while this is not possible in [10].

1.2   Models of Mobile Computation

One can distinguish various types of mobile computation, which depend on the way the environment is treated under migration.

Following Cardelli [7], we regard a *closure* as the run-time description of a running procedure, i.e. the code plus the context of its execution. In general this context may include data, active network connections which are preserved on transmission, and new connections that are created to keep the closure in touch with the site that it has left behind.

With respect to the notion of closure, we can distinguish three increasingly richer models of mobility:

1. Code mobility only.
2. Mobility of *agents*, which are closures with contexts which lack link information. These agents do not communicate remotely with other agents, but move to some location and communicate locally there.

3. Mobility of general closures which include network connections (links), like in Obliq [8].

In this paper we focus on the agent mobility only. At the end of Section 3 we discuss possible extensions towards the last, most general model.

1.3   Distributed Concurrent Constraint Programming

To our knowledge, there have been only two previous proposals for distributed extensions of ccp: Distributed Oz [18] and Distributed ccp [13].

The proposal in [13] is based on the notion of agents computing within their local stores of constraints, and exchanging constraint abstractions through channels. A process receiving an abstraction applies it to its local variables, thus making a sort of local version of the received constraint. The dependency on global information is avoided by a static analysis of the program, giving the sufficient conditions under which the store of two agents can be divided in two local (independent) stores.

In [18] the notion of global and local information coexist: the computation of an agent mainly depend on local data, but the bindings on the shared logical variables are global and require handling by a distributed constraint solving algorithm. The main kind of mobility is cell mobility, namely the information content of a cell (a sort of imperative variable) can be exchanged between agents.

Neither [18] nor [13] deal with distribution and agent migration in our sense, i.e. by using an explicit notion of site, in a network organized hierarchically, and by transferring environment and store along with the code.

1.4   Structure of the Paper

The next section presents an abstract paradigm for the description of process migration between any two sites within a hierarchical network. Section 3 shows how the paradigm can be enriched to cope with the concepts of environment and constraint store, thus laying the foundations of concurrent constraint programming with process migration. Section 4 presents a simple (centralized) interpreter for the paradigm described in Section 3, and Section 5 discusses future work.

2   The Basic Paradigm for Migration

In this section we present our methodology for describing migrating agents within a hierarchically organized network. Our basic assumption is that the topology of such a network can be described as a tree, where each node is associated with a name n and contains an agent A. Names are unique only amongst peer nodes (sharing the same parent), and the unique address (*location*) of a node is given by the string π formed by concatenating the names of the nodes on the direct path from the root to that node. Thus we permit the same name to be used more than once in a system, and our calculus ensures that no ambiguity concerning addresses can raise when an agent migrates within the network.

An agent A in a node n can migrate to any other node m in the network. In this migration A is relocated together with all its subnodes and is inserted in m together with the agent B of m. The structure of the network can change as a result of this migration, for instance when a process which contains nested nodes migrates to a leaf node.

We assume two basic actions for migration: *go* and *fetch*. The first sends an agent to a node n at a specified location; the second gets a copy of an agent from a node n at a specified location, leaving the agent available for another request. We think that this naturally formulates "go" instructions and "fetch" requests. In both cases we specify the location by giving the path to n starting from the first (i.e. lowest in the tree) common ancestor of n and the node m which is performing the action. We will call this path the *relative address* from the point of view of m, and the *sub-address* from the point of view of the ancestor.

The syntax of our basic calculus is specified by the following grammar, where the symbol $\|$ represents the usual parallel operator and $\mathbf{0}$ represents inaction:

$$Agents \ A ::= \mathbf{0} \mid node(n, A) \mid go(\pi, A) \mid fetch(\pi) \mid A \parallel A$$

We assume the usual structural equivalences for the parallel operator:

$$A \parallel \mathbf{0} \equiv A$$
$$A_1 \parallel A_2 \equiv A_2 \parallel A_1$$
$$(A_1 \parallel A_2) \parallel A_3 \equiv A_1 \parallel (A_2 \parallel A_3)$$

The operational semantics is defined by a labeled transition systems whose configurations are agents and labels have the following form, where A is an agent:

- $s(\pi_f, \pi_t, A)$: send A from sub-address π_f to relative address π_t
- $r(\pi_f, \pi_t, A)$: receive A from relative address π_f to sub-address π_t
- $vs(\pi_f, \pi_t, A)$: virtual send A from sub-address π_f to relative address π_t
- $vr(\pi_f, \pi_t, A)$: virtual receive A from relative address π_f to sub-address π_t
- $as(\pi_f, \pi_t, A)$: actual send A from sub-address π_f to sub-address π_t
- $ar(\pi_f, \pi_t, A)$: actual receive A from sub-address π_f to sub-address π_t
- $migrate(\pi_f, \pi_t, A)$: relocate A from sub-address π_f to sub-address π_t

The last three kinds of labels correspond to transitions that can be performed only by the first common ancestor of the nodes m and n between which the migration takes place. Basically, the idea is the following: when a node m executes an action $go(\pi_t, A)$, it performs a send transition $s(m, \pi_t, A)$. Correspondingly, the node n at the relative address π_t performs a virtual receive transition $vr(\pi_f, n, A)$, where π_f is the relative address of m from the point of view of n. This virtual transition is a "spontaneous initiative", i.e. it is generated by the agent $\mathbf{0}$ (always present in a node because of the equivalence $A \equiv A \parallel \mathbf{0}$).

These transitions propagate upwards in the tree until they hit a common ancestor. At this point the send becomes an actual send, matches with the virtual receive, and the migration takes place.

Table 1. Specification of labels and conditions for the propagation rule. The function hd gives the first element of a string.

ℓ	$Cond$	ℓ'
$s(\pi_f, \pi_t, B)$	$hd(\pi_t) \neq n$	$s(n\pi_f, \pi_t, B)$
$s(\pi_f, \pi_t, B)$	$hd(\pi_t) = n$	$as(n\pi_f, \pi_t, B)$
$r(\pi_f, \pi_t, B)$	$hd(\pi_f) \neq n$	$r(\pi_f, n\pi_t, B)$
$r(\pi_f, \pi_t, B)$	$hd(\pi_f) = n$	$ar(\pi_f, n\pi_t, B)$
$vs(\pi_f, \pi_t, B)$	$-$	$vs(n\pi_f, \pi_t, B)$
$vr(\pi_f, \pi_t, B)$	$-$	$vr(\pi_f, n\pi_t, B)$
$migrate(\pi_f, \pi_t, B)$	$-$	$migrate(n\pi_f, n\pi_t, B)$

During the upward propagation of $vr(\pi_f, \pi, A)$ the sub-address π of the virtual receiver is incrementally constructed, until it becomes π_t. Analogously, during the upward propagation of $s(\pi', \pi_t, A)$, the sub-address π' of the sender is constructed, until it becomes π_f. The actual send and the virtual receive can match only if the sub-addresses correspond, i.e. only if they are of the form $as(\pi_f, \pi_t, A)$ and $vr(\pi_f, \pi_t, A)$ respectively. Note that, strictly speaking, only one of these constructed address is necessary to test if the two actions match; we do it this way just for the sake of symmetry.

The mechanism for the $fetch(\pi)$ action is analogous: in this case its node will perform a receive transition and the node at the relative address π will perform a corresponding virtual send transition. Note however that $fetch$ and go are not symmetric to each other: go does not cause a duplication of the agent, while $fetch$ does.

The above ideas are formalized by the following rules, which specify the transition relation. λ represents the empty string.

The following four axioms introduce the send and receive, and their virtual counterparts.

$$(send) \quad go(\pi_t, A) \xrightarrow{s(\lambda, \pi_t, A)} \mathbf{0}$$
$$(receive) \quad fetch(\pi_f) \xrightarrow{r(\pi_f, \lambda, A)} A$$
$$(virtual \ send) \qquad A \xrightarrow{vs(\lambda, \pi_t, A)} A$$
$$(virtual \ receive) \qquad \mathbf{0} \xrightarrow{vr(\pi_f, \lambda, A)} A$$

The following rule specifies the upwards propagation of transitions in the tree structure:

$$(propagation) \quad \frac{A \xrightarrow{\ell} A'}{node(n, A) \xrightarrow{\ell'} node(n, A')} \quad Cond$$

In this rule, ℓ' and the side condition $Cond$ depend on ℓ as specified in Table 1.

The following two symmetric rules describe the actual migration:

$$(\textit{migrate}_{go}) \quad \frac{A_1 \xrightarrow{as(\pi_f,\pi_t,B)} A_2 \quad A_2 \xrightarrow{vr(\pi_f,\pi_t,B)} A_3}{A_1 \xrightarrow{migrate(\pi_f,\pi_t,B)} A_3}$$

$$(\textit{migrate}_{fetch}) \quad \frac{A_1 \xrightarrow{ar(\pi_f,\pi_t,B)} A_2 \quad A_2 \xrightarrow{vs(\pi_f,\pi_t,B)} A_3}{A_1 \xrightarrow{migrate(\pi_f,\pi_t,B)} A_3}$$

Note that, if the two nodes between which the relocation takes place are *not* along the same branch, then one can use more elegant rules for migration, modeling it as *handshaking* between the real and the virtual actions. More formally, the *migrate*$_{go}$ could be replaced by the following:

$$(\textit{migrate}'_{go}) \quad \frac{A_1 \xrightarrow{s(\pi_f,n\pi_t,B)} A'_1 \quad A_2 \xrightarrow{vr(n\pi_f,\pi_t,B)} A'_2}{node(n, A_1 \parallel A_2) \xrightarrow{migrate(n\pi_f,n\pi_t,B)} node(n, A'_1 \parallel A'_2)}$$

and analogously for the *migrate*$_{fetch}$.

This rule however does not cover the case of relocation between ancestor and descendant, because that situation cannot be described, in our paradigm, by using the parallel operator.

Finally, the rule for the parallel operator is the standard interleaving rule, refined by a condition intended to maintain the uniqueness of names among sibling nodes:

$$(\textit{parallel}) \quad \frac{A_1 \xrightarrow{\ell} A'_1}{A_1 \parallel A_2 \xrightarrow{\ell} A'_1 \parallel A_2} \quad names\,A'_1 \cap names\,A_2 = \emptyset$$

where the function *names*(A) gives all the names of top-level nodes in A. Formally:

$$\begin{aligned}
names(0) &= \emptyset \\
names(node(n, A)) &= \{n\} \\
names(go(\pi, A)) &= \emptyset \\
names(fetch(\pi)) &= \emptyset \\
names(A_1 \parallel A_2) &= names(A_1) \cup names(A_2)
\end{aligned}$$

We conclude this section with some examples illustrating how our model works.

Examples

In the following examples, for the sake of simplicity we omit null agents and represent the agent $node(n, 0)$ by $node(n)$, or (in the figures) by n:

(1) Reorganising a Branched Network to a Linear Network

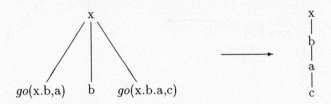

There is only one (strict) order of migrations:

$$node(x, node(x, go(x.b, node(a)) \parallel node(b) \parallel go(x.b.a, node(c))))$$
$$\xrightarrow{migrate(x,x.b,node(a))}$$
$$node(x, node(b, node(a) \parallel go(x.b.a, node(c))))$$
$$\xrightarrow{migrate(x,x.b.a,node(c))}$$
$$node(x, node(b, node(a, node(c))))$$

(2) Using Fetch

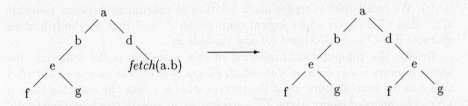

Again the reader can verify that there is only one order for migration commands to be executed

(3) Swapping Children Nodes Using Two Agents

In this case two different migration histories are possible:

1. $\xrightarrow{migrate(a.b,a.c,node(d))}$ ... $\xrightarrow{migrate(a.c,a.b,node(e))}$

2. $\xrightarrow{migrate(a.c,a.b,node(e))}$ ... $\xrightarrow{migrate(a.b,a.c,node(d))}$

3   Enhancing ccp with Migration

In the previous section we have dealt with the simple case of agents without environment or store. Of course, this is a very simplistic assumption. One of the main issues about migration is the formalization of the way a migrating process is inserted in to the environment of the host, how it interacts with the resources of the host, what are the scoping rules, etc.

In this section we investigate how the basic calculus for migration can be enriched with the notions of environment and constraint store, laying the foundations for concurrent constraint programming with process mobility.

Let us first recall the definition of ccp [16]:

$$\text{Agents } A ::= \mathbf{0} \mid tell(c) \mid \sum_{i=1}^{n} ask(c_i) \rightarrow A_i \mid A \parallel A \mid p(x) \mid \exists_x A$$

The c and c_i's are *constraints*, i.e. elements of a given constraint system $(C, \vdash)$. We recall that $\vdash$ represents a relation of entailment between elements of C, that C is closed under logical conjunction $\wedge$, and that a cylindrification operator $\exists_x : C \rightarrow C$ is defined for any variable x.

Briefly, the computational meaning of this paradigm is the following: the agents interact via a common *store* which ranges over C. The execution of $tell(c)$ adds c to the current store, i.e. if the current store is s then the resulting store is $s \wedge c$. The *guarded choice* agent $\sum_{i=1}^{n} ask(c_i) \rightarrow A_i$ selects nondeterministically one j such that $ask(c_j)$ is enabled in the current store s, i.e. $s \vdash c_j$, and then behaves like A_j. The agent $\exists_x A$ behaves like A, with x considered *local* to A. Finally, the agent $p(x)$ is a procedure call. Its meaning is given by a declaration of the form $p(y) :- A$.

In this presentation, taken from [16], there is a unique global set of declarations. Furthermore, although in the course of the computation some agents might obtain a local store, initially there is only a unique global store (this assumption makes it easier to describe the semantics). Since our purpose here is to study agent migration in the presence of a structure of environments and stores, we will enrich this paradigm with the possibility of associating local declarations and a local store with an agent (besides a local variable). More precisely, we will substitute the hiding construct $\exists_x A$ with the more general block construct:

$$block(D, X, s, A)$$

where D is a (possibly empty) set of local procedure declarations, X is a (possibly empty) set of local variables, and s is the initial (possibly empty) local store.

Thus the syntax of this extended ccp, enhanced with the migration constructs, will be:

$$Agents\ A ::= \mathbf{0} \mid tell(c) \mid \sum_{i=1}^{n} ask(c_i) \to A_i \mid A \parallel A \mid p(x) \mid$$
$$block(D, X, s, A) \mid node(n, A) \mid go(\pi, A) \mid fetch(\pi)$$

The operational semantics is defined via a labeled transition system as follows: the basic configurations are the blocks, the labels are only those introduced in Section 2, plus τ, which will label the transitions corresponding to the standard (unlabeled) ccp transitions. The transition rule for tell is similar to the one for standard ccp:

$$block(D, X, s, tell(c)) \xrightarrow{\tau} block(D, X, s \sqcup c, \mathbf{0})$$

The symbol $\sqcup$ here represents concatenation, and will be interpreted as logical conjunction when the store is checked for entailment. In [16] the corresponding rule uses logical conjunction directly. We need to distinguish the contribution made by an agent essentially to deal with the presence of an initial local store. This will become apparent in the rule for nested blocks.

The guarded choice rule is just the same as in standard ccp.

$$block(D, X, s, \sum_{i=1}^{n} ask(c_i) \to A_i) \xrightarrow{\tau} block(D, X, s, A_j) \quad s \vdash c_j$$

For the parallel operator, we have to add the condition on uniqueness of sibling names. The function $names$ extends to ccp in the obvious way (for the procedure call it gives the empty set and for the choice it gives the union of the names of all branches).

$$\frac{block(D,X,s,A_1) \xrightarrow{\ell} block(D,X,s',A_1')}{block(D,X,s,A_1 \| A_2) \xrightarrow{\ell} block(D,X,s',A_1' \| A_2)} \quad names(A_1') \cap names(A_2) = \emptyset$$

The procedure call is just the same as in standard ccp. In this rule, Δ_y^x is an elegant mechanism which links the formal and the actual parameter, and avoids clashes with other variable names in the network. See [16] for details. In our case, we will have to enrich it so that it also avoids clashes with sibling node names

$$block(D, X, s, p(x)) \xrightarrow{\tau} block(D, X, s, \Delta_y^x(A)) \quad p(y) :\text{-} A \in D$$

The rule for the block construct enriches the rule for hiding in [16] with the treatment of definitions in nested blocks, and with the distinction of the agent's contribution to the store, which is necessary for coping with the possibility of an initial (non empty) local store.

$$block(D_1 \lhd D_2, X_2, (\exists_{X_2} s_1) \sqcup s_2, A)$$
$$\xrightarrow{\ell}$$
$$\frac{block(D_1 \lhd D_2, X_2, (\exists_{X_2} s_1) \sqcup s_3, A)}{block(D_1, X_1, s_1 \sqcup \exists_{X_2} s_2, block(D_2, X_2, s_2, A))}$$
$$\xrightarrow{\ell}$$
$$block(D_1, X_1, s_1 \sqcup \exists_{X_2} s_3, block(D_2, X_2, s_3, A))$$

Here, $D_1 \lhd D_2$ represents the hierarchical union of D_1 and D_2, i.e. in case p is defined both in D_1 and in D_2, the declarations for p in D_2 override those in D_1.

The intuition behind the above rule is the following: In the internal block, the procedure declarations D_1 of the external block are visible, except for those which are "shadowed" by local declarations of the same procedure name (standard rule of scoping). The external store (s_1) is also entirely visible, except for the constraints involving variables with the same name as the local ones (X_2). The information about the shadowed external variables (X_2) is be filtered away by using the cylindrification operator $\exists_{X_2}$. Conversely, in the external block the information produced in the internal block $(s_2$ and $s_3)$ is entirely visible, except for the constraints involving the local variables. Again, this information is filtered away by using $\exists_{X_2}$. This way of treating the store is inspired by [16].

The rule for the node expresses that the environment of an agent in a node is the same as the environment of the node[1]:

$$\frac{node(n, block(D, X, s, A)) \xrightarrow{\ell} node(n, block(D, X, s', A'))}{block(D, X, s, node(n, A)) \xrightarrow{\ell} block(D, X, s', node(n, A'))}$$

Note that the premise of this rule is a transition between node agents. These will be considered auxiliary configurations and the rules for their transitions are the rules *propagation*, *migrate$_{go}$* and *migrate$_{fetch}$* of Section 2. The rule *parallel* is not needed.

Finally we have to adapt the rules *send*, *receive*, and their virtual counterparts. The following definitions formalize migration with dynamic scope, i.e. when a migrating agent brings with it only its internal environment, not its external one:

$$block(D, X, s, go(\pi_t, A)) \xrightarrow{s(\lambda, \pi_t, A)} block(D, X, s, \mathbf{0})$$
$$block(D, X, s, fetch(\pi)) \xrightarrow{r(\pi_f, \lambda, A)} block(D, X, s, A)$$
$$block(D, X, s, A) \xrightarrow{vs(\lambda, \pi_t, A)} block(D, X, s, A)$$
$$block(D, X, s, \mathbf{0}) \xrightarrow{vr(\pi_f, \lambda, A)} block(D, X, s, A)$$

---

[1] We could have simplified the syntax and the semantics by unifying the concept of node and block, i.e. we could have considered only one construct containing a node name, local declarations, local variables, local store and an agent. The reason why we did not do this is because we think of a node as a physical site which can host many parallel agents, each one with its own environment.

Note that we could model a more lexical kind of scoping rule by modifying the label of the send and the receive actions. For instance, the send rule would be written as

$$block(D, X, s, go(\pi_t, A)) \overset{s(\lambda, \pi_t, block(D, X, s, A))}{\longrightarrow} block(D, X, s, \mathbf{0})$$

In this way we export also the local environment and the store of the father. However note that this is a mixture of dynamic and lexical scope: to represent a purely lexical scoping rule, we would need closures.

3.1 An Example

We illustrate now our extension of ccp with an example. We assume dynamic scope, although in this example it does not really matter.

Assume that a seller, at address *root.a*, is willing to sell a certain good to the best offerer, by auction. Three potential buyers, at nodes *root.b*, *root.c*, and *root.d* respectively, are willing to buy the product, but are too busy to participate directly in the auction process. Instead, they send an agent to the site where the auction takes place. The agent will have certain parameters specified, like the increment for raising the bidding each time, and the maximum price the buyer is willing to pay. At the end, the auctioneer will send an agent back to each buyer to tell whether he has won the bidding or not.

The following process represents the auctioneer. For simplicity, we assume a very simple kind of auction, with only one round: all the offers are collected, compared, and the best one wins. We use $ask_X(c) \to A$ to represent the agent $ask(\exists_X c) \to tell(c) \parallel A$.

The following process represents the potential buyer at site *root.b*. The other buyers are similar, except possibly for the price offered (100) and the continuation process (A).

> *node*(*root.b*,
>   *block*($\emptyset$, {*price, answer*}, {*price* = 100},
>   *go*(*root.a, offer*(*b, price*))   ∥   *ask*(*winner*(*answer*) → *A*))

Note that, thanks to the mobility of the store, the information can be transmitted from the buyer to the auctioneer and viceversa. Thanks to the locality of the stores, there is no need of distributed constraint solving, and we can also ensure a certain privacy of the information; for instance, the winner's identity will not be available to the other buyers.

$$
\begin{aligned}
node(&root.a, \\
&block(\emptyset, \{pb, pc, pd\}, \emptyset, \\
&\quad ask(offer(b, pb) \wedge offer(c, pc) \wedge offer(d, pd)) \rightarrow \\
&\quad\quad ask_{pb,pc,pd}(pb \geq pc \wedge pb \geq pd) \rightarrow \\
&\quad\quad\quad go(root.b, tell(winner(yes))) \\
&\quad\quad\quad \| \\
&\quad\quad\quad go(root.c, tell(winner(no))) \\
&\quad\quad\quad \| \\
&\quad\quad\quad go(root.d, tell(winner(no))) \\
&\quad + \\
&\quad\quad ask_{pb,pc,pd}(pc \geq pb \wedge pc \geq pd) \rightarrow \\
&\quad\quad\quad go(root.b, tell(winner(no))) \\
&\quad\quad\quad \| \\
&\quad\quad\quad go(root.c, tell(winner(yes))) \\
&\quad\quad\quad \| \\
&\quad\quad\quad go(root.d, tell(winner(no))) \\
&\quad + \\
&\quad\quad ask_{pb,pc,pd}(pd \geq pb \wedge pd \geq pc) \rightarrow \\
&\quad\quad\quad go(root.b, tell(winner(no))) \\
&\quad\quad\quad \| \\
&\quad\quad\quad go(root.c, tell(winner(no))) \\
&\quad\quad\quad \| \\
&\quad\quad\quad go(root.d, tell(winner(yes))))))
\end{aligned}
$$

4   Interpreter

We have implemented an interpreter in SICStus Prolog based on the operation semantics defined in previous sections; the interpreter can be obtained over the Web at http://www.soi.city.ac.uk/~drg/migration. The software has been used as part of an undergraduate module on Software Agents given to final year Computing and Software Engineering students at City University.

Our implementation technique involves representing a transition rule in the form:

$$
\frac{A1 \xrightarrow{l_1} A_1' \ \dots \ A_n \xrightarrow{l_n} A_n'}{A_1 \xrightarrow{l} A_n'} \quad Condition
$$

by the Prolog clause

```
trans(A1,Label,name(Label,ObsA1,...,ObsAn),An'):-
    trans(A1,L1,ObsA1,A1'), ..., trans(An,Ln,ObsAn,An'),
    Condition.
```

Thus, for instance, the axiom

$$go(\pi_t, A) \; \overset{s(\lambda, \pi_t, A)}{\longrightarrow} \; \mathbf{0}$$

is represented by the unit clause

```
trans(go(To,A), s([],To,A), send(s([],To,A)),0).
```

and the rule

$$\frac{A_1 \overset{as(\pi_f, \pi_t, B)}{\longrightarrow} A_2 \qquad A_2 \overset{vr(\pi_f, \pi_t, B)}{\longrightarrow} A_3}{A_1 \overset{migrate(\pi_f, \pi_t, B)}{\longrightarrow} A_3}$$

is represented by the clause

```
trans(A1,migrate(Fr,To,B),migrate_go(migrate(Fr,To,B),OA,OB),A3):-
      trans(A1,as(Fr,To,B),OA,A2),
      trans(A2,vr(Fr,To,B),OB,A3).
```

Users can input an agent description as a Prolog term at the prompt; the interpreter will process this term and output a trace of

$agent_0 \; migration\_action_1 \; agent_1 \; \dots \; migration\_action_n \; agent_n$

and will offer to display alternative traces and final states (if these exist). The final state of the agent is also reported, which can be either *inactive* (contains no migration instructions) or *stuck* (contains migration instructions which cannot be processed, for example references to addresses which do not exist).

For instance, Example 3 of Section 2 is represented by the term

```
node(a,node(b,go([a,c],node(d,0)))//node(c,go([a,b],node(e,0))))
```

where the symbol "//" represents parallel composition.

If we give this term to the prompt, the interpreter responds in the following way:

```
History:
Scene:1 node(a,node(b,go([a,c],node(d,0)))//
                              node(c,go([a,b],node(e,0))))
Move: 2 migrate([a,b],[a,c],node(d,0))
Scene:3 node(a,node(b,0)//node(c,node(d,0)//go([a,b],node(e,0))))
Move: 4 migrate([a,c],[a,b],node(e,0))
Scene:5 node(a,node(b,node(e,0))//node(c,node(d,0)//0))
Inactive final state
New Network=node(a,node(b,node(e,0))//node(c,node(d,0)))
More solutions? ;
```

```
History:
Scene:1 node(a,node(b,go([a,c],node(d,0))))//
                                node(c,go([a,b],node(e,0))))
Move: 2 migrate([a,c],[a,b],node(e,0))
Scene:3 node(a,node(b,node(e,0)//go([a,c],node(d,0)))//node(c,0))
Move: 4 migrate([a,b],[a,c],node(d,0))
Scene:5 node(a,node(b,node(e,0)//0)//node(c,node(d,0)))
Inactive final state
New Network=node(a,node(b,node(e,0))//node(c,node(d,0)))
More solutions? ;

No (more) solutions
```

5 Future Work

In the present proposal names are "static entities". One might want to relax the side condition of the parallel rule and provide instead a renaming mechanism that renames a migrating node when it is going to be inserted in parallel with another node having the same name.

In our approach the paths contained in an agent do not change during migration. This means that the relative address specified by a path inside an agent will refer, after migration, to a location different than the one before migration. This might be regarded as undesirable. One direction of future work is to enrich the calculus so to ensure location invariance during migration.

One of the advantages of SOS semantics is that it helps in developing an algebraic theory of the language, based on the concept of bisimulation. This task is particularly facilitated when the rules are in the so-called De-Simone format [9, 11], or similar formats [4], since such formats ensures that bisimulation is a congruence. In our case the labels of the transitions contain agents and therefore we need to consider a sort of higher-order extension of the De-Simone format along the lines of [2]. In the future we intend to check whether the format of our rules is in some sort of extended De-Simone format for which the congruence theorem holds, and then try to determine the algebraic laws of the language following similar work done in first-order process algebras [1].

References

1. Luca Aceto, Bard Bloom, and Frits Vaandrager. Turning SOS rules into equations. *Information and Computation*, 111(1):1–52, 1994.
2. Karen L. Bernstein. A congruence theorem for structured operational semantics of higher-order languages. In *Thirteenth Annual IEEE Symposium on Logic in Computer Science*, pages 153–164, 1998.
3. K. Bharat and L. Cardelli. Migratory applications. In J. Vitek and C. Tschudin, editors, *Mobile Object Systems: Towards the Programmable Internet*, LNCS 1222, pages 131–148. Springer-Verlag, 1997.

4. Bard Bloom, Sorin Istrail, and Albert R. Meyer. Bisimulation can't be traced. *Journal of the ACM*, 42(1):232–268, 1995.
5. Chiara Bodei, Pierpaolo Degano, and Corrado Priami. Names of the π-calculus agents handled locally. *Theoretical Computer Science*.
6. G. Boudol, I. Castellani, M. Hennessy, and A. Kiehn. Observing localities. *TCS*, 114(1):31–61, June 1993.
7. L. Cardelli. Mobile computation. In J. Vitek and C. Tschudin, editors, *Mobile Object Systems: Towards the Programmable Internet*, LNCS 1222, pages 3–6. Springer-Verlag, 1997.
8. Luca Cardelli. A Language with Distributed Scope. *Computing Systems*, 8(1):27–59, Winter 1995.
9. R. de Simone. Higher-level synchronising devices in MEIJE-SCCS. *Theoretical Computer Science*, 37(3):245–267, 1985.
10. C. Fournet, G. Gonthier, JJ. Levy, L. Maranget, and D. Remy. A Calculus of Mobile Agents. In U. Montanari and V. Sassone, editors, *Proc. CONCUR'97*, LNCS 1119, pages 406–421, Pisa, Italy, August 1996. Springer-Verlag.
11. Jan Friso Groote and Frits Vaandrager. Structured operational semantics and bisimulation as a congruence. *Information and Computation*, 100(2):202–260, 1992.
12. R. Milner, J. Parrow, and D Walker. A Calculus of Mobile Processes. *Information and Control*, 100:1–77, 1992.
13. Jean-Hugues Réty. Distributed concurrent constraint programming. *Fundamenta Informaticae*, 34(3):323–346, 1998.
14. Davide Sangiorgi. *Expressing Mobility in Process Algebras: First-Order and Higher-Order Paradigms*. PhD thesis, Department of Computer Science, Edinburgh University, 1993.
15. Davide Sangiorgi. π-Calculus, Internal Mobility and Agent-Passing Calculi. *TCS*, 167(1,2):235–274, 1996.
16. Vijay Saraswat, Martin Rinard, and Prakash Panangaden. Semantic Foundations of Concurrent Constraint Programming. In *POPL 91*, pages 333–352. ACM Press, 1991.
17. Bent Thomsen. Plain CHOCS. A second generation calculus for higher order processes. *Acta Informatica*, 30(1):1–59, 1993.
18. Peter Van Roy, Seif Haridi, Per Brand, Gert Smolka, Michael Mehl, and Ralf Scheidhauer. Mobile objects in distributed Oz. *ACM Transactions on Programming Languages and Systems*, 19(5):804–851, 1997.

A System for Tabled Constraint Logic Programming

Baoqiu Cui and David S. Warren

Department of Computer Science
SUNY at Stony Brook
Stony Brook, NY 11794-4400, U.S.A.
{cbaoqiu,warren}@cs.sunysb.edu

Abstract. As extensions to traditional logic programming, both tabling and Constraint Logic Programming (CLP) have proven powerful tools in many areas. They make logic programming more efficient and more declarative. However, combining the techniques of tabling and constraint solving is still a relatively new research area. In this paper, we show how to build a *Tabled Constraint Logic Programming* (*TCLP*) system based on XSB — a tabled logic programming system. We first discuss how to extend XSB with the fundamental mechanism of constraint solving, basically the introduction of attributed variables to XSB, and then present a general framework for building a TCLP system. An interface among the XSB tabling engine, the corresponding constraint solver, and the user's program is designed to fully utilize the power of tabling in TCLP programs.

1 Introduction

As two separate research directions within the area of Logic Programming (LP), tabling and Constraint Logic Programming (CLP) have long been studied. Both of them have proven to be powerful tools and have made logic programming more efficient and more declarative.

Since its introduction in logic programming [21], tabling (also called *memoing*) has been used in many areas [23]. It can not only avoid redundant computations and many infinite loops, but can also, through tabled aggregation [20], give an easy way to find the optimal solutions for some problems. Tabling for pure logic programming has been implemented in the XSB system [19,4].

CLP is a natural extension of LP, and has gained much success since the late 1980's. Stemming from LP, CLP is a new class of programming languages which applies efficient constraint solving techniques to increase the power and declarativity of LP. Just like a classic logic programming system, a CLP system can also benefit from the power of tabling — the ability to avoid redundant computations and infinite loops and to find the optimal solutions. In other words, tabling can further increase the declarativity of a CLP system. Some mostly theoretical work has been done to combine tabling and constraint solving. For example, tabling has been applied to the constraint extensions of Datalog in

J. Lloyd et al. (Eds.): CL 2000, LNAI 1861, pp. 478–492, 2000.
© Springer-Verlag Berlin Heidelberg 2000

[22] and to CLP in [12], a general scheme for the evaluation of constraint logic programs based on a tabling mechanism has been given in [2], and a tabling algorithm for CLP has been designed in [14]. However, no practical general framework for building a *Tabled Constraint Logic Programming* (*TCLP*) system has been constructed.

Having the best tabling engine, XSB is a very good candidate system to be extended to a TCLP system. However, prior to version 2.0, XSB did not have the features necessary to incorporate constraint solving. This motivated to the introduction of *attributed variables* to XSB.

In the early stage of constraint logic programming, constraint solving was "hard-wired" into a built-in constraint solver over a specific constraint domain. This implementation strategy makes it difficult to modify an existent constraint solver to build a new solver over a new domain. To build a constraint solver over a new domain, one has to start everything from scratch. This situation changed with the introduction of attributed variables. Attributed variables [11, 5, 6] are a new logic programming data type that associates variables with arbitrary attributes and supports extensible unification [7]. Because of the ability to store attributes, attributed variables can be used to represent user-defined constraints on the variables (usually a whole constraint store can be represented by a set of attributed variables). Attributed variables can extend the default unification algorithm in that, when an attributed variable is to be unified with a term (which can be another attributed variable), a user-defined *unification handler* (in a high-level language, like Prolog) is called to process the two objects to be unified and possibly change the attributes of the involved attributed variable(s).

Attributed variables have proven to be a flexible and powerful mechanism to extend a classic logic programming system with the ability to solve constraints, and they have been implemented in many constraint logic programming systems, e.g. SICStus [13] and ECL^iPS^e [1]. Based on attributed variables, logic programming systems have been enhanced by constraint solvers over rational and real numbers [8] and feature trees [16]. Also, attributed variables have been recently used in the implementation of a high level language to write constraint solvers — Constraint Handling Rules (CHR) [9, 10], where constraints are compiled into clauses and stored in attributed variables. Compared to CHR, using attributed variables to directly implement constraint solvers is as "constraint assembler" programming [10].

The flexibility of the attributed variable mechanism is the major reason why we chose it to introduce constraints to XSB. Another reason is that we want to make XSB a conservative extension of CLP, so that standard CLP programs run (reasonably) well on XSB. XSB is a conservative extension of Prolog in that it includes all functionality of Prolog: Prolog programs run well on XSB. For this reason we took relatively standard implementation techniques from CLP as a basis for our implementation of constraints in XSB. However, the interesting, important, and challenging aspect of the integration is the interaction between the tabling mechanisms and the constraint mechanisms, and whether this approach can result in a (reasonably) efficient TCLP system. This paper concentrates on the interaction of the implementation of the two mechanisms: constraints and tabling: the representation of constraints through attributed variables and the representation of tables as tries.

To introduce attributed variables to XSB, a new data type and a new type of interrupt have to be added to XSB (see [3]). More importantly, in order to copy constraints into and out of tables, we need to modify parts of the basic data structure of the tabling engine, namely the *tabling tries* and the *substitution factor* [17, 18], to support attributed variables. Tabling tries provide an efficient way to look up terms in a table or insert terms into a table, and the whole table space of XSB is divided into two parts: subgoal tables (a.k.a. *subgoal tries*) and answer tables (a.k.a. *answer tries*). Subgoal tables contain all the subgoal calls, while answer tables contain only the answer substitutions of the corresponding subgoal calls. (We call the answer substitutions the "substitution factor" since they are the only parts of the entire answer subgoal that need to be stored.) In a TCLP system, a subgoal call is associated with a set of constraints, and an answer is associated with a set of answer constraints. The two sets of constraints are normally represented by the same set of attributed variables, whose attributes in the call might be updated in the answer. Therefore, we have to keep the update information of attributed variables in the subgoal table and answer table. This requires the substitution factor to be extended to contain not only regular variables in the call, but also attributed variables in the call.

Having introduced attributed variables to XSB, it is possible to simply apply tabling to a CLP program in the same way we table a normal LP program: a subgoal (or answer), together with the constraints involved, is saved into or retrieved from the table as a regular XSB subgoal (or answer). The *identical* subgoal call (with the *identical* constraints) will never be computed twice. However there exist two drawbacks in this naive tabling. First, since only identical calls (or answers) are checked when they are saved into or retrieved from the table, in order to get any reasonable reuse of tables, constraints must be represented in a canonical form. Second, when a new call is made, only looking up the table for the equivalent call and then consuming the existing answers in the table cannot fully utilize the power of tabling, and the amount of table space required can be extremely large. In many cases, a new subgoal call can consume the answers of an old call in the table if the old call subsumes the new one. Allowing this kind of subsumption tabling can make more use of the tables and further reduce the amount of redundant computation [2].

In this paper, we shall present a general framework for building a TCLP system based on XSB using the idea of subsumption tabling. In this framework, an interface among XSB's tabling engine, the constraint solver, and the CLP programs is designed, which gives the user more control on how the tabling engine works on the tabled predicates. The interface is divided into two parts: one is at the point when a subgoal call is to be put into the subgoal table; the other is at the point when an answer is put into the answer table. In the first part, we can define what form of subgoals should be stored in the subgoal table: for example a goal more general than the specific call might be specified. In the second part, we can define what kind of answers to a certain subgoal should be considered new and stored into the answer table. This is done in a similar way in which table aggregation [20] is implemented.

The remainder of the paper is organized as follows: In Sect. 2, we explain how to extend XSB with attributed variables. We concentrate more on the modifications of tabling tries and substitution factor to efficiently support attributed variables. In Sect. 3, we discuss some new issues when constraints and tabling are combined. Then, we present the general framework for building a TCLP system in Sect. 4. An example of the application of this framework is shown in Sect. 5. Finally, we give the conclusion and future work.

2   Extending XSB with Attributed Variables

2.1   Basic Changes to the System

Since attributed variables are a new data type in XSB, a new cell tag, ATTV, is added to the system. An attributed variable is represented as a pair of words (as a list): the first word is a free variable, which can be further bound to another term; the second word is a regular Prolog term, which is the attribute of this attributed variable. A new type of interrupt, *attributed variable interrupt*, is added to XSB, so that whenever an attributed variable is to be unified with a non-variable term, an attributed variable interrupt is triggered, and then the high-level user-defined unification handler is called to finish the unification.

In this paper, we focus on how to extend tabling tries and substitution factor to support attributed variables. Other more detailed information about the implementation can be found in [3].

2.2   Modifications of Tabling Engine for Attributed Variables

In XSB, tabling tries are used as the basic data structure of the table. They provide an efficient way for term lookup and insertion. As constraints are stored in attributed variables, we have to extend tabling tries to support attributed variables in order to copy constraints into and out of tables. Moreover, being variables, attributed variables must be stored in the substitution factor. Since they have certain patterns of use, optimizations can be done for them. Thus we treat them specially in the substitution factor.

As attributed variables are represented as lists, they can be copied into tries as lists: the first word (the free variable) can be copied as a regular variable, and the second word (the attribute) can be copied as a normal Prolog term. However, this representation could store the attributes of an attributed variable multiple times if it appeared in a term multiple time. This could waste a lot table space if the size of the attribute is very big (say this attributed variable is involved in many complicated constraints). Basically, to support attributed variables in tries, two problems have to be considered. First, since attributed variables are treated as variables, they (including their attributes) have to be kept shared when copied into and out of tables. Second, because an attributed variable in the call might often not be updated in the answer, it is important not to construct its attribute again in the answer table. We need to find a way to share the unchanged attributed variables between the subgoal table and answer table.

In XSB without attributed variables, an array called *VarEnumerator* and a counter called *var_ctr* are used to keep track of all the variables encountered when we copy a term into a trie, so that variables are numbered and kept shared in tries. When a variable is encountered for the first time, it is bound to *VarEnumerator*[*var_ctr*] (and trailed) and *VarEnumerator*[*var_ctr*] itself is set to be a free variable. Then a node, $\overline{v_i}$ ($i = var\_ctr$), is put into the trie and *var_ctr* is increased by one. Later, if this variable is encountered again, it will be dereferenced to *VarEnumerator*[*i*]. Thus we can tell that it is an old variable, and a node, v_i, is inserted into the trie. Here, nodes $\overline{v_i}$ and v_i are two different types of trie nodes, which represent the first and a later occurrence of the *i*th variable in the term respectively.

Carefully designed, *VarEnumerator* and *var_ctr* can also be used efficiently to handle attributed variables in a similar way. The basic idea is that attributed variables and regular variables are numbered together and they share the use of *VarEnumerator*. To distinguish an attributed variable and regular variable in tries, a new type of trie node is added. When an attributed variable, X (see Fig. 1(a)), is encountered for the first time, its first word (the free variable) is bound to *VarEnumerator*[*var_ctr*] (and trailed) and *VarEnumerator*[*var_ctr*] is set to be a free variable (shown in Fig. 1(b)). Then a node, $\widehat{v_i}$ ($i = var\_ctr$), is put into the trie and *var_ctr* is increased by one. Node $\widehat{v_i}$ is the newly added type of trie node, which denotes the first occurrence of an attributed variable (the *i*th variable in the term). Following $\widehat{v_i}$, the attribute of X (pointed to by the cs cell) is copied into the trie as a normal term. Now, if this attributed variable is encountered again (from X' in Fig. 1(b)), it will be dereferenced to *VarEnumerator*[*i*] and treated as a later occurrence of a *regular* variable, so only one node, v_i, is inserted into the trie. The attribute of X is *not* copied into the trie again.

As we can see, the same type of trie node, v_i, is used for the later occurrence of a variable, no matter it is a regular variable or an attributed variable. This does not cause any confusion when a term is copied out of the table. We can tell whether a node v_i is a later occurrence of a regular variable or an attributed variable by the index *i*, because the first occurrence of this variable (saved in the trie as $\overline{v_i}$ or $\widehat{v_i}$) has been built in the heap and a tagged pointer to it has been saved in an array (similar to *VarEnumerator*).

The above described algorithm can be used directly to construct the subgoal trie. The numbering and sharing of attributed variables is shown in the following example.

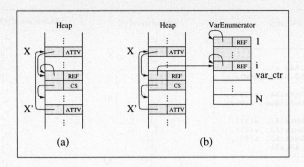

Fig. 1. How to number attributed variables and keep them shared in tries: (a) Before the new attributed variable X is processed; (b) After X is processed.

Example 1. Suppose we have a program and a query as shown in Fig. 2(a)[1]. After the query has been executed, the subgoal trie of p/5 contains only one subgoal and is shown in Fig. 2(b). In this subgoal, attributed variable A2 appears twice: the first occurrence is saved as $\hat{v_3}$ (since it is the third variable in the call) followed by the attribute a(2), while the second occurrence is saved as only one node, v_3.

Constructing the answer trie (e.g. the one shown in Fig. 2(c)) is more complex than constructing the subgoal trie. Because some attributed variables (e.g. A3 in Fig. 2(a)) in a subgoal call might not be changed in the answer, there is no need to construct these attributed variables again in the answer trie. Instead, we want to share them between the subgoal trie and answer trie. This can be achieved by initializing the array *VarEnumerator* and *var_ctr* in a special way before we copy an answer into the answer trie (see [3]). We reserve the first k elements of *VarEnumerator* for all the attributed variables in the call (assuming there are a total of k attributed variables in the call), and number all the new variables in the answer starting from $k + 1$. By doing so, we can use only one node, say v_i ($1 \leq i \leq k$), to represent an unchanged attributed variable in the call.

For example, in the program and query shown in Fig. 2, there are three attributed variables in the call of p(X,A1,A2,A3,A2): A1, A2, A3, among which A3 is not changed in the answer. Therefore, the first 3 elements of *VarEnumerator* are reserved for the three attributed variables, and *var_ctr* is initialized as 3. New variables in the answer, A2 (= A4) and New, are numbered 4 and 5 respectively (see the nodes $\hat{v_4}$ and $\hat{v_5}$ in Figure 2(c)). The unchanged attributed variable A3 is numbered 3 in the answer trie (since it is the third attributed variable in the call) and represented by a single node v_3.

---

[1] The predicate put_attribute(+ *Var*,+*Attr*) is a newly added built-in predicate. It changes *Var* to an attributed variable with attribute *Attr* if *Var* is a regular variable, or updates the attribute of *Var* to *Attr* if *Var* is already an attributed variable.

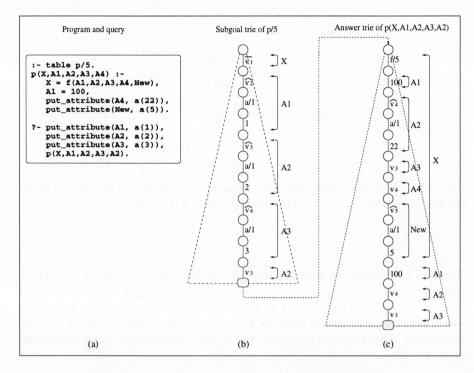

Fig. 2. An example of a subgoal trie and answer trie

3 Tabling and Constraints: Necessary Operations

To efficiently apply tabling to constraint logic programs, some general operations on constraints are needed from the constraint solver, e.g *projection* (or *approximate projection* [2]) and *entailment checking*, though they are not so important in a normal CLP system. Currently we only consider *ideal* CLP systems [14], i.e. we assume that complete algorithm are available for operations of satisfiability checking, projection, and entailment checking. For the constraint solvers in which projection operation is hard (or impossible) to get (e.g. the constraint solver over finite domains), approximate projection can be used but the completeness is not guaranteed [2].

3.1 Projection

In the execution of a query Q in a TCLP program, each call of a subgoal G (an atom) is associated with a set of constraints, a subset of constraints of the current constraint store which includes all the constraints accumulated so far since the beginning of the execution of Q. The basic idea of tabling is to try to avoid recomputing the subgoal G if it has been called in the same (or similar) environment before, where the environment of G is the related constraint set. Each call of a subgoal and the associated constraint set are stored in the table and act as an index. Therefore, the need for the projection of a set of constraints onto a finite set of variables appears. This operation is indeed necessary whenever putting a call or putting an answer into the table. When putting a call into the table, we want to restrict the constraint set to contain only related constraints, the constraints which contain only the variables in the called subgoal; when putting an answer into the table, it is also necessary to project out variables and constraints introduced during the subcomputation.

3.2   Entailment Checking

In a TCLP system, the operation to check if a set of constraints is entailed by another set of constraints is required for several purposes. Firstly, before a call is put into the table, we have to make sure that no call in the table is equivalent to this call, i.e., their associated constraint sets are not equivalent. Two sets of constraints are equivalent if they can be entailed by each other[2].

Secondly, when a subgoal is called, only checking if it has been called in *exactly the same* environment as before cannot fully utilize the power of tabling. It not only requires more table space, but also forces some unnecessary redundant computation. This is because, if a previous call can be entailed by the current call (i.e., the previous call subsumes the current call), then the answer of this previous call can be consumed by the current call, and it is possible that there is no need to recompute the current call. For example, if a call $p(X) \wedge \{X > 5\}$ is already in the table and an answer, $X = 10$, has been returned, then a new call like $p(X) \wedge \{X > 7\}$ can immediately use the answer $X = 10$ in the table, since the constraint $\{X > 5\}$ is entailed by $\{X > 7\}$.

Thirdly, before a new answer of a call is saved into the table, it has to be guaranteed that no duplicate answers are stored in the table. More generally, if there is already an answer in the table and it is entailed by the new answer, then the new answer can be discarded.

4   Our Solution: A General Framework

Given the necessary operations on constraints, we construct a general framework for building a TCLP system. This framework is domain independent and is parameterized by the constraint operations. The implementations of the domain dependent operations themselves are left to the developers of the different constraint solvers.

Basically this framework sets up an interface among the tabling engine of XSB, the constraint solver, and the CLP programs, and the purpose is to give the user more control over the tabling engine. Generally, this interface can be

---

[2] In some constraint solvers which always keep constraints in a canonical form, this operation may not be required, since two equivalent constraints are always identical.

divided into two parts. In the first part, the user tells the XSB engine what kind of calls should be stored in the subgoal table. The user could generalize a call even if it has not been seen before. If a more general call has been called before, a new call which is subsumed by this old call should, in general, not be put into the subgoal table. Instead it should consume the answers for the more general call. In the second part, the constraint solver tells the XSB engine what kind of answers should be considered new and put into the answer table. This can be done in a similar way in which tabled aggregation is implemented (we assume some familiarity with the implementation of aggregation in XSB, see [20]).

The interface consists of three *interface predicates*. The first two of them are provided by the constraint solver:

1. `projection(+TargetVars)`
   This is the constraint projection operation. It projects the current constraint store over a set of variables, `TargetVars`.
2. `entail(+Answer1, +Answer2)`
   This predicate is defined using the entailment checking operation of the constraint solver. Given two answers, `Answer1` and `Answer2`, to the call of a tabled predicate, this predicate checks if the first one entails the second one. We assume that answer constraints are represented within the answers using attributed variables.

The third interface predicate is:

3. `abstract(+OrigCall, −NewCall, −Constraints)`

which is the most complicated one. It controls what kind of calls of a tabled predicate should be stored in the subgoal tables, i.e., it abstracts the call, `OrigCall`, of a tabled predicate *Pred* to a more general call, `NewCall` (which has a new predicate, *TPred*), and only stores `NewCall` in the subgoal tables. Basically `abstract/3` relaxes the constraints related to `OrigCall`, and stores the constraints that are not passed to `NewCall` into `Constraints`. In other words, `OrigCall` is equivalent to the conjunction of `NewCall` and `Constraints`.

Just as XSB performs variant tabling and subsumptive tabling on pure Prolog [20], our framework supports two different kinds of basic call abstractions. The first one is called *variant abstraction*, which is the default one and does not actually do any useful abstraction. In this case, the arguments of `NewCall` are the same as the arguments of `OrigCall`, and `Constraints` is an empty list `[]`. So every different call pattern of *Pred* is stored in the table. The second kind of abstraction is called *subsumptive abstraction*. In this case, whenever a call, `OrigCall`, of predicate *Pred* is made, `abstract/3` looks up the current subgoal table of *TPred* to see if a more general call than `OrigCall` has been called before (using the projection and entailment checking operations from the constraint solver). If there is, then the more general call is returned in `NewCall`. Otherwise, `NewCall` just takes the arguments of `OrigCall`, and `NewCall` is saved into the subgoal table.

As long as projection and entailment checking operations from the constraint solver are correct and complete, these two kinds of call abstraction guarantee the correctness and completeness of user's programs. However, they are not always the best call abstraction, and sometimes the user might want to overwrite the system defined `abstract/3` if she knows more about the call patterns of some predicates. This is allowed in our framework, but the user must be aware that it is the user's responsibility to keep the correct semantics and the correctness of the programs.

Having the three interface predicates defined, we can transform the user's program so that it can make more use of the table. The transformation and how the interface works can be explained by the following example:

Example 2. Given a tabled constraint logic program P as shown in Fig. 3, which contains only one tabled predicate `p/n` and has two clauses for it, we can transform it into the program shown in Fig. 4. Without losing generality, we assume X1, ..., Xn are (attributed) variables.

In the new program, we introduce a new tabled predicate `'_$tabled_p'/n`, and rewrite the clause of `p/n`, so that the call of `p/n` is abstracted by `abstract/3` first (line 04), and then the abstracted new call (of predicate `'_$tabled_p'/n`) is called. The constraints abstracted out by `abstract/3` are put back into the constraint store and solved (by `solve/1`, line 07) before any answer is returned to the original call of `p/n`.

The new predicate `'_$tabled_p'/n` is defined similar to the tabled aggregation predicate `bagPO/3` in XSB. Lines 10 and 11 are two internal predicates to get the return skeleton (the substitution factor) of the current call. The predicate `entail/2` is used as a partial order operator to keep only the most general answers in the answer table (some older answers might be reduced by the new answer). Also, before a new answer is put into the answer table, the projection operation is called (by `projection/1`, line 25) so that only related constraints are stored in the answer table.

We have to point out that, in some programs, especially those to search the optimal solution of some problems, there is only one (i.e. the best) answer for a call, which is returned by combining the old answer in the table with the new answer. In this case, the predicate `'_$tabled_p'/n` can be defined similar to `bagReduce/4` in XSB [20], and the interface predicate `entail/2` has to be substituted by a predicate like `reduce/3`.

5   A Real Example

Based on the above design, we have built a tabled constraint logic programming system over the domain of real numbers. The constraint solver is the partially ported version of clp(Q,R) written by Christian Holzbaur [8], which is implemented using attributed variables.

In this section, by giving the example of the shortest distance problem, we show how to write a tabled constraint program in this TCLP system, and how the user's program is transformed.

```
:- table p/n.

p(X1,...,Xn) :- Body1.
p(X1,...,Xn) :- Body2.
```

Fig. 3. Original program P

```
01   :- table '_$tabled_p'/n.
02
03   p(X1,...,Xn) :-
04           abstract(p(X1,...,Xn),
05                    '_$tabled_p'(NewX1,...,NewXn), Constraints),
06           '_$tabled_p'(NewX1,...,NewXn),
07           solve(Constraints).
08
09   '_$tabled_p'(X1,...,Xn) :-
10           '_$savecp'(Breg),
11           breg_retskel(Breg,n,Skel,Cs),
12           copy_term(p(X1,...,Xn,Skel), p(OldX1,...,OldXn,OldSkel)),
13           '_$orig_p'(X1,...,Xn),
14           ((get_returns(Cs,OldSkel,Leaf),
15             entail(p(OldX1,...,OldXn),p(X1,...,Xn)))
16           ->      fail
17           ;       (findall(t(Cs,OldX1,...,OldXn,Leaf),
18                            (get_returns(Cs,OldSkel,Leaf),
19                             entail(p(X1,...,Xn),p(OldX1,...,OldXn))),
20                            List),
21                    member(t(Cs,_,...,_,Leaf),List),
22                    delete_return(Cs,Leaf),
23                    fail
24                   ;
25                    projection([X1,...,Xn]),
26                    true
27                   )
28           ).
29
30   '_$orig_p'(X1,...,Xn) :- Body1.
31   '_$orig_p'(X1,...,Xn) :- Body2.
```

Fig. 4. New program transformed from the program in Fig. 3

Problem: *Given two nodes, X and Y, in the directed weighted graph of Fig. 5(a) (each edge is associated with a weight, the distance between the two nodes of the edge), find the shortest distance between X and Y.*

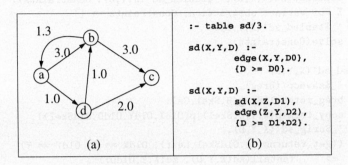

(a)

```
:- table sd/3.

sd(X,Y,D) :-
        edge(X,Y,D0),
        {D >= D0}.

sd(X,Y,D) :-
        sd(X,Z,D1),
        edge(Z,Y,D2),
        {D >= D1+D2}.
```

(b)

Fig. 5. Shortest distance problem

This problem can be solved by a TCLP program over the domain of real numbers shown in Fig. 5(b) (we omit the facts of `edge/3`). A call of `sd(+X,+Y,-Dist)` will return a sequence of answers, $D_1, \ldots, D_n$, for `Dist`, where each D_k ($1 \leq k \leq n$) is a constraint of the form `Dist >=` N_k. Each N_k is the *current achievable shortest* distance from X to Y, so we have $N_1 > N_2 > \ldots > N_n$, and finally N_n is the shortest distance from X to Y.

Since the call pattern of `sd/3` is general enough (see the second clause of Fig. 5(b), where the third argument `D1` is always a free variable), we can simply use the variant call abstraction. So the program shown in Fig. 5(b) is transformed to the program shown in Fig. 6 (the clause of `'_$tabled_sd'/3` is optimized for better performance).

Some running results of the transformed program are shown in Fig. 7. We can see that the shortest distance from a to c is 3.0, and the shortest distance from a to b is 2.0, all returned in the second answer. The shortest distance from d to a is 2.3, which is returned in the very first answer.

6   Conclusion and Future Work

As presented in this paper, we have introduced attributed variables into XSB and extended XSB with the basic mechanism to support constraint solving. By changing the data structure of subgoal table and answer table in XSB to support attributed variables, constraints can now be copied into and out of tables.

Based on such fundamental changes to the system, we constructed a general framework for building a Tabled Constraint Logic Programming System extending the tabling engine of XSB. This framework is domain independent, and it provides an interface among the XSB engine, the constraint solver, and the user's

```
:- table '_$tabled_sd'/3.

sd(X,Y,D) :-
        abstract(sd(X,Y,D),'_$tabled_sd'(X,Y,D), Constraints),
        % For variant abstraction, Constraints == []
        '_$tabled_sd'(X,Y,D),
        solve(Constraints).

'_$tabled_sd'(X,Y,D) :-
        '_$savecp'(Breg),
        breg_retskel(Breg,3,Skel,Cs),
        copy_term(p(X,Y,D,Skel),p(OldX,OldY,OldD,OldSkel)),
        '_$orig_sd'(X,Y,D),
        ((get_returns(Cs,OldSkel,Leaf), OldX == X, OldY == Y)
         ->     (entail(sd(X,Y,D), sd(X,Y,OldD))
                ->      delete_return(Cs,Leaf)
                ;       fail
                )
         ;      projection([D]),
                true
        ).

'_$orig_sd'(X,Y,D) :-
        edge(X,Y,D0),
        {D >= D0}.
'_$orig_sd'(X,Y,D) :-
        sd(X,Z,D1),
        edge(Z,Y,D2),
        {D >= D1+D2}.
```

Fig. 6. Transformed version of the program in Fig. 5(b)

| ?- sd(a,c,Dist).	| ?- sd(a,b,Dist).	| ?- sd(d,a,Dist).
Dist >= 6.0000;	Dist >= 3.0000;	Dist >= 2.3000;
Dist >= 3.0000;	Dist >= 2.0000;	no
no	no	

Fig. 7. Running results of the shortest distance program

programs. The user's programs are transformed at the source code level using the interface predicates, so that the transformed programs can make more use of the tables. Experiments have been done on the domain of real numbers (using the clp(Q,R) [8]), and this framework has been proven to work.

Future work includes:

1. Integrate the framework with constraint solvers over other domains;
2. Explore better ways to represent constraints using attributed variables over different domains, so that constraints can be stored more efficiently in tries;
3. Move some of the program transformation work into the engine level to improve the performance;
4. Apply our system to symbolic bisimulation of infinite-state systems, a formal verification problem requiring tabling and constraints [15].

Acknowledgements

This work is partially supported by NSF Grants CCR-9702681, CCR-9705998, and CCR-9711386.

References

1. P. Brisset, et al. *ECL^{i}PS^e 4.0 User Manual*. IC-Parc at Imperial College, London, July 1998.
2. Philippe Codognet. A tabulation method for constraint logic programs. In *Proceedings of INAP'95, 8th Symposium and Exhibition on Industrial Applications of Prolog*, Tokyo, Japan, October 1995.
3. Baoqiu Cui and David S. Warren. Attributed variables in XSB. In *Proceedings of Workshop on Parallelism and Implementation Technology for (Constraint) Logic Programming Languages*, pages 61–74, Las Cruces, New Mexico, USA, December 1999.
4. The XSB Group. The XSB logic programming system, version 2.0, 1999. Available from http://www.cs.sunysb.edu/~sbprolog.
5. Christian Holzbaur. *Specification of Constraint Based Inference Mechanisms through Extended Unification*. PhD thesis, Department of Medical Cybernetics and Artificial Intelligence, University of Vienna, 1990.
6. Christian Holzbaur. Metastructures vs. attributed variables in the context of extensible unification. In *International Symposium on Programming Language Implementation and Logic Programming*, LNCS 631, pages 260–268. Springer Verlag, August 1992.
7. Christian Holzbaur. Extensible unification as basis for the implementation of CLP languages. In Baader F. and et al., editors, *Proceedings of the Sixth International Workshop on Unification*, TR-93-004, pages 56–60, Boston University, MA, 1993.
8. Christian Holzbaur. *OFAI clp(q,r) Manual, Edition 1.3.3*. Austrian Research Institute for Artificial Intelligence, Vienna, TR-95-09, 1995.
9. Christian Holzbaur and Thom Frühwirth. Compiling constraint handling rules. In *ERCIM/COMPULOG Workshop on Constraints*, CWI, Amsterdam, The Netherlands, 1998.

10. Christian Holzbaur and Thom Frühwirth. Compiling constraint handling rules into Prolog with attributed variables. In *Proceedings of the 1999 International Conference on Principles and Pratice of Declarative Programming*, LNCS, Paris, France, September 1999. Springer Verlag.

11. S. L. Huitouze. A new data structure for implementing extensions to Prolog. In P. Deransart and J. Maluszyński, editors, *International Symposium on PLILP*, LNCS 456, pages 136–150. Springer, Berlin, Germany, August 1990.

12. Mark Johnson. Memoization in constraint logic programming. In *Proceedings of PPCP'93, First Workshop on Principles and Practice of Constraint Programming*, Rhode Island, Newport, April 1993.

13. The Intelligent Systems Laboratory. *SICStus Prolog User's Manual Version 3.7.1.* Swedish Institute of Computer Science, October 1998.

14. Fred Mesnard and Sèbastien Hoarau. A tabulation algorithm for CLP. In *Proceedings of International Workshop on Tabling in Logic Programming*, pages 13–24, 1997.

15. Madhavan Mukund, C. R. Ramakrishnan, I. V. Ramakrishnan, and Rakesh Verma. Symbolic bisimulation using tabled constraint logic programming. Submitted to TAPD'2000. Available from http://www.cs.sunysb.edu/~cram/papers/.

16. Bernhard Pfahringer and Johannes Matiasek. A CLP schema to integrate specialized solvers and its application to natural language processing. Technical report, Austrian Research Institute for Artificial Intelligence, Vienna, 1992.

17. P. Rao, I. V. Ramakrishnan, K. Sagonas, T. Swift, and D. S. Warren. Efficient table access mechanisms for logic programs. In L. Sterling, editor, *ICLP*, pages 697–711, 1995.

18. Prasad Rao. *Efficient data structures for tabled resolution.* PhD thesis, SUNY at Stony Brook, 1997.

19. K. Sagonas, T. Swift, and D. S. Warren. XSB as an efficient deductive database engine. In *ACM SIGMOD Conference*, 1994.

20. K. Sagonas, T. Swift, D. S. Warren, J. Freire, and P. Rao. *The XSB Programmer's Manual: version 1.9*, 1998.

21. H. Tamaki and T. Sato. Old resolution with tabulation. In *Proceedings of the 3rd ICLP*, pages 84–98, 1986.

22. D. Toman. Top-down beats bottom-up for constraint extensions of datalog. In *Proceedings of International Logic Programming Symposium ILPS'95*. MIT Press, 1995.

23. D. S. Warren. Memoing for logic programs with applications to abstract interpretatino and partial deduction. *Communications of the ACM*, 1992.

Finding Tractable Formulas in NNF

Edgar Altamirano and Gonçal Escalada-Imaz

Artificial Intelligence Research Institute (IIIA)
Spanish Scientific Research Council (CSIC), Campus UAB, s/n
08193 Bellaterra, Barcelona (Spain)
{ealtamir,gonzalo}@iiia.csic.es

Abstract. Many applications in Computer Science require to represent knowledge and to reason with non normal form formulas. However, most of the advances in tractable reasoning are applied only to CNF formulas. In this paper, we extend tractability to several classes of non normal formulas which are of high practical interest. Thus, we first define three non normal Horn-like classes of formulas $F_1 \wedge F_2 \wedge \ldots \wedge F_n$ where each F_i is constituted by a disjunction of two optional terms $F_i = NNF_i^- \vee C_i^+$: the first one is in Negation Normal Form (NNF) composed exclusively with negative literals and the second one is a conjunction of positive propositions. These formulas codify the same problems that the Horn formulas but with significantly, even exponentially, less propositional symbols. Second, we define sound and refutational complete inference rule sets for each class. Our third contribution consists in the design of a sound, complete and strictly linear running time algorithm for each class. As a result, the time required by our linear algorithms running on the defined non normal Horn-like formulas can be exponentially less than that required by the existing linear Horn-SAT algorithms.

1 Introduction

In some practical applications of Computer Science, the well-known Normal Forms CNF and DNF do not provide a natural framework to represent knowledge and to reason. In fact, performing inferences efficiently with formulas whose forms are non restricted to the classical ones is a matter of major interest in many practical applications inside very heterogeneous areas such as Expert Systems, Deductive Data Bases, Hardware Design, Automated Software Verification, Symbolic Optimisation, Logic Programming, Automated Theorem Proving, Petri Nets, Truth Maintenance Systems, etc.

However, most of the existing efficient proof methods are designed to work with CNF formulas. So, it is a common practice to translate knowledge representations from general forms to CNF's [10,36]. This transformation was originally proposed in 1970 by Tseitin [39] who published the first algorithm, later [25] included the case for first-order logic, [30] covered the cases for modal and intuitionistic logics, finally, Hähnle [22] investigated the problem of translating arbitrary finitely valued logics to short CNF signed formulas.

J. Lloyd et al. (Eds.): CL 2000, LNAI 1861, pp. 493–507, 2000.
© Springer-Verlag Berlin Heidelberg 2000

The translation procedure is in polynomial time if auxiliary propositions are allowed in the CNF formula but it takes exponential time otherwise. Thus, the principle of transforming a WFF in a CNF formula and then applying a CNF-based inference method has two important drawbacks [23]. First, translations procedures take several computational steps and easily can create an exponential growth of symbols even before inference procedures are applied. Second, there exist some efficient transformations methods based on substitutions of sub-formulas by literals preserving only the satisfiability relation but no other relations of practical interest, e.g. the logical equivalence relation.

In addition, interesting structures as Horn-like, that could exist in the original formulas can be lost in the transformed formula [38].

1.1   Our NNF Tractability Contribution

In spite of the large number of potential applications, few attention has been devoted to non-clausal reasoning. Thus, we present new results related to this field and more precisely to tractability with formulas in Negation Normal Form (NNF).

In this paper, we identify NNF formulas $F_1 \wedge F_2 \wedge \ldots \wedge F_n$ having a Horn-like structure. Each F_i is a disjunction of two optional terms, i.e. $F_i = NNF_i^- \vee C_i^+$: the first one is a NNF formula with only negated propositions, noted NNF^-, and the second one is a conjunction of non-negated atomic propositions, noted C^+.

The three classes of formulas we are proposing vary according to the expressiveness allowed to the NNF^- term from the simplest one, where the NNF^- is a disjunction of negative literals (clause form), noted D^-, the second, where the NNF^- is a disjunction of conjunctions of negative literals, i.e. $C_1^- \vee \ldots \vee C_k^-$ or DNF^- and the third class, with the NNF^- being a conjunction of disjunctions of negative literals, i.e. $D_1^- \wedge \ldots \wedge D_k^-$ or CNF^-.

The three classes of formulas can arise from an original non-clausal representation of the problem. These formulas are compact representations of Horn formulas given that they require less symbols than Horn formulas to codify identical problems; this reduction can be in an exponential rate.

Afterwards, we define sound and refutational complete inference rule sets for each class of formulas. Finally, we detail algorithms in pseudo-code with suitable data structures to resolve SAT-problems expressed in this kind of specified formulas. These algorithms are formally analysed and showed to be sound, refutational complete and a strictly linear running time. They are extensions of the pure Horn algorithms such as [14,29,21].

Although one could think that an alternative way to solve Horn problems would be to transform the Horn formulas to our class of factorised Horn formulas and then, to apply the algorithms exposed here, firstly the cost of the transformations should be analysed, which is beyond the scope of this paper. Thus, we stress the fact that the proposed algorithms are more appropriate for many real problems that require a non canonical representation.

Conversely, one possibility to solve non-clausal Horn-like problems consists in introducing artificial literals for transforming original problems in pure Horn problems and then applying Horn algorithms. But as mentioned previously, the logical equivalence property is lost and also, the cost of the transformations is not warranted to be done in strictly linear time.

This paper is structured as follows. In the next section we briefly review the research about tractable reasoning and related issues. In section three we define the ϕ class of non normal formulas which is our first extension of the class of Horn formulas. In sections four and five we deal with σ and ω classes which include as a particular case the ϕ class. For each of the mentioned classes, we specify a sound and complete set of inference rules and a strictly linear algorithm is detailed.

2   Related Work

Next, we revise the main works published concerning tractable reasoning. Thus, we review successively the existing results with CNF and NNF formulas.

2.1   CNF Tractability

The propositional satisfiability (CNF-SAT) problem is fundamental at the core in Computer Science. It was the first NP-complete problem found [12]. Since then, a rather big effort has been done do determine some CNF-SAT islands of tractability with significant repercussions in applications. The most important classes that can be resolved in deterministic polynomial time are: 2-CNF, for which linear algorithms were designed in [5,19,17], and Horn-SAT, that admits also linear algorithms as showed in [26,14,29,21,34,20]. Several variants of the Horn-SAT problem have been also found out to be solvable in polynomial time: renamable Horn [4,28], extended Horn [11], CC-balanced [13], SLUR [35] and q-Horn [9,8].

The Horn-SAT problem is polynomially solvable since the work of Karp [27]. After that, Henschen and Wos [24] showed that if a Horn formula is unsatisfiable, then, there exists a refutation proof employing unit propagation only. Jones and Laaser [26] showed that a direct implementation of this principle leads to an algorithm of quadratic complexity. Later, Dowling and Gallier [14] presented two linear algorithms to resolve the Horn-SAT problem: one with a forward chaining strategy and the second one based on backward chaining. In [34] and [20] it is proved that the backward algorithm is incomplete and not linear respectively. In [29,21,15,2] were proposed different linear versions, all of them based on a forward chaining strategy. A linear and complete algorithm with backward chaining strategy is described in [20].

2.2   NNF Tractability

Several methods have been developed to infer with formulas in NNF. This is the case of Matings [3], Matrix Connection [6,7], Dissolution [31,32], and TAS [1]. These methods give a step forward to show that deduction could be performed on formulas in non-clausal form avoiding thus, the transformation to normal forms. However, no studies relative to NNF tractability employing one of these methods have been carried out.

To our knowledge, the first published results concerning non-clausal tractability comes from [16,15,18] where a strictly linear forward chaining algorithm to test for the satisfiability of certain NNF formulas subclass is detailed. Such a class embeds the Horn case as a particular case. In [20] a linear backward algorithm is given for the same NNF subclass of formulas.

New results concerning NNF tractability are reported in [33] where a method called Restricted Fact Propagation is presented which is a quadratic, incomplete non-clausal inference procedure.

More recently, in [37,38] a significant advance in NNF tractability has been accomplished. The author define a class of formulas by extending the Horn formulas to the field of NNF. Such extension relies on the concept of polarity. A method to make inferences and potentially to detect refutational formulas is designed. In [37], a SLD-resolution variant with the property of being refutationally complete is showed but its computational complexity is not studied. In [38] a method for propositional NNF Horn-like formulas is described and it is stated that the method is sound, incomplete and linear. However, concerning the last issue, no algorithm is specified, indeed the steps of the method are described as different propagations of some truth values in a sparse tree. Then, although it seems that the number of inferences of the proposed method is linear, it is not proved the resulting complexity (w.r.t. the number of computer instructions) of a linear number of truth value propagations on the employed sparse trees.

A preliminary version of the contain of our current article has been presented in [2].

3 ϕ-Formulas

The ϕ-formulas are a direct extension of the Horn formulas in the sense that a Horn clause (disjunction of negative literals and at most one positive literal) is extended to include one conjunction of positive propositions instead of a positive proposition. The ϕ-formulas, permit us to represent a real problem with many less symbols, whereas keeping the good computational properties of Horn-like structure formulas

3.1   Syntax and Semantics

Firstly, we recall the required definitions of classical logic before introducing the first non normal class of formulas, denoted ϕ-formulas.

Definition 1. *A* literal *L is either an atomic proposition $p \in \mathbf{P}$, noted L^{+} or its negation $\neg p$, noted L^{-}.*

Definition 2. *A* classical clause *is a finite disjunction of literals: $(L_1 \vee \ldots \vee L_k)$. A* unit clause *$(L)$ includes only one literal. We denote the empty clause by $\square$.*

Definition 3. *A* Horn *clause is a classical clause with at most one positive literal. A* Horn formula *is a conjunction of Horn clauses.*

Notation. From now on, D stands for a disjunction of literals $(L_1 \vee \ldots \vee L_k)$ and C denotes a conjunction of literals $(L_1 \wedge \ldots \wedge L_k)$. D^{+} and C^{+} (D^{-} and C^{-}) include only positive (negative) literals.

Definition 4. *A* CNF *formula is a conjunction of disjunctions of literals $(D_1 \wedge \ldots \wedge D_m)$ and DNF is a disjunction of conjunction of literals $(C_1 \vee \ldots \vee C_m)$. Also, CNF^{+} and DNF^{+} (CNF^{-} and DNF^{-}) includes only positive (negative) literals.*

Definition 5. *A* clause *C^{ϕ} is a disjunction of two optional terms $C^{\phi} = D^{-} \vee C^{+}$: D^{-} is a negative disjunction and C^{+} is a positive conjunction. Clauses with only the D^{-} (C^{+}) term are said negative (positive) clauses.*

Remark. A clause $C^{\phi} = D^{-} \vee C^{+}$ is a Horn clause if $C^{+} = (p)$.

Definition 6. *A* ϕ-formula *is a finite conjunction of clauses C^{ϕ}.*

An interpretation I assigns to each formula ϕ one value in the set $\{0, 1\}$.

Definition 7. *An interpretation I satisfies:*

- *A literal p ($\neg p$) iff $I(p) = 1$ ($I(p) = 0$).*
- *A disjunction $D = L_1 \vee \ldots \vee L_k$, iff $I(L_i) = 1$, for at least one L_i.*
- *A conjunction $C = L_1 \wedge \ldots \wedge L_k$, iff $I(L_i) = 1$ for every L_i.*
- *A clause $C^{\phi} = D^{-} \vee C^{+}$, iff $I(D^{-}) = 1$ or $I(C^{+}) = 1$.*
- *A ϕ-formula if I satisfies all clauses C^{ϕ} of the formula.*

An interpretation I is a model *of a ϕ-formula if satisfies the formula. We say that ϕ is* satisfiable *if it has at least one model, otherwise, it is* unsatisfiable.

3.2 Inference Rules

In this section we introduce the two required inference rules to process ϕ-formulas: The Variable Truth Assignment (VTA) and the And Elimination (AE) and we show that both together form a sound and complete logical calculi.

Henceforth, ϕ and $\phi_{\square}$ represent respectively any ϕ-formula and any ϕ-formula containing the empty clause $\square$.

Definition 8. Variable Truth Assignment (VTA).
It consists in assigning true to a variable p. More specifically, if $(p) \in \phi$ then VTA derives a formula ϕ' obtained from ϕ by removing (p) and the occurrences of $\neg p$.

Definition 9. And Elimination (AE).
Inference rule AE derives from a positive conjunction clause $(p_1 \wedge \ldots \wedge p_i \wedge \ldots \wedge p_n)$, the unit clauses $(p_1), \ldots, (p_i), \ldots, (p_n)$.

Definition 10. Clause Proof.
A refutation of a formula ϕ, is a succession of formulas $< \phi_1, \phi_2, \ldots, \phi_n >$ such that $\phi_1 = \phi, \phi_n = \phi_\square$ and for each $1 \leq i \leq n-1$, either $\phi_{i+1} = TVA(\phi_i)$ or $\phi_{i+1} = AE(\phi_i)$.

Example 1. Let us $\phi = \{(p_1), (p_3), (\neg p_1 \vee (p_2 \wedge p_4)), (\neg p_2 \vee \neg p_3 \vee (p_1 \wedge p_5)), (\neg p_2 \vee \neg p_5)\} = \{(p_1), (p_3), C_1, C_2, C_3\}$. The inference chaining to get a formula with the empty clause is as follows:

$\{(p_1), (p_3), (\neg p_1 \vee (p_2 \wedge p_4)), C_2, C_3\}$
$\vdash_{TVA} \{(p_3), (p_2 \wedge p_4), C_2, C_3\}$
$\vdash_{AE} \{(p_3), (p_2), (p_4), (\neg p_2 \vee \neg p_3 \vee (p_1 \wedge p_5)), C_3\}$
$\vdash_{TVA} \{(p_2), (p_4), (\neg p_2 \vee (p_1 \wedge p_5)), C_3\}$
$\vdash_{TVA} \{(p_4), (p_1 \wedge p_5), (\neg p_5)\}$
$\vdash_{AE} \{(p_4), (p_1), (p_5), (\neg p_5)\}$
$\vdash_{TVA} \{(p_4), (p_1), \square\} = \phi_\square$

Theorem 1. Soundness. $\phi \vdash_{VTA+AE} \phi' \Rightarrow \phi \models \phi'$.

The proofs of the soundness of each rule are trivial and the proof of the theorem follows straightforwardly from those proofs.

Theorem 2. Completeness. *If ϕ is unsatisfiable then $\phi \vdash_{VTA+AE} \phi_\square$.*

The proof is by induction on the length of ϕ, i.e. the number of occurrences of literals in ϕ. The following theorem extends completeness to atomic clauses.

Theorem 3. Completeness. $\phi \models (L) \Rightarrow \phi \vdash_{VTA+AE} (L)$.

3.3 Algorithm Description

Initially, if ϕ has no positive unit clauses then it is satisfiable because all the clauses have at least one negative literal. So, assume that $(p) \in \phi$. Thus ϕ is satisfiable iff $\phi.\{p \leftarrow 1\}$ is satisfiable. In other words ϕ is satisfiable if the formula ϕ' resulting of removing (p) from ϕ and the occurrences of $\neg p$ is satisfiable. This operation is performed for each positive unit clause in ϕ. Now, observe that some clauses in the initial formula can become positive because of the removals of negative literals. Also due to these removals, a pure negative clause can become empty. Thus, at this stage, three situations can arise:

1. An empty clause is produced. The algorithm ends by determining that the original formula is unsatisfiable.
2. No positive clauses have emerged. The algorithm ends by determining that the formula is satisfiable.
3. A positive clause is produced. Then, the algorithm applies the And-Elimination rule and adds new unit clauses to the formula. Thus, a new iteration of the described operations above are carried out with these new unit clauses.

We begin the description of the algorithm by a very simple version in order to help the reader to understand it. Afterwards, we shall advance progressively towards the definitive version which is more elaborated but it warrants a strictly linear worst case complexity.

(VTA ϕ p): It applies the VTA rule returning the formula ϕ' resulting of removing from ϕ the clause (p) and the occurrences of $\neg p$ and possibly, adding some conjunctions C^+ among which could be the empty clause $\square$.

(AE ϕ C^+): It applies the And-Elimination rule returning the formula ϕ' resulting of removing C^+ from ϕ and adding the unit clauses (p) for each conjunct p in C^+.

Notation. We note ϕ^+ the set of positive clauses in ϕ which can be empty.

VTA-AE-Propagation(ϕ)
>   If $\phi^+ = \{\}$ then return(sat)
>   If $\square \in \phi$ then return(unsat)
>   If $(p) \in \phi$ then return(VTA-AE-Propagation (VTA ϕ (p))))
>   If $C^+ \in \phi$ then return(VTA-AE-Propagation (AE ϕ C^+))
End

Theorem 4. *The previous algorithm returns sat iff the input formula ϕ is satisfiable.*

Theorem 5. *The maximal number of recursions is at most in $O(size(\phi))$.*

The previous algorithm is correct but not very efficient. Its efficiency is similar to that of the method proposed in [37,38] and [33]. Although the number of recursions is bounded by O(n), the complexity of each line is clearly not constant and so, the algorithm's complexity measured in computer instructions number is not linear.

One can check that searching for the clauses including some occurrence of $\neg p$ without a suitable data structure has $O(size(\phi))$ computational cost. Hence, the real complexity of the algorithms in number of computer instructions is at least in $O(n^2)$.

To improve this complexity, we shall use the following data structures:
$Neg(p)$: Set of pointers to the C^ϕ clauses in ϕ which include $\neg p$.
$Neg.Counter(C^\phi)$: it is a counter of the remaining negative literals $\neg p \in C^\phi$ such that the corresponding propositions p have not been derived yet.

With this data structures, the procedure VTA firstly obtains by means of Neg(p) the clauses C^ϕ containing $\neg p$. Then, instead of removing physically $\neg p$ in each C^ϕ, the counter Neg.Counter(C^ϕ) is decremented. Thus, although no information of which negative literals have been removed from C^ϕ is maintained, the necessary information of how many negative literals there still left in C^ϕ is furnished by Neg.Counter(C^ϕ) at each moment of the inference process. If this counter is set to 0 means that a positive conjunctive clause C^+, maybe empty, has been deduced from the initial clause C^ϕ. With the described data structure, the procedure VTA is the following.

VTA (ϕ (p))
  Remove (p) from ϕ
  for $\forall C^\phi \in Neg(p)$ **do:**
    Decrement Neg.Counter(C^ϕ)
    if Neg.Counter(C^ϕ) $= 0$ **then do:**
      Add C^+ to ϕ
  Return(ϕ)

Now, remark that a same proposition p can be deduced in more than one conjunction C^+, and then the counter Neg.counter(C^ϕ) such that $pointer(C^\phi)$ $\in Neg(p)$ could be decremented more than once. To disallow these multiple decrements, we use a boolean variable as follows: $Val(p) = 1$ iff p has already been derived from ϕ. So, the truth propagation of variable p is allowed only when the flag $Val(p)$ is 0, and once the propagation has been performed, the flag is set to 1 disallowing further propagations. Also, a list C^+ of non-negated propositions in C^ϕ is required. Thus, the procedure AE becomes:

AE (ϕ C^+)
  Remove C^+ from ϕ
  $\forall p \in C^+$ **do:**
  if $Val(p) = 0$ **then do:**
    Add (p) to ϕ
    $Val(p) \leftarrow 1$
  Return(ϕ)

Following with the improvements of the algorithm, we remark that to know whether $\square \in \phi$ takes a computational cost in $O(|\phi|)$. But this cost can be reduced if each time that a positive conjunction C^+ is going to be added to ϕ is tested whether $C^+ = \square$ or not. In the affirmative case, the algorithm stops the process and it returns 'unsatisfiable'.

A last point consists in avoiding the search throughout the complete formula of (1) the unit clauses and (2) the positive conjunction. For this purpose, (1) we store unit clauses in a stack and (2) we will call the procedure AE each time that a C^+ conjunction is going to be added to ϕ.

In order to get a more efficient algorithm we shall apply iteratively, instead of recursively, the VTA and the AE inference rules. Thus the definitive algorithm is the following:

while $Stack \neq \emptyset$ **do:**
    $p \leftarrow pop(Stack)$ **{PROCEDURE VTA}**
    for $\forall C^\phi \in Neg(p)$ **do:**
        Decrement $Neg.Counter(C^\phi)$
        if $Neg.Counter(C^\phi) = 0$ **then do:**
            if $C^+ = \{\}$ **return** 'Unsatisfiable'
            $\forall p \in C^+$ **do:**   **{PROCEDURE AE}**
                if $Val(p) = 0$ **then do:**
                    $push(p, Stack)$
                    $Val(p) \leftarrow 1$
return 'Satisfiable'

The initialisation of the data structures is carried out in the following procedure:

$Stack \leftarrow \emptyset$;
for $\forall p \in Prop(\phi)$ **do:** $Val(p) \leftarrow 0$, $Neg(p) \leftarrow \{\}$;
for $\forall C^\phi \in \phi$ **do:**
    If $C = \{\}$ then return('unsatisfiable')
    Else $C = \{\neg p_1, \ldots, \neg p_k, C^+\}$ **do:**
    If $k \neq 0$ **do:**
        $Neg.Counter(C^\phi) \leftarrow k$
        for $1 \leq i \leq k$ **do:** Add C^ϕ to $Neg(p_i)$
    Else for $\forall p \in C^+$ **do:**
        if $Val(p) = 0$ **then do:** $Val(p) \leftarrow 1$, $push(p, Stack)$

Theorem 6. Correctness. *The previous algorithm is correct: it returns unsatisfiable iff ϕ is unsatisfiable.*

Theorem 7. Complexity. *The last algorithm is strictly in $O(size(\phi))$.*

Proof.
(1) It is trivial to check that the initialisation of the data structures takes at most $O(size(\phi))$.
The following two statements derive straightforwardly from the construction design of the algorithm:
(2) Each VTA procedure is done at most once for each proposition.
(3) Each AE procedure is executed at most once for each positive conjunction.
(4) By (2), the total number of operations in the VTA procedure is

$$O(\sum_{p \in \phi} | Neg.Counter(C^\phi) |) \leq O(size(\phi))$$

(5) By (3), the total number of operations in the AE procedure is limited to

$$O(\sum_{C \in \phi} | C^+ |) \leq O(size(\phi))$$

(6) By (1), (4) and (5), the algorithm is in $O(size(\phi))$.

4 σ-Formulas

The σ-formulas include ϕ-formulas as a particular case. The σ-formulas require exponentially less symbols than ϕ-formulas to represent the same logical problem.

Definition 11. *A clause C^σ, is a disjunction of two optional terms $C^\sigma = DNF^- \vee C^+ = C_1^- \vee C_2^- \vee \ldots \vee C_n^- \vee C^+$. Two particular cases are noted: clauses with only negative (positive) literals are called negatives (positives).*

Definition 12. *A σ-formula is a finite conjunction of clauses C^σ.*

Interpretations, models and other semantic concepts are easily defined from the previous class of ϕ-formulas and the definition of the σ-language here above.

As before, σ and $\sigma_\square$ stand for respectively any σ-formula and any σ-formula containing the empty clause $\square$.

Definition 13. Variable Truth Assignment VTA2.
If $(p) \in \sigma$ then VTA2 obtains the formula σ' resulting of removing from σ, the unit clause (p) and the conjunctions $(\neg p \wedge \neg p_1 \wedge \ldots \wedge \neg p_k)$.

Theorem 8. Soundness. *VTA2 is sound, namely $\sigma \vdash_{VTA2} \sigma' \Rightarrow \sigma \models \sigma'$.*

Theorem 9. Completeness. *If σ is unsatisfiable then $\sigma \vdash_{VTA2+AE} \sigma_\square$.*

The proofs of both theorems are immediate from the same proofs for the ϕ-formulas and the definition above of the σ-formulas language.

Example 2. Let the following unsatisfiable formula: $\sigma = \{(p_1), (p_3), (\neg p_1 \wedge \neg p_2) \vee (\neg p_3 \wedge \neg p_4) \vee (p_5 \wedge p_6), (\neg p_5 \wedge \neg p_6) \vee (p_7 \wedge p_8), (\neg p_7 \wedge \neg p_9)\} = \{(p_1), (p_3), C_1, C_2, C_3\}$

A proof sequence of the unsatisfiability of σ is:

$\{(p_1), (p_3), (\neg p_1 \wedge \neg p_2) \vee (\neg p_3 \wedge \neg p_4) \vee (p_5 \wedge p_6), C_2, C_3\}$
$\vdash_{VTA2} \{(p_3), (\neg p_3 \wedge \neg p_4) \vee (p_5 \wedge p_6), C_2, C_3\}$
$\vdash_{VTA2} \{(p_5 \wedge p_6), C_2, C_3\}$
$\vdash_{AE} \{(p_5), (p_6), (\neg p_5 \wedge \neg p_6) \vee (p_7 \wedge p_8), C_3\}$
$\vdash_{VTA2} \{(p_6), (p_7 \wedge p_8), (\neg p_7 \wedge \neg p_9)\}$
$\vdash_{AE} \{(p_6), (p_7), (p_8), (\neg p_7 \wedge \neg p_9)\}$
$\vdash_{VTA2} \{(p_6), (p_8), \square\} = \sigma_\square$

Algorithm's Principle. The principle of the VTA2-AE-deduction algorithm is similar to that of the first VTA-AE-deduction algorithm, namely the rules VTA2 and AE are applied until giving rise to one of the two following situations: (1) the empty clause is derived (the original formula is unsatisfiable), or (2) no more new clauses are derived (the original formula is satisfiable).

Data Structures. The data structures vary slightly.
(1) Now a *Flag First*(C_i^-) is associated with each conjunction C_i^- in the term $DNF^- = C_1^- \vee C_2^- \vee \ldots \vee C_n^-$ of a clause $C^\sigma = DNF^- \vee C^+$. This is due to

the fact that $Neg.counter(C^\sigma)$ now counts the number of negative conjunctions (and not atomic literals) C_i^- in DNF^- not falsified by the propositions p already deduced. These conjunctions C_i^- are falsified as soon as one of the propositions in the conjunction is derived.

But, notice that further deductions of the same negative conjunction must not provoke decrements of the counter. Indeed, only one decrement for each conjunction can be enabled. Otherwise, the following error could be committed. Assume that $C^\sigma = DNF^- \vee C^+$ and $DNF^- = C_1^- \vee C_2^- \vee \ldots C_i^- \vee \ldots \vee C_n^-$. In order to have DNF^- falsified at least one proposition p_i in each conjunction C_i^- must be deduced. However notice that n propositions deduced, not distributed in the n conjunctions, do not falsify DNF^-.

To ensure that the counter is decremented only once per each negative conjunction, we require a flag $First(C_i^-)$ which indicates whether any proposition whose negation is in C_i^- has been already derived. Thus, the meaning of the aforementioned flag is $First(C_i^-) = F$ iff no proposition in C_i^- has been deduced. Once the first proposition is deduced $First(C_i^-)$ is set to T.

(2) Another small modification is related to the Neg(p) data structure. Neg(p) must point to the conjunctions $C_i^- = (\neg p \wedge \neg p_1 \wedge \ldots \wedge \neg p_k)$ containing $\neg p$ (instead of pointing to the $\neg p$ occurrences themselves). Thus, Neg(p) is a list of couples (C_i^-, C^σ) of pointers to each C_i^- containing $\neg p$ and to the clause C^σ containing C_i^-.

Algorithm. The algorithm for σ-formulas is supported on the same structure that the algorithm for the ϕ-formulas. As AE inference works well for both types of formulas no modification of the AE-Deduction is required. Thus, only VTA procedure is modified as follows:

> **VTA2 (σ (p))**
> Remove (p) from σ
> **for** $\forall (C^-, C^\sigma) \in Neg(p)$ **do:**
>   **if** $First(C^-) = F$ **then do:**
>   Decrement $Neg.Counter(C^\sigma)$
> $First(C^-) \leftarrow T$
>   **if** $Neg.Counter(C^\sigma) = 0$ **then do:**
>   **if** $C^+ = \Box$ return Unsatisfiable
>   Else $C^+ = (p_1 \wedge p_2 \ldots \wedge p_n)$
>   Begin PROCEDURE AE with C^+

The algorithm VTA2-AE-Deduction is obtained from the VTA-AE-Deduction by replacing in it the VTA procedure by the new VTA2 procedure defined here above.

Theorem 10. Algorithm Correctness. *VTA2-AE-Deduction(σ) returns* Unsatisfiable *iff σ is unsatisfiable.*

Theorem 11. Algorithm Complexity. *VTA2-AE-Deduction(σ) is strictly in* $O(size(\sigma))$.

Proofs of both theorems follow from the corresponding theorems for ϕ-formulas and the slight differences between σ-formulas and ϕ-formulas.

5 ω-Formulas

Like σ-formulas, ω-formulas includes Horn and ϕ-formulas as particular cases.

Definition 14. *A clause C^ω is a disjunction of two optional terms $C^\omega = CNF^- \vee C^+$: CNF^- is a conjunctive normal form with only negative literals and C^+ is a positive conjunction. A ω-formula is a finite conjunction of clauses of kind C^ω.*

Notation. ω-formulas are denoted by ω. Any ω-formula containing the empty clause will be noted $\omega_\square$.

Definition 15. Variable Truth Assignment VTA3. *If $(p) \in \omega$ then VTA3 derives a new formula ω' resulting of removing from ω the unit clause (p), the conjunctions $(\neg p \wedge D_2^- \wedge \ldots \wedge D_m^-)$ and all the occurrences of $\neg p$.*

Interpretation, Model, other semantic concepts and clause proof definition are extended from the ϕ-formulas case without difficulty.

Example 3. Let the unsatisfiable formula $\omega = \{(p_1), (p_2), (((\neg p_1 \vee \neg p_2) \wedge (\neg p_3 \vee \neg p_4)) \vee (p_5 \wedge p_6)), ((\neg p_5 \vee \neg p_6) \vee (p_7 \wedge p_8)), (\neg p_8)\} = \{(p_1), (p_2), C_1, C_2, C_3\}$

A proof sequence of the unsatisfiability of ω is:

$\{(p_1), (p_2), (((\neg p_1 \vee \neg p_2) \wedge (\neg p_3 \vee \neg p_4)) \vee (p_5 \wedge p_6)), C_2, C_3\}$
$\vdash_{VTA3} \{(p_2), ((\neg p_2 \wedge (\neg p_3 \vee \neg p_4)) \vee (p_5 \wedge p_6)), C_2, C_3\}$
$\vdash_{VTA3} \{(p_5 \wedge p_6)), C_2, C_3\}$
$\vdash_{AE} \{(p_5), (p_6), ((\neg p_5 \vee \neg p_6) \vee (p_7 \wedge p_8)), C_3\}$
$\vdash_{VTA3} \{(p_6), (\neg p_6 \vee (p_7 \wedge p_8)), C_3\}$
$\vdash_{VTA3} \{(p_7 \wedge p_8), (\neg p_8)\}$
$\vdash_{AE} \{(p_7), (p_8), (\neg p_8)\}$
$\vdash_{VTA3} \{(p_7), \square\} = \omega_\square$

Theorem 12. Soundness. $\omega \vdash_{VTA3} \omega' \Rightarrow \omega \models \omega'$.

Theorem 13. Completeness. *Let ω being an unsatisfiable formula; then $\omega \vdash_{VTA3+AE} \omega_\square$.*

The proofs of both theorems are analogous to the same proofs for the ω-formulas.

The principle of the iterative algorithm for ω-formulas is similar to the precedent ones. It applies the inference rules while unit clauses (p) are deduced. This process runs until the empty clause is deduced, or no more positive clauses are derived.

The data structures for these new classes of formulas require only one modification which is related to the employed counter. Given that the CNF^- term of each clause C^ω is a finite conjunction of disjunctions of negative literals, i.e.

$CNF^- = (D_1^- \wedge D_2^- \wedge \ldots \wedge D_m^-)$ we need one counter $Neg.Counter(D_i^-)$ of negative literals for each disjunction D_i^-. All the other data structures defined for the ϕ-formulas are kept for the current algorithm.

In order to design an algorithm to test the satisfiability of ω-formulas we need to modify only the procedure VTA associated with the VTA inference rule. This procedure is very similar to the previous one. Now, instead of having one counter for each clause, we use so many counters as negative disjunctions D^- exist in a clause C^ω. If one of these counters is set to 0 means that the CNF^- has been falsified. Thus, the new VTA3 procedure is as follows.

VTA3 (ω (p))
Remove (p) from ω
    for $\forall(D^-, C^\omega) \in Neg(p)$ **do:**
        Decrement $Neg.Counter(D^-)$
        if $Neg.Counter(D^-) = 0$ **then do:**
            if $C^+ \in C^\omega$ is $C^+ = \square$ **then return** 'Unsatisfiable'
            Else $C^+ = (p_1 \wedge p_2 \wedge \ldots \wedge p_n)$
            Begin procedure AE with C^+

The algorithm VTA3-AE-Deduction for the ω-formulas is obtained by replacing the VTA procedure in the algorithm for the ϕ-formulas with this new VTA3 procedure.

Theorem 14. Correctness. *The algorithm VTA3-AE-Deduction(ω) returns unsatisfiable iff ω is unsatisfiable.*

Theorem 15. Complexity. *VTA3-AE-Deduction is strictly in $O(size(\omega))$.*

The Proofs of both theorems are similar to the previous 10 and 11 theorems for the σ-formulas language.

6 Conclusions

On the theoretical side, our contribution described here aims at pushing further the frontiers of non clausal tractability. Thus, we firstly have defined three classes of formulas in Negation Normal Form having a Horn-like shape. Secondly, we have established a set of inference rules which are sound and refutationally complete for each one of the three classes. In third place, we have designed strictly linear algorithms to solve the satisfiability problem in each class of formulas.

On the practical side, as the formulas keep a Horn-like structure, they are of relevant interest in such applications as for instance those based in Rule Based Systems. Indeed, the rules and the questions of many real applications require to represent and to reason with a richer language than the Horn formulas language. In this sense, the proposed formulas absorb the Horn language as a particular case. In addition, the proposed formulas represent logically equivalent pure Horn problems but with exponentially less symbols. Hence, as the described algorithms runs in linear time on these classes, the gain of time can be of an exponential order with respect to the known linear algorithms running on the Horn formulas.

Acknowledgements

We are grateful to the anonymous referees for their helpful comments. This research was developed under a bilateral collaboration framework between the IIIA-CSIC and the CINVESTAV-IPN and was partially financed by the CSIC, the CONACyT and the Universidad Autónoma de Guerrero (Mexico).

References

1. Aguilera, G., de Guzman, I.P., Ojeda, M.: Increasing the efficiency of automated theorem proving. Journal of Applied Non-classical Logics, 5:1 (1995) 9–29
2. Altamirano, E., Escalada-Imaz G.: Efficient algorithms for several factorized Horn theories (in Spanish). 2nd Congress Catala d'Intel.ligencia Artificial, Girona, Spain (1999) 31–38
3. Andrews, P.B.: Theorem proving via general matings. Journal of Association Computing Machinery, 28 (1981)
4. Aspvall, B.: Recognising disguised NR(1) instances of the satisfiability problem. Journal of Algorithms, 1 (1980) 97–103
5. Aspvall B., Plass M.F., Tarjan R.E.: A linear-time algorithm for testing the truth of certain quantified Boolean formulas. Information Processing Letters, 8:3 (1979) 121–132
6. Bibel, W.: Automated theorem proving. Fiedr, Vieweg and Sohn. (1982)
7. Bibel W.: Mating in matrices. Communications of the ACM, 26:11 (1983)
8. Boros E., Crama Y., Hammer P.L., Saks M.: A complexity index for satisfiability problems SIAM Journal on Computing, 23 (1994) 45–49
9. Boros E., Hammer P.L., Sun X.: Recognition of q-Horn formulae in linear time. Discrete Applied Mathematics, 55 (1994) 1–13
10. Boy de la Tour, T.: Minimising the number of clauses by renaming. In: CADE-10, (1990) 558–572
11. Chandru V., Hooker, J.N.: Extended Horn sets in propositional logic. Journal of ACM, 38 (1991) 205–221
12. Cook S.A.: The complexity of theorem-proving procedures. Third ACM Symposium on theory of Computing, (1971) 151–158
13. Conforti M., Cornuéjols G., Kapoor A., Vusković K., Rao M.R.: Balanced matrices. In: J.R. Birge and K.G. Murty, Mathematical Programming: State of the Art, (1994)
14. Dowling W.F., Gallier J.H.: Linear-time algorithms for testing the satisfiability of propositional Horn formulae. Journal of Logic Programming, 3 (1984) 267–284
15. Escalada-Imaz G.: Optimisation d'algorithmes d'inference monotone en logique des propositions et du premier ordre. Université Paul Sabatier, Toulouse, France (1989)
16. Escalada-Imaz G.: Linear forward inferences engines for a class of rule systems (in French). Laboratoire D'Automatique et Analyse des Systemes, Toulouse, France, (1989) LAAS-89172
17. Escalada-Imaz G.: A quadratic algorithm and a linear algorithm for 2-CNF (in French). Laboratoire D'Automatique et Analyse des Systemes, Toulouse, France, (1989) LAAS-89378
18. Escalada-Imaz G., Martínez-Enríquez A.M.: Forward chaining inference engines of optimal complexity for several classes of rule based systems (in Spanish). Informática y Automática, 27:3 (1994) 23–30

19. Even S., Itai A., Shamir A.: On the complexity of timetable and multicommodity flow problems. SIAM J. of Computing, 5 (1976) 691–703
20. Ghallab M., Escalada-Imaz, G.: A linear control algorithm for a class of rule-based systems. Journal of Logic Programming, 11 (1991) 117–132
21. Gallo, G., Urbani, G.: Algorithms for testing the satisfiability of propositional formulae. Journal of Logic Programming, 7 (1989) 45–61
22. Hähnle, R.: Short conjunctive normal forms in finitely-valued logics. Journal of Logic and Computation, 4:6 (1994) 905–927
23. Hähnle R., Murray N.V., Rosenthal, E.: Completeness for linear regular negation normal form inference systems. In: Proceedings ISMIS'97, (1997)
24. Henschen L., Wos L.: Unit refutations and Horn sets. Journal of the Association for Computing Machinery, 21:4 (1974) 590–605
25. Henschen L., Lusk E., Overbeek R., Smith B.T., Veroff R., Winker S., Wos L.: Challenge problem 1. SIGART Newsletter, 72 (1980) 30–31
26. Jones N., Laaser W.: Complete problems for deterministic polynomial time. Theoretical Computer Science, 3 (1977) 105–117
27. Karp R.M.: Reducibility among combinatorial problems. In: Miller, R. E., Thatcher, J. W. (eds): Complexity of Computer Computations. Plenum Press. N.Y. (1972) 85–103
28. Lewis H.R.: Renaming a set of clauses as a Horn set. Journal of the ACM, 25 (1978) 134–135
29. Minoux, M.: LTUR: A simplified linear-time unit resolution algorithm for Horn formulae and computer implementation. Information Processing Letters, 29 (1988) 1–12
30. Mints, G.: Gentzen-type systems and resolution rules, part 1: Propositional logic. In: Proc. COLOG-88, Tallin. Lecture Notes in Computer Science, 417. Springer, (1990) 198–231
31. Murray N.V., Rosenthal, E.: Dissolution: making paths vanish. Journal of the ACM, 3 (1993) 504–535
32. Ramesh, A.G.: Some applications of non-Clausal deduction. Department of Computer Science, State University of new York at Albany, (1995)
33. Roy, R., Chowdhury, Dalal: Model theoretic semantics and tractable algorithm for CNF-BCP, In: Proc. of the AAAI-97, (1997) 227–232
34. Scutellà M.G.: A note on Dowling and Gallier's top-down algorithm for propositional Horn satisfiability. Journal of Logic Programming, 8 (1990) 265–273
35. Schlipf J.S., Annextein F., Franco J., Swaminathan, R.P.: On finding solutions for extended Horn formulas. Information Processing Letters, 54 (1995) 133–137
36. Socher, R.: Optimising the clausal normal form transformation. Journal of Automated Reasoning, 7 (1991) 325–336
37. Stachniak, Z.: Non-clausal reasoning with propositional definite theories. In: International Conference on Artificial Intelligence and Symbolic Computation. Lecture Notes in Computer Science, 1476. Springer Verlag, (1998) 296–307
38. Stachniak, Z.: Polarity guided tractable reasoning. In: International American Association on Artificial Intelligence, AAAI-99 (1999) 751–758
39. Tseitin, G.: On the complexity of proofs in propositional logics. In: Siekmann, J., Wrightson, G. (eds.): Automation of Reasoning 2: Classical Papers on Computational Logic, Springer, (1983) 466–483

The Taming of the (X)OR

Peter Baumgartner[1] and Fabio Massacci[2*]

[1] Institut für Informatik, Universität Koblenz-Landau
D-56073 Koblenz, Germany
peter@uni-koblenz.de http://www.uni-koblenz.de/~peter/
[2] Dip. di Ingegneria dell'Informazione
Università di Siena, 53100 Siena, Italy
massacci@dii.unisi.it, http://www.dii.unisi.it/~massacci/

Abstract. Many key verification problems such as bounded model-checking, circuit verification and logical cryptanalysis are formalized with combined clausal and affine logic (i.e. clauses with xor as the connective) and cannot be efficiently (if at all) solved by using CNF-only provers.

We present a decision procedure to *efficiently* decide such problems. The Gauss-DPLL procedure is a tight integration in a unifying framework of a Gauss-Elimination procedure (for affine logic) and a Davis-Putnam-Logeman-Loveland procedure (for usual clause logic).

The key idea, which distinguishes our approach from others, is the full interaction bewteen the two parts which makes it possible to maximize (deterministic) simplification rules by passing around newly created unit or binary clauses in either of these parts. We show the correctness and the termination of Gauss-DPLL under very liberal assumptions.

1 Introduction

In many application areas such as formal verification [Cla90,BCC+99], logical cryptanalysis [Mas99,MM00], planning [KS96,GMS98], and AI in general [SKM97] the traditional formulation of a logical inference problem as a satisfiability problem in clausal normal form (CNF) is becoming unsatisfactory.

"Real world" problems are seldomly formulated in CNF and must always be converted to it. The natural formulations of real problems make use of many logical connectives: definitions (e.g. gates in circuit verifications), exclusive or (e.g. Feistel-operations in logical cryptanalysis), disjunctions (e.g. non-deterministic actions in planning) etc.

When such formulae are transformed into CNF the performance of the system is not very impressive, unless special heuristic information on the problem domain is used (see e.g. [GMS98] on planning and [WvM99] on the DIMACS parity bit problems).

Our motivating application was logical cryptanalysis, the encoding of cryptographic problems as SAT problems [Mas99,MM00]. Known plaintext attacks to the US Data Encryption Standard can be encoded as a SAT problem with formulae of increasing complexity. The experimental analysis in [Mas99,MM00] showed that the performance of state-of-the-art CNF solvers such as rel_sat [BS97], sato [Zha97], ntab [CA96], and

---

* F. Massacci acknowledges the support of a STM CNR grant.

satz [Li99] degraded as soon as formulae containing exclusive-or appeared in the original formulation. Thus, solving real crypto-problems with CNF-provers looks unlikely.

A similar situation is found in circuit verification where the usage of successful BDD-packages [BRB90] has proven to be utterly ineffective when coping with fairly basics circuits such as multipliers. Parity bit problems, based on logically simple formulae, proved to be extremely hard for CNF based provers [SKM97,WvM99,JT96,Li00].

"The taming of the xor" has therefore become one of the major research efforts in the SAT community to tackle real world applications. The first solution is to cast the problem into CNF using advanced translations beyond Teitsin definitional translation [Wil90,GW00]. Otherwise one can use a dual-phase algorithm that solves the xor-part separately [WvM99], or more complex algorithms using multiple polynomials [WvM00]. Other researchers have focused on direct handling of xors as a black box subroutine of classical DPLL algorithms [Li00]. In the BDD community a number of "*DD" (where "*" may be instantiated to almost any alphabetic string) decision diagrams has been proposed to solve this problem [BDW95,DBR97].

Most of these works start from the observation that satisfiability of affine logic – sets of xor-clauses, i.e. clauses made up with xor as the connective – can be decided in polynomial time [Sch78]. In particular, one can use a Gaussian Elimination procedure (GE procedure) to decide a given affine logic problems in quadratic time.

It seems therefore possible to include GE as a black-box subroutine in a procedure for a more general logic, and this is indeed done in [Li00,WvM99,WvM00]. We will not directly do so, because the problems in our application domain (logical cryptanalysis), are beyond affine clause logic: after an appropriate transformation we end up with *two* sets of clauses, a set of usual or-clauses, and a set of xor-clauses. Our task is to decide the satisfiability of the combined problem, and, if satisfiable, output a model.

The experimental analysis reported by [Li00,WvM99,WvM00] showed that incorporating the GE procedure as a black-box subroutine definitely pays off if the affine logic part is overwhelming. This is the case for artificial DIMACS problems such as the bit parity problem or Pretolani's encoding of Urquhart's formulae [JT96,Li00,WvM99]. However, they also all agree that this is not sufficient when the affine logic part is only a part of the overall formula. This is indeed the case for DES encodings whereas xor clauses are just the hard core part (4% of whole) [Mas99,Li00]. This is true for many other problems such as model checking [BCC$^+$99,Li00].

So we want to have affine-logic reasoning in our calculus and, at the same time, we do not want to abandon the good, old and after all extremely efficient DPLL procedure. Our contribution is a revised DPLL where or-clauses and xor-clauses mutually co-exist.

In order to achieve a homogeneous architecture, we treat xor-clauses by more traditionally styled inference rules. In this way, the inferences carried out on either or-clauses or xor-clauses can heavily influence each other. This allows for performance optimizations by passing around newly created unit or binary clauses in the or-clause logic part to the xor-clause logic part (and vice versa). In both parts they can be used to *simplify* the currently derived clauses. By giving preference to simplifications, branching of the search space due to the or-logic part is delayed until unavoidable or even prevented.

Of course, our inference-rule based mechanism specializes to a variant of the GE procedure when restricted to affine logic. When applied to a pure inclusive-or clause logic problem, the method instantiates to the (propositional version of the) well-known Davis-Putnam-Logeman-Loveland (DPLL) procedure [DLL62]. This choice is motivated by the nice properties of DPLL: its conceptual simplicity, space efficiency, few inference rules, efficient and adaptable implementations (the most efficient systematic propositional methods are based on DPLL [BS97,Zha97,CA96,Li99]), and the possibility to immediately extract a model in case that no refutation exists.

The suggested calculus in this paper can also be understood as an attempt to "lift" these properties to the case of a combined inclusive/exclusive-or logic. The underlying inference rules can roughly be divided in three classes: *Resolution*-type inferences to implement GE (however, one parent clause is *always* deleted), *simplification* inference rules (which do not cause branching) and the *cut* rule (aka split) to force a case analysis $A - \neg A$ to advance the derivation when other rules are no longer applicable.

This is only part of the story: one major difference between ours and the classical DPLL procedure is that we do not insist on explicitly computing a model; instead, we allow our procedure to terminate earlier, once a *functional description of a model* is computed. For instance, an equivalence like $A \equiv B$ is not subject to further case analysis to actually compute truth assignments for A and B. Instead it serves a functional description of our model. If we really want to have a truth assignment, we can choose a random value for, say, B and then the value of A can be easily calculated.

The rest of this paper is structured as follows: we start with some preliminary definitions. Then we introduce the basic ingredients of our calculus (simplification and GE inference rules). These are then combined with some more inference rules in a single calculus called Gauss-DPLL. Finally, we sketch its correctness.

2   Preliminaries

We apply the usual notions of propositional logic, in a way consistent to [CL73].

An *atom* is either a propositional variable or the symbol $\top$ (*"true"*). A *literal* is an atom or a negated atom. For a literal L, its *complement* $\overline{L}$ is the atom A, if one has $L = \neg A$, or else $\overline{L}$ is $\neg L$. For a literal L we denote by $|L|$ the atom of L, i.e. $|A| = A$ and $|\neg A| = A$ for any atom A.

An *assignment* is a pair A/L, where A is an atom different from $\top$, and L is a literal.

An *or-clause* is a possibly empty multiset $\{L_1, \ldots, L_n\}$ of literals, usually written as $L_1 \vee \cdots \vee L_n$ if $n > 0$, and $\square$ if $n = 0$. Similarly, a *xor-clause* is a possibly empty multiset $\{L_1, \ldots, L_n\}$ of literals, usually written as $L_1 \oplus \cdots \oplus L_n$ if $n > 0$, and $\square$ if $n = 0$. The atoms of a clause C, denoted by $|C|$ are computed in the obvious way as $|C| = \{|L| : L \in C\}$. A *clause* refers to an or-clause or a xor-clause.

Remark 1 (Special Cases). A clause with exactly one literal (i.e. a unit clause) can be seen as an or-clause, as a xor-clause or as an assignment where the value $\top$ or $\neg\top$ is assigned to the atom of the literal according the sign of the literal in the obvious way. A xor-clause with two literals can also be seen as an assignment. For instance $\neg A$ can be seen as the assignment $A/\neg\top$, whereas $A \oplus \neg B$ can be seen as the assignment B/A or the assignment A/B. The calculus below contains rules for such transitions.

In the sequel we use $A, B, \ldots$ for atoms, $K, L, \ldots$ for literals and $C, D, \ldots$ for clauses. The calligraphic letters $\mathcal{A}$, $\mathcal{C}$ and $\mathcal{X}$ are reserved to denote sets of assignment, sets of or-clauses, and sets of xor-clauses, respectively. When writing down or-clauses, we use the notation $L \vee C$ to denote $\{L\} \vee C$, and $C \vee D$ to denote $C \cup D$ (and similarly for xor-clauses by using $\oplus$). Also, we write "C, C" instead of "$\{C\} \cup C$", where C is a (x)or-clause set.

Literal occurrences in xor-clauses can be flagged as *selected*. Selection is indicated by underlining, as in $\underline{L} \oplus C$. The purpose is to state C as a "definition" of L.

Quite frequently, we need the *set of selected atoms of* X, which is $\mathrm{sel}(X) = \{|L| \mid L$ is selected in C, for some $C \in X\}$.

Translation to normal form. We have a strict separation in our clause sets: in the one part, only "$\vee$" occurs, and in the other part only "$\oplus$" occurs. Treating arbitrary propositional formulae is conceivable as well. However, due to the presence of xor-clauses, we can transform the initial formula into two separate sets, in a much simpler way than with CNF transformations.

For instance the formula $A \vee B \vee (C \oplus D \oplus E)$ can be transformed into the two clauses $A \vee B \vee F$ and $\neg F \oplus C \oplus D \oplus E$ introducing the new symbol F. It is easy to see that this is a satisfiability preserving transformation. Even with optimized CNF transformation we cannot get away with less than 6 clauses.

In our target application [MM00] we have only formulae of the form $L \leftrightarrow L_1 \oplus \cdots \oplus L_n$ or $L = L_1 \vee \cdots \vee L_n$. So, a transformation into normal form will be definitely easy. Hence we assume as given a clause-normal-form transformation that transforms the given formula φ (containing arbitrary connectives) equivalently into a set of or-clauses and a set of xor-clauses (read conjunctively).

3   Simplification by Boolean Reduction

Simplification by boolean reduction means to transform a clause into normal form by exploiting trivial boolean reductions. This is achieved by the inference rules $\mathcal{R}_{\mathsf{Bool}}$ shown in Figure 1; they are also used in the preprocessing step of the encoding of DES in [MM00], and they extend to the xor-case the rules given in [Mas98,HS98].

More precisely, *reduction of a clause C by the $\mathcal{R}_{\mathsf{Bool}}$ inference rules* means to repeatedly replace C by the result of a single application of an inference rule from $\mathcal{R}_{\mathsf{Bool}}$ to C, resulting finally in a normal form of C.

Proposition 1. *The reduction of a clause C by the $\mathcal{R}_{\mathsf{Bool}}$ inference rules terminates.*

The proof is straightforward and is omitted (the proof of Lemma 2 below makes the ordering explicit that guarantees termination).

Remark 2 (Transparent Selection). In the reduction process, the inference rules are applied to xor-clauses *transparently* wrt. selected literals according to the following rules: (i) selection within C (referring to the actual instance of the meta-variable in the inference rules $\mathcal{R}_{\mathsf{Bool}}$) is preserved. (ii) selection of L, A, $\neg A$, B or $\neg B$ carries over to the resulting clause, if the respective literal still is present (in complemented form, however) in the conclusion.

The reason to preserve selection is to make in the calculus a re-orientation of a definition impossible, where e.g. $\neg A$ is just as good a definition name as A.

Elimination of logical constants

$$L \oplus \top \oplus C \to \overline{L} \oplus C$$

$$\neg \top \oplus C \to C$$

$$\top \vee C \to \top$$

$$\neg \top \vee C \to C$$

Elimination of redundancies

$$L \oplus L \oplus C \to C$$

$$A \oplus \neg A \oplus C \to \top \oplus C$$

$$\neg A \oplus \neg B \oplus C \to A \oplus B \oplus C$$

$$L \vee L \vee C \to L \vee C$$

$$A \vee \neg A \vee C \to \top$$

Fig. 1. The inference rules $\mathcal{R}_{\mathsf{Bool}}$ for boolean reduction; in "$\varphi \to \psi$" the left hand side φ is the premise and the right hand side ψ is the conclusion. The case $C = \square$ is permitted in all rules, except of $\top \vee C \to \top$.

In general, a normal form derived in the way just described is not unique. Still, all normal forms are logically equivalent and this is what we are interested in. Thus we let $C\!\downarrow$ denote some arbitrary normal form of C.

For instance, $\neg \underline{A} \oplus \neg B \oplus \neg C$ has three normal forms and $\neg \underline{A} \oplus \neg B \oplus \neg C\!\downarrow$ may be $\underline{A} \oplus B \oplus \neg C$ (notice how selection carries over). The single normal form of $\underline{A} \oplus A \oplus B$ is B (however, such cyclic definitions are impossible to construct in the calculus).

4   Simplification by Boolean Assignments

The device introduced here is comparable to the uniform substitution rule by Teitsin. It has been already introduced in [Mas98,HS98].

Remark 3 (Assumptions about Sets of Assignments). From now on, when considering a set $\mathcal{A}$ of assignments, we insist that whenever $A/L \in \mathcal{A}$ and $A/K \in \mathcal{A}$ then $L = K$ (functionality), and whenever $A/L \in \mathcal{A}$ then $|L|/K \notin \mathcal{A}$, for every literal K (idempotency).

Notice that idempotency guarantees in particular $A/A \notin \mathcal{A}$ and $A/\neg A \notin \mathcal{A}$.

Definition 1 (Simplification by Assignments). *The simplification of a clause C by a set of assignments $\mathcal{A} = \{A_1/L_1, \ldots A_n/L_n\}$, denoted by $C /\!/ \mathcal{A}$, is obtained by simultaneous substitution of each occurrence of A_i (resp. $\neg A_i$) in C by L_i (resp. $\overline{L_i}$), for $1 \le i \le n$.*

Simplification is applied transparently to selected literals in a "destructive" way: if A (or $\neg A$) is selected in a xor-clause C and a simplification $C /\!/ \{A/L, \ldots\}$ is performed, the literal occurrence L (resp. $\overline{L}$) in the resulting clause does not get selected.

Definition 2. *An atom A is defined in a set of assignments $\mathcal{A}$ iff $A/L \in \mathcal{A}$, for some literal L. It is undefined iff it is not defined.*

Definition 3 (Extending a Set of Assignments). *Let $\mathcal{A}$ be a set of assignments and A/L be an assignment such that both A and $|L|$ are undefined in $\mathcal{A}$. Then, the extension of $\mathcal{A}$ by A/L, denoted by $\mathcal{A} \circ (A/L)$, is the set of assignments $\{B/(K /\!/ \{A/L\}) \mid B/ K \in \mathcal{A}\} \cup \{A/L\}$. In this definition the literal K is read as a unit clause.*

If the atom A is undefined in $\mathcal{A}$, then $\mathcal{A} \circ A = \mathcal{A} \circ (A/\top)$, and $\mathcal{A} \circ \neg A = \mathcal{A} \circ (A/\neg \top)$

Lemma 1 (Preservation of Properties). *If $\mathcal{A}$ is functional and idempotent, then, under the conditions stated in Def. 3, both $\mathcal{A} \circ (A/L)$ and $\mathcal{A} \circ L$ are functional and idempotent.*

Proof. (Sketch) Consider the general case $\mathcal{A} \circ (A/L)$. Since A is undefined in $\mathcal{A}$ and only the right hand sides are modified by extension, functionality is preserved. $\mathcal{A} \circ (A/L)$ is idempotent because the right hand sides in $\mathcal{A}$ are subject to substitution by the new assignment A/L and that $|L|$ is undefined in $\mathcal{A}$. This makes non-idempotency impossible.

5 Gauss Resolution Rules

The Gauss Elimination (GE) procedure can be represented by two resolution-like rules:

$$\text{Gauss}^- \ \frac{L \oplus C \qquad \bar{L} \oplus D}{C \oplus D} \qquad \text{Gauss}^+ \ \frac{L \oplus C \qquad L \oplus D}{\top \oplus C \oplus D}$$

For the Gauss$^-$ rule, we say that $C \oplus D$ is the *Gauss-resolvant of* $L \oplus C$ *on* L *into* $\bar{L} \oplus D$, and similarly for Gauss$^+$ rule.

As for resolution, these rules are sound, i.e. the conclusion is a consequence of the premises. However, in sharp contrast to resolution, in both rules each premise is a consequence of the conclusion and the other premise:

Proposition 2. *All of the following hold:*

1. $\{L \oplus C, \bar{L} \oplus D\} \models C \oplus D$ *and* $\{L \oplus C, C \oplus D\} \models \bar{L} \oplus D$
2. $\{L \oplus C, L \oplus D\} \models \top \oplus C \oplus D$ *and* $\{L \oplus C, \top \oplus C \oplus D\} \models L \oplus D$

Using proposition 2 we can delete one of the premises once the Gauss-resolvant has been added to the xor-clause set *without loosing completeness*, because it is an equivalence preserving transformation. The intuition is that the deleted clause can always be restored by applying the inference rules. Thus one can avoid the exponential explosion of resolution: the number of clauses never grows more than the initial set of clauses. If we apply boolean reduction rules, one can eliminate duplicated literals in a clause, and hence the length of each clause never exceeds the number of available atoms.

These two rules, together with a deletion strategy, describe a Gauss-Elimination procedure as known from high-school which has a quadratic complexity. Take the given xor-clauses $X = \{C_1, \ldots, C_n\}$ as a system of linear equations in a boolean ring $\oplus C_1 = 1, \ldots, \oplus C_n = 1$, where each variable is assigned a value 0 or 1, $\oplus$ is addition modulo 2, and $\neg A$ is $A \oplus 1$. In this view, the overall strategy to determine whether X is satisfiable is first to derive (if possible) a triangular form of X. For this, select a clause with a literal, say L, and eliminate with the two rules all occurrences of L and $\bar{L}$ from the remaining clauses. This is possible by design of the inference rules, as the conclusion contains neither L nor $\bar{L}$. If necessary, we apply boolean reduction rules until each clause contains at most one occurrence of L or $\bar{L}$. Next, the clause containing L is put aside and the variable elimination process continues in this way until all clauses are processed.

If the empty clause comes up, the xor-clause set is unsatisfiable. If a triangular matrix results, a unique model can be computed by propagating the assignments forced by the shorter clauses towards the longer clauses. For a non-triangular form, the system is under-determined and more than one model exists.

Unfortunately, unrestricted application of the Gauss$^-$ and Gauss$^+$ rules to a set of xor-clauses may be a non-terminating process. The system might cycle among a finite set of logically equivalent forms without reaching a fix point.

As an example consider $X = \{A \oplus C, \neg A \oplus D\}$. Resolving $A \oplus C$ on A into $\neg A \oplus D$ yields $X' = \{A \oplus C, C \oplus D\}$. Next, resolving $A \oplus C$ on C into $C \oplus D$ results in X again (after reduction).

This problem is solved by using the strategy described above to derive a triangular form. It would be acceptable if the xor-clause set is fixed, but this is not our case: first, new unary or binary xor-clauses may come up as the derivation proceeds, and it can be advantageous to delay the decision on the variables to eliminate. Second, the initial xor-clause set is undetermined in most cases [Li00], and the value of many "independent" variables is determined only by the constraints expressed by the or-clauses.

6   Gauss-DPLL

In this section we introduce the inference rules which are at the basis of a generalization of the Davis-Putnam-Logeman-Loveland Procedure, which we call *Gauss*-DPLL.

The inference rules, but one, are of the form

$$\text{Name } \frac{\mathcal{A} \quad C \quad X}{\mathcal{A}' \quad C' \quad X'} \text{ Condition}$$

where $\mathcal{A}$ is a set of assignments, C is a set of or-clauses, X is a set of xor-clauses, possibly with some selected literals. The primed versions are the sets derived by the rule.

The intuition is that in $\mathcal{A}$ we store the definitions A/L which say how to set the value of an atom A on the basis of the value of another atom or a logical constant. The sets C and X contain the (x)or-clauses that have not been completely processed yet.

The main idea behind selected literals is that a xor-clause C containing a selected literal L can be seen as a definition of the corresponding atom $|L|$ in terms of the value of the other literals of C. For the whole system to be consistent, the clause C can only be used as the definition of *only one* atom. Further, the calculus achieves that there is only one such definition – be it in just one single xor-clause or as an assignment.

The twist to implement the GE procedure in this way is, that, when no rule is applicable, the set X and the selected literals in it implicitly describe a triangular form of the linear modulo 2 equations in X. For instance, if $X = \{\underline{A} \oplus B, \underline{C} \oplus B\}$ this implicitly describe a triangular form which is (partly) undetermined: A and C have been "solved" as functions of B. In terms of linear equation this is obvious: we have two equations and three variables.

We are now turning to the inference rules of *Gauss*-DPLL.

The following inference rules are used to reduce clauses; to avoid trivial loops, the applicability condition $C \neq C \downarrow$ is assumed:

$$\text{V-Red } \frac{\mathcal{A} \quad C, C \quad X}{\mathcal{A} \quad C\downarrow, C \quad X} \qquad \oplus\text{-Red } \frac{\mathcal{A} \quad C \quad C, X}{\mathcal{A} \quad C \quad C\downarrow, X}$$

The following inference rules simplify a clause by the current assignments; the applicability condition $C \neq C /\!/ \mathcal{A}$ is assumed:

$$\text{V-Simp} \quad \frac{\mathcal{A} \quad C, C \quad X}{\mathcal{A} \quad C /\!/ \mathcal{A}, C \quad X} \qquad \oplus\text{-Simp} \quad \frac{\mathcal{A} \quad C \quad C, X}{\mathcal{A} \quad C \quad C /\!/ \mathcal{A}, X}$$

An inference rule for the simplification of $\mathcal{A}$ wrt. $\mathcal{A}$ is not necessary, because $\mathcal{A}$ is both functional and idempotent (cf. Remark 3) as being constructed.

Now we turn to the inference rules to implement the GE procedure as described in Section 5. First, we need a rule to select a literal L for elimination.

$$\text{Select} \quad \frac{\mathcal{A} \quad C \quad L \oplus C, X}{\mathcal{A} \quad C \quad \underline{L} \oplus C, X} \qquad \begin{cases} \text{if } \text{sel}(\{L \oplus C\} \cup X) \cap \text{atoms}(L \oplus C) = \{\} \\ \text{and } |L| \neq \top \end{cases}$$

The intuition behind the applicability condition is that we can use a xor-clause as definition of only one literal at a time, i.e. $\text{sel}(L \oplus C) \cap \text{atoms}(L \oplus C) = \{\}$. To guarantee that no trivially cyclic definition as in $\underline{A} \oplus A \oplus B$ comes up, the $\oplus$-Red inference rule must be preferred to Select (all the required preferences are stated in Def. 4 below). The subcondition $\text{sel}(X) \cap \text{atoms}(L \oplus C) = \{\}$ states that the new definition must not depend from other definitions. If it were absent, a cyclic situation as in $\{\underline{A} \oplus B, A \oplus \neg B\}$ comes up easily.

Then we have the proper Gauss-Resolution rule:

$$\text{Gauss} \quad \frac{\mathcal{A} \quad C \quad \underline{L} \oplus C, D, X}{\mathcal{A} \quad C \quad \underline{L} \oplus C, D', X} \qquad \begin{cases} \text{if } D' \text{ is Gauss resolvent of } L \oplus C \\ \text{on } L \text{ into } D \end{cases}$$

Intuitively, this rule says that we take $\underline{L} \oplus C$ as a definition of L and replace in D the literal L (or $\overline{L}$) by its definition. To guarantee that there is no occurrence of L (or $\overline{L}$) left in D', the $\oplus$-Red inference rule must be preferred to Gauss. The Gauss rule is applied transparently wrt. selected literals, i.e. a possibly selected literal in D remains selected in D' (the literal L (or $\overline{L}$) in D' cannot be selected anyway, cf. invariant (ii) in Lemma 2).

Example 1. Consider the following derivation where $\mathcal{A}$ and C have been removed for readability and numbers are for reference:

(1) $\quad A \oplus B \oplus E, A \oplus C, B \oplus C \quad$ start
(2) $\quad A \oplus B \oplus E, \underline{A} \oplus C, B \oplus C \quad$ by Select
(3) $\quad C \oplus B \oplus E \oplus \top, \underline{A} \oplus C, B \oplus C \quad$ by Gauss$^+$ of $A \oplus C$ on A into $A \oplus B \oplus E$
(4) $\quad \neg C \oplus B \oplus E, \underline{A} \oplus C, B \oplus C \quad$ by $\oplus$-Red on $C \oplus B \oplus E \oplus \top$
(5) $\quad \neg C \oplus B \oplus E, \underline{A} \oplus C, B \oplus \underline{C} \quad$ by Select
(6) $\quad B \oplus B \oplus E, \underline{A} \oplus C, B \oplus \underline{C} \quad$ by Gauss$^-$ of $B \oplus C$ on C into $\neg C \oplus B \oplus E$
(7) $\quad E, \underline{A} \oplus C, B \oplus \underline{C} \quad$ by $\oplus$-Red on $B \oplus B \oplus E$
(8) $\quad E, \underline{A} \oplus B \oplus \top, B \oplus \underline{C} \quad$ by Gauss$^+$ of $B \oplus C$ on C into $A \oplus C$
(9) $\quad E, \underline{A} \oplus \neg B, B \oplus \underline{C} \quad$ by $\oplus$-Red on $\underline{A} \oplus B \oplus \top$
(10) $\quad \underline{E}, \underline{A} \oplus \neg B, B \oplus \underline{C} \quad$ by Select

Now we can apply neither Gauss, nor Select, and indeed we terminated with an undetermined set of equations where A and C are defined in terms of B.

This example explains well the importance of giving precedence to the $\oplus$-Red rule over the Gauss rule. Consider step (6): without simplifying the two Bs we will not be able to eliminate them: Gauss alone will introduce two Cs, or two As etc.

To see the importance of the applicability condition of Select, let us look at the last step. Without it, we could have continued as follows:

$$(11')\quad E,\ \underline{A}\oplus\neg B,\ \underline{B}\oplus\underline{C}\quad \text{bySelect}$$
$$(12)\quad E,\ \underline{A}\oplus\underline{C},\ \underline{B}\oplus\underline{C}\quad \text{byGauss}^-$$
$$(13)\quad E,\ \underline{A}\oplus\underline{B}\oplus\top,\ \underline{B}\oplus\underline{C}\ \text{byGauss}^+$$
$$(14)\quad E,\ \underline{A}\oplus\neg\underline{B},\ \underline{B}\oplus\underline{C}\quad \text{by}\oplus\text{-Red}$$

So we are using $A \oplus C$ sometimes as a definition of A and sometimes as a definition of C. This will clearly lead to a non-terminating sequence.

The rules presented so far constitute the core of the GE procedure as described in Section 5. The next set of inference rule transforms unit (x)or-clauses into assignments, with the purpose to trigger new simplification steps.

$$\vee\text{-Unit}\ \dfrac{\mathcal{A}\quad L,\ C\quad X}{\mathcal{A}\circ L\quad C\quad X}\qquad \oplus\text{-Unit}\ \dfrac{\mathcal{A}\quad C\quad L,\ X}{\mathcal{A}\circ L\quad C\quad X}$$

Here, L may or may not be selected.

Remark 4. Since we give preference to Red and Simp over the Unit rules, the extension of $\mathcal{A}$ to $\mathcal{A}\circ L$ is defined, i.e. $|L|$ is undefined in $\mathcal{A}$. Thus, functionality and idempotency are preserved by Lemma 1, and the set of assignments strictly increases.

Now, the well-known DPLL splitting rule is introduced. The purpose is to advance a derivation once no other rule is applicable.

$$\text{Split}\ \dfrac{\mathcal{A}\quad C\quad X}{\mathcal{A}\circ A\quad C\quad X\qquad \mathcal{A}\circ\neg A\quad C\quad X}\quad \text{if } A\in\text{atoms}(C),\text{ for some } C\in\mathcal{C}$$

This is the sole rule with two consequences. Observe that the splitting in the two cases A and $\neg A$ is expressed in our notation as two respective assignments $A/\top$ and $A/\neg\top$.

Remark 5. Once again we have no condition such as "A is undefined in $\mathcal{A}$" because we give preference to Red and Simp over Split, and therefore the same reasoning as in Remark 4 applies.

The applicability condition in Split is not necessary for completeness, but is useful for stopping the search without going to compute explicitly any of the models that would be possible by assigning all combinations of $\top$ and $\neg\top$ to the "independent" atoms occurring in definitions represented by the X. However, for the atoms occurring in C, applying Split is mandatory as the last resort to make progress in processing C.

Remark 6 (Explicit Models). If we arrive at a stage where no rule is applicable, and the empty clause has not been found, we have a functional description of a model. To obtain a model as a set of assignments of logical constants to atoms, we can add to $\mathcal{A}$ an arbitrary truth value assignment for each atom that is not selected in a xor-clause in X. The exhaustive application of the Simp, Red and Unit rules leads to the desired result in $\mathcal{A}$ then.

The next rules for equivalences are not necessary for completeness but they allow for a substantial speed-up as they correspond to powerful forms of pruning: some hard DIMACS problems are solved by using rules of equivalent form alone in [Li00].

$$\text{V-Eqv-1} \quad \frac{\mathcal{A} \qquad A \vee B, \neg A \vee \neg B, C \qquad X}{\mathcal{A} \circ (A/\neg B) \qquad C \qquad X} \quad \text{if } B \notin \text{sel}(X)$$

$$\text{V-Eqv-2} \quad \frac{\mathcal{A} \qquad A \vee \neg B, \neg A \vee B, C \qquad X}{\mathcal{A} \circ (A/B) \qquad C \qquad X} \quad \text{if } B \notin \text{sel}(X)$$

$$\oplus\text{-Eqv} \quad \frac{\mathcal{A} \qquad C \qquad A \oplus L, X}{\mathcal{A} \circ (A/\overline{L}) \qquad C \qquad X} \quad \text{if } |L| \notin \text{sel}(\{A \oplus L\} \cup X)$$

Remark 7. Similarly as said above in Remark 4 for the Split rule, we insist to prefer the Simp and Red rules over the Eqv rules. Therefore, all stated extensions of $\mathcal{A}$ in the Eqv rules are defined, thus both functionality and idempotency are preserved (cf. Lemma 1), and also A is undefined in $\mathcal{A}$.

To avoid loops, the turning of (x)or-clauses into assignments by the Eqv rules must not contradict the implicit ordering of literals as determined by the selected literals in X (this ordering is made explicit in the proof of Lemma 2). This is what the stated applicability conditions are good for.

The $\oplus$-Eqv rule is formulated general enough, because any binary xor-clause of the form $\neg A \oplus \neg B$ can be turned into $A \oplus B$ by boolean reduction.

7 An Effective Calculus for Proof Search

Finally, it has to be said how to combine the inference rules of Section 6:

Definition 4 (Affine Logic Tree (ALT)). *We consider (incomplete) binary trees where every node N is labelled with a tuple $(\mathcal{A}, C, X)$. The label of N is denoted by $\lambda(N)$.*

Affine logic trees, ALTs, for C and X, where C (resp. X) is an or-clause set (resp. xor-clause set) are defined inductively in the following way:

Initialization Step: *the tree $\mathcal{T}$ consisting of a root node N only and such that $\lambda(N) = (\{\}, C, X)$ is an ALT for C and X.*

Non-branching Extension Step: *if N' is a leaf of an ALT $\mathcal{T}'$ for C and X, and one of the non-branching inference rules is applicable to $\lambda(N')$, then $\mathcal{T}$ is an ALT for C and X, where $\mathcal{T}$ is obtained from $\mathcal{T}'$ by attaching one new child node N below N', and $\lambda(N)$ is obtained by a single application of one of the non-branching inference rules to $\lambda(N')$. Applicability of these inference rules is given preference as follows:*
- $\oplus$-Simp *and* $\oplus$-Red *must be applied before* Gauss *and* Select
- $\oplus$-Simp *and* $\oplus$-Red *must be applied before* $\oplus$-Unit *and* $\oplus$-Eqv
- $\vee$-Simp *and* $\vee$-Red *must be applied before* $\vee$-Unit, $\vee$-Eqv-1 *and* $\vee$-Eqv-2.

Branching Extension Step: *if N' is a leaf of an ALT $\mathcal{T}'$ for C and X, and non-branching extension steps are not applicable to N', and Split is applicable to $\lambda(N')$, then $\mathcal{T}$ is an ALT for C and X, where $\mathcal{T}$ is obtained from $\mathcal{T}'$ by attaching two new child nodes N_l and N_r below N', and $\lambda(N_l)$ and $\lambda(N_r)$ are obtained by a single application of Split to $\lambda(N')$.*

We abbreviate "ALT for C and X" as "ALT" if context allows.

Definition 5 (Open, Closed, Derivation, Finishedness, Fairness). *A branch $\mathcal{B}$ in an ALT $\mathcal{T}$ is closed iff for some node N of $\mathcal{B}$ it holds $\square \in C \cup X$, where $\lambda(N) = (\mathcal{A}, C, X)$. Otherwise it is open. An ALT $\mathcal{T}$ is closed iff every branch of $\mathcal{T}$ is closed, otherwise it is open. The branch $\mathcal{B}$ is finished iff $\mathcal{B}$ is closed or no extension step is applicable to the leaf of $\mathcal{B}$. An ALT $\mathcal{T}$ is finished iff every branch of $\mathcal{T}$ is finished. The term unfinished means not "not finished". A derivation $\mathcal{D}$ (for given C and X) is a sequence $\mathcal{T}_0, \mathcal{T}_1, \ldots, \mathcal{T}_n, \ldots$ of ALTs, such that $\mathcal{T}_0$ is obtained by an initialization step, and for $i > 0$, $\mathcal{T}_i$ is obtained by an extension step applied to $\mathcal{T}_{i-1}$. A derivation $\mathcal{D}$ is fair iff it does not end in an unfinished ALT.*

Remark 8. The ALTs are the objects that are actually computed with. Observe that a *fair* derivation either ends in a closed ALT (which means that the set $C \cup X$ is unsatisfiable), or ends in an open ALT with at least one open and finished branch (which, as will be shown, represents a *functional description* of a model for $C \cup X$), or does not terminate (which will be shown to be impossible in Lemma 2).

An *effective proof procedure* can be constructed by the simplest greedy strategy: start with an ALT for C and X by an initialization step, and apply extension steps as long as possible. Thereby, one would actually pursue only one branch at a time, not further extend closed branches and delete closed branches from memory as soon as derived. Under these regime, only polynomial space is consumed.

We do not specify a sophisticated proof procedure here, in particular since the design of an *efficient* proof procedure that takes advantage of good strategies for the unspecified parameters (selection of literals, actual preference of inference rules) depends from practical experiments which have not been carried out yet. For instance, it seems natural to choose, among the possible selections of literals in xor-clauses, those that maximize the future application of the Eqv or Unit rules. Fortunately, the correctness proof in the next section guarantees that any setting within the inference rule preferences stated in Definition 4 is complete.

8 Correctness

The *soundness* proof – that any closed ALT for C and X indicates unsatisfiability of $C \cup X$ – is done by standard means and is omitted. To show *completeness*, we first show that exhaustive application of the inference rules always terminates:

Lemma 2 (Termination). *Any derivation $\mathcal{D}$ for given C and X is finite.*

Proof. It suffices to show that no branch can be endlessly extended. At the heart of this proof are well-founded, strict partial orderings $\gg_N$ on clauses associated to the nodes N of the constructed ALTs. As a preliminary step, let $>_N$ be a binary relation over atoms associated to node N, which is defined inductively as follows:

$$>_N = \begin{cases} \{(A, \top) \mid A \text{ is an atom}\}, \text{ if } N \text{ is the root node} \\ >_{N'} \cup \{(A/L) \mid (A/L) \in \mathcal{A}\} \\ \quad \cup \{(|K|, |L_1|), \ldots, (|K|, |L_k|) \mid \underline{K} \oplus L_1 \oplus \cdots \oplus L_k \in X\} \ , \\ \text{where } \lambda(N) = (\mathcal{A}, C, X), \text{ if } N \text{ has the immediate ancestor node } N'. \end{cases}$$

That is, $>_N$ starts in a trivial way, and gets enlarged as new assignments come up or selections are done when going down the branches. An important detail is that $>_N$ monotonically increases in this process.

The transitive closure of $>_N$ is denoted by $\succ_N$. In order to compare clauses take the usual multiset extension $\succ\!\!\succ_N$ of the literal ordering in which L_1 is strictly greater than L_2 iff $|L_1| \succ_N |L_2|$ or else $L_1 = \neg L_2$ (i.e. $\neg A$ is greater than A). It is well-known that if $\succ_N$ is a strict, well-founded ordering (on atoms), as will be shown below, so is $\succ\!\!\succ_N$ (on clauses).

We need several *invariants* to hold for each node N, where $\lambda(N) = (\mathcal{A}, C, X)$:

(i) If $|K| >_N |L|$, then (a) $|K|$ is the left hand side of an assignment in $\mathcal{A}$, or (b) K or $\overline{K}$ is the selected literal in some xor-clause in X.

(ii) For each selected atom $A \in \mathrm{sel}(X)$ there is exactly one xor-clause $C \in X$ such that A or $\neg A$ is a selected literal in C. Furthermore, this literal is the only selected literal occurrence in C.

(iii) If N has an immediate ancestor node N' and $\mathrm{sel}(X) \subset \mathrm{sel}(X')$, where $\lambda(N') = (\mathcal{A}', C', X')$, then either the $\oplus$-Simp rule or the $\oplus$-Unit rule or the $\oplus$-Eqv rule is applied to N' to obtain N (but no other rule). That is, if a selection is lost, these are the only possible sources.

(iv) The relation $\succ_N$ is a strict partial ordering on atoms.

(v) If N has an immediate ancestor node N' and Select is applied to N', then $>_N \supset >_{N'}$.

The proof of the invariants is omitted here for space reasons; it can be found in the full version. They are used now to argue for termination. We feel no need for a completely formal presentation of the lexicographic ordering underlying the following argumentation.

Suppose, to the contrary, there is an infinite sequence of branches $\mathcal{B}_0, \mathcal{B}_1, \ldots$ such that, for $j \geq 0$, $\mathcal{B}_j$ is a branch of some $\mathcal{T}_i$ of the given derivation (written as in Def. 5), and that an extension step is applied to the leaf of $\mathcal{B}_j$, and $\mathcal{B}_{j+1}$ is a branch resulting from this application. We are now investigating possible sources for this branch sequence to be infinite.

First, from some point in time on, the $>_N$-relation is the same (referring to the leaves of the branches in the considered branch sequence), because only finitely many literals are at disposal, and $>_{N_j} \subseteq >_{N_{j+1}}$ by construction of $>_N$, where N_j is the leaf of $\mathcal{B}_j$.

Consequently, together with invariant (v), the Select rule is applied a *last* time along the considered branch sequence.

Second, each of $\vee$-Unit, $\oplus$-Unit, and Split is applied a last time, because each of them *strictly* increases the set of assignment it modifies. This was argued for in Remarks 4 and 5. Clearly, this strictness suffices as a proof for the claim.

Third, each Eqv rule is applied a last time. The arguments are the same is in "second", by using Remark 7.

Fourth, the rules mentioned at "second" and "third" are the only ones to extend assignments. Hence, from some point in time on, the set of assignments is the same in each leaf of the considered branch sequence.

Fifth, from "fourth" and the idempotency of assignments (cf. again Remarks 4, 5 and 7) it follows immediately that the Simp rules are applied a last time.

Sixth, hence, only the Gauss and Red rules remain as sources for infiniteness of the branch sequence. To show this impossibility, observe that with "first" the ordering $\gg_N$ is the same from some point in time on (invariant (iv) guarantees that $\gg_N$ is indeed a well-founded, strict partial ordering). Further, the ordering $\gg_N$ is made such that the Gauss and Red rules both work strictly decreasing. More precisely, the Gauss rule refers to the Gauss$^-$ and Gauss$^+$ rules. These are applied with a left premise, in which L is the only selected literal (cf. the applicability condition of Gauss and invariant (ii)) and which is strictly larger than each of the rest literals (by construction of the ordering). Hence, the right premise strictly decreases wrt. $\gg_N$. For the Red rules it is straightforward to check that they work strictly decreasing wrt. $\gg_N$, provided they are applicable. An important detail is to make $\neg A$ bigger than A.

Hence, in sum, with Gauss and Red working strictly decreasing wrt. $\gg_N$, which is the same from some point in time on, both of them are applied a last time.

All inference rules are now shown to be applied a last time along the considered branch sequence. Hence it must be finite, and thus the lemma is proven.

Theorem 1 (Completeness). *Let $\mathcal{D}$ be a fair derivation for a set of or-clauses C and a set of xor-clauses X. Then, $\mathcal{D}$ is finite, and if the last ALT $\mathcal{T}$ in $\mathcal{D}$ is open, then $C \cup X$ is satisfiable.*

This is our main result. Observe that in the contrapositive direction it just expresses refutation completeness.

Proof. Finiteness of $\mathcal{D}$ is given by Lemma 2. Therefore suppose that $\mathcal{T}$ is the last ALT in $\mathcal{D}$, and that $\mathcal{T}$ is open. We are concentrating on an open and finished branch $\mathcal{B}$ in $\mathcal{T}$, which must exist according to Remark 8. Let N be the leaf of $\mathcal{B}$, and $\lambda(N) = (\mathcal{A}, C, X)$. The first observation is that $C = \{\}$ or $C = \{\top\}$ (which is equivalent). The proof is by contradiction: the case that C contains the empty clause is impossible, because then $\mathcal{B}$ would be closed. Also, if C would consist of clauses containing the symbol $\top$ only (with the single exception of the clause $\top$), it would would have been simplified to either $C = \{\}$, $C = \{\top\}$ or $C = \{\square\}$ (contradicting the finishedness of $\mathcal{B}$). Hence C contains at least a clause with a literal different from $\top$. Let L be such a literal. But then, Split with $|L|$ would have been applied, contradicting finishedness of $\mathcal{B}$ again. This completes the proof that $C = \{\}$ or $C = \{\top\}$.

Thus, to construct a model, we have to consider $\mathcal{A}$ and X only. We use the strategy indicated in Remark 6: we give an arbitrary value to the variables that are not selected in X, and we show how to extend to a model.

Fact: in each clause $C \in X$ there is exactly one occurrence of a selected literal, and all the selected literals are pairwise different (modulo sign). This is due to invariant (ii) in the proof of Lemma 2, and the finishedness of $\mathcal{B}$. For, if in some $C \in X$ no literal would be selected, and Select is not applicable to C, then some literal in C is selected in a different clause (modulo sign), and thus Gauss would be applicable, contradicting finishedness.

Now take any literal L occuring in X but such that $|L| \notin \text{sel}(X)$. Add it as an assignment $|L|/\top$ (or $|L|/\neg\top$) to $\mathcal{A}$. $\mathcal{A}$ must still be idempotent and functional, because as a consequence of finishedness, $|L|$ must be undefined in $\mathcal{A}$, and so Lemma 1 is applicable. Repeat this, until all non-selected literals receive an explicit (arbitrary) truth value in $\mathcal{A}$.

Finally, only the selected literals in X do not have explicit truth values in $\mathcal{A}$. Since each of them occurs only once in a clause in X (by the above *fact*), their truth values can be chosen locally to the containing clauses as the appropriate parity for the rest clause, which has been completely specified by the arbitrary assignments. Furthermore, by the *fact* again, this can be done for *every* xor-clause in X. Hence, for each such selected literal L and its appropriate truth value, add a respective assignment $|L|/\top$ (or $|L|/\neg\top$) to $\mathcal{A}$. This is possible, because, by finishedness again, L must be undefined in $\mathcal{A}$ (by the $\oplus$-Simp rule). Finally, explicit truth assignments for all the literals occuring as right hind sides in $\mathcal{A}$ are added arbitrarily. This procedure results in a functional assignment to either $\top$ or $\neg\top$ for all atoms, which is just a model.

9   Conclusions

In this paper we have presented a decision procedure called Gauss-DPLL for combined clausal and affine logic (i.e. clauses with xor as the connective).

We have argued that procedures to solve such problems are needed to *efficiently* decide respective problems, which occur frequently in real-world applications like circuit verification and logical cryptanalysis. Gauss-DPLL is a tight integration in a unifying framework of a Gauss-Elimination procedure (for affine logic) and a Davis-Putnam-Logeman-Loveland procedure (for usual clause logic).

The main ideas, which distinguishes our approach from other approaches in the literature, are the following: at first, we provide a coherent approach of the treatment of both or and xor-clauses which specialized to optimized decision procedures when the input is restricted to either of them. Second we allow for a heavy interleaving of the two parts with the purpose to maximize (deterministic) simplification by passing around newly created unit or binary clauses in either of these parts. Last, but not least, we are able to stop the search and output a functional description of the model rather than a completely specified model.

As noted in [Li00], the explicit handling of equivalences makes it possible to transform exponentially long proofs of hard DIMACS benchmarks by Dubois and Pretolani [JT96,Li00] using classical DPLL into short polynomial proofs. This result is accomplished by Li using rules corresponding to restricted versions of boolean reduction, simplifications and equivalences. The Gauss-DPLL procedure also inherits that speedup over classical DPLL.

The calculus is not implemented yet, but we plan to do so in the near future.

References

[BCC+99] A. Biere, A. Cimatti, E. Clarke, M. Fujita, and Y. Zhu. Symbolic model checking using SAT procedures instead of BDDs. In *Proc. of ACM/IEEE DAC-99*, pages 317–320. ACM Press, 1999.

[BDW95] B. Becker, R. Drechsler, and R. Werchner. On the relation between BDDs and FDDs. *Inf. and Comp.*, 123(2):185–197, 1995.

[BRB90] K. Brace, R. Rudell, and R. Bryant. Efficient implementation of a BDD package. In *Proc. of ACM/IEEE DAC-90*, pages 40–45. IEEE Press, 1990.

[BS97] R. Bayardo and R. Schrag. Using CSP look-back techniques to solve real-world SAT instances. In *Proc. of AAAI-97*, pages 203–208. AAAI Press/The MIT Press, 1997.

[CA96]   J. Crawford and L. Auton. Experimental results on the crossover point in random 3SAT. *AIJ*, 81(1-2):31–57, 1996.

[CL73]   C. Chang and R. Lee. *Symbolic Logic and Mechanical Theorem Proving*. Academic Press, 1973.

[Cla90]   L. Claesen, ed. *Formal VLSI Correctness Verification: VLSI Design Methods*, volume II. Elsevier, 1990.

[DBR97]   R. Drechsler, B. Becker, and S. Ruppertz. Manipulation algorithms for K*BMDs. In *Proc. of TACAS-97*, LNCS 1217, pages 4–18. Springer-Verlag, 1997.

[DLL62]   M. Davis, G. Logeman, and D. Loveland. A machine program for theorem proving. *CACM*, 5(7), 1962.

[GMS98]   E. Giunchiglia, A. Massarotto, and R. Sebastiani. Act and the rest will follow: Explit-ing nondeterminism in planning as satisfiability. In *Proc. of AAAI-98*, pages 948–952. The MIT Press, 1998.

[GW00]   J. Groote and J. Warners. The propositional formula checker HeerHugo. *JAR*, 2000. To appear.

[HS98]   U. Hustadt and R. Schmidt. Simplification and backjumping in modal tableau. In *Proc. of TABLEAUX-98*, LNAI 1397 , pages 187–201. Springer-Verlag, 1998.

[JT96]   D. Johnson and M. Trick, eds. *Cliques, Coloring, satisfiability: the second DIMACS implementation challenge*, volume 26 of *AMS Series in Discr. Math. and TCS*. AMS, 1996.

[KS96]   H. Kautz and B. Selman. Pushing the envelope: Planning, propositional logic and stocastic search. In *Proc. of AAAI-96*, pages 1194–1201. The MIT Press, 1996.

[Li99]   Chu-Min Li. A constraint-based approach to narrow search trees for satisfiability. *IPL*, 71(2):75–80, 1999.

[Li00]   Chun-Min Li. Integrating equivalency reasoning into Davis-Putnam procedure. To appear in *Proc. of AAAI-00*.

[Mas98]   Fabio Massacci. Simplification: A general constraint propagation technique for propositional and modal tableaux. In *Proc. of TABLEAUX-98*, LNAI 1397, pages 217–231. Springer-Verlag, 1998.

[Mas99]   Fabio Massacci. Using Walk-SAT and Rel-sat for cryptographic key search. In *Proc. of IJCAI-99*, pages 290–295. Morgan Kaufmann, 1999.

[MM00]   Fabio Massacci and Laura Marraro. Logical cryptanalysis as a SAT-problem: Encoding and analysis of the u.s. Data Encryption Standard. *JAR*, 2000. To appear.

[Sch78]   T. Schaefer. The complexity of satisfiability problems. In *Proc. of STOC-78*, pages 216–226. ACM Press, 1978.

[SKM97]   Bart Selman, Henry Kautz, and David McAllester. Ten challenges in propositional resoning and search. In *Proc. of IJCAI-97*, pages 50–54. Morgan Kaufmann, 1997.

[Wil90]   J. Wilson. Compact normal forms in propositional logics and integer programming formulations. *Comp. and Op. Res.*, 17(3):309–314, 1990.

[WvM99]   J. Warners and H. van Maaren. A two phase algorithm for solving a class of hard satisfiability problems. *Op. Res. Lett.*, 23(3-5):81–88, 1999.

[WvM00]   J. Warners and H. van Maaren. Recognition of tractable satisfiability problems through balanced polynomial representations. *Discr. Appl. Math.*, 2000.

[Zha97]   H. Zhang. SATO: An Efficient Propositional Theorem Prover. In *Proc. of CADE 97*, LNAI 1249, pages 272–275, 1997. Springer-Verlag.

On an ω-Decidable Deductive Procedure for Non-Horn Sequents of a Restricted FTL

Regimantas Pliuškevičius

Institute of Mathematics and Informatics
Akademijos 4, Vilnius 2600, Lithuania
regis@ktl.mii.lt

Abstract. A new deduction-based procedure is presented for non-Horn, so-called DR-sequents with repetitions of a restricted first-order linear temporal logic with temporal operators "next" and "always". The main part of the proposed deductive procedure is automatic generation of the inductive hypothesis. The proposed deductive procedure consists of three separate decidable deductive procedures replacing the infinitary omega-type rule for the operator "always". These three decidable parts cannot be joined. Therefore the proposed deductive procedure (by analogy with ω-completeness) is only ω-decidable. The specific shape of DR-sequents allows us in all the three parts of the proposed deductive procedure to construct: (1) a deduction tree in some linear form , i.e., with one "temporal" branch; (2) length-preserving derivations, i.e., the lengths of generated sequents are the same.

1 Introduction

Temporal logic has been found valuable for the specification of various computer systems and multi-agent systems (see, e.g., [3]). To use such specifications, however, it is necessary to have techniques for reasoning on temporal logic formulas. Model-checking methods are effective and automatic for temporal formulas that are propositional. For more complex systems, however, it is necessary or convenient to employ a first-order temporal logic (FTL, in short). FTL is a very expressive language (see, e.g., [1]). Unfortunately, FTL is incomplete, in general (see, e.g., [1, 10]). But it becomes complete (see, e.g., [5, 11]) after adding an ω-type rule (which we present in the sequent version):

$$\frac{\Gamma \to \Delta, A; \ldots; \Gamma \to \Delta, \bigcirc^k A; \ldots}{\Gamma \to \Delta, \square A}(\to \square_\omega),$$

where $\bigcirc^k A$ means "k-time next A". So, FTL is ω-complete, in general. In some particular cases, the FTL (and, of course, in the propositional case) is finitary complete and/or decidable (see, e.g., [4]).

The deductive procedure Sat_ω, proposed here, is based on a revised version of saturation-type [6, 7] calculi devoted to consider some complete classes of FTL. The object of consideration of Sat_ω is the so-called DR-sequents with

J. Lloyd et al. (Eds.): CL 2000, LNAI 1861, pp. 523–537, 2000.

repetitions, that are a certain skolemized version of M. Fisher's normal form [2]. The shape of DR-sequents allows us to construct decidable "loop-free" calculi for "induction-free" DR-sequents, i.e., without positive occurrence of $\square$ and for DR-sequents "with induction", i.e., containing positive occurrence of $\square$. The proposed deductive procedure Sat_ω for DR-sequents consists of three separate decidable parts. The goal of the first part of Sat_ω is to obtain (from a given DR-sequent S) a so-called elementary DR-sequent S^*. The problem of generating an elementary DR-sequent is decidable, i.e., after the finite number of steps we get either $Sat_\omega \vdash S^*$ (if the given DR-sequent S is valid) or $Sat_\omega \nvdash S^*$ (if S is invalid). The goal of the second part of Sat_ω is to construct the so-called similarity substitution σ (each component of which is periodic, for example, $x^* \leftarrow f_1(\ldots(f_n(x^*))\ldots)$ and the sequent S_p, which is identical to $S^*\sigma$ where $S^*\sigma$ differs from S^* only by values of the variables, which are determined by the similarity substitution σ. The problem of generating the similarity substitution σ and the sequent S_p such that $S_p = S^*\sigma$ is decidable, i.e., after the finite number of steps we get either $Sat_\omega \vdash S_p$ (if the given DR-sequent S is valid), or $Sat_\omega \nvdash S^*\sigma$ (if S is invalid). With the aid of the obtained similarity substitution σ the *inductive hypothesis of the shape* $S^*\sigma^n (n \in \omega)$ is constructed directly. Then the generated inductive hypothesis $S^*\sigma^n$ is verified, i.e., it is checked that $Sat_\omega \vdash S^*\sigma^n$ $(n \in \omega)$. This verification is carried out by induction on n. The basis case, i.e., that $Sat_\omega \vdash S^*\sigma$, is the same as the second stage of Sat_ω. The step of induction, i.e., that $Sat_\omega \vdash S^*\sigma^n \Rightarrow Sat_\omega \vdash S^*\sigma^{n+1}$, is realized in the third stage of Sat_ω. If all the three parts are successful, then $Sat_\omega \vdash S$, i.e., the given DR-sequent S is valid. The second and third parts of Sat_ω cannot be connected: we cannot deduce the sequent $S^*\sigma^n$. We can only automatically test that from the assumption $S^*\sigma^n$ it is possible (or not) to deduce a sequent S_p such that $S_p = S^*\sigma^{n+1}$. The second and third parts make up the main stage of the proposed deductive procedure Sat_ω. In common they replace the ω-rule $(\rightarrow \square_\omega)$ for DR-sequents. The specific shape of DR-sequents enables us in all the three parts of Sat_ω to construct: (1) a deduction tree in some linear form , i.e., with one "temporal" branch; (2) length-preserving derivations, i.e., the lengths of generated sequents are the same. These properties demonstrate a high degree of mechanization of the proposed deductive procedure. Since all the three parts of Sat_ω are decidable (but not joinable!), by analogy with the ω-completeness, we can say that the deductive procedure Sat_ω is ω-decidable.

In general, we call a *deductive procedure for an ω-complete logic ω-decidable, if it consists of $n > 1$ separate, not joinable, decidable deductive procedures.* Let P_ω be an ω-decidable deductive procedure and D_ω be the objects (sequents or formulas) of consideration of P_ω. Then D_ω compose an *ω-decidable class.* Therefore, the ω-decidability is a natural extension of the traditional decidability which is applied to a complete logic or a subset of the complete logic.

The paper is organized as follows. Section 2 introduces a loop-free infinitary (i.e., with the ω-rule $(\rightarrow \square_\omega)$) calculus $G^*_{L\omega}$ containing instead of the traditional loop rule $(\square \rightarrow)$ a non-traditional, nonlocal loop-free rule and an induction-free (i.e., without the ω-rule $(\rightarrow \square_\omega)$) decidable calculus G^*. The infinitary calculus is sound and complete with respect to DR-sequents. In section 3, the three separate decidable parts consisting of the proposed deductive procedure Sat_ω are described and founded. The equivalence between the proposed procedure Sat_ω and the infinitary calculus $G^*_{L\omega}$ is sketched. In section 4, conclusions, related works and future investigations are described briefly.

2   Infinitary Calculus $G^*_{L\omega}$ and Induction-Free Calculus G^*

The proposed deductive procedure Sat_ω is founded using the infinitary, loop-free infinitary calculus $G^*_{L\omega}$ containing a non-traditional, non-local loop-free rule instead of the traditional loop rule ($\square \rightarrow$). Since of the objects of consideration of the calculus $G^*_{L\omega}$ are DR-sequents (see below), the calculus $G^*_{L\omega}$ does not contain any logical rules. For simplicity, we consider only one-place predicate and function symbols, also, we assume that all the predicate symbols are flexible (i.e., change their value in time), and all function symbols are rigid (i.e., with time-independent meanings). We consider only skolemized formulas.

In the first-order linear temporal logic we have that $\bigcirc(A \odot B) \equiv \bigcirc A \odot \bigcirc B (\odot \in \{\supset, \wedge, \vee\})$ and $\bigcirc \sigma A \equiv \sigma \bigcirc A (\sigma \in \{\neg, \square, \forall x, \exists x\})$. Relying on these equivalences we can consider occurrences of the "next" operator $\bigcirc$ only entering the formula $\bigcirc^k E$ (where E is an *elementary formula*, i.e., the expression of the shape $P(t)$, where P is a predicate symbol, t is a term). For the sake of simplicity, we "eliminate" the "next" operator and the formula $\bigcirc^k E$ is abbreviated as E^k (i.e., as an elementary formula with the index k). We also use the notation A^k for an arbitrary formula A in the following meaning.

Definition 1 (Index, Atomic Formula). *1) If E is an elementary formula, $i, k \in \omega$, $k \neq 0$, then $(E^i)^k := E^{i+k}$ $(E^0 := E)$; $E^l (l \geqslant 0)$ is called an atomic formula, and E^l becomes elementary if $l = 0$; 2) $(A \odot B)^k := A^k \odot B^k$ if $\odot \in \{\supset, \wedge, \vee\}$; $(\sigma A)^k := \sigma A^k$ if $\sigma \in \{\square, \forall x, \neg, \exists x\}$. For example, the expression $\forall x(P^1(x) \supset Q^3(f(x)))^1$ means the formula $\forall x(P^2(x) \supset Q^4(f(x)))$.*

Definition 2 (Sequent). *A sequent is an expression of the form $\Gamma \rightarrow \Delta$, where we assume that Γ, Δ are arbitrary finite multisets (i.e., not sequences or sets) of formulas.*

Definition 3 (Kernel Formula). *Formulas of the shape $\square \forall x(Q^l(\bar{f}(x)) \supset E^k(x))$ are called the kernel formulas, if $E^k(x)$ is an atomic formula without function symbols (called the conclusion of the kernel formula); if $k = 0$, then the kernel formula is called the elementary one; $Q^l(\bar{f}(\bar{x}))$ is an atomic formula (called the premise formula of the kernel), where $\bar{f}(x) = f_1(f_2 \ldots (f_n(x)) \ldots)$, ($f_i$ $(1 \leqslant i \leqslant n)$ is one-place function symbol) called an eigen-term of the kernel premise.*

Definition 4 (DR-Sequents, Induction-Free DR-Sequents, Elementary DR-Sequents). *A sequent S is a DR-sequent if S has the shape $\square \Omega \rightarrow \Sigma, \Pi^1$, $\square^0 A$, where $\square^0 \in \{\emptyset, \square\}$; $\Sigma = \emptyset$ or consists of elementary formulas, $\Pi^1 = \emptyset$ or* *consists of atomic formulas of the form* E^l $(l > 0)$ $(\Sigma, \Pi^1$ *is the parametrical part of a DR-sequent);* $\Box\Omega$ *consists of kernel formulas;* $A = \exists y_1, \ldots, y_n \overset{m}{\underset{i=1}{\vee}} \neg E_i(y_i)$ $(m \leqslant n)$, *where* $E_i(y_i)$ *is an atomic formula. If* $\Box^0 = \varnothing$, *i.e., if* $S = \Box\Omega \rightarrow \Sigma, \Pi^1, A$, *then* S *is called an induction-free DR-sequent. A DR-sequent is an elementary one if all kernel formulas are elementary ones. We assume that all eigen-terms of kernel premises are different. Besides a DR-sequent must satisfy the following conditions:*

(1) *let* E^l *be a parametrical formula, then* $E^l = E_i^l(\bar{f}_i(x^*))$, *where* $E_i^k(\bar{f}_i(x))$ *is the premise of a kernel formula and* $l < k$ *(saturation condition);*

(2) *for any kernel formula* $\Box\forall x(Q^l(\bar{f}(x)) \supset E^k(x))$ *there must be* $k < l$ *(kernel index condition);*

(3) *for each kernel conclusion there exists a kernel premise having the same predicate symbol and vice versa (bounded connectivity condition);*

(4) *there exist at least two kernel conclusions with the same predicate symbol (kernel conclusion repetitions condition).*

From the bounded connectivity condition and the notion of sequent we get the following

Lemma 1. *Let* $S = \Box\Omega \rightarrow \Sigma, \Pi^1, \Box A$ *be a DR-sequent, then the kernel* $\Box\Omega$ *can be "ordered" in the following way* $\Box\forall x_1(E_1^{k_1}(\bar{f}_1(x_1)) \supset E^{l_1}(x_1))$, $\Box\forall x_2$ $(E_2^{k_2}(\bar{f}_2(x_2)) \supset E_1^{l_2}(x_2)), \ldots, \Box\forall x_n(E_n^{k_n}(\bar{f}_n(x_n)) \supset E_{n-1}^{l_n}(x_n))$ $k_i > l_i$, $1 \leqslant i \leqslant n$ *and* $E = E_n$.

Remark 1. (a) Since we consider *DR*-sequents with repetitions (see the kernel conclusion repetitions condition), the same *DR*-sequent might have different ordered kernels. For example, let $\Box\Omega^1 = \Box\forall x_1(E^3(f(x_1)) \supset E^1(x_1))$, $\Box\forall x_2(E^4(h(x_2))) \supset E^1(x_2))$, $\Box\forall x_3(E^5(g(x_3)) \supset E^1(x_3))$. The kernel $\Box\Omega^1$ has the shape indicated in Lemma 1, therefore $\Box\Omega^1$ is an ordered kernel. It is easy to present another ordered kernel of the following shape: $\Box\forall x_1(E^3(f(x_1)) \supset E^1(x_1))$, $\Box\forall x_2(E^5(g(x_2)) \supset E^1(x_2))$, $\Box\forall x_3(E^4(h(x_3)) \supset E^1(x_3))$. It should be stressed that, if we choose some ordering of the kernel, then this ordering must be fixed forever, i.e., after fixed ordering we consider the kernel $\Box\Omega$ *not as a multiset but as a list.*

(b) A Horn-like version (so-called *D*-sequents) of *DR* -sequents is of the following shape $\Sigma, \Pi^1, \Box\Omega \rightarrow \Box^0 A$, where $\Sigma(\Pi^1)$ consists of elementary (atomic, respectively), formulas, $\Box^0 \in \{\varnothing, \Box\}$; $A = \exists y_1, \ldots, y_n \overset{m}{\underset{i=1}{\vee}} E_i(y_i)$ $(m \leq n)$ $(E_i(y_i)$ is an atomic formula); the kernel $\Box\Omega$ consists of formulas of the shape $\Box\forall x(E^k(x) \supset Q^l(\bar{f}(x)))$, where $k < l$. The ω-decidable deductive procedure for Horn-like *D*-sequents is described and founded in [9].

Definition 5 (Fixed-Ordered *DR*-Sequents: *FODR*-Sequents). *A DR-sequent with a fixed ordered kernel is a fixed-ordered DR-sequent (in short: FODR-sequent).*

Definition 6 (Compatible Kernel and Parametrical Formulas). *Let $S = \square\Omega \;\to\; \Sigma, \Pi^1, \square A$ be a FODR-sequent and $\square\Omega \;=\; \square\forall x_1(E_1^{k_1}(\bar{f}_1(x_1)) \supset E^{l_1}(x_1))$, $\square\forall x_2(E_2^{k_2}(\bar{f}_2(x_2)) \supset E_1^{l_2}(x_2))$, ..., $\square\forall x_{i+1}(E_{i+1}^{k_{i+1}}(\bar{f}_{i+1}(x_{i+1})) \supset E_i^{l_{i+1}}(x_{i+1}))$, ..., $\square\forall x_n(E_n^{k_n}(\bar{f}_n(x_n)) \supset E_{n-1}^{l_n}(x_n))$ (where $E = E_n$). Let $1 \leqslant i \leqslant n-2$, $E_i(\bar{f}_i(x_i^*))$ be any elementary formula from Σ, then the elementary kernel formula $\square\forall x_{i+1}(E_{i+1}^{k_{i+1}}(\bar{f}_{i+1}(x_{i+1})) \supset E_i(x_{i+1}))$ is compatible with $E_i(\bar{f}_i(x_i^*))$. The elementary kernel formula $\square\forall x_1(E_1^{k_1}(\bar{f}_1(x_1)) \supset E(x_1))$ is compatible with $E_n(\bar{f}_n(x_n^*))$ (where $E_n = E$).*

Definition 7 (Operation $(+)$). *Let $S = \square\Omega \;\to\; \Sigma, \Pi^1, \square^0 A$ be a FODR-sequent. Let $E_i(\bar{f}_i(x_i^*))$ (where $1 \leqslant i \leqslant n-1$) be any elementary formula from Σ and the elementary kernel formula $\square\forall x_{i+1}(E_{i+1}^{k_{i+1}}(\bar{f}_{i+1}(x_{i+1})) \supset E_i(x_{i+1}))$ from the sequent S is compatible with $E_i(\bar{f}_i(x_i^*))$. Then operation $(+)$ is defined as follows: $(E_i(\bar{f}_i(x_i^*)))^+ := E_{i+1}^{k_{i+1}-1}(\bar{f}_{i+1}(x_{i+1}^*))$ (where x_{i+1}^* is a new variable such that $x_{i+1}^* \leftarrow \bar{f}_i(x_i^*)$. Let $i = n$, then $(E_n(\bar{f}_n(x_n^*)))^+ := E_1^{k_1-1}(\bar{f}_1(x_1^*))$, where x_1^* is a new variable such that $x_1^* \leftarrow \bar{f}_n(x_n^*)$. Let $\Sigma = E_1(t_1), \ldots, E_n(t_n)$, then $(\Sigma)^+ := (E_1(t_1))^+, \ldots, (E_n(t_n))^+$.*

Example 1. Let $\Sigma = E(f(x_1^*))$, $E(h(x_2^*))$, $E(g(x_3^*))$; $\square\Omega = \square\forall x_1(E^2(f(x_1)) \supset E(x_1))$, $\square\forall x_2(E^3(h(x_2)) \supset E(x_2))$, $\square\forall x_3(E^4(g(x_3)) \supset E(x_3))$. Then $E(f(x_1^*))$ is compatible with the elementary kernel formula $\square\forall x_2(E^3(h(x_2)) \supset E(x_2))$; $E(h(x_2^*))$ is compatible with the elementary kernel formula $\square\forall x_3(E^4(g(x_3)) \supset E(x_3))$; $E(g(x_3^*))$ is compatible with the elementary kernel formula $\square\forall x_1 (E^2(f(x_1)) \supset E(x_1))$. Therefore $(\Sigma)^+ := E^2(h(x_{21}))$, $E^3(g(x_{31}))$, $E^1(f(x_{11}))$, where $x_{21} \leftarrow f(x_1^*)$, $x_{31} \leftarrow h(x_2^*)$, $x_{11} \leftarrow g(x_3^*)$.

Derivations in the calculus $G_{L\omega}^*$ are constructed in the bottom-up manner in the form of an infinite tree. The values of variables in the separation rule $(ISIF)$ (see below) will be indicated alongside with the premise of the rule in the form of substitutions $x^* \leftarrow t$, where x^* is a new variable, t is a corresponding term. According to that, the axiom of the calculus $G_{L\omega}^*$ will be enriched by the corresponding substitution. The shape of $FODR$-sequents allows us to specify, in a simple way, the axiomatic substitution using the matching methodology which is more efficient than the universal unification methodology. To specify the axiomatic substitution, let us introduce the following definitions.

Definition 8 (Solution of the Substitution). *Let $\sigma := \{x_n \leftarrow \bar{f}_n(x_{n-1}); x_{n-1} \leftarrow \bar{f}_{n-1}(x_{n-2}); \ldots; x_1 \leftarrow \bar{f}_1(x_0)\}$. Then the substitution $\sigma^* := \{x_n \leftarrow \bar{f}_n(\bar{f}_{n-1} (\ldots(\bar{f}_1(x_0))\ldots))\}$ is called the solution of the substitution σ.*

Definition 9 (Superterm of a Term). *Let $p = f_1(\ldots(f_i \ldots(f_n(x))\ldots)\ldots)$ (where x is a constant or a variable) and $q = f_1(\ldots(f_i(y))\ldots)$ (y is a variable) $(1 \leqslant i \leqslant n)$ (in a separate case, $n = 0$), then the term p is called a superterm of the term q (in symbols $p \succeq q$).*

Definition 10 (Matching Terms). *Let p, q be terms, σ be a substitution. We say that the term p matches the term q if $p\sigma \succeq q$.*

Definition 11 (Calculi $G^*_{L\omega}$, G^*). *The calculus $G^*_{L\omega}$ is defined by the following postulates.*

The axiom $(\exists)$: $\Box\Omega \to \Gamma, E_i(\bar{f}(x^*)), \exists y_1, \ldots, y_m \overset{n}{\underset{j=1}{\vee}} \neg E_j(\bar{f}_j(y_j))$ $(m \leqslant n,$

$m \geqslant 0,\ 1 \leqslant i \leqslant n)$, *where* $\bar{f}(x^*)\sigma^* \succeq \bar{f}_j(y_j)$; σ^* *is the solution of* σ_1, *where* σ_1 *starts from the substitution* $x^* \leftarrow t$ *and* $\sigma_1 \subseteq \sigma, \sigma$ *is the list of substitution obtained during the generation of the axiom* $(\exists)$.

The rules consist of the ω-type rule: $\dfrac{\{\Gamma \to \Delta, A^k\}_{k \in \omega}}{\Gamma \to \Delta, \Box A}$ $(\to \Box_\omega)$ *and the following (loop-free) integrated separation induction-free rule:*

$$\dfrac{\Box\Omega, \Box\Omega_1 \to (\Sigma)^+, \Pi, B^{k-1}}{\Box\Omega, \Box\Omega_1^1 \to \Sigma, \Pi^1, B^k}\ (ISIF), \quad k > 0,$$

where $\Sigma = \varnothing$ *or consists of elementary formulas;* $(\Sigma)^+$ *means the same as in Definition 7;* $\Pi^1 = \varnothing$ *or consists of atomic formulas of the shape* E^l $(l > 0)$; $\Box\Omega = \varnothing$ *or consists of elementary kernel formulas;* $\Box\Omega^1 = \varnothing$ *or consists of non-elementary kernel formulas;* $B = \exists y_1, \ldots, y_n \overset{m}{\underset{i=1}{\vee}} \neg E_i(y_i)$ $(m \leqslant n)$, $E_i(y_i)$ *is an atomic formula.*

The calculus G^* is obtained from $G^*_{L\omega}$ by dropping the ω-type rule $(\to \Box_\omega)$.

Analogously as in [5], using [8], we get the following

Theorem 1. *The calculus $G^*_{L\omega}$ is sound and complete for FODR-sequents.*

Lemma 2. *The calculus G^* is decidable.*

Proof. Follows from the decidability of the axiom $(\exists)$ and the shape of the rule $(ISIF)$.

Remark 2. The saturation and bounded connectivity conditions are non-essential for the construction of the proposed deductive procedure Sat_ω. The restrictions that only a one-place predicate and function symbols are considered and that a conclusion of the kernel formula does not contain function symbols are also non-essential. All these restrictions allow us only to simplify the components of Sat_ω. But the kernel index condition is essential for correctness of the rule $(ISIF)$. Indeed, let $S = \Box\forall x(P^1(f(x)) \supset P(x)), \Box\forall y(P(g(y)) \supset P^1(y)) \to P(c),$ $\exists y \neg P^1(f(g(y)))$. For the sequent S the kernel index condition is destroyed. It is easy to verify that $G^* \nvdash S$, but $G \vdash S$ (where G is obtained from G^* replacing the rule $(ISIF)$ by traditional loop-rules $(\Box \to), (\forall \to))$.

3 Description of the Deductive Procedure Sat_ω

Let us define the generalized integrated separation rule (GIS) which is the main tool of the proposed deductive procedure Sat_ω and which is applied to any non-induction-free FODR-sequent.

Definition 12 (Generalized Integrated Separation Rule: (GIS), Successful Application of (GIS)). *Let $S = \Box\Omega, \Box\Omega_1^1 \rightarrow \Sigma, \Pi^1, \Box A$ be a FODR-sequent. Let $(\Sigma)^+$ mean the same as in Definition 7, then the generalized integrated separation rule (GIS) is as follows:*

$$\frac{\Box\Omega, \Box\Omega_1^1 \rightarrow \Sigma, \Pi^1, B; \Box\Omega, \Box\Omega_1 \rightarrow (\Sigma)^+, \Pi, \Box B}{\Box\Omega, \Box\Omega_1^1 \rightarrow \Sigma, \Pi^1, \Box B} \ (GIS).$$

If the left premise of (GIS), i.e., the sequent $S_1 = \Box\Omega, \Box\Omega_1^1 \rightarrow \Sigma, \Pi^1, B$ is such that $G^* \vdash S_1$ we say that bottom-up application of (GIS) is successful.

To define the first deductive procedure of Sat_ω, let us define the kernel conclusion complexity of $FODR$-sequent $S : \pi(S)$, which serves as a halting test for the first deductive procedure of Sat_ω.

Definition 13 (Kernel Conclusion Complexity of $FODR$-Sequent S : $\pi(S)$, Elementary $FODR$-Sequent). *Let $S = \Box\Omega, \Box\Omega_1^1 \rightarrow \Sigma, \Pi^1, \Box B$ be a FODR-sequent, where $\Box\Omega$ $(\Box\Omega_1^1)$ consists of elementary (non-elementary, respectively) kernel formulas. Let $P_1^{k_1}, \ldots, P_n^{k_n}$ be the list of all kernel conclusions, then the kernel conclusion complexity of the FODR-sequent S (denoted as $\pi(S)$) is defined as $\max(k_1, \ldots, k_n)$. If $\pi(S) = 0$, then the FODR-sequent S is an elementary one.*

Now, let us define the first deductive procedure of Sat_ω, named the preliminary k-th resolvent (denoted by $PRe^k(S)$). The aim of $PRe^k(S)$ is to generate (from a given $FODR$-sequent S) the elementary $FODR$-sequent S^*.

Definition 14 (Preliminary k-th Resolvent: $PRe^k(S)$). *Let S be a FODR-sequent, then the preliminary k-th resolvent of the FODR-sequent S (in symbols: $PRe^k(S)$) is defined in the following way: $PRe^0(S) = S$. Let $PRe^k(S) = S_k = \Box\Omega, \Box\Omega_1^1 \rightarrow \Sigma, \Pi^1, \Box B$. Then $PRe^{k+1}(S)$ is defined in the following way:*

1. Let us bottom-up apply the rule (GIS) to S_k and S_{k1}, S_{k2} be the left and right premise of the application of (GIS).

2. If $G^* \nvdash S_{k1}$, then $PRe^{k+1}(S) = \bot$ (false) and the calculation of $PRe^{k+1}(S)$ is stopped.

3. Let $G^* \vdash S_{k1}$ (i.e., the bottom-up application of (GIS) is successful), then $PRe^{k+1}(S) = S_{k2}$.

4. If $PRe^{k+1}(S) = S_{k2}$ and $k+1 = \pi(S)$, then the calculation of $PRe^{k+1}(S)$ is finished.

Using the decidability of the calculus G^* we get the following

Lemma 3. *For a given FODR-sequent S the problem of generating the elementary sequent S^* is decidable.*

Example 2. Let $S = \Box\Omega^1 \rightarrow E^2(f(x_1^*)), E^3(h(x_2^*)), E^3(g(x_2^*)), E^4(g(x_3^*)), \Box A$, where $\Box\Omega^1$ is the same as in Remark 1(a), i.e., $\Box\Omega^1 = \Box\forall x_1(E^3(f(x_1)) \supset E^1(x_1)), \Box\forall x_2(E^4(h(x_2)) \supset E^1(x_2)), \Box\forall x_3(E^5(g(x_3)) \supset E^1(x_3)); A = \exists y(\neg\exists(y) \vee$

$\neg E^1(y) \vee \neg E^2(y))$. Let us construct the elementary $FODR$-sequent S^* using the procedure $PRe^k(S)$. Since $S_{11} = \Box\Omega^1 \rightarrow E^2(f(x_1^*)), E^3(h(x_2^*)), E^4(g(x_3^*))$, A is the axiom $(\exists)$, $G^* \vdash S_{11}$. Therefore, by definition, $PRe^1(S) = S^* = \Box\Omega \rightarrow E^1(f(x_1^*)), E^2(h(x_2^*)), E^3(g(x_3^*)), \Box A$ which is the elementary $FODR$-sequent, where $\Box\Omega = \Box\forall x_1(E^2(f(x_1)) \supset E(x_1)), \Box\forall x_2(E^3(h(x_2)) \supset E(x_2))$, $\Box\forall x_3(E^4(g(x_3)) \supset E(x_3))$.

Now we are going to define the basis part of Sat_ω – the saturated k-th resolvent (in symbols: $SRe^k(S^*)$). The aim of $SRe^k(S^*)$ is to generate (from the elementary $FODR$-sequent S^* obtained, by means of $PRe^k(S^*)$) the similarity substitution σ and an elementary $FODR$-sequent S_p such that $S_p = S^*\sigma$, i.e., S_p is coincidental with $S^*\sigma$, where $S^*\sigma$ differs from S^* only by the values of the variables which are determined by the "similarity" substitution σ. To define $SRe^k(S)$, let us define the halting test for $SRe^k(S^*)$, namely, the similarity index.

Definition 15 (Similarity Index). *Let $S = \Box\Omega \rightarrow \Sigma, \Pi^1, \Box B$ be an elementary $FODR$-sequent and $p_1, \ldots, p_n$ be indices of kernel premise formulas of S. Then $p(S) = \sum_{i=1}^{n} p_i$ is the similarity index of S. For example, let S^* be the elementary $FODR$-sequent obtained in Example 2, then $p(S^*) = 2 + 3 + 4 = 9$.*

Definition 16 (Saturated k-th Resolvent: $SRe^k(S^*)$). *Let S^* be an elementary $FODR$-sequent. Then the definition of $SRe^k(S^*)$ is obtained from the definition of $PRe^k(S^*)$ replacing $PRe^k(S^*)$ by $SRe^k(S^*)$ and replacing the point (4) by a new point (4): If $SRe^{k+1}(S^*) = S_{k2}$ and $k + 1 = p(S^*)$, then the calculation of $SRe^{k+1}(S^*)$ is completed.*

The notation $SRe^k(S) \neq \bot$ $(k \in \omega)$ means that all the possible bottom-up applications of (GIS) in constructing $SRe^k(S)$ are successful.

Lemma 4 (Composition of $SRe^k(S)$). *Let $SRe^n(S) = S_n, SRe^m(S_n) = S^*$ and $SRe^n(S) \neq \bot$, $SRe^m(S_n) \neq \bot$ $(n, m \in \omega)$, then $SRe^l(S) = S^*$, where $l = n + m$.*

Proof. By induction on l.

Lemma 5 (Decomposition of $SRe^k(S)$). *Let $SRe^{n+m}(S) = S^*$ and $SRe^{n+m}(S) \neq \bot$, then for each n and m there exists a sequent S_n such that $SRe^n(S) = S_n$ and $SRe^m(S_n) = S^*$.*

Proof. By induction on $n + m$.

Lemma 6 ("Length-Preserving" of $SRe^k(S)$). *Let S be an elementary $FODR$-sequent, i.e., $S = \Box\Omega \rightarrow \Sigma, \Pi^1, \Box A$ and $SRe^k(S) = S^*$, then $S^* = \Box\Omega \rightarrow \Sigma_1, \Pi_1^1, \Box A$, where $|\Sigma, \Pi^1| = |\Sigma_1, \Pi_1^1|$, i.e., the lengths of parametrical parts of S and S^* are the same.*

Proof. By induction on k. If $k = 0$, then $S = S^*$. Let $k \geqslant 1$ and let us consider the construction of $SRe^1(S) = S_1$. Let $\square\Omega = \square\forall x(E_1^{k_1}(\bar{f}_1(x_1)) \supset E(x_1)), \ldots, \square\forall x_i(E_i^{k_i}(\bar{f}_i(x_i)) \supset E_{i-1}(x_i)), \square\forall x_{i+1}(E_{i+1}^{k_{i+1}}(\bar{f}_{i+1}) \supset E_i(x_{i+1})), \ldots, \square\forall x_n(E_n^{k_n}(\bar{f}_n(x_n)) \supset E_{n-1}(x_n))$, where $E_n = E$. Let us consider an atomic formula E^l from the parametrical part of S. Assume $E^l \in \Pi^1$ (where $l > 0$), then by definition of (GIS) we have that the descendant of the atomic formula E^l in S_1 is of the shape E^{l-1}. Let $E^l = E_i(\bar{f}(x_i^*)) \in \Sigma$ (where $1 \leqslant i \leqslant n + 1$), then, by definition of the operation $(+)$, see Definition 7, the descendant of the elementary formula $E_i(\bar{f}_i(x_i))$ in S_1 is of the shape $E_{i+1}^{k_{i+1}-1}(\bar{f}_{i+1}(x_{i+1}^*))$ (where $x_{i+1}^* \leftarrow \bar{f}(x_i^*)$); if $i = n$, then $E_{i+1}^{k_{i+1}-1}(\bar{f}_{i+1}(x_{i+1}^*)) = E_1^{k_1-1}(\bar{f}_1(x_1^*))$. Therefore $S_1 = \square\Omega \to \Sigma_{11}, \Pi_{11}^1, \square A$, where $|\Sigma_{11}, \Pi_{11}^1| = |\Sigma, \Pi^1|$ (∗). If $k = 1$, then $S^* = S_1$. Let $k > 1$, then, relying on Lemma 5, we get $SRe^{k-1}(S_1) = S^*$. Using the induction hypothesis we have that $S^* = \square\Omega \to \Sigma_1, \Pi_1^1, \square A$ and $|\Sigma_1, \Pi_1^1| = |\Sigma_{11}, \Pi_{11}^1|$(∗∗). Using Lemma 4 and (∗), (∗∗) we get $SRe^k(S) = S^* = \square\Omega \to \Sigma_1, \Pi_1^1, \square A$ and $|\Sigma_1, \Pi_1^1| = |\Sigma, \Pi^1|$.

Lemma 7 (Accessibility of a Kernel Premise). *Let $S = \square\Omega \to \Sigma, \Pi^1, \square A$ be an elementary FODR-sequent, where $\square\Omega$ is a fixed ordered kernel of the shape $\square\forall x(E_1^{k_1}(\bar{f}_1(x_1)) \supset E(x_1)), \ldots, \square\forall x_i(E_i^{k_i}(\bar{f}_i(x_i)) \supset E_{i-1}(x_i)), \square\forall x_{i+1}(E_{i+1}^{k_{i+1}}(\bar{f}_{i+1}) \supset E_i(x_{i+1})), \ldots, \square\forall x_n(E_n^{k_n}(\bar{f}_n(x_n)) \supset E_{n-1}(x_n))$, where $E = E_n$. Let $E_i^l(\bar{f}_i(x_i^*))$ $(1 \leqslant i \leqslant n)$ be any member of the parametrical part Σ, Π^1, i.e., $\Delta = E_i^l(\bar{f}_i(x_i^*)), \Delta_1$, where $\Delta = \Sigma, \Pi^1$; let $SRe^k(S) \neq \bot (k \in \omega)$. Then $SRe^q(S) = \square\Omega \to E_{i+m}^{k_{i+m}-1}(\bar{f}_{i+m}(x_{i+m}^*)), \Delta_1^*, \square A$, where $1 \leqslant m \leqslant n - i$, if $i < n$; if $i = n$, then $m = 0$ and $E_{i+m}^{k_{i+m}-1}(\bar{f}_{i+m}(x_{i+m}^*)) = E_1^{k_1-1}(\bar{f}_1(x_1^*))$; moreover, $q = l + k_{i+1} + \ldots + k_{i+m-1} + 1$ if $m > 1$, and $q = l + 1$ if $m \leqslant 1$; besides, $x_{i+m}^* \leftarrow \bar{g}_i(x_i^*)$, where $\bar{g}_i(x_i^*) = g_{i1}(\ldots(g_{in}(x_i^*)\ldots))$, $g_{ir} = f_{jr}$ $(1 \leqslant r \leqslant n)$ and $f_{jr} \in \bar{f}_j(1 \leqslant j \leqslant n)$.*

Proof. By induction on m. Let $m = 0$, i.e., $i = n$. Since $SRe^k(S) \neq \bot(k \in \omega)$, applying (GIS) $q = (l + 1)$-time we get $SRe^q(S) = E_1^{k_1-1}(\bar{f}_1(x_1^*))$, where $x_1^* \leftarrow \bar{f}_n(x_n^*)$. Let $m = 1$. Since $SRe^k(S) \neq \bot$ $(k \in \omega)$, applying (GIS) $(l + 1)$-time we get $SRe^{l+1}(S) = S_1 = \square\Omega \to E_{i+1}^{k_{i+1}-1}(\bar{f}_{i+1}(x_{i+1}^*)), \Delta_{11}, \square A$ (where $x_{i+1}^* \leftarrow \bar{f}_i(x_i^*).$ (∗)). Let $m > 1$. Since $SRe^k(S) \neq \bot$ $(k \in \omega)$, we have that $SRe^k(S_1) \neq \bot$ $(k \in \omega)$. Applying the induction assumption to the sequent S_1, we get $SRe^\rho(S_1) = \square\Omega \to E_{i+m}^{k_{i+m}-1}(\bar{f}_{i+m}(x_{i+m}^*)), \Delta_1^*, \square A$, where $\rho = k_{i+1} - 1 + \ldots + k_{i+m-1} + 1$ and $x_{i+m}^* \leftarrow (\bar{h}_i(x_{i+1}^*)(∗∗)(\bar{h}_i(x_{i+1}^*) = h_{i1}(\ldots(x_{i+1}^*)\ldots)$ $h_{ir} = f_{jr}$, $f_{jr} \in \bar{f}_j$, $1 \leqslant j \leqslant n)$. Applying Lemma 4 to (∗), (∗∗) we get $SRe^q(S) = \square\Omega \to E_{i+m}^{k_{i+m}-1}(\bar{f}_{i+m}(x_{i+m}^*)), \Delta_1^*, \square A$, where $q = l + 1 + \rho = l + k_{i+1} + \ldots + k_{i+m-1} + 1$, $x_{i+m}^* \leftarrow \bar{h}_i(\bar{f}_i(x_i^*))$, and $\bar{h}_i(\bar{f}_i(x_i^*)) = \bar{g}_i(x_i^*) = g_{i1}(\ldots(g_{in}(x_i^*))\ldots)$, $g_{ir} = f_{jr}$, $1 \leqslant r \leqslant n$.

Lemma 8 (Generating a σ-Similar Sequent). *Let S^* be an elementary FODR-sequent, $SRe^k(S^*) \neq \bot$ $(k \in \omega)$, $p = p(S^*)$ be the similarity index of S^*, then $SRe^p(S^*) = S_p$ such that $S^*\sigma = S_p$, where σ is called the similarity substitution and the sequent S_p is called σ-similar to S^*.*

Proof. Let $S^* = \Box\Omega \to \Sigma, \Pi^1, \Box A$ be an elementary $FODR$-sequent, where $\Box\Omega = \Box\forall x(E_1^{k_1}(\bar{f}_1(x_1)) \supset E(x_1)), \ldots \Box\forall x_i(E_i^{k_i}(\bar{f}_i(x_i)) \supset E_{i-1}(x_i)), \Box\forall x_{i+1}$ $(E_{i+1}^{k_{i+1}}(\bar{f}_{i+1}) \supset E_i(x_{i+1})), \ldots, \Box\forall x_n(E_n^{k_n}(\bar{f}_n(x_n)) \supset E_{n-1}(x_n))$, and $E_n = E$. Let $1 \leqslant i \leqslant n-1$ and $E_i^l(\bar{f}_i(x_i^*))$ be any member of the parametrical part Σ, Π^1, i.e., $\Delta = E_i^l(\bar{f}_i(x_i^*)), \Delta_1$, where $\Delta = \Sigma, \Pi^1$. Let us take $i = i + m$, $n = i + m$ and apply Lemma 7 to the sequent S^*: we get $SRe^q(S^*) = S_q = \Box\Omega \to E_n^{k_n-1}(\bar{f}_n(x_n^*)), \Delta_{1q}, \Box A$ (where $q = l + k_{i+1} + \cdots + k_{n-1} + 1$ and $x_n^* \leftarrow \bar{g}_i(x_i^*)$) (*). Since $SRe^k(S^*) \neq \bot$ ($k \in \omega$), we can successfully continue the calculation of $SRe^k(S^*)$. Applying (GIS) k_n-time from the sequent S_q, we get $SRe^{q_1}(S_q) = S_{q_1} = \Box\Omega \to E_1^{k_1-1}(\bar{f}_1(x_1^*)), \Delta_{1q_1}, \Box A$ (where $q_1 = k_n$, $x_1^* \leftarrow \bar{f}_n(x_n^*) = x_1^* \leftarrow \bar{f}_n(\bar{g}_i(x_i^*))$) (**). Let us take $i = 1, i + m$, and apply Lemma 7 to the sequent S_{q_1}: we get $SRe^{q_2}(S_{q_1}) = S_{q_2} = \Box\Omega \to E_i^{k_i-1}(\bar{f}_i(x_{ip}^*)), \Delta_{1q_2}, \Box A$ (where $q_2 = k_1 - 1 + k_2 + \cdots + k_{i-1} + 1$ and $x_{i1}^* \leftarrow \bar{h}_i(x_1^*) = x_{ip}^* \leftarrow \bar{h}_i(\bar{f}_n(\bar{g}_i(x_i^*)))$) (***). Applying Lemma 4 to (*), (**), (***), we get $SRe^{q_3}(S^*) = S_{q_3} = \Box\Omega \to E_i^{k_i-1}(\bar{f}_i(x_{ip}^*)), \Delta_{1q_3}, \Box A$, where $q_3 = q + q_1 + q_2 = l + k_{i+1} + \cdots + k_{n-1} + 1 + k_n + k_1 - 1 + k_2 + \cdots + k_{i-1} + 1 = l + k_1 + \cdots + k_{i-1} + k_{i+1} + \cdots + k_n + 1$ (+). Applying (GIS) $(k_i - 1 - l)$-time beginning with the sequent S_{q_3}, we get $SRe^{q_4}(S_{q_3}) = \Box\Omega \to E_i^l(\bar{f}_i(x_{i1}^*)), \Delta_1^*, \Box A$ (where $q_4 = k_i - 1 - l$ (++). Applying Lemma 4 to (+), (++) we get $SRe^p(S^*) = \Box\Omega \to E_i^l(\bar{f}_i(x_{ip}^*)), \Delta_1^*, \Box A$, where $p = k_1 + \cdots + k_n = p(S^*)$ (i.e., the similarity index of the sequent S^*) and $x_{ip}^* \leftarrow \bar{h}_i(\bar{f}_n(\bar{g}_i(x_i^*))) \oplus$. The substitution $\oplus$ expresses the relation between the variable $x_i^* \in S^*$ and the variable $x_{ip}^* \in S_p$ and this relation is got from the substitutions obtained during the calculation of $SRe^p(S^*)$ by eliminating intermediate variables between x_i^* and x_{ip}^*. Adding the equality $x_{ip}^* = x_i^*$ to $\oplus$, we get the substitution $x_i^* \leftarrow \bar{h}_i(\bar{f}_n(\bar{g}_i(x_i^*)))$.

Now, let us consider the transformation of the parametrical formula of the shape $E_n^l(\bar{f}_n(x_n^*))$ (i.e., the case where $i = n$). Since $SRe^k(S^*) \neq \bot$ ($k \in \omega$), we can successfully apply (GIS) $(l + 1)$-time and get $SRe^{l+1}(S^*) = S_1 = \Box\Omega \to E_1^{k_1-1}(\bar{f}_1(x_1^*)), \Delta_{11}, \Box A$ (where $x_1^* \leftarrow \bar{f}_n(x_n^*)$) (*). Let us now take $i = 1$, $i + m = n$ and apply Lemma 7 to the sequent S_1: $SRe^q(S_1) = S_2 = \Box\Omega \to E_n^{k_n-1}(\bar{f}_n(x_{n1}^*)), \Delta_{12}, \Box A$ (where $q = k_1 - 1 + k_2 + \cdots + k_{n-1} + 1 = k_1 + \cdots + k_{n-1}$; $x_{n1}^* \leftarrow \bar{h}_n(x_1^*) = x_{n1}^* \leftarrow \bar{h}_n(\bar{f}_n(x_n^*))$) (**). Applying (GIS) $(k_n - 1 - l)$-time from the sequent S_2, we get $SRe^{q_1}(S_1) = S_3 = \Box\Omega \to E_n^l(\bar{f}_n(x_{n1}^*)), \Delta_{12}, \Box A$ (where $q_1 = k_n - 1 - l$) (***). Applying Lemma 4 to (*), (**), (***) we get $SRe^p(S^*) = \Box\Omega \to E_n^l(\bar{f}_n(x_{n1}^*)), \Delta_1^*, \Box A$, where $p = l + 1 + q + q_1 = l + 1 + k_1 + \cdots + k_{n-1} + k_n - 1 - l = k_1 + \cdots + k_n = p(S^*)$ (i.e., the similarity index of the sequent S^*) and $x_{np}^* \leftarrow \bar{h}_n(\bar{f}_n(x_n^*)) \oplus\oplus$. Adding the equality $x_{np}^* = x_n^*$ to $\oplus\oplus$, we get the substitution $x_n^* \leftarrow \bar{h}(\bar{f}_n(x_n^*))$.

Therefore, we get that each parametrical member $E_i^l(\bar{f}_i(x_i^*))$ ($1 \leqslant i \leqslant n$) after $p = p(S^*)$ steps is transformed into the atomic formula $E_i^l(\bar{f}_i(x_{ip}^*))$, where $x_{ip}^* \leftarrow \bar{g}_i(x_i^*)$ ($+^*$). The substitution ($+^*$) expresses the relation between the variables $x_i^* \in S^*$ and $x_{ip}^* \in S_p$ and this relation is got from the substitutions obtained during the calculation of $SRe^p(S^*)$ by eliminating intermediate variables between x_i^* and x_{ip}^*. Adding the equality $x_{ip}^* = x^*$ to ($+^*$) we get the substitution $x_i^* \leftarrow \bar{g}_i(x_i^*)$. Therefore, $S^*\sigma = SRe^p(S^*) = S_p$, where

$\sigma := \{x_1^* \leftarrow \bar{g}_1(x_1^*); \ldots x_n^* \leftarrow \bar{g}_n(x_n^*)\}$. Hence, after $p = p(S^*)$ steps, we get the sequent S_p such that $S^*\sigma = S_p$. The Lemma is proved.

The proof of Lemma 8 presents an implicit way for constructing the similarity substitution σ. Now we present the explicit way for constructing the similarity substitution σ.

Algorithm (SS) (algorithm for constructing the similarity substitution).

Let $S^* = \Box\Omega \rightarrow E_1(x_1^*), \ldots, E_r(x_r^*), \Box A$ be an elementary $FODR$-sequent and let $p(S^*) = n$, and $SRe^k(S^*) = S_n = \Box\Omega \rightarrow E_1(x_{n,1}), \ldots, E_n(x_{n,r}), \Box A$. Let σ_1 be a sequence of substitutions obtained during the construction of $SRe^k(S^*) = S_n$, i.e., $\sigma_1 = x_{11} \leftarrow t_{11}(x_1^*), \ldots, x_{r1} \leftarrow t_{r1}(x_r^*); \ldots; x_{1,r-1} \leftarrow t_{1,r-1}(x_{1,r-2}); \ldots;$ $x_{r,r-1} \leftarrow t_{r,r-1}(x_{r,n-2}); x_{1,r} \leftarrow t_{1,r}(x_{1,r-1}); \ldots; x_{r,r} \leftarrow t_{r,r}(x_{r,r-1})$. Let us, subsequently, eliminate from σ_1 the intermediate variables $x_{i1}, \ldots x_{i,r-1} (1 \leqslant i \leqslant r)$, i.e., replace these variables by the corresponding values. Continue these transformations until the sequence σ_n that contains r substitutions of the shape $x_{ni} \leftarrow t_{ni}(\ldots(t_{1i}(x_i^*))\ldots)(1 \leqslant i \leqslant r)$ is obtained. Add the equalities of the shape $x_{ni} = x_i^* \; (1 \leqslant i \leqslant r)$ to σ_n. Then the desired similarity substitution σ has the shape $\sigma := \{x_1^* \leftarrow t_{n1}(\ldots(t_{11}(x_1^*))\ldots); \ldots; x_r^* \leftarrow t_{nr}(\ldots(t_{1r}(x_r^*))\ldots)\}$.

Lemma 9 (Correctness of the Algorithm (SS)). *Let S^* be an elementary $FODR$-sequent, and $SRe^p(S) = S_p$, where $p = p(S^*)$, then, using the algorithm (SS), we can construct a substitution σ such that $S^*\sigma = S_p$.*

Proof. Using Lemma 8 and decidability of G^*.

Lemma 10 (Decidability of $S\sigma$). *The problem of generating a σ-similar sequent $S\sigma$ is decidable.*

Proof. Using Lemma 8 and Algorithm (SS).

Now we present examples showing how simply the sequent S_p (σ-similar to the given elementary $FODR$-sequent S^*) and similarity substitution σ are generated.

Example 3. (a) Let S^* be the same elementary $FODR$-sequent as in Example 2, i.e., $S^* = \Box\Omega \rightarrow E^1(f(x_1^*)), E^2(h(x_2^*)), E^3(g(x_3^*)), \Box A$, where $\Box\Omega = \Box\forall x_1(E^2(f(x_1)) \supset E(x_1)), \Box\forall x_2(E^3(h(x_2)) \supset E(x_2)), \Box\forall x_3(E^4(g(x_3)) \supset E(x_3));$ $A = \exists y(\neg E(y) \vee \neg E^1(y) \vee \neg E^2(y))$. The similarity index $p(S^*) = 2 + 3 + 4 = 9$ and the construction of $SRe^k(S^*)$ stops when $k = 9$. It is easy to verify that all the applications of (GIS) are successful, therefore we indicate only the temporal branch of application of (GIS) and the substitutions generated by means of operation $(+)$ (see Definition 7):

$$
\begin{array}{c}
\begin{array}{r}
x_{13} \leftarrow g(x_{32}) \\
x_{23} \leftarrow f(x_{12})
\end{array} \\
S_9 = \quad \Box\Omega \rightarrow E^1(f(x_{13})), E^2(h(x_{23})), E^3(g(x_{33})), \Box A; \quad x_{33} \leftarrow h(x_{22}) \\
\hline
\Box\Omega \rightarrow E(g(x_{32})), E(f(x_{12})), E(h(x_{22})), \Box A; \\
\hline
\Box\Omega \rightarrow E^1(g(x_{32})), E^1(f(x_{12})), E^1(h(x_{22})), \Box A; \quad x_{12} \leftarrow g(x_{31})
\end{array}
\qquad
\begin{array}{c}
(9) \\[1.5em]
(8)
\end{array}
$$

$$\frac{}{\Box\Omega \to E^2(g(x_{32})), E(g(x_{31})), E^2(h(x_{22})), \Box A;\ x_{22} \leftarrow f(x_{11})} \ (7)$$

$$\frac{}{\Box\Omega \to E^3(g(x_{32})), E^1(g(x_{31})), E(f(x_{11})), \Box A;\ x_{32} \leftarrow h(x_{21})} \ (6)$$

$$\frac{}{\Box\Omega \to E(h(x_{21})), E^2(g(x_{31})), E^1(f(x_{11})), \Box A;\ x_{11} \leftarrow g(x_3^*)} \ (5)$$

$$\frac{}{\Box\Omega \to E^1(h(x_{21})), E^3(g(x_{31})), E(g(x_3^*)), \Box A;\ x_{31} \leftarrow h(x_2^*)} \ (4)$$

$$\frac{}{\Box\Omega \to E^2(h(x_{21})), E(h(x_2^*)), E^1(g(x_3^*)), \Box A;\ x_{21} \leftarrow f(x_1^*)} \ (3)$$

$$\frac{}{\Box\Omega \to E(f(x_1^*)), E^1(h(x_2^*)), E^2(g(x_3^*)), \Box A} \ (2)$$

$$S^* = \frac{}{\Box\Omega \to E^1(f(x_1)), E^2(h(x_2^*)), E^3(g(x_3^*)), \Box A} \ (1)$$

Let us construct now the similarity substitution σ. First, we construct a substitution of the shape $\{x_{13} \leftarrow \overline{\tau}_1(x_1^*);\ x_{23} \leftarrow \overline{\tau}_2(x_2^*);\ x_{33} \leftarrow \overline{\tau}_3(x_3^*)\}$, where $\overline{\tau}_i$ $(1 \leqslant i \leqslant 3)$ is a sequence of function symbols f, h, g, i.e., expressing the relations between the variables from S_9 and that from S^*. Let σ_1 be a sequence of substitutions obtained during the construction of $SRe^9(S^*)$, i.e., $\sigma_1 = x_{21} \leftarrow f(x_1^*)$; $x_{31} \leftarrow h(x_2^*);\ x_{11} \leftarrow g(x_3^*);\ x_{32} \leftarrow h(x_{21});\ x_{22} \leftarrow f(x_{11});\ x_{12} \leftarrow g(x_{31})$; $x_{13} \leftarrow g(x_{32});\ x_{23} \leftarrow f(x_{12});\ x_{33} \leftarrow h(x_{22})$. Let us eliminate intermediate variables x_{i2} $(1 \leqslant i \leqslant 3)$ replacing the variables x_{i2} by the corresponding values of these variables. So instead of the sequence σ_1 we get $\sigma_2 = x_{13} \leftarrow g(h(x_{21}))$; $x_{23} \leftarrow f(g(x_{31}));\ x_{33} \leftarrow h(f(x_{11}))$. In the same manner, let us eliminate the variables x_{i1} $(1 \leq i \leq 3)$. So instead of σ_2, we get $\sigma = x_{13} \leftarrow g(h(f(x_1^*)))$; $x_{23} \leftarrow f(g(h(x_2^*)));\ x_{33} \leftarrow h(f(g(x_3^*)))$. Now, by adding $x_i^* = x_{i3}$ $(1 \leq i \leq 3)$ to σ_3, we get the desired similarity substitution $\sigma := \{x_1^* \leftarrow g(h(f(x_1^*)));\ x_2^* \leftarrow f(g(h(x_2^*)));\ x_3^* \leftarrow h(f(g(x_3^*)))\}$.

(b) Let $S_1^* = \Box\Omega \to E^1(f(x_1^*)),\ E^2(h(x_3^*)),\ E^3(g(x_2^*)),\ \Box A$, where A is the same as in part (a) and $\Box\Omega = \Box\forall x_1(E^2(f(x_1)) \supset E(x_1)),\ \Box\forall x_2(E^4(g(x_2)) \supset E(x_2)),\ \Box\forall x_3(E^3(h(x_3)) \supset E(x_3))$. It is easy to see that the sequent S_1^* is equivalent to the sequent S^* from part (a) of the example. The similarity index $\nu(S_1^*) = 2+3+4 = 9$ and the construction of $SRe^k(S_1^*)$ stops when $k = 9$. As in part (a), all the applications of (GIS) are successful, therefore we indicate only the temporal branch of application of (GIS) and the substitutions generated by means of operation $(+)$ (see Definition 7):

$$S_9 = \frac{}{\Box\Omega \to E^1(f(x_{13})), E^2(h(x_{33})), E^3(g(x_{23})), \Box A;\ \begin{matrix} x_{13} \leftarrow h(x_{32}) \\ x_{23} \leftarrow f(x_{12}) \\ x_{33} \leftarrow g(x_{22}) \end{matrix}}$$

$$\frac{}{\Box\Omega \to E(h(x_{32})), E(g(x_{22})), E(f(x_{12})), \Box A;} \ (9)$$

$$\frac{}{\Box\Omega \to E^1(h(x_{32})), E^1(g(x_{22})), E^1(f(x_{12})), \Box A;\ x_{12} \leftarrow h(x_{31})} \ (8)$$

$$\frac{}{\Box\Omega \to E^2(h(x_{32})), E^2(g(x_{22})), E(h(x_{31})), \Box A;\ x_{32} \leftarrow g(x_{21})} \ (7)$$

$$\frac{}{\Box\Omega \to E(g(x_{21})), E^3(g(x_{22})), E^1(h(x_{31})), \Box A;\ x_{22} \leftarrow f(x_{11})} \ (6)$$

$$\frac{\qquad\qquad\qquad\qquad\qquad\qquad\qquad\qquad\qquad\qquad}{\Box\Omega \to E^1(g(x_{21})), E(f(x_{11})), E^2(h(x_{31})), \Box A; \ x_{31} \leftarrow g(x_2^*)} \quad (5)$$

$$\frac{}{\Box\Omega \to E^2(g(x_{21})), E^1(f(x_{11})), E(g(x_2^*)), \Box A; \ x_{11} \leftarrow h(x_3^*)} \quad (4)$$

$$\frac{}{\Box\Omega \to E^3(g(x_{21})), E(h(x_3^*)), E^1(g(x_2^*)), \Box A; \ x_{21} \leftarrow f(x_1^*)} \quad (3)$$

$$\frac{}{\Box\Omega \to E(f(x_1^*)), E^1(h(x_3^*)), E^2(g(x_2^*)), \Box A} \quad (2)$$

$$\frac{}{\qquad\qquad\qquad\qquad\qquad\qquad\qquad\qquad\qquad\qquad} \quad (1)$$

$$S_1^* = \ \Box\Omega \to E^1(f(x_1^*)), E^2(h(x_3^*)), E^3(g(x_2^*)), \Box A$$

Analogously as in part (a) of this example, we find the similarity substitution of the following shape $\sigma^* := \{x_1^* \leftarrow h(g(f(x_1^*))); \ x_2^* \leftarrow f(h(g(x_2^*)));$ $x_3^* \leftarrow g(f(h(x_3^*)))\}$. Therefore, in spite of the fact that the $FODR$-sequent S_1^* is equivalent to the $FODR$-sequent S^* from part (a) of this example, we get different similarity substitutions, i.e., $\sigma \neq \sigma^*$.

Therefore, using the elementary sequent S^*, the similarity substitution σ (generated by means of calculation of $SRe^k(S^*)$ and Algorithm (SS)), we can construct the sequent S_p such that $S_p = S^*\sigma$. Let us construct the substitution σ^n in the following way. Let $\sigma = \{x_1^* \leftarrow \overline{f}_1(x_1^*), \dots, x_m^* \leftarrow \overline{f}_m(x_m^*)\}$, then $\sigma^n = \{x_1^* \leftarrow \overline{f}_1^n(x_1^*), \dots, x_m^* \leftarrow \overline{f}_m^n(x_m^*)\}$, where $\overline{f}_i(x_i^*) = \varnothing; \overline{f}_i^n(x_i^*) = \overline{f}_i(\overline{f}_i^{n-1}(x_i^*))$. Therefore $\sigma^0 = \varnothing$ and $\sigma^1 = \sigma$. For example, if $\sigma = x^* \leftarrow f(g(x^*))$, then $\sigma^2 = x^* \leftarrow f(g(f(g(x^*))))$.

We want to use the calculation of elementary k-th resolvents to deduce (from sequent $S^*\sigma^n$) the sequent S_p such that $S_p = S^*\sigma^{n+1}$ (for each $n \in \omega$). The foundation of this possibility is carried out by induction on n. The basis case (i.e., when $n = 0$) is carried out by calculating $SRe^p(S^*)$ and by Algorithm (SS). To found the step of induction, let us introduce the notion of a hypothetical k-th resolvent of the elementary $FODR$-sequent $S^*: HRe^k(S^*)$. The deductive procedure $HRe^k(S^*)$ is the third part of Sat_ω. The aim of $HRe^k(S^*)$ is as follows: assuming that we can generate an elementary $FODR$-sequent $S^*\sigma^n$, to verify the possibility of deducing the elementary $FODR$-sequent S_p such that $S_p = S^*\sigma^{n+1}$. The halting test of $HRe^k(S^*)$ is the same as for $SRe^k(S^*)$, namely, the similarity index of the elementary $FODR$-sequent S^*.

Definition 17 (Hypothetical k-th Resolvent: $HRe^k(S)$). *Let S be an elementary $FODR$-sequent, σ – the similarity substitution, m be an arbitrary natural number, then $HRe^0(S) = S\sigma^m$. Let $HRe^k(S) = S_k$, then $HRe^{k+1}(S)$ is defined in the following way. 1. Let us bottom-up apply (GIS) to S_k and S_{k1}, S_{k2} be the left and right premise of the application of (GIS). 2. If $G^* \nvdash S_{k1}$, then $HRe^{k+1}(S) = \perp$ (false) and the calculation of $HRe^{k+1}(S)$ is stopped. 3. Let $G^* \vdash S_{k1}$, then $HRe^{k+1}(S) = S_{k2}$. 4. If $HRe^{k+1}(S) = S_{k2}$ and $k + 1 = p(S)$, then the calculation of $HRe^{k+1}(S)$ is finished.*

Just like in Lemma 10 we get the following

Lemma 11 (Decidability of $HRe^k(S)$). *Let $HRe^0(S) = S\sigma^m$, then the problem of generating the sequent S_p such that $S_p = S\sigma^{m+1}$ is decidable.*

Now we can define the proposed deductive procedure Sat_ω.

Definition 18 (Deductive Procedure Sat_ω, $FODR$-Sequent Derivable by Means of Sat_ω). *The deductive procedure Sat_ω consists of three decidable procedures: (1) $PRe^k(S)$ (where S is a given $FODR$-sequent); (2) $SRe^k(S^*)$ (where S^* is an elementary $FODR$-sequent obtained by means of $PRe^k(S)$); (3) $HRe^k(S^*)$. $FODR$-sequent S is derivable using Sat_ω (in symbols: $Sat_\omega \vdash S$) if three conditions are satisfied: (1) $PRe^n(S) = S^*$ (where $n = \pi(S)$, $\pi(S)$ is the kernel conclusion complexity of S); (2) $SRe^p(S^*) = S_p = S^*\sigma$ ($p = p(S^*)$, $p(S^*)$ is the similarity index of S^*; σ is the similarity substitution); (3) $HRe^0(S) = S^*\sigma^m \Rightarrow HRe^p(S^*) = S_p = S^*\sigma^{m+1}$ (m is an arbitrary natural number); otherwise, $Sat_\omega \nvdash S$.*

Example 4. Let S be the $FODR$-sequent from Example 2. In Example 2, the sequent S was reduced by means of $PRe(S)$ to the elementary $FODR$-sequent S^*. In Example 3(a), the similarity substitution σ was constructed and the sequent S_9 generated such that $S_9 = S^*\sigma$. Now, using $HRe^k(S)$ let us verify the possibility to generate (from $S^*\sigma^m$) a sequent S_p such that $S_p = S^*\sigma^{m+1}$. So, assume that $HRe^0(S^*) = S^*\sigma^m$. Analogously as in Example 3(a), we get that $HRe^9(S^*) = S_9 = S^*\sigma^{m+1}$. Therefore $Sat_\omega \vdash S^*\sigma^k$ ($k \in \omega$) and hence $Sat_\omega \vdash S$. In the same way we get $Sat_\omega \vdash S_1^*\sigma^{*k}$ ($k \in \omega$), where S_1^* and σ^* are the same as in Example 3(b).

Remark 3. The procedures $SRe^k(S)$ and $HRe^k(S)$ of Sat_ω cannot be joined: we cannot deduce the sequent $S\sigma^n$. We can only test that from the assumption $S\sigma^n$ it is possible (or not) to generate the sequent S_p such that $S_p = S\sigma^{n+1}$.

Lemma 12. *Let S be a $FODR$-sequent and $Sat_\omega \vdash S = \square\Omega \to \Sigma, \Pi^1, \square A$, then $G_{L\omega}^* \vdash S$.*

Proof. From $Sat_\omega \vdash S$ it follows that all the possible bottom-up applications of (GIS) in all the three parts of Sat_ω are successful. From this fact (and using admissibility of the rule (GIS) in $G_{L\omega}^*$), by induction on n we can prove that $G^* \vdash S_n = \square\Omega \to \Sigma, \Pi^1, A^n$ ($n \in \omega$). Applying $(\to \square_\omega)$ to S_n, we get $G_{L\omega}^* \vdash S$.

Lemma 13. *Let S be a $FODR$-sequent and $G_{L\omega}^* \vdash S$, then $Sat_\omega \vdash S$.*

Proof. From $G_{L\omega}^* \vdash S$ we can prove that all the possible bottom-up applications of (GIS) in all the three parts of Sat_ω are successful. Using this fact we can get $Sat_\omega \vdash S$.

From Lemma 12, 13 we get the following

Theorem 2. *Let S be a $FODR$-sequent, then $G_{L\omega}^* \vdash S \iff Sat_\omega \vdash S$.*

Having in mind the definition of ω-decidability (see the end of Introduction), using Remark 3, Theorem 2 and Lemmas 3, 10, 11, we get the following

Theorem 3. *The deductive procedure Sat_ω is ω-decidable and $FODR$-sequents compose an ω-decidable class.*

4   Conclusions, Related Works, and Future Investigations

We have presented the new effective deduction-based ω-decidable procedure Sat_ω for the DR-sequents of a restricted first-order linear temporal logic with temporal operators $\bigcirc$ ("next") and $\square$ ("always"). The DR-sequents allow us to express a variety of safety properties of programs. The objects of consideration of Sat_ω are non-Horn DR-sequents. The calculus Sat_ω consists of three decidable parts (that replace the infinitary rule $(\to \square_\omega)$) possessing a high degree of mechanization.

There are few interesting results (see, e.g. [4]) referring to traditional decidability of fragments of FTL. As far as we know, the proposed deductive procedure Sat_ω and deductive procedure described in [9] are the first results on ω-decidability of a restricted FTL.

DR-sequents are a certain skolemized version of M.Fisher's normal form [2]. Basing on the seminal paper [2], an interesting project "Mechanizing First-Order Temporal Logic" is realized at the Manchester Metropolitan University (Department of Computing and Mathematics).

In future investigations we are going to extend the proposed ω-decidable procedure for more general sequents than DR-sequents, including also other temporal operators and other temporal models, e.g., past\branching time cases.

References

1. Abadi M.: The power of temporal proofs. *Theoretical Comp. Sci.* 64 (1989) 35–84.
2. Fisher M.: A normal form for temporal logics and its applications in theorem proving and execution. *Journal of Logic and Computation* 7(4) (1997).
3. Fisher M., Wooldridge M.: On the formal specification and verification of multi-agent systems. *Intern. Journal of Cooperative Information Systems* 6(1) (1997) 37–65.
4. Hodkinson I., Wolter F., Zakharyaschev M.: Decidable fragments of first-order temporal logics. (To appear in: *Annals of Pure and Applied Logic*).
5. Kawai H.: Sequential calculus for a first-order infinitary temporal logic. *Zeitchr. fur Math. Logic und Grundlagen der Math.* 33 (1987) 423–452.
6. Pliuškevičius R.: The saturated tableaux for a linear miniscoped Horn-like temporal logic. *Journal of Automated Reasoning* 13 (1994) 51–67.
7. Pliuškevičius R.: Replacement of induction by similarity saturation in a first-order linear temporal logic. *Journal of Applied Non-Classical Logics* 8 (1–2) (1998) 141–169.
8. Pliuškevičius R.: Infinitary calculus for a restricted first-order linear temporal logic without contraction of quantified formulas. *Lithuanian Mathematical Journal* 39(3) (1999) 378–397.
9. Pliuškevičius R.: An effective deductive procedure for a restricted first-order linear temporal logic. (Submitted to *Annals of Pure and Applied Logic*).
10. Szalas A.: Concerning the semantic consequence relation in first-order temporal logic. *Theoretical Comput. Sci.* 47 (1986) 329–334.
11. Szalas A.: A complete axiomatic characterization of first-order temporal logic of linear time. *Theoretical Comput. Sci.* 54 (1987) 199–214.

Representing Object Code

Marco Benini

Dipartimento di Scienze dell'Informazione
Università degli Studi di Milano
via Comelico 39/41 — 20135, Milano, Italy
benini@dsi.unimi.it

Abstract. In this paper, a logical representation of object code programs is presented. The coding is particularly well-suited for mechanization, and it enjoys interesting properties with respect to some relevant approaches to program synthesis, program derivation and formal verification [FD93,LO94,KLO96,FLO97a,LO98]. The paper describes both the representation with its properties, and a tool which permits to translate object programs for the MC68000 microprocessor into the formalism of the ISABELLE logical framework.

1 Introduction

In a verification system it is very important to be able to mechanically represent programs in the formal language used to reason on them. In fact, if the representation of code is left to the human verifier, there is no guarantee that the represented program and the original code describe the same computational process. In this paper, object code programs are considered because they constitute an important area in the application of formal methods as remarked, e.g., in [Yu93,BKN98].

A logical representation of an object code program should meet three conditions with respect to the formal verification task:

- it must be *faithful*, that is, it has to admit a standard interpretation which maps to the same computational process as the original code;
- it must be *meaningful*, that is, it has to allow the full exploitation of the power of the formal system used to reason about programs;
- it must be *intelligible*, so that the relation between the original code and its representation is as plain as possible.

The first point reduces to say that the represented code is equivalent to the original program; to meet this goal, usually, one requires that the representation has to be as close as possible to the original program, under the standard interpretation. Hence, one uses the third point, intelligibility, in addition to the formal semantics of the logical system, to fulfill the requirement for a faithful representation. In this case, simplicity of representation is not a fault, but, on the contrary, it is a benefit because it highly enhances the confidence in the formal proofs.

J. Lloyd et al. (Eds.): CL 2000, LNAI 1861, pp. 538–552, 2000.

The second requirement, significance, has the same importance as the others, in fact, a *poor* representation of object code does not permit to use the formal system to its full power, with the result that a correctness proof is harder to obtain, and it appears longer and trickier than necessary.

The proposed representation is very simple, and very close to the description of the MC68000 assembly language one can find in the data book of the microprocessor, thus clearly meeting the requirements of intelligibility and faithfulness. Moreover, the proposed representation admits a standard schema for correctness proofs, which inductively unfolds the possible computations of the program; this fact shows that the representation is meaningful. Furthermore, the proposed representation assumes a distinguished relevance when coupled with a constructive formal system.

In this respect, it is worth noticing that most correctness proofs have been developed using higher-order classical logic, e.g., [Cam88,BG90,Cho94,BP97], or using first-order classical theories extended by computational logics, see, e.g., [Man69,Dij75,BM85,Yu93]. However, as one can easily check by looking at the previously mentioned proofs, most formal verification tasks are developed according to constructive guidelines: as a matter of facts, most correctness proofs do not focus on showing that a program cannot produce but the intended behavior, but, on the contrary, they prove that a program *computes* a specification.

The idea is to assign a meaning to specifications as requests for computations. Nevertheless, this view is reductive: the meaning of a specification may also be prescriptive, that is, the specification acts like a constraint the program is not allowed to violate. These different meanings of specifications are referred to with the words *liveness* for the computational reading, and *safety* for the constraint-oriented view, as customary in the field.

In a constructive approach, the computational reading of a formula is defined by induction on the structure of the formula:

- every atomic formula represents a request for an elementary computation;
- the formula $A \wedge B$ represents a request for a computation which satisfies both A and B, thus, it represents a request for both the computations represented by A and B;
- the formula $A \vee B$ represents a request for a computation which decides between A and B, that is, a computation for $A \vee B$ is either a computation for A or a computation for B;
- the formula $A \to B$ represents a request for a computation which translates any computation for A into a computation for B;
- the formula $\forall x. A(x)$ represents a request for a computation of $A(t)$ with an arbitrary input t;
- the formula $\exists x. A(x)$ represents a request for a computation of an output t which satisfies the computation requirement represented by $A(t)$.

A definition of the negation case depends on the particular constructive logic: in the intuitionistic case, a specification of the form $\neg A$ requires that the constraint

A is not satisfied by the program, in other words, negation is the way to specify safety properties[1].

The *computational reading* of formulas can be developed only in a constructive framework, because it relies on the ability to formally derive *witnesses* for disjunctive and existential specifications. For a detailed formal treatment of the computational readings for formulas and proofs the reader is referred to [MO81,MMO88,MMO91,LO94,KLO96,FLO97a,FLO97b,FFM99,Ben00].

In a very natural way, liveness properties are modeled as theorems of a constructive logical system, since their proofs require the unfolding of the computations performed by the examined program. On the contrary, safety properties are best modeled in a classical environment, and their proof often requires the use of the *tertium non datur* principle.

Therefore, the ultimate purpose of this paper is to describe a logical representation for object code programs which is compatible with a constructive approach to formal verification, while remaining efficient in a classical approach.

The requirement of efficiency justifies an analysis of compression techniques, which, discarding information which may appear as non relevant to the development of a correctness proof, make the representation more compact, more understandable, and thus, more manageable by a semiautomatic theorem prover.

2   Translating Object Code into Logic

The notion of object code is slightly ambiguous; in fact, it may be interpreted in four different ways:

1. The object code of a program is the content of the computer memory when the operative system passes it the control;
2. The object code of a program is the content of an executable file;
3. The object code of a program is the output of a compiler, in other words, the content of an *object* (.o) file;
4. The object code is the symbolic representation of the output of a compiler, i.e., it is an assembly program.

All these possibilities are right, to some extent, and all of them are supported by the translation tool, OCT (Object Code Translator).

The OCT tool is divided into two parts, the *preprocessor* and the *translation procedure*; the former transforms an executable file or an object file into an assembly program; the latter takes an assembly program as input and produces a logical theory suitable for reasoning with ISABELLE [Pau94].

The preprocessor reconstructs an assembly program where every address is *resolved*, that is, the assembly code is allocated in memory from a given address.

---

[1] More precisely, one may express a safety property A by means of its double negation, $\neg\neg A$. To maintain compatibility with the classical interpretation of logical symbols, it is necessary to work in Kuroda logic [Gab81,AFMM96,MMO97], that is, **IL** (intuitionistic first-order logic) plus the Kuroda axiom, $(\forall x. \neg\neg A(x)) \to \neg\neg\forall x. A(x)$.

Thus, the output of the preprocessor is equivalent to the symbolic (assembly) representation of the content of the memory when the program will be executed.

The translation procedure takes as input an assembly source code where no macros are present and where every address is resolved, and it translates this code into a logical representation.

The target assembly language is the one of the MC68000 microprocessor; the main reason behind the choice of this particular architecture is that several case studies for formal verification problems have been developed starting from the MC68000 microprocessor; in particular, the translation tool benefits from the good work in [Yu93], where many functions from the standard libc library have been proven correct, providing a consistent set of test cases.

The translation algorithm operates on the language of first-order intuitionistic logic plus the theory of modular arithmetic where the types byte, word and longword are integers modulo 2^8, integers modulo 2^{16} and integers modulo 2^{32}, respectively. Modular arithmetic is available in the ISABELLE framework, and there are reasoners which can efficiently deal with it, see [Sho79,CLS96,BNP98].

The output of the translation procedure is an ISABELLE theory containing a series of axioms, one per instruction, encoding the program. This theory file inherits the necessary type declarations as well as the constants representing registers and memory from the theory of the microprocessor.

The theory of the microprocessor has three roles:

- it provides the minimal set of instruments to reason about object code programs;
- it declares the types which are needed to represent the code;
- it declares the constants which constitute the world the microprocessor operates on.

The set of instruments is given by the logical system, the theory of identity, the set of provers, such as the *Simplifier* [Pau97] which allows equational reasoning, the *Computer Arithmetic Toolkit* [BNP98], to deal with modular arithmetic, and the *Classical Reasoner* [Pau97], to cope with purely logical problems.

The types byte, word and longword are specializations of modular numbers. In practice, both signed and unsigned numbers are used. Their coding is declared in the modular arithmetic package. Hence, the microprocessor theory declares three versions for every type; for instance, it defines pure bytes, denoted by the type byte, which is the set of integer numbers quotiented by the relation (mod 2^8), signed bytes, denoted by sbyte and representing the range of numbers from -128 to 127, and unsigned bytes, denoted by ubyte and representing the range of numbers from 0 to 255.

The type time, following the fact that the microprocessor clock is discrete, is equivalent to Int, that is, time is modeled by integer numbers.

In the microprocessor theory, the constants for memory and registers are declared. Specifically, the MC68000 microprocessor[2] provides sixteen 32-bit user registers, eight of them (the d registers) being data registers, the others (denoted

---

[2] The details of the MC68000 architecture can be found in [Mot89].

by a) being address registers. The program counter register is indicated with pc. Since registers change their values over time, they have been modeled as functions from time to values:

$$d_i : \texttt{time} \rightarrow \texttt{slongword} \qquad , 0 \leq i \leq 7$$
$$a_i : \texttt{time} \rightarrow \texttt{slongword} \qquad , 0 \leq i \leq 7$$
$$\texttt{pc}: \texttt{time} \rightarrow \texttt{ulongword}$$

A particular case is the status register which is modeled by a set of functions, one for each flag in the register:

$$\texttt{Zflag}: \texttt{time} \rightarrow \texttt{bool} \qquad (* \text{ zero } *)$$
$$\texttt{Nflag}: \texttt{time} \rightarrow \texttt{bool} \qquad (* \text{ negative } *)$$
$$\texttt{Cflag}: \texttt{time} \rightarrow \texttt{bool} \qquad (* \text{ carry } *)$$
$$\texttt{Vflag}: \texttt{time} \rightarrow \texttt{bool} \qquad (* \text{ overflow } *)$$
$$\texttt{Xflag}: \texttt{time} \rightarrow \texttt{bool} \qquad (* \text{ extension } *)$$

The memory is represented as a function from addresses and times to values:

$$\texttt{memory}: \texttt{ulongword} \times \texttt{time} \rightarrow \texttt{byte}$$

The general format of the logical representation of an instructions I is

$$\forall t: \texttt{time}. \, \text{pc}(t) = A \rightarrow B \wedge C$$

where A is the absolute address of the instruction I, B specifies the value of the program counter at time $t + 1$, and C specifies the value of every register, flag and memory cell at time $t+1$, depending on the instruction operands, the status of memory at time t, and the values of registers and flags at time t.

The format of the B part can be either

$$\text{pc}(t + 1) = H(\text{pc}(t))$$

or

$$(f(t) \rightarrow \text{pc}(t + 1) = H_1(\text{pc}(t))) \wedge (\neg f(t) \rightarrow \text{pc}(t + 1) = H_2(\text{pc}(t)))$$

where H, H_1 and H_2 are arithmetical expressions depending on the current value of the program counter and calculating the address of the next instruction to execute; $f(t)$ is a formula, depending on the time t, and usually, it is a literal representing a flag, but, in general it may be a conjunction of (negations of) flag predicates.

For example: the instruction

$$64: \texttt{MOVE} \ \#1, \text{d}_0$$

which puts the value 1 into the d_0 register[3], is translated into

$$\forall t.\, \text{pc}(t) = 64 \rightarrow \text{pc}(t+1) = \text{pc}(t) + 2 \wedge$$
$$\wedge\, d_0(t+1) = 1 \wedge$$
$$\wedge\, d_1(t+1) = d_1(t) \wedge \ldots \wedge d_7(t+1) = d_7(t) \wedge$$
$$\wedge\, a_0(t+1) = a_0(t) \wedge \ldots \wedge a_7(t+1) = a_7(t) \wedge$$
$$\wedge\, \neg\text{Vflag}(t+1) \wedge \neg\text{Cflag}(t+1) \wedge \neg\text{Zflag}(t+1) \wedge$$
$$\wedge\, \neg\text{Nflag}(t+1) \wedge \neg\text{Xflag}(t+1) \wedge$$
$$\wedge\, \forall a.\, \texttt{memory}(a, t+1) = \texttt{memory}(a, t) \ .$$

Also, the instruction

$$72 : \texttt{BEQ} \ 8$$

which represents a conditional branch 8 positions forward if the zero flag is set, is translated into

$$\forall t.\, \text{pc}(t) = 72 \rightarrow (\text{Zflag}(t) \rightarrow \text{pc}(t+1) = \text{pc}(t) + 8) \wedge$$
$$\wedge\, (\neg\text{Zflag}(t) \rightarrow \text{pc}(t+1) = \text{pc}(t) + 2) \wedge$$
$$\wedge\, d_0(t+1) = d_0(t) \wedge \ldots \wedge d_7(t+1) = d_7(t) \wedge$$
$$\wedge\, a_0(t+1) = a_0(t) \wedge \ldots \wedge a_7(t+1) = a_7(t) \wedge$$
$$\wedge\, (\text{Vflag}(t+1) \leftrightarrow \text{Vflag}(t)) \wedge$$
$$\wedge\, (\text{Zflag}(t+1) \leftrightarrow \text{Zflag}(t)) \wedge$$
$$\wedge\, (\text{Nflag}(t+1) \leftrightarrow \text{Nflag}(t)) \wedge$$
$$\wedge\, (\text{Cflag}(t+1) \leftrightarrow \text{Cflag}(t)) \wedge$$
$$\wedge\, (\text{Xflag}(t+1) \leftrightarrow \text{Xflag}(t)) \wedge$$
$$\wedge\, \forall a.\, \texttt{memory}(a, t+1) = \texttt{memory}(a, t) \ .$$

Some remarks on the proposed representation are needed:

- The simplicity of the representation makes evident its correctness, since it is very adherent to the description found in the data book.
- The preprocessor takes care of eliminating the dependency on the system architecture. Then the translation procedure transforms a symbolic equivalent of the memory image of the program into a logical representation which is faithful. Thus, the result is really equivalent to what will be executed.
- The theory of the microprocessor and the output of the translation procedure are Harrop theories.

An important point, anticipated in the introduction, is that the representation naturally imposes a structure on correctness proofs. In fact, in order to prove that the program P has the property ϕ, a proof of ϕ which unfolds the possible computations of P is required. The general format of that proof is

$$\Gamma, R$$
$$\vdots$$
$$\phi$$

,

---

[3] The set of instructions of the MC68000 microprocessor is documented in [Mot89].

where R is the representation of P and Γ is a set of assumptions specifying, at least, the initial state before the execution of P.

The proof $\dfrac{\Gamma, R}{\phi}$ has a canonical form, since every step in the computation of P can be simulated by a proper application of inference rules; for example, if $\mathrm{pc}(t_0) = n$ and n is a location belonging to the program P, then the execution of the instruction of P at address n is simulated by the following proof schema

$$\dfrac{\mathrm{pc}(t_0) = n \quad \dfrac{\forall t.\, \mathrm{pc}(t) = n \to B(t) \land C(t)}{\mathrm{pc}(t_0) = n \to B(t_0) \land C(t_0)}}{B(t_0) \land C(t_0)}$$

where $B(t_0)$ gives the possible values of the program counter at time $t_0 + 1$, and $C(t_0)$ computes the values of registers, flags and memory at time $t_0 + 1$.

As soon as no loops are involved, a combination of instances of the preceding proof schema and applications of the substitution rule really unfolds any possible computation of the program.

When a loop is present in the program, necessarily there is a branching instruction which assigns a value n to the program counter such that the instruction located at n has already been executed. In this case, when composing instances of the preceding proof schema, it always appears a schema of the form

$$\Gamma, R, \mathrm{pc}(t) = n$$
$$\vdots$$
$$\mathrm{pc}(t + k) = n$$

which naturally suggests to use an induction principle. In the case of structured (non-interleaving) cycles, a convenient choice is the *bounded chain principle*[4]:

$$\dfrac{\exists x.\, x \leq b \land P(x) \quad \begin{array}{c} [p \leq b],\, [P(p)] \\ \vdots \\ B \lor (\exists y.\, p < y \leq b \land P(y)) \end{array}}{B}$$

which is applied instantiating $P(x)$ to $\mathrm{pc}(x) = n$, and B to $\exists t.\, \mathrm{pc}(t) = m$, where m is the location reached when the loop finishes its execution. The bound b has to be guessed, and corresponds to an upper bound for the computational complexity of the loop.

It is possible to mechanically generate the proof schema which inductively unfolds every possible computation of a program; however, the details of this construction, whose pieces have been sketched above, and the proof of its adherence to the microprocessor's semantics are too complex to be presented here.

Essential to remark is the fact that a correctness proof schema can be generated for a program either in a constructive logical system, or in a classical

---

[4] This induction schema formalizes a specialization of the *descending chain principle* [MO81,MMO88,MMO91,Fer97,Ben00], and is valid in every discrete ordering.

environment. So, in both cases the representation is really meaningful, providing a strong guideline in the development of correctness proofs.

The importance of being an Harrop theory cannot be appreciated without introducing some details on constructive systems. A formal system is said to be *uniformly constructive* [Fer97] when

- if Π is a proof of $A \vee B$, then either there is a proof Π' of A, or there is a proof Π' of B, and Π' is an instance of a combination of subproofs of Π;
- if Π is a proof of $\exists x. A(x)$, then there is a proof Π' of $A(t)$, and Π' is an instance of a combination of subproofs of Π.

When a proof Π' is required to be an instance of a combination of subproofs of another proof Π, it amounts to demand that the conclusion D of Π' is implicitly proven by Π, or, in other words, that D is in the *truth content* of Π. Actually, one can prove that the truth content of a proof can be algorithmically generated, see [MO81,Fer97,Ben00] for details.

A well-known fact is that, when a set of Harrop axioms is added to an uniformly constructive formal system, the result is another uniformly constructive system, see, e.g., [ST96,Fer97,FFM99], so the discussed representation preserves applicability of the instruments that make use of the truth content of a correctness proof to analyze the corresponding program [Ben00].

The importance of constructive systems in formal verification appears also from the fact that, in an uniformly constructive system, one can assign a *computational meaning* to specifications [MMO88,MMO91,FLO97b,Ben00], as briefly illustrated in the introduction. An important consequence of this fact is related to the possibility to extract information from correctness proofs by generating the associated truth content, and to ensure that the extracted information is enough to symbolically compute the program on an input [MO81].

Henceforth, the proposed representation takes a deeper meaning in a constructive framework, where it admits a computational reading which formally proves that the representation is faithful.

3   Compressing the Representation

The representation of object code as described in the previous section is satisfactory for the purposes illustrated in the introduction, but it suffers from being quite redundant.

In fact, most of the information contained in the formula which encodes an instruction, proves to be useless in practice. For example, considering the fragment

$$40: \text{ MOVE } \#7, d_0$$
$$42: \text{ ADD } \#1, d_0$$
$$44: \text{ MOVE } d_0, (a_1)$$

when a correctness proof is developed, in most cases, the fragment encoding in a logical form can be reduced to

$$\forall t. \, pc(t) = 40 \rightarrow pc(t+3) = 46 \wedge d_0(t+3) = 8 \wedge \text{memory}(a_1(t), t+3) = 8$$

In this section some techniques are presented which can be used to mechanically compress the logical representation.

The *enveloping* technique is based on the fact that compilers produce object code with a peculiar structure; in particular, a procedure is compiled in a way which can be represented as

E
C
E

the C part is the code which implements the procedure, while the E part, the *envelope*, takes care of retrieving the parameters and returning the result.

For example, the following function in the C language:

```
int f( int x )
{
    return (x + 1) ;
}
```

is compiled by the gcc compiler into the following object code

```
 0 : LINK #0, a6
 2 : MOVE 0(a7), d0
 5 : ADD #1, d0
 7 : MOVE d0, −8(a7)
10 : UNLK a6
12 : RTS
```

the parts which constitute the body of the function and its envelope are marked.

The envelope compression technique takes apart the representation for the envelope, proves that it correctly passes through parameters, and proves that it correctly returns the result; these proofs are routine and they can be efficiently mechanized. In such a way, the human verifier has only to prove that the body of the procedure is correct.

The drawback of the enveloping compression technique is that it requires that the object code is organized according the envelope pattern, which is not always the case for human-produced or highly optimized code.

Very important to remark is the fact that this compression technique does not discard information, thus, when applicable, it is safe.

The analysis of the flow of control of a program is probably the most important technique for compressing the logical representation. It is based on the grouping of sequential blocks of instructions.

The algorithm which performs this kind of compression is complex because of the amount of details, but its main structure can be described as a transformation on graphs: given an assembly program P, a graph is constructed whose nodes are the instructions of P and whose directed edges are drawn from an instruction I to any instruction J which may be executed just after I. The compression of sequential blocks can be formulated as a transformation on this graph which collapses two nodes A and B if there is an edge from A to B, and no edges of the form A to C, or C to B, for any node C.

For example, the fragment of code at the beginning of this section, after the compression, is represented by the formula

$$\forall\, t.\, \mathrm{pc}(t) = 40 \rightarrow \mathrm{pc}(t+3) = \mathrm{pc}(t) + 6 \,\wedge$$
$$\wedge\, \mathrm{d_0}(t+3) = 8 \,\wedge$$
$$\wedge\, \mathrm{d_1}(t+3) = \mathrm{d_1}(t) \wedge \ldots \wedge \mathrm{d_7}(t+3) = \mathrm{d_7}(t) \,\wedge$$
$$\wedge\, \mathrm{a_0}(t+3) = \mathrm{a_0}(t) \wedge \ldots \wedge \mathrm{a_7}(t+3) = \mathrm{a_7}(t) \,\wedge$$
$$\wedge\, \neg\mathtt{Vflag}(t+3) \wedge \neg\mathtt{Zflag}(t+3) \,\wedge$$
$$\wedge\, \neg\mathtt{Nflag}(t+3) \wedge \neg\mathtt{Cflag}(t+3) \wedge \neg\mathtt{Xflag}(t+3) \,\wedge$$
$$\wedge\, \mathtt{memory}(\mathrm{a_1}(t), t+3) = 8 \,\wedge$$
$$\wedge\, \forall\, x.\, x\neg = \mathrm{a_1}(t) \rightarrow \mathtt{memory}(x, t+3) = \mathtt{memory}(x, t) \ .$$

An important point about the compression of sequential code is the fact that the compressed representation is again an Harrop theory, thus preserving uniform constructivity and, more general, the benefits of the chosen representation.

Moreover, the algorithm which generates the compressed representation can be easily employed to compute a proof schema for the program, starting from the general correctness proof schema and reducing it to use just the compressed representation.

However, although the compression of sequential code does not reduce the amount of information about what the original program computes, it destroys the information on the order in which sequential computations are performed. Occasionally this matters, especially when dealing with safety properties. Nevertheless, if ϕ is a formula which does not contain explicit references to values of time not appearing in the compressed representation, and, moreover, if ϕ does not contain existentially quantified subformulas over time variables, then the following theorem holds in **CL** (classical first-order logic):

Theorem 1. *Let R be the theory which contains the representation of a program P, let R_c be the theory containing the representation of P where sequential blocks are compressed, and let ϕ be a formula as above, then, if $\mathbf{CL}, R, \Gamma \vdash \phi$, then $\mathbf{CL}, R_c, \Gamma \vdash \phi$.*

This theorem constitutes a preservation result for a large subclass of liveness specifications, remarking the importance of the compression algorithm. The proof of the theorem is laborious, so it is omitted for the sake of brevity; it is based on the subformula property of the normalization theorem for **CL** [ST96].

The previous theorem can be strengthened when working in a constructive system which contains the intuitionistic logic plus the Kuroda principle: in that case, in fact, the formula ϕ is required not to contain explicit references to values of time not appearing in the compressed representation, and, ϕ is required not to contain an occurrence of an existentially quantified subformula $\exists\, t.\, A(t)$ over a time variable t, *unless* the witness $A(t)$ appearing[5] in the truth content of **IL**, $R, \Gamma \vdash \phi$ meets the conditions on ϕ, too. In practice, most of the times, it is evident form the program that a witness $A(t)$ exists and that t is in the time domain of the compressed representation.

The analysis of the flow of control of a program naturally gives raise to another compression technique: the idea is to maintain in the representation just what is or was or will be changed inside the program. In practice, the equalities stating that a register (memory cell, flag) retains the same value since it is neither read, nor written by the program, are deleted from the representation.

The algorithm which performs the compression of equalities is a variant of the algorithm which compresses sequential blocks. In fact, it is modeled by a transformation on a labelled version of the graph of a program as previously defined. Being G the graph associated to the program P; every node N is labelled with the set C_N of registers, flags and memory cells that are changed by the execution of the instruction the node represents; moreover, every node N of G is labelled with the set R_N of registers, flags and memory cells which are read by the instruction in N, that is, the registers, flags and cells which are on the right-hand side of equalities whose left-hand side is in C_N. The transformation that performs the compression operates as follows: let N and M be two nodes connected by an arc from N to M, the labels of N are updated as $C'_N = C_N \cup R_M$ and $R'_N = R_N \cup (R_M \setminus C_N)$. The least fixed point of this transformation produces a graph G^* such that, for every node N in G^*, the label C_N contains exactly the left-hand side of the equalities which must be retained in the compressed representation of the instruction associated with N.

Furthermore, the two compression techniques derived from the analysis of the flow of control may be combined in a single compression algorithm. In the example from the beginning of this section, the combined algorithm produces

$$\forall t.\, \mathrm{pc}(t) = 40 \to \mathrm{pc}(t+3) = 46 \wedge \mathrm{d}_0(t+3) = 8 \wedge \mathtt{memory}(\mathrm{a}_1(t), t+3) = 8$$

for the whole sequential block.

As before, the result of the compression of equalities, as well as, the result of the combined algorithm, is an Harrop theory, thus preserving significance of the representation. Moreover, as before, a correctness proof schema for the program can be generated by the compression algorithm.

On the other hand, the compression of equalities discards more information than the compression of sequential blocks, and, as a result, the previous preservation theorem does not hold anymore. Still, there is a characterization of formulas whose provability is preserved under the compression of equalities. However, the combined compression algorithm is usually preferred, hence a preservation result for the single compression technique is not shown, in favor of a characterization of the formulas preserved by the combined transformation.

Let ϕ be a formula such that:

---

[5] Being constructive, the system guarantees the appearance of such a witness in the truth content of the proof, see [MO81].

1. it does not contain explicit references to values of time non appearing in the compressed representation;
2. it does not contain occurrences of timed registers, timed flags and timed memory locations non appearing in the compressed representation;
3. it does not contain existentially quantified subformulas over a time variable;

then, the following preservation theorem holds

Theorem 2. *Let R be the theory which contains the representation of a program P, let R_c be the theory containing the representation of P compressed according to the combined algorithm, and let ϕ be a formula as above, then, if $\mathbf{CL}, R, \Gamma \vdash \phi$, then $\mathbf{CL}, R_c, \Gamma \vdash \phi$.*

The proof follows the same pattern as the previous preservation result, thus, it heavily uses the subformula property and the normalization theorem for $\mathbf{CL}$. As in the previous case, the conditions on ϕ can be relaxed in Kuroda logic, allowing existentially quantified subformulas on time, whose witnesses are in the time domain to the compressed representation.

It is evident that the class of formulas whose provability is preserved by the combined algorithm is a proper subclass of those preserved by the compression of sequential blocks. In this respect, the combined algorithm is stronger, as remarked before.

On the other hand, it should be clear that the class of formulas preserved by the combined algorithm is *natural*, since the requirements it has to satisfy is, intuitively, that the formulas do not contain references to objects (registers, flags, memory cells and times) which have been discarded in the compression process.

An apparently interesting variation on the previous combined algorithm is given by considering a specification S of the form $\exists\, t.\, \mathrm{pc}(t) = x \wedge A$, which constitutes an usual pattern for liveness properties, and compressing the code with respect to S, that is, to keep in the representation only the objects (registers, flags and memory cells) which are referred in S.

The algorithm which computes a compressed representation for a program P, according to this requirement is a variant of the algorithm which performs the compression of equalities: being G the labelled graph for the program P constructed as above, being S the specification, which, by assumption, has the form $\exists\, t.\, \mathrm{pc}(t) = x \wedge A$, and calling N the node corresponding to the instruction at the address x, a new labelled graph G' is constructed, where G' is equal to G except for the node N, where the label C_N is substituted with the set of all registers, flags and memory cells occurring in S. The result of the compression algorithm is the result on running the combined compression procedure on G'.

It is evident that the result is a representation which is the minimal one computing just the values mentioned in the specification. But the resulting representation may be (and it is often the case) too poor to allow to prove the specification itself.

In fact, no *natural* preservation result is known at the moment being, and there is the strong belief that no reasonable preservation theorem can be proven. In fact, characterizing the class of formulas whose provability is preserved by this kind of compression procedure appears to be hopeless. However, it is possible to describe some restricted classes of formulas which enjoy the mentioned preservation property, but none of them is significantly large, or representative of a wide class of specifications.

However, although in general the previous claim holds, in a constructive setting some preliminary results give an hope. Precisely, a compression algorithm which operates as above, but takes additional information on unsuccessful proof attempts in account is currently being studied. This approach uses information extraction algorithms from a partial proof, the failed attempt, to analyze the lack of information which prevented the completion of the correctness proof. The lacking information, which is part of the full representation of the program, is added to the set of objects the compression algorithm has to retain, and the partial correctness proof is redone, up to the point where it failed; since new information is available, new inference steps can be performed, and more chances for a success are gained. Unfortunately, no definitive result on what is preserved by this approach is currently available.

4   Conclusions

In this paper a simple way to represent object code programs has been introduced, and it has been made clear that it is suitable for mechanization. Moreover, the chosen representation can be compressed with various techniques, without affecting the provability of wide classes of specifications.

The novelty of the contribution lies in three points:

1. A general proof schema for correctness proofs can be generated along with the representation. It corresponds to a proof by induction on the paths of computation of the represented program.
2. The provability in both classical and Kuroda logic of a wide class of specifications is not affected by two important compressions of the representation of a program.
3. In a proper constructive framework, the addition of the theory of the microprocessor and the theory containing the program representation generates an enlarged logical system which is still constructive. Moreover, in a constructive system the preservation results on the compression algorithms can be slightly extended.

About the last point, it is worth remarking that, although constructive systems are not usually employed in formal verification, most correctness proofs have a constructive flavor, because this is what a human reader asks for to be convinced by the proof itself. More important, proving techniques based on constructive methods allow deeper kinds of analysis of the resulting correctness proofs, as discussed in [Ben00]. Thus the presented work is also a first effort to introduce these novel techniques to the formal verification community.

References

[AFMM96] A. Avellone, C. Fiorentini, P. Mantovani, and P. Miglioli. On maximal intermediate predicate constructive logics. *Studia Logica*, 57:373–408, 1996.

[Ben00] M. Benini. *Verification and Analysis of Programs in a Constructive Environment*. PhD thesis, Dipartimento di Scienze dell'Informazione, Università degli Studi di Milano, January 2000.

[BG90] G. Birtwistle and B. Graham. Verifying SECD in HOL. In J. Staunstrup, editor, *Proceedings of the IFIP TC10/WG10.5 Summer School on Formal Methods for VLSI Design*. North Holland, 1990.

[BKN98] M. Benini, S. Kalvala, and D. Nowotka. Program abstraction in a higher-order logic framework. In J. Grundy and M. Newey, editors, *Proceedings of Theorem Proving in Higher-Order Logic '98 International Conference*, volume 1479 of *Lecture Notes in Computer Science*, pages 33–48. Springer Verlag, 1998.

[BM85] R.S. Boyer and J.S. Moore. Program verification. *Journal of Automated Reasoning*, 1(1):17–23, 1985.

[BNP98] M. Benini, D. Nowotka, and C. Pulley. Computer arithmetic: Logic, calculation and rewriting. In D.M. Gabbay and M. De Rijke, editors, *Frontiers of Combining Systems 2*, Series in Logic and Computation, pages 77–93. Research Studies Press, 1998.

[BP97] G. Bella and L.C. Paulson. Using Isabelle to prove properties of the Kerberos authentication system. In H. Orman and C. Meadows, editors, *Workshop on Design and Formal Verification of Security Protocols*. DIMACS, September 1997.

[Cam88] A.J. Camilleri. *Executing Behavioural Definitions in Higher-Order Logic*. PhD thesis, Cambridge University, February 1988. Technical Report No 140, Computer Laboratory, Cambridge University.

[Cho94] C.T. Chou. Mechanical verification of distributed algorithms in higher-order logic. In T.F. Melham and J. Camilleri, editors, *Higher-Order Logic Theorem Proving and Its Applications*, volume 859 of *Lecture Notes in Computer Science*, pages 158–176. Springer Verlag, September 1994.

[CLS96] D. Cyrluk, P. Lincoln, and N. Shankar. On Shostak's decision procedure for combinations of theories. In M.A. McRobbie and J.K. Slaney, editors, *Automated Deduction — CADE-13*, volume 1104 of *Lecture Notes in Computer Science*, pages 463–477. Springer Verlag, 1996.

[Dij75] E.W. Dijkstra. Guarded commands, non determinacy and formal derivation of programs. *Communications of the ACM*, 18(8):453–458, 1975.

[FD93] P. Flener and Y. Deville. Logic program synthesis from incomplete specifications. *Journal of Symbolic Computation*, 15(5–6):775–806, 1993.

[Fer97] M. Ferrari. *Strongly Constructive Formal Systems*. PhD thesis, Dipartimento di Scienze dell'Informazione, Università degli Studi di Milano, 1997.

[FFM99] M. Ferrari, C. Fiorentini, and P. Miglioli. Extracting information from intermediate T-systems. In *Intuitionistic Modal Logics and Applications*, Trento, Italy, 1999. Federated Logic Conference.

[FLO97a] P. Flener, K.K. Lau, and M. Ornaghi. Correct-schema-guided synthesis of steadfast programs. In *Proceedings XIIth IEEE International Automated Software Engineering Conference*, pages 153–160, 1997.

[FLO97b] P. Flener, K.K. Lau, and M. Ornaghi. On correct program schemas. In N.E. Fuchs, editor, *Proceedings of the 7th International Workshop on Logic-Based Program Synthesis and Transformation*, Lecture Notes in Computer Science. Springer Verlag, 1997.

[Gab81]   D.M. Gabbay. *Semantical Investigations in Heyting Intuitionistic Logic*. D. Reidel Publishing Company, Dordrecht, 1981.

[KLO96]   C. Kreitz, K.K. Lau, and M. Ornaghi. Formal reasoning about modules, reuse and their correctness. volume 1085 of *Lecture Notes in Artificial Intelligence*. Springer Verlag, 1996.

[LO94]   K.K. Lau and M. Ornaghi. A formal view of specification, deductive synthesis and transformation of logic programs. In Y. Deville, editor, *Logic Program Synthesis and Transformation. Proceedings of LOPSTR'93*, Workshops in Computing, pages 10–31. Springer Verlag, 1994.

[LO98]   K.K. Lau and M. Ornaghi. Isoinitial models for logic programs: A preliminary study. In J.L. Freire-Nistal, M. Falaschi, and M. Vilares-Ferro, editors, *Proceedings of the 1998 Joint Conference on Declarative Programming*, pages 443–455, 1998.

[Man69]   Z. Manna. Properties of programs and the first order predicate calculus. *Journal of the Association for Computing Machinery*, 16(2), 1969.

[MMO88]   P. Miglioli, U. Moscato, and M. Ornaghi. Constructive theories with abstract data types for program synthesis. In D. Skordev, editor, *Mathematical Logic and its Applications*, pages 293–302. Plenum Press, 1988.

[MMO91]   P. Miglioli, U. Moscato, and M. Ornaghi. Program specification and synthesis in constructive formal systems. In K.K. Lau and T.P. Clement, editors, *Logic Program Synthesis and Transformation, Manchester 1991*, pages 13–26. Springer Verlag, 1991.

[MMO97]   P. Miglioli, U. Moscato, and M. Ornaghi. Avoiding duplications in tableau systems for intuitionistic and Kuroda logics. *Logical Journal of the IGPL*, 1(5):145–167, 1997.

[MO81]   P. Miglioli and M. Ornaghi. A logically justified model of computation. *Fundamenta Informaticæ*, IV(1,2), 1981.

[Mot89]   Motorola Inc., editor. *MC68020 32-bit Microprocessor User's Manual*. Prentice Hall, New Jersey, 1989.

[Pau94]   L.C. Paulson. *Isabelle: A Generic Theorem Prover*, volume 828 of *Lecture Notes in Computer Science*. Springer Verlag, 1994.

[Pau97]   L.C. Paulson. Generic automatic proof tools. In R. Veroff, editor, *Automated Reasoning and its Applications*, chapter 3. The MIT Press, 1997. Also, Report No 396, Computer Laboratory, Cambridge University.

[Sho79]   R.E. Shostak. A practical decision procedure for arithmetic with function symbols. *Journal of the Association for Computing Machinery*, 26(2):351–360, 1979.

[ST96]   H. Schwichtenberg and A.S. Troelstra. *Basic Proof Theory*, volume 43 of *Cambridge Tracts in Theoretical Computer Science*. Cambridge University Press, 1996.

[Yu93]   Y. Yu. Automated proofs of object code for a widely used microprocessor. Technical Report 114, Digital Equipment Corporation, Systems Research Center, October 1993.

Towards an Efficient Tableau Method for Boolean Circuit Satisfiability Checking

Tommi A. Junttila and Ilkka Niemelä

Helsinki University of Technology
Dept. of Computer Science and Engineering
Laboratory for Theoretical Computer Science
P.O.Box 5400, FIN-02015 HUT, Finland
{Tommi.Junttila,Ilkka.Niemela}@hut.fi

Abstract. Boolean circuits offer a natural, structured, and compact representation of Boolean functions for many application domains. In this paper a tableau method for solving satisfiability problems for Boolean circuits is devised. The method employs a direct cut rule combined with deterministic deduction rules. Simplification rules for circuits and a search heuristic attempting to minimize the search space are developed. Experiments in symbolic model checking domain indicate that the method is competitive against state-of-the-art satisfiability checking techniques and a promising basis for further work.

1 Introduction

Propositional satisfiability checkers have been applied successfully to many interesting domains such as planning [11] and model checking of finite state systems [1, 3, 2]. The success has built on recent significant advances in the performance of SAT checkers based both on stochastic local search algorithms and on complete systematic search.

In this paper we are interested in developing SAT checking methodology especially for symbolic model checking purposes. Most work on symbolic model checking [6] has been based on binary decision diagrams (BDDs) [5]. However, BDD-based methods suffer from the fact that a BDD representation of a Boolean expression can require exponential space. Recent research has shown that this problem can be overcome by using state-of-the-art SAT checking methods which work in polynomial space in the size of the input [1, 3, 2].

Most successful satisfiability checkers assume that the input formulae are in conjunctive normal form (CNF). This sometimes makes efficient modeling of an application challenging because natural non-clausal formalizations can lead to significant blow-up when the formulae are transformed to CNF. An example of the CNF transformation problem is a formula of the form

$$(P_1 \wedge Q_1) \vee \cdots \vee (P_n \wedge Q_n)$$

whose equivalent CNF is of exponential size. If it is enough to preserve satisfiability, the size of the CNF can be decreased to linear by introducing a new atom

J. Lloyd et al. (Eds.): CL 2000, LNAI 1861, pp. 553–567, 2000.
© Springer-Verlag Berlin Heidelberg 2000

for each conjunction and transforming the formula to

$$(R_1 \vee \cdots \vee R_n) \wedge (R_1 \leftrightarrow (P_1 \wedge Q_1)) \wedge \cdots \wedge (R_n \leftrightarrow (P_n \wedge Q_n))$$

whose CNF is

$$(R_1 \vee \cdots \vee R_n) \wedge \cdots \wedge (R_n \vee \neg P_n \vee \neg Q_n) \wedge (\neg R_n \vee P_n) \wedge (\neg R_n \vee Q_n) \quad .$$

Notice, however, that now the number of atomic formulae has increased by n and the search space (and running time) of typical SAT checkers could increase exponentially.

In this paper we study an alternative approach to solving propositional satisfiability problems which is not based on representing the input in CNF but as a *Boolean circuit*. This allows a compact and natural representation in many domains. Using Boolean circuits as the input format makes it possible to simplify the representation by sharing common subexpressions and by preserving natural structures and concepts of the domain.

Our idea is to combine advantages of a compact representation based on Boolean circuits and polynomial space requirements of CNF-based search procedures and devise a satisfiability checking algorithm for Boolean circuits, i.e., a procedure for finding truth assignments for a circuit given some constraints on its output values or for determining that none such exists.

There is a lot of previous research on theorem proving and satisfiability checking methods working with arbitrary (non-clausal) formulae. The work is mainly based on tableaux and sequent calculi, see e.g. [13] for a technique to make this approach more amenable to real applications using simplification methods. A commercial SAT-checking system, Prover [4], is also working with non-CNF input. Also SAT checking systems basically working with CNF input have been extended to handle more general formulae. This has been done both for complete SAT checkers, e.g. in [8], as well as for local search methods [10, 17].

In this paper we develop a tableau method that works directly with Boolean circuits. Instead of standard (cut free) tableau techniques we employ a direct cut rule combined with deterministic (non-branching) deduction rules. The aim is to achieve high performance and to avoid some computational problems in cut free tableaux [7]. In order make the method more efficient we devise simplification rules and a search heuristic which attempts to minimize the search space of the algorithm. The heuristic is inspired by the search technique used in a system for computing stable models [15, 18]. Experimental results indicate that the cut-based tableau method combined with suitable deduction and simplification rules and the search space minimizing heuristic has promising performance, e.g., in symbolic model checking applications.

The rest of the paper is structured as follows. We start by introducing Boolean circuits. Then we develop a tableau method for circuits. In Section 4 we identify transformation rules for simplifying circuits and then we describe an experimental implementation of the tableau method. Section 6 provides a simple translation of circuits to CNF used in the experiments presented in the following section where our tableau method is compared to state-of-the-art satisfiability checkers using symbolic model checking benchmarks.

2   Boolean Circuits

A *Boolean circuit* C is an acyclic directed graph where the nodes are called the *gates* of C. The gates with no outgoing edges are the *output gates* and the gates with no incoming edges and no Boolean function are the *input gates* of C. Each non-input gate is associated with a Boolean function and "calculates" its value from the values of its children. In this paper we represent Boolean circuits as *Boolean equation systems*. Such systems offer a convenient way of writing down circuits and of describing transformations on them. For more on Boolean circuits, see e.g. [16].

Given a finite set $\mathcal{V}$ of Boolean variables, a *Boolean equation system* (a *system* for short) $\mathcal{S}$ over $\mathcal{V}$ is a set of equations of the form $v = f(v_1, \ldots, v_k)$, where $v, v_1, \ldots, v_k \in \mathcal{V}$ and f is an arbitrary Boolean function. Boolean circuits can be seen as Boolean equation systems of a certain form where each variable has at most one equation and the equations are not recursive. More precisely this can be characterized as follows. Given a Boolean equation system $\mathcal{S}$ over $\mathcal{V}$ such that for each variable $v \in \mathcal{V}$ there is at most one equation in $\mathcal{S}$, we define the directed graph $G(\mathcal{S}) = \langle \mathcal{V}, E \rangle$, where $E = \{\langle v', v \rangle \mid v = f(\ldots, v', \ldots) \in \mathcal{S}\} \subseteq \mathcal{V} \times \mathcal{V}$. The graph $G(\mathcal{S})$ describes the variable dependencies in $\mathcal{S}$ and if $G(\mathcal{S})$ is acyclic, then $G(\mathcal{S})$ can be seen as a Boolean circuit. See Fig. 1 for an example. The variables of $\mathcal{S}$ correspond to the gates of the circuit and the variables for which there is no equation are the input gates of the circuit. A variable defined by an equation of form $v = \top$ ($v = \bot$) in turn corresponds to a constant gate "true" ("false").

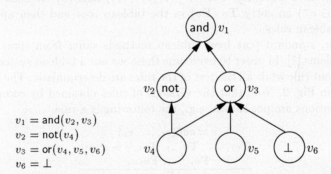

$$v_1 = \text{and}(v_2, v_3)$$
$$v_2 = \text{not}(v_4)$$
$$v_3 = \text{or}(v_4, v_5, v_6)$$
$$v_6 = \bot$$

Fig. 1. A system over $\{v_1, \ldots, v_6\}$ and the corresponding Boolean circuit.

A *truth valuation* for $\mathcal{S}$ is a function $\tau : \mathcal{V} \rightarrow \{\text{true}, \text{false}\}$. Valuation τ is *consistent* if $\tau(v) = f(\tau(v_1), \ldots, \tau(v_k))$ holds for each equation $v = f(v_1, \ldots, v_k)$ in $\mathcal{S}$. A system $\mathcal{S}$ is *satisfiable* if there exists a consistent valuation for it. The question of whether a system is satisfiable is obviously an **NP**-complete problem under the plausible assumption that each Boolean function appearing in the system can be computed in deterministic polynomial time. However, note that each Boolean equation system describing a Boolean circuit has exactly 2^n

consistent truth assignments, where n is the number of input gates in the circuit (the system only describes the *structure* of the circuit). Therefore, in case of Boolean circuits, we are interested in the *constrained satisfaction problem*: given that variables in $c^+ \subseteq \mathcal{V}$ must be true and those in $c^- \subseteq \mathcal{V}$ false (the *constraints*), is there a consistent valuation that respects these constraints? Again, this is obviously an **NP**-complete problem.

In the rest of the paper we consider the class of Boolean circuits where the following Boolean functions are allowed in the gates (equations).

- $\top$ (a constant function) is always true. The constant $\bot$ is always false.
- $\mathsf{equiv}(v_1, \ldots, v_n) = \mathrm{true}$ iff all v_i, $1 \leq i \leq n$, are true or all v_i, $1 \leq i \leq n$, are false.
- $\mathsf{or}(v_1, \ldots, v_n) = \mathrm{true}$ iff at least one v_i, $1 \leq i \leq n$, is true.
- $\mathsf{and}(v_1, \ldots, v_n) = \mathrm{true}$ iff all v_i, $1 \leq i \leq n$, are true.
- $\mathsf{even}(v_1, \ldots, v_n) = \mathrm{true}$ iff an even number of v_is, $1 \leq i \leq n$, are true.
- $\mathsf{odd}(v_1, \ldots, v_n) = \mathrm{true}$ iff an odd number of v_is, $1 \leq i \leq n$, are true.
- $\mathsf{not}(v) = \mathrm{true}$ iff v is not true.

3   A Tableau Method

In this section we develop a tableau method for solving satisfiability problems for constrained Boolean circuits. A straightforward approach would be to interpret each equation $v = f(v_1, \ldots, v_k)$ as an equivalence $v \leftrightarrow f(v_1, \ldots, v_k)$. We could thus use a traditional tableau method [14] by setting (i) for each equation $v = f(v_1, \ldots, v_k)$ in $\mathcal{S}$ an entry $\mathbf{T}(v \leftrightarrow f(v_1, \ldots, v_k))$ and (ii) for each constraint $v \in c^+$ ($v \in c^-$) an entry $\mathbf{T}v$ ($\mathbf{F}v$) in the tableau root and then applying the standard tableau rules.

However, standard (cut free) tableau methods suffer from some computational problems [7]. In order to overcome these we use a tableau system that has an explicit cut rule while all the rest of the rules are deterministic. The basic rules are shown in Fig. 2. Note that the versions of rules obtained by commutativity of the operations are not shown, e.g., the following is a rule:

$$
\frac{\begin{array}{c} v = \mathsf{odd}(v_1, \ldots, v_k) \\ \mathbf{T}v_1, \ldots, \mathbf{T}v_{j-1}, \mathbf{T}v_k, \; j \text{ is even} \\ \mathbf{F}v_j, \ldots, \mathbf{F}v_{k-1} \end{array}}{\mathbf{F}v}
$$

Given a system $\mathcal{S}$, the root of the tableau consists of the equations in $\mathcal{S}$ and the constraints. The rules appearing in Fig. 2 are then applied as in the standard tableau method. A branch in the tableau is *contradictory* if it contains both $\mathbf{F}v$ and $\mathbf{T}v$ entries for a variable in $v \in \mathcal{V}$. A branch is *complete* if it contains an $\mathbf{F}v$ or $\mathbf{T}v$ entry for each $v \in \mathcal{V}$ and no application of rules in Fig. 2(b)–(f) leads to contradiction.

Theorem 1. *The above tableau system is sound and complete in the sense that a complete branch gives a satisfying truth assignment for $\mathcal{S}$ while the absence of a complete branch indicates that the system is unsatisfiable.*

$$\frac{v \in \mathcal{V}}{Tv \mid Fv} \qquad \frac{v = \top}{Tv} \quad \frac{v = \bot}{Fv} \qquad \frac{v = \mathsf{not}(v_1)}{\begin{array}{c} Fv_1 \\ \hline Tv \end{array}} \quad \frac{v = \mathsf{not}(v_1)}{\begin{array}{c} Tv_1 \\ \hline Fv \end{array}}$$

(a) The explicit cut rule (b) Constant rules   (c) Negation rules

$$\frac{v = \mathsf{or}(v_1, \dots, v_k)}{\begin{array}{c} Fv_1, \dots, Fv_k \\ \hline Fv \end{array}} \quad \frac{v = \mathsf{and}(v_1, \dots, v_k)}{\begin{array}{c} Tv_1, \dots, Tv_k \\ \hline Tv \end{array}} \quad \frac{v = \mathsf{or}(v_1, \dots, v_k)}{\begin{array}{c} Tv_i, i \in \{1, \dots, k\} \\ \hline Tv \end{array}} \quad \frac{v = \mathsf{and}(v_1, \dots, v_k)}{\begin{array}{c} Fv_i, i \in \{1, \dots, k\} \\ \hline Fv \end{array}}$$

(d) "Up" rules for or and and

$$\frac{v = \mathsf{equiv}(v_1, \dots, v_k)}{\begin{array}{c} Tv_1, \dots, Tv_k \\ \hline Tv \end{array}} \qquad \frac{v = \mathsf{equiv}(v_1, \dots, v_k)}{\begin{array}{c} Fv_1, \dots, Fv_k \\ \hline Tv \end{array}} \qquad \frac{v = \mathsf{equiv}(v_1, \dots, v_k)}{\begin{array}{c} Tv_i, i \in \{1, \dots, k\} \\ Fv_j, i \in \{1, \dots, k\} \\ \hline Fv \end{array}}$$

(e) "Up" rules for equiv

$$\frac{v = \mathsf{even}(v_1, \dots, v_k)}{\begin{array}{c} Tv_1, \dots, Tv_j, \ j \text{ is even} \\ Fv_{j+1}, \dots, Fv_k \\ \hline Tv \end{array}} \qquad \frac{v = \mathsf{even}(v_1, \dots, v_k)}{\begin{array}{c} Tv_1, \dots, Tv_j, \ j \text{ is odd} \\ Fv_{j+1}, \dots, Fv_k \\ \hline Fv \end{array}}$$

$$\frac{v = \mathsf{odd}(v_1, \dots, v_k)}{\begin{array}{c} Tv_1, \dots, Tv_j, \ j \text{ is odd} \\ Fv_{j+1}, \dots, Fv_k \\ \hline Tv \end{array}} \qquad \frac{v = \mathsf{odd}(v_1, \dots, v_k)}{\begin{array}{c} Tv_1, \dots, Tv_j, \ j \text{ is even} \\ Fv_{j+1}, \dots, Fv_k \\ \hline Fv \end{array}}$$

(f) "Up" rules for even and odd

Fig. 2. Basic rules.

Notice that for Boolean circuits it would be sufficient to apply the cut rule to the input gates only: other gates are functionally fully dependent on input (and constant) gates. Therefore the values of all gates can be evaluated by using the rules in Fig. 2(b)–(f) once the values of input gates are assigned.

The size of a tableau depends essentially on the branching of the tableau, i.e., on the number of times that the *cut rule* in Fig. 2(a) is applied. In order to avoid the use of the cut rule we devise a set of additional rules which complement the basic rules. These rules given in Fig. 3 can be used in the tableau construction without affecting its soundness or completeness. In the following, the rules in Fig. 2(b)–(f) and Fig. 3 are called the *deterministic deduction rules*.

$$\frac{v = \mathsf{not}(v_1)}{\mathbf{T}v} \qquad \frac{v = \mathsf{not}(v_1)}{\mathbf{F}v}$$
$$\frac{\phantom{v = \mathsf{not}(v_1)}}{\mathbf{F}v_1} \qquad \frac{\phantom{v = \mathsf{not}(v_1)}}{\mathbf{T}v_1}$$

(a) "Down" rules for not

$$\frac{\begin{array}{c} v = \mathsf{or}(v_1,\dots,v_k) \\ \mathbf{F}v \end{array}}{\mathbf{F}v_1,\dots,\mathbf{F}v_k} \quad \frac{\begin{array}{c} v = \mathsf{and}(v_1,\dots,v_k) \\ \mathbf{T}v \end{array}}{\mathbf{T}v_1,\dots,\mathbf{T}v_k} \quad \frac{\begin{array}{c} v = \mathsf{equiv}(v_1,\dots,v_k) \\ \mathbf{T}v_i,\ i \in \{1,\dots,k\} \\ \mathbf{T}v \end{array}}{\mathbf{T}v_1,\dots,\mathbf{T}v_k} \quad \frac{\begin{array}{c} v = \mathsf{equiv}(v_1,\dots,v_k) \\ \mathbf{F}v_i,\ i \in \{1,\dots,k\} \\ \mathbf{T}v \end{array}}{\mathbf{F}v_1,\dots,\mathbf{F}v_k}$$

(b) "Down" rules for or, and and equiv

$$\frac{\begin{array}{c} v = \mathsf{or}(v_1,\dots,v_k) \\ \mathbf{F}v_1,\dots,\mathbf{F}v_{k-1} \\ \mathbf{T}v \end{array}}{\mathbf{T}v_k} \qquad \frac{\begin{array}{c} v = \mathsf{equiv}(v_1,\dots,v_k) \\ \mathbf{T}v_1,\dots,\mathbf{T}v_{k-1} \\ \mathbf{T}v \end{array}}{\mathbf{T}v_k} \qquad \frac{\begin{array}{c} v = \mathsf{equiv}(v_1,\dots,v_k) \\ \mathbf{T}v_1,\dots,\mathbf{T}v_{k-1} \\ \mathbf{F}v \end{array}}{\mathbf{F}v_k}$$

$$\frac{\begin{array}{c} v = \mathsf{and}(v_1,\dots,v_k) \\ \mathbf{T}v_1,\dots,\mathbf{T}v_{k-1} \\ \mathbf{F}v \end{array}}{\mathbf{F}v_k} \qquad \frac{\begin{array}{c} v = \mathsf{equiv}(v_1,\dots,v_k) \\ \mathbf{F}v_1,\dots,\mathbf{F}v_{k-1} \\ \mathbf{T}v \end{array}}{\mathbf{F}v_k} \qquad \frac{\begin{array}{c} v = \mathsf{equiv}(v_1,\dots,v_k) \\ \mathbf{F}v_1,\dots,\mathbf{F}v_{k-1} \\ \mathbf{F}v \end{array}}{\mathbf{T}v_k}$$

(c) "Last undetermined child" rules for or, and and equiv

$$\frac{\begin{array}{c} v = \mathsf{even}(v_1,\dots,v_k) \\ \mathbf{T}v_1,\dots,\mathbf{T}v_j,\ j \text{ is even} \\ \mathbf{F}v_{j+1},\dots,\mathbf{F}v_{k-1} \\ \mathbf{T}v \end{array}}{\mathbf{F}v_k} \quad \frac{\begin{array}{c} v = \mathsf{even}(v_1,\dots,v_k) \\ \mathbf{T}v_1,\dots,\mathbf{T}v_j,\ j \text{ is even} \\ \mathbf{F}v_{j+1},\dots,\mathbf{F}v_{k-1} \\ \mathbf{F}v \end{array}}{\mathbf{T}v_k} \quad \frac{\begin{array}{c} v = \mathsf{odd}(v_1,\dots,v_k) \\ \mathbf{T}v_1,\dots,\mathbf{T}v_j,\ j \text{ is odd} \\ \mathbf{F}v_{j+1},\dots,\mathbf{F}v_{k-1} \\ \mathbf{T}v \end{array}}{\mathbf{F}v_k}$$

$$\frac{\begin{array}{c} v = \mathsf{even}(v_1,\dots,v_k) \\ \mathbf{T}v_1,\dots,\mathbf{T}v_j,\ j \text{ is odd} \\ \mathbf{F}v_{j+1},\dots,\mathbf{F}v_{k-1} \\ \mathbf{T}v \end{array}}{\mathbf{T}v_k} \quad \frac{\begin{array}{c} v = \mathsf{even}(v_1,\dots,v_k) \\ \mathbf{T}v_1,\dots,\mathbf{T}v_j,\ j \text{ is odd} \\ \mathbf{F}v_{j+1},\dots,\mathbf{F}v_{k-1} \\ \mathbf{F}v \end{array}}{\mathbf{F}v_k} \quad \frac{\begin{array}{c} v = \mathsf{odd}(v_1,\dots,v_k) \\ \mathbf{T}v_1,\dots,\mathbf{T}v_j,\ j \text{ is odd} \\ \mathbf{F}v_{j+1},\dots,\mathbf{F}v_{k-1} \\ \mathbf{F}v \end{array}}{\mathbf{T}v_k}$$

$$\frac{\begin{array}{c} v = \mathsf{odd}(v_1,\dots,v_k) \\ \mathbf{T}v_1,\dots,\mathbf{T}v_j,\ j \text{ is even} \\ \mathbf{F}v_{j+1},\dots,\mathbf{F}v_{k-1} \\ \mathbf{T}v \end{array}}{\mathbf{T}v_k} \qquad \frac{\begin{array}{c} v = \mathsf{odd}(v_1,\dots,v_k) \\ \mathbf{T}v_1,\dots,\mathbf{T}v_j,\ j \text{ is even} \\ \mathbf{F}v_{j+1},\dots,\mathbf{F}v_{k-1} \\ \mathbf{F}v \end{array}}{\mathbf{T}v_k}$$

(d) "Last undetermined child" rules for even and odd

Fig. 3. Additional deduction rules.

Example 1. Consider the circuit in Fig. 1 and the constrained satisfaction problem where variable v_1 must be true. Below is a tableau solving this problem

$$
\begin{array}{ll}
1. & v_1 = \mathsf{and}(v_2, v_3) \\
2. & v_2 = \mathsf{not}(v_4) \\
3. & v_3 = \mathsf{or}(v_4, v_5, v_6) \\
4. & v_6 = \bot \\
5. & \mathbf{T}v_1 \\
6. & \mathbf{F}v_6 \qquad\qquad\qquad (4) \\
\end{array}
$$

$$
\begin{array}{ll}
7. \ \mathbf{T}v_4 \ (\text{cut}) & 8. \ \ \mathbf{F}v_4 \ (\text{cut}) \\
9. \ \mathbf{F}v_2 \ (2,7) & 11. \ \mathbf{T}v_2 \ (2,8) \\
10. \ \mathbf{F}v_1 \ (1,9) & 12. \ \mathbf{T}v_3 \ (1,5,11) \\
\quad\times \ \ (5,10) & 13. \ \mathbf{T}v_5 \ (3,6,8) \\
\end{array}
$$

where expressions 1–4 represent the circuit and expression 5 the constraint. For each other expression we give in parentheses the expressions from which it is derived using the tableau rules. Notice that the left hand branch (1–7,9,10) is contradictory and does not provide a solution but the right hand branch (1–6,8,11–13) is complete and yields a satisfying truth assignment where $\tau(v_1) = \tau(v_2) = \tau(v_3) = \tau(v_5) = \text{true}$ and $\tau(v_4) = \tau(v_6) = \text{false}$.

The use of the cut rule can be further limited by employing stronger deterministic deduction rules. There is an interesting trade-off between the computational complexity involved in implementing a deduction rule and its ability to derive further truth values. We consider as an interesting compromise a deduction rule that we call *one-step lookahead*.

One-Step Lookahead: Consider a branch B and an expression $\mathbf{T}v$ ($\mathbf{F}v$). If a complementary pair of variables $\mathbf{T}w, \mathbf{F}w$ can be derived using the deterministic deduction rules from $B \cup \{\mathbf{T}v\}$ (from $B \cup \{\mathbf{F}v\}$), deduce $\mathbf{F}v$ ($\mathbf{T}v$).

For instance, in the example above one-step lookahead could be applied to the branch containing expressions 1–6 and for $\mathbf{T}v_4$. Now $\mathbf{T}v_1, \mathbf{F}v_1$ can be derived and, hence, $\mathbf{F}v_4$ can be deduced. After that the branch can be completed using the deterministic deduction rules and a solution is found without any cuts (branching). The one-step lookahead rule is similar to the failed literal rule [12] in Davis-Putnam procedures for CNF satisfiability checking and the lookahead rule in Smodels system [18] computing stable models. Notice that examining whether the lookahead rule is applicable for a given expression $\mathbf{T}v$ ($\mathbf{F}v$) can be done in linear time in the size of the branch (given appropriate implementation techniques). Hence, determining the applicability of the rule is more expensive than for the other deterministic deduction rules. However, the lookahead rule is quite powerful in decreasing the number of cut rule applications needed to determine the existence of a solution. Experimental results indicate that often the additional overhead is worth the effort.

4 Satisfiability Preserving Simplifications

In order to simplify the structure of a circuit, some efficiently implementable, simple satisfiability preserving simplifications can be applied to a circuit. Actually, some of these simplifications require that the value of a gate is assigned and should thus be applied to a constrained circuit (where $\mathbf{T}v$ and $\mathbf{F}v$ provide the information).

1. Common subexpressions can be *shared*, i.e., if a system has two similar equations, $v = f(v_1, \ldots, v_k)$ and $v' = f(v_1, \ldots, v_k)$, then $v' = f(v_1, \ldots, v_k)$ can be removed from the system and all the occurrences of v' are substituted with v.
2. If a gate has a child whose value is determined, the connection to the child can be removed by the rewriting rules shown in Fig. 4(b)–(c). Figure 4 also shows some other simplification rewriting rules. One simplification that deserves special attention is the "input gate under true equivalence"-simplification in Fig. 4(d). It can detect that an input gate is functionally fully depended on other gates and removes it.
3. A *cone of influence* reduction can be performed: if a variable is not constrained and no other equation refers to it (i.e. it is an output gate in the circuit), it can be removed, that is, gates that cannot influence constrained gates can be removed.

5 An Experimental Implementation

We have made an experimental implementation called BCSat [9] of the tableau method described in Sec. 3 for Boolean circuits. In the following we briefly discuss the implementation.

After parsing in the circuit, some simple preprocessing steps are applied to it. First, we set the constraints in the tableau root. We then apply the deterministic deduction rules, one-step lookahead and the satisfiability preserving simplifications of Sec. 4 until nothing new can be deduced. Naturally, if any step here leads to a contradiction, the circuit is unsatisfiable and the procedure is stopped.

After this the tableau is built one branch at a time using a chronological backtracking procedure. At each search level, we first apply the deterministic rules and the one-step lookahead rule as long as they produce new information. We then choose the next undetermined *cut variable* for which the cut rule is applied, after which the search branches to the next level. The cut variable is selected by using the following heuristic. For each undetermined variable v the following question is considered: if v is set to false (true), how many values of other undetermined variables can be deduced by using the deterministic rules? Call these numbers $v^{\perp}$ and $v^{\top}$, respectively. A variable for which $\min\{v^{\perp}, v^{\top}\}$ is largest is then selected as the cut variable. The reasoning behind this choice of cut variable is that choosing a maximum of the minimum minimizes the sum of the remaining search space (the number of still possible variable assigments) left

$$\frac{v = \mathsf{and}()}{v = \mathsf{T}} \qquad \frac{v = \mathsf{or}()}{v = \perp} \qquad \frac{v = \mathsf{equiv}()}{v = \mathsf{T}} \qquad \frac{v = \mathsf{even}()}{v = \mathsf{T}} \qquad \frac{v = \mathsf{odd}()}{v = \perp}$$

$$\frac{v = \mathsf{and}(v')}{v = v'} \qquad \frac{v = \mathsf{or}(v')}{v = v'} \qquad \frac{v = \mathsf{equiv}(v')}{v = \mathsf{T}} \qquad \frac{v = \mathsf{even}(v')}{v = \mathsf{not}(v')} \qquad \frac{v = \mathsf{odd}(v')}{v = v'}$$

(a) Simplification rules for 0-ary and 1-ary gates

$$\frac{\begin{array}{c} v = \mathsf{or}(v_1, \ldots, v_{i-1}, v_i, v_{i+1}, \ldots, v_k) \\ \mathbf{F}v_i \end{array}}{\begin{array}{c} v = \mathsf{or}(v_1, \ldots, v_{i-1}, v_{i+1}, \ldots, v_k) \\ \mathbf{F}v_i \end{array}} \qquad \frac{\begin{array}{c} v = \mathsf{or}(v_1, \ldots, v_{i-1}, v_i, v_{i+1}, \ldots, v_k) \\ \mathbf{T}v_i \end{array}}{\begin{array}{c} v = \mathsf{T} \\ \mathbf{T}v_i \end{array}}$$

$$\frac{\begin{array}{c} v = \mathsf{and}(v_1, \ldots, v_{i-1}, v_i, v_{i+1}, \ldots, v_k) \\ \mathbf{T}v_i \end{array}}{\begin{array}{c} v = \mathsf{and}(v_1, \ldots, v_{i-1}, v_{i+1}, \ldots, v_k) \\ \mathbf{T}v_i \end{array}} \qquad \frac{\begin{array}{c} v = \mathsf{and}(v_1, \ldots, v_{i-1}, v_i, v_{i+1}, \ldots, v_k) \\ \mathbf{F}v_i \end{array}}{\begin{array}{c} v = \perp \\ \mathbf{F}v_i \end{array}}$$

$$\frac{\begin{array}{c} v = \mathsf{even}(v_1, \ldots, v_{i-1}, v_i, v_{i+1}, \ldots, v_k) \\ \mathbf{T}v_i \end{array}}{\begin{array}{c} v = \mathsf{odd}(v_1, \ldots, v_{i-1}, v_{i+1}, \ldots, v_k) \\ \mathbf{T}v_i \end{array}} \qquad \frac{\begin{array}{c} v = \mathsf{even}(v_1, \ldots, v_{i-1}, v_i, v_{i+1}, \ldots, v_k) \\ \mathbf{F}v_i \end{array}}{\begin{array}{c} v = \mathsf{even}(v_1, \ldots, v_{i-1}, v_{i+1}, \ldots, v_k) \\ \mathbf{F}v_i \end{array}}$$

$$\frac{\begin{array}{c} v = \mathsf{odd}(v_1, \ldots, v_{i-1}, v_i, v_{i+1}, \ldots, v_k) \\ \mathbf{T}v_i \end{array}}{\begin{array}{c} v = \mathsf{even}(v_1, \ldots, v_{i-1}, v_{i+1}, \ldots, v_k) \\ \mathbf{T}v_i \end{array}} \qquad \frac{\begin{array}{c} v = \mathsf{odd}(v_1, \ldots, v_{i-1}, v_i, v_{i+1}, \ldots, v_k) \\ \mathbf{F}v_i \end{array}}{\begin{array}{c} v = \mathsf{odd}(v_1, \ldots, v_{i-1}, v_{i+1}, \ldots, v_k) \\ \mathbf{F}v_i \end{array}}$$

(b) "Determined child"-simplification rules for or, and, even and odd

$$\frac{\begin{array}{c} v = \mathsf{equiv}(v_1, \ldots, v_{i-1}, v_i, v_{i+1}, \ldots, v_k) \\ \mathbf{T}v_i \end{array}}{\begin{array}{c} v = \mathsf{and}(v_1, \ldots, v_{i-1}, v_{i+1}, \ldots, v_k) \\ \mathbf{T}v_i \end{array}} \qquad \frac{\begin{array}{c} v = \mathsf{equiv}(v_1, v_2, \ldots, v_n) \\ \mathbf{T}v \\ v_1 \text{ is an input gate} \\ v_2 \text{ is an input or a constant gate} \end{array}}{\begin{array}{c} v = \mathsf{equiv}(v_2, \ldots, v_n) \\ \mathbf{T}v \\ v_1 = v_2 \end{array}}$$

(c) A "determined child"-simplification   (d) "Input gate under true equivalence"-
    rule for equiv   simplification

$$\frac{\begin{array}{c} v = \mathsf{not}(v') \\ v' = \mathsf{not}(v'') \end{array}}{\begin{array}{c} v = v'' \\ v' = \mathsf{not}(v'') \end{array}} \qquad \frac{v = \mathsf{and}(\ldots, v', \ldots, v_1, \ldots)}{\begin{array}{c} v_1 = \mathsf{not}(v') \\ \hline v = \perp \\ v_1 = \mathsf{not}(v') \end{array}} \qquad \frac{v = \mathsf{or}(\ldots, v', \ldots, v_1, \ldots)}{\begin{array}{c} v_1 = \mathsf{not}(v') \\ \hline v = \mathsf{T} \\ v_1 = \mathsf{not}(v') \end{array}}$$

(e) Double negation and "$v/\neg v$" simplifications

Fig. 4. Satisfiability preserving simplification *rewriting* rules for constrained circuits (an equation of form $v = v'$ means that occurrences of v are substituted with v').

in both search branches: if the number of undetermined variables is N, then after the cut and deterministic rules the search space left is $\mathcal{O}(2^{N-v^{\perp}}+2^{N-v^{\top}})$. This is minimized by our heuristic and we have thus chosen a *balancing* heuristic rather than a greedy one. As a small improvement we do not count the determined not-gates into $v^{\perp}$ or $v^{\top}$ since not is a fully deterministic operation w.r.t. to its only argument. Our experiments so far indicate that counting in all the variables when computing $v^{\perp}$ and $v^{\top}$ leads to smaller tableaux than when considering only the undetermined input variables.

The lookahead and computation of $v^{\perp}$ and $v^{\top}$ are implemented simply by first assigning an undetermined variable v to false and then applying the deterministic rules. The number $v^{\perp}$ is then stored and the effects of the assignment and application of deterministic rules are undone. The same procedure is repeated for true. If it is found out that assigning a variable to false (true) leads to a contradiction but assignment to true (false) does not, the variable is assigned to true (false), and the deterministic rules are applied. If both assignments lead to contradiction, backtracking to the previous search level occurs. This kind of lookahead and its use was inspired by the one used in the Smodels system [18].

6   Translating Circuits into CNF

In order to compare our tool to some satisfiability checkers requiring the input to be in CNF, we now present a very simple translation from Boolean circuits to CNF. We do not treat here equiv-, even- or odd-gates with more than 2 inputs (this would require more than a linear number of clauses or additional variables). Furthermore, the experimental cases we consider do not have such gates. The CNF translation is the conjunction of clauses obtained from the gates by the translation rules in Table 1. Input gates (variables with no definitions) are

Table 1. Boolean circuit to CNF translation rules.

Gate	CNF clause(s)
$v = \top$	v
$v = \bot$	$\neg v$
$v = \mathsf{not}(v_1)$	$(v \vee v_1) \wedge (\neg v \vee \neg v_1)$
$v = \mathsf{or}(v_1, \ldots, v_n)$	$(v \vee \neg v_1) \wedge \cdots \wedge (v \vee \neg v_n) \wedge (\neg v \vee v_1 \vee \cdots \vee v_2)$
$v = \mathsf{and}(v_1, \ldots, v_n)$	$(\neg v \vee v_1) \wedge \cdots \wedge (\neg v \vee v_n) \wedge (v \vee \neg v_1 \vee \cdots \vee \neg v_2)$
$v = \mathsf{even}(v_1, v_2)$ and $v = \mathsf{equiv}(v_1, v_2)$	$(v \vee v_1 \vee v_2) \wedge (v \vee \neg v_1 \vee \neg v_2) \wedge$ $(\neg v \vee v_1 \vee \neg v_2) \wedge (\neg v \vee \neg v_1 \vee v_2)$
$v = \mathsf{odd}(v_1, v_2)$	$(v \vee v_1 \vee \neg v_2) \wedge (v \vee \neg v_1 \vee v_2) \wedge$ $(\neg v \vee v_1 \vee v_2) \wedge (\neg v \vee \neg v_1 \vee \neg v_2)$

translated into $(v \vee \neg v)$. The constraints in the constrained satisfaction problem are simply translated into corresponding unit clauses (like the constant gates).

7   Some Experiments

We use the bounded model checking examples of Biere et al [1]. For each problem instance we use two different input sources. First one is the DIMACS CNF output produced directly by the bounded model checker tool **BMC** [1]. We will call this format **BMC**-CNF. We were also able to reconstruct Boolean circuits from the Prover output format files produced by **BMC**. These circuits were used as such or translated into CNF as described in Sec. 6.

We used the following solvers: BCSat described in this paper, CGrasp [8], Satz [12] and Sato [19]. BCSat and CGrasp both work on Boolean circuit input formats (we made a straightforward translation from our format to that of CGrasp). These tools were thus ran only on the Boolean circuit input. Since Satz and Sato expect DIMACS CNF as input format, we ran these tools in both **BMC**-CNF and CNF translated from circuits. All solvers were used "as is", no engineering work was put on trying to find suitable parameter settings. Unfortunately, we did not have access to the Prover tool [4].

The tests were run on 450 MHz Pentium machines running the Linux operating system. The times shown are the user times measured with the `time` command. The times do not include neither the generation of input files with the **BMC** tool nor translations between formats.

As the first test case we used the barrel shifter, with results shown in Table 2. The parameter $|r|$ in the first column indicates the number of registers in the shifter and also the number of time steps in **BMC**. The next two columns show the times of CNF solvers Sato and Satz when ran on **BMC**-CNF. The next four columns show the solver times when ran on unsimplified Boolean circuit input (translated into CNF in case of Sato and Satz). The last column shows the running time of the BCSat tool when allowed to make simplifications described in Sec. 4. The striking difference in the performance is due to the "input gate under true equivalence"-simplification in Fig. 4(d): BCSat finds out during the simplification that the circuit is not satisfiable and does thus not perform any actual search. This observation also explains the good results of the Prover tool as described in [1]: Prover simplifies the equivalences, too.

Table 2. Barrel shifter ($|r|$ = number of registers).

	BMC-CNF		Circuit, no red.				BCSat
$|r|$	Sato	Satz	BCSat	CGrasp	Sato	Satz	red.
4	0	0	0	0	5	0	0
5	13	465	302	135	≥1h	44	0
6	73	≥1h	≥1h	≥1h	-	224	0
7	280	-	-	-	-	1369	0
8	613	-	-	-	-	≥1h	0
9	≥1h	-	-	-	-	-	0
10	-	-	-	-	-	-	0

Table 3 shows our next example in which a counter-example of length k has to be found in a buggy design of a mutual exclusion algorithm under fairness. Unlike in other examples, the instances here are satisfiable. Again, the solvers are run on **BMC**-CNF, circuit input and then on simplified circuit input (the simplification times for solvers other than BCSat are not included in their running times).

Table 3. Counterexample for liveness in a buggy DME with 2 cells.

| | BMC-CNF | | Circuit, no red. | | | | Circuit, red. | | | |
k	Sato	Satz	BCSat	CGrasp	Sato	Satz	BCSat	CGrasp	Sato	Satz
10	0	1	104	17	1	1	4	4	0	0
11	1	3	3	28	3	$\geq$1h	3	6	0	$\geq$1h
12	0	6	4	61	5	4	3	9	0	$\geq$1h
13	$\geq$1h	$\geq$1h	5	126	136	3	4	11	0	-
14	2	$\geq$1h	6	152	6	3	6	23	0	-
15	249	-	223	150	152	4	6	21	0	-
16	$\geq$1h	-	8	129	$\geq$1h	5	13	36	7	-
17	$\geq$1h	-	8	178	$\geq$1h	5	8	94	1	-
18	-	-	13	201	-	6	10	57	3	-
19	-	-	10	1255	-	7	19	99	4	-
20	-	-	14	445	-	8	514	110	23	-
21	-	-	16	369	-	8	13	161	1	-
22	-	-	22	1253	-	10	17	190	$\geq$1h	-
23	-	-	24	412	-	11	15	210	3185	-
24	-	-	26	891	-	11	19	349	23	-
25	-	-	27	867	-	11	20	666	2	-
26	-	-	30	2573	-	14	26	666	11	-
27	-	-	28	892	-	16	30	3091	$\geq$1h	-
28	-	-	38	1356	-	24	34	2941	$\geq$1h	-
29	-	-	34	937	-	35	34	2815	-	-
30	-	-	47	$\geq$1h	-	46	38	3159	-	-

Our two last examples concern the same mutual exclusion algorithm, this time a correct one (thus there are no counter-examples and the instances are unsatisfiable). Table 4 shows results in the case of two users, parameterized w.r.t. the number of time steps. This means that we parameterize over the circuit depth since the greater the number of time steps, the greater the circuit depth. On the other hand, Table 5 depicts results when the number of time steps is kept as 10 but the number of users is parameterized. This corresponds to parameterization over circuit width. When comparing these two parameterization dimensions, we notice that the circuit depth seems to be a more crucial dimension for solver efficiency.

Admittedly, in order to draw any firm conclusions on the behavior of different solvers, more experiments should be conducted, especially on other types of Boolean circuits. However, we make some preliminary observations: (i) BCSat

Table 4. Liveness in DME with 2 cells, parameterized w.r.t. the number of time steps.

	BMC-CNF		Circuit, no red.				Circuit, red.			
k	Sato	Satz	BCSat	CGrasp	Sato	Satz	BCSat	CGrasp	Sato	Satz
10	1322	1	2	43	178	1	1	18	1	0
11	≥1h	1	3	159	≥1h	1	3	17	≥1h	0
12	≥1h	2	3	113	≥1h	2	4	48	12	1
13	-	5	5	193	-	3	5	68	7	1
14	-	15	6	280	-	4	6	72	27	3
15	-	52	9	380	-	8	8	95	6	3
16	-	≥1h	23	1859	-	10	12	105	159	7
17	-	≥1h	37	641	-	25	14	188	23	10
18	-	-	47	858	-	34	17	245	166	21
19	-	-	55	1010	-	78	343	428	≥1h	37
20	-	-	117	2010	-	32	524	400	≥1h	67
21	-	-	341	3457	-	211	1054	633	-	326
22	-	-	3461	1682	-	≥1h	≥1h	2496	-	≥1h
23	-	-	≥1h	3591	-	≥1h	≥1h	1274	-	≥1h
24	-	-	≥1h	3495	-	-	-	2254	-	-
25	-	-	-	2621	-	-	-	≥1h	-	-
26	-	-	-	≥1h	-	-	-	1962	-	-
27	-	-	-	≥1h	-	-	-	≥1h	-	-
28	-	-	-	-	-	-	-	2939	-	-
29	-	-	-	-	-	-	-	≥1h	-	-
30	-	-	-	-	-	-	-	≥1h	-	-

Table 5. Liveness in DME with 10 time steps, parameterized w.r.t. the number of cells.

	BMC-CNF		Circuit, no red.				Circuit, red.			
cells	Sato	Satz	BCSat	CGrasp	Sato	Satz	BCSat	CGrasp	Sato	Satz
2	1322	1	2	43	178	1	1	18	1	0
3	≥1h	4	4	82	≥1h	2	4	36	1	1
4	≥1h	18	7	340	≥1h	4	8	59	124	1
5	-	73	13	364	-	5	14	125	≥1h	1
6	-	≥1h	20	691	-	7	20	129	25	2
7	-	≥1h	28	1058	-	13	34	88	≥1h	6
8	-	-	35	1891	-	10	39	204	≥1h	3
9	-	-	47	1678	-	16	50	166	-	4
10	-	-	67	2053	-	20	63	178	-	5
11	-	-	81	2567	-	22	83	381	-	5
12	-	-	93	≥1h	-	31	98	416	-	7
13	-	-	101	≥1h	-	26	107	781	-	7
14	-	-	119	-	-	46	126	872	-	19
15	-	-	139	-	-	43	165	817	-	9
16	-	-	160	-	-	44	183	926	-	15
17	-	-	192	-	-	56	218	1059	-	12
18	-	-	232	-	-	94	239	1035	-	13
19	-	-	242	-	-	85	260	584	-	42
20	-	-	275	-	-	112	295	1653	-	19

and Satz seem to work quite similarly: this is probably because they both use lookahead and their heuristics are somewhat similar. (ii) All solvers seem to be a bit input syntax sensitive: there are cases when simplifications help but also counter-cases.

Finally, note that since our Boolean circuits were reconstructed from the output generated for the Prover tool, the circuits are probably not equal to those that would be generated should the BMC tool support Boolean circuit formalism directly. However, we assume that the circuits we have are quite close to those.

8   Conclusions

We have developed a tableau method for solving Boolean circuit satisfiability problems. The method works directly on Boolean circuits and does not require any clausal form translation of the circuit. Our method differs from standard tableau techniques. It uses an explicit cut rule together with deterministic (non-branching) deduction rules. In addition to typical deduction rules propagating truth values, our method employs a one-step lookahead rule which is computationally more expensive than standard propagation rules but which enables stronger propagation and reduces the need to use the cut rule. Furthermore, we identify simplification rules which preserve satisfiability but reduce the size and the form of a circuit. We have developed a prototype implementation of the method which applies the simplification rules and builds a tableau one branch at the time using backtracking search and a search heuristic based on the lookahead rule. We have tested the method on symbolic model checking benchmarks against state-of-the-art satisfiability checkers. The experiments indicate that the tableau method provides a promising basis for solving Boolean satisfiability problems. Interesting topics of further research include the development of refined search heuristics that take better into account the circuit structure, intelligent backtracking methods and simplification techniques.

Acknowledgements

The authors wish to thank Patrik Simons for discussing the implementation of the Smodels system and to gratefully acknowledge the financial aid of the Academy of Finland (projects no. 43963 and 47754). Tommi Junttila is grateful for the support from Helsinki Graduate School in Computer Science and Engineering (HeCSE) and Tekniikan Edistämissäätiö ("Foundation of Technology").

References

1. A. Biere, A. Cimatti, E. Clarke, and Y. Zhu. Symbolic model checking without BDDs. In W. R. Cleaveland, editor, *Tools and Algorithms for the Construction and Analysis of Systems (TACAS'99)*, volume 1579 of *LNCS*, pages 193–207. Springer, 1999.
2. A. Biere, A. Cimatti, E. M. Clarke, M. Fujita, and Y. Zhu. Symbolic model checking using SAT procedures instead of BDDs. In *Proceedings of the 36th ACM/IEEE Design Automation Conference (DAC'99)*, pages 317–320. ACM, 1999.
3. A. Biere, E. Clarke, R. Raimi, and Y. Zhu. Verifying safety properties of a PowerPC microprocessor using symbolic model checking without BDDs. In N. Halbwachs and D. Peled, editors, *Computer Aided Verification: 11th International Conference (CAV'99)*, volume 1633 of *LNCS*, pages 60–71. Springer, 1999.
4. A. Borälv. The industrial success of verification tools based on Stålmarck's method. In *Proceeding of the 9th International Conference on Computer Aided Verification (CAV'97)*, volume 1254 of *LNCS*, pages 7–10, Haifa, Israel, June 1997. Springer.
5. R. Bryant. Graph-based algorithms for boolean function manipulation. *IEEE Transactions on Computers*, 35(8):677–691, 1986.
6. J. Burch, E. Clarke, K. McMillan, D. Dill, and L. Hwang. Symbolic model checking: 10^{20} states and beyond. *Information and Computation*, 98(2):142–170, 1992.
7. M. D'Agostino and M. Mondadori. The taming of the cut. *Journal of Logic and Computation*, 4:285–319, 1994.
8. L. Guerra e Silva, L. M. Silveira, and J. Marques-Silva. Algorithms for solving Boolean satisfiability in combinatorial circuits. In *Design, Automation and Test in Europe (DATE'99)*, pages 526–530. IEEE, 1999.
9. T. Junttila. BCSat — a satisfiability checker for Boolean circuits. Available at http://www.tcs.hut.fi/~tjunttil/bcsat.
10. H. Kautz, D. McAllester, and B. Selman. Exploiting variable dependency in local search. A draft available at http://www.cs.cornell.edu/home/selman/papers-ftp/papers.html, 1997.
11. H. Kautz and B. Selman. Pushing the envelope: Planning, propositional logic, and stochastic search. In *Proceedings of the 13th National Conference on Artificial Intelligence*, Portland, Oregon, July 1996.
12. C. Li and Anbulagan. Look-ahead versus look-back for satisfiability problems. In *Principles and Practice of Constraint Programming – CP97*, volume 1330 of *LNCS*, pages 341–355. Springer, 1997.
13. F. Massacci. Simplification — a general constraint propagation technique for propositional and modal tableaux. In H. de Swart, editor, *Proceedings of the International Conference on Automated Reasoning with Analytic Tableaux and Related Methods (TABLEAUX-98)*, pages 217–231. Springer, May 1998.
14. A. Nerode and R. A. Shore. *Logic for Applications*. Text and Monographs in Computer Science. Springer-Verlag, 1993.
15. I. Niemelä and P. Simons. Efficient implementation of the well-founded and stable model semantics. In M. Maher, editor, *Proceedings of the Joint International Conference and Symposium on Logic Programming*, pages 289–303. The MIT Press, 1996.
16. C. H. Papadimitriou. *Computational Complexity*. Addison-Wesley, 1995.
17. R. Sebastiani. Applying GSAT to non-clausal formulas. *Journal of Artificial Intelligence Research*, 1:309–314, 1994.
18. P. Simons. Towards constraint satisfaction through logic programs and the stable model semantics. Research report A47, Helsinki University of Technology, Helsinki, Finland, August 1997. Available at http://www.tcs.hut.fi/pub/reports/A47.ps.gz.
19. H. Zhang. SATO: An efficient propositional prover. In *Automated Deduction – CADE-14*, volume 1249 of *LNCS*, pages 272–275. Springer, 1997.

Certification of Compiler Optimizations Using Kleene Algebra with Tests

Dexter Kozen[1][*] and Maria-Cristina Patron[2]

[1] Computer Science Department, Cornell University
Ithaca NY 14853-7501, USA
kozen@cs.cornell.edu
[2] Center for Applied Mathematics, Cornell University, Ithaca NY 14853-7501, USA
mpatron@cam.cornell.edu

Abstract. We use Kleene algebra with tests to verify a wide assortment of common compiler optimizations, including dead code elimination, common subexpression elimination, copy propagation, loop hoisting, induction variable elimination, instruction scheduling, algebraic simplification, loop unrolling, elimination of redundant instructions, array bounds check elimination, and introduction of sentinels. In each of these cases, we give a formal equational proof of the correctness of the optimizing transformation.

1 Introduction

Kleene algebra (KA) is the algebra of regular expressions. It was first introduced by Kleene in 1956 [6] and further developed in the 1971 monograph of Conway [4]. It has reappeared in many contexts in mathematics and computer science; see [7] and references therein.

In [8], an extension of KA called Kleene algebra with tests (KAT) was introduced. This system combines programs and assertions in a simple, purely equational system. In [10] it was shown that KAT strictly subsumes propositional Hoare logic, is of no greater complexity, and is deductively complete over relational models (Hoare logic is not). Moreover, KAT requires nothing beyond the constructs of classical equational logic, in contrast to Hoare logic, which requires a specialized syntax involving partial correctness assertions.

KAT has been applied successfully in various low-level verification tasks involving communication protocols, basic safety analysis, source-to-source program transformation, and concurrency control [1–3,8]. A useful feature of KAT in this regard is its ability to accommodate certain basic equational assumptions regarding the interaction of atomic instructions. This feature makes KAT ideal for reasoning about the correctness of low-level code transformations.

In this paper we show how KAT can be used to verify a variety of common compiler optimizations: dead code elimination, common subexpression elimination, copy propagation, loop hoisting, induction variable elimination, instruction

---

[*] Supported by National Science Foundation grant CCR-9708915.

J. Lloyd et al. (Eds.): CL 2000, LNAI 1861, pp. 568–582, 2000.
© Springer-Verlag Berlin Heidelberg 2000

scheduling, algebraic simplification, loop unrolling, elimination of redundant instructions, array bounds check elimination, and introduction of sentinels. In each of these cases, we give a formal, machine-verifiable equational proof of the correctness of the optimizing transformation.

The verification of compiler optimizations is more than just a theoretical exercise. We were led to these investigations by recent work in typed assembly language (TAL) [12], proof-carrying code (PCC) [13], and efficient code certification (ECC) [9]. These are systems that provide a means for an untrusted compiler to convince a trusted verifier that the object code it produces meets certain safety requirements.

PCC is the most powerful of these systems. It is quite flexible in the security policies it can express, but a significant problem is the size of certificates [14]. ECC addresses this issue by taking advantage of compiler conventions, giving a significant reduction in certificate size. In ECC, the production and verification of certificates is very efficient and invisible to both the code producer and consumer. However, these savings come only at a cost of reduced expressiveness and compiler dependence. In particular, whereas TAL and PCC deal well with optimizing transformations, ECC, being more dependent on the form of the object code produced by the compiler, is less robust with respect to code motion. To verify optimized code, ECC would require the certificate to include a concise description of the sequence of optimizing transformations that were performed, along with a machine-verifiable justification of these transformations. Such an extension might be based on the system KAT as described here.

In the last section, we discuss an interesting paradox that arises in connection with *dead variables*, those whose current value will never be used. This paradox is the source of a potentially dangerous pitfall in informal reasoning. A formal treatment in KAT helps to illuminate this pitfall.

2   Kleene Algebra and Kleene Algebra with Tests

In this section we briefly review the definitions of Kleene algebra and Kleene algebra with tests; see [7] for a more thorough introduction.

2.1   Kleene Algebra (KA)

The following axiomatization is from [7]. A Kleene algebra $(K, +, \cdot, {}^*, 0, 1)$ is an idempotent semiring under $+, \cdot, 0, 1$ satisfying

$$1 + pp^* = p^* \tag{1}$$

$$1 + p^*p = p^* \tag{2}$$

$$q + pr \leq r \rightarrow p^*q \leq r \tag{3}$$

$$q + rp \leq r \rightarrow qp^* \leq r, \tag{4}$$

where $\leq$ refers to the natural partial order on K:

$$p \leq q \stackrel{\text{def}}{\Longleftrightarrow} p + q = q.$$

These axioms say essentially that * behaves like the reflexive transitive closure operator of relational algebra or the Kleene asterate operator of formal languages. The operation $+$ gives the supremum with respect to $\leq$. All the operators are monotone with respect to $\leq$.

Besides basic properties of * such as $1 \leq a^*$, $a \leq a^*$, $a^*a^* = a^*$, and $a^{**} = a^*$, we will find the following two identities particularly useful:

$$p(qp)^* = (pq)^*p \tag{5}$$
$$(p+q)^* = p^*(qp^*)^* = (p^*q)^*p^*. \tag{6}$$

These identities are called the *sliding rule* and the *denesting rule*, respectively. In addition, the following result will prove useful:

Lemma 1. *In any Kleene algebra, $xy = xyx \rightarrow xy^* = x(yx)^*$.*

Proof. We show independently that

$$xy \leq xyx \rightarrow xy^* \leq x(yx)^* \tag{7}$$
$$xyx \leq xy \rightarrow x(yx)^* \leq xy^*. \tag{8}$$

To show (7), by (4) it is enough to show $xy \leq xyx \rightarrow x + x(yx)^*y \leq x(yx)^*$. Reasoning under the assumption $xy \leq xyx$, we have

$$
\begin{aligned}
x + x(yx)^*y &= x + (xy)^*xy &&\text{by the sliding rule (5)} \\
&\leq x + (xy)^*xyx &&\text{by the assumption } xy \leq xyx \\
&= (1 + (xy)^*xy)x &&\text{distributivity} \\
&= (xy)^*x &&\text{by (2)} \\
&= x(yx)^* &&\text{by the sliding rule (5).}
\end{aligned}
$$

For (8), reasoning under the assumption $xyx \leq xy$, we have by distributivity and (1) that $x + xyxy^* \leq x + xyy^* = x(1 + yy^*) = xy^*$, thus by (3), $(xy)^*x \leq xy^*$. The right-hand side of (8) then follows from the sliding rule (5).

2.2   Kleene Algebra with Tests (KAT)

A Kleene algebra with tests is a Kleene algebra with an embedded Boolean subalgebra. Formally, it is a two-sorted structure $(K, B, +, \cdot, ^*, ^-, 0, 1)$ such that

- $(K, +, \cdot, ^*, 0, 1)$ is a Kleene algebra;
- $(B, +, \cdot, ^-, 0, 1)$ is a Boolean algebra; and
- $B \subseteq K$.

The Boolean complementation operator $^-$ is defined only on B.

The elements of B are called *tests*. We will denote arbitrary elements of K by the letters $p, q, r, s, t, u, v, \ldots$ and tests by $a, b, c, d, \ldots$.

When applied to arbitrary elements of K, the operators $+, \cdot, 0, 1$ refer to non-deterministic choice, composition, fail and skip, respectively. Applied to tests, they take on the additional meaning of Boolean disjunction, conjunction, falsity and truth, respectively. These two usages do not conflict—for example, sequentially testing b and c is the same as testing their conjunction bc—and their coexistence permits considerable economy of expression.

For applications in program verification, the standard interpretation would be a KA of binary relations on a set and the Boolean algebra of subsets of the identity relation. One can also consider trace models in which the Kleene elements are sets of traces (sequences of states) and the boolean elements are sets of states (traces of length 0).

The encoding of the while program constructs is as in Propositional Dynamic Logic [5]:

$$p \, ; \, q \overset{\text{def}}{=} pq$$
$$\textbf{if } b \textbf{ then } p \textbf{ else } q \overset{\text{def}}{=} bp + \bar{b}q$$
$$\textbf{while } b \textbf{ do } p \overset{\text{def}}{=} (bp)^* \bar{b}.$$

The following result, also observed in [8], follows directly from Lemma 1. Intuitively, if the execution of the program q does not affect the value of the test b, then neither does q^*.

Lemma 2. *In any* KAT*, if* $bq = qb$, *then* $bq^* = (bq)^* b = q^* b = b(qb)^*$.

Proof. If $bq = qb$, then by Boolean algebra $bq = bbq = bqb$, thus $bq^* = b(qb)^*$ by Lemma 1. The other equations follow from the sliding rule (5) and symmetry.

2.3   KAT and Hoare Logic

Hoare logic is a system for deriving partial correctness properties of compound programs compositionally from properties of their constituent parts. Traditionally, these properties are expressed by *partial correctness assertions* (PCAs) of the form $\{b\} \, p \, \{c\}$, where b and c are assertions in the underlying assertion language and p is a program. Intuitively, the PCA $\{b\} p \{c\}$ says that if the property b holds at the start of execution of p, and if p halts, then c must be true in the halting state.

As mentioned in the introduction, KAT subsumes Hoare logic [10]. The PCA $\{b\} p \{c\}$ is expressed $bp\bar{c} = 0$, or equivalently, $bp = bpc$. Intuitively, $bp\bar{c} = 0$ says that there is no halting computation of p satisfying precondition b and postcondition $\bar{c}$, and $bp = bpc$ says that testing c after executing p with precondition b is always redundant.

In traditional Hoare logic, atomic programs are assignments $x := e$ and the only atomic assumption is the *assignment rule* $\{P[x/e]\} \, x := e \, \{P\}$. Hoare logic operates by deriving PCAs involving compound programs inductively, using the assignment rule as an axiom. The operation of KAT is analogous, except that the assumptions and conclusions are equations between programs, and the form of the assumptions can be more general. Theorems of KAT are universally quantified Horn formulas of the form $(\bigwedge_i p_i = q_i) \to p = q$. In our applications below, the

$p_i = q_i$ are typically premises that involve atomic instructions and tests that are immediately self-evident, and the conclusion $p = q$ is the equivalence of the unoptimized and optimized code fragments.

In our optimization examples, there are certain kinds of premises that occur frequently. For example, we often need to know that two atomic instructions that do not affect each other can occur in either order. This would be expressed in KAT by a commutativity condition of the form $pq = qp$. We would take this assertion as a premise on the left-hand side of the Horn formula above. Another common example is the fact that after loading a register with a value, that register contains that value. This is expressed by an equation of the form $p = pa$, where p is the load instruction and a is the assertion that the register contains the value. This assertion allows us to introduce new assertions into an annotated program and delete them when they are no longer needed. As a final example, the fact that if a register already contains a value, then there is no need to load it again would be encoded as an equation of the form $ap = a$. This premise allows us to delete redundant instructions.

We use such atomic premises extensively in the derivations of Section 3. In all cases the truth of the premise is directly evident. Moreover, it has been observed that in the decision procedure for KAT, premises of the form $p = 0$ can be eliminated without loss of efficiency [1, 11].

3   Verifying Optimizations in KAT

In this section we consider several examples of common compiler optimizations and show how they can be encoded and verified in KAT. In each case, we give the program fragments before and after the optimizations, their translations into the language of KAT, and an equational proof that the two fragments are equivalent.

3.1   Dead Code Elimination

Dead code elimination is a code transformation that removes unreachable instructions. Let us start with a very simple example. Consider the program p; **if** a **then** q. This is expressed in KAT as $p(aq + \bar{a})$. The $\bar{a}$ in this expression represents the implicit **else** clause. Suppose we know that the test a is always false after the execution of p. This would imply that the test of the **if** statement is false in the program above, so q would never be executed. We could remove it to obtain the optimized fragment p.

The assumption that the test a is always false after the execution of p is expressed in KAT by the identity $p = p\bar{a}$, or equivalently $pa = 0$. Intuitively, immediately after the execution of p, we must always be in a state in which $\bar{a}$ holds. In this case, executing the guard $\bar{a}$ after p is always redundant; equivalently, executing the guard a after p aborts the computation.

Reasoning in KAT under the assumption $p = p\bar{a}$, we have

$$p(aq + \bar{a}) = p\bar{a}(aq + \bar{a}) = p\bar{a}aq + p\bar{a}\,\bar{a} = p0q + p\bar{a} = 0 + p\bar{a} = p\bar{a} = p.$$

Thus the KAT expressions representing the two program fragments are equal.

For the case of a **while** loop, consider the fragment p ; **while** a **do** q, which is encoded in KAT as the expression $p(aq)^*\bar{a}$. Again, suppose that the test a is always false after the execution of p; that is, $p\bar{a} = p$. This means that the **while** loop will never be executed, and we should again be able to obtain the optimized fragment p.

As above, reasoning in KAT under the assumption $p = p\bar{a}$, we have

$$p(aq)^*\bar{a} = p\bar{a}(aq)^*\bar{a} = p\bar{a}(1 + aq(aq)^*)\bar{a} = p\bar{a}\bar{a} + p\bar{a}aq(aq)^*\bar{a}$$
$$= p\bar{a} + p0q(aq)^*\bar{a} = p\bar{a} + 0 = p\bar{a} = p.$$

Both of these cases give examples of how assumptions about atomic programs and tests (here $p = p\bar{a}$) are used to derive the equivalence of the unoptimized and optimized programs. We have essentially given purely equational proofs of the universal Horn formulas $p = p\bar{a} \to p(aq + \bar{a}) = p$ and $p = p\bar{a} \to p(aq)^*\bar{a} = p$.

3.2 Common Subexpression Elimination

Common subexpression elimination is a code transformation that avoids redundant evaluation of the same expression by using the result of the first computation. For example, consider the program fragment $i := expr$; $j := expr$, where $expr$ is an expression not containing i. We wish to show that this can be replaced by $i := expr$; $j := i$.

Consider the following programs and tests:

$$p \stackrel{\text{def}}{=} i := expr \qquad\qquad w \stackrel{\text{def}}{=} \text{make } j \text{ undefined}$$
$$q \stackrel{\text{def}}{=} j := expr \qquad\qquad a \stackrel{\text{def}}{\iff} i = expr$$
$$r \stackrel{\text{def}}{=} j := i \qquad\qquad b \stackrel{\text{def}}{\iff} i = j.$$

We wish to prove that $pq = pr$. We can postulate the following premises:

$1p = 1pa$ atomic PCA $\{expr = expr\}\, i := expr\, \{i = expr\}$

$aq = aqb$ atomic PCA $\{i = expr\}\, j := expr\, \{i = j\}$

$br = b$ there is no need to assign $j := i$ if $i = j$ already

$r = wr$ j is dead immediately before the assignment $j := i$

$qw = w$ an assignment to a dead variable is redundant.

The first two of these are both instances of the Hoare assignment rule. Under these premises, we can reason equationally as follows:

$$pq = 1pq = 1paq = 1paqb = 1paqbr = 1paqr$$
$$= 1pqr = pqr = pqwr = pwr = pr.$$

3.3   Copy Propagation

Copy propagation is a code transformation that eliminates an assignment of the form $j := i$ and replaces all further references to j by references to i. For example, consider the program fragment

$$i := expr \; ; \; j := expr \; ; \; k := 4 * j + 2$$

where i and j do not occur in $expr$. By common subexpression elimination (Section 3.2), the second assignment can be replaced by $j := i$.

First we argue that we can replace the last assignment by $k := 4 * i + 2$. Letting $p, q, r,$ and s denote the assignments $i := expr$, $j := i$, $k := 4 * j + 2$, and $k := 4 * i + 2$ respectively, we wish to show that $pqr = pqs$. It suffices to show that $qr = qs$. Consider the program and tests

$$a \stackrel{\text{def}}{\Longleftrightarrow} 4 * j + 2 = 4 * i + 2$$
$$b \stackrel{\text{def}}{\Longleftrightarrow} k = 4 * i + 2$$
$$w \stackrel{\text{def}}{=} \text{make } k \text{ undefined.}$$

As above, we postulate the following premises:

$1q = 1qa$	atomic PCA $\{4 * i + 2 = 4 * i + 2\}\, j := i \,\{4 * j + 2 = 4 * i + 2\}$
$ar = arb$	atomic PCA $\{4 * j + 2 = 4 * i + 2\}\, k := 4 * j + 2 \,\{k = 4 * i + 2\}$
$bs = b$	there is no need to assign $k := 4 * i + 2$ if $k = 4 * i + 2$ already
$s = ws$	k is dead immediately before the assignment $k := 4 * i + 2$
$rw = w$	an assignment to a dead variable is redundant.

The first two of these are instances of the Hoare assignment rule. Using these assumptions, we can reason as follows:

$$qr = 1qr = 1qar = 1qarb = 1qarbs = 1qars$$
$$= 1qrs = qrs = qrws = qws = qs.$$

Moreover, if we know that j is a dead variable, we can optimize further by removing the assignment to j, obtaining the optimized code ps. Letting $v \stackrel{\text{def}}{=}$ "make j undefined", we wish to show that $pqsv = psv$. We have $sv = vs$, since j does not occur in s, and $qv = v$, since if j is dead, the assignment is redundant. This allows us to conclude $pqsv = pqvs = pvs = psv$.

3.4   Loop Hoisting

Loop hoisting is a transformation that involves moving code out of loops. It can take one of two forms: in the first form, an expression whose value does not depend on the number of times through the loop need not be evaluated inside the loop, but can be evaluated once before the first execution of the body of the loop. In the second, an expression whose value is not used anywhere inside the loop need not be evaluated inside the loop, but can be evaluated once after the loop.

As an example of the first type of transformation, consider the following program fragment:

$$
\begin{array}{ll}
sum := 1\,; & p \\
\textbf{while } 1 \leq i \leq n \textbf{ do } \{ & \\
\quad sum := sum + i * expr\,; & q \\
\quad i := i + 1\,; & s \\
\} &
\end{array}
$$

where $expr$ is an expression not containing i or sum. Let k be a new variable. This fragment is equivalent to the fragment

$$
\begin{array}{ll}
sum := 1\,; & p \\
k := expr\,; & u \\
\textbf{while } 1 \leq i \leq n \textbf{ do } \{ & \\
\quad sum := sum + i * k\,; & r \\
\quad i := i + 1\,; & s \\
\} &
\end{array}
$$

Formally, "k is a new variable" is captured by saying that k does not appear in any expression in the first fragment and that k can be made undefined immediately after the execution of the fragment.

Define the program and tests

$$
a \overset{\text{def}}{\Longleftrightarrow} 1 \leq i \leq n
$$
$$
b \overset{\text{def}}{\Longleftrightarrow} k = expr
$$
$$
w \overset{\text{def}}{=} \text{ make } k \text{ undefined.}
$$

We would like to show $p(aqs)^*\bar{a}w = pu(ars)^*\bar{a}w$. Postulating the assumptions

$u = ub$	$k = expr$ after $k := expr$, since k does not occur in $expr$
$b = bu$	if $k = expr$ already, no need to assign $k := expr$
$bq = qb$	since sum does not occur in $expr$
$bs = sb$	since i does not occur in $expr$
$br = rb$	since sum does not occur in $expr$,

using Lemma 2 and copy propagation (Section 3.3) we can argue as follows:

$$
pu(ars)^* = pub(ars)^* = pub(abrs)^* = pub(aburs)^*
$$
$$
= pub(abqs)^* = pub(aqs)^* = pu(aqs)^*.
$$

Now since w commutes with a, $\bar{a}$, q, and s, we have by Lemma 2 that $w(aqs)^* = (aqs)^*w$. Also, $uw = w$ since there is no need to assign to a dead variable. Thus

$$
pu(aqs)^*\bar{a}w = puw(aqs)^*\bar{a} = pw(aqs)^*\bar{a} = p(aqs)^*\bar{a}w.
$$

In conclusion, $pu(ars)^*\bar{a}w = p(aqs)^*\bar{a}w$, which is what we had to prove.

As an example of the second type of transformation, consider the following program in which the computation p inside the loop and the test a do not use i:

$$
\begin{array}{ll}
\textbf{while } a \textbf{ do } \{ & \\
\quad i := r\,; & u \\
\quad p\,; & p \\
\quad r := r + 1\,; & q \\
\} & \\
i := r\,; & u
\end{array}
$$

Since i is assigned a different expression each time the loop is executed, the previous example does not apply. Nevertheless, since i is not used in the rest of the loop, we still obtain the optimized code:

$$
\begin{array}{ll}
\textbf{while } a \textbf{ do } \{ & \\
\quad p\,; & p \\
\quad r := r + 1\,; & q \\
\} & \\
i := r\,; & u
\end{array}
$$

We would like to prove $(aupq)^*\bar{a}u = (apq)^*\bar{a}u$. Defining the atomic program $w \overset{\text{def}}{\Longleftrightarrow}$ "make i undefined", we have the following postulates:

$$
\begin{array}{ll}
u = wu & i \text{ is dead just before the assignment } i := r \\
wpq = pqw & p \text{ and } q \text{ do not refer to } i \\
wa = aw & a \text{ does not refer to } i \\
w\bar{a} = \bar{a}w & a \text{ does not refer to } i \\
uw = w & \text{an assignment to a dead variable is redundant.}
\end{array}
$$

Reasoning under these assumptions using the sliding rule (5) and Lemma 2,

$$
(aupq)^*\bar{a}u = (awupq)^*\bar{a}wu = (waupq)^*w\bar{a}u = w(aupqw)^*\bar{a}u = w(auwpq)^*\bar{a}u
$$
$$
= w(awpq)^*\bar{a}u = (apq)^*w\bar{a}u = (apq)^*\bar{a}wu = (apq)^*\bar{a}u.
$$

3.5   Induction Variable Elimination

This is a loop optimization that replaces multiplicative operations inside the loop with less expensive additive ones. This type of optimization might arise in matrix algorithms. For example, consider the program

$$
\begin{array}{ll}
i := init\,; & u \\
j := i * expr_2\,; & q \\
\textbf{while } a \textbf{ do } \{ & \\
\quad i := i + expr_1\,; & p \\
\quad j := i * expr_2\,; & q \\
\} &
\end{array}
$$

where i and j do not occur in $expr_1$ and $expr_2$. Note that whenever i is increased by $expr_1$, j is increased by $expr_1 * expr_2$. The optimized code is

$$
\begin{aligned}
&i := init \,; & &u\\
&j := i * expr_2 \,; & &q\\
&\textbf{while } a \textbf{ do } \{\\
&\quad i := i + expr_1 \,; & &p\\
&\quad j := j + expr_1 * expr_2 \,; & &r\\
&\}
\end{aligned}
$$

Using the transformation of Section 3.4, we can further optimize to obtain

$$
\begin{aligned}
&i := init \,;\\
&j := i * expr_2 \,;\\
&m := expr_1 \,;\\
&n := expr_1 * expr_2 \,;\\
&\textbf{while } a \textbf{ do } \{\\
&\quad i := i + m \,;\\
&\quad j := j + n \,;\\
&\}
\end{aligned}
$$

To establish the equivalence of the first two programs, we need to prove

$$uq(apq)^*\bar{a} = uq(apr)^*\bar{a}.$$

It suffices to prove $q(apq)^* = q(apr)^*$. Consider the tests

$$
\begin{aligned}
b &\stackrel{\text{def}}{\Longleftrightarrow} j = i * expr_2,\\
b' &\stackrel{\text{def}}{\Longleftrightarrow} j + expr_1 * expr_2 = (i + expr_1) * expr_2\\
c &\stackrel{\text{def}}{\Longleftrightarrow} j + expr_1 * expr_2 = i * expr_2
\end{aligned}
$$

We have the assumptions $q = qb$; $b = bq$; $b = b'$ from basic number-theoretic reasoning; $cr = crb$, an instance of the Hoare assignment rule; and $bp = bpc$, which follows from $b = b'$ and the instance $\{b'\}\, p \,\{c\}$ of the Hoare assignment rule. In addition, we have $cq = cr$, which is an instance of the property that if two expressions have the same value, then the assignment of either expression to the variable j has the same effect. This would hold even if j occurred in both expressions. Here, j does not occur in the expression $i * expr_2$, and using $w \stackrel{\text{def}}{\Longleftrightarrow}$ "make j undefined" along with the premises $wq = q$ and $rw = w$, $cq = cr$ can be proved by

$$cr = crb = crbq = crbwq = crwq = cwq = cq.$$

The property $cq = cr$ holds even in the more general case in which j can occur in both expressions. We do not know how to prove this in Hoare logic or Kleene algebra from more primitive assumptions without introducing new symbols into the underlying programming or assertion language. However, we are content to take $cq = cr$ as a primitive assumption.

We have $bpq = bpcq = bpcqb = bpcrb = bpcr = bpr$. Since $bpq = bpqb$, it follows that $bapq = bapqb$ and $bapr = baprb$. Using the sliding rule (5) and Lemma 1, we then have

$$q(apq)^* = qb(apqb)^* = q(bapq)^*b = q(bapr)^*b = qb(aprb)^* = q(apr)^*.$$

3.6   Instruction Scheduling

Unrelated instructions can be reordered so as to maximize the throughput of a processor pipeline. For example, $p\,;\,q$ and $q\,;\,p$ are equivalent if there is no dependency between the instructions p and q. The nondependency assumption is expressed in KAT by the equation $pq = qp$. These assumptions can be used to reorder instructions arbitrarily as long as no dependencies are violated.

3.7   Algebraic Simplification

This transformation eliminates statements corresponding to trivial algebraic identities, which occasionally arise due to constant propagation and other previous transformations. For example, any assignment of the form $i := i + 0$ or $i := i * 1$ can be eliminated. This is simply an application of an assumption of the form $ap = a$ and the Kleene algebra axiom $1q = q$.

3.8   Loop Unrolling

Sometimes it is possible to reduce the number of tests and jumps executed in a loop by unrolling the loop. We can unroll the loop **while** a **do** p once to obtain **while** a **do** $\{p\,;\,$**if** a **then** $p\}$. We have to prove $(ap)^*\bar{a} = (ap(ap + \bar{a}))^*\bar{a}$. The following lemma of pure KAT captures the essence of this transformation.

Lemma 3. *In any Kleene algebra,* $u^* = (1 + u)(uu)^*$.

Proof. For the direction $\geq$, by monotonicity, distributivity, idempotence, denesting (6), and the basic properties of *, we have

$$(1 + u)(uu)^* = (uu)^* + u(uu)^* \leq u^*(uu^*)^* = (u + u)^* = u^*.$$

For the direction $\leq$, by (3) it is enough to prove $1 + u(1+u)(uu)^* \leq (1+u)(uu)^*$. By (1) and distributivity, we have

$$1 + u(1 + u)(uu)^* = u(uu)^* + 1 + uu(uu)^* = u(uu)^* + (uu)^* = (1 + u)(uu)^*.$$

We can now prove the equivalence of the two programs using sliding (5), denesting (6), the basic axioms, and Lemma 3.

$$(ap(ap + \bar{a}))^*\bar{a} = (apap + ap\bar{a})^*\bar{a} = ((ap\bar{a})^*apap)^*(ap\bar{a})^*\bar{a}$$
$$= ((1 + (ap\bar{a})^*ap\bar{a})apap)^*(ap\bar{a})^*\bar{a} = (apap + (ap\bar{a})^*ap\bar{a}apap)^*(ap\bar{a})^*\bar{a}$$
$$= (apap)^*(ap\bar{a})^*\bar{a} = (apap)^*(1 + ap\bar{a}(ap\bar{a})^*)\bar{a}$$
$$= (apap)^*(1 + ap\bar{a} + ap\bar{a}ap\bar{a}(ap\bar{a})^*)\bar{a} = (apap)^*(1 + ap\bar{a})\bar{a}$$
$$= (apap)^*\bar{a} + ap(apap)^*\bar{a} = (1 + ap)(apap)^*\bar{a} = (ap)^*\bar{a}.$$

3.9 Redundant Loads and Stores

In the instruction sequence **load** r, i ; **store** r, i, the store instruction is redundant, since the first ensures that the value of i is the same as the contents of register r. We obtain the optimized code **store** r, i. Letting $p \overset{\text{def}}{=} $ **load** r, i, $q \overset{\text{def}}{=} $ **store** r, i, and $a \overset{\text{def}}{\Longleftrightarrow} r = i$, we can postulate $p = pa$, since after loading i into register r, the test $r = i$ is redundant; and $aq = a$, since storing r in i is redundant if the value is already there. Under these assumptions, we have $pq = paq = pa = p$.

3.10 Array Bounds Check Elimination

Consider the following program to initialize the elements of an array:

$$i := 0 \; ; \; \textbf{while } i < x.length \textbf{ do } \{x[i] := e(i) \; ; \; i := i + 1\}$$

A compiler has to check that array accesses fall within bounds:

$$
\begin{array}{ll}
\quad i := 0 & u \\
\alpha : \textbf{test } i \geq x.length & \\
\quad \textbf{jtrue } \beta & \\
\quad \textbf{compute } e(i) & p \\
\quad \textbf{if } i \textbf{ in bounds then } x[i] := e(i) & q \\
\quad \quad \textbf{else error} & s \\
\quad i := i + 1 & v \\
\quad \textbf{goto } \alpha & \\
\beta : \ldots &
\end{array}
$$

The bounds check inside the loop is redundant. The optimized code is

$$
\begin{array}{ll}
\quad i := 0 & u \\
\alpha : \textbf{test } i \geq x.length & \\
\quad \textbf{jtrue } \beta & \\
\quad \textbf{compute } e(i) & p \\
\quad x[i] := e(i) & q \\
\quad i := i + 1 & v \\
\quad \textbf{goto } \alpha & \\
\beta : \ldots &
\end{array}
$$

Consider also the tests

$$a \overset{\text{def}}{\Longleftrightarrow} 0 \leq i$$

$$b \overset{\text{def}}{\Longleftrightarrow} i < x.length$$

$$c \overset{\text{def}}{\Longleftrightarrow} ab \quad \Longleftrightarrow \quad i \text{ is in bounds.}$$

We have to prove $u(bp(cq + \bar{c}s)v)^* \bar{b} = u(bpqv)^* \bar{b}$. We see that if a is true at the beginning of the loop, it remains true after one iteration; that is, $a(bp(cq+\bar{c}s)v) =$

$a(bp(cq + \bar{c}s)v)a$. Reasoning under the assumptions $u = ua$, $ab = c$, $pc = cp$, and $a(bpqv) = (bpqv)a$ and using dead code elimination (Section 3.1), and Lemma 2, we have

$$\begin{aligned}
u(bp(cq + \bar{c}s)v)^*\bar{b} &= ua(bp(cq + \bar{c}s)v)^*\bar{b} = ua(abp(cq + \bar{c}s)v)^*\bar{b} \\
&= ua(cp(cq + \bar{c}s)v)^*\bar{b} = ua(pc(cq + \bar{c}s)v)^*\bar{b} = ua(pcqv)^*\bar{b} \\
&= ua(abpqv)^*\bar{b} = ua(bpqv)^*\bar{b} = u(bpqv)^*\bar{b}.
\end{aligned}$$

Note that **KAT** does *not* contain explicit machinery for number-theoretic reasoning; that is a separate issue. However, as shown in this example, it does reduce the correctness of the optimizing code transformation to a set of basic number-theoretic assumptions on atomic programs and tests that justify the transformation.

3.11   Introduction of Sentinels

Our last example is also related to arrays. Suppose we want to check if a certain element, say T, is among the elements of a nonempty array x of length n. This can be done by:

$$\begin{array}{ll}
i := 0\,; & p \\
\textbf{while } i < n \textbf{ and } x[i] \neq T \textbf{ do } \{ & \\
\quad i := i + 1\,; & q \\
\} & \\
\textbf{if } i < n \textbf{ then } \text{found} = \text{true}\,; & t \\
\textbf{else } \text{found} = \text{false}\,; & s
\end{array}$$

In order to eliminate one of the tests of the **while** loop, we introduce a *sentinel*: we extend the array x by a new element initialized with T. The optimized program is

$$\begin{array}{ll}
x[n] := T\,; & u \\
i := 0\,; & p \\
\textbf{while } x[i] \neq T \textbf{ do } \{ & \\
\quad i := i + 1\,; & q \\
\} & \\
\textbf{if } i < n \textbf{ then } \text{found} = \text{true}\,; & t \\
\textbf{else } \text{found} = \text{false}\,; & s
\end{array}$$

To prove that the two programs are equivalent, consider the tests

$$a \stackrel{\text{def}}{\iff} i < n \qquad\qquad c \stackrel{\text{def}}{\iff} x[n] = T$$
$$b \stackrel{\text{def}}{\iff} x[i] \neq T \qquad\qquad d \stackrel{\text{def}}{\iff} i \leq n.$$

Since $x[n]$ will not be used further in the program, we can also use $w \stackrel{\text{def}}{\iff}$ "make $x[n]$ undefined". We want to prove

$$p(abq)^*\bar{a}b(at + \bar{a}s)w = up(bq)^*\bar{b}(at + \bar{a}s)w. \tag{9}$$

Since $uw = w$ and u commutes with the programs p, q, s, t and the tests a and ab, we can introduce u on the left-hand side of (9) and move it to the front of the expression using Lemma 2. It therefore suffices to prove

$$up(abq)^* \bar{a}b(at + \bar{a}s)w = up(bq)^* \bar{b}(at + \bar{a}s)w.$$

Since $u = uc$, $cp = pc$, and $p = pd$, we have $up = upcd$, thus it suffices to prove

$$cd(abq)^* \bar{a}b = cd(bq)^* \bar{b}. \tag{10}$$

Now note that $cdb \leq a$, or in other words $cdb = cdba$, $cq = qc$, and $aq = aqd$. Then

$$cdbq = cdbaq = cdbaqd = ccdbaqd = cdbaqcd = cdbqcd.$$

Using Lemma 1 variously with $x = cd$ and $y = abq$ and with $x = cd$ and $y = bq$, sliding (5), and the properties $cd\bar{a} \leq \bar{b}$ and $cdba = cdb$, we have

$$cd(abq)^* \bar{a}b = cd(abqcd)^* \bar{a}b = (cdabq)^* cd(\bar{a} + \bar{b}) = (cdabq)^* (cd\bar{a} + cd\bar{b})$$
$$= (cdabq)^* cd\bar{b} = (cdbq)^* cd\bar{b} = cd(bqcd)^* \bar{b} = cd(bq)^* \bar{b}.$$

This proves (10).

4   The Dead Variable Paradox

We conclude with some remarks about an interesting paradox concerning dead variables (variables whose values will never be used). This paradox is the source of a potentially dangerous pitfall that can arise when reasoning informally about the liveness of variables. A formal treatment in KAT helps to illuminate this issue.

The reader will have noticed that we have made extensive use of the construct

$$w \stackrel{\text{def}}{=} \text{make } i \text{ undefined,}$$

along with the atomic assertions $pw = w$ and $wp = p$, where p is an assignment to i of an expression not containing i, and may have wondered why we did not use the test

$$d \stackrel{\text{def}}{\Longleftrightarrow} i \text{ is a dead variable}$$

and the assertions $pd = d$ and $dp = p$ instead. For example, if $p \stackrel{\text{def}}{=} i := 1$ and $q \stackrel{\text{def}}{=} j := 2$, we could postulate the atomic premises

$$p = dp \quad i \text{ is dead immediately before the assignment } p$$
$$qd = dq \quad \text{the assignment } q \text{ does not affect } i$$
$$pd = d \quad \text{an assignment to a dead variable is redundant,}$$

then eliminate the first assignment to i in the program $i := 1 \,;\, j := 2 \,;\, i := 1$ by arguing $pqp = pqdp = pdqp = dqp = qdp = qp$.

The problem is that the proposition "i is a dead variable" is not a property of the local state of the computation. It does not commute with other tests involving i, which it must do in order to be a Boolean element of a Kleene algebra with tests, and its use as a test in the context of KAT can lead to paradoxical results.

To illustrate, consider the following calculation. Defining $a \overset{\text{def}}{\Longleftrightarrow} i = 1$, we have $p = pa$, since $i = 1$ immediately after the assignment, and $ap = a$, since the assignment is redundant if $i = 1$ already. We also have $ad = da$ by commutativity. But then $pp = padp = pdap = da$, which is clearly an erroneous conclusion.

Our solution to this paradox is to use w instead of d. The program w can be regarded as an assignment of an undefined value to i. As such, it is a transformation of the local state, much like an ordinary assignment. Since w is a program and not a test, it is not required by the axioms of KAT to commute with tests.

References

1. Ernie Cohen. Hypotheses in Kleene algebra. Available as
   ftp://ftp.bellcore.com/pub/ernie/research/homepage.html, April 1994.
2. Ernie Cohen. Lazy caching. Available as
   ftp://ftp.bellcore.com/pub/ernie/research/homepage.html, 1994.
3. Ernie Cohen. Using Kleene algebra to reason about concurrency control. Available as ftp://ftp.bellcore.com/pub/ernie/research/homepage.html, 1994.
4. John Horton Conway. *Regular Algebra and Finite Machines*. Chapman and Hall, London, 1971.
5. Michael J. Fischer and Richard E. Ladner. Propositional dynamic logic of regular programs. *J. Comput. Syst. Sci.*, 18(2):194–211, 1979.
6. Stephen C. Kleene. Representation of events in nerve nets and finite automata. In C. E. Shannon and J. McCarthy, editors, *Automata Studies*, pages 3–41. Princeton University Press, Princeton, N.J., 1956.
7. Dexter Kozen. A completeness theorem for Kleene algebras and the algebra of regular events. *Infor. and Comput.*, 110(2):366–390, May 1994.
8. Dexter Kozen. Kleene algebra with tests. *Transactions on Programming Languages and Systems*, 19(3):427–443, May 1997.
9. Dexter Kozen. Efficient code certification. Technical Report 98-1661, Computer Science Department, Cornell University, January 1998.
10. Dexter Kozen. On Hoare logic and Kleene algebra with tests. *Trans. Computational Logic*, 1(1), July 2000. To appear.
11. Dexter Kozen and Frederick Smith. Kleene algebra with tests: Completeness and decidability. In D. van Dalen and M. Bezem, editors, *Proc. 10th Int. Workshop Computer Science Logic (CSL'96)*, volume 1258 of *Lecture Notes in Computer Science*, pages 244–259, Utrecht, The Netherlands, September 1996. Springer-Verlag.
12. Greg Morrisett, David Walker, Karl Crary, and Neal Glew. From System F to typed assembly language. In *25th ACM SIGPLAN/SIGSIGACT Symposium on Principles of Programming Languages*, pages 85–97, San Diego California, USA, January 1998.
13. George C. Necula. Proof-carrying code. In *Proc. 24th Symp. Principles of Programming Languages*, pages 106–119. ACM SIGPLAN/SIGACT, January 1997.
14. George C. Necula and Peter Lee. The design and implementation of a certifying compiler. In *Proc. Conf. Programming Language Design and Implementation*, pages 333–344. ACM SIGPLAN, 1998.

An Application of Model Building in a Resolution Decision Procedure for Guarded Formulas

Michael Dierkes

Laboratoire LEIBNIZ - IMA Grenoble
46, av. Félix Viallet; 38 031 Grenoble Cedex, France
Michael.Dierkes@imag.fr

Abstract. Semantic resolution refinements are a very efficient way to restrict the resolution rule. Their principle is to avoid resolution between clauses that are true in a certain interpretation. In this way, the number of deduced clauses can be decreased drastically, and deduction can be restricted to clauses that are interesting from a semantic point of view. In this article, we present a semantic refinement of a resolution decision procedure for formulas of the *guarded fragment* (without equality). This fragment of first-order logic was introduced in [1] in order to explain the nice properties (in particular decidability) of propositional modal logics. In fact, many modal logics can be translated into the guarded fragment. Guarded clauses, defined in [8], are a generalization of guarded formulas in clausal form and decidable by resolution. The method presented in this article uses a model building procedure for guarded clauses which contain a positive maximal literal. A set of such clauses can be derived from the guarded clause set under consideration.

1 Introduction

Semantic resolution refinements are very efficient refinements of the resolution rule as far as the number of deducible clauses is concerned. Their principle is to use semantic information about the present predicate symbols in order to filter resolution inferences. In general, an interpretation I is given, and then it is avoided to resolve two clauses that are both true in I. This idea is due to Slagle [12]. Examples for theorem provers using semantic approaches are SATCHMO [9] and SCOTT [13]. Another method using semantic reasoning was presented in [4], and a framework for semantic resolution methods can be found in [7].

Since the number of the clauses that can be deduced by resolution from a given clause set may drastically decrease if semantic restrictions are applied to the resolution rule, such restrictions should allow to find proofs that are easier to understand for a human user. Additionally, the deduced clauses are more relevant from a semantic point of view.

If the interpretation I that is used for the restriction is a model for a subset of the clause set S under consideration, I can be seen as a model hypothesis

J. Lloyd et al. (Eds.): CL 2000, LNAI 1861, pp. 583–597, 2000.

for S. If a clause from S is false in I, further resolution steps are performed in order to deduce clauses that allow to adapt I. This is the approach we adopted in this article to get a semantic refinement of a resolution decision procedure for guarded formulas. In order to obtain a model for a subset of S, we must of course have a model building procedure at our disposal. Therefore, we will define a model building procedure for a certain class of guarded formulas.

The *guarded fragment* of first order logic was introduced in [1] in order to explain the nice properties of modal logics, as for example decidability. In fact, many modal logics can be translated into the guarded fragment. Formulas of this fragment are called *guarded*, and it has been shown that every formula of the guarded fragment admits a finite model.

Transformation of guarded formulas into clausal form has inspired the class of *guarded clauses*, whose definition imposes very strong syntactic restrictions on variable occurrences: every non-ground functional term that occurs in a guarded clause C must contain all the variables that occur in C. Additionally, a guarded clause must contain a *guard* literal, which is a negative literal in which all the variables of the clause occur as arguments, and that does not contain any non-ground functional term. Sets of guarded clauses are decidable by saturation under ordered resolution which has been shown using a non-liftable [11] and a liftable ordering [8].

The model building method we define in this article allows to transform a given satisfiable set S of guarded clauses (without equality) in which every clause contains a positive greatest literal into a set S' of so-called *primitive guarded Horn clauses* such that the $\subseteq$-least Herbrand model $\mathcal{M}_{S'}$ of S' is a model of S. Since it is possible to evaluate guarded clauses in $\mathcal{M}_{S'}$, we consider S' as the representation of a (infinite) model of S.

This article is structured as follows: first, we review some notions in order to settle our notation. In Section 3, we review the resolution decision procedure presented in [10]. In Section 4, we present the model building procedure, and in Section 5 we show how to integrate it into the decision procedure for guarded formulas. We discuss a generalization of our method in Section 6, and conclude in Section 7.

2   Preliminaries

We assume the reader to be familiar with the standard logic notions as term, formula, clause, Herbrand interpretation, etc.

Throughout this article, if not stated otherwise, we will mean *finite set of clauses* if we write *set of clauses*. Furthermore, we will always assume that for two different clauses, there is no variable that occurs in both of them.

We consider clauses over a signature $(\mathcal{C}, \mathcal{F}, \mathcal{P}, \mathcal{V})$ where $\mathcal{C}$ is a finite set of constant symbols, $\mathcal{F}$ is a finite set of function symbols, $\mathcal{P}$ is a finite set of predicate symbols, and $\mathcal{V}$ is a countably infinite set of variables.

We denote by $\doteq$ *syntactic* equality, i.e. $\doteq$ is always interpreted as equality w.r.t the empty equational theory. Syntactic equality will be introduced by a transformation step of our method, and we assume that $\doteq$ does not occur in a clause set for which we want to build a model.

For a literal L, we denote by $\text{args}(L)$ the n-tuple of arguments of L, and by L^c the complementary of L (so if $L = A$ for an atom A, then $L^c = \neg A$, and vice versa). For a set of literals S, we denote by S^c the set $\{L^c \mid L \in S\}$.

A literal L is *flat* iff all of its arguments are variables or constant symbols. A set of literals is flat iff all of its literals are flat. For a set of literals S, S^+ (S^-) is the set of all positive (negative) literals in S. A clause is a set of literals interpreted as disjunction. A clause C for which $C = C^+$ ($C = C^-$) is called *positive* (*negative*). A clause C is *Horn* if $|C^+| \le 1$.

Substitutions are defined as usual. For a substitution σ, we denote $\text{dom}(\sigma)$ (resp. $\text{codom}(\sigma)$) the domain (resp. co-domain) of σ. A substitution with the domain $\{x_1, \ldots, x_n\}$ that maps each x_i to a t_i is denoted by $\{x_i \leftarrow t_i \mid 1 \le i \le n\}$. For a set of variables V, we denote by $\sigma|_V$ the restriction of σ to variables in V, i.e. the substitution $\{x \leftarrow t \in \sigma \mid x \in V\}$. For a substitution $\sigma = \{x_1 \leftarrow t_1, \ldots, x_n \leftarrow t_n\}$, we denote by $eq(\sigma)$ the set of equations $\{x_1 \doteq t_1, \ldots, x_n \doteq t_n\}$.

Let $\mathcal{S}$ be a set of clauses over the signature $(\mathcal{C}, \mathcal{F}, \mathcal{P})$. Then, the *Herbrand base* of $\mathcal{S}$, denoted by $HB_\mathcal{S}$, is the set of all ground atoms over $(\mathcal{C}, \mathcal{F}, \mathcal{P})$. A Herbrand interpretation I for a clause set $\mathcal{S}$ is identified with a subset of $HB_\mathcal{S}$. Then, $I \models A$ iff $A \in I$, and $I \models \neg A$ iff $A \notin I$ for every atom A over $(\mathcal{C}, \mathcal{F}, \mathcal{P})$.

The *depth* of a term is defined as follows: if t is a constant or a variable, then $\text{depth}(t) = 0$. Else, t is a functional term $f(t_1, \ldots, t_n)$, and $\text{depth}(t) = 1 + \max(\text{depth}(t_1), \ldots, \text{depth}(t_n))$. The depth of an atom is the maximal depth of its arguments, and the depth of a literal the depth of its atom.

Let $\prec$ be an ordering on ground literals. Then, $\prec$ is extended to non-ground literals by $L_1 \prec L_2$ iff $L_1\sigma \prec L_2\sigma$ for all ground substitutions σ. A literal L is *maximal* in a clause C iff there is no $L' \in C$ with $L \prec L'$. L is the $\prec$-*greatest* literal of C iff $L' \prec L$ for all $L' \in C \setminus \{L\}$.

2.1   Rules

A *rule* has the form $r = L_1, \ldots, L_n \rightarrow H_1, \ldots, H_m$, where the L_i are (possibly negative) literals, and the H_i are positive literals. We call the set $\{L_1, \ldots, L_n\}$ the *body* of r and denote it by $\text{body}(r)$. The set $\{H_1, \ldots, H_m\}$ is called the *head* of r and denoted by $\text{head}(r)$. As usual, the head is interpreted as a disjunction, whereas the body is interpreted as a conjunction. If the head of a rule contains only one literal, we will identify it with this literal.

A Herbrand interpretation I is called a *model* of a set of rules $\mathcal{R}$ iff for all $r \in \mathcal{R}$ and for all ground substitutions σ, $I \models \text{body}(r\sigma)$ implies $I \models \text{head}(r\sigma)$. A model I of $\mathcal{R}$ is called *well-supported* if there is a literal ordering $<$ such that for every ground atom $A \in I$, there is a ground substitution σ and rule $A_1, \ldots, A_l, \neg B_1, \ldots, \neg B_m \rightarrow C_1, \ldots C_n \in \mathcal{R}$ such that $A = C_k\sigma$ for some k with $1 \le k \le n$, $I \not\models \{\neg A_1, \ldots, \neg A_l, B_1, \ldots, B_m, C_1, \ldots, C_n\}\sigma \setminus \{A\}$, and $A_i\sigma < A$ for $1 \le i \le l$. If we want to make the ordering $<$ explicit, we say that I is a $<$-well-supported model.

For a clause $C = \{\neg A_1, \ldots, \neg A_l, B_1, \ldots, B_m, C_1, \ldots C_n\}$ and a literal ordering $<$ such that C_i is $<$-maximal in C for $1 \leq i \leq n$ and B_i is not $<$-maximal in C for $1 \leq i \leq m$, we denote by $r_C^<$ the rule $A_1, \ldots, A_l, \neg B_1, \ldots, \neg B_m \to C_1, \ldots C_n$. For a set of clauses $\mathcal{S}$, we denote by $\mathcal{R}_{\mathcal{S}}^<$ the set of rules: $\{r_C^< \mid C \in \mathcal{S}\}$. Clearly, a well-supported model of $\mathcal{R}_{\mathcal{S}}^<$ is a model of $\mathcal{S}$. We will often write clauses in rule form since this allows to make maximal literals explicit.

2.2   Covering Literals

A literal L is *covering* if every functional subterm of L contains all the variables in $\mathrm{var}(L)$.

Example 1. $P(x, f(x, y), a)$, $Q(f(x, y), h(x, x, y))$ and $Q(f(a, b), a)$ are covering literals, whereas $Q(f(x, y), h(x, y, z))$ and $R(x, f(a, b))$ are not covering.

For two unifiable covering literals, there exists an mgu that has a special form as stated by the following lemma:

Lemma 1 ([6]). *Let L_1 and L_2 be two non-ground, variable disjoint, unifiable covering literals with $\mathrm{depth}(L_1) \leq \mathrm{depth}(L_2)$. Then there exists an mgu σ such that $\mathrm{var}(L_1) \subseteq \mathrm{dom}(\sigma)$ and for all $x \leftarrow t \in \sigma$,*

- *if $x \in \mathrm{var}(L_1)$, then $\mathrm{var}(t) \subseteq \mathrm{var}(L_2)$, and*
- *if $x \in \mathrm{var}(L_2)$, then t is ground or $t \in \mathrm{var}(L_2)$.*

We denote an mgu of two literals L_1 and L_2 as in Lemma 1 by $\overline{\mathrm{mgu}}(L_1, L_2)$.

Corollary 1. *Let L_1 and L_2 be two unifiable covering literals of the same depth, and $\sigma = \mathrm{mgu}(L_1, L_2)$. Then, $\mathrm{codom}(\sigma)$ does not contain any functional term.*

2.3   Guarded Clauses

We adopt the definition of guarded clauses of [8]:

Definition 1. *A clause C is called* guarded *if all its literals are of depth less than or equal to 1, and if it satisfies the following additional conditions:*

1. *every functional term in C contains all the variables of C, and*
2. *if C is non-ground then it contains a negative literal (the guard) which has the form $\neg P(t_1, \ldots, t_n)$ such that for $1 \leq i \leq n$, t_i is a variable or a constant, and all variables of C occur among the t_i.*

Note that this definition implies that all the literals of a guarded clause are covering. As shown in [8], every formula of the guarded fragment can be transformed into a set of guarded clauses.

Example 2. The following two clauses are guarded: $\{\neg P(x, y), P(x, f(x, y))\}$ and $\{\neg Q(a, x, y), \neg P(f(x, y), h(x, x, y)), Q(a, b, a), \neg P(x, x)\}$.
The clauses $\{P(x, f(x, y)), \neg Q(x, h(x, y, x), y)\}$, $\{\neg P(x, y), Q(x, y, h(x, y, z))\}$ and $\{\neg P(x, y), Q(x, f(a, b), y)\}$ are not guarded.

We call the rule r a *guarded rule* iff $C = \text{body}(r)^c \cup \text{head}(r)$ is a guarded clause.

Definition 2. *A Horn clause is a primitive guarded Horn clause if it is ground and positive, or it is a guarded clause of form $\{\neg P(x_1, \ldots, x_n), Q(t_1, \ldots, t_m)\}$ where the x_i are variables, $x_i \neq x_j$ if $i \neq j$ and $1 \leq i, j \leq n$, and for the positive literal it holds that $depth(Q(t_1, \ldots, t_m)) > 0$.*

Primitive guarded Horn clauses (PGHC) have been introduced in [6] in order to represent Herbrand interpretations. The interpretation represented by a set of primitive guarded Horn clauses is its $\subseteq$-least Herbrand model.

3   Deciding Sets of Guarded Clauses

In [8], it is shown that sets of guarded clauses with equality can be decided using the superposition calculus defined in [2] with an appropriate choice of a reduction ordering $\prec$ and a selection function Σ: the ordering $\prec$ has to be an admissible literal ordering (see [2] for details) in which the term ordering is a lexicographic path ordering based on a precedence $\prec$ for which $P \prec c \prec f$ for all $P \in \mathcal{P}$, $c \in \mathcal{C}$, and $f \in \mathcal{F}$. The selection function Σ is such that (i) if a clause is non-ground and contains no functional term, then one of its guards is selected, and (ii) if a clause is ground or contains a functional term, then no literal is selected.

Since we do not deal with equality in this work, we only need the resolution and factoring rules. A literal is called *eligible* in a clause C if either it is selected in C by Σ, or it is $\prec$-maximal in C and no other literal in C is selected.

- **Resolution**: from $\{A_1\} \cup R_1$ and $\{\neg A_2\} \cup R_2$, derive $R_1\sigma \cup R_2\sigma$ if A_1 and $\neg A_2$ are eligible in their respective clauses and unifiable with mgu σ.
- **Factoring**: from $\{A_1, A_2\} \cup R$, derive $\{A_1\theta\} \cup R\theta$ if A_1 is eligible and unifiable with A_2 with mgu θ.

Using these two rules, only finitely many new clauses can be deduced from a given set of guarded clauses. Since the calculus is refutationally complete, it is a decision procedure for sets of guarded clauses.

4   The Model Building Procedure

In this section we describe the method used to build a model for a set of guarded clauses in which every clause contains a positive, non-flat $\prec$-greatest literal (this implies that no literal is selected). For such a set $\mathcal{S}$, our method allows to find a set $\mathcal{S}'$ of primitive guarded Horn clauses such that the $\subseteq$-least Herbrand model of $\mathcal{S}'$ is a model for $\mathcal{S}$.

In this section, we will use the rule form $\mathcal{R}_{\mathcal{S}}^{\prec}$ of the set $\mathcal{S}$ under consideration. Since the head of a rule $r \in \mathcal{R}_{\mathcal{S}}^{\prec}$ contains exactly one literal, we will refer to this literal as the head of the rule.

For a set $\mathcal{R}$ of guarded rules in which the head is the $\prec$-greatest literal, we denote by $\mathcal{M}_\mathcal{R}$ its unique well-supported model. It is possible to evaluate ground atoms in $\mathcal{M}_\mathcal{R}$: a ground atom A is true in $\mathcal{M}_\mathcal{R}$ iff there is a rule $r \in \mathcal{R}$ such that A is unifiable with head(r) by mgu σ, and all $L \in$ body(r)σ are true in $\mathcal{M}_\mathcal{R}$. Since all $L \in$ body(r)σ are ground and $\prec$-smaller than A, we get an effective evaluation procedure in this way.

4.1   Flattening of Positive Body Literals

In order to flatten positive body literals, we use a transformation based on saturation under resolution. To do this, we define the following deduction rule:

Definition 3. *Let $\mathcal{R}$ be a set of guarded rules in which the head is non-flat and the $\prec$-greatest literal. Then, $RES_\mathcal{R}$ is the inference rule defined as follows: let $r_1 = R_1 \cup \{L_1\} \to M$ and $r_2 = R_2 \to L_2$ be two guarded rules in which the head is non-flat and the $\prec$-greatest literal, and*

- $\sigma = mgu(L_1, L_2)$,
- $depth(L_1) = 1$,
- *all positive literals in R_2 are flat.*

Then, two cases are distinguished:

1. if $R_1\sigma \cup R_2\sigma$ is not ground,

$$\frac{R_1 \cup \{L_1\} \to M \quad R_2 \to L_2}{R_1\sigma \cup R_2\sigma \to M\sigma}$$

2. if $R_1\sigma \cup R_2\sigma$ is ground and true in $\mathcal{M}_\mathcal{R}$,

$$\frac{R_1 \cup \{L_1\} \to M \quad R_2 \to L_2}{\to M\sigma}$$

Lemma 2. *Let $\mathcal{R}$ be a set of guarded rules in which the head is non-flat and the $\prec$-greatest literal, and $\mathcal{R}'$ be the saturation of $\mathcal{R}$ under $RES_\mathcal{R}$. Let*

$$\mathcal{R}'' = \{r \in \mathcal{R}' \mid body(r) \text{ does not contain any non-flat positive literal}\}.$$

Then, $\mathcal{R}'$ is a set of guarded rules in which the head is the $\prec$-greatest literal, and $\mathcal{M}_\mathcal{R} = \mathcal{M}_{\mathcal{R}''}$. Furthermore, if the rules in $\mathcal{R}$ do not contain any non-flat negative body literal, the clauses in $\mathcal{R}''$ neither do so.

Proof. Let $r_1, r_2 \in \mathcal{R}$ and σ be as in Definition 3. If the rule deduced by $RES_\mathcal{R}$ is ground, then clearly the head is non-flat and the greatest literal, so let us assume that the deduced rule is not ground. Since $depth(L_1) = depth(L_2) = 1$, codom($\sigma$) does not contain any functional term (Corollary 1). Therefore, the deduced rule is a guarded rule. Clearly, $M\sigma$ is the $\prec$-greatest literal in $r_1\sigma$, so for $L \in (R_1 \cup \{\neg L_1\})$, we have that $L \prec M\sigma$. For $L \in R_2\sigma$, we have that $L \prec L_2\sigma = L_1\sigma \prec M\sigma$. So, $M\sigma$ is the $\prec$-greatest literal in the deduced rule d.

Now we show that $\mathcal{M}_\mathcal{R} = \mathcal{M}_{\mathcal{R}'}$. Let θ be a ground substitution such that $\mathcal{M}_\mathcal{R} \models \text{body}(d\theta) = (R_1\sigma \cup R_2\sigma)\theta$. Then, $\mathcal{M}_\mathcal{R} \models L_2\sigma\theta$, and $\mathcal{M}_\mathcal{R} \models (R_1 \cup \{L_1\})\sigma\theta$. So $\mathcal{M}_\mathcal{R} \models M\sigma\theta = \text{head}(d\theta)$. Therefore, adding d to $\mathcal{R}$ does not modify the well-supported model $\mathcal{M}_\mathcal{R}$.

Finally we show that for every ground atom A, $\mathcal{M}_{\mathcal{R}'} \models A$ iff $\mathcal{M}_{\mathcal{R}''} \models A$ by induction, using the induction hypothesis that for all literals $L \prec A$, $\mathcal{M}_{\mathcal{R}'} \models L$ iff $\mathcal{M}_{\mathcal{R}''} \models L$.

Let $A \in \mathcal{M}_{\mathcal{R}'}$. Then, there is a ground substitution σ and a rule $r \in \mathcal{R}'$ such that $A = \text{head}(r\sigma)$, $L \prec A$ for $L \in \text{body}(r\sigma)$, and $\mathcal{M}_{\mathcal{R}'} \models \text{body}(r\sigma)$ (note that $\text{body}(r\sigma)$ may be the empty conjunction).

Let $\{B_1, \ldots, B_l\}$ be exactly those positive literals in $\text{body}(r)$ that have depth 1 (this set may be empty). From the induction hypothesis, it follows that $\mathcal{M}_{\mathcal{R}''} \models \{B_1\sigma, \ldots, B_l\sigma\}$. So for $1 \leq i \leq l$, there is $r_i \in \mathcal{R}''$ such that $B_i\sigma = \text{head}(r_i\theta_i)$ and $\mathcal{M}_{\mathcal{R}''} \models \text{body}(r_i\theta_i)$ for some ground substitution θ_i.

Since $\mathcal{R}'' \subseteq \mathcal{R}'$, we have that $r_i \in \mathcal{R}'$. Since $\mathcal{R}'$ is saturated under $\text{RES}_\mathcal{R}$, it must contain the rule d obtained by consecutively resolving r on B_i with r_i using mgu σ_i for $1 \leq i \leq l$. Since $\text{body}(r_i)$ does not contain any non-flat positive literal and the co-domain of σ_i does not contain any functional term for $1 \leq i \leq n$, $\text{body}(d)$ cannot contain any non-flat positive literal. Therfore, $d \in \mathcal{R}''$. If d is ground, then $d = \rightarrow A$, so $A \in \mathcal{M}_{\mathcal{R}''}$. Otherwise, let τ be such that $\text{head}(d\tau) = \text{head}(r\sigma)$. Then, $\mathcal{M}_{\mathcal{R}''} \models \text{body}(d\tau)$. Since d is true in $\mathcal{M}_{\mathcal{R}''}$, it must be that $\mathcal{M}_{\mathcal{R}''} \models \text{head}(d\tau) = A$.

Now assume that $A \in \mathcal{M}_{\mathcal{R}''} \setminus \mathcal{M}_{\mathcal{R}'}$. Then, there is a ground substitution σ and a rule $r \in \mathcal{R}''$ such that $A = \text{head}(r_\sigma)$, $L \prec A$ for $L \in \text{body}(r\sigma)$, and $\mathcal{M}_{\mathcal{R}'} \models \text{body}(r\sigma)$. If $\text{body}(r\sigma) = \emptyset$, then $\rightarrow A \in \mathcal{R}''$, which implies that $\rightarrow A \in \mathcal{R}'$. Otherwise, since $\mathcal{R}'' \subseteq \mathcal{R}'$, there must be a $L \in \text{body}(r\sigma)$ such that $\mathcal{M}_{\mathcal{R}'} \not\models L$. But this is in contradiction to the induction hypothesis.

Since the co-domains of all the unifiers that occur during the saturation process do not contain any functional term, all the negative body literals in the resulting set are flat.

□

We will denote by $flatten\_positive\_body\_literals(\mathcal{R})$ the set $\mathcal{R}''$, where $\mathcal{R}$ and $\mathcal{R}''$ are as in the above lemma.

4.2   Flattening of Negative Body Literals

The idea for flattening negative body literals is the following: a ground instance $\neg A\theta$ of a literal $\neg A$ is true in a well-supported model $\mathcal{M}$ of a rule set $\mathcal{R}$ iff for all $r \in \mathcal{R}$, either $A\theta$ cannot be unified with $head(r)$, or there is a literal L in $\text{body}(r)$ such that $L^c\sigma$ is true in $\mathcal{M}$, where $\sigma = mgu(A, \text{head}(r))$. In order to express that A cannot be unified with the head of a rule r, we have to introduce literals built with the syntactic equality predicate $\doteq$. The algorithm implementing this technique is shown in Figure 1.

Lemma 3. *Let $\mathcal{R}$ be a set of guarded rules not containing $\doteq$, in which the head is non-flat and the $\prec$-greatest literal and such that all positive literals in the rule* *bodies are flat, and let r be a guarded rule with non-flat $\prec$-greatest head and in which all equational literals are flat. Then, for every ground substitution θ,*

$$\mathcal{M_R} \models body(r\theta) \quad iff \quad \mathcal{M_R} \models body(r'\theta)$$
$$for\ an\ r' \in flatten\_negative\_body\_literals(r, \mathcal{R}),$$

and for all $r' \in flatten\_negative\_body\_literals(r, \mathcal{R})$, r' is a guarded rule, all negative literals in $body(r')$ are flat, and $head(r')$ is non-flat and the $\prec$-greatest literal in r'.

Proof. Let $\neg A_j$ be a non-ground, negative covering literal of depth 1 that is contained in the body of the rule r (if no such A_j exists, the claim is trivial), and let θ be a ground substitution such that $\mathcal{M_S} \models \neg A_j\theta$. Let $\{r_1, \ldots, r_n\} = \{r \in \mathcal{R} \mid head(r)$ is unifiable with $A_j\}$, and $\sigma_i = \overline{\mathrm{mgu}}(head(r_i), A_j)$ for $1 \leq i \leq n$. Let Φ_j be defined as in Figure 1.

Then, $\mathcal{M_S} \models \neg A_j\theta$ iff for $1 \leq i \leq n$, eihter $head(r_i)$ is not unifiable with $A_j\theta$, or $\mathcal{M_S} \not\models body(r_i\sigma_i\theta)$ iff for every i with $1 \leq i \leq n$, either a $x\theta \doteq t\theta \in eq(\sigma_i \mid_{\mathrm{var}(A_j)})$ is false, or all $L \in eq(\sigma_i \mid_{\mathrm{var}(A_j)})\theta$ are true and $\mathcal{M_S} \not\models K\theta$ for a $K \in body(r_i\sigma_i)$ iff there is a conjunction $D \in \Phi_j$ such that $\mathcal{M_S} \models D\theta$. Now, the claim follows from the fact that in the set of rules generated by the procedure *flatten_negative_body_literals*, there is a rule r' in which $\neg A$ has been replaced by D.

For the σ_i in the for-loop, $codom(\sigma_i)$ does not contain any functional term for $1 \leq i \leq n$ according to Corollary 1. Therefore, $body(r_i\sigma_i)^+ \cup eq(\sigma_i|_{\mathrm{var}(A_j)})$ contains only flat literals for $1 \leq j \leq m$, and so all negative literals in the resulting rules are flat. Since the σ_i are mgus as in Lemma 1, we have that for every $L \in body(r_i\sigma_i) \cup eq(\sigma_i|_{\mathrm{var}(A_j)})$, $\mathrm{var}(L) \subseteq \mathrm{var}(A_j)$. Since variables that occur in A_j, but not in $A_j\sigma_i$ are instanciated according to σ_i (if possible) in the second for-loop, the resulting rules are guarded rules. Finally, since the literals in D_i are either flat equational literals or body literals of a rule whose head is equal to $A_j\sigma_i$, the head is the $\prec$-maximal literal in every resulting rule. $\square$

We give an example to show how the transformation works:

Example 3. Let

$$\mathcal{R} = \{R(x) \rightarrow R(f(x, a)); Q(x, y), T(x) \rightarrow R(f(x, y))\}, \text{ and}$$
$$r = P(x, y), \neg R(f(x, y)) \rightarrow S(f(x, y)).$$

Then, *flatten_negative_body_literals*$(r, \mathcal{R}) =$

$$P(x, a), \neg Q(x, a), \neg R(x) \rightarrow S(f(x, a))$$
$$P(x, y), \neg Q(x, y), \neg y \doteq a \rightarrow S(f(x, y))$$
$$P(x, a), \neg T(x), \neg R(x) \rightarrow S(f(x, a))$$
$$P(x, y), \neg T(x), \neg y \doteq a \rightarrow S(f(x, y))$$

procedure *flatten_negative_body_literals* $(r, \mathcal{R})$
begin
let $\{\neg A_1, \ldots, \neg A_m\} = \{L \in \text{body}(r) \mid L \text{ is non-flat and negative}\}$
for $j = 1$ to m **do**
  let $\{r_1, \ldots, r_n\} = \{r' \in \mathcal{R} \mid \text{head}(r') \text{ is unifiable with } A_j\}$
  for $1 \le i \le n$, let $\sigma_i = \overline{\text{mgu}}(\text{head}(r_i), A_j)$ and $E_i = eq(\sigma_i|\text{var}(A_j))$
  and $S_i = \{\{L^c\} \cup E_i \mid L \in \text{body}(r_i \sigma_i)\} \cup \{\{L^c\} \mid L \in E_i\}$
  $\Phi_j = \{\bigcup_{i=1}^n K_i \mid K_i \in S_i\}$
end for
$\mathcal{R}' = \{(\text{body}(r) \setminus \{\neg A_1, \ldots, \neg A_m\}) \cup D_1 \cup \ldots \cup D_m \to \text{head}(r) \mid D_i \in \Phi_i\}$
for all $r \in \mathcal{R}'$ **do**
  while there is $x \doteq t \in \text{body}(r)$ where x is a variable **do**
    $r = (\text{body}(r) \setminus \{x \doteq t\} \to \text{head}(r))\{x \leftarrow t\};$ **end while**
  if there is $a \doteq b \in \text{body}(r)$ where a and b are different constant symbols **then**
    delete r from $\mathcal{R}'$; **end if**
  delete all $a \doteq a \in \text{body}(r)$ where a is a constant
end for all
result $= \mathcal{R}'$
end procedure

Fig. 1. The *flatten_negative_body_literals* procedure

Lemma 4. *Let $\mathcal{R}$ be a set of guarded rules not containing $\doteq$, in which the head is non-flat and the $\prec$-greatest literal, and in which all positive body literals are flat. Let*

$$\mathcal{R}' = \bigcup_{r \in \mathcal{R}} \text{flatten\_negative\_body\_literals}(r, \mathcal{R}).$$

Then, all negative literals in the bodies of the rules in $\mathcal{R}'$ are flat, and $\mathcal{M}_{\mathcal{R}} = \mathcal{M}_{\mathcal{R}'}$.

Proof. By Lemma 3, all the negative body literals of the rules in $\mathcal{R}'$ are flat. Now we show that for every ground atom A, $A \in \mathcal{M}_{\mathcal{R}}$ iff $A \in \mathcal{M}_{\mathcal{R}'}$ by induction, using the induction hypothesis that for all $B \prec A$, $B \in \mathcal{M}_{\mathcal{R}}$ iff $B \in \mathcal{M}_{\mathcal{R}'}$.

$\mathcal{M}_{\mathcal{R}} \subseteq \mathcal{M}_{\mathcal{R}'}$: Let $A \in \mathcal{M}_{\mathcal{R}}$. Then, there is a rule $r \in \mathcal{R}$ such that for some ground substitution σ, $A = \text{head}(r)\sigma$, $B \prec A$ for all $B \in \text{body}(r)\sigma$, and $\mathcal{M}_{\mathcal{R}} \models \text{body}(r)\sigma$. There is an $r' \in \text{flatten\_negative\_body\_literals}(r, \mathcal{R})$ such that $\mathcal{M}_{\mathcal{R}} \models \text{body}(r')\sigma$ (Lemma 3). Since for all $B \in \text{body}(r')\sigma$, it holds that $B \prec \text{head}(r')\sigma = \text{head}(r)\sigma = A$, it follows from the induction hypothesis that $\mathcal{M}_{\mathcal{R}'} \models \text{body}(r')\sigma$. But then $A \in \mathcal{M}_{\mathcal{R}'}$.

$\mathcal{M}_{\mathcal{R}'} \subseteq \mathcal{M}_{\mathcal{R}}$: by reversing the above. $\qquad\qquad\qquad\qquad\qquad\qquad\qquad\square$

4.3   Transformation into Primitive Guarded Horn Clauses

Now, we will show that it is possible to compute for a given set $\mathcal{R}$ of guarded rules with non-flat $\prec$-greatest heads a set $\mathcal{S}$ of primitive guarded Horn clauses such that the well-supported model of $\mathcal{R}$ coincides with the $\subseteq$-least Herbrand model of $\mathcal{S}$ on predicate symbols that occur in $\mathcal{R}$. For the sake of simplicity, we will indentify a PGHC with its rule form, and call a rule which corresponds to a PGHC *primitive*.

As a first step, we flatten all body literals using the procedures in 4.1 and 4.2. Now, the idea of this transformation is to take the body of a rule r which is not primitive, and to define a fresh predicate symbol Q by $\text{body}(r) \rightarrow Q(x_1, \ldots, x_n)$ where $\{x_1, \ldots, x_n\} = \text{var}(r)$. Then, we unfold the new rule on all positive literals, and finally, we flatten the negative literals in the resulting rules.

If the rules we obtain in this way are not primitive, we apply the same operation to those rules. Since the number of predicate symbols that may occur in the rule bodies is finite and the rule bodies are flat, there is only a finite number of different rule bodies, so we have to introduce only a finite number of new predicate symbols. As a last step, the the rule bodies are replaced by the corresponding flat literal.

The procedure used to unfold flat rules on their positive literals is shown in Figure 2. If we unfold a rule that contains an equality literal, the variables of this equality literal might be instanciated. In order to deal with non-flat equational literals, we use the simplification rules shown in Figure 3.

Lemma 5. *Let r be a flat guarded rule, and let $\mathcal{R}$ be a set of guarded rules in which all body literals are flat and the head is non-flat and the $\prec$-greatest literal. Then, every rule $r' \in unfold\_and\_simplify(r, \mathcal{R})$ is a guarded rule, and all $L \in body(r')$ which are positive or built with $\doteq$ are flat.*

Proof. Since sets of guarded rules are closed under resolution, the resulting clauses are guarded rules. Since body literals in $\mathcal{R}$ are flat and never instanciated with non-ground functional terms by a resolution step, positive literals in the bodies of the resulting rules are flat.

Now we show that non-flat equational clauses can always be flattened using the rules in Figure 3. Let $L = \neg x \doteq t$ be a literal in a flat guarded rule r. Then, either t is a variable in $\text{var}(r)$ or a constant. Suppose that t is a constant. If r is resolved using mgu σ and $x\sigma$ is a variable, $L\sigma$ is flat. Otherwise, $L\sigma$ can be reduced to *true* or *false*. Now suppose that t is a variable. If neither $x\sigma$ nor $t\sigma$ are a variable, we can reduce L to *true*, *false* or a disjunction of flat equational literals. If both are variables or constants, $L\sigma$ is flat. If one of them is a variable and the other one a functional term, $L\sigma$ can be reduced to *true*, since a non-ground functional term in a guarded rule contains all the variables of the rule, and there are no non-ground functional terms in non-ground rules.   □

Finally, the procedure that implements the transformation into PGHC is shown in Figure 4.

Theorem 1. *The procedure transform_to_PGHC terminates for every set $\mathcal{R}$ of guarded rules with non-flat $\prec$-greatest heads, and furnishes a set $\mathcal{R}'$ of primitive guarded Horn clauses such that $\mathcal{M}_\mathcal{R} = \mathcal{M}_{\mathcal{R}'} \cap HB_\mathcal{R}$.*

Proof. Termination is guaranteed by the fact that the number of different flat rule bodies is finite, since the set $\mathcal{P}$ of predicate symbols is finite (new predicate symbols are introduced into rule bodies only after the while loop).

procedure *unfold_and_simplify* $(r, \mathcal{R})$
begin
$\mathcal{R}' = \emptyset$; let $\{A_1, \ldots, A_n\} = \text{body}(r)^+$
for all $(r_1, \ldots, r_n) \in \mathcal{R}^n$ s.th. $\theta = \text{mgu}((A_1, \ldots, A_n), (\text{head}(r_1), \ldots, \text{head}(r_n)))$ exists
do
$\quad r' = \bigcup_{i=1}^n \text{body}(r_i\theta) \cup \text{body}(r\theta)^- \rightarrow \text{head}(r\theta)$
$\quad$ **if** r' is ground and $\mathcal{M}_\mathcal{R} \models \text{body}(r')$ **then** $\mathcal{R}' = \mathcal{R}' \cup \{\rightarrow \text{head}(r')\}$ **end if**
$\quad$ **if** $\text{body}(r')$ contains no contradiction and is not ground **then**
$\quad\quad \mathcal{R}' = \mathcal{R}' \cup \{r'\}$; **end if**
end for all
apply the simplification rules in Figure 3 exhaustively to the rules in $\mathcal{R}'$
result $= \mathcal{R}'$
end procedure

Fig. 2. The *unfold_and_simplify* procedure

$$\Gamma \cup \{\neg t \doteq t\} \rightarrow H \Rightarrow$$
$$\Gamma \cup \{\neg f(t_1, \ldots, t_n) \doteq g(s_1, \ldots, s_m)\} \rightarrow H \Rightarrow \Gamma \rightarrow H \text{ if } f \neq g$$
$$\Gamma \cup \{\neg x \doteq f(t_1, \ldots t_n)\} \rightarrow H \Rightarrow \Gamma \rightarrow H$$
$$\Gamma \cup \{\neg f(t_1, \ldots, t_n) \doteq f(s_1, \ldots, s_n)\} \rightarrow H \Rightarrow \Gamma \cup \{\neg t_1 \doteq s_1\} \rightarrow H$$
$$\vdots$$
$$\Gamma \cup \{\neg t_n \doteq s_n\} \rightarrow H$$

Fig. 3. Rules for the simplification of equational literals

As a first step, we flatten all positive body literals as described in Section 4.1. Then, we flatten the negative body literals, using the procedure *flatten_negative_body_literals*. Since this procedure may re-introduce non-flat positive body literals, we possibly have to flatten positive body literals again. Since flattening of positive body literals cannot introduce non-flat negative literals, $\mathcal{R}'$ contains only clauses with flat bodies.

If a new predicate symbol Q is introduced by a rule $r = \Gamma \rightarrow Q(x_1, \ldots, x_n)$, then Γ is true in well-supported model of $\mathcal{R} \cup \{r\}$ iff $Q(x_1, \ldots, x_n)$ is true in it. Therefore, Γ can be replaced by $Q(x_1, \ldots, x_n)$. Clearly, the unfolding in *unfold_and_simplify* does not modify the well-supported model, and neither does *flatten_negative_body_literals* as stated by Lemma 4. Therefore $\mathcal{M}_\mathcal{R} = \mathcal{M}_{\mathcal{R}'} \cap HB_\mathcal{R}$. $\qquad\square$

4.4   Evaluation of Guarded Clauses

The evaluation of a given guarded clauses in a model built by our method can be done in the following way: Let $\mathcal{S}$ be a set of primitive guarded Horn clauses generated by our method from a given set of guarded clauses containing a positive greatest literal. Then, $\mathcal{S}$ is also a set of guarded clauses.

procedure *transform_to_PGHC* ($\mathcal{R}$)
begin
$\mathcal{R}_1 = $ flatten_positive_body_literals($\mathcal{R}$)
$\mathcal{R}_2 = \bigcup_{r \in \mathcal{R}_1}$ flatten_negative_body_literals($r, \mathcal{R}_1$)
$\mathcal{R}' = $ flatten_positive_body_literals($\mathcal{R}_2$)
$\mathcal{A} = \mathcal{R}'; \mathcal{R}'' = \emptyset; Repl = \emptyset$
while $\mathcal{A} \neq \emptyset$ **do**
  choose $r \in \mathcal{A}; \mathcal{A} = \mathcal{A} \setminus \{r\}; \mathcal{R}'' = \mathcal{R}'' \cup \{r\}$
  if r is not primitive and no $r' \in Repl$ exists such that body(r) = body(r')**then**
    let Q be a fresh predicate symbol with $P \prec Q$ for all $P \in \mathcal{P}$
    let $\{x_1, \ldots, x_n\} = $ var(body(r))
    let $r' = $ body(r) $\rightarrow Q(x_1, \ldots, x_n)$
    $Repl = Repl \cup \{r'\}$
    $\mathcal{D} = $ unfold_and_simplify($r', \mathcal{R}'$)
    $\mathcal{A} = \mathcal{A} \cup \bigcup_{r \in \mathcal{D}}$ flatten_negative_body_literals($r, \mathcal{R}'$)
  end if
end while
for all $r \in \mathcal{R}''$ that are not primitive **do**
  let $r' \in Repl$ be such that body(r) = body(r')
  body(r) = {head(r')}
end for all
result = $\mathcal{R}''$
end procedure

Fig. 4. The procedure *transform_to_PGHC*

Let C be the guarded clause we want to evaluate, and let $\{x_1, \ldots, x_n\} = $ var(C). Let Q be a fresh predicate symbol such that $P \prec Q$ for all $P \in \mathcal{P}$, and let f be a fresh n-ary function symbol. Let $C' = C \cup \{Q(f(x_1, \ldots, x_n))\}$. Then, $Q(f(x_1, \ldots, x_n))$ is the $\prec$-greatest literal in C'. Now, we only have to transform $\mathcal{S} \cup \{C'\}$ into a set $\mathcal{S}'$ of PGHC, and then to test whether $\mathcal{S}' \cup \{\neg Q(x)\}$ is satisfiable. Clearly, this is the case iff C is true in $\mathcal{M}_{\mathcal{S}}$.

5   Integration of the Model Building Procedure into the Decision Procedure

We integrate the model building procedure into the decision procedure for guarded clauses in the following way (let $<$ be a total literal ordering):
while the empty clause is not found and $\mathcal{S}$ is not saturated,

- let $\mathcal{S}' = \{C \in \mathcal{S} \mid$ all $\prec$-maximal literals in C are positive$\}$
- for all $C \in \mathcal{S}'$, delete all $\prec$-maximal literals in C except the $<$-maximal
- build a model $\mathcal{M}$ for $\mathcal{S}'$
- deduce (one or more) new clauses from $\mathcal{S}$ using factoring and resolution as defined in Section 3, with the semantic restriction w.r.t $\mathcal{M}$ (i.e. at least one of the parent clauses must be false in $\mathcal{M}$), and add them to $\mathcal{S}$.

So, after each iteration of the while-loop, $\mathcal{M}$ is possibly modified, taking into account the new clauses. Since only finitely many new clauses can be deduced, the model can be modified only finitely many times before a definite model $\mathcal{M}$ is found. The refutational completeness is guaranteed by the fact that semantic resolution is complete, in particular using $\mathcal{M}$. We need the ordering $<$ to ensure that always the same maximal literal is chosen from a clause containing more than one maximal literals. Note that we can only find a model for the initial set if the clauses in $\mathcal{S}'$ always contain a $\prec$-greatest literal (i.e. not more than one maximal literal).

We give a simple example to show how our method works.

Example 4. Consider the satisfiable set of clauses $\mathcal{S} =$

$\{(1)\,\{P(a,b)\},\ (2)\,\{T(a,b)\}\ (3)\,\{\neg S(x,y), P(f(x,y), g(x,y))\},$
$(4)\,\{\neg P(x,y), P(f(x,y), g(x,y)), S(f(x,y), g(x,y))\},$
$(5)\,\{\neg Q(x,y), R(f(x,y), g(x,y))\},\ (6)\,\{\neg R(x,y), T(f(x,y), g(x,y))\},$
$(7)\,\{\neg T(x,y), Q(f(x,y), g(x,y))\},\ (8)\,\{\neg P(x,y) \vee \neg Q(x,y)\}\}$

From this set of clauses, the Bliksem theorem prover [3] that uses special techniques to deal with guarded clauses deduces about 15 new clauses (depending on the used ordering). In the best case, our method can do with 3 new clauses: we assume that $T \prec S \prec P \prec Q$. Then, the subset of clauses without maximal negative literal contains the clauses (1) to (7), whose rule form is $\mathcal{R} =$

$\{\rightarrow P(a,b);\quad \rightarrow T(a,b);\ P(x,y), \neg S(f(x,y), g(x,y)) \rightarrow P(f(x,y), g(x,y));$
$S(x,y) \rightarrow P(f(x,y), g(x,y));\ Q(x,y) \rightarrow R(f(x,y), g(x,y))$
$R(x,y) \rightarrow T(f(x,y), g(x,y));\ T(x,y) \rightarrow Q(f(x,y), g(x,y))$

Transformation to Horn clauses results in replacing the third rule by $P(x,y) \rightarrow P(f(x,y), g(x,y))$, since the literal $\neg S(f(x,y), g(x,y))$ is true in $\mathcal{M}_{\mathcal{R}}$. The clause (8) is false in $\mathcal{M}_{\mathcal{R}}$, since for example the atom $P(f(a,b), g(a,b))$ as well as the atom $Q(f(a,b), g(a,b))$ is true in $\mathcal{M}_{\mathcal{R}}$. So we can deduce the following clauses:

$(9)\{\neg T(x,y), \neg P(f(x,y), g(x,y))\}$ from (7),(8)
$(10)\{\neg S(x,y), \neg T(x,y)\}$ from (3),(9)
$(11)\{\neg P(x,y), \neg T(x,y), S(f(x,y), g(x,y))\}$ from (4),(9)

Now, a model for the clauses (1) to (7) and (11) is built, so that we get the set of rules (after deletion of rules whose bodies are true) $\mathcal{R}' =$

$\{\rightarrow P(a,b);\quad \rightarrow T(a,b);\quad \rightarrow N_3(a,b);\ S(x,y) \rightarrow P(f(x,y), g(x,y));$
$Q(x,y) \rightarrow R(f(x,y), g(x,y));\ R(x,y) \rightarrow T(f(x,y), g(x,y));$
$T(x,y) \rightarrow Q(f(x,y), g(x,y));\ N_1(x,y) \rightarrow P(f(x,y), g(x,y));$
$N_2(x,y) \rightarrow N_1(f(x,y), g(x,y));\ N_3(x,y) \rightarrow N_2(f(x,y), g(x,y));$
$N_1(x,y), R(x,y) \rightarrow N_3(f(x,y), g(x,y))$

Now, all clauses are true in $\mathcal{M}_{\mathcal{R}'}$, so no further inferences are possible.

6   Generalization to Loosely Guarded Clauses

Our model building method can be generalized to so-called *loosely guarded clauses*, which are a generalization of guarded clauses. In order to define them, the second condition of Definition 1 has to be replaced by

2. if C is non-ground then it contains a set of negative literals $\neg A_1, \ldots, \neg A_n$ (the *loose guard*) which do not contain functional terms and such that every pair of variables from $var(C)$ occurs together in one of the $\neg A_i$.

The main difference is that the decision procedure for loosely guarded formulas uses a certain kind of hyperresolution for the literals of the loose guard (see [10]). Concerning our model building method, the only difference is that in the *unfold_and_simplify* procedure, instead of resolving on *all* positive body literals, only a certain body literals are resolved upon (due to space limitations, we will not go into detail). The other procedures can be applied as they are.

7   Conclusion and Future Work

We have presented a method for the semantic refinement of a resolution decision procedure for guarded formulas. This refinement is based on a automated model building procedure for sets of guarded clauses in which every clause contains a positive greatest literal.

In general, model building is a more complex task than deciding satisfiability. Therefore, our method does not necessarily have an efficiency advantage. But in any case semantic restrictions might help to find proofs that are easier to understand for human users, since human reasoning usually uses semantic considerations. Already the smaller number of deduced clauses should be helpful for this purpose, but also the fact that the new clauses are deduced under semantic guide-lines, so they are more "meaningful".

In the case where a given set S of guarded clauses is satisfiable, our method can sometimes build a model for S. This is the case if every clause in S and that can be deduced from S by resolution contains not more than one positive maximal literal. In [5], it has been shown that for any set S of guarded clauses (without equality), a set S' of guarded clauses can be found in which every clause has a positive greatest literal and such that $M_{S'}$ is a model for S. Therefore, by applying the transformation method in [5] first and then the model building method presented in this article, a model can be built for any guarded clause set (without equality).

Models built by our method are expressed by primitive guarded Horn clauses, which is a relatively simple mechanism that is likely to be understandable for humans. Furthermore, primitive guarded Horn clauses might be useful to find finite models for guarded formulas, since the represented Herbrand model can easily be enumerated. In order to find a finite model, we first try to find for each enumerated ground atom A a smaller ground atom A' such that we can put $A = A'$ without loosing satisfiability. Only if such an atom does not exist, A

is used to generate greater ground atoms. This algorithm gives good results in practice, but its termination is an open problem. However, if the initial guarded formula is a translation of a modal formula, a Kripke model for the modal formula can be obtained from a finite model of the guarded formula (every element of the domain of the finite model corresponds to a world).

The decision procedure for guarded clauses in [8] can treat clauses containing equality. Therefore, our method could possibly extended to such clauses. Another possible extension is the treatment of guarded clauses as defined in [11], where equality literals are not permitted, but literals may contain functional ground terms, and have a depth greater than 1. This might be possible using decomposition techniques as in [6].

An implementation of the presented method will be ready soon.

References

1. Hajnal Andréka, Johan van Benthem, and István Nemeti. Modal logics and bounded fragments of predicate logic. *Journal of Philosophical Logic*, 27(3):217–274, 1998.
2. L. Bachmair and H. Ganzinger. On restrictions of ordered paramodulation with simplification. In *Proceedings of CADE-10*, volume 449 of *LNCS*. Springer, 1990.
3. Homepage of the Bliksem theorem prover. http://www.mpi-sb.mpg.de/~bliksem/.
4. R. Caferra and N. Peltier. Extending semantic resolution via automated model building: applications. In *Proceeding of IJCAI'95*, pages 328–334. Morgan Kaufman, 1995.
5. M. Dierkes. Defining a unique Herbrand model for sets of guarded clauses. Accepted for International Workshop on First Order Theorem Proving FTP'2000.
6. M. Dierkes. Simplification of Horn clauses that are clausal forms of guarded formulas. In *Proceedings of LPAR'99*, volume 1705 of *LNAI*. Springer, 1999.
7. H. Ganzinger, Ch. Meyer, and Ch Weidenbach. Soft typing for ordered resolution. In *Proceedings of CADE-14*, volume 1249 of *LNAI*. Springer, 1997.
8. H. Ganzinger and H. de Nivelle. A superposition decision procedure for the guarded fragment with equality. In *Proc. 14th IEEE Symposium on Logic in Computer Science*. IEEE Computer Society Press, 1999.
9. Rainer Manthey and François Bry. SATCHMO: A theorem prover implemented in Prolog. In *Proc. of CADE-9*, pages 415–434. Springer, LNCS 310, 1988.
10. Hans de Nivelle. Resolution decides the guarded fragment. Research Report CT-1998-01, ILLC, 1998.
11. Hans de Nivelle. A resolution decision procedure for the guarded fragment. In *Automated Deduction - CADE-15*, volume 1421 of *LNCS*, 1998.
12. James R. Slagle. Automatic theorem proving with renamable and semantic resolution. *Journal of the ACM*, 14(4):687–697, October 1967.
13. J. Slaney. SCOTT: a model-guided theorem prover. In *Proceedings IJCAI-93*, volume 1, pages 109–114. Morgan Kaufmann, 1993.

Model Checking for Timed Logic Processes

Supratik Mukhopadhyay and Andreas Podelski

Max-Planck-Institut für Informatik
Im Stadtwald, 66123 Saarbrücken, Germany
{supratik,podelski}@mpi-sb.mpg.de

Abstract. We apply techniques from logic programming and constraint databases to verify real time systems. We introduce *timed logic processes* (TLPs) as a fragment of constraint query languages over reals. We establish a formal connection between TLPs and timed automata, and between the procedure of the UPPAAL model checker for restricted temporal-logic properties of timed automata and the top-down query evaluation of TLPs (with tabling in the XSB style). This connection yields an alternative implementation of the UPPAAL procedure. Furthermore, we can extend that procedure in order to accommodate more expressive properties...

1 Introduction

Some software and hardware components meet the tasks for which they have been designed only if they relate properly to the passage of time. Behaviors of such computing systems operating in real time are difficult to predict by "inspection". Therefore real-time systems have become a prime target of formal specification and verification methods [AD94,DT98,LPY95,SS95]. In this paper, we start investigating how techniques from logic programming [TS86,CW96] and constraint databases [KKR95,Rev90,JM94] can be used to explain and to enhance these methods.

We single out a fragment of constraint query languages [JM94,KKR95] over reals that allows us to model real-time systems operating over dense time. We call the programs expressed in this fragment *timed logic processes* (abbreviated TLPs). We establish a formal connection of TLPs with timed automata, a standard model for timed systems [AD94]. We use this connection to design a model checking procedure for the temporal logic $\mathcal{L}_s$ [LPY95] ("logic of safety and bounded liveness") as the top-down query evaluation of TLPs; this gives a direct account of the procedure used in the UPPAAL model checker [LPY95,BLL+96]. More precisely, we reduce the model checking problem for $\mathcal{L}_s$ properties of timed automata to the membership problem for the model-theoretic semantics of a TLP obtained by a product construction. The *local* model checking procedure of UPPAAL [LPY95,BLL+96] (originally defined via tree rewriting) is a special case of OLDT resolution [TS86,CW96] over arithmetic constraints. We have implemented a prototype model checker for timed systems based on OLDT resolution with constraints using the CLP($\mathcal{R}$) [JMSY92] system of Sicstus 3.7, and

J. Lloyd et al. (Eds.): CL 2000, LNAI 1861, pp. 598–612, 2000.
© Springer-Verlag Berlin Heidelberg 2000

we have applied it to several standard benchmark examples, and have obtained reasonable timings for these examples.

The logic $\mathcal{L}_s$ contains only a restricted version of disjunction which, in our setup, corresponds to queries without conjunction. Since our evaluation procedure applies to general queries, we readily obtain a model checking procedure for the extension of $\mathcal{L}_s$ where the disjunction of is not restricted (i.e., where the temporal-logic formulas can be formed using disjunction in the usual way).

The forward analysis of timed systems, as implemented in UPPAAL, is generally non-terminating. It can be turned into a terminating procedure by introducing the *splitting* operation on constraints in [SS95]. As an alternative, we propose a new operation called *trim*. In contrast with splitting, trimming is defined on the logical semantics of constraints and yields a (finite) transition system that is bisimilar to the one for the timed automaton. Trimming can be combined directly with our procedure based on OLDT resolution with constraints, which turns it into a terminating procedure.

Unbounded liveness properties are not expressible in $\mathcal{L}_s$ (and cannot be handled by UPPAAL). Model checking for such properties amounts to computing the greatest model of a TLP in our setup. In order to obtain a *local* model checker for unbounded liveness properties, we introduce a new method that we call *greatest model resolution*. As a consequence, we can now verify *receptiveness* properties of timed logic processes.

2 Timed Logic Processes

We identify a fragment of constraint query languages over reals (in the sense of [KKR95,Rev90,BS91]) that will allows us to model real-time systems. Furthermore, as we will see below, it allows us to express the product constructions that come up in the course of model checking for formulas in the temporal logic $\mathcal{L}_s$ [LPY95]. We call the programs expressed in this fragment as *timed logic processes* (abbreviated TLPs). A TLP is a set of *clauses* of one of the following four forms:

$$(1) \quad p(\boldsymbol{x}) \longleftarrow \varphi, p'(\boldsymbol{x'})$$
$$(2) \quad p(\boldsymbol{x}) \longleftarrow p_1(\boldsymbol{x}), p_2(\boldsymbol{x}),$$
$$(3) \quad p(\boldsymbol{x}) \longleftarrow \gamma$$
$$(4) \quad init \longleftarrow p(\boldsymbol{x}), \boldsymbol{x} = 0$$

where the constraints φ are of one of the two forms (here n is the length of the tuple $\boldsymbol{x} \equiv \langle x_1, \ldots, x_n \rangle$ of variables)

$$(1.1) \quad \gamma_1(\boldsymbol{x}) \wedge \bigwedge_{i=1}^{n} x_i' = x_i + z \wedge z \geq 0 \wedge \gamma_2(\boldsymbol{x'}) \quad (\text{``time transitions''})$$
$$(1.2) \quad \gamma_1(\boldsymbol{x}) \wedge \bigwedge_{i \in S} x_i' = 0 \wedge \bigwedge_{i \notin S} x_i' = x_i \wedge \gamma_2(\boldsymbol{x'}) \quad (\text{``edge transitions''})$$

where $S \subseteq \{1, \ldots, n\}$ and the syntax of the constraints γ is defined by

$$\gamma ::= true \mid x_i > c \mid x_i < c \mid x_i \geq \ \mid x_i \leq c \mid \gamma \wedge \gamma$$

where $c \in \mathcal{N}$, the set of non-negative integers. We call these constraints the guards of the clauses. The variable z in (1.1) is called *increment variable*.

A first motivation for TLPs is that this model subsumes the timed automata [AD94] model; i.e., we can translate timed automata to timed logic processes. These translations use only clauses of the form (1) with constraints φ of the form (1.1) (for *time transitions*) or (1.2) (for *edge transitions*) and clauses of the form (4) (for expressing the initial position). Clauses of the form (2) are used for expressing alternation (compare [DW99]) in product constructions used in model checking. Clauses of the form (3) are used to rewrite an agent to a nil agent (in this respect there is a strong similarity with process algebras; thus $p(\boldsymbol{x}) \longleftarrow \gamma$ states that the agent p can rewrite to the nil agent if the values of the variables $\boldsymbol{x}$ satisfy the formula γ). These clauses can also be used to express assertions about processes (e.g., by rewriting an agent to the nil agent if the values of the variables $\boldsymbol{x}$ violate a safety property). We will see later that clauses of the form (3) can also used for expressing $\mathcal{L}_s$ properties. Thus the TLP framework not only allows modeling a system, but also allows writing assertions about the behaviors of the system.

3   Translation of Timed Automata into TLPs

We will next translate a timed automaton U into a TLP P. Let

$$U = \langle AP, X_n, L, E, P, \ell^0, inv \rangle$$

be a timed automaton. Here, AP is a set of atomic propositions, X_n is a set of n clocks (whose values are referred to by the variables $x_1, \ldots, x_n$), L is a set of locations, E is a set of edges, P is a labeling function that labels each location with a set of atomic propositions, $\ell^0 \in L$ is the initial location and inv is a function that assigns to each location an invariant constraint (see [AD94] for more details).

For each location $\ell \in L$, we introduce an n-ary predicate $\ell(\boldsymbol{x})$. For each location $\ell \in L$, the TLP $\mathcal{P}$ contains a clause of the form (1) with a constraint φ of the form (1.1) where $\gamma_1(\boldsymbol{x})$ and $\gamma_2(\boldsymbol{x}')$ are both the invariant $inv(\ell)$ of the location ℓ. That is, $\gamma_2(\boldsymbol{x}')$ is obtained from $\gamma_1(\boldsymbol{x})$ by renaming all variables tuple $\boldsymbol{x}$ to their primed versions $x_1', \ldots, x_n'$ in the tuple $\boldsymbol{x}'$.

For each edge $\langle \ell, \theta, Reset, \ell' \rangle \in E$ leading from the location ℓ to the location ℓ', where θ is the guard of the edge and $Reset$ is the set of clocks reset in that edge, the TLP $\mathcal{P}$ contains a clause of the form (1) with a constraint φ of the form (1.2) with head predicate $\ell(\boldsymbol{x})$ and body predicate $\ell'(\boldsymbol{x})$, where $\gamma_1 \equiv \theta \wedge inv_\ell(\boldsymbol{x})$, $\gamma_2 \equiv inv_{\ell'}$ and $S = Reset$ (here inv_ℓ and $inv_{\ell'}$ are respectively the invariants of locations ℓ and ℓ'). We also add a clause $init \longleftarrow \ell^0(\boldsymbol{x}) \wedge \boldsymbol{x} = 0$.

The semantics of a timed automaton is defined in terms of *traces* that are sequences of *positions* starting with the position $\langle \ell^0, 0, \ldots, 0 \rangle$ in the initial location with all n clocks set to 0. The semantics of a TLP is defined by its *ground derivations* that start with the *ground atom* $\ell^0(0, \ldots, 0)$. Identifying positions and ground atoms, we obtain the following statement.

Theorem 1 (Adequacy of Translation). *The timed automaton U and the TLP $\mathcal{P}$ obtained by the translation outlined above have the same semantics.*

In our definition, the semantics of a timed automaton contains also *convergent* traces. Unbounded liveness properties, however, refer only to *divergent* traces.

4   Logic of Safety and Bounded Liveness ($\mathcal{L}_s$)

The syntax of formulas Φ in the logic $\mathcal{L}_s$ (*Logic of Safety and Bounded Liveness*) [LPY95] is given as follows:

$$\Phi \ ::= \ \theta \mid q \mid q \vee \Phi \mid \theta \vee \Phi \mid \Phi_1 \wedge \Phi_2 \mid [\![\Phi \mid \forall \Phi \mid x.\Phi \mid Z$$

where θ is an atomic constraint of the form $x_i \sim c$ with $\sim \in \{=, <, >, \geq, \leq\}$, c is a non-negative integer, q is an atomic proposition and $Z \in Id$ is an identifier (identifiers are called variables in the mu-calculus). The meaning of the identifiers Z is specified by a unique declaration $\mathcal{D}(Z) : Z = \Phi$ for each identifier assigning a formula Φ of $\mathcal{L}_s$ to that identifier Z.

The satisfaction relation $\models$ for $\mathcal{L}_s$ is the largest relation satisfying a number of conditions that are formulated in terms of timed automata in [LPY95] and that we here formulate for a TLP $\mathcal{P}$ and an atom $p(v)$ standing for one of its 'states'.

- $\mathcal{P}, p(v) \models \theta$ implies $v \models \theta$.
- $\mathcal{P}, p(v) \models q$ implies $q \in P(p)$. (where P is a function that assigns to each predicate in $\mathcal{P}$ a set of atomic propositions).
- $\mathcal{P}, p(v) \models q \vee \Phi$ implies $\mathcal{P}, p(v) \models q$ or $\mathcal{P}, p(v) \models \Phi$.
- $\mathcal{P}, p(v) \models \theta \vee \Phi$ implies $\mathcal{P}, p(v) \models \theta$ or $\mathcal{P}, p(v) \models \Phi$.
- $\mathcal{P}, p(v) \models \Phi_1 \wedge \Phi_2$ implies $\mathcal{P}, p(v) \models \Phi_1$ and $\mathcal{P}, p(v) \models \Phi_2$.
- $\mathcal{P}, p(v) \models [\![\Phi$ implies $\mathcal{P}, p'(v') \models \Phi$ for all ground resolvents $p'(v')$ of $p(v)$ through clauses of the form (1.2).
- $\mathcal{P}, p(v) \models \forall \Phi$ implies $\mathcal{P}, p'(v') \models \Phi$ for all ground resolvents $p'(v')$ of $p(v)$ through clauses of the form (1.1).
- $\mathcal{P}, p(v) \models x.\Phi$ implies $\mathcal{P}, p(v)[0/x] \models \Phi$ (where the ground atom $p(v)[0/x]$ is obtained from $p(v)$ by reseting 'place' in v corresponding to the variable x to zero).
- $\mathcal{P}, p(v) \models Z$ implies $\mathcal{P}, p(v) \models \mathcal{D}(Z)$.
- $\mathcal{P}, p_1(v_1) \wedge \ldots \wedge p_m(v_m) \models \Phi$ implies $\mathcal{P}, p_1(v_1) \models \Phi, \ldots, \mathcal{P}, p_m(v_m) \models \Phi$.

We call a variable that does not occur on the right hand side of any declaration in an $\mathcal{L}_s$ formula the root variable for that formula. An $\mathcal{L}_s$ formula is a set of declarations having a root variable. Note that we take the greatest fixpoint of the set of declarations (viewed as a set of equations). For a TLP $\mathcal{P}$ and an $\mathcal{L}_s$ formula Φ, we say that $\mathcal{P} \models \Phi$ iff $\mathcal{P}, init \models \Phi$.

An example of a bounded liveness specification in $\mathcal{L}_s$ is as follows: let $\mathcal{C}$ be an atomic constraint. Then the formula $X = [\![(z.Z)$ where $Z = \mathcal{C} \vee (z < i \wedge \forall Z \wedge [\![Z)$ asserts that $\mathcal{C}$ should be satisfied within i time units of resolving through a clause of the form (1.2) (for timed automata, this amounts to the statement that $\mathcal{C}$

should be satisfied within i time units of taking an edge transition). We call the variables $\boldsymbol{x}$ the *real variables*.

In order to specify properties about TLPs, it is useful to consider the dual of the logic $\mathcal{L}_s$. So before introducing the model checking method, we first introduce the syntax of $\widetilde{\mathcal{L}_s}$ which expresses the dual of $\mathcal{L}_s$ formulas. The syntax of $\widetilde{\mathcal{L}_s}$ is given as follows:

$$\widetilde{\Phi} \ ::= \ \theta \mid q \mid q \wedge \widetilde{\Phi} \mid \theta \wedge \widetilde{\Phi} \mid \widetilde{\Phi_1} \vee \widetilde{\Phi_2} \mid \Diamond\widetilde{\Phi} \mid \exists\widetilde{\Phi} \mid x.\widetilde{\Phi} \mid Z$$

where θ is an atomic constraint and q is an atomic proposition. An $\widetilde{\mathcal{L}_s}$ formula is a set of declarations with a root variable. Note that we take the least fixpoint of the set of declarations (viewed as a set of equations). For every formula Φ of $\mathcal{L}_s$, we can define a formula $\widetilde{\Phi}$ in $\widetilde{\mathcal{L}_s}$ such that for a TLP $\mathcal{P}$, $\mathcal{P} \models \widetilde{\Phi}$ iff $\mathcal{P} \not\models \Phi$. We do not provide the semantics of $\widetilde{\mathcal{L}_s}$ formulas which are easily understood from those of $\mathcal{L}_s$ formulas (dual of those of $\mathcal{L}_s$ formulas).

5   Product Program

Given a TLP $\mathcal{P}$, and an $\widetilde{\mathcal{L}_s}$ formula $\widetilde{\Phi}$, we construct the product TLP $\mathcal{P}^{\widetilde{\Phi}}$, in which the arity of each predicate is n (assuming that the arity of each predicate in $\mathcal{P}$ is k and the corresponding $\mathcal{L}_s$ formula Φ has $n-k$ real variables), such that $\mathcal{P} \models \widetilde{\Phi}$ iff the predicate $\langle init, \widetilde{Z} \rangle$ (see below) is in the least model of $\mathcal{P}^{\widetilde{\Phi}}$. Here $\widetilde{Z}$ is the root variable of $\widetilde{\Phi}$. The construction is as follows. For the root variable $\widetilde{Z}$ we create the (0-ary predicate) $\langle init, \widetilde{Z} \rangle$. For each predicate $\langle p, X \rangle$ created, expand (i.e., create a rule(s) defining that predicate) using the following rules if the predicate is not already expanded (depending on the declaration $X = \Psi$ defining X in $\widetilde{\Phi}$.):

- $X = q$: $\langle p, X \rangle(\boldsymbol{x}) \longleftarrow true$ if $q \in P(p)$ (where P is a function assigning to each predicate symbol a set of atomic propositions).
- $X = \theta$: $\langle p, X \rangle(\boldsymbol{x}) \longleftarrow \theta$.
- $X = q \wedge X'$: $\langle p, X \rangle(\boldsymbol{x}) \longleftarrow \langle p, X' \rangle(\boldsymbol{x})$ if $q \in P(p)$.
- $X = \theta \wedge X'$: $\langle p, X \rangle(\boldsymbol{x}) \longleftarrow \langle p, X' \rangle(\boldsymbol{x}) \wedge \theta$.
- $X = X_1 \vee X_2$: $\langle p, X \rangle(\boldsymbol{x}) \longleftarrow \langle p, X_1 \rangle(\boldsymbol{x})$ and $\langle p, X \rangle(\boldsymbol{x}) \longleftarrow \langle p, X_2 \rangle(\boldsymbol{x})$.
- $X = \Diamond X'$: For each clause C in $\mathcal{P}$ of the form (1.2) such that the predicate p stands on the head of the clause create a clause of the form $\langle p, X \rangle(\boldsymbol{x}) \longleftarrow \langle p', X' \rangle(\boldsymbol{x}') \wedge \varphi \wedge \varphi'$ where φ is the constraint in the body of the clause C and $\varphi' \equiv \bigwedge_{i=k+1}^{n} x_i' = x_i$.
- $X = \exists X'$: For each clause C of the form (1.1) such that the predicate p stands on its head, create a clause of the form $\langle p, X \rangle(\boldsymbol{x}) \longleftarrow \langle p', X' \rangle(\boldsymbol{x}') \wedge \varphi \wedge \varphi'$, where φ is the constraint in C and φ' is given by $\bigwedge_{i=k+1}^{n} x_i' = x_i + z$.
- $X = x_i.X'$: $\langle p, X \rangle(\boldsymbol{x}) \longleftarrow \langle p, X' \rangle(\boldsymbol{x}') \wedge x_i = 0 \wedge \bigwedge_{j \neq i} x_j' = x_j$.

Theorem 2. *Given a TLP $\mathcal{P}$ and an $\mathcal{L}_s$ formula Φ, $\mathcal{P} \models \Phi$ if and only if the atom $\langle init, \widetilde{Z} \rangle$ is not in the least model of $\mathcal{P}^{\widetilde{\Phi}}$ (as created above) where $\widetilde{\Phi}$ is the dual of the $\mathcal{L}_s$ formula Φ and Z is the root variable of Φ (i.e., $\widetilde{Z}$ is the root variable of $\widetilde{\Phi}$).*

Implementation. To prove $\mathcal{P} \models \Phi$, we try to prove $\mathcal{P} \not\models \widetilde{\Phi}$ where $\widetilde{\Phi}$ is the $\widetilde{\mathcal{L}_s}$ formula corresponding to Φ (i.e., the dual of Φ). This is proved by proving that $\langle init, \widetilde{Z} \rangle$ is not in the least model of $\mathcal{P}^{\widetilde{\Phi}}$ (where Z is the root variable of Φ). We can either compute the least model of $\mathcal{P}^{\widetilde{\Phi}}$ using the least fix point of the immediate consequence operator (see [JM94] for a definition of the immediate consequence operator) resulting in a global model checker. Alternately we can extend XSB-style tabling [CW96,TS86,Vie87] with constraints to prove that $\langle init, \widetilde{Z} \rangle$ does not succeed in the tabled resolution using the non-ground transition system. To be precise, our method extends with constraints the OLDT resolution of [TS86]. Extending standard results from logic programming [TS86] we get, the state $\langle init, \widetilde{Z} \rangle$ succeeds iff it succeeds in the derivation tree obtained by using tabled resolution. Note that the tabling strategy produces a local model checker for $\widetilde{\mathcal{L}_s}$ ($\mathcal{L}_s$). To guarantee termination of the model checking procedure, we can use the trim operation on constraints, described below, along with the tabling strategy mentioned above.

Providing a Counter Example. To provide a counter example, we follow the following method. With each non-ground goal we keep the following information: the constraints encountered so far (including the mgus, i.e., most general unifiers, which are also regarded as constraints), a list of the numbers of clauses encountered so far (we assume that the clauses are numbered) and a list of increment variables encountered so far (assuming that they are suitably renamed). Thus a non-ground goal will take the form of a five-tuple $\langle Q, \varphi_1, \varphi_2, L_1, L_2 \rangle$ where Q is a conjunction of predicates, φ_1 is the constraint store, φ_2 is the concatenation of all the constraints of all the clauses (and the mgus) encountered thus far, L_1 is a list of the numbers of the clauses encountered so far, L_2 is the list of the increment variables of the clauses encountered so far. Now the "earliest" (with respect to time) ground counter example (i.e., a ground derivation acting as a witness to the success) can be provided in the following way. First project φ_2 on the set of variables in the list L_2. Let the constraint obtained be φ. Now minimize $\Sigma_{z_i \in L_2} z_i$ with respect to φ. The solutions of z_i obtained in this method can be used in providing a ground counter example. The counter example can now be generated from the sequence of clauses and the values of the corresponding increment variables.

6   The Trim Operation on Constraints

We first start with the observation the model checking procedure described above is possibly non-terminating. The counter example is provided by the translation to TLP of the timed automaton in figure 2.

Our aim is to define an equivalence relation $\approx_M$ on the set of non-ground states of $\mathcal{P}$ (i.e., states of the form $\langle p(x), \varphi \rangle$ where p is a predicate symbol and φ is the constraint store in which the free variables are x) such that the following conditions hold:

- The quotient (in the standard sense) of the non-ground transition system of $\mathcal{P}$, induced by $\approx_M$, denoted by $\mathcal{P}/\approx_M$, has a finite index, i.e., a finite number of "states" or equivalence classes (see [JM94] for a definition of non-ground transition system induced by a constraint query language program).
- The transition system induced by $\mathcal{P}/\approx_M$ (in the standard sense) bisimulates [Mil89] the non-ground transition system induced by $\mathcal{P}$.

The suffix M denotes the maximal constant occurring in the guards of the TLP $\mathcal{P}$ (this suffix is kept since the equivalence relation $\approx_M$ involves M).

Let $\mathcal{P}$ be a TLP with M as the maximal constant occurring in the guards of the clauses. Let s be any non-ground state. Let $sol(s)$ denote the set of ground instances of s. Now we define an equivalence relation $\approx_M$ on the set of non-ground states of $\mathcal{P}$ as follows: $\approx_M$ is the smallest equivalence relation satisfying the following:

- $\langle p(\boldsymbol{x}), \varphi \rangle \approx_M \langle p(\boldsymbol{x}), \varphi' \rangle$ if for all $p(\boldsymbol{v}) \in sol(\langle p(\boldsymbol{x}), \varphi \rangle)$ there exists $p(\boldsymbol{w}) \in sol(\langle p(\boldsymbol{x}), \varphi' \rangle)$ such that $\forall i \in \{1, \ldots, n\}$ either $(v_i = w_i)$ or $(v_i > M \wedge w_i > M)$ and vice versa.

From now on, we view the non-ground transition system induced by $\mathcal{P}$ as a labeled transition system in which the clauses act as labels.

Proposition 1. *The non-ground transition system of $\mathcal{P}$ and the quotient of the non-ground transition system of $\mathcal{P}$ induced by $\approx_M$ are bisimilar.*

Now we show how to decide whether two nonground states are equivalent using the trim operation described below.

Below, by a reachable nonground state $\langle p(\boldsymbol{x}), \varphi \rangle$, we mean that there is a non-ground derivation from *init* to $\langle p(\boldsymbol{x}), \varphi \rangle$ using the clauses in $\mathcal{P}$. Given a "reachable" non-ground state $\langle p(\boldsymbol{x}), \varphi \rangle$, we convert it to a state $\langle p(\boldsymbol{x}), \varphi' \rangle$ such that $\langle p(\boldsymbol{x}), \varphi \rangle = \langle p(\boldsymbol{x}), \varphi' \rangle$, where φ' is in a normalized form where we allow constraints of the form $x_i \sim c$ or $x_i - x_j \, relop \, a$ where $\sim \in \{>, \geq, <, \leq\}$, $relop \in \{>, \geq\}$, c is a natural number and a is an integer (note that it can be easily shown that for reachable nonground states the constraint store can be converted into normalized form; it can also be shown that there exists an algorithm for doing this). In what follows we deal with constraints in normalized form.

Definition 1 (Trim). *We define an operator trim, which given a satisfiable constraint φ, produces a constraint $\varphi' = trim(\varphi)$, by the method given below. The constraint $trim(\varphi)$ is obtained from the normalized form of φ by the following operations:*

- *Remove all constraints of the form $x_j - x_i > a$ or $x_j - x_i \geq a$, for each pair of variables $x_i, x_j, i \neq j$, such that $\varphi \wedge x_i > M$ is satisfiable and $\exists_{-x_j}(\varphi)$ is equivalent to $\exists_{-x_j}(\varphi \wedge x_i > M)$ and $(\varphi \wedge x_j > M)$ is not equivalent to φ, where a is an integer and the existential quantifier is over all variables but x_j.*
- *Remove all constraints of the form $x_i < c$ or $x_i \leq c$ where c is an integer and $c > M$.*
- *For each i, such that $(\varphi \wedge x_i > M)$ is equivalent to φ, replace all the constraints of the form $x_i - x_j \sim a$ or $x_i \sim c$ by the constraint $x_i > M$, where a and c are integers and $c > M$ and $\sim \in \{>, \geq\}$.*

Lemma 1. *For reachable non-ground states* $\langle p(\boldsymbol{x}), \varphi \rangle$ *and* $\langle p(\boldsymbol{x}), \varphi' \rangle$, $\langle p(\boldsymbol{x}), \varphi \rangle$ $\approx_M \langle p(\boldsymbol{x}), \varphi' \rangle$ *iff* $\langle p(\boldsymbol{x}), trim(\varphi) \rangle = \langle p(\boldsymbol{x}), trim(\varphi') \rangle$.

In the above, we identify two nonground states iff they have the same ground instances. At a high level, the trim operation can be viewed as an accurate widening operation, i.e., it does not lose precision with respect to model checking for the properties that we are concerned with here. The removal and replacement of constraints in the definition of trim can be seen as constraint widening operations. The basic intuition is as follows: once the value of a real variable goes above the maximal constant, it does not matter what the value is. Hence, if a constraint has a solution in which the value of a variable is above the maximal constant, then the constraint can be widened to incorporate all "similar tuples". Logically, the relation $\approx_M$ can be viewed as a symbolic bisimulation. Thus, the relation $\approx_M$ provides a logical characterization of the trim operation on constraints. Note that the definition of trim itself provides with an algorithm for trimming.

Lemma 2. *The equivalence relation* $\approx_M$ *produces a finite number of reachable equivalence classes (i.e., equivalence classes containing reachable nonground states).*

Proposition 2. *Given two reachable non-ground states* $\langle p(\boldsymbol{x}), \varphi \rangle$ *and* $\langle p(\boldsymbol{x}), \varphi' \rangle$, *where both* φ *and* φ' *are in normalized form, it is effectively decidable whether* $\langle p(\boldsymbol{x}), \varphi \rangle \approx_M \langle p(\boldsymbol{x}), \varphi' \rangle$.

The trim operation described above can be combined with the tabling strategy described above to provide a termination guarantee for the model checking procedure. If $\langle p'(\boldsymbol{x}), \varphi' \rangle$ is the resolvent of $\langle p(\boldsymbol{x}), \varphi \rangle$ through a clause C, then we add the goal $\langle p'(\boldsymbol{x}), trim(\varphi') \rangle$ as the table entry. The details are described in the full version of the paper [MP99]. By lemma 2, termination of the algorithm is guaranteed. From the proof of lemma 2 (see [MP99]), it can be seen that the model checking procedure described above requires polynomial space in the worst case.

We have implemented a prototype local model checker based on the method given above. Though the implementation is still very much sub optimal (no fine tuning has been done) the performance of the model checker seems to be encouraging. We used our model checker to verify the safety property of several well known benchmark examples taken from literature. The experimental results are summarized in table in Figure 1. All the results are obtained on PC (200 MHz Pentium Pro). All the timings denote the total time needed.

7   Full Disjunction

Note that the logic $\mathcal{L}_s$ [LPY95] described above allows only restricted disjunction. In this subsection, we show that in our framework we can allow for full disjunction. Note that it is stated in [LPY95] that their model checking technique based on the rewrite tree cannot be extended to a logic with general

Example	time (seconds)
Example in figure 2	1.5
Fischer's Protocol (Two Processes) [LPY95]	4.2
Rail-road Crossing	1.8
Audio Protocol [HWT95]	7.2

Fig. 1. Experimental Results

disjunction. We call the extension of the logic $\mathcal{L}_s$ with full disjunction $\mathcal{XL}_s$. Dually, we call the the extension of the logic $\mathcal{L}_s$ with full conjunction as $\widetilde{\mathcal{XL}}_s$ (i.e., the dual of $\mathcal{XL}_s$). The satisfaction relation for $\mathcal{XL}_s$ is the satisfaction relation for $\mathcal{L}_s$ augmented with the clause:

- $\mathcal{P}, p(v) \models \Phi_1 \vee \Phi_2$ implies $\mathcal{P}, p(v) \models \Phi_1$ or $\mathcal{P}, p(v) \models \Phi_2$.

For an $\mathcal{XL}_s$ formula Φ we can obtain an $\widetilde{\mathcal{XL}}_s$ formula $\widetilde{\Phi}$ in the similar way as above ($\widetilde{\mathcal{XL}}_s$ is the corresponding extension of $\widetilde{\mathcal{L}}_s$). Given a TLP $\mathcal{P}$ and a $\widetilde{\mathcal{XL}}_s$ formula $\widetilde{\Phi}$, we can construct a product program $\mathcal{P}^{\widetilde{\Phi}}$ using an extension of the product construction given above by the following "alternating" clause.

- $X = X_1 \wedge X_2 \colon \langle p, X \rangle(x) \longleftarrow \langle p, X_1 \rangle(x) \wedge \langle p, X_2 \rangle(x)$.

Theorem 3. *Given a TLP $\mathcal{P}$ and an $\mathcal{XL}_s$ formula Φ, $\mathcal{P} \models \Phi$ if and only if $\langle init, \widetilde{Z} \rangle$ is not in the least model of $\mathcal{P}^{\widetilde{\Phi}}$ where $\widetilde{\Phi}$ is the $\widetilde{\mathcal{XL}}_s$ formula corresponding to Φ and Z is the root variable of Φ.*

Note that we do not have to change the implementation for this extension – we can reuse the implementation described above.

Note that the rewrite tree based model checking procedure [LPY95] implemented in the model checker UPPAAL [BLL+96] can be viewed as a special case of our derivation tree using tabled resolution with constraints as described above. Use of tabled resolution with constraints allows us to increase the expressiveness of the underlying logic ([LPY95] allows only restricted disjunction). Also note that the model checking procedure in [LPY95] may not terminate (consider the timed automaton given in Figure 2 and the formula $X = x2 < 2 \wedge [\![X \wedge \forall X$ where $x2$ refers to the clock $x2$ of the timed automaton; this asserts that always the value of the clock $x2$ will be less than 2). In contrast our model checking procedure combined with the trim operation is guaranteed to terminate. Like the model checking procedure in [LPY95], our model checking procedure is also local (only the reachable portion of the state space is explored and the state space is explored in a demand-driven fashion).

8   Unbounded Liveness Properties

We now look at unbounded liveness properties. An unbounded liveness property is a declaration of the form $X = q \vee \forall [\![X$ (this is actually the dual of the property

$X = q \wedge \exists \Diamond X$, where we take the least fixpoint of the declaration) where q is an atomic proposition and we take the greatest fixpoint of the declaration (viewed as an equation). This asserts that for all (infinite) ground derivations (starting from $init$) using resolutions through clauses of the form (1.1) immediately followed by a resolution through a clause of the form (1.2), there exists a ground atom in that satisfies q (for timed automata this is the same as the assertion that for all (infinite) traces starting from the initial position using time transitions followed by edge transitions, i.e., first taking a time transition and then following it up with an edge transition and so on, there exists a position that satisfies q). Note that this is the negation of the specification which there exists a (infinite) ground derivation (starting from $init$) using resolutions through clauses of the form (1.1) immediately followed by a resolution through a clause of the form (1.2), such that every ground atom in the derivation satisfies the atomic proposition q.

Given an unbounded liveness specification Ψ ($\Phi \equiv \widetilde{\Psi}$; $\widetilde{\Psi}$ is the negation of Ψ; $\mathcal{P} \models \Psi$ iff $\mathcal{P} \not\models \Phi$), and a TLP $\mathcal{P}$, we construct a TLP $\mathcal{P}^{\Phi}$ such that $\mathcal{P} \models \Phi$ iff the atom $\langle init, X \rangle$ is in the greatest model of $\mathcal{P}^{\Phi}$, where X is the root variable of Φ. The construction of a product program is same as that shown in case of $\widetilde{\mathcal{L}_s}$.

Theorem 4. *Given a TLP $\mathcal{P}$ and an unbounded liveness specification Ψ, we have $\mathcal{P} \models \Psi$ if and only if the atom $\langle init, X \rangle$ is not in the greatest model of $\mathcal{P}^{\Phi}$, where $\Phi = \widetilde{\Psi}$ and X is the root variable of Φ.*

9   Implementation

Since model checking $\mathcal{P}$ for an (unbounded) liveness property Ψ reduces to checking whether $\langle init, X \rangle$ is contained in the greatest model of $\mathcal{P}^{\Phi}$ (as constructed above), it can be done by computing the greatest fixpoint of the immediate consequence operator for $\mathcal{P}^{\Phi}$. This results in a global model checker. Alternately, since the clauses in $\mathcal{P}^{\Phi}$ have at most one predicate in the body (from the construction of the program), we introduce a new greatest model resolution with tabling[1] prove that $\langle init, X \rangle$ is in the greatest model of $\mathcal{P}^{\Phi}$. To the best of the knowledge of the authors, this is the first time any kind of tabling (without negation) is used for the greatest model of a constraint query language program. The greatest model resolution algorithm with tabling is given in Figure 3. In Figure 3, by $\langle pred(\boldsymbol{x}), \varphi \rangle \xrightarrow{C} \langle pred'(\boldsymbol{x}), \varphi' \rangle$, we mean that $\langle pred'(\boldsymbol{x}), \varphi' \rangle$ is the resolvent of $\langle pred(\boldsymbol{x}), \varphi \rangle$ and the clause C where $pred$ denotes a predicate symbol. In step 4(b)i of the algorithm we check whether there exists a goal $\langle pred'(\boldsymbol{x}), \varphi'' \rangle$ in the table such that φ'' entails the constraint store φ' of the newly generated goal $\langle pred'(\boldsymbol{x}), \varphi' \rangle$. In this case, we do not need to register the solutions into the table. We will terminate at the first instance of a success leaf or the first instance when a newly generated goal contains a goal already in the table (whichever occurs earlier). Note that in the above implementation, use of negation along with

---

[1] Note that the tabling used here is different from that used in section 5 as well as those in [CW96,TS86].

tabled resolution for least model would have resulted in splitting of constraints which is prohibitively expensive in practice.

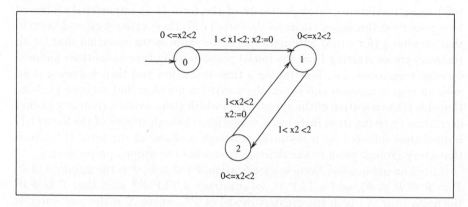

Fig. 2. An example timed automaton

Theorem 5 (Soundness). *If procedure in Figure 3 terminates then* $\langle init, X \rangle$ *is contained in the greatest model of* $\mathcal{P}^{\Phi}$ *if and only if it returns 'yes'.*

Note that procedure in Figure 3 may not terminate. To ensure the termination of the model checking procedure, as in the previous section, we can combine the trim operation described above along with the procedure. The combined algorithm requires polynomial space in the worst case. The details are straightforward. We refer the reader to [MP99] for the details. Using our method, we have been able to verify the unbounded liveness property $X = at\_2 \vee \forall [\![ ] \!] X$ for the example of timed automaton shown in Figure 2 (TLP corresponding to that timed automaton), where the atomic proposition at_2 is satisfied only by the location 2.

The local model checking algorithm given in section 5 and the model checking algorithm for unbounded liveness properties given above can be combined effectively to model check for receptiveness[2] properties. A receptiveness property is a formula of the form $\Phi_1; \Phi_2$, where Φ_1 is a declaration of the form $X = X_1 \vee \exists \Diamond X \vee \exists X$ and Φ_2 is a declaration of the form $X_1 = q \wedge \exists \Diamond X_1$, where we take the least fixpoint for the first declaration and the greatest fixpoint for the second declaration. This asserts that there exists a reachable ground atom p such that there exists an infinite derivation (using resolutions through clauses of the form (1.1) immediately followed by a resolution through a clause of the form (1.2)) starting from p in which every ground atom satisfies q (for timed automata, this amounts to the specification that there exists a reachable position $\tilde{p}$ such that there exists an (infinite) trace starting from $\tilde{p}$ using time transitions followed by edge transitions, i.e., first taking a time transition and then

---

[2] Note that our definition of receptiveness is different from that in [AH97].

Procedure Greatest Model Resolution
Input Program $\mathcal{P}^{\Phi}$ and the atom (0-ary predicate) $\langle init, X \rangle$
Output A yes/no answer whether the atom is in the greatest model of $\mathcal{P}^{\Phi}$
Data Structures
Stack *Table*
Boolean *Flag* = *false*
begin
Push $\langle init, X \rangle$ in *Table*.
repeat

1. Let $\langle pred(x), \varphi \rangle$ be the non-ground goal at the top of the stack *Table*. If $\langle pred(x), \varphi \rangle$ fails (i.e., there does not exist a clause through which it resolves), pop it from *Table* and go to the end of the **repeat-until** loop to check if *Table* is empty. (end **If**)
2. If $\langle pred(x), \varphi \rangle$ succeeds through a clause, make *Flag true*. (end **If**)

3. If *Flag* is *true* return yes.

4. **else**
    (a) Succ:=$\{\langle pred'(x), \varphi' \rangle \mid \langle pred(x), \varphi \rangle \xrightarrow{C} \langle pred'(x), \varphi' \rangle\}$ where C is a clause in $\mathcal{P}^{\Phi}$.
    (b) **for** each element $\langle pred'(x), \varphi' \rangle$ in *Succ* **do**
        i. If there exists $\langle pred'(x), \varphi'' \rangle$ in *Table* such that $\varphi'' \models \varphi'$, make *Flag true*.
        ii. **else** push $\langle pred'(x), \varphi' \rangle$ to *Table*. (end **If**)
    (c) **end for** (end **If**)
5. If *Flag* is *true* return yes. (end **If**)

until *Table* is empty (end of **repeat until**)
return no.
end

Fig. 3. Greatest Model Resolution (GMR) Procedure

following it up by an edge transition and so on, such that every position in that trace satisfies q). Using the combination mentioned above, we have been able to falsify the receptiveness property for the example in Figure 2 with $q = \neg at\_2$. The model checker UPPAAL [BLL+96] does not seem to be able to verify receptiveness properties. We leave the details of model checking for receptiveness properties to the full paper.

10   Related Work

Logic-based methods for specification and verification are slowly gaining popularity. In the past few years there has been a lot of work on model checking using deductive methods [RRR+97,GGV99]. While most of these works have been focussed on finite state systems, there has also been substantial work on verification of integer-valued and parameterized systems using methods based on logic [FR96,FP93,RKR+00]. Bjorner et.al. [BBC+96] use the theorem prover STEP to verify real time systems.

The works from the logic programming, theorem proving and database community that come closest to our work are [CDD+98,GP97,Fri98,Urb96]. In [CDD+98], real time systems were translated into constraint logic programs. But no detailed model checking results based on such a translation has been provided. Gupta and Pontelli in [GP97] have been able to verify several interesting properties of real time systems. In contrast with automated model checking methods, they rely on the programmer to write a "driver" routine to identify the finite number of finite repeating patterns in the infinite strings accepted by a timed automaton. In a recent paper, Gupta and Pontelli [GP99] describe definite clause grammar for the model checker UPPAAL. In an interesting approach, they use Horn logic denotational semantics framework for specifying, implementing and automatically verifying real time systems. But in their approach, they have to make sure that the verification of properties leads to finite computations. Gupta [Gup99] extends the methods of [GP97] to more general settings.

Fribourg in [Fri98] verifies real time systems specified by logic programs with gap constraints. This work only considers reachability problems for real time systems. Termination is always guaranteed here because a backward analysis is used (industrial-scale tools like UPPAAL use forward analysis in spite of a missing termination guarantee [LPY95]).

Urbina in [Urb96] baptizes a class of CLP programs hybrid automata without, however, establishing a formal connection with the standard model for timed systems. In fact, the semantics results in [Urb96] cannot be connected with liveness properties of timed automata, in contrast to our work on TLPs.

The works from the verification community that come closest to our work are [LPY95,DT98,SS95]. The model checking method in [LPY95] based on the rewrite tree can be viewed as a special case of our model checking procedure based on OLDT resolution extended to constraints. We have been able to model check for a logic which is strictly more expressive than that in [LPY95]. Also, the model checker UPPAAL [BLL+96] does not seem to be able to model check for receptiveness properties that we have been able to model check for. In [DT98] Daws and Tripakis present a global model checking procedure for real time systems. In contrast, ours is a local one. Also, their method can be used only for model checking "reachability" properties like safety while we have given methods to deal with unbounded liveness properties. Sokolsky and Smolka [SS95] present a local model checker for real time systems. But, as mentioned in the Introduction, their method for ensuring termination is based on an expensive "splitting" of constraints. We have also not received any report on the performance of their model checker on any practical example. Du, Ramakrishnan and Smolka [DRS99] extend XSB with the POLINE constraint library to verify real time systems. But they follow the same techniques as [SS95] and hence they also ensure termination using expensive splitting of constraints.

References

[AD94]   R. Alur and D. Dill. A theory of timed automata. *Theoretical Computer Science*, 126(2):183–236, 1994.

[AH97]   R. Alur and T. A. Henzinger. Modularity for timed and hybrid systems. In A. Mazurkiewicz and J. Winkowski, editors, *CONCUR'97: Concurrency Theory*, volume 1243 of *LNCS*, pages 74–88. Springer-Verlag, 1997.

[BBC+96] N. Bjorner, A. Browne, E. Chang, M. Colon, A. Kapur, Z. Manna, H. Sipma, and T. Uribe. Step: Deductive-algorithmic verification of reactive and real-time systems. In R. Alur and T. A. Henzinger, editors, *CAV'96: Computer Aided Verification*, volume 1102 of *LNCS*, pages 415–418. Springer-Verlag, 1996.

[BLL+96] Johan Bengtsson, Kim. G. Larsen, Fredrik Larsson, Paul Petersson, and Wang Yi. Uppaal in 1995. In T. Margaria and B. Steffen, editors, *TACAS*, LNCS 1055, pages 431–434. Springer-Verlag, 1996.

[BS91]   A. Brodsky and Y. Sagiv. Inference of inequality constraints in logic programs. In *PODS: Principles of Database Systems*, pages 227–240. ACM Press, 1991.

[CDD+98] B. Cui, Y. Dong, X. Du, K. N. Kumar, C. R. Ramakrishnan, I. V. Ramakrishnan, A. Roychoudhury, S. A. Smolka, and D. S. Warren. Logic programming and model checking. In *PLAP/ALP98*, volume 1490 of *LNCS*, pages 1–20. Springer-Verlag, 1998.

[CW96]   W. Chen and D. S. Warren. Tabled evaluation with delaying for general logic programs. *JACM*, 43(1):20–74, 1996.

[DRS99]   Xiaoqun Du, C. R. Ramakrishnan, and Scott. A. Smolka. Tabled resolution + constraints: A recipe for model checking real-time systems, 1999. Submitted.

[DT98]   C. Daws and S. Tripakis. Model checking of real-time reachability properties using abstractions. In Bernhard Steffen, editor, *TACAS98: Tools and Algorithms for the Construction of Systems*, LNCS 1384, pages 313–329. Springer-Verlag, March/April 1998.

[DW99]   M. Dickhöfer and T. Wilke. Timed alternating tree automata: The automata-theoretic solution to the tctl model checking problem. In J. Widermann, P. van Emde Boas, and M. Nielsen, editors, *ICALP: Automata, Languages and Programming*, volume 1644 of *LNCS*, pages 281–290. Springer-Verlag, 1999.

[FP93]   Laurent Fribourg and Marcos Veloso Peixoto. Concurrent constraint automata. Technical Report LIENS 93-10, ENS Paris, 1993.

[FR96]   L. Fribourg and J. Richardson. Symbolic verification with gap-order constraints. In J. P. Gallagher, editor, *LOPSTR'96: Logic Based Program Synthesis and Transformation*, volume 1207 of *LNCS*, pages 20–37. Springer-Verlag, 1996.

[Fri98]   Laurent Fribourg. A closed-form evaluation for extended timed automata. Technical report, ENS Cachan, 1998.

[GGV99]   G. Gottlob, E. Grädel, and H. Veith. Datalog lite: A deductive approach to verification. Technical report, Technische Universität Wien, 1999.

[GP97]   G. Gupta and E. Pontelli. A constraint-based approach for the specification and verification of real-time systems. In Kwei-Jay Lin, editor, *IEEE Real-Time Systems Symposium*, pages 230–239. IEEE Press, 1997.

[GP99]   Gopal Gupta and Enrico Pontelli. A horn logic denotational framework for specification, implementation, and verification of domain specific languages, March 1999.

[Gup99]   Gopal Gupta. Horn logic denotations and their applications. In *The Logic Programming Paradigm: A 25 year perspective*. Springer-Verlag, 1999.

[HWT95]   Pei-Hsin Ho and Howard Wong-Toi. Automated analysis of an audio control protocol. In P. Wolper, editor, *the Seventh Conference on Computer-Aided Verification*, pages 381–394, Liege, Belgium, 1995. Springer-Verlag. LNCS 939.

[JM94]   J. Jaffar and M. J. Maher. Constraint logic programming: A survey. *The Journal of Logic Programming*, 19/20:503–582, May-July 1994.

[JMSY92]   J. Jaffar, S. Michaylov, P.J. Stuckey, and R.H.C. Yap. The clp(r) language and system. *ACM Transactions on Programming Languages and Systems*, 14(3):339–395, 1992.

[KKR95]   P. C. Kanellakis, G. M. Kuper, and P. Z. Revesz. Constraint query languages. *Journal of Computer and System Sciences*, 51:26–52, 1995. (Preliminary version in *Proc. 9th ACM PODS*, 299–313, 1990.).

[LPY95]   K. G. Larsen, P. Peterson, and W. Yi. Model-checking for real-time systems. In Horst Reichel, editor, *Fundamentals of Computation Theory*, volume 965 of *LNCS*, pages 62–88. Springer-Verlag, 1995.

[Mil89]   Robin Milner. *Communication and Concurrency*. Prentice Hall, 1989.

[MP99]   Supratik Mukhopadhyay and Andreas Podelski. Model checking for timed logic processes, 1999. Available at http://www.mpi-sb.mpg.de/~supratik/.

[Rev90]   Peter Revesz. A closed form for datalog queries with integer order. In S. Abiteboul and P. C'. Kanellakis, editors, *ICDT: the International Conference on Database Theory*, volume 470 of *LNCS*, pages 187–201. Springer-Verlag, 1990.

[RKR+00]   A. Roychoudhury, K. N. Kumar, C. R. Ramakrishnan, I. V. Ramakrishnan, and S. A. Smolka. Verification of parameterized systems using logic program transformations. In *TACAS'00: Tools and Algorithms for the Construction and Analysis of Systems*, volume 1785 of *LNCS*, pages 172–187. Springer, 2000.

[RRR+97]   Y. S. Ramakrishna, C. R. Ramakrishnan, I. V Ramakrishnan, S. A. Smolka, T. W. Swift, and D. S. Warren. Efficient model checking using tabled resolution. In O. Grumberg, editor, *the 9th International Conference on Computer-Aided-Verification*, pages 143–154. Springer-Verlag, July 1997.

[SS95]   Oleg Sokolsky and Scott. A. Smolka. Local model checking for real-time systems. In Pierre Wolper, editor, *7th International Conference on Computer-Aided Verification*, volume 939 of *LNCS*, pages 211–224. Springer-Verlag, July 1995.

[TS86]   Hisao Tamaki and Taisuke Sato. Old resolution with tabulation. In *International Conference on Logic Programming*, LNCS, pages 84–98. Springer-Verlag, 1986.

[Urb96]   L. Urbina. Analysis of hybrid systems in clp(r). In *Principles and Practice of Constraint Programming, CP96*, Lectures Notes in Computer Science 1118, pages 451–467. Springer-Verlag, 1996.

[Vie87]   L. Vielle. A database-complete proof procedure based on sld-resolution. In *Fourth International Conference on Logic Programming*. MIT Press, 1987.

Perfect Model Checking
via Unfold/Fold Transformations

Alberto Pettorossi[1] and Maurizio Proietti[2]

[1] DISP, University of Roma Tor Vergata, Roma, Italy
adp@iasi.rm.cnr.it
[2] IASI-CNR, Roma, Italy
proietti@iasi.rm.cnr.it

Abstract. We show how unfold/fold program transformation techniques may be used for proving that a closed first order formula holds in the perfect model of a logic program with locally stratified negation. We present a program transformation strategy which is a decision procedure for some given classes of programs and formulas.

1   Introduction

One of the main motivations of this paper is to better understand the relationship between unfold/fold program transformation [4, 20] and theorem proving. It is usually recognized that folding steps during program transformation correspond to applications of inductive hypotheses during proofs by induction, and goal replacements correspond to lemma applications.

Some transformational techniques for proving equivalence properties of functional and logic programs have already been presented in [8, 11] and [13, 17], respectively. In this paper we extend these techniques by introducing a method for proving that a closed first order formula φ holds in the perfect model $M(P)$ [1, 15] of a locally stratified logic program P. This property is denoted by $M(P) \models \varphi$.

Our proof method for showing that $M(P) \models \varphi$ holds, consists of two steps:
Step 1: we use a variant of the Lloyd-Topor transformation [12] for transforming a statement of the form: $f \leftarrow \varphi$ where f is a new predicate symbol, into a conjunction $F(f, \varphi)$ of clauses such that $P \wedge F(f, \varphi)$ is locally stratified and $M(P) \models \varphi$ iff $M(P \wedge F(f, \varphi)) \models f$, and
Step 2: we show that $M(P \wedge F(f, \varphi)) \models f$ holds by applying transformation rules which preserve perfect models, and deriving from $P \wedge F(f, \varphi)$ a new program of the form: $Q \wedge f$.

We illustrate our proof method by means of the following example.
Example. [*Semaphore*] Consider the following program P, where $s \ldots s0$ with n occurrences of the successor function s, denotes the natural number n:

1. $down(sx) \leftarrow \neg down(x)$		3. $up(sx, 0) \leftarrow down(x)$
2. $up(0, 0)$		4. $up(sx, sy) \leftarrow up(sx, y), x > y$

This program describes a semaphore which as time progresses, alternates between the states *up* and *down*. When the semaphore goes *up* for the n-th time, it stays *up* for a period of $2n$ time-units, and when it goes *down*, it stays

J. Lloyd et al. (Eds.): CL 2000, LNAI 1861, pp. 613–628, 2000.

down for one time-unit only. We want to prove the following property of the semaphore: (A) $\forall x, y\,((x > y,\ up(x, y)) \rightarrow up(ssx, 0))$, which states that if the semaphore is *up* then it will be *up* again in the future. We start from the statement: $f \leftarrow (\forall x, y\,(x > y,\ up(x, y)) \rightarrow up(ssx, 0))$. By applying a variant of the Lloyd-Topor transformation (see Section 3), we get the clauses:

5. $f \leftarrow \neg g$ 6. $g \leftarrow x > y,\ up(x, y),\ \neg up(ssx, 0)$

This concludes Step 1 of our proof method. Step 2 is realized by applying transformation rules which preserve perfect models (see Section 4). We proceed by introducing the following two definitions: (i) $h \leftarrow x > y,\ up(sx, y),\ \neg up(sssx, 0)$ and (ii) $k(n) \leftarrow x > z,\ plus(y, n, z),\ up(sx, y),\ \neg up(sssx, 0)$.

By positive and negative unfolding, folding, and goal replacement, we get the program $Q :\ f \leftarrow \neg g,\ g \leftarrow h,\ h \leftarrow k(s0),\ k(n) \leftarrow k(sn)$. Now, since k is a useless predicate being defined by the recursive clause $k(n) \leftarrow k(sn)$ without a base case, we may apply the clause deletion rule (see rule R6 in Section 4) and we get the program $R :\ f \leftarrow \neg g,\ g \leftarrow h,\ h \leftarrow k(s0)$. This step is correct because in the perfect model of program R there are no atoms with predicate k.

Then, since the definition of the predicate k in program R is empty, we delete clause $h \leftarrow k(s0)$ by unfolding it w.r.t. $k(s0)$. Analogously, we delete the clause $g \leftarrow h$ by unfolding it w.r.t. h. Thus, the derived program consists of clause $f \leftarrow \neg g$ only. Finally, by unfolding $f \leftarrow \neg g$ w.r.t. $\neg g$ we get f, because the definition of g in the derived program is empty. This completes our transformational proof of Property (A).   □

The tight correspondence between program transformation and theorem proving can also be exploited to turn program transformation strategies into proof strategies. In particular, at Step 2 of our proof method, in order to direct the transformation rules, we may use the so called UFS strategy (see Section 5) which is an enhancement of a transformation strategy proposed in [14]. When our UFS strategy terminates, it derives from $P \wedge F(f, \varphi)$ *either* (i) a new program of the form $Q \wedge f$, in which case $M(P) \models \varphi$, *or* (ii) a program R where no clause has head predicate f, in which case $M(P) \not\models \varphi$, because $M(P) \models \varphi$ iff $M(P \wedge F(f, \varphi)) \models f$ iff $M(R) \models f$ and f does not hold in the perfect model of R. We will show that the UFS strategy terminates for some classes of properties and some classes of logic programs with locally stratified negation, and thus, it can be used as a decision procedure for those classes.

2   Preliminaries

In this section we recall some basic definitions used in the paper. For notions not defined here and, in particular, for those of *stratum, locally stratified logic program*, and *perfect model*, the reader may refer to [1, 12, 15].

The formulas and programs we consider are constructed by using a fixed first-order language $\mathcal{L}$. Logic programs are conjunctions of clauses which may have negated atoms in their bodies. A goal is a conjunction of literals. The empty goal is *true*. The *head* and the *body* of a clause C are denoted by $hd(C)$ and $bd(C)$, respectively. The predicate symbol of the atom $hd(C)$ is called the *head predicate* of C. Given a term t we denote by $vars(t)$ the set of all variables occurring in t. Similar notations will be used for the variables occurring in formulas. Given a clause C, a variable in $bd(C)$ is said to be *existential* iff it belongs to $vars(bd(C)) - vars(hd(C))$. Given a formula φ we denote by $freevars(\varphi)$ the set of all free variables of φ. A literal is said to be *propositional* iff its predicate symbol is nullary, that is, it has arity 0. A goal (or a clause, or a program) is propositional iff all its literals are propositional. A formula is said to be *function-free* iff no function symbols occur in it.

We say that a predicate p *depends on* a predicate q in P iff either there exists in P a clause of the form: $p(\ldots) \leftarrow B$ such that q occurs in the goal B or there exists in P a predicate r such that p depends on r in P and r depends on q in P. The *definition* of a predicate p in a program P, denoted by $Def(p, P)$, is the conjunction of all clauses of P whose head predicate is p. We say that p *is defined in* P iff $Def(p, P)$ is not empty. The *extended definition* of a predicate p in a program P, denoted by $Def^*(p, P)$, is the conjunction of the definition of p and the definitions of all the predicates on which p depends in P. The set of the *useless* predicates of a program P is the maximal set U of predicates of P such that a predicate p is in U iff the body of each clause of $Def(p, P)$ has a positive literal whose predicate is in U. For instance, p and q are useless and r is not useless in the program $(p \leftarrow q, r) \wedge (q \leftarrow p) \wedge (r \leftarrow)$.

3   From First-Order Formulas to Logic Programs

In this section we present a method that given a locally stratified program P and a closed first order formula φ in the language $\mathcal{L}$, introduces a new predicate f and constructs a locally stratified program $P \wedge F(f, \varphi)$ such that $M(P) \models \varphi$ iff $M(P \wedge F(f, \varphi)) \models f$.

In order to construct $F(f, \varphi)$ we need to consider a class of formulas, called *statements* [12], of the form $A \leftarrow \beta$ where A is an atom and β, called the body of the statement, is a (possibly open) first-order logic formula. We write $C[\gamma]$ to denote a first-order formula where the subformula γ occurs as a conjunct 'at top level', that is, $C[\gamma] = \rho_1 \wedge \ldots \wedge \rho_r \wedge \gamma \wedge \sigma_1 \wedge \ldots \wedge \sigma_s$ for some first-order formulas $\rho_1, \ldots, \rho_r, \sigma_1, \ldots, \sigma_s$, and some $r \geq 0$ and $s \geq 0$. When we say that the formula $C[\gamma]$ is transformed into the formula $C[\delta]$, we mean that $C[\delta]$ is obtained from $C[\gamma]$ by replacing the top level conjunct γ by the new top level conjunct δ.

Given a conjunction of statements the following LT transformation, similar to the one proposed in [12], terminates and it produces a locally stratified program. **The LT Transformation.**

Given a conjunction of statements, perform the following transformations:

(A) Eliminate from the body of every statement all occurrences of logical constants, connectives, and quantifiers other than $true, \neg, \wedge$, and $\exists$. For every statement st, rename the bound variables of st so that none of them occurs in $freevars(st)$ and all of them are distinct.

(B) Apply *as long as possible* the following rules:

(B.1) $A \leftarrow C[\neg true]$ is deleted

(B.2) $A \leftarrow C[\neg\neg\varphi]$ is transformed into $A \leftarrow C[\varphi]$

(B.3) $A \leftarrow C[\neg(\varphi \wedge \psi)]$ is transformed into $A \leftarrow C[\neg newp(y_1, \ldots, y_k)] \wedge$
$$newp(y_1, \ldots, y_k) \leftarrow \varphi \wedge \psi$$

where $\varphi \neq true$, $\psi \neq true$, $newp$ is a new predicate symbol, and
$\{y_1, \ldots, y_k\} = freevars(\varphi \wedge \psi)$.

(B.4) $A \leftarrow C[\neg \exists x\, \varphi]$ is transformed into $A \leftarrow C[\neg newp(y_1, \ldots, y_k)] \wedge$
$$newp(y_1, \ldots, y_k) \leftarrow \varphi$$

where $newp$ is a new predicate symbol and $\{y_1, \ldots, y_k\} = freevars(\exists x\, \varphi)$.

(B.5) $A \leftarrow C[\exists x\, \varphi]$ is transformed into $A \leftarrow C[\varphi]$ □

Given a locally stratified program P and a closed first-order formula φ, we denote by $F(f, \varphi)$ the conjunction of the clauses derived by applying the LT transformation to the statement $f \leftarrow \varphi$, where f is a new predicate symbol occurring neither in φ nor in P. We assume that the new predicates introduced during the construction of $F(f, \varphi)$ do not occur in P.

The reader may verify that in the Semaphore Example of Section 1, clauses 5 and 6 have been derived by applying the LT transformation starting from the following statement: $f \leftarrow \forall x, y\,((x > y,\, up(x, y)) \rightarrow up(ssx, 0))$. The following result states that the LT transformation is correct w.r.t. the perfect model semantics, thereby extending the result by Lloyd and Topor, who showed that their transformation is correct w.r.t. the Clark completion semantics. Thus, Step 1 of our proof method is sound.

Theorem 1. [Correctness of LT Transformation w.r.t. Perfect Models]
Let P be a locally stratified program, φ be a closed first-order formula, and f be a predicate symbol occurring neither in φ nor in P. If $F(f, \varphi)$ is obtained from $f \leftarrow \varphi$ by the LT transformation, then (i) $P \wedge F(f, \varphi)$ is a locally stratified program, and (ii) $M(P) \models \varphi$ iff $M(P \wedge F(f, \varphi)) \models f$.   □

4   Transformation Rules

In this section we present our transformation rules and we provide a sufficient condition under which they preserve perfect models. We extend the results in [19] which refers to the definition, positive unfolding, and folding rules only.

A *transformation sequence* is a sequence of programs $P_0, \ldots, P_n$, where, for $0 \leq k \leq n-1$, program P_{k+1} is derived from program P_k by the application of a transformation rule as indicated below. We assume that the set of predicate symbols of the language is partitioned into two categories: *basic* predicates and *non-basic* predicates. Atoms, literals, and goals which have occurrences of basic predicates only, are called *basic atoms*, *basic literals*, and *basic goals*, respectively. We assume that each basic atom is in a strictly smaller stratum w.r.t. any non-basic atom. The partition of the set of predicates into basic or non-basic predicates is arbitrary.

For $0 \leq k \leq n$, we also consider the conjunction $Defs_k$ of *definitions*, constructed as follows:

(1) $Defs_0$ is the conjunction of every clause C in program P_0 of the form $p(x_1, \ldots, x_m) \leftarrow L_1, \ldots, L_n$, with $n > 0$ such that: (i) $x_1, \ldots, x_m$ are distinct variables (possibly not all variables) occurring in the goal $L_1, \ldots, L_n$, (ii) at least one literal among $L_1, \ldots, L_n$ is a non-basic positive literal, (iii) no predicate symbol occurring in the goal $L_1, \ldots, L_n$ depends on p in P_0, and (iv) $C = Def(p, P_0)$; (2) for $k > 0$, $Defs_k$ is the conjunction of the clauses in $Defs_0$ and those introduced by the definition rule R1 during the transformation sequence $P_0, \ldots, P_k$.

R1. Definition Rule. We get program P_{k+1} by adding to program P_k a clause C of the form: $newp(x_1, \ldots, x_m) \leftarrow L_1, \ldots, L_n$, with $n > 0$, such that: (i) $x_1, \ldots, x_m$ are distinct variables occurring in $L_1, \ldots, L_n$, (ii) at least one literal among $L_1, \ldots, L_n$ is a non-basic positive literal, and (iii) the predicate symbol $newp$ is a non-basic predicate occurs neither in $P_0, \ldots, P_k$ nor in the goal $L_1, \ldots, L_n$.

R2. Positive Unfolding Rule. Let C be a renamed apart clause in P_k of the form $H \leftarrow G_1, A, G_2$, where A is an atom, and G_1 and G_2 are (possibly empty) goals. Suppose that: (1) $D_1, \ldots, D_m$, with $m \geq 0$, are all clauses of program P_k, such that A is unifiable with $hd(D_1), \ldots, hd(D_m)$, with most general unifiers $\theta_1, \ldots, \theta_m$, respectively, and (2) C_i is the clause $(H \leftarrow G_1, bd(D_i), G_2)\theta_i$, for $i = 1, \ldots, m$. By *unfolding* C w.r.t. A we derive program P_{k+1} by replacing C in program P_k by $C_1, \ldots, C_m$.

In particular, if $m = 0$ then we derive P_{k+1} by deleting clause C from P_k.

R3. Negative Unfolding Rule. Let C be a renamed apart clause in P_k of the form $H \leftarrow G_1, \neg A, G_2$, where A is an atom, and G_1 and G_2 are (possibly empty) goals. Let $D_1, \ldots, D_m$, with $m \geq 0$, be all clauses of program P_k, such that A is unifiable with $hd(D_1), \ldots, hd(D_m)$, with most general unifiers $\theta_1, \ldots, \theta_m$, respectively. Assume that: (1) $A = hd(D_1)\theta_1 = \cdots = hd(D_m)\theta_m$, that is, for $i = 1, \ldots, m$, A is an instance of $hd(D_i)$, (2) for $i = 1, \ldots, m$, D_i has no existential variables, and (3) from $G_1, \neg(bd(D_1)\theta_1 \vee \ldots \vee bd(D_m)\theta_m), G_2$ we get an equivalent disjunction $Q_1 \vee \ldots \vee Q_r$ of goals, with $r \geq 0$, by first pushing $\neg$ inside and then pushing $\vee$ outside. By *unfolding* C w.r.t. $\neg A$ we derive program P_{k+1} by replacing C in program P_k by $C_1, \ldots, C_r$, where for $i = 1, \ldots, r$, clause C_i is $H \leftarrow Q_i$.

In particular: (i) if $m = 0$ then we get the new program P_{k+1} by deleting $\neg A$ from the body of clause C, and (ii) if for some $i \in 1, \ldots, m$, $bd(D_i) = true$ then we derive program P_{k+1} by deleting clause C from P_k.

R4. Folding Rule. Let D be a renamed apart definition in $Defs_k$ and C be a clause in P_k of the form $H \leftarrow G_1, B, G_2$, where B, G_1, and G_2 are (possibly empty) goals. Suppose that for some substitution θ: (i) $B = bd(D)\theta$, and (ii) for every variable x in the set $vars(D) - vars(hd(D))$, we have that $x\theta$ is a variable which occurs neither in $\{H, G_1, G_2\}$ nor in the term $y\theta$, for any variable y occurring in $bd(D)$ and different from x. By *folding* clause C w.r.t. B using clause D we derive the clause $E : H \leftarrow G_1, hd(D)\theta, G_2$ and we get program P_{k+1} by replacing C in P_k by E.

R5. Tautology Rule. We get the new program P_{k+1} by replacing in P_k a conjunction of clauses by the corresponding equivalent conjunction of clauses,

according to the following equivalences, where G and R denote (possibly empty) goals, and H and A denote atoms: 1. $(H \leftarrow A, \neg A, G) \leftrightarrow true$
2. $(H \leftarrow G, \quad H \leftarrow G, R) \leftrightarrow (H \leftarrow G)$ 3. $(H \leftarrow H, G) \leftrightarrow true$
4. $(H \leftarrow A, G, R, \quad H \leftarrow \neg A, G) \leftrightarrow (H \leftarrow G, R, \quad H \leftarrow \neg A, G)$

R6. Clause Deletion Rule. We get the new program P_{k+1} by removing from P_k the definitions of the useless predicates of P_k.

R7. Goal Replacement Rule. Let C be a renamed apart clause in P_k of form $H \leftarrow G_1, Q, G_2$, where Q, G_1, and G_2 are (possibly empty) goals. Suppose that, for some goal R, we have: $M(P_0) \models \forall x_1 \ldots x_u (\exists y_1 \ldots y_v \ Q \leftrightarrow \exists z_1 \ldots z_w \ R)$ where: (i) $\{y_1, \ldots, y_v\} = vars(Q) - vars(H, G_1, G_2)$, (ii) $\{z_1, \ldots, z_w\} = vars(R) - vars(H, G_1, G_2)$, and (iii) $\{x_1, \ldots, x_u\} = vars(Q, R) - \{y_1, \ldots, y_v, z_1, \ldots, z_w\}$. Suppose also that Q and R are basic goals and H is a non-basic atom. Then we derive program P_{k+1} by replacing C in P_k by the clause $H \leftarrow G_1, R, G_2$.

Theorem 2. [Correctness of the Transformation Rules] Let $P_0, \ldots, P_n$, be a transformation sequence such that the following holds: *if* for some k with $1 \leq k < n$, we have applied rule R4 for folding clause C in P_k using clause D in $P_0 \wedge Defs_k$, *then* there exists i, with $0 \leq i < k$ such that D occurs in P_i and P_{i+1} is derived from P_i by positive unfolding of D w.r.t. a non-basic atom. Then we have that $M(P_0 \wedge Defs_n) = M(P_n)$.   □

Notice that the statement obtained from Theorem 2 by replacing 'positive unfolding' by 'negative unfolding' is not a theorem, as shown by the following example. Let P_0 be the program $(p \leftarrow \neg q(x)) \wedge (q(x) \leftarrow q(x)) \wedge (q(x) \leftarrow r)$. By negative unfolding w.r.t. $\neg q(x)$ we get program P_1: $(p \leftarrow \neg q(x), \neg r) \wedge (q(x) \leftarrow q(x)) \wedge (q(x) \leftarrow r)$. Then by folding we get program P_2: $(p \leftarrow p, \neg r) \wedge (q(x) \leftarrow q(x)) \wedge (q(x) \leftarrow r)$. We have that $M(P_0) \models p$, while $M(P_2) \models \neg p$.

5   A Strategy for Unfold/Fold Proofs

In order to verify whether or not $M(P) \models \varphi$ holds, Step 2 of our unfold/fold proof method requires the construction of a transformation sequence from program $P \wedge F(f, \varphi)$ to a new program, say T, such that *either* (i) $Def(f, T)$ is f, and in this case we infer that $M(P) \models \varphi$, or (ii) T is a program where $Def(f, T)$ is the empty conjunction, and in this case we infer that $M(P) \not\models \varphi$. To construct this transformation sequence we need a strategy for guiding the application of the transformation rules. In this section we present such a strategy, called UFS (short for Unfold/Fold proof Strategy). The UFS strategy is an extension of the strategy introduced in the case of definite logic programs for eliminating existential variables [14]. The basic idea is that by eliminating existential variables, from $P \wedge F(f, \varphi)$ we may derive a program, say S, such that $Def^*(f, S)$ is a *propositional* program. Then, we can transform S by using the clause deletion, unfolding, tautology, and goal replacement rules, into a program T satisfying either (i) or (ii) above. Obviously, since in general $M(P) \models \varphi$ is an undecidable property, our UFS strategy may fail to produce a propositional program.

For specifying the UFS strategy, we need the following definition [12].

Definition 1. A *level mapping* of a program P is a mapping from the set of predicate symbols occurring in P to the set of natural numbers. The *level* of predicate p is the value of p under this mapping.

By the definition of the LT transformation there exists a level mapping of $P \wedge F(f, \varphi)$ such that: (i) the level of every predicate defined in P is 0, (ii) the level of every predicate defined in $F(f, \varphi)$ is greater than 0, (iii) for each clause $p(\ldots) \leftarrow B$ in $F(f, \varphi)$ the level of every predicate in B is strictly smaller than the level of p, and (iv) the predicate f has the highest level, say K. For instance, in the Semaphore Example we may choose the level mapping m as follows: $m(down) = m(up) = m(>) = 0$, $m(g) = 1$, and $m(f) = 2$ (thus, $K = 2$).

The UFS strategy requires three substrategies: (1) UNFOLD, (2) TAUTOLOGY & REPLACE, and (3) DEFINE & FOLD, which we will specify below for the classes of programs and formulas for which the UFS strategy terminates.

The Unfold/Fold Proof Strategy UFS.

Input: (i) $P \wedge F(f, \varphi)$, where P is a locally stratified program and φ is a closed first order formula, and (ii) a set *Laws* of equivalences of the form: $M(P) \models \forall x_1 \ldots x_u (\exists y_1 \ldots y_v \, Q \leftrightarrow \exists z_1 \ldots z_w \, R)$, where Q and R are basic goals.
Output: A program T such that: (i) $M(T) \models f$ iff $M(P \wedge F(f, \varphi)) \models f$, and (ii) $Def(f, T)$ is either f or the empty conjunction.

Let $P \wedge F(f, \varphi)$ be $P \wedge P^1 \wedge \ldots \wedge P^K$, where for $i = 1, \ldots, K$, program P^i is the conjunction of the clauses whose head predicate has level i. $T := P$;
for $i = 1, \ldots, K$ **do**
Let *Pos* be the conjunction of the clauses of P^i whose body has at least one non-basic positive literal, and *Neg* be the conjunction of the clauses of P^i which are not in *Pos*. Let *Defs* be *Pos* and *Out* be the empty conjunction.
while *Pos* is not the empty conjunction **do**   (†)
(1) UNFOLD(T, *Pos*, U): From program $T \wedge Pos$ we derive $T \wedge U$ by a finite sequence of applications of the positive or negative unfolding rules to the clauses in *Pos*. We require that:
[*Progression*] the positive unfolding rule is applied at least once to each clause in *Pos*.
(2) TAUTOLOGY & REPLACE(T, *Laws*, U, R): From program $T \wedge U$ we derive $T \wedge R$ by a finite sequence of applications of the tautology and goal replacement rules to the clauses in U, using the equivalences in the set *Laws*.
(3) DEFINE & FOLD(T, R, *Defs*, *OutClauses*, *NewDefs*): From program $T \wedge R$ we derive $T \wedge OutClauses \wedge NewDefs$ by: (i) a finite sequence of applications of the definition rule by which we introduce the (possibly empty) conjunction *NewDefs* of clauses, followed by (ii) a finite sequence of applications of the folding rule to the clauses in R, using clauses occurring in *Defs* $\wedge$ *NewDefs*. We assume that the following conditions are satisfied:
(3.1) [*Positive definitions*] The body of each clause in *NewDefs* has at least one non-basic positive literal.
(3.2) [*No existential variables*] Each clause in *OutClauses* which has been derived by folding has no existential variables.

(3.3) [*Full Folding*] Each predicate in the body of each clause in *OutClauses* which has been derived by folding, occurs in $Defs \wedge NewDefs$.

$Out := Out \wedge OutClauses$; $Pos := NewDefs$; $Defs := Defs \wedge NewDefs$ **od**;

Delete from Out the definitions of useless predicates, thereby deriving Out';

$T := T \wedge Out' \wedge Neg$;

Initialize D to the conjunction of all definitions of nullary predicates in T;

Initialize Q to the conjunction of all definitions of non-nullary predicates in T;

while D is a not a conjunction of unit clauses **do**   (‡)

UNFOLD(Q, D, U): From program $Q \wedge D$ we derive $Q \wedge U$ by a (possibly empty) sequence of applications of the positive or negative unfolding rules to the clauses in D. (Here the Progression requirement need not be satisfied.)

TAUTOLOGY & REPLACE$(Q, Laws, U, R)$; $D := R$ **od**;

Unfold the clauses of Q w.r.t. their propositional literals, thereby deriving Q';   (‡‡‡)

$T := Q' \wedge D$ **end for**   □

Our UFS strategy proceeds by iterating over levels (from level 1 to level K) a sequence of transformations on the program T, which initially is P. For $i = 1, \ldots, K$, the conjunction of the clauses defining the predicates with level i, that is, program P^i, is processed by the UFS strategy, and the WHILE loop (†) generates from program $T \wedge P^i$ (which is $T \wedge Neg \wedge Pos$) the new program T. The objective of the WHILE loop (†) is: (i) to ensure that positive unfolding steps w.r.t. non-basic atoms are performed before folding, and (ii) to avoid existential variables via definition and folding steps. Then useless predicates are deleted. Finally, the WHILE loop (‡) performs unfolding, tautology, and goal replacement steps on the definitions of nullary predicates so to reduce each of them, if possible, either to the empty definition (in which case the corresponding predicate is *false*) or to a unit clause (in which case the corresponding predicate is *true*). The truth values of the propositional predicates are then propagated by the unfolding steps (‡‡‡). When the last program level K has been processed, we get for the predicate f either the empty definition or the clause f. Thus, we may establish whether or not $M(P \wedge F(f, \varphi)) \models f$ holds.

The soundness of our proof strategy follows from the fact that the transformation rules are used in such a way that the hypothesis of the Correctness Theorem of Section 4 holds. The UFS strategy may not terminate, because in general $M(P \wedge F(f, \varphi)) \models f$ is undecidable. Indeed, (i) during the execution of the WHILE loop (†) we may introduce by applying the definition rule, an infinite number of new clauses, and thus, *Pos* never becomes the empty conjunction, and (ii) the WHILE loop (‡) may not terminate for nullary predicates which depend on non-nullary predicates.

The reader may check that our introductory Semaphore Example has indeed been worked out using the UFS proof strategy.

6   Decision Procedures Based on Unfold/Fold Proofs

Now we present two classes of formulas, called *tree-typed formulas* and *tree-typed clausal formulas*, and two classes of programs, called *MR programs* and

DL programs, for which a deterministic version of the UFS strategy, called dUFS strategy, terminates. Thus, the dUFS strategy is a decision procedure for establishing whether or not $M(P) \models \varphi$ holds, when φ and P are in the given classes.

In this section we assume that all predicates are non-basic. The tree-typed formulas are function-free formulas whose variables range over sets of trees denoted by *tree programs* which we now define.

Definition 2. [Tree Programs] A *tree program* is a conjunction of tree clauses. A *tree clause* is a clause of the form: $r_0(t(x_1, \ldots, x_n)) \leftarrow r_1(x_1), \ldots, r_n(x_n)$, with $n \geq 0$, where t is a function symbol and $x_1, \ldots, x_n$ are distinct variables. A *tree atom* is an atom whose predicate is defined by a tree program.

Definition 3. [Tree-Typed Formulas] A *tree-typed formula* over a program P is a first-order formula φ, defined as follows:
$$\varphi ::= p(x_1, \ldots, x_n) \mid \neg\varphi \mid \varphi_1 \wedge \varphi_2 \mid \varphi_1 \vee \varphi_2 \mid \forall x \, (r(x) \rightarrow \varphi) \mid \exists x \, (r(x) \wedge \varphi)$$
where: (i) $x_1, \ldots, x_n$, with $n \geq 0$, are distinct variables, (ii) all predicates occurring in φ are defined in P, and (iii) $Def^*(r, P)$ is a tree program.

Example. [Even-Odd Paths] Let us consider the following *Even-Odd* program:

1. $bin(leaf)$ 4. $even(t(x, y)) \leftarrow \neg even(x)$
2. $bin(t(x, y)) \leftarrow bin(x), bin(y)$ 5. $even(t(x, y)) \leftarrow \neg even(y)$
3. $even(leaf)$ 6. $odd(t(x, y)) \leftarrow \neg odd(x), \neg odd(y)$

Clauses 1 and 2 are tree clauses. The formula $\forall x \, (bin(x) \rightarrow even(x) \vee odd(x))$ is a tree-typed formula over *Even-Odd*. Informally, the formula means that in every binary tree there exists a path of even length or all paths have odd length. Thus, we expect that $M(P) \models \varphi$ holds, as we will formally prove below.   □

The Tree-Typed LT Transformation.
In order to construct the locally stratified program $F(f, \varphi)$ for a given tree-typed formula φ, we apply the so called *tree-typed LT transformation,* which is a variant of the LT transformation (see Section 3) obtained by replacing rules (B.3) and (B.4) by the following ones:

(B.3)* $A \leftarrow C[\neg(\varphi \wedge \psi)]$ is transformed into $A \leftarrow C[\neg newp(y_1, \ldots, y_k)] \wedge$
$$newp(y_1, \ldots, y_k) \leftarrow \rho \wedge \varphi \wedge \psi$$

where *newp* is a new predicate symbol, $\{y_1, \ldots, y_k\} = freevars(\varphi \wedge \psi)$, and ρ is the conjunction of all tree atoms $r(y)$ occurring as conjuncts at top level in $C[\neg(\varphi \wedge \psi)]$ and such that $y \in \{y_1, \ldots, y_k\}$.

(B.4)* $A \leftarrow C[\neg \exists x \, (r(x) \wedge \varphi)]$ is transformed into $A \leftarrow C[\neg newp(y_1, \ldots, y_k)] \wedge$
$$newp(y_1, \ldots, y_k) \leftarrow \rho \wedge r(x) \wedge \varphi$$

where *newp* is a new predicate symbol, $\{y_1, \ldots, y_k\} = freevars(\exists x \, (r(x) \wedge \varphi))$, and ρ is the conjunction of all tree atoms $r(y)$ occurring as conjuncts at top level in $C[\neg \exists x \, (r(x) \wedge \varphi)]$ and such that $y \in \{y_1, \ldots, y_k\}$.

Example. [Even-Odd Paths. Continued] For the tree-typed formula $\varphi \colon \forall x \, (bin(x) \rightarrow even(x) \vee odd(x))$, the corresponding $F(f, \varphi)$ obtained by tree-typed LT transformation is the conjunction of the following two clauses:

7. $f \leftarrow \neg g$ 8. $g \leftarrow bin(x), \neg even(x), \neg odd(x)$ □

Theorem 3. [Correctness of the Tree-Typed LT Transformation w.r.t. Perfect Models] For every locally stratified logic program P and closed tree-typed formula φ over P, if $F(f,\varphi)$ is obtained from φ by the tree-typed LT transformation, then (i) $P \wedge F(f,\varphi)$ is a locally stratified program and $M(P) \models \varphi$ iff $M(P \wedge F(f,\varphi)) \models f$, and (ii) for each clause C in $F(f,\varphi)$ we have that: (ii.1) C is of the form $newp(x_1,\ldots,x_m) \leftarrow r_1(x_1),\ldots,r_n(x_n),G$, where $r_1(x_1),\ldots,r_n(x_n)$ are tree atoms, (ii.2) $vars(C) = \{x_1,\ldots,x_n\}$, (ii.3) G is a function-free goal, and (ii.4) $C = Def(newp, P \wedge F(f,\varphi))$. $\qquad\square$

Definition 4. [Monadic Regular Programs] A *monadic regular program* is a conjunction of monadic regular clauses. A *monadic regular clause* (or an *MR clause*, for short) is a locally stratified clause of the form:

$$p_0(t(x_1,\ldots,x_n)) \leftarrow p_1(y_1),\ldots,p_k(y_k),\neg p_{k+1}(y_{k+1}),\ldots,\neg p_m(y_m)$$

with $n, m \geq 0$, where t is a function symbol, $x_1,\ldots,x_n$ are distinct variables, and $y_1,\ldots,y_m$ are (not necessarily distinct) variables occurring in $\{x_1,\ldots,x_n\}$.

Tree programs are MR programs.

We now describe the deterministic version of the UFS strategy, called dUFS.

The Unfold/Fold Proof Strategy dUFS.

The dUFS strategy is obtained from the UFS strategy defined in Section 5, by replacing the substrategies: (1) UNFOLD, (2) TAUTOLOGY & REPLACE, and (3) DEFINE & FOLD by the following ones, respectively:

(1d) BREADTH-FIRST UNFOLD(T,Pos,U): From program $T \wedge Pos$ we derive $T \wedge U$ by: (i) one application of positive unfolding w.r.t. each positive literal occurring in the body of a clause in Pos, followed by (ii) one application of negative unfolding w.r.t. each negative literal occurring in the body of a clause in Pos.

(2d) TAUTOLOGY(T,U,R): From program $T \wedge U$ we derive $T \wedge R$ by a sequence of applications of the tautology rule, constructed by rewriting as long as possible an instance of the left hand side of an equivalence of Rule R5 by the corresponding instance of the right hand side.

(3d) BLOCK-DEFINE & FOLD$(T, R, Defs, OutClauses, NewDefs)$: From program $T \wedge R$ we derive program $T \wedge OutClauses \wedge NewDefs$ as follows:
for each non-unit clause C in R
(i) we partition $bd(C)$ into subconjunctions, called *blocks*, such that $bd(C) = B_1 \wedge \ldots \wedge B_m$, and two literals occur in the same subconjunction B_i, for some $i, 1 \leq i \leq m$, iff they share a variable,
(ii) for $i = 1,\ldots,m$, we apply the definition rule and we add to $NewDefs$ a clause of the form $Newp \leftarrow B_i$, where $vars(Newp) = vars(B_i) \cap vars(hd(C))$, unless a variant clause modulo the head predicate symbol, already occurs in $Defs$, and
(iii) we fold C w.r.t. B_1, and we fold the resulting clause w.r.t. B_2, and so on, until we fold w.r.t. B_m. $\qquad\square$

We have that:
- the BREADTH-FIRST UNFOLD substrategy fulfills the Progression requirement,
- in the TAUTOLOGY substrategy we have omitted the *Laws* argument because goal replacements are not performed, and
- the BLOCK-DEFINE & FOLD substrategy fulfills the conditions (3.1), (3.2), and (3.3) of the DEFINE & FOLD substrategy of Section 5. Indeed, Condition (3.1) is fulfilled, because each variable occurring in the body of a clause generated

by the strategy dUFS also occurs in a tree atom, and therefore, each block has at least one non-basic positive literal. Moreover, by Points (ii) and (iii) in (3d) above, also Conditions (3.2) and (3.3) are fulfilled.

Example. [*Even-Odd Paths. Continued*] The proof that $\forall x \, (bin(x) \rightarrow even(x) \vee odd(x))$ holds in the perfect model of the *Even-Odd* program is as follows. We have that program P is made out of clauses from 1 to 6, program P^1 (at level 1) is made out of clause 8, and program P^2 (at level 2) is made out of clause 7. We start from level 1. Initially Pos = clause 8. By breadth-first unfolding, from clause 8 we get the following clauses:

   9. $g \leftarrow bin(x), bin(y), even(x), even(y), odd(x)$

   10. $g \leftarrow bin(x), bin(y), even(x), even(y), odd(y)$

By the tautology rule R5.2 we delete clause 10 (it is subsumed by clause 9). Then we apply the BLOCK-DEFINE & FOLD substrategy by introducing the following two definitions: 11. $h_{eo} \leftarrow bin(x), even(x), odd(x)$ and   12. $h_e \leftarrow bin(y), even(y)$ and by folding clauses 9 we get: 9.f $g \leftarrow h_{eo}, h_e$

Now Pos = clause 11 $\wedge$ clause 12, and we have to execute once more the body of the WHILE loop (†) of the dUFS strategy. By unfolding clauses 11 and 12 we get:

   11.1 $h_{eo} \leftarrow bin(x), bin(y), \neg even(x), \neg odd(x), \neg odd(y)$

   11.2 $h_{eo} \leftarrow bin(x), bin(y), \neg even(y), \neg odd(x), \neg odd(y)$

   12.1 h_e

   12.2 $h_e \leftarrow bin(x), bin(y), \neg even(x)$

   12.3 $h_e \leftarrow bin(x), bin(y), \neg even(y)$

By the tautology rule R5.2 we delete clause 11.2 (it is subsumed by clause 11.1) and we also delete clauses 12.2 and 12.3 (they are subsumed by clause 12.1). Then we apply the BLOCK-DEFINE & FOLD substrategy by introducing the following definition: 13. $h_o \leftarrow bin(x), \neg odd(x)$ and by folding clause 11.1 we get: 11.1f $h_{eo} \leftarrow g, h_o$

Now Pos = clause 13. By unfolding clause 13 we get:

   13.1 h_o 13.2 $h_o \leftarrow bin(x), bin(y), \neg odd(x), \neg odd(y)$

By the tautology rule R5.2 we delete clause 13.2 (it is subsumed by clause 13.1). No application of the BLOCK-DEFINE & FOLD substrategy is required. Now Pos is empty, and Out is the conjunction of the following clauses: 12.1 h_e and 13.1 h_o together with clauses 9.f and 11.1f. We then delete clauses 9.f and 11.1f because they are the definitions of the predicates g and h_{eo} which are useless in Out. The WHILE loop (‡) does not change D. Since $Q = Q'$, we have that T is made out of the clauses of P together with the clauses 12.1 and 13.1.

We can now start processing level 2, that is, program P^2. Since Pos is the empty conjunction, the body of the WHILE loop (†) is never executed. Neg is clause 7, and before the execution of the WHILE loop (‡), program T is made out of the clauses in P together with the following clauses:

   7. $f \leftarrow \neg g$ 12.1 h_e 13.1 h_o

After the WHILE loop (‡) and the statement (†††) we get the new program T made out of the clauses in P and the clause: 7.1 f together with clauses 12.1 and 13.1. Now, since $M(T) \models f$, we have that $M(P) \models \varphi$.   □

Obviously, the BREADTH-FIRST UNFOLD, TAUTOLOGY, and BLOCK-DEFINE &
FOLD substrategies terminate. Also the dUFS proof strategy terminates for tree-
typed formulas and MR programs, as stated by the following theorem.

**Theorem 4. [Termination of the dUFS Proof Strategy for MR
Programs]** Let P be an MR program and φ be a tree-typed formula over P.
Then the dUFS proof strategy with input program $P \wedge F(f, \varphi)$ terminates with
output program T. Moreover, $Def(f, T)$ is f iff $M(P) \models \varphi$ and $Def(f, T)$ is the
empty conjunction iff $M(P) \not\models \varphi$.   □

Thus, dUFS is a decision procedure for $M(P) \models \varphi$ when P is an MR program and φ is a tree-typed formula over P. Although very restricted, the classes
of MR programs and tree-typed formulas allow us to express some interesting
properties, such as the equivalence of finite tree automata (see, for instance,
[10]), as shown in the following example.

Example. [*Equivalence of Tree Automata*] The tree language recognized by a
(nondeterministic top-down) finite tree automaton $T = (Q, \Sigma, \delta, q0, F)$ corresponds to a subset of the perfect model of a tree program P_T (which is also its
least Herbrand model) defined as follows:
- for each state $q \in Q$ we define a unary predicate p_q,
- for each symbol $a \in \Sigma$ of arity k we define a k-ary function symbol f_a,
- for each tuple $(q, a, q1, \ldots, qk)$ in the transition relation δ, where a is a k-ary
symbol with $k \geq 1$, P_T has the clause: $p_q(f_a(x_1, \ldots, x_k)) \leftarrow p_{q1}(x_1), \ldots, p_{qk}(x_k)$
- for each state $q \in F \subseteq Q$ and 0-ary symbol b such that q is a final state for b,
P_T has the unit clause: $p_q(f_b)$
Then the tree language recognized by the tree automaton T with initial state $q0$,
is the set $\{t \mid M(P_T) \models p_{q0}(t)\}$. Given another tree automaton U with initial
state $r0$ and represented by program P_U, we have that T and U recognize the
same language iff $M(P_T \wedge P_U) \models \forall x\, (p_{q0}(x) \rightarrow p_{r0}(x)) \wedge \forall x\, (p_{r0}(x) \rightarrow p_{q0}(x))$.
Thus, the equivalence of T and U can be reduced to the verification of a tree-
typed formula over the tree program $P_T \wedge P_U$ (recall that each tree program is
also an MR program).   □

We now introduce a second class of formulas, called *tree-typed clausal formulas*, and a second class of programs, called *deterministic linear programs* (or *DL
programs*, for short) for which the unfold/fold proof strategy dUFS terminates.
Thus, given a tree-typed clausal formula φ, and a DL program P, we can decide
whether or not $M(P) \models \varphi$ holds by using the proof strategy dUFS.

Definition 5. [Tree-Typed Clausal Formulas] Let P be any program and
R be a tree program. A *tree-typed clausal formula* over a program $P \wedge R$ is a
closed first-order formula φ generated by the following grammar:
$$\varphi ::= \forall x\, (r(x) \rightarrow \varphi) \mid \delta \qquad \delta ::= p(x_1, \ldots, x_n) \mid \neg p(x_1, \ldots, x_n) \mid \delta \vee \delta$$
where: (i) $x_1, \ldots, x_n$, with $n \geq 0$, are distinct variables, (ii) all predicates oc-
curring in φ are defined in $P \wedge R$, (iii) for each predicate p, $Def^*(p, P \wedge R)$ is a
subconjunction of P, (iv) for each predicate r, $Def^*(r, P \wedge R)$ is a subconjunction
of R, and (v) no predicate is defined in both P and R.

Definition 6. [Deterministic Linear Programs] A *linear clause* is a locally
stratified clause of one of these three forms:

$$p(t_1(x_1, \ldots, x_m), \ldots, t_n(x_u, \ldots, x_v))$$
$$p(t_1(x_1, \ldots, x_m), \ldots, t_n(x_u, \ldots, x_v)) \leftarrow q(y_1, \ldots, y_k)$$
$$p(t_1(x_1, \ldots, x_m), \ldots, t_n(x_u, \ldots, x_v)) \leftarrow \neg q(y_1, \ldots, y_k)$$

with $n \geq 0$, where: (i) $t_1, \ldots, t_n$ are function symbols, (ii) $x_1, \ldots, x_m, \ldots, x_u, \ldots, x_v$ are distinct variables, and (iii) $y_1, \ldots, y_k$ are distinct variables occurring in $\{x_1, \ldots, x_m, \ldots, x_u, \ldots, x_v\}$. A *deterministic linear program* (or *DL program*, for short) is a conjunction of linear clauses such that no two clause heads are unifiable.

There are MR programs which are not DL programs and vice versa.

Theorem 5. [Termination of the dUFS Proof Strategy for DL Programs] Let P be a DL program, R be a tree program, and φ be a tree-typed clausal formula over $P \wedge R$. Then the dUFS strategy with input program $P \wedge F(f, \varphi)$ terminates with output program T. Moreover, $Def(f, T)$ is f iff $M(P) \models \varphi$ and $Def(f, T)$ is the empty conjunction iff $M(P) \not\models \varphi$.   □

Example. [Clausal wMSnS] The clausal fragment of the weak monadic second order theory of two successor functions (cwMS2S) [16] is the set of closed formulas φ such that $\mathcal{W} \models \varphi$, where: (i) φ is a closed formula generated by the following grammar:

$$\varphi ::= \forall w \, (word(w) \to \varphi) \mid \forall x \, (set(x) \to \varphi) \mid \delta$$
$$\delta ::= member(w, x) \mid \neg member(w, x) \mid \delta \vee \delta$$

(ii) $\mathcal{W}$ is the structure $\mathcal{P}_{fin}(\{0, 1\}^*)$ of finite sets of words over $\{0, 1\}$, where: (ii.1) the successor functions s_0 and s_1 are interpreted as $s_0(w) = w0$ and $s_1(w) = w1$, respectively, (ii.2) the predicates *word* and *set* hold of all words and finite sets of words, respectively, and (ii.3) $member(w, x)$ is interpreted as membership of word w to set x.

We may define the *word*, *set*, and *member* predicates by means of the following *Member* program, which is $P \wedge R$, where:

P:

$member(emptyword, leaf(n)) \leftarrow acceptlabel(n)$
$member(emptyword, t(x_0, n, x_1)) \leftarrow acceptlabel(n)$
$member(s_0(w), t(x_0, n, x_1)) \leftarrow member(w, x_0)$
$member(s_1(w), t(x_0, n, x_1)) \leftarrow member(w, x_1)$
$acceptlabel(accept)$

R:

$word(emptyword)$
$word(s_0(w)) \leftarrow word(w)$
$word(s_1(w)) \leftarrow word(w)$
$set(leaf(n)) \leftarrow label(n)$
$set(t(x_0, n, x_1)) \leftarrow set(x_0),$
$\qquad label(n), set(x_1)$
$label(accept)$
$label(refuse)$

Every finite set of words is represented as a finite tree, and (1) t (of arity 3) and *leaf* (of arity 1) are the tree constructors, (2) both the internal nodes and the leaf nodes are labeled by either the constant *accept* or the constant *refuse*, and they are called *accept nodes* or *refuse nodes*, respectively, and (3) left arcs are labeled by 0 and right arcs are labeled by 1. The empty word is represented by the constant *emptyword*. The *accept paths* of a tree x are the sequences of labels from an accept node to the root. A word w is member of a set x iff w is an accept path of x. For instance, the set $\{0, 01\}$ is represented by the tree $t(leaf(accept), refuse, t(leaf(accept), refuse, leaf(refuse)))$.

We have that the structure $\mathcal{W}$ corresponds to the perfect model (equal to the least Herbrand model) of *Member*, in the sense that: $\mathcal{W} \models \varphi$ iff $M(\textit{Member}) \models \varphi$. Since (1) P is a DL program, (2) R is a tree program, and (3) every formula φ which is generated by the grammar of Point (i) above is a tree-typed clausal formula over $P \wedge R$, by Theorem 5 we have that by using our dUFS proof strategy we can test whether or not $M(\textit{Member}) \models \varphi$ holds. Thus, dUFS is a decision procedure for cwMS2S. The extension from cwMS2S to cwMSnS (with n successors, instead of 2) can be obtained by a straightforward modification of the *Member* program.   □

7   Conclusions and Related Work

The idea of using unfold/fold transformations for proving program properties goes back to [11], where it was advocated as a method for proving the equivalence of functional terms. The present paper extends the techniques proposed in [13] for showing equivalences of definite programs w.r.t. least Herbrand models and, in particular, (i) we consider logic programs with locally stratified negation and perfect model semantics, (ii) we prove first-order formulas, and (iii) we present an automated strategy for performing proofs. A different extension of [13] has been recently presented in [17], where the authors prove equivalences of definite programs w.r.t. least Herbrand models by using a more powerful folding rule.

Our transformational method for proving properties of the perfect model of a locally stratified logic program is related to other methods for theorem proving as we now illustrate.

(i) The method based on the Clark completion [6, 12] amounts to prove that $M(P) \models \varphi$ by showing that $comp(P) \vdash \varphi$, where $comp(P)$ denotes the Clark completion of program P. Notice that for some program P and formula φ, such as the ones introduced in our Semaphore and Even-Odd Paths Examples, the relation $M(P) \models \varphi$ can be proved by our unfold/fold proof method and yet $comp(P) \nvdash \varphi$.

(ii) Several enhancements of the resolution method have been proposed in the literature for verifying properties of logic programs with negation w.r.t. the perfect model semantics. Among those we recall the SLDNF-resolution [12] which is based on the *negation as finite failure* rule, but it is unable to deal with infinitely failed derivations and moreover, it is not complete w.r.t. the Clark completion. We also recall the SLS-resolution [1, 15] which enhances the resolution method by using the *negation as* (finite or infinite) *failure* rule. In the absence of *floundering* [12], SLS-resolution is sound and complete w.r.t. the perfect model semantics. However, it is not an effective inference rule, in the sense that the set of consequences of the perfect model of a logic program is not recursively enumerable. Finally, we recall the SLG-resolution [5], which combines resolution and *tabling*. SLG is an effective method and it is more powerful than the SLDNF-resolution for dealing with infinitely failed derivations. SLG-resolution can be used for efficiently verifying CTL properties of finite-state transition system [9, 18]. Notice that, however, our folding rule is more powerful than tabling, because it allows us to tabulate a conjunction of literals, instead of one literal only.

(iii) Brass and Dix [3] have proposed a query evaluation algorithm for disjunctive logic programs based on transformation rules. These rules include the positive unfolding and tautology rules, and they preserve several semantics including the perfect model semantics for the class of locally stratified logic programs. However, Brass and Dix do not take into consideration the folding and goal replacement rules, which play a crucial role in our technique.

(iv) The satisfaction relation $M(P) \models \varphi$ may also be proved by adding to $comp(P)$ a set of formulas, or *induction schemata*, that formalize an induction principle over terms of the Herbrand universe. Thus, one may use standard techniques for inductive theorem proving [2]. The main difference between this method and our unfold/fold proof method is that the latter does not require any induction schema.

(v) The unfold/fold proof method is related to methods for *proof by consistency* (also called *inductionless induction* method) of equational formulas by using term rewriting systems (see [7] for a recent revisitation). This relationship is based on the ability of the unfold/fold proof method of proving inductive properties without using an explicit induction schema. However, the proofs by consistency are refutational proofs, they work by finding minimal counterexamples, and they require suitable well-founded orderings on terms, while the unfold/fold proof method does not require such term orderings.

References

1. K. R. Apt and R. N. Bol. Logic programming and negation: A survey. *Journal of Logic Programming*, 19, 20:9–71, 1994.
2. R.S. Boyer and J.S. Moore. *A Computational Logic*. Academic Press, New York, 1979.
3. S. Brass and J. Dix. Semantics of (disjunctive) logic programs based on partial evaluation. *Journal of Logic Programming*, 40:1–46, 1999.
4. R. M. Burstall and J. Darlington. A transformation system for developing recursive programs. *JACM*, 24(1):44–67, January 1977.
5. W. Chen and D. S. Warren. Tabled evaluation with delaying for general logic programs. *JACM*, 43(1), 1996.
6. K. L. Clark. Negation as failure. In H. Gallaire and J. Minker (eds.) *Logic and Data Bases*, 293–322. Plenum Press, New York, 1978.
7. H. Comon and R. Nieuwenhuis. Induction = I-axiomatization + first-order consistency. *Information and Computation*. (To appear).
8. B. Courcelle. Equivalences and Transformations of Regular Systems – Applications to Recursive Program Schemes and Grammars. *Theo. Comp. Sci.*, 42:1–122, 1986.
9. E. A. Emerson. Temporal and modal logic. In J. van Leuveen (ed.) *Handbook of Theoretical Computer Science*, volume B, 997–1072. Elsevier, 1990.
10. J. Engelfriet. Tree Automata and Tree Grammars. DAIMI FN-10, Department of Computer Science, University of Aarhus, Denmark, April 1975.
11. L. Kott. Unfold/fold program transformation. In M. Nivat and J.C. Reynolds (eds.) *Algebraic Methods in Semantics*, 411–434. Cambridge University Press, 1985.
12. J. W. Lloyd. *Foundations of Logic Programming*. Springer-Verlag, 1987. 2nd Ed.

13. A. Pettorossi and M. Proietti. Synthesis and transformation of logic programs using unfold/fold proofs. *Journal of Logic Programming*, 41(2&3):197–230, 1999.
14. M. Proietti and A. Pettorossi. Unfolding-definition-folding, in this order, for avoiding unnecessary variables in logic programs. *Theo. Comp. Sci.*, 142(1):89–124, 1995.
15. T. C. Przymusinski. On the declarative and procedural semantics of logic programs. *Journal of Automated Reasoning*, 5:167–205, 1989.
16. M. O. Rabin. Decidability of second-order theories and automata on infinite trees. *Transactions of the American Mathematical Society*, 141:1–34, July 1969.
17. A. Roychoudhury, K. Narayan Kumar, C.R. Ramakrishnan, I.V. Ramakrishnan, and S. A. Smolka. Verification of parametrized systems using logic program transformations. In *Proc. TACAS 2000*, LNCS 1785, 172–187. Springer, 2000.
18. Y. S. Ramakrishna, C. R. Ramakrishnan, I. V. Ramakrishnan, S. A. Smolka, T. Swift, and D. S. Warren. Efficient model checking using tabled resolution. In *Proc. CAV '97*, LNCS 1254, 143–154. Springer, 1997.
19. H. Seki. Unfold/fold transformation of stratified programs. *Theo. Comp. Sci.*, 86:107–139, 1991.
20. H. Tamaki and T. Sato. Unfold/fold transformation of logic programs. In *Proceedings of ICLP'84*, 127–138. Uppsala University, Sweden, 1984.

Automatic Derivation and Application of Induction Schemes for Mutually Recursive Functions*

Richard J. Boulton[1][**] and Konrad Slind[2]

[1] Division of Informatics, University of Edinburgh
80 South Bridge, Edinburgh EH1 1HN, UK
[2] University of Cambridge Computer Laboratory
New Museums Site, Pembroke Street, Cambridge CB2 3QG, UK

Abstract. This paper advocates and explores the use of *multi-predicate* induction schemes for proofs about mutually recursive functions. The *interactive* application of multi-predicate schemes stemming from datatype definitions is already well-established practice; this paper describes an *automated* proof procedure based on multi-predicate schemes. Multi-predicate schemes may be formally derived from (mutually recursive) function definitions; such schemes are often helpful in proving properties of mutually recursive functions where the recursion pattern does not follow that of the underlying datatypes. These ideas have been implemented using the HOL theorem prover and the *Clam* proof planner.

1 Introduction

The abstract syntax of programming languages is usually represented formally as recursive types. For example, a type of boolean expressions might be declared in the following ML-like style:[1]

```
datatype prop = var of string | not of prop
              | and of prop × prop | or of prop × prop
```

Parsing maps text in the concrete syntax of the language into elements of these recursive types. Early stages of compilers may map the types into other recursive types that represent a simpler internal language from which it is easier to generate machine instructions. Thus they are recursive functions (or procedures) operating over the recursive types. Code generators and interpreters will also typically be recursive functions defined over these types. In declarative languages the original source programs are often recursive functions or predicates.

---

* Research supported by the Engineering and Physical Sciences Research Council of Great Britain under grants GR/L03071 and GR/L14381. The authors thank Alan Bundy, Ian Green and Christoph Walther for their feedback on this work.
** Address from January 2000: Department of Computing Science, University of Glasgow, 17 Lilybank Gardens, Glasgow G12 8QQ, UK.
[1] The constructors and and or will be treated as infixes.

J. Lloyd et al. (Eds.): CL 2000, LNAI 1861, pp. 629–643, 2000.
© Springer-Verlag Berlin Heidelberg 2000

Many impressive examples of machine-assisted formal reasoning about languages and programs can be found in the literature. The basis of such proofs is typically a structural induction theorem (*scheme*). For example, the scheme for the **prop** type is:

$$\forall P. \ ((\forall s. \ P(\mathbf{var}(s))) \ \wedge \ (\forall e. \ P(e) \supset P(\mathbf{not}(e))) \ \wedge$$
$$(\forall e_1 \ e_2. \ P(e_1) \wedge P(e_2) \supset P(e_1 \ \mathbf{and} \ e_2)) \ \wedge$$
$$(\forall e_1 \ e_2. \ P(e_1) \wedge P(e_2) \supset P(e_1 \ \mathbf{or} \ e_2)) \ \supset$$
$$\forall e. \ P(e) \ .$$

There are, however, fundamental features for which effective automation techniques have not yet been developed. One such feature is mutual recursion. In real-world examples mutual recursion is quite common because if there are mutually dependent syntactic categories, the types representing them will be mutually recursive and hence functions defined over those types will usually be mutually recursive too. For example, Standard ML [10] has a mutually dependent block of 7 syntactic categories involving at least 28 clauses and 4 cycles, the largest of which has 4 categories in it.

In this paper we present an approach to automating induction for mutually recursive functions. The essence of the approach is to use induction schemes that have one predicate for each of the mutually recursive functions. Such schemes have been applied before in interactive proofs (where the instances for all the predicates are provided by the user) but previous research on automating induction has only considered schemes with a single predicate.

An important subsidiary issue is how mutually recursive definitions and multi-predicate schemes are obtained: we demonstrate how simple manipulations allow us to reduce mutual recursion to single recursion, and how multi-predicate schemes are likewise produced from single-predicate schemes. These manipulations thus allow us to build on previous work [13, 12]. Our work differs from previous work on generating multi-predicate schemes (e.g. [15, Appendix A]) in that our schemes follow the recursion pattern of the mutually recursive *functions* rather than the recursion pattern of the *types*.

Example 1. As an example of our approach consider the following functions defined by Paulson [10, page 167] for computing the negation normal form of **prop**:

$$nnf(\mathbf{var}(x)) = \mathbf{var}(x)$$
$$nnf(\mathbf{not}(\mathbf{var}(x))) = \mathbf{not}(\mathbf{var}(x))$$
$$nnf(\mathbf{not}(\mathbf{not}(p))) = nnf(p)$$
$$nnf(\mathbf{not}(p \ \mathbf{and} \ q)) = nnf(\mathbf{not}(p)) \ \mathbf{or} \ nnf(\mathbf{not}(q))$$
$$nnf(\mathbf{not}(p \ \mathbf{or} \ q)) = nnf(\mathbf{not}(p)) \ \mathbf{and} \ nnf(\mathbf{not}(q))$$
$$nnf(p \ \mathbf{and} \ q) = nnf(p) \ \mathbf{and} \ nnf(q)$$
$$nnf(p \ \mathbf{or} \ q) = nnf(p) \ \mathbf{or} \ nnf(q)$$

$$nnfpos(\mathbf{var}(x)) = \mathbf{var}(x) \qquad nnfpos(p \ \mathbf{and} \ q) = nnfpos(p) \ \mathbf{and} \ nnfpos(q)$$
$$nnfpos(\mathbf{not}(p)) = nnfneg(p) \qquad nnfpos(p \ \mathbf{or} \ q) = nnfpos(p) \ \mathbf{or} \ nnfpos(q)$$
$$nnfneg(\mathbf{var}(x)) = \mathbf{not}(\mathbf{var}(x)) \quad nnfneg(p \ \mathbf{and} \ q) = nnfneg(p) \ \mathbf{or} \ nnfneg(q)$$
$$nnfneg(\mathbf{not}(p)) = nnfpos(p) \qquad nnfneg(p \ \mathbf{or} \ q) = nnfneg(p) \ \mathbf{and} \ nnfneg(q)$$

The definition of *nnf* has been modified to be more efficient than the first version given by Paulson but, as he describes, the mutually recursive functions are more efficient still. Now suppose we wish to prove the equivalence of the two versions:

$$\forall p. \; nnf(p) = nnfpos(p)$$

Using the *structural* induction scheme for **prop** given above leads to difficulties. The first case of the induction (for **var**) is simple. In the case for **not**, however, we have $nnf(p) = nnfpos(p)$ (where p is fixed) as a hypothesis and the formula to be proved (the conclusion) is:

$$nnf(\text{not}(p)) = nnfpos(\text{not}(p))$$

The right-hand side rewrites using the definition of *nnfpos* to $nnfneg(p)$ but none of the clauses of the definition of *nnf* apply to the left-hand side. The solution is to do a case-split on the form of p. This works when p is a **var** form but there is again trouble in the **not** case which rewrites as follows:

$$nnf(\text{not}(\text{not}(p'))) = nnfneg(\text{not}(p'))$$
$$nnf(p') = nnfpos(p')$$

This is not matched by the hypothesis $nnf(p) = nnfpos(p)$ because p and p' are different. In fact, $p = \text{not}(p')$, so the hypothesis is $nnf(\text{not}(p')) = nnfpos(\text{not}(p'))$ which rewrites to $nnf(\text{not}(p')) = nnfneg(p')$. However one looks at it, the hypothesis cannot be used to prove the conclusion. The problem is that the induction has gone only one step through the mutually recursive cycle for *nnfpos* and *nnfneg*.

The solution proposed in this paper is to use an induction scheme that follows the recursion of the mutually recursive functions:

$$\forall P \, Q. \; ((\forall s. \; P(\text{var}(s))) \wedge (\forall e. \; Q(e) \supset P(\text{not}(e))) \wedge$$
$$(\forall e_1 \, e_2. \; P(e_1) \wedge P(e_2) \supset P(e_1 \text{ and } e_2)) \wedge$$
$$(\forall e_1 \, e_2. \; P(e_1) \wedge P(e_2) \supset P(e_1 \text{ or } e_2)) \wedge$$
$$(\forall s. \; Q(\text{var}(s))) \wedge (\forall e. \; P(e) \supset Q(\text{not}(e))) \wedge \qquad (1)$$
$$(\forall e_1 \, e_2. \; Q(e_1) \wedge Q(e_2) \supset Q(e_1 \text{ and } e_2)) \wedge$$
$$(\forall e_1 \, e_2. \; Q(e_1) \wedge Q(e_2) \supset Q(e_1 \text{ or } e_2)) \supset$$
$$(\forall v_1. \; P(v_1)) \wedge (\forall v_2. \; Q(v_2)) \; .$$

Observe that the scheme has two conclusions. Only one of these is used to match against the formula to be proved. This means that initially only one of P and Q will be instantiated. The main role of our procedure is to instantiate the other predicate during the proof. The example in Section 3 shows this in action. For the example at hand, if P matches to the original conjecture, Q eventually becomes instantiated to $\forall p. \; nnf(\text{not}(p)) = nnfneg(p)$. By this means, the proof works out very smoothly.

It is also possible to prove the proposition using a single-predicate induction scheme derived from the definition of *nnf*. This avoids the case-split and also allows the proof to go through but it is not so smooth and hence would be more of a challenge for an automatic prover. Of course, in examples where *nnf* does not occur, *e.g.*, showing the result of *nnfpos* is in normal form, the induction scheme for *nnf* would not be available, and (1) is essential.

2 Deriving Multi-predicate Schemes from Definitions

Our approach to deriving induction schemes requires some background information on how mutually recursive functions are defined. The definition of mutually recursive functions $f_1 \ldots f_n$ is handled by mapping the original recursion equations to recursive equations for a single 'union' function $\mathcal{U}$; after $\mathcal{U}$ is defined, the originally specified equations can be achieved by defining each f_i in terms of $\mathcal{U}$, and then rewriting $\mathcal{U}$ with these definitions. In the same spirit, our induction schemes are derived by manipulating the induction scheme for $\mathcal{U}$. The validity of the derived definitions and induction scheme is assured because they are constructed by deductive steps in a sound logic [6]. For lack of space, we have omitted a formal description of these algorithms; the interested reader can find them in [14].

Sums. We use a sum type to help represent $\mathcal{U}$. The datatype (α, β) **sum** is built from the `inl` and `inr` constructors. A type (τ, δ) **sum** is more usually rendered as $\tau + \delta$. The usual facts about constructors hold, *i.e.*, `inl` and `inr` are injective and distinct. We also use 'case' expressions over sums:

$$sum\_case\ f\ g\ (\texttt{inl}\ x) = f\ x \qquad sum\_case\ f\ g\ (\texttt{inr}\ y) = g\ y\ .$$

Returning to our example, the union function $\mathcal{U} : \texttt{prop+prop} \to \texttt{prop}$ for *nnfpos* and *nnfneg* is formulated as follows: the arguments to *nnfpos* are injected into the sum with `inl`, and similarly, arguments to *nnfneg* are injected into the sum with `inr`. In this example, the range of $\mathcal{U}$ is just `prop`; however, when the range types of $f_1 \ldots f_n$ do not coincide, the range type of the union function is a sum.

$$
\begin{aligned}
\mathcal{U}(\texttt{inl}(\texttt{var}\ x)) &= \texttt{var}\ x \\
\mathcal{U}(\texttt{inl}(\texttt{not}\ x)) &= \mathcal{U}(\texttt{inr}\ x) \\
\mathcal{U}(\texttt{inl}(x\ \texttt{and}\ y)) &= \mathcal{U}(\texttt{inl}\ x)\ \texttt{and}\ \mathcal{U}(\texttt{inl}\ y) \\
\mathcal{U}(\texttt{inl}(x\ \texttt{or}\ y)) &= \mathcal{U}(\texttt{inl}\ x)\ \texttt{or}\ \mathcal{U}(\texttt{inl}\ y) \\
\mathcal{U}(\texttt{inr}(\texttt{var}\ x)) &= \texttt{not}\ (\texttt{var}\ x) \\
\mathcal{U}(\texttt{inr}(\texttt{not}\ x)) &= \mathcal{U}(\texttt{inl}\ x) \\
\mathcal{U}(\texttt{inr}(x\ \texttt{and}\ y)) &= \mathcal{U}(\texttt{inr}\ x)\ \texttt{or}\ \mathcal{U}(\texttt{inr}\ y) \\
\mathcal{U}(\texttt{inr}(x\ \texttt{or}\ y)) &= \mathcal{U}(\texttt{inr}\ x)\ \texttt{and}\ \mathcal{U}(\texttt{inr}\ y)
\end{aligned}
\tag{2}
$$

The function specified by the recursion equations for $\mathcal{U}$ is defined by invoking the *relationless* definition algorithm described in [12].[2] Now the desired functions can be defined:

$$nnfpos(x) = \mathcal{U}\ (\texttt{inl}\ x) \qquad nnfneg(x) = \mathcal{U}\ (\texttt{inr}\ x)\ .$$

---

[2] Termination is subsequently proved automatically, but validity is not threatened if it isn't.

Finally, the definitions of *nnfpos* and *nnfneg* can be used (from right to left) to rewrite the definition of $\mathcal{U}$ to derive the originally specified recursion equations.

What about induction? The following induction scheme has been automatically derived for $\mathcal{U}$, by the algorithm detailed in [13], which uses deductive steps to manipulate the wellfounded induction theorem into the desired form:

$$\forall P.\ (\forall x.\ P\,(\mathtt{inl}(\mathtt{var}\ x)))\ \wedge\ (\forall x.\ P\,(\mathtt{inr}\ x) \supset P\,(\mathtt{inl}(\mathtt{not}\ x)))\ \wedge \qquad (3)$$
$$(\forall x\ y.\ P\,(\mathtt{inl}\ x) \wedge P\,(\mathtt{inl}\ y) \supset P\,(\mathtt{inl}(x\ \mathtt{and}\ y)))\ \wedge$$
$$(\forall x\ y.\ P\,(\mathtt{inl}\ x) \wedge P\,(\mathtt{inl}\ y) \supset P\,(\mathtt{inl}(x\ \mathtt{or}\ y)))\ \wedge$$
$$(\forall x.\ P\,(\mathtt{inr}(\mathtt{var}\ x)))\ \wedge\ (\forall x.\ P\,(\mathtt{inl}\ x) \supset P\,(\mathtt{inr}(\mathtt{not}\ x)))\ \wedge$$
$$(\forall x\ y.\ P\,(\mathtt{inr}\ x) \wedge P\,(\mathtt{inr}\ y) \supset P\,(\mathtt{inr}(x\ \mathtt{and}\ y)))\ \wedge$$
$$(\forall x\ y.\ P\,(\mathtt{inr}\ x) \wedge P\,(\mathtt{inr}\ y) \supset P\,(\mathtt{inr}(x\ \mathtt{or}\ y)))$$
$$\supset \forall x.\ P\ x\ .$$

It is easy to manipulate (3) into the desired multi-predicate scheme. The derivation starts by instantiating $P : \mathtt{prop} + \mathtt{prop} \to \mathtt{bool}$ in (3) to $sum\_case\ Q_1\ Q_2$. This opens up the possibility to reduce with the definition of sum_case at each (former) occurrence of P. The result is

$$(\forall x.\ Q_1(\mathtt{var}\ x))\ \wedge\ (\forall x.\ Q_2\ x \supset Q_1(\mathtt{not}\ x))\ \wedge$$
$$(\forall x\ y.\ Q_1\ x \wedge Q_1\ y \supset Q_1(x\ \mathtt{and}\ y))\ \wedge$$
$$(\forall x\ y.\ Q_1\ x \wedge Q_1\ y \supset Q_1(x\ \mathtt{or}\ y))\ \wedge$$
$$(\forall x.\ Q_2(\mathtt{var}\ x))\ \wedge\ (\forall x.\ Q_1\ x \supset Q_2(\mathtt{not}\ x))\ \wedge \qquad (4)$$
$$(\forall x\ y.\ Q_2\ x \wedge Q_2\ y \supset Q_2(x\ \mathtt{and}\ y))\ \wedge$$
$$(\forall x\ y.\ Q_2\ x \wedge Q_2\ y \supset Q_2(x\ \mathtt{or}\ y))$$
$$\supset \forall s.\ sum\_case\ Q_1\ Q_2\ s\ .$$

Now all that is necessary is to instantiate s, once with $\mathtt{inl}\ v_1$, and once with $\mathtt{inr}\ v_2$. Simplifying again with the definition of sum_case and then performing some trivial tidying-up steps gives the desired result, in which the antecedant is that of (4) and the conclusion is $(\forall v_1.\ Q_1\ v_1) \wedge (\forall v_2.\ Q_2\ v_2)$.

3   An Example Proof

It is not possible in the space available to present a real-world example and cut-down versions do not display the range of features we wish to illustrate. Thus the example given below, concerning annotated trees, is somewhat contrived. The general idea of restructuring trees is, however, reminiscent of operations on abstract syntax trees in compilers. The types involved are:

```
datatype atree = annotate of string × atree | node of utree
and utree = leaf | branch of num × utree × utree | anode of atree
```

The types `atree` and `utree` are of annotated trees and unannotated trees, respectively, where the constructors `node` and `anode` allow switching between the two. The functions used are:

$$amerge(\mathtt{annotate}(s, at)) = concat(s, at)$$
$$amerge(\mathtt{node}(t)) = \mathtt{node}(merge(t))$$

$$concat(s_1, \mathtt{annotate}(s_2, at)) = concat(strcat(s_1, s_2), at)$$
$$concat(s, \mathtt{node}(t)) = \mathtt{annotate}(s, \mathtt{node}(merge(t)))$$

$$merge(\mathtt{leaf}) = \mathtt{leaf}$$
$$merge(\mathtt{branch}(n, t_1, t_2)) = \mathtt{branch}(n, merge(t_1), merge(t_2))$$
$$merge(\mathtt{anode}(at)) = \mathtt{anode}(amerge(at))$$

where *strcat* concatenates two strings. The example illustrates a number of important features with reasonable simplicity and brevity:

- a recursion pattern in the functions that differs from the recursion pattern of the types, and hence an induction scheme that differs from the standard structural induction;
- functions with different argument types;
- functions with different result types;
- functions that cannot be unwound to a single recursive function;
- more than two mutually recursive functions and hence more than two induction predicates.

The induction scheme derived by the approach outlined in Sect. 2 is:

$\forall P_1\ P_2\ P_3.$
$(\forall s\ at.\ P_2(s, at) \supset P_1(\mathtt{annotate}(s, at)))\ \wedge\ (\forall t.\ P_3(t) \supset P_1(\mathtt{node}(t)))\ \wedge$
$(\forall s_1\ s_2\ at.\ P_2(strcat(s_1, s_2), at) \supset P_2(s_1, \mathtt{annotate}(s_2, at)))\ \wedge$
$(\forall s\ t.\ P_3(t) \supset P_2(s, \mathtt{node}(t)))\ \wedge$
$P_3(\mathtt{leaf})\ \wedge\ (\forall n\ t_1\ t_2.\ P_3(t_1) \wedge P_3(t_2) \supset P_3(\mathtt{branch}(n, t_1, t_2)))\ \wedge$
$(\forall at.\ P_1(at) \supset P_3(\mathtt{anode}(at)))\quad\supset$
$(\forall v_1 : \mathtt{atree}.\ P_1(v_1)) \wedge (\forall v_2 : \mathtt{string} \times \mathtt{atree}.\ P_2(v_2)) \wedge (\forall v_3 : \mathtt{utree}.\ P_3(v_3))$

Although this scheme is perfectly useful, it does not fit well with our current proof-planning technology which cannot handle the induction hypothesis $P_2(strcat(s_1, s_2), at)$, since it involves a function application. However, an acceptable version is simple to obtain, by instantiating P_2 with $\lambda(s, v).\ Q(v)$ and beta-reducing. This yields, with some renaming of the induction predicates,

$\forall P\ Q\ R.\ (\forall s\ at.\ Q(at) \supset P(\mathtt{annotate}(s, at)))\ \wedge\ (\forall t.\ R(t) \supset P(\mathtt{node}(t)))\ \wedge$
$(\forall s_1\ s_2\ at.\ Q(at) \supset Q(\mathtt{annotate}(s_2, at)))\ \wedge$
$(\forall s\ t.\ R(t) \supset Q(\mathtt{node}(t)))\ \wedge$
$R(\mathtt{leaf})\ \wedge\ (\forall n\ t_1\ t_2.\ R(t_1) \wedge R(t_2) \supset R(\mathtt{branch}(n, t_1, t_2)))\ \wedge$
$(\forall at.\ P(at) \supset R(\mathtt{anode}(at)))\quad\supset$
$(\forall v_1 : \mathtt{atree}.\ P(v_1)) \wedge (\forall v_2 : \mathtt{atree}.\ Q(v_2)) \wedge (\forall v_3 : \mathtt{utree}.\ R(v_3))\ .$

The property to be proved is the idempotency of *amerge*:

$$\forall at.\ amerge(amerge(at)) = amerge(at)$$

The first step is to match this goal with one of the conjuncts of the conclusion of the induction scheme. Type constraints mean it has to be either the first or second conjunct. The first is more appropriate but the second could be tried if the proof attempt using the first fails. So, the induction predicate P is instantiated to $\lambda at.\ amerge(amerge(at)) = amerge(at)$ and Q and R remain uninstantiated. Beta-reduction yields the following goal (with the v's renamed to something more meaningful for this presentation):

$$(\forall at.\ amerge(amerge(at)) = amerge(at))\ \wedge\ (\forall at.\ Q(at))\ \wedge\ (\forall t.\ R(t))$$

A proof procedure for induction would now normally attempt to prove all the hypotheses of the instantiated induction scheme. However, since Q and R have not yet been instantiated, only the hypotheses whose consequent involves P should be attempted.

Case $Q(at) \supset P(\mathtt{annotate}(s, at))$. The initial form of the first case of the proof is:[3]

$$Q(at)\ \vdash_?\ amerge(amerge(\mathtt{annotate}(s, at))) = amerge(\mathtt{annotate}(s, at))$$

Using the definition of *amerge* the conclusion reduces as follows:

$$Q(at)\ \vdash_?\ amerge(concat(s, at)) = concat(s, at)$$

If we were using the structural induction scheme we would be stuck at this point because the hypothesis would be $P(at)$, i.e., $amerge(amerge(at)) = amerge(at)$ which is no use in proving the conclusion. Using the scheme derived from the functions, however, the hypothesis is $Q(at)$ which we can use by (second-order) matching it to the residual conclusion. This instantiates Q to:

$$\lambda at.\ \forall s.\ amerge(concat(s, at)) = concat(s, at)$$

This λ-abstraction can be formed in a straightforward manner from the conclusion of the goal. The λ-bound variables are the arguments of Q in the hypothesis (In this case there is only one.) and the other variables in the conclusion are universally quantified. Having made this instantiation, the truth of this case of the proof follows immediately by beta-reduction in the hypothesis.

Case $R(t) \supset P(\mathtt{node}(t))$. This case proceeds in a similar way and serves to instantiate R. The initial goal is reduced using the definitions as follows:

$$R(t)\ \vdash_?\ amerge(amerge(\mathtt{node}(t))) = amerge(\mathtt{node}(t))$$
$$R(t)\ \vdash_?\ amerge(\mathtt{node}(merge(t))) = \mathtt{node}(merge(t))$$
$$R(t)\ \vdash_?\ \mathtt{node}(merge(merge(t))) = \mathtt{node}(merge(t))$$

---

[3] The $\vdash_?$ symbol is used to separate the hypotheses and conclusion of the conjecture. The question mark indicates that we do not yet know that the conjecture is a theorem.

We now apply the injectivity of the **node** constructor to reduce the goal further:

$$R(t) \vdash_? \ merge(merge(t)) = merge(t)$$

(Actually, the fact that **node** is a function is sufficient to justify this step but it is a safer step when the function in question is injective because there is then an equality between the two forms rather than just an implication.) Instantiating R to $\lambda t.\ merge(merge(t)) = merge(t)$ completes this case of the proof.

Now that both Q and R have been instantiated the remaining induction cases can be attempted. Actually, even if only Q (or only R) had been instantiated during the proofs of the cases for P, it would still be possible to proceed with the cases for Q, during which R would become instantiated. This is a property of the induction schemes generated from mutually recursive functions and is made more formal in Sect. 4.

Case $Q(at) \supset Q(\text{annotate}(s, at))$. Having renamed the s from the scheme to avoid a conflict, the goal in this case is:

$$\forall s.\ amerge(concat(s, at)) = concat(s, at)$$
$$\vdash_? \ amerge(concat(s, \text{annotate}(s', at))) = concat(s, \text{annotate}(s', at))$$

The conclusion rewrites using the definition of *concat* to:

$$amerge(concat(strcat(s, s'), at)) = concat(strcat(s, s'), at)$$

Instantiating s in the hypothesis to $strcat(s, s')$ completes this case.

The remaining cases of the proof are straightforward using the definitions and the injectivity of the type constructors.

The formula used to instantiate Q could be used in another way, namely to strengthen the original conjecture by adding it as another conjunct and then restart the proof. Indeed this could be done even if the structural induction scheme for the types were used. A structural induction using the strengthened goal is, however, more tricky, requiring an automated procedure to do such things as: use one of the conjuncts of the hypothesis twice and detect that the two conjuncts of the conclusion are identical. These things are easy for a human to see but are challenging for an automatic procedure to do in general. Using the scheme generated from the functions is considerably simpler.

4   A Proof Procedure for Using Multi-predicate Schemes

The example proof in Sect. 3 motivates a proof procedure `induction_mutual` for multi-predicate induction schemes. The procedure takes a scheme S, a goal term t, and a matching induction predicate P_k as arguments.

Definition 1. *The scheme S has the general form:*

$$P_{1,1}(v_{1,1}) \wedge \ldots \wedge P_{1,n_1}(v_{1,n_1}) \wedge C_1 \supset P_{1,0}(f_1[v_{1,1}, \ldots, v_{1,n_1}])$$

$$\vdots$$

$$\frac{P_{m,1}(v_{m,1}) \wedge \ldots \wedge P_{m,n_m}(v_{m,n_m}) \wedge C_m \supset P_{m,0}(f_m[v_{m,1}, \ldots, v_{m,n_m}])}{(\forall v_1.\ P_1(v_1)) \wedge \ldots \wedge (\forall v_r.\ P_r(v_r))}$$

with the following properties (where $[x]$ denotes the set $\{1, \ldots, x\}$):

1. *$m > 0$, $\forall i \in [m]$. $n_i \geq 0$, $r > 0$.*
2. *The P's are induction predicates.*
3. *The v's are vectors of one or more variables.*
4. *The C's are additional conditions.*
5. *$\forall i \in [m]$. $f_i[v_{i,1}, \ldots, v_{i,n_i}]$ denotes a vector of terms involving variables in $v_{i,1}, \ldots, v_{i,n_i}$.*
6. *$\forall i \in [r]$. $\exists j \in [m]$. $P_i = P_{j,0}$.*
7. *$\forall i \in [m]$. $\forall j \in [n_i]$. $\exists k \in [m]$. $P_{i,j} = P_{k,0}$.*
8. *The free variables appearing in $\{v_{i,1}, \ldots, v_{i,n_i}, C_i, f_i[v_{i,1}, \ldots, v_{i,n_i}]\}$ are assumed to be universally quantified in hypothesis i.*

The consequent *of hypothesis i of the scheme is $P_{i,0}(f_i[v_{i,1}, \ldots, v_{i,n_i}])$ and the* antecedants *are $\{P_{i,1}(v_{i,1}), \ldots, P_{i,n_i}(v_{i,n_i}), C_i\}$. If h denotes hypothesis i then let $pred(h)$ denote $P_{i,0}$.*

It is not necessary for all the $P_{i,j}$ predicates $(1 \leq i \leq m, 0 \leq j \leq n_i)$ to appear in the conclusion of the scheme (i.e., be equal to one of the P_k $(1 \leq k \leq r)$).

Property 6 of Definition 1 says that each of the induction predicates in the conclusion must appear as the consequent of at least one of the hypotheses. Property 7 says that each of the predicates in the antecedants of the hypotheses must be the consequent of one of the hypotheses.

Definition 2. *A predicate is* native *in the antecedants of a hypothesis if it is equal to the predicate that appears in the consequent. Otherwise it is* foreign.

For the proof procedure it is useful to distinguish cases of the induction that involve foreign predicates in the antecedants. This motivates the following definition.

Definition 3. *A hypothesis*

$$P_{i,1}(v_{i,1}) \wedge \ldots \wedge P_{i,n_i}(v_{i,n_i}) \wedge C_i \supset P_{i,0}(f_i[v_{i,1}, \ldots, v_{i,n_i}])$$

of a scheme is said to be a base case *if $n_i = 0$. Otherwise it is a* step case *if there is a $j \in [n_i]$ such that $P_{i,j} = P_{i,0}$, and a* cycle case *if there is a $j \in [n_i]$ such that $P_{i,j} \neq P_{i,0}$. So, a hypothesis may be both a step case and a cycle case.*

Let us now assume that P_k has been selected as the induction predicate for the goal term t and that variables $\{x_1, \ldots, x_{l_k}\}$ in t have been matched up to v_k.

Without loss of generality, t can be assumed to have the form $\forall x_1 \ldots x_{l_k} \, y_1 \ldots y_u$. $F[x_1, \ldots, x_{l_k}, y_1, \ldots, y_u]$ (universal quantifiers can be commuted).

The `induction_mutual` procedure is shown in Fig. 1. The procedure is non-deterministic and may fail at various points. The intention is that it should backtrack at points of failure and try alternative execution paths (see below). The subroutine `use_hypotheses` assumes that the goal has been rewritten to a conjunction of formulas and tries to match hypotheses to the conjuncts. It goes beyond the procedures typically found in inductive provers in that it can instantiate predicate variables in the hypotheses during the matching process.

Some remarks about the procedure:

- The x's and y's are vectors of variables.
- The function $frees$ computes the free variables of a term.
- ϕ is a substitution and $(p\phi)_\beta$ denotes the result of applying ϕ to p and beta-reducing (including redexes from previous calls of `use_hypotheses`).
- $\text{match}(p,t)$ is true if and only if p can be made syntactically equal to t by instantiating the universal quantifiers in p.
- The subroutines `base_case` and `step_case` are as they might be in a procedure for induction using a single-predicate scheme. Specifically, `base_case` reduces using the definitions of the functions in the goal and performs standard logical simplifications, while `step_case` manipulates the induction conclusion using the definitions and lemmas to get it into a form in which (some of) the hypotheses can be used. It then uses the hypotheses and simplifies. Both subroutines are allowed to leave a residual goal. For simple examples it would suffice for these subroutines to do exhaustive rewriting with the function definitions but for more complex examples it is beneficial to use heuristic procedures such as those in *Clam* [5].
- The syntactic form '(`base_case` then `use_hypotheses`)(h)' means "apply the `base_case` subroutine to h and then apply the `use_hypotheses` subroutine to any residual goals".

The choice points in the procedure are:

1. The selection of an instantiated predicate;
2. Within the `base_case` and `step_case` subroutines;
3. The selection and ordering of the antecedants Γ' in `use_hypotheses`.

Failure of a conjunction of antecedents (the induction hypotheses) to match the residual term causes backtracking which drives a search through the different combinations and permutations of antecedents at choice point 3. The search terminates if a match is found. If no combination of antecedents produces a match then `use_hypotheses` fails. This may cause backtracking at point 2 to yield a different residual term. If that is not successful the induction predicates may be processed in a different order (point 1) but this is unlikely to help the proof because the cases for the originally chosen predicate must be processed eventually. Further backtracking might cause earlier instantiations of predicates to be undone and a different choice to be made at point 3 for an earlier invocation of `use_hypotheses`, but undoing instantiations may be difficult to implement.

For a discussion of the termination properties of the procedure see [2].

```
procedure induction_mutual(S, t, P_k);

    procedure matches(p, t);
        p_1 ∧ ... ∧ p_u := p;    t_1 ∧ ... ∧ t_u := t;
        I := {i ∈ [u] | p_i has the form P_i(x_i)};
        for i ∈ I do begin y_i := frees(t_i) − x_i;  Λ_i := λx_i. ∀y_i. t_i end;
        φ := {Λ_i/P_i | i ∈ I};
        if ∀i ∈ [u]. match((p_iφ)_β, t_i) then
            begin
                for i ∈ I do instantiate P_i to Λ_i;
                return true
            end
        else return false
    end procedure;

    procedure use_hypotheses(Γ ⊃ t);
        if (∃Γ' ⊆ Γ. (Γ' = {a_1, ..., a_u}) ∧ u > 0 ∧ matches(a_1 ∧ ... ∧ a_u, t))
        then return
        else fail
    end procedure;

    H := the hypotheses of S;
    instantiate P_k to λx_1 ... x_{l_k}. ∀y_1 ... y_u. F[x_1, ..., x_{l_k}, y_1, ..., y_u];
    while H ≠ {} do
        begin
            P := any pred(h) (for h ∈ H) that has been instantiated;
            Cases := {h ∈ H | pred(h) = P};
            beta-reduce applications of instantiated induction predicates in Cases;
            H := H − Cases;
            Base := {h ∈ Cases | h is a base case};
            Cycle := {h ∈ Cases | h is a cycle case and not a step case};
            Step := {h ∈ Cases | h is a step case and not a cycle case};
            StepAndCycle := {h ∈ Cases | h is both a step case and a cycle case};
            for h ∈ Base do base_case(h);
            for h ∈ Cycle do (base_case then use_hypotheses)(h);
            for h ∈ Step do step_case(h);
            for h ∈ StepAndCycle do (step_case then use_hypotheses)(h)
        end

end procedure
```

Fig. 1. The induction procedure for multi-predicate induction schemes

5   Implementation and Results

The algorithm described in Sect. 2 for generating induction schemes from mutually recursive function definitions has been implemented in the HOL theorem prover [6]. The `induction_mutual` procedure of Sect. 4 has been implemented in the *Clam* proof planner [5] and the resulting proof plans can be turned into a tactic for use in HOL via an interface between the two systems [1]. Although it would in principle be possible to do everything in HOL, *Clam*, which is based on Prolog, has good support for the meta-variables needed for the uninstantiated induction predicates and for more complex examples offers sophisticated heuristics for controlling the rewriting stages.

For the step cases of `induction_mutual` (using the terminology of Definition 3), the rippling method [4] is used to guide the proof. Rippling takes place with respect to the hypotheses that correspond to the native induction predicate (Definition 2). For non-step cases reduction (symbolic evaluation) and simplification are used. Currently, the instantiation of induction predicates works for cases in which reduction or "rippling out" are used. Another form of rippling, called "rippling in", guides the proof to a point at which a universally quantified variable in the hypothesis can be instantiated in a non-trivial way (cf. the third case of the proof in Sect. 3). This form of rippling is typically required where one of the functions has an "accumulator" argument.

The `induction_mutual` procedure was developed using a simple example about mutually recursive *even* and *odd* predicates plus an example involving a type of arbitrarily branching trees:

```
datatype tree = leaf of int | node of (tree)list
```

Here, the recursive type is nested under a type constructor (`list`). Functions defined over such nested recursive types are naturally mutually recursive. The example involves two functions, *flatten_tree* and *fringe*, that construct a list of the leaf nodes of a tree but in different ways. The function *flatten_tree* uses a second-order *map* function, while *fringe* has a mutually recursive counterpart, *fringes*, for dealing with the list of subtrees. The conjecture is that the two definitions are equivalent.

The procedure of Fig. 1 has been used to automatically prove both of the development examples, the example presented in Sect. 3, and the other formulas listed in Table 1.

The function *reverse_tree* reverses the order of the leaf nodes and is defined in a similar way to *flatten_tree* using *map*. Since *reverse_tree* is not mutually recursive, Example 4 does not involve mutually recursive functions but a multi-predicate scheme is still used because the `tree` type is nested recursive. The proof requires lemmas for the distributivity of *map*, *reverse*, and *flatten* (which flattens a list of lists and is used in the definition of *flatten_tree*) over *app* (which concatenates two lists), and the lemma $app(x, \mathtt{nil}) = x$. In addition, Example 5 requires the associativity of *app*, and Example 6 requires Example 5 as a lemma.

Our implementation is also capable of generating the induction scheme for the *exp*/*exhelp* example discussed in [8] and successfully plans all but one case.

Table 1. Theorems proved using the *Clam* implementation

	Conjecture	No. of lemmas
1	$\forall n.\ even(n) \supset \neg odd(n)$	0
2	$\forall n.\ even(n) \vee even(suc(n))$	0
3	$\forall t.\ flatten\_tree(t) = fringe(t)$	0
4	$\forall t.\ flatten\_tree(reverse\_tree(t)) = reverse(flatten\_tree(t))$	4
5	$\forall x\ y.\ fringes(app(x, y)) = app(fringes(x), fringes(y))$	1
6	$\forall t.\ fringe(reverse\_tree(t)) = reverse(fringe(t))$	3
7	$\forall at.\ amerge(amerge(at)) = amerge(at)$	0

The case that cannot be handled involves nested recursive function calls, which are currently out of the scope of *Clam*. The proof procedure does get as far as synthesizing the instantiation for the second induction predicate. In fact, an interactive proof in HOL is very simple once this instantiation has been found, involving merely an application of the instantiated induction scheme, followed by conditional rewriting using the definitions of the functions. (Of course, such a freewheeling approach would be problematic as a fully automatic procedure because of concerns about termination of rewriting.)

6 Related Work

The procedure presented here for induction using multi-predicate schemes is in some respects similar to so-called *middle-out reasoning* [7]. The proof of the original conjecture proceeds simultaneously with finding suitable instances for the induction predicates, with each assisting the other. The formulas used to instantiate the predicates can be seen as intermediate lemmas or as extra conjuncts that generalise the original conjecture. Like middle-out reasoning, the procedure uses meta-variables to stand for some initially unknown term structure.

Also related is Protzen's lazy generation of induction hypotheses [11]. Protzen generates the actual induction scheme during the proof rather than instances for its predicate(s). This allows hypotheses to be used that would not be suggested by recursion analysis. His work is in a destructor-style setting and it is not obvious how it would transpose to the constructor-style we use. There appears to be an implicit assumption that only one induction predicate is required so his work would not immediately be applicable to functions defined over mutually recursive types. It is conceivable that his approach would provide a good way to control the rewriting prior to instantiation of our additional induction predicates.

Kapur and Subramaniam describe a technique for automating induction over mutually recursive functions using cover sets [8]. Their approach is to unroll the mutual recursion to obtain a cover set that captures the recursive dependencies. It is not clear from their paper how their algorithm generalises to more than two mutually recursive functions or that it works in general for two functions that are each defined in terms of both functions. Our approach can handle both of these situations.

Liu and Chang [9] deal with mutual recursion by generating strong induction schemes, i.e., ones in which the property is assumed to hold for a chain of smaller values rather than just the next smallest. The hypotheses for the smaller values are captured by defining auxiliary recursive functions which follow the recursion pattern of the mutually recursive functions but with predicates in place of the original expressions. By this means, all the necessary hypotheses for the proof are obtained. Liu and Chang's paper is mainly about generating the schemes, saying little about how they are used in proofs.

7   Conclusions and Future Work

This paper makes two contributions: a procedure for automating proofs about mutually recursive functions and a procedure for deriving the multi-predicate induction schemes used by the first procedure. The latter goes beyond previous work on generating multi-predicate schemes from mutually recursive datatypes and single-predicate schemes from non-mutual functions by deriving multi-predicate schemes from mutually recursive functions. The procedures have been implemented and tested in the *Clam* proof planner and the HOL theorem prover, respectively. The implemented proof procedure makes use of *Clam*'s infrastructure but it is essentially independent of the details of *Clam*, and hence could be re-used in other systems.

The induction schemes have one predicate for each of the mutually recursive functions. This avoids the need for techniques such as unwinding the functions into a single function (which tends to cause a quadratic increase in size and is not always possible anyway). One induction predicate is matched against the initial goal and the instantiations for the other predicates are synthesized as part of the proof procedure. An important point is that the induction scheme follows the recursion pattern of the functions rather than of the types over which they are defined (though these do coincide in many cases).

An item for future work is to investigate examples where there is more than one occurrence of an uninstantiated predicate in the hypotheses, *e.g.*:

$$\forall x \ y. \ Q(x) \wedge Q(y) \supset P(\mathsf{C}(x, y))$$

In such cases, it becomes more difficult to find an instantiation. Also, if there is more than one recursive function involved in a conjecture it may be necessary to combine induction schemes as is done, for example, by Boyer and Moore [3], Liu and Chang [9], and by Walther [16].

References

1. R. Boulton, K. Slind, A. Bundy, and M. Gordon. An interface between CLAM and HOL. In *Proceedings of the 11th International Conference on Theorem Proving in Higher Order Logics (TPHOLs'98)*, volume 1479 of *Lecture Notes in Computer Science*, pages 87–104, Springer, 1998.
2. R. J. Boulton. Multi-predicate induction schemes for mutual recursion. Informatics Research Report EDI-INF-RR-0014, Division of Informatics, University of Edinburgh, April 2000.
3. R. S. Boyer and J S. Moore. *A Computational Logic*. ACM Monograph Series. Academic Press, New York, 1979.
4. A. Bundy, A. Stevens, F. van Harmelen, A. Ireland, and A. Smaill. Rippling: A heuristic for guiding inductive proofs. *Artificial Intelligence*, 62:185–253, 1993.
5. A. Bundy, F. van Harmelen, C. Horn, and A. Smaill. The OYSTER-CLAM system. In *Proceedings of the 10th International Conference on Automated Deduction*, volume 449 of *Lecture Notes in Artificial Intelligence*, pages 647–648, Springer, 1990.
6. M. J. C. Gordon and T. F. Melham, editors. *Introduction to HOL: A theorem proving environment for higher order logic*. Cambridge University Press, 1993.
7. J. T. Hesketh. *Using Middle-Out Reasoning to Guide Inductive Theorem Proving*. PhD thesis, University of Edinburgh, 1991.
8. D. Kapur and M. Subramaniam. Automating induction over mutually recursive functions. In *Proceedings of the 5th International Conference on Algebraic Methodology and Software Technology (AMAST'96)*, volume 1101 of *Lecture Notes in Computer Science*, Springer, 1996.
9. P. Liu and R.-J. Chang. A new structural induction scheme for proving properties of mutually recursive concepts. In *Proceedings of the 6th National Conference on Artificial Intelligence*, volume 1, pages 144–148. AAAI, July 1987.
10. L. C. Paulson. *ML for the Working Programmer*. Cambridge University Press, 2nd edition, July 1996.
11. M. Protzen. Lazy generation of induction hypotheses. In *Proceedings of the 12th International Conference on Automated Deduction (CADE-12)*, volume 814 of *Lecture Notes in Artificial Intelligence*, pages 42–56, Springer, 1994.
12. K. Slind. Function definition in higher-order logic. In *Proceedings of the 9th International Conference on Theorem Proving in Higher Order Logics (TPHOLs'96)*, volume 1125 of *Lecture Notes in Computer Science*, pages 381–397, Springer, 1996.
13. K. Slind. Derivation and use of induction schemes in higher-order logic. In *Proceedings of the 10th International Conference on Theorem Proving in Higher Order Logics (TPHOLs'97)*, volume 1275 of *Lecture Notes in Computer Science*, pages 275–290, Springer, 1997.
14. K. Slind. Reasoning about Terminating Functional Programs. PhD Thesis, Institut für Informatik, Technische Universität München, 1999. Accessible at http://www.cl.cam.ac.uk/users/kxs/papers.
15. M. VanInwegen and E. Gunter. HOL-ML. In *Proceedings of the 6th International Workshop on Higher Order Logic Theorem Proving and its Applications (HUG'93)*, volume 780 of *Lecture Notes in Computer Science*, pages 61–74, Springer, 1994.
16. C. Walther. Combining induction axioms by machine. In *Proceedings of the Thirteenth International Joint Conference on Artificial Intelligence (IJCAI-93)*, volume 1, pages 95–100, Morgan Kaufmann Publishers, Inc.

Proof Planning with Multiple Strategies

Erica Melis and Andreas Meier

Universität des Saarlandes, Fachbereich Informatik
66041 Saarbrücken, Germany
{melis,ameier}@ags.uni-sb.de

Abstract. Humans have different problem solving strategies at their disposal and they can flexibly employ several strategies when solving a complex problem, whereas previous theorem proving and planning systems typically employ a single strategy or a hard coded combination of a few strategies. We introduce multi-strategy proof planning that allows for combining a number of strategies and for *switching* flexibly between strategies in a proof planning process. Thereby proof planning becomes more robust since it does not necessarily fail if one problem solving mechanism fails. Rather it can *reason* about preference of strategies and about failures. Moreover, our strategies provide a means for structuring the vast amount of knowledge such that the planner can cope with the otherwise overwhelming knowledge in mathematics.

1 Introduction

The choice of an appropriate problem solving strategy is a crucial human skill and is typically guided by some meta-level reasoning. Trained mathematicians use different problem solving strategies. For instance, a theorem can be solved by analogy to another previously solved theorem, by forward reasoning, or by backward reasoning. For teaching mathematics this has been described in [20]. Schoenfeld [21] too investigates strategies and advocates the teaching of their heuristic control.

For automated theorem proving the situation is quite different currently. Traditional automated theorem provers (ATPs) such as OTTER or SPASS either blindly search for a proof in a rather unmanageable search space or use a search heuristic determined by parameter settings to traverse the search space. As a result, these systems cannot recognize mathematically promising search paths or combine several search strategies. Their performance depends on whether the ATP's search heuristic is appropriate for proving the particular problem. Indeed, experience has shown that no one theorem prover or heuristic is best for any problem.

As a reaction to these difficulties several approaches combine different problem solving strategies: (1) different systems are combined in a way that allocates certain time slices to each system in a row until one of the systems solves the problem [1]; (2) different instances of the same system with different parameter

J. Lloyd et al. (Eds.): CL 2000, LNAI 1861, pp. 644–659, 2000.

settings are successively tried for completely solving a problem [24]; (3) cooperation of different systems by exchanging specific intermediate results has been realized in [9].

As we discuss below, these solutions are insufficient at least for the problems arising in proof planning. Moreover, there is another problem rarely addressed in automated theorem proving that we shall tackle in this paper. In ATPs the search space is largely determined by the axioms included into the problem formalization. Thus, the success of an ATP depends extremely on the problem formalization including the selected axioms. This is problematic in a realistic setting for proving many theorems, where all mathematical knowledge is available in principle.

An alternative technique for theorem proving is proof planning. It differs from traditional automated theorem proving in that it considers a theorem to be proved as a planning problem [6, 18]. A partial plan is refined by introducing new steps or adding new constraints until the proof plan is fully instantiated and complete, i.e., it has no open goals anymore. A step is represented by a (instantiated) method such as induction, diagonalization, or estimations.

Typically, the search space in proof planning differs from that of ATPs because proof planning tries to solve a problem at the level of methods most of which are more abstract than the logical inference steps of ATPs. Even more important for restricting the search space is the meta-level reasoning that guides the selection of methods. Currently, this meta-level reasoning is encoded by a list of control rules [13] or by variations of the difference reduction search heuristic called rippling [7].

However, when the class of theorems to be proved with the same methods and control rules grows, the search heuristics might prove to be inappropriate for new theorems. There are at least two reasons for this phenomenon. First, mathematics is very knowledge-intensive and all the knowledge (methods, axioms) has to be used indeed. If all the methods are potentially available, then the search space becomes unmanageable. Secondly, in order to be able to prove nontrivial mathematical theorems, different subproblems have to be attacked in different ways. For instance, a certain subgoal (e.g., a tautology) may be hard to prove by proof planning but proved easily by an ATP.

The above mentioned approaches to combine several ATP strategies are not sufficient for proof planning since they are not flexible enough: (1) They do not offer the possibility to switch flexibly between strategies during the planning process and cannot make use of explicit meta-reasoning at the level of strategies. (2) None of the approaches provides any means for managing and structuring the overwhelming amount of knowledge that realistic theorem proving is faced with.

To solve the mentioned problems of proof planning we introduce multi-strategy proof planning that can *switch flexibly* between different strategies in the same planning process and can use knowledge in a structured way. We extend the notion of a strategy such that different strategies can employ different refinement or modification algorithms and different search heuristics. The strategy choices in our multi-strategy planning are subject to strategic control by meta-level reasoning.

The paper is organized as follows. First, we briefly review previous proof planning in the ΩMEGA system. Then we introduce multi-strategy proof planning and describe how it is realized in MULTI, the multi-strategy planner of the ΩMEGA system. Finally, we provide evidence that MULTI is more powerful than the previous proof planner of ΩMEGA and discuss examples of the limit domain which are provable only by MULTI.

2   Basics of Knowledge Based Proof Planning

Proof planning considers mathematical theorems as planning problems. A planning problem is defined by an initial partial plan (specified by the proof assumptions and the open goal given by the theorem to be proved) and a set of methods. A *partial plan* π is a tuple $(T, \prec, CS)$, where T is a set of steps that are instantiated methods, $\prec$ is a partial order over T, and CS is a collection of constraints (the constraint store) for general and for domain-specific constraints such as inequality constraints and set constraints, respectively. A simple planner searches for a (partially instantiated) method M whose application proves a goal g. It introduces M into the plan. The subgoals needed for the application of M replace g in the planning state. The planner continues to search for methods applicable to a subgoal and terminates when a solution is found.

We illustrate proof planning in the limit domain for which a typical problem is: 'show that the limit of the sum of two real functions is equal to the sum of their limits' whose formalization is

$$\lim_{x \to a} f(x) = l_1 \wedge \lim_{x \to a} g(x) = l_2 \vdash \lim_{x \to a} (f(x) + g(x)) = l_1 + l_2.$$

Since the limit is defined by

$$\lim_{x \to a} h(x) = l \Leftrightarrow$$
$$\forall \epsilon (0 < \epsilon \to \exists \delta (0 < \delta \wedge \forall x (x \neq a \wedge |x - a| < \delta \to |h(x) - l| < \epsilon))),$$

we need to show that

$$\forall \epsilon (0 < \epsilon \to \exists \delta (0 < \delta \wedge \forall x (x \neq a \wedge |x - a| < \delta \to |(f(x) + g(x)) - (l_1 + l_2)| < \epsilon)))$$

holds under the assumptions

$$\forall \epsilon_1 (0 < \epsilon_1 \to \exists \delta_1 (0 < \delta_1 \wedge \forall x_1 (x_1 \neq a \wedge |x_1 - a| < \delta_1 \to |f(x_1) - l_1| < \epsilon_1)))$$
$$\forall \epsilon_2 (0 < \epsilon_2 \to \exists \delta_2 (0 < \delta_2 \wedge \forall x_2 (x_2 \neq a \wedge |x_2 - a| < \delta_2 \to |g(x_2) - l_2| < \epsilon_2))).$$

An epsilon-delta-proof of this problem as well as similar theorems constructs a real number δ (dependent on ϵ) that satisfies the inequalities in the theorem. Epsilon-delta-proofs require proof planning with the general methods QuantifierElim*, AndElim*, QuantifierIntro*, AndIntro*, =subst, and Focus and the domain-specific methods Solve, Solve*, and ComplexEstimate. QuantifierElim*, AndElim*, QuantifierIntro*, and AndIntro* iteratively apply certain natural deduction rules. For instance, `AndIntro*` closes an open goal $A_1 \wedge A_2 \ldots \wedge A_n$ and introduces the new subgoals A_1, $A_2 \ldots$, and A_n. `AndElim*` decomposes an assumption $A_1 \wedge A_2 \ldots \wedge A_n$ into assumptions A_1, $A_2 \ldots$, and A_n. `Focus` marks subformulas or terms whose position is provided as a parameter of the method. The method `=subst` reduces a goal $t[a]$ which contains an occurrence of a formula a to the new goal $t[b]$ where the occurrence of a is replaced by an occurrence of b, if there is a proved equation $a = b$. The `Solve` method satisfies inequalities between simple terms such as $x < c$ by passing it to a constraint solver that collects consistent constraints in a constraint store CS [14]. `Solve*` reduces a goal $a_1 < b_1$ to a subgoal $b_2\sigma \leq b_1\sigma$ in case an assumption $a_2 < b_2$ exists and a_1, a_2 can be unified by the substitution σ. Finally, `ComplexEstimate` reduces inequality goals $b < e$ with a complex term b to simpler inequality subgoals, see [15].

The previous proof planner of ΩMEGA, PLANNER, refines a partial plan by applying different operations refining or modifying the partial plan until a solution, i.e., a sequence of steps that transforms the initial state into a goal state and satisfies the constraints, is found. PLANNER has refinement and modification operations for backward and forward planning, for the expansion of complex methods, for the instantiation of meta-variables[1], and backtracking. These operations are invoked in a default order: First, backward and forward planning and backtracking is employed until no open goal is left. Then complex methods are expanded and the constraint solver is employed to compute instantiations for the meta-variables from the set of collected constraints. Backtracking is used only if a situation is reached where none of the selected methods can be applied to an open goal.

When proof planning limit theorems, PLANNER behaves as follows: It *backwardly* decomposes the goal formula to (in)equality subgoals (by applying methods such as `QuantifierIntro*` and `AndIntro*`). Then simple (in)equality goals are closed by `Solve`. In order to satisfy more complex goals, *forward* planning is necessary before the backward planning can be continued. The forward planning decomposes an assumption (by applying methods such as `QuantifierElim*` and `AndElim*`) in order to obtain a new assumption that can be used to further tackle a goal by `Solve*` or `ComplexEstimate`. When no open goal is left and all constraints are collected, the constraint solver computes instantiations for the meta-variables that are consistent with the collected constraints. Then the meta-variables are instantiated everywhere in the proof.

3   Multi-strategy Proof Planning

In the following, we introduce multi-strategy proof planning. First, an example (exercise 4.1.3 in the analysis textbook [2]) illustrates that and why the proof planning with a fix combination of refinement and modification operations that

---

[1] A meta-variable is a place holder for a term or a formula. In the following, meta-variables are denoted by capital letters.

works for many examples is insufficient as a general technique. Then we introduce proof planning with multiple strategies and its implementation, MULTI. In Section 4 we shall show how multi-strategy proof planning overcomes these problems. (This example is just one, see, e.g., [17] for other examples.)

3.1   A Motivating Example

Exercise 4.1.3. Let $f : \mathbf{R} \to \mathbf{R}$ and let $c \in \mathbf{R}$. Show that $\lim_{x_1 \to c} f(x_1) = l$ if and only if $\lim_{x \to 0} f(x + c) = l$.

Two implications have to be proof planned for solving this exercise:

$$\lim_{x_1 \to c} f(x_1) = l \Rightarrow \lim_{x \to 0} f(x + c) = l \tag{1}$$

and

$$\lim_{x \to 0} f(x + c) = l \Rightarrow \lim_{x_1 \to c} f(x_1) = l \tag{2}$$

Since the limit $\lim_{x \to a}$ is defined as described in the previous section we need to show for (1) that

$$\forall \epsilon (0 < \epsilon \to \exists \delta (0 < \delta \wedge \forall x (x \neq 0 \wedge |x - 0| < \delta \to |f(x + c) - l| < \epsilon)))$$

holds under the assumption

$$\forall \epsilon_1 (0 < \epsilon_1 \to \exists \delta_1 (0 < \delta_1 \wedge \forall x_1 (x_1 \neq c \wedge |x_1 - c| < \delta_1 \to |f(x_1) - l| < \epsilon_1))).$$

PLANNER evaluates a list of control rules to determine which method to apply next. When planning for (1), first the complex goal formula is (backwardly) decomposed. This creates the new subgoals $0 < D$ and $|f(x' + c) - l| < e$.[2] The simple goal $0 < D$ can be closed by Solve that passes the inequality to CS. The goal $|f(x' + c) - l| < e$ is too complex to be send to the constraint solver. An appropriate assumption that can be used to further simplify this goal is the subformula $|f(x_1) - l| < \epsilon_1$ of the original assumption. This subformula is highlighted ('focused') by the method Focus and then unwrapped by forward planning. This unwrapping yields the new assumption $|f(X_1) - l| < E_1$ and the additional goal $|X_1 - c| < d_1$. Now $|f(x' + c) - l| < e$ can be closed by the method Solve*. This yields the new goals $E_1 \leq e$ and $X_1 = x' + c$ which can be closed by Solve. The goal $|X_1 - c| < d_1$ should be closed by the method Solve* using the assumption $|x' - 0| < D$. However, Solve* is not applicable because $(X_1 - c)$ and $(x' - 0)$ are not unifiable and hence proof planning is blocked. If we could use the information $X_1 = (x' + c)$ available in the constraint store, an *eager instantiation* of X_1 by $(x' + c)$ would unblock the planning because the goal would be instantiated to $|x' + c - c| < d_1$ which could be simplified to $|x'| < d_1$. For this simplified goal Solve* would be applicable (using the assumption $|x'| < D$ that is implied by the assumption $|x' - 0| < D$).

---

[2] The universally quantified variables x, ϵ in the goal are replaced by new constants x', e, whereas the existentially quantified δ is replaced by a new meta-variable D.

Planning for (2) works similarly, except that a goal $|f(x_1') - l| < e_1$ arises which can potentially be closed by the method Solve* using the assumption $|f(X + c) - l| < E$. Again, Solve* is not applicable in this situation because x_1' and $(X + c)$ are not unifiable and hence proof planning is blocked. In this case no helpful information is available in the constraint store. The problem is that the unification has a residuum $X + c = x_1'$. If we could prove this equation we could apply it to rewrite the goal and the proof planning became unblocked.

In both cases, (1) and (2), PLANNER fails to find a proof plan. In (1) PLANNER fails since its fix order to plan first until no open goals are left and to instantiate the meta-variables afterwards excludes an instantiations of meta-variables while there are still open goals. In (2) PLANNER fails since backtracking is the only reaction to blocked planning as opposed to reasoning about failures and repair.

Designing more elaborate methods that perform the (failure) reasoning implicitly does not solve this problem in general since methods should not encapsulate and hide the control because then the control cannot be modified, extended, adapted to new situations (see [18] for a discussion). Moreover, methods should be the building blocks of a plan rather than executing several algorithms.

3.2 Strategies

In order to make proof planning more robust and flexible we allow to combine the common planning algorithm with other *algorithms* also refining or modifying partial proof plans such as case-based planning, call of traditional ATPs, expansion of complex steps, and instantiation of meta-variables. In addition, the behavior of these algorithms can be influenced by different parameter settings. For instance, there are particular parameter settings for ATPs to make them appropriate to tackle particular problems. Similarly, a planner is equipped with parameters determining a list of methods and control rules to specify which methods and which control rules it can use. Rippling [7] is such an algorithm and constitutes a strategy together with parameters for its direction and for the measure of annotations. In general, we define each instantiation of an algorithm by parameters to be a *strategy*.

Multi-strategy planning can employ different strategies during one proof process and can switch flexibly between strategies to tackle different subproblems by different strategies. In particular,

- several strategies can cooperate for planning a proof of a theorem,
- this cooperation can be guided by strategic meta-reasoning.

Below, algorithms are indicated by italic fond and strategies (more generally, knowledge sources) by bold face, while methods and control rules are in typewriter fond.

3.3 Realization in MULTI

In MULTI, strategies are implemented as data structures with three slots: (1) an application condition stating which kind of problems/tasks the strategy can tackle, (2) the modification or refinement algorithm which is employed by the strategy, and (3) the parameter setting with that the algorithm is employed. Among the algorithms which are employed in MULTI are *PPlanner* for partial order planning, *Exp* for the expansion of complex methods, *InstMeta* for refining a partial plan by instantiating certain meta-variables in the partial plan, *ATP* which tries to close an open goal by calling a traditional ATP such as OTTER [12], *CPlanner* for case-based planning [19], and *BackTrack* for removing steps introduced by other algorithms.

In MULTI, not only an open goal is a task but other kinds of tasks can be created and solved by strategies too. For instance, each introduction of a meta-variable creates the task to instantiate this meta-variable and each introduction of a complex method into the plan creates the task to expand this method. Different tasks can be tackled by different algorithms and strategies.

This paper describes the strategies of *PPlanner* and *InstMeta* needed to accomplish epsilon-delta-proofs. The parameters of *PPlanner* are a list of methods, a list of control rules, and a termination condition specifying when the strategy application should terminate; a parameter of *InstMeta* is the function that determines how the instantiation is found. In particular, we need the strategies **NormalizeGoal**, **UnwrapHyp**, **SolveLinearInequality**, and **=SubstApply** which are instantiations of *PPlanner* and the strategy **InstFromCS** which is an instantiation of *InstMeta*. By **NormalizeGoal**, **SolveLinearInequality**, and **UnwrapHyp** the methods and control rules needed to find epsilon-delta-proofs are structured such that those methods and control rules are grouped together which are needed to tackle certain classes of subproblems.

The strategy **SolveLinearInequality** (see Table 1) is applicable to prove inequality goals. Its list of methods consists of `Solve`, `Solve*`, `ComplexEstimate`, and `Focus`. Its list of control rules contains `stop-with-focus` and `eager-instantiate`. **SolveLinearInequality** terminates when there are no further inequality goals. Note that it is the chosen parameterization of *PPlanner* that makes **SolveLinearInequality** appropriate to tackle inequality goals as stated in its application condition.

Table 1. The **SolveLinearInequality** strategy

Strategy: SolveLinearInequality		
Appl-condition	Linear-Inequality	
Algorithm	*PPlanner*	
Parameters	Methods	`Solve, Solve*, ComplexEstimate, Focus, ...`
	C-Rules	`stop-with-focus, eager-instantiate, ...`
	Termination	No-Linear-Inequalities

The parameters of **NormalizeGoal** determine that the strategy plans backwardly and can decompose goals that contain logical connectives or quantifiers. For instance, it contains the method `AndIntro*` that can decompose a goal that is a conjunction.

The task of **UnwrapHyp** is to unwrap a focused, i.e., highlighted, subformula of an assumption in order to make it available for proving a goal. The list of methods in the strategy **UnwrapHyp** determines that *PPlanner* plans forward, e.g., with the method `AndElim*`. The control rules determine that if **UnwrapHyp** is called, the available methods can only be applied to an assumption that carries a focus and if the method application does not destroy the focused subformula. For instance, if the assumptions $B_1 \wedge B_2$ and $A_1 \wedge A_2 \wedge focus(A_3 \wedge A_4)$ are in the planning state, the method `AndElim*` can only be used to decompose the second assumption into assumptions A_1, A_2, and $A_3 \wedge A_4$ but not to A_3 and A_4. **UnwrapHyp** terminates when the focused subformula is fully unwrapped.

The strategy **=SubstApply** is applicable on every goal. It introduces a (or few) new equation as a goal which is closed either by applying theory-specific equational reasoning or by constraint solving. Then this equation is used to rewrite the original goal by the method `=subst`. **=SubstApply**'s purpose is to repair failed proof attempts caused by a slightly failed unification whose residuum is an equation (or a few equations).

How could we achieve the same refinement of the partial plan without using a strategy? If we employed the method `=subst` inside the strategy **SolveLinearInequalities**, then we would need a control rule that chooses, say as the last method, `=subst`. If we represented this failure reasoning by control rules inside a strategy, the choice of the method `=subst` and its parameter required to reason about the failed proof attempt *before* it was actually attempted. Since the evaluation of the control rules is not repeated when some of the selected methods are not applicable, the only way to determine whether `=subst` should really be tried, is to encode the failure of applying the previously tried method (because of a failed unification) into the application-conditions of `subst`. We think that this is not conceptually clean. Moreover, the parameter of the method `=subst` (the residuum of the unification) can be chosen only when the previously failed proof attempt is analyzed. This is, however, not the task of application-conditions of a method but (meta-)reasoning about the proof. The control and usage of **=SubstApply** are explained in the next section.

The strategy **InstFromCS** instantiates meta-variables which occur in constraints collected by the constraint solver. **InstFromCS** specifies that *InstMeta* replaces a meta-variable by a term that is computed by the constraint solver and that satisfies the currently collected constraints.

MULTI employs a blackboard architecture because this is an established means to organize the cooperation of several independent components – so-called knowledge sources – for solving a complex problem. The information about the status of the problem solving process is stated on a blackboard that can be accessed and changed by the knowledge sources. MULTI's architecture is similar to the *BB1* blackboard system [10]. The architecture of MULTI is summarized in the following and described in more detail in [16]. The architecture has two blackboards, one for the solution problem and one for the control problem. The solution blackboard contains the partial proof plan and a store which contains the status of the execution of strategies. The strategies are the knowledge sources which work on this solution blackboard. A strategy component contains all the strategies that can be used. The control blackboard contains job offers and demands. The **MetaReasoner** is the knowledge source working on the control blackboard. A scheduler looks up the control blackboard, takes the highest ranked job offer, and executes it.

Table 2. Cycle of MULTI

Job Offer. Strategies whose application condition is true put a job offer onto the control blackboard.

Guidance. The MetaReasoner evaluates strategic control knowledge with information from the blackboards. It orders the set of job offers accordingly.

Invocation. The scheduler invokes the first strategy from the list of job offers and deletes that strategy from the list.

Execution. The invoked strategy refines or modifies the solution blackboard objects and may place demands onto the control blackboard.

In a nutshell, MULTI operates according to the outline in Table 2. A strategy can change the solution blackboard by refining or modifying the partial plan and saving information to the store. If a strategy's condition part is satisfied, a strategy posts its applicability information, i.e., a job offer to tackle a certain task, onto the control blackboard. Strategies can also post demands onto the control blackboard. For instance, if the currently executed strategy S can only continue, if another strategy S' is executed first, then S is interrupted, its status saved to the store, and a demand for S' is placed onto the control blackboard. After the execution of S' the strategy S can be reinvoked again from the store.

In order to rank the job offers the **MetaReasoner** evaluates strategic control knowledge represented by *strategic control rules*. The meta-reasoning at the strategy-level can prefer a strategy or can cause a switch to another strategy if the current one is not appropriate. For instance, as a consequence of a failed proof attempt **MetaReasoner** should prefer a strategy that avoids the failure. Other instances of meta-reasoning include reasoning about demands.

Since demands originate from interrupted and blocked strategies it makes sense to prefer job offers for a demand. This preference is expressed in the strategic control rule `prefer-demand-satisfying`. The rule `prefer-demand-satisfying` has a higher priority than the rule `delay-instantiations-from-cs` that delays the instantiation of meta-variables. This means that if there is a demand for **InstFromCS**, then **InstFromCS** can be applied even when there are still open goals.

Now we illustrate MULTI's proof planning for epsilon-delta-proofs. First **NormalizeGoal** is called to decompose backwardly the goal formula. Then **SolveLinearInequality** is called on the produced inequality subgoals. If a goal is not solvable with one of the present assumptions, an appropriate subformula of an assumption is highlighted using the method **Focus**. After this focus is set

SolveLinearInequality is interrupted. This is controlled by the control rule `stop-with-focus` which states that if a focus is set, then the current computation should be interrupted and first the focused subformula should be unwrapped by **UnwrapHyp**. This flexible switch is performed as follows.

- The current status of the **SolveLinearInequality** execution is saved in the store and a demand is placed onto the control blackboard to call **UnwrapHyp**.
- After the execution of **UnwrapHyp** the demand is removed from the control blackboard.
- Then the interrupted execution of **SolveLinearInequality** can be reinvoked again from the store.

4   Results and Experiences with MULTI

A comparison of MULTI's performance with traditional ATPs such as OTTER would make little or no sense because even relatively simple limit theorems cannot be solved by them. A comparison with the proof planner *CIAM* [8] is not a good idea either because it does not have domain-specific methods and cannot solve most of these problems. A comparison with Bledsoe's work [5] is not possible, mainly because his system was not tried with the larger variety of limit theorems that would include the problematic examples. The limit domain's methods have been designed in a way that PLANNER would have at least the strength of Bledsoe's system. For these reasons we compare MULTI's performance with PLANNER only.

4.1   Experiments

Experiments with proving many theorems on convergent sequences, convergence of functions, and continuity have shown that MULTI performs better than PLANNER. In particular, MULTI can prove more problems than PLANNER with its default combination of refinement operations. Table 3 contains some typical examples from the fourth chapter of the textbook [2] that can be solved by MULTI but not by PLANNER.

Below we shall examine 4.1.3(1) and (2) in more detail. The mathematical content of some other examples from Table 3 is spelled out here to give an impression beyond the table's information.

Theorem 4.1.8. (Sequential Criterion) Let $f : A \to \mathbf{R}$ and let c be a cluster point of A; then:

(i) $\lim_{x \to c} f = L$ if and only if

(ii) for every sequence (x_n) in A that converges to c such that $x_n \neq c$ for all $n \in \mathbf{N}$, the sequence $(f(x_n))$ converges to L.

Exercise 4.1.12. Suppose the function $f : \mathbf{R} \to \mathbf{R}$ has limit L at 0, and let $a > 0$. If $g : \mathbf{R} \to \mathbf{R}$ is defined by $g(x) := f(ax)$ for $x \in \mathbf{R}$, show that $\lim_{x \to 0} g = L$.

Table 3. Some problems provable with MULTI but not with PLANNER.

Name of problem	success reason
exercise 4.1.3 first part	Eager Instantiation
exercise 4.1.3 second part	Reasoning about Failure
exercise 4.1.12	Eager Instantiation
theorem 4.1.8	Reasoning about Failure
example 4.2.8.(a)	Theorem Application
exercise 4.2.2.(a)	Theorem Application
exercise 4.2.9.(a)	ATP Application
exercise 4.2.9.(b)	ATP Application

Example 4.2.8.(a). (Show that) $\lim_{x \to 0} x^{\frac{3}{2}} = 0$ $(x > 0)$

Exercise 4.2.2.(a). (Show the existence of the limit) $\lim_{x \to 2} \sqrt[2]{\frac{2x+1}{x+3}}$ $(x > 0)$

Exercise 4.2.9.(a). Let f, g be defined on A to $\mathbf{R}$ and let c be a cluster point of A. Show that if both $\lim_{x \to c} f$ and $\lim_{x \to c}(f + g)$ exists, then $\lim_{x \to c} g$ exists.

In Table 3 the left column names theorems, examples, and exercises from [2] that exhibit failures in proof planning with PLANNER. The right column contains a shorthand of the reason for the success of MULTI. Here, Eager Instantiation means the possibility to instantiate certain meta-variables eagerly; Reasoning about Failure means the ability to reason about failures of method applications; ATP Application labels problems for which some subgoals are solvable by an ATP strategy; Theorem Application labels problems solvable by switching to a strategy that applies previously proved limit theorems rather than using the strategies for epsilon-delta-proofs.

Since the knowledge engineering for proof planning is pretty difficult, the number of theorems that have been successfully proof planned so far is growing only slowly. However, if not quantitatively then at least qualitatively, there is striking evidence for the need to reason about the choice of strategies and their combination in mathematics since the newly solved examples exhibit common features in mathematics.

Generally speaking, the main practical results are (i) a *greater robustness* of MULTI's proof planning in the sense that if one strategy does not succeed in planning a proof, MULTI can switch to another one; (ii) the use of strategic meta-level reasoning allows to *flexibly guide* the proof planning; (iii) the integration of independent theorem provers.

As a side effect of multi-strategy proof planning, a new abstraction level of proof plans is introduced that can be used for the presentation of proof ideas like, e.g., 'we unwrap the assumption X and then prove inequalities'. Moreover, the refinement of a partial plan by a human user can be integrated easily within MULTI since one of the strategies represents the user and via the interface the user can directly choose one of the offers from the control blackboard thereby overwriting the automatic meta-level reasoning.

4.2   Explanation of MULTI's Success

In the following, MULTI's success is explained and illustrated in more detail.

Meta-reasoning at the Level of Strategies. A great deal of the power of proof planning stems from its strategic meta-reasoning. While control rules in *PPlanner* (and in PLANNER) allow to reason at the level of methods, MULTI allows for meta-reasoning at the level of strategies. The meta-reasoning can deal, e.g., with avoiding proof failures, different ways to backtrack, determine in which situation a complex method should be expanded, or when to call case-based planning [19].

Lets have a look at meta-reasoning about failed proof attempts. PLANNER cannot reason about failure and repair. It can only find an applicable method to close the goal or backtrack. MULTI, however, can reason about failures.

The idea behind it is as follows. Planning can be blocked if a unification required in the application condition of the method does not succeed but has a residuum $t_1 = t_2$. If we knew $t_1 = t_2$, or could prove it, then the equality could be applied eagerly and proof planning became unblocked. The strategic control rule `prefer-repair-unify` checks whether a failure is caused by blocked unification and whether this unification could be enabled by additional equality constraints or equational reasoning. If this is the case, no backtracking is performed but the last strategy execution is stored and the strategy =**SubstApply** is called. It introduces the needed equality constraint as a new goal, solves it, and then applies the method =**subst** to the original goal such that the unification will work later on. Then the interrupted strategy execution is reinvoked.

To illustrate, in exercise 4.1.3(2) the planning became unblocked if we knew $X + c = x_1'$. Then =**SubstApply** introduces the equality constraint $X + c = x_1'$ as a new goal. The new equation $X + c = x_1'$ is used to replace the x_1' in $|f(x_1') - l|$ by $(X + c)$. When **SolveLinearInequality** is reinvoked, `Solve*` is applicable to the changed goal $|f(X + c) - l| < e$ with the assumption $|f(X + c) - l| < E$ since the unification is possible now. `Solve` closes the new goal $X + c = x_1'$ and passes this constraint to the constraint solver.

Flexible Combination of Algorithms. MULTI allows to switch between strategies during the planning process. The necessity of this feature was indicated for exercise 4.1.3.(1) in § 3.1, where an eager instantiation of a meta-variable had to be performed to unblock the proof planning.

To allow for an eager instantiation of a meta-variable the list of control rules of the strategy **SolveLinearInequality** contains the rule `eager-instantiate`.

```
(control-rule eager-instantiate
    (IF (instantiation-determined-for-mv ?MV))
    (THEN (interrupt (InstFromCS ?MV))))
```

This control rule states that if the current constraint store fully determines the instantiation for a meta-variable, then the current strategy should be interrupted and a demand for instantiating the meta-variable should be placed onto the control blackboard.

For instance, in planning exercise 4.1.3(1), `Solve*` closes the goal $|f(x' + c) - l| < e$ with assumption $|f(X_1) - l| < E_1$. Thereby the constraint $X_1 = x' + c$ arises from unifying $|f(x' + c) - l|$ and $|f(X_1) - l|$ and is added to the constraint store. This constraint determines the instantiation of X_1. Therefore, the strategic control rule `eager-instantiate` fires and requests the interruption of **SolveLinearInequality** together with a demand for instantiating X_1. Guided by the strategic control rule `prefer-demand-satisfying` the **MetaReasoner** prefers the job offer of **InstMetaCS** which then instantiates X_1 by $(x' + c)$. Then the interrupted execution of **SolveLinearInequality** is continued and simplifies the instantiated goal $|x' + c - c| < d_1$ to $|x'| < d_1$ which can be closed with `Solve*`.

Structuring Knowledge. Since the parameters of *PPlanner* allow to configure strategies, different behaviors can be simulated that correspond to proving in different theory contexts, e.g., proving in a particular chapter of a book. In this way, the natural structure of mathematical books can be used. Imagine, e.g., a problem in which the limit of a composite function has to be found. This problem could be solved by speculating a limit and proving it by an epsilon-delta-proof which requires to expand the definition of the limit. Knowing the basic limit theorems, this problem could also be solved by decomposing the function and applying the limit theorems to the non-decomposable functions. The second proof will be shorter and more abstract than the first one but it relies on other theorems. The decision which collection of methods to choose from may largely depend on the context in which a problem should be solved. The context determines the resources that can be use, e.g., the prior knowledge of theorems.

Currently, some of the examples and exercises from [2] are provable only with the second kind of proof, e.g., example 4.2.8.(a) or exercise 4.2.2.(a). The reason is that their epsilon-delta-proofs that would require estimations of non-polynomial functions like *square root* or *sinus* which require more theory-specific knowledge in addition to the commonly successful estimation methods. After reducing the goal (e.g., $\lim_{x \to 0} sin(x) + 1 = 1$) by the strategy applying general limit theorems to three subgoals $\lim_{x \to 0} sin(x) = X_1$, $\lim_{x \to 0} = X_2$, and $X_1 + X_2 = 1$, the subgoals can be tackled by general or theory-specific estimations (such as $sin(x) \leq 1$, or $\lim_{x \to 0} sin(x) = 0$).

Integrating ATP Systems. When the strategies performing epsilon-delta-proofs fail, other strategies are available in MULTI, e.g., strategies with an ATP as algorithm. A multi-strategy proof planner can employ a traditional ATP to solve problems that are simple enough such that the ATP can find a complete proof. Then this prover is a refinement algorithm that does not produce new subgoals.

In MULTI, a strategy calling OTTER [12] with parameters is employed. These parameters are ATP-specific and control the search of the ATP. For certain classes of problems it is known which parameter setting is appropriate to find a proof. The application condition of the strategy checks whether a problem belongs to one of these classes. If not, then the ATP strategy is called with a default setting.

For instance, certain subproofs of the exercises 4.2.9.(a) and 4.2.9.(b) are solvable by OTTER but not with the epsilon-delta-proof strategy. Despite the general observation that ATPs cannot solve most limit theorems, they can prove certain subproblems. The reason for the success on the subproblems of 4.2.9.(a) and (b) is OTTER's strength in low-level inferences.

5   Conclusion and Related Work

We have presented multi-strategy proof planning that combines several strategies and thereby leverages the strength of different problem solving strategies. Note that our definition of a strategy extends the common notion of a strategy that determines how to traverse a search space.

Proof planning with multiple strategies integrates several refinement and modification mechanisms and search strategies in a flexible way. Such an approach is necessary in proof planning because

1. more often than not, a mathematical problem cannot be solved by a single strategy
2. a fix control of functionalities of a proof planner may be too rigid
3. in a *realistic* mathematical scenario, a vast amount of existing mathematical knowledge is available in principle which requires means that help structuring the knowledge.

The power of our multi-strategy proof planning stems from the collaboration of different strategies, its guidance by strategic meta-reasoning, and from the design of strategies that include different problem solving algorithms and a parameterization that may reflect mathematical knowledge structure. In particular, the reasoning about failed problem solving attempts is a precious source of guidance —at least in mathematics. Therefore, an important result is the discovery of a pattern of meta-reasoning about a class of failed proof attempts in mathematics. In addition to being more powerful, multi-strategy proof planning provides an appropriate framework for integrating user interaction and stand-alone ATPs into proof planning.

We implemented multi-strategy proof planning in a system, MULTI, which is a component of the proof assistant ΩMEGA [3]. The design of MULTI decouples the plan refinement and modification from the search control. This has been useful in AI-planning, as discussed, e.g., in [22].

We have compared the performance of MULTI with the previous proof planner of ΩMEGA. First experiments have shown a better performance of the multi-strategy proof planner MULTI in a realistic mathematical domain as compared with the otherwise similar proof planner. Now there are two levels where decisions are made, the strategic and the method level. This structures and changes the search spaces. As opposed to our approach an encoding of more control into single methods would hide the control and its structure and thus open the door to more arbitrarily designed methods. Therefore, the separation of methods from (most of) the control is a good idea because of extensibility and modifiability.

Related and Future Work. Another contribution to greater robustness and certain 'strategic' guidance has been the failure reasoning by critics [11]. With the introduction of critics Ireland and Bundy also separate the proof methods from a particular and common kind of meta-reasoning, failure reasoning. These critics typically suggest repairs in order to continue with rippling. While critics are an beautiful first step towards more flexibility, multi-strategy planning extends and generalizes the failure reasoning of critics to general meta-reasoning about several other strategies and introduces the blackboard mechanism for communication.

For planning in complex domains that differ considerably from the proof planning domains, Wilkins and Myers [23] describe a multi-agent planning architecture (MPA) that integrates a meta-reasoning component (meta-planning cell) and various stand-alone problem solving components for the same reasons explained above. [4] propose a multi-agent architecture to combine ATPs and proof planning. They propose to develop and employ a resource management that will evaluate single agents as well as the society of agents. The goal of this project is to model human proof search behavior as a mixture of the activities of several agents.

We demonstrated how proof planning benefits from the flexibility and structure of multi-strategy proof planning. The strategy level introduces new choice points and changes the potential search space, e.g., by structuring the knowledge. With a large number of problems we shall test the influence of the new structure of the search spaces and of the additional evaluation of control knowledge on the overall performance.

References

1. Gandalf. In *CASC-14* http://www.cs.jcu.edu.au/~tptp/casc-14/, 1997.
2. R.G. Bartle and D.R. Sherbert. *Introduction to Real Analysis*. John Wiley& Sons, New York, 1982.
3. C. Benzmüller, L. Cheikhrouhou, D. Fehrer, A. Fiedler, X. Huang, M. Kerber, M. Kohlhase, K. Konrad, A. Meier, E. Melis, W. Schaarschmidt, J. Siekmann, and V. Sorge. OMEGA: Towards a mathematical assistant. In *Proc. CADE-14*, pages 252–255. Springer-Verlag, 1997.
4. C. Benzmüller, M. Jamnik, M. Kerber, and V. Sorge. Agent Based Mathematical Reasoning? In *7th CALCULEMUS Workshop*, pages 21–32, 1999.
5. W.W. Bledsoe, R.S. Boyer, and W.H. Henneman. Computer proofs of limit theorems. *Artificial Intelligence*, 3(1):27–60, 1972.
6. A. Bundy. The use of explicit plans to guide inductive proofs. In *Proc. of CADE-9*, pages 111–120, 1988.
7. A. Bundy, A. Stevens, F. Van Harmelen, A. Ireland, and A. Smaill. A heuristic for guiding inductive proofs. *Artificial Intelligence*, 63:185–253, 1993.
8. A. Bundy, F. van Harmelen, J. Hesketh, and A. Smaill. Experiments with proof plans for induction. *Journal of Automated Reasoning*, 7:303–324, 1991.

9. J. Denzinger and M. Fuchs. Cooperation of heterogeneous provers. In *Proc. of IJCAI*, pages 10 – 15. Morgan Kaufmann, 1999.

10. B. Hayes-Roth. A blackboard architecture for control. *Artificial Intelligence*, pages 251–321, 1985.

11. A. Ireland and A. Bundy. Productive use of failure in inductive proof. *Journal of Automated Reasoning*, 16(1-2):79–111, 1996.

12. W.W. McCune. Otter 2.0 users guide. Technical Report ANL-90/9, Argonne National Laboratory, 1990.

13. E. Melis. AI-techniques in proof planning. In *Proc. of European Conference on Artificial Intelligence*, pages 494–498. Kluwer, 1998.

14. E. Melis. Combining proof planning with constraint solving. In *Proc. of Calculemus and Types'98*, 1998.

15. E. Melis. The "limit" domain. In *Proc. of the Fourth International Conference on Artificial Intelligence in Planning Systems (AIPS'98)*, pages 199–206, 1998.

16. E. Melis and A. Meier. Proof planning with multiple strategies. Seki report SR-99-06, Universität des Saarlandes, FB Informatik, 1999.

17. E. Melis and A. Meier. Proof planning with multiple strategies II. In *FLoC'99 workshop on Strategies in Automated Deduction*, pages 61–72, 1999.

18. E. Melis and J.H. Siekmann. Knowledge-based proof planning. *Artificial Intelligence*, 1999.

19. E. Melis and C. Ullrich. Flexibly interleaving processes. In K.-D. Althoff and R. Bergmann, editors, *International Conference on Case-Based Reasoning*, volume 1650 of *Lecture Notes in Artificial Intelligence*, pages 263–275. Springer, 1999.

20. G. Polya. *How to Solve it*. Princeton University Press, Princeton, 1945.

21. A.H. Schoenfeld. *Mathematical Problem Solving*. Academic Press, New York, 1985.

22. D.S. Weld. An introduction to least committment planning. *AI magazine*, 15(4):27–61, 1994.

23. D.E. Wilkins and K.L. Myers. A multiagent planning architecture. In *Proc. of the Fourth International Conference on AI Planning Systems (AIPS'98)*, pages 154–162, 1998.

24. A. Wolf. Strategy selection for automated theorem proving. In *Proc. of AIMSA'98*, pages 452–465, 1998.

The Theory of Total Unary RPO Is Decidable

Paliath Narendran[1] and Michael Rusinowitch[2]

[1] Institute of Programming and Logics, Department of Computer Science
State University of New York at Albany, Albany, NY 12222, USA
`dran@cs.albany.edu`
[2] LORIA-INRIA Lorraine, 615, rue du jardin botanique, BP 101
54602 Villers les Nancy cedex, France
`rusi@loria.fr`

Abstract. The Recursive Path Ordering (*rpo*) is a syntactic ordering on terms that has been widely used for proving termination of term-rewriting systems [7, 20]. How to combine term-rewriting with ordered resolution and paramodulation is now well-understood and it has been successfully applied in many theorem-proving systems [11, 16, 21]. In this setting an ordering such as rpo is used both to orient rewrite rules and to select maximal literals to perform inferences on. In order to further prune the search space the ordering requirements on conditional inferences are better handled when they are treated as constraints [12, 18]. Typically a non-orientable equation $s = t$ will be split as two constrained rewrite rules: $s \rightarrow t \mid s > t$ and $t \rightarrow s \mid t > s$. Such constrained rules are useless when the constraint is unsatisfiable. Therefore it is important for the efficiency of automated reasoning systems to investigate decision procedures for the theory of terms with ordering predicates.

Other types of constraints can be introduced too such as disunification constraints [1]. It is often the case that they can be expressed with ordering constraints (although this might be inefficient).

We prove that the first-order theory of the recursive path ordering is decidable in the case of unary signatures with total precedence. This solves a problem that was mentioned as open in [6]. The result has to be contrasted with the undecidability results of the lexicographic path ordering [6] for the case of symbols with arity ≥ 2 and total precedence and for the case of unary signatures with partial precedence. We recall that lexicographic path ordering (lpo) and the recursive path ordering and many other orderings such as [13, 10] coincide in the unary case.

Among the positive results it is known that the existential theory of total lpo is decidable [3, 17]. The same result holds for the case of total rpo [8, 15].

The proof technique we use for our decidability result might be interesting by itself. It relies on encoding of words as trees and then on building a tree automaton to recognize the rpo relation.

Keywords: Recursive path ordering, first-order theory, ground reducibility, tree automata, ordered rewriting.

J. Lloyd et al. (Eds.): CL 2000, LNAI 1861, pp. 660–672, 2000.
© Springer-Verlag Berlin Heidelberg 2000

1   The Recursive Path Ordering on Words

We assume that A is a finite alphabet, A^* the set of words on A and ϵ is the empty word. We shall often identify a letter with the corresponding word of length one. There is a correspondance between words and terms on a unary alphabet: every letter can be considered as a unary function and every word $a_1, a_2, \ldots, a_n$ can be considered as a term $a_1(a_2(\ldots a_n(x)\ldots))$ where x is an element of the set of variables X.

The *Recursive Path Ordering* (*rpo*) originally introduced by Dershowitz [7] is defined as follows on words:

Given a finite total precedence $\succ^A$ on A,

$$s \succ_{rpo}^A t$$

if and only if one of the following holds:

1. $s \neq \epsilon$ and $t = \epsilon$
2. $s = as'$ and $t = bt'$ and either
   (a) $a \succ^A b$ and $s \succ_{rpo}^A t'$ or
   (b) $a = b$ and $s' \succ_{rpo}^A t'$ or
   (c) $b \succ^A a$ and $s' \succeq_{rpo}^A t$

where $s' \succeq_{rpo}^A t$ is an abbreviation for $s' \succ_{rpo}^A t$ or $s' = t$.

The following properties of rpo are well-known and their proofs can be found in the literature (e.g. [7]). We omit the superscript A when it is clear from context.

Proposition 1. *The relation $\succ_{rpo}$ is antireflexive, transitive, monotonic (i.e. $aw \succ_{rpo} aw'$ if $w \succ_{rpo} w'$), total, well-founded and has the subterm property (i.e. $w \succ_{rpo} w'$ when w' is a proper subterm of w).*

When the precedence is not total, all properties but totality of $\succ_{rpo}$ remain valid.

We now give a few properties that will be useful in the sequel.

Lemma 1. *If $s \succ_{rpo} t$ then for all $w \in A^*$, $ws \succ_{rpo} wt$.*

Proof: by induction on the length of w and by the monotonicity property.   □

Lemma 2. *If $a \in A$ and $w \succ_{rpo} w'$ then for all $w'' \in A^*$ such that $a \succ_{rpo} w''$, we have $aw \succ_{rpo} w''aw'$.*

Proof: by induction on the length of w''. If w'' is empty it is obvious. If $w'' = bu$ where $b \in A$, then by definition of rpo we must have $a \succ^A b$ and $a \succ_{rpo} u$. Since u is shorter than w'', by induction hypothesis we have $aw \succ_{rpo} uaw'$. By the definition of rpo, we also have $aw \succ_{rpo} buaw'$ and the result follows.   □

The next lemma shows that when terms s, t have the same number of maximal symbols a then the comparison can be done by considering only the rightmost (innermost) occurrence of a whose arguments are different in s and t.

Lemma 3. *Let* $w_1, w_2, \ldots, w_k, u_1, u_2, \ldots, u_k$ *be two sequences of words such that each letter in each word is strictly smaller than* $a \in A$. *If* $w \succ_{rpo} w'$ *then we have:*

$$aw_1 aw_2 \ldots aw_k aw \succ_{rpo} au_1 au_2 \ldots au_k aw'$$

Proof: By induction hypothesis we can assume that:

$$aw_2 \ldots aw_k aw \succ_{rpo} au_2 \ldots au_k aw'$$

by the previous lemma we have:

$$aw_2 \ldots aw_k aw \succ_{rpo} u_1 au_2 \ldots au_k aw'$$

by the subterm property and transitivity we have:

$$w_1 aw_2 \ldots aw_k aw \succ_{rpo} u_1 au_2 \ldots au_k aw'$$

The result follows by monotonicity. □

We denote by $max(w, A)$ the maximal letter of A that occurs in word w and by $mul(w, A)$ the number of occurrences of this letter in w. As a consequence of the previous lemmas we get:

Lemma 4. $w \succ_{rpo} w'$ *iff one of the following holds:*

1. $max(w, A) \succ max(w', A)$
2. $max(w, A) = max(w', A)$ *and* $mul(w, A) > mul(w', A)$
3. $a = max(w, A) = max(w', A)$, $mul(w, A) = mul(w', A)$, $w = w_0 aw_1 aw_2 \ldots aw_k$, $w' = u_0 au_1 au_2 \ldots au_k$ *and there exists* $0 \leq i \leq k$ *such that* $w_i \succ_{rpo} u_i$ *and for all* $j > i$ *we have* $w_j = u_j$.

A first idea would be to try to use word automata in order to recognize the relation $\succ_{rpo}$. However this is not possible. Consider $A = \{a, b\}$ with $a \succ b$. We introduce the product alphabet $A^2 = \{(u, v) \mid u, v \in A \cup \{\bot\}\}$, where $\bot$ is a new symbol. Classically we can associate to every couple of words $U = u_1.u_2 \ldots u_m \in A^*$ and $V = v_1.v_2 \ldots v_n \in A^*$ a word $U \otimes V = (u_1, v_1), (u_2, v_2), \ldots$ on A^2 by completing the shortest word (if any) by some $\bot$'s in order to get two words of the same length. Assume that the relation $R = \{U \otimes V \mid U, V \in A^* \text{ and } U \succ V\}$ is recognizable on A^2 by an automaton $\mathcal{A}$ with N states. Then $b^N a^{N+1} \otimes a^N b^{N+1}$ belongs to R. By a pigeon-hole argument the automaton will enter twice the same state when reading the second half of the word. Then by pumping between the corresponding positions, $\mathcal{A}$ should accept also $b^N a^m \otimes a^N b^m$, with $m \leq N$. Since $a^N b^m \succ b^N a^m$, this raises a contradiction.

2   Coding Words as Trees

We shall now define a tree representation of words so that comparison of words can be performed by an automaton. Our goal is to represent a word

$w = w_1 a w_2 \ldots a w_k a w_{k+1}$ by a binary tree $a(t_{k+1}, a(t_k, \ldots, a(t_1, \epsilon) \ldots))$, where t_i represents w_i and $a \in A$ is maximal in w w.r.t. $\succ^A$. First we introduce a new signature F that contains a binary symbol for each element of the alphabet A. The binary symbol associated with $a \in A$ will be denoted also a, by abuse of notation. We shall introduce also a constant symbol ϵ_a for each $a \in A$. We shall denote by a' the successor of a with respect to the total precedence $\succ^A$ of A. We denote by o (resp. m) the minimal (resp. maximal) element of A.

The translation function τ from A^* to $T(F)$ is defined using auxiliary functions τ_a, $a \in A$.

$$\tau_{a'}(w_1 a' w_2) = a'(\tau_a(w_2), \tau_{a'}(w_1)) \quad \text{when } a' \notin w_2$$
$$\tau_{a'}(w) = a'(\tau_a(w), \epsilon_{a'}) \quad\quad \text{when } a' \notin w$$
$$\tau_o(w.o) = o(\epsilon_o, \tau_o(w))$$
$$\tau_o(\epsilon) = o(\epsilon_o, \epsilon_o)$$

Now we define $\tau(w) = \tau_m(w)$.

Example 1. Assume $A = \{a, b, c\}$ with $a \succ^A b \succ^A c$. Then $\tau(\epsilon) = a(b(c(\epsilon_c, \epsilon_c), \epsilon_b), \epsilon_a)$.

Example 2. Assume $A = \{a, b, c\}$ with $a \succ^A b \succ^A c$. Then $\tau(caacb) =$

$a(b(c(\epsilon_c, \epsilon_c), b(c(\epsilon_c, c(\epsilon_c, \epsilon_c)), \epsilon_b))), a(b(c(\epsilon_c, \epsilon_c), \epsilon_b), a(b(c(\epsilon_c, c(\epsilon_c, \epsilon_c)), \epsilon_b), \epsilon_a)))$

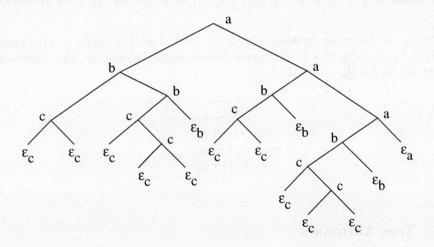

Note that τ is a real encoding. In other terms, two different words are never coded as the same tree.

Lemma 5. *The function τ is injective.*

Proof: Let $I_a = \{c \preceq^A a\}$. We prove by induction on a that τ_a is injective on I_a^*. Since $I_m = A$ this will imply the result. If $a = o$ then $\tau_o(o^k) = \tau_o(o^j)$ clearly entails $j = k$. Now we assume by induction hypothesis that I_a is injective. Consider two words $w_1, w_2 \in I_{a'}$ such that $\tau_{a'}(w_1) = \tau_{a'}(w_2)$. If neither of w_1, w_2 contains a' we have $a'(\tau_a(w_1), \epsilon_{a'}) = a'(\tau_a(w_2), \epsilon_{a'})$ and therefore $\tau_a(w_1) = \tau_a(w_2)$ which implies $w_1 = w_2$ by the induction hypothesis. The case when $w_1 = u_1 a' v_1$ (for some words $u_1 \in I_{a'}, v_1 \in I_a$) and a' does not occur in w_2 is impossible since $\tau_{a'}(w_1)$ should contain in that case more a' that $\tau_{a'}(w_2)$. Now assume that $w_1 = u_1 a' v_1$ and $w_2 = u_2 a' v_2$ with $u_1, u_2 \in I_{a'}, v_1, v_2 \in I_a$. We prove by induction on the sum of the lengths of w_1 and w_2 that $\tau_{a'}(w_1) = \tau_{a'}(w_2)$ implies $w_1 = w_2$. The base case is trivial. $a'(\tau_a(v_1), \tau_{a'}(u_1)) = a'(\tau_a(v_2), \tau_{a'}(u_2))$ which implies by decomposition $\tau_a(v_1) = \tau_a(v_2)$ and $\tau_{a'}(u_1) = \tau_{a'}(u_2)$. From the induction hypothesis we have $v_1 = v_2$, $u_1 = u_2$ and therefore $w_1 = w_2$. $\qquad \square$

A *finite tree automaton* over a signature $\mathcal{F}$ is a tuple $\mathcal{A} = (Q, Q_f, \Delta)$ where Q is a finite set of states, $Q_f \subseteq Q$ is a subset of accepting states and Δ is a set of transition rules of type:

$$f(q_1, \ldots, q_n) \to q$$

where $n \geq 0$, f is symbol of $\mathcal{F}$ of arity n and $q, q_1, \ldots, q_n \in Q$. We consider here bottom-up tree automata: they are applied to ground terms inductively from the leaves to the root. A ground term t is accepted by $\mathcal{A}$ if $t \to^*_\Delta q$ for some state $q \in Q_f$.

For more details about tree automata a recent reference is [4].

Lemma 6. *The set of trees $\{\tau(w) | \ w \in A^*\}$ is recognizable by a tree automaton $\mathcal{C}$.*

Proof: The following automaton does the work. Let $Q = \{q_a | \ q \in A\} \cup \{qs_o\}$, $Q_f = \{q_m\}$ where m is the maximal element in the precedence. The transitions are, for all $a \in A$:

$$
\begin{aligned}
\epsilon_a &\to q_a, \quad a \neq o \\
\epsilon_o &\to qs_o \\
o(qs_o, qs_o) &\to q_o \\
o(qs_o, q_o) &\to q_o \\
a(q_a, q_{a'}) &\to q_{a'}
\end{aligned}
$$

$\qquad \square$

3 Tree Automata

We define now a tree automaton for comparing two words. First let us extend F with a constant $\perp$. By abuse of notation we denote by fg a new function symbol associated with the couple $(f, g) \in (F \cup \{\perp\}) \times (F \cup \{\perp\})$. We denote by F^2 the signature $\{fg \mid f, g \in F \cup \{\perp\}\}$ (product alphabet), where the arity of fg is equal to the maximum of the arities of f and g ($\perp$ has arity 0). The automaton will traverse in a bottom-up way the tree obtained by gluing together the tree structures associated to the two words.

The coding of a couple of trees $(t_1, t_2) \in T(F)^2$ as a tree $t_1 \otimes t_2$ on the product alphabet F^2 is defined recursively as follows:

$$f(s_1, s_2) \otimes g(r_1, r_2) = fg(s_1 \otimes r_1, s_2 \otimes r_2)$$
$$f(s_1, s_2) \otimes \epsilon_a = f\epsilon_a(s_1 \otimes \bot, s_2 \otimes \bot)$$
$$\epsilon_a \otimes f(s_1, s_2) = \epsilon_a f(\bot \otimes s_1, \bot \otimes s_2)$$
$$f(s_1, s_2) \otimes \bot = f\bot(s_1 \otimes \bot, s_2 \otimes \bot)$$
$$\bot \otimes f(s_1, s_2) = \bot f(\bot \otimes s_1, \bot \otimes s_2)$$

Lemma 7. *The set of trees* $\{\tau(w) \otimes \tau(v)| \ w, v \in A^*\}$ *is recognizable by a tree automaton.*

Proof: We just need to take the product of two copies of the automaton in Lemma 6. □

Theorem 1. *The set of trees* $\{\tau(w) \otimes \tau(v) \mid w \succ_{rpo} v\}$ *is recognizable by a tree automaton.*

Proof: let $Q = \{q_+^a, q_-^a, q_>^a, q_<^a, q_=^a \mid a \in A\}$ be the set of states. The set of accepting states is $Q_f = \{q_+^m, q_>^m\}$ where m is the maximum element of the alphabet. The meaning of q_+^a (resp. q_-^a) is that on the right branch we have encountered more (resp. less) a's in $\tau(w)$ than in $\tau(v)$. The meaning of $q_>^a$ (resp. $q_<^a$, resp. $q_=^a$) is that the number of a's is the same but some a-free subword tips the balance in favour of w (resp. v, resp. equality).

The transitions of the bottom-up tree automaton include, for all $a, b \in A$ with $a = b'$:

$aa(-, q_+^a) \rightarrow q_+^a$	$aa(q_>^b, q_=^a) \rightarrow q_>^a$
$aa(-, q_-^a) \rightarrow q_-^a$	$aa(q_>^b, q_<^a) \rightarrow q_>^a$
$a\epsilon_a(-, -) \rightarrow q_+^a$	$aa(q_>^b, q_>^a) \rightarrow q_>^a$
$\epsilon_a a(-, -) \rightarrow q_-^a$	$aa(q_+^b, q_=^a) \rightarrow q_>^a$
$\bot a(-, -) \rightarrow q_-^a$	$aa(q_+^b, q_<^a) \rightarrow q_>^a$
$a\bot(-, -) \rightarrow q_+^a$	$aa(q_+^b, q_>^a) \rightarrow q_>^a$
$\epsilon_a \epsilon_a \rightarrow q_=^a$	$aa(q_-^b, q_=^a) \rightarrow q_<^a$
$\bot \epsilon_a \rightarrow q_-^a$	$aa(q_-^b, q_<^a) \rightarrow q_<^a$
$\epsilon_a \bot \rightarrow q_+^a$	$aa(q_-^b, q_>^a) \rightarrow q_<^a$
$aa(q_=^b, q_=^a) \rightarrow q_=^a$	$aa(q_<^b, q_=^a) \rightarrow q_<^a$
$aa(q_=^b, q_>^a) \rightarrow q_>^a$	$aa(q_<^b, q_<^a) \rightarrow q_<^a$
$aa(q_=^b, q_<^a) \rightarrow q_<^a$	$aa(q_<^b, q_>^a) \rightarrow q_<^a$

In order to complete the automaton we may add a failure state and transitions for detecting trees that do not stand for a couple of words. We call $\mathcal{A}$ the automaton we get finally.

We now show that if $w \succ_{rpo} u$ then $\tau(w) \otimes \tau(u)$ is accepted by $\mathcal{A}$. For this we show the more general result:

Claim: *If a is the maximal letter in w then $\tau_a(w) \otimes \tau_a(u) \to_\Delta q \in \{q_+^a, q_>^a\}$.*

We proceed by induction on a (w.r.t. $\succ^A$). The base case when $w \in \{o\}^*$ is left to the reader. Assume that the result is true for all $c \prec a$. Consider now the words w, u and $a \in A$ such that $a = max(w, A)$ and $w \succ_{rpo} u$.

Let t be $\tau_a(w) \otimes \tau_a(u)$. By Lemma 4 there are three ways to get $w \succ_{rpo} u$:

If $a = max(w, A) \succ d = max(u, A)$ then $\tau_a(t) = aa(t_1, a\epsilon_a(t_2, t_3))$ for some terms t_1, t_2, t_3. It can be checked that $t \to_\Delta q_+^a$.

The case when $a = max(w, A) = max(u, A)$ and $mul(w, A) > mul(u, A)$ is similar.

Assume now that $w = w_0 a w_1 a w_2 \ldots a w_k a w_k$, $u = u_0 a u_1 a u_2 \ldots a u_k a u_k$ and a is larger than every symbol in w_i, u_j where $i, j = 0, \ldots, k$. Let b be the predecessor of a: $b' = a$. By Lemma 4, $w \succ_{rpo} u$ iff there exists j such that $w_j \succ_{rpo} u_j$ and $l > j$ implies $w_l = u_l$. Let us denote $\tau_b(w_j) \otimes \tau_b(u_j)$ by s_j.

Then $t = aa(s_k, aa(s_k, aa(\ldots, aa(s_j, \ldots, aa(s_0, \epsilon_a) \ldots)))$. Running the automaton on t one can get, after some steps, $aa(s_k, \ldots aa(q', q) \ldots)$ for some $q \in \{q_=^a, q_<^a, q_>^a\}$. By the induction hypothesis (since $b \prec a$) $s_j \to_\Delta^* q'$. where q' is either q_+^b or $q_>^b$. Hence applying one more rule of the automaton we also have: $aa(q', q) \to_\Delta q_>^a$. Since s_l codes a couple of identical words, we have $s_l \to_\Delta^* q_=^b$, for $l > j$. Applying several times the rule $aa(q_=^b, q_>^a) \to q_>^a$ allows one to conclude. By symmetry we can show that $\tau(w) \otimes \tau(u) \to_\Delta q \in \{q_-^m, q_<^m\}$ whenever $w \prec_{rpo} u$.

For the converse one needs to show that whenever $\tau(w) \otimes \tau(u) \to_\Delta q \in Q_f$ we have $w \succ_{rpo} u$. Since the ordering $\succ_{rpo}$ is total either $w \prec_{rpo} u$ or $w \succ_{rpo} u$. In the first case $q \in \{q_-^m, q_<^m\}$ and in the second, $q \in \{q_+^m, q_>^m\} = Q_f$. Now since the automaton $\mathcal{A}$ is deterministic if $q \in Q_f$ then necessarily $w \succ_{rpo} u$. □

The first-order theory we will show decidable has both inequality interpreted as $\succ_{rpo}$ and equality interpreted as identity. When $a \in A$ we shall reduce the satisfiability of a formula $au \succ_{rpo} v$ (resp. $u \succ_{rpo} av$) to the satisfiability of $w \succ_{rpo} v \wedge w = au$ (resp. $u \succ_{rpo} w \wedge w = au$). This motivates the next theorem.

Note that the set $\{av \otimes v | v \in A^*\}$ is recognizable by a word automaton. However we have now adopted a tree representation for the words to handle inequalities and we cannot mix different representations of the same word. Hence we have to prove:

Theorem 2. *The set of trees $\{\tau(av) \otimes \tau(v) \mid v \in A^*\}$ (where $a \in A$) is recognizable by a tree automaton.*

Proof: Note that adding a letter a to a word w amounts to replacing a leaf by a node of the tree representation of w. There is a unique position where this node can be inserted: it is at the position of the rightmost occurrence of ϵ_a. Let $Q = \{q_0, q_1, q_2\}$ be the set of states. The state q_1 recognizes the trees on F^2 obtained as the product of two identical trees. The accepting state is q_0. The transitions of the bottom-up tree automaton include, for all $b \in A$:

$$
\begin{array}{rcl}
\epsilon_a \bot & \to & q_0 \\
\epsilon_b \epsilon_b & \to & q_1 \\
bb(q_1, q_1) & \to & q_1 \\
a\epsilon_a(q_1, q_0) & \to & q_0 \\
bb(q_1, q_0) & \to & q_0
\end{array}
$$

□

4   RPO Theory

An *RPO formula* is a first-order formula constructed from terms on the unary signature A and the binary predicate symbols "$\succ$" and "$=$". The formula is interpreted in $T(A)$, with $\succ$ as $\succ_{rpo}$ and $=$ as identity. We denote by $\phi(x_1, \dots, x_n)$ an RPO formula with free variables $x_1, \dots, x_n$.

A *flat formula* is an RPO formula whose atoms are of type: $x = y, x = ay, x = a, x \succ y, a \succ x$ or $x \succ a$, where x, y are variables. Hence terms in flat formulas are restricted to types x, ax, a, where $a \in A, x \in X$.

Using transformations that preserve solutions we can reduce the decision of RPO formulas to the decision of flat formulas. These transformations include the following abstraction rules, where $a, b \in A$:

$$au \succ_{rpo} v \quad \vdash \quad \exists u'(u' \succ_{rpo} v \wedge u' = au) \tag{1}$$

$$u \succ_{rpo} av \quad \vdash \quad \exists v'(u \succ_{rpo} v' \wedge v' = av) \tag{2}$$

$$abu = v \quad \vdash \quad \exists u'(au' = v \wedge u' = bu) \tag{3}$$

$$u = abv \quad \vdash \quad \exists v'(av' = v \wedge v' = bv) \tag{4}$$

These rules are completed by the decomposition rules derived from the definition of $\succ_{rpo}$, and the decomposition and clash rules for the predicate $=$ in $T(A)$.

Theorem 3. *Given an RPO formula $\phi(x_1, \dots, x_n)$ there exists an automaton that recognizes*

$$\{u_1 \otimes \dots \otimes u_n \mid u_1, \dots, u_n \text{ is a solution of } \phi\}.$$

Proof: We can assume the formula ϕ is flat. The proof will be by induction on the structure of ϕ. The technique is classical ([4]). Let $\mathcal{U}$ be an automaton that recognizes all terms. We first remark that given two automata $\mathcal{A}_1, \mathcal{A}_2$ for the solutions of $\phi_1(\overline{xz})$ and $\phi_2(\overline{zy})$, where $\overline{x}, \overline{y}, \overline{z}$ are disjoint sets of variables, the set of solutions of $\phi_1(\overline{xz}) \wedge \phi_2(\overline{zy})$ is the intersection of the regular languages recognized by $\mathcal{A}_1 \otimes (\otimes_{|y|}\mathcal{U})$ and $(\otimes_{|x|}\mathcal{U}) \otimes \mathcal{A}_2$.

Base case: assume that $\phi(x_1, \dots, x_n)$ is atomic. Its satisfiability is equivalent to the conjunction of flat atomic formulas obtained by replacing (repeatedly) every strict maximal subterm t in every atom by a fresh variable x_t. Automata recognizing the solutions of formula of type $x \succ y$ (resp. $x = ay$) can be constructed thanks to Theorem 1 (resp. 2). For the other cases $(x = y, x = a, a \succ x, x \succ a)$ automata are easily obtained too.

Step case: i) Suppose $\phi(x_1, \ldots, x_n) = \neg\psi(x_1, \ldots, x_n)$. By taking the intersection of the complement automaton for $\psi(x_1, \ldots, x_n)$ with $\otimes_n \mathcal{C}$ (product of n copies of $\mathcal{C}$) we get an automaton for ϕ. ii) If $\phi(x_1, \ldots, x_n) = \exists x_1 \, \psi(x_1, \ldots, x_n)$. then by projection (i.e. forgetting first component) one get an automaton for ϕ. $\square$

We can now conclude with the main result which is a direct consequence of the previous theorem:

Theorem 4. *The first-order theory of rpo is decidable when the signature is built from a finite set of constants and unary symbols.*

5 On Normal Forms and Ordered Rewriting

5.1 The Recursive Path Ordering on Terms

We assume that F is a finite set of function symbols given with their arity. $T(F, V)$ is the set of finite terms built on F and an alphabet V of (first-order) *variable symbols*. $\equiv$ denotes syntactic equality of terms. $T(F)$ is the set of terms which do not contain any variables. A multiset over a set X is a function M from X to the natural numbers. Any ordering $>$ on X can be extended to an ordering $\gg$ on finite multisets over X as follows: $M \gg N$ if a) $M \neq N$ and b) whenever $N(x) > M(x)$ then $M(y) > N(y)$ for some $y > x$. Note that if $>$ is well-founded so is $\gg$.

Given a finite total precedence $\succ^F$ on functions,

$$s = f(s_1, \ldots, s_m) \succ^F_{rpo} g(t_1, \ldots, t_n) = t$$

if and only if one of the following holds:

1. $f \succ^F g$ and $s \succ^F_{rpo} t_i$ for all $1 \leq i \leq n$
2. $f = g$, $m = n$ and $\{s_1, \ldots, s_m\} \gg^F_{rpo} \{t_1, \ldots, t_m\}$
3. There exists a j, $1 \leq j \leq m$, such that $s_j \succ^F_{rpo} t$ or $s_j \sim_{rpo} t$.

where $\sim_{rpo}$ is defined as *permutatively equal*, or, in other words, the terms are treated as *unordered* trees. The set $t/\sim_{rpo}$ is the equivalence class of t for $\sim_{rpo}$. The multiset extension of $\succ_{rpo}$ used above, namely $\gg_{rpo}$, is defined in terms of this equivalence.

5.2 Ordered Rewriting

An *ordered* term rewrite system (TRS) is a pair $(E, \succ)$, where E is a set of equations, and $\succ$ is an ordering on terms. The *ordered rewriting relation* defined by $(E, \succ)$ is the smallest monotonic binary relation $\rightarrow_{E,\succ}$ on terms such that $s\sigma \rightarrow_{E,\succ} t\sigma$ whenever $s = t \in E$ and $s\sigma \succ t\sigma$.

Let us recall that a term t is *ground reducible* w.r.t. a rewrite system $\mathcal{R}$ iff all instances $t\sigma \in T(F)$ of t are reducible by $\mathcal{R}$. This definition extends to ordered rewriting, replacing $\mathcal{R}$ with $\rightarrow_{E,>}$ when E is a finite set of (unconstrained) equations.

Ground reducibility is decidable for arbitrary finite term rewriting systems [19]. It is undecidable for finite sets of *equations* [9].

We show it is decidable in the special case where all symbols occcurring in the set of equations E have arity 0 or 1, (in that case we say that the equations are *unary*) and the ordering is $\succ_{rpo}$ with a total precedence. In fact, we can state a slightly more general result. An equation is said to be *semiground* if at least one member is a ground term.

Theorem 5. *Given a term t, and system of equations E such each element of E is either unary or semiground it is decidable whether t is ground reducible by $\rightarrow_{E,\succ_{rpo}}$.*

Given set of terms $G_1, \ldots, G_n$ and a function symbol f of arity n we denote by $f(G_1, \ldots, G_n)$ the set of terms $\{f(g_1, \ldots, g_n) \mid g_1 \in G_1, \ldots, g_n \in G_n\}$.

Lemma 8. $\{u \in T(F) \mid s(u) \succ_{rpo} t(u)\}$, *for unary terms s, t is either empty or* $T(F)$.

Proof: Applying the rpo definition we have that $s(x) \succ_{rpo} t(x)$ is either equivalent to $v(x) \succ_{rpo} x$ or $x \succ_{rpo} v(x)$ for some term v. $\quad\Box$

Lemma 9. $\{w \in T(F) \mid \exists v : s(w) \succ_{rpo} t(v)\}$ *is either equal to $T(F)$ or to* $\{x \in T(F) \mid x \succ_{rpo} u\}$, *where u is a ground term.*

Proof: $s(x) \succ_{rpo} t(y)$ for some y iff $s(x) \succ_{rpo} t(\bot)$ where $\bot$ is the minimal constant in the signature. By decomposition we get the result. $\quad\Box$

Lemma 10. $\{u \in T(F) \mid u \succ_{rpo} t\}$ *where t is a ground term, is recognizable by a tree automaton.*

Proof: It is by simple induction on t w.r.t. $\succ_{rpo}$. If t is $\bot$ this is trivial. Otherwise assume by the induction hypothesis that for all $t' \prec_{rpo} t$, $L_{t'} = \{u \in T(F) \mid u \succ_{rpo} t'\}$ is a regular tree language.

Let $t = f(t_1, \ldots, t_n)$. Assume w.l.o.g. that $t_1 \succeq_{rpo} t_2, \ldots, \succeq_{rpo} t_n$. Then $x \succ_{rpo} f(t_1, \ldots, t_n)$ iff either

1. $x = g(x_1, \ldots, x_m)$ and $f \succ g$ and for some i: $x_i \succ_{rpo} t$.
2. $x = g(x_1, \ldots, x_m)$ and $f \prec g$ and for all j: $x \succ_{rpo} t_j$.
3. $x = f(x_1, \ldots, x_n)$ and $\{x_1, \ldots, x_n\} \gg_{rpo} \{t_1, \ldots, t_n\}$

The language L_t is regular since it can be defined as a component of the least solution of the following system of equations:

$$L_t = L_1 \cup L_2 \cup L_3$$

$$L_1 = \bigcup_{g \prec f,\ 1 \leq j \leq m} g(h_1, \ldots, h_i, \ldots, h_m) \text{ where } h_i = \begin{cases} L_t & \text{if } i = j, \\ T(F) & \text{otherwise} \end{cases}$$

$$L_2 = \bigcup_{f \prec g} \left(g(T(F), \ldots, T(F)) \cap \bigcap_{1 \leq i \leq n} L_{t_i} \right)$$

$$L_3 = \bigcup_{1 \leq j \leq n,\ \sigma \in \mathcal{S}_n} f(l^j_{\sigma(1)}, \ldots, l^j_{\sigma(n)}) \text{ where } l^j_k = \begin{cases} t_k / \sim_{rpo} & \text{if } k < j, \\ L_{t_j} & \text{if } k = j, \\ T(F) & \text{if } k > j. \end{cases}$$

and where $\mathcal{S}_n$ is the permutation group of $\{1, \ldots, n\}$. Note that L_2 and L_3 are regular by induction hypothesis since they are obtained by composition of languages of type L_u with $u \prec_{rpo} t$.   □

Since $\{u \in T(F) \mid t \succ_{rpo} u\}$ is the complement in $T(F)$ of the language $\{u \in T(F) \mid u \succ_{rpo} t\} \cup \{t\}$ which is regular we also have:

Lemma 11. $\{u \in T(F) \mid t \succ_{rpo} u\}$ where t is a ground term, is recognizable by a tree automaton.

Now given a set of equations E satisfying the hypothesis of Theorem 5 it can be decomposed as a set of orientable unary equations E_1 union a set E_2 of non-orientable unary ones union E_3 a set of semiground equations.

Hence by Lemma 8 and Lemma 9 the set of ground and reducible terms for E is the set of ground terms that have a subterm in the set:

$$\{l(t) \mid l(x) = r(x) \in E_1, l(x) \succ_{rpo} r(x), t \in T(F)\}$$
$$\cup \{l(t) \mid l(x) = r(y) \in E_2, l(t) \succ_{rpo} r(\bot), t \in T(F)\}$$
$$\cup \{s \mid s = t \in E_3, s \succ_{rpo} t, t \in T(F)\}$$
$$\cup \{s \mid s = t \in E_3, s \succ_{rpo} t, s \in T(F)\} \quad (5)$$

By Lemma 10 and Lemma 11 this set is a regular tree language. We denote it by RED_E.

Given a term t of $T(F, X)$ it can be decided whether it is ground reducible by the ordered rewrite system E since in this special case it amounts to checking whether t belongs to a regular tree language. This may be obtained as a consequence of stronger results [2]. We give here a simple direct proof.

Let $\mathcal{A} = (Q, Q_f, \Delta)$ be the automaton for RED_E. We may assume that all states are reachable. And $Q_f = \{q_f\}$. Assume that t has m variables $x_1, \ldots, x_m$ with possibly repeated occurrences. Let $t(q_1, \ldots, q_m)$ be the term (on an extended signature $F \cup Q$) obtained by replacing every variable x_i with a state q_i. We can compute the result of applying the automaton to it. Let

$SUC = \{\langle q_1, \ldots, q_m \rangle \mid t(q_1, \ldots, q_m) \rightarrow_\Delta^* q_f\}$. Now it suffices to show that for every m-tuples of ground terms $\langle t_1, \ldots, t_m \rangle$ we have

$$\langle t_1, \ldots, t_m \rangle \rightarrow_{\Delta^m}^* \langle q_1, \ldots, q_m \rangle \in SUC$$

This is a reachability problem on the product automaton Δ^m and therefore is decidable.

Remark: The result also holds for lexicographic path orderings.

Conclusion

Using a non-standard coding of words as trees and tree automata techniques we have been able to show decidability of the theory of total unary rpo. A question that remains open is whether the existential theory of rpo with *partial* precedence is decidable.

Acknowledgements

We thank Hubert Comon, Florent Jacquemard and Pierre Lescanne for their comments.

References

1. R. Caferra and N. Peltier. Disinference rules, model building and abduction. *Logic at work: Essays dedicated to the memory of Helena Rasiowa* (Part 5: Logic in Computer Science, Chap. 20). Physica-Verlag, 1998.
2. A-C. Caron, J-L. Coquide, and M. Dauchet. Encompassment properties and automata with constraints. In C. Kirchner, editor, *Proceedings 5th Conference on Rewriting Techniques and Applications, Montreal (Canada)*, volume 690 of *Lecture Notes in Computer Science*, pages 328–342. Springer-Verlag, 1993.
3. H. Comon. Solving inequations in term algebras. In *Proc. 5th IEEE Symposium on Logic in Computer Science (LICS)*, Philadelphia, June 1990.
4. H. Comon, M. Dauchet, R. Gilleron, F. Jacquemard, D. Lugiez, S. Tison, M. Tommasi. *Tree Automata Techniques and Applications.* http://www.grappa.univ-lille3.fr/tata/
5. H. Comon, P. Narendran, R. Nieuwenhuis, and M. Rusinowitch. Decision problems in ordered rewriting. In Proc. 13th IEEE Symp. Logic in Computer Science (LICS'98), Indianapolis, IN, USA, June 1998, pages 276-286, 1998.
6. H. Comon and R. Treinen. The first-order theory of lexicographic path orderings is undecidable. *Theoretical Computer Science* 176, April 1997.
7. N. Dershowitz. Orderings for term-rewriting systems. *Theoretical Computer Science* 17(3): 279–301. 1982.
8. J.-P. Jouannaud and M. Okada. Satisfiability of systems of ordinal notations with the subterm ordering is decidable. In *18th International Colloquium on Automata, Languages and Programming (ICALP)*, volume 510 of *Lecture Notes in Computer Science*, pages 455-468, Madrid, Spain, July 1991. Springer-Verlag.

9. D. Kapur, P. Narendran, D. Rosenkrantz and H. Zhang. Sufficient Completeness, Ground-Reducibility and Their Complexity. *Acta Informatica* 28 (1991) 311-350.
10. D. Kapur, P. Narendran and G. Sivakumar. A path ordering for proving termination of term rewriting systems. In H. Ehrig (ed.), *10th CAAP*, volume 185 of *Lecture Notes in Computer Science*, pages 173-187, Berlin, March 1985.
11. D. Kapur and H. Zhang. An Overview of Rewrite Rule Laboratory (RRL), J. of Computer and Mathematics with Applications, 29, 2, 1995, 91-114.
12. C. Kirchner, H. Kirchner, and M. Rusinowitch. Deduction with symbolic constraints. *Revue Franaise d'Intelligence Artificielle*, 4(3):9–52, 1990. Special issue on automatic deduction.
13. P. Lescanne. Some properties of the Decomposition Ordering, a simplification ordering to prove termination of rewriting systems. RAIRO, 16(4):331–347, 1982.
14. U. Martin and E. Scott. The order types of termination orderings on monadic terms, strings and multisets. J. Symbolic Logic 62 (1997) 624–635.
15. P. Narendran, M. Rusinowitch and R. Verma. RPO constraint solving is in NP. In: Computer Science Logic (CSL 98), Brno, Czech Republic. August 1998. 12p. LNCS 1584, Springer-Verlag, 1999.
16. W. McCune and R. Padmanabhan. Automated Deduction in Equational Logic and Cubic Curves, Springer-Verlag LNCS 1095 (1996)
17. R. Nieuwenhuis. Simple LPO constraint solving methods. *Inf. Process. Lett.* 47(2):65–69, Aug. 1993.
18. R. Nieuwenhuis and A. Rubio. Theorem proving with ordering constrained clauses. In D. Kapur, editor, Proceedings of 11th Conf. on Automated Deduction, Saratoga Springs, NY, 1992, volume 607 of *Lecture Notes in Artificial Intelligence*, pages 477–491, June 1992, Springer-Verlag.
19. D. Plaisted. Semantic confluence tests and completion methods. *Information and Control*, 65:182–215, 1985.
20. J. Steinbach. Extensions and comparison of simplification orderings. Proceedings of 3rd RTA, Chapel Hill, NC, volume 355 of *Lecture Notes in Computer Science*, pages 434-448, 1989, Springer-Verlag.
21. C. Weidenbach. SPASS: Combining Superposition, Sorts and Splitting in A. Robinson and A. Voronkov, editors, Handbook of Automated Reasoning, Elsevier, 1999. To appear.

On the Problem of Computing the Well-Founded Semantics

Zbigniew Lonc* and Mirosław Truszczyński

Department of Computer Science, University of Kentucky
Lexington KY 40506-0046, USA
{lonc, mirek}@cs.engr.uky.edu

Abstract. The well-founded semantics is one of the most widely studied and used semantics of logic programs with negation. In the case of finite propositional programs, it can be computed in polynomial time, more specifically, in $O(|At(P)| \times size(P))$ steps, where $size(P)$ denotes the total number of occurrences of atoms in a logic program P. This bound is achieved by an algorithm introduced by Van Gelder and known as the alternating-fixpoint algorithm. Improving on the alternating-fixpoint algorithm turned out to be difficult. In this paper we study extensions and modifications of the alternating-fixpoint approach. We then restrict our attention to the class of programs whose rules have no more than one positive occurrence of an atom in their bodies. For programs in that class we propose a new implementation of the alternating-fixpoint method in which false atoms are computed in a top-down fashion. We show that our algorithm is faster than other known algorithms and that for a wide class of programs it is linear and so, asymptotically optimal.

1 Introduction

Well-founded semantics was introduced in [16] to provide 3-valued interpretations to logic programs with negation. Since its introduction, the well-founded semantics has become one of the most widely studied and most commonly accepted approaches to negation in logic programming [1, 9, 5, 6, 17, 3]. It was implemented in several top-down reasoning systems, most prominent of which is XSB [13].

Well-founded semantics is closely related to the stable-model semantics [10], another major approach to logic programs with negation. The well-founded semantics approximates the stable-model semantics [16, 8]. Moreover, computing the well-founded model of propositional programs is polynomial [15] while computing stable models is NP-hard [11]. Consequently, evaluating the well-founded semantics can be used as an effective preprocessing technique in algorithms to compute stable models [14]. In addition, as demonstrated by smodels [12], at present the most advanced and most efficient system to compute stable models of DATALOG⁻ programs, the well-founded semantics can be used as a powerful lookahead mechanism.

---

* On leave from Warsaw University of Technology.

J. Lloyd et al. (Eds.): CL 2000, LNAI 1861, pp. 673–687, 2000.
© Springer-Verlag Berlin Heidelberg 2000

Despite the importance of well-founded semantics, the question of how fast it can be computed has not attracted significant attention. Van Gelder [15] described the so called *alternating-fixpoint* algorithm. Van Gelder's algorithm runs in time $O(|At(P)| \times size(P))$, where $At(P)$ is the set of atoms occurring in a logic program P, —$At(\mathrm{P})$— denotes the cardinality of $At(P)$, and $size(P)$ is the size of P. Improving on this algorithm turned out to be difficult. The first progress was obtained in [2]. The algorithm described there, when restricted to programs whose rules contain at most two positive occurrences of atoms in their bodies, runs in time $O(|At(P)|^{4/3}|P|^{2/3})$, where $|At(P)|$ stands for the number of atoms in $At(P)$ and $|P|$ — for the number of rules in P. For programs whose rules have no more than one positive atom in the body a better estimate of $O(|At(P)|^{3/2}|P|^{1/2})$ was obtained. For some classes of programs this is an asymptotically better estimate than the $O(|At(P)| \times size(P))$ estimate that holds for the algorithm by Van Gelder. A different approach to computing the well-founded model was proposed in [17,4]. It is based on the notion of a program transformation [3]. The resulting algorithm is an improvement on the alternating-fixpoint algorithm. However, no formal analysis of the running time is offered in [17,4] and it is not clear whether the algorithm proposed there is asymptotically faster than the algorithm by Van Gelder.

The alternating-fixpoint algorithm works by successively improving lower approximations T and F to the sets of atoms that are true and false, respectively, with respect to the well-founded semantics. The algorithm starts with $T = \emptyset$. Using this estimate, it computes the first estimate for F. Using this estimate, it computes now a better estimate for T. The algorithm continues this process until further improvements are not possible and returns the sets T and F as the well-founded semantics. The most time-consuming part of this algorithm is in computing estimates to the set of atoms that are false. In the Van Gelder algorithm, the best possible approximation (given the current estimate for T) is always computed by using a bottom-up approach. Let us also mention that a dual version of the alternating-fixpoint algorithm is possible. We start with $F = \emptyset$, and then alternatingly compute approximations to T and F.

In this paper we show that new false atoms can be computed by means of a top-down approach by finding atoms that do not have a proof. Moreover, we show that it is not necessary to find *all* atoms that can be established to be false at a given stage. Finding a proper subset (as long as it is not empty) is also sufficient and results in a correct algorithm.

We apply this approach to the class of programs that have at most one positive atom in the body. We denote this class of programs by $\mathcal{LP}_1$. In the main contribution of the paper, we describe an algorithm that correctly computes the well-founded semantics for programs in that class. Our algorithm alternatingly computes estimates for the sets for atoms that are true and false. Estimates for the set of false atoms are computed in a top-down fashion. In addition, while each new estimate for the set of false atoms may not be optimal, we show that over all iterations the total time needed to compute the set of atoms that are false with respect to the well-founded semantics is asymptotically better than in the case of the original Van Gelder algorithm. Specifically, we show that our algorithm runs in time $O(|At(P)|^2 + size(P))$. Thus, for programs with $size(P) \geq |At(P)|^2$, our algorithm runs in linear time and is asymptotically optimal! It is also easy to see that when $|P| > |At(P)|$, the asymptotic estimate of the running time of our algorithm is better than that of algorithms by Van Gelder [15] and Berman et al. [2].

The paper is organized as follows. In the next section we provide a brief review of the key notions and terminology. In Section 3 we describe several modifications to the original Van Gelder algorithm, we show their correctness and estimate their running time. The ultimate effect of our considerations there is a general template for an algorithm to compute the well-founded semantics. Any algorithm computing some (not necessarily all) atoms that can be established as false given a current estimate to the well-founded can be used with it. One such algorithm, for programs from the class $\mathcal{LP}_1$, is described and analyzed in Section 4. It constitutes the main contribution of the paper and yields a new, currently asymptotically most efficient algorithm for computing the well-founded semantics for programs in $\mathcal{LP}_1$. The last section contains conclusions.

2   Preliminaries

We start by reviewing basic concepts and notation related to logic programs and the well-founded semantics, as well as some simple auxiliary results. In the paper we consider the propositional case only.

Let P be a normal logic program. By $At(P)$ we denote the set of atoms occurring in P. Let $M \subseteq At(P)$ (throughout the paper we often drop a reference to P from our notation, whenever there is no danger of ambiguity). By P_M we denote the program obtained from P by removing all rules whose bodies contain negated literals of the form $\mathbf{not}(a)$, where $a \in M$. Further, by P^h we denote the program obtained from P by removing from the bodies of its rules *all* negative literals. Clearly, the program P_M^h coincides with the *Gelfond-Lifschitz* reduct of P with respect to M. The *Gelfond-Lifschitz* operator on the algebra of all subsets of At, GL (following our convention, we omit the reference to P from the notation), is defined by

$$GL(M) = LM(P_M^h),$$

where $LM(Q)$ stands for a least model of a Horn program Q.

We now present characterizations of the well-founded semantics. We phrase them in the language of operators and their fixpoints. All operators considered here are defined on the algebra of subsets of $At(P)$. We denote a least fixpoint (if it exists) of an operator O by $lfp(O)$.

It is well known that GL is antimonotone. Consequently, $GL^2 = GL \circ GL$ is monotone and has a least fixpoint. The set of atoms that are true with respect to the well-founded semantics of a program P, denoted by T_{wfs}, is precisely the least fixpoint of the operator GL^2, that is, $T_{wfs} = lfp(GL^2)$ [15,8]. The set of atoms that are false with respect to the well-founded semantics of a program P, denoted by F_{wfs}, is given by $\overline{GL(T_{wfs})}$ (throughout the paper, $\overline{X}$ denotes the complement of a set X with respect to $At(P)$).

One can define a dual operator to GL^2 by

$$A(M) = \overline{GL(GL(\overline{M}))}.$$

It is easy to see that A is monotone and that its least fixpoint is F_{wfs}. Thus, $F_{wfs} = lfp(A)$ and $T_{wfs} = GL(\overline{F_{wfs}})$.

We close this section by discussing ways to compute $GL(M)$ for a given finite propositional logic program P and a set of atoms $M \subseteq At(P)$. A straightforward approach is to compute the Gelfond-Lifschitz reduct P_M^h and then to compute its least model. The resulting algorithm is asymptotically optimal as it runs in time linear in the size of the program. However, in this paper we will use a different approach, more appropriate for the computation of the well-founded semantics. Let P be a logic program with negation. We define $At^-(P) = \{\textbf{not}(a): a \in At(P)\}$. For every set $M \subseteq At(P) \cup At^-(P)$, we define $true(M) = M \cap At(P)$. If we interpret literals of $At^-(P)$ as new *atoms*, then for every set $M \subseteq At(P)$, the program $P \cup \textbf{not}(M)$ can be viewed as a Horn program. Thus, it has a least model. It is easy to see that

$$GL_P(M) = true(LM(P \cup \textbf{not}(\overline{M}))).$$

Here, P appearing at the left-hand side of the equation stands for the original logic program, while P appearing at the right-hand side of the equation stands for the same program but interpreted as a Horn program. Thus, using the algorithm of Dowling and Gallier [7], the Gelfond-Lifschitz reduct can be computed in time $O(size(P) + |M|) = O(size(P))$ (since $M \subseteq At(P)$, $|M| = O(size(P))$).

3   Algorithms

The departure point for our discussion of algorithms to compute the well-founded semantics is the *alternating-fixpoint* algorithm from [15]. Using the terminology introduced in the previous section it can be formulated as follows.

Algorithm 1 (Van Gelder)
   $F := \emptyset$;
   repeat
      $T := true(LM(P \cup \textbf{not}(F)))$; (* or equivalently: $T := GL(\overline{F})$; *)
      $F := \overline{LM(P_T^h)}$; (* or equivalently: $\overline{GL(T)}$; *)
   until no change in F;
   return T and F.

Let F' and F'' be the values of the set F just before and just after an iteration of the **repeat** loop in Algorithm 1. Clearly,

$$F'' = \overline{GL(GL(\overline{F'}))} = A(F').$$

Thus, after iteration i of the **repeat** loop, $F = A^i(\emptyset)$. Consequently, it follows from our earlier remarks that when Algorithm 1 terminates, the set F that is returned satisfies $F = F_{wfs}$. Since there is no change in F in the last iteration, when the algorithm terminates, we have $T = T_{wfs}$. That is, Algorithm 1 is correct.

We will now modify Algorithm 1. The basis for Algorithm 1 is the operator A. This operator is not *progressive*. That is, M is not necessarily a subset of $A(M)$. We will now introduce a related progressive operator, say B, and show that it can be used to replace A. Let P be a logic program and let T, F be two subsets of $At(P)$. By $P_{F,T}$ we denote the program obtained from P by removing

1. all rules whose heads are in F
2. all rules whose bodies contain a positive occurrence of an atom from F
3. all rules whose bodies contain a negated literal of the form $\mathbf{not}(a)$, where $a \in T$.

Clearly, $P_{F,T} \subseteq P_T$.

We define an operator $B(F)$ as follows:

$$B(F) = \overline{LM(P^h_{F,T})}, \quad \text{where } T = GL(\overline{F}).$$

The following result gathers key properties of the operator B.

Theorem 1. *Let P be a normal logic program. Then:*

1. *B is monotone*
2. *For every $F \subseteq At(P)$, $A(F) \subseteq B(F)$*
3. *For every $F \subseteq F_{wfs}$, $B(F) \subseteq F_{wfs}$*
4. *$lfp(B) = F_{wfs}$*
5. *For every $F \subseteq At(P)$, $B(F) = F \cup (\overline{F} \setminus LM(P^h_{F,T}))$, where $T = GL(\overline{F})$.*

Proof: (1) Assume that $F_1 \subseteq F_2$. Set $T_i = GL(\overline{F_i})$, $i = 1, 2$. Clearly, $\overline{F_2} \subseteq \overline{F_1}$ and, by antimonotonicity of GL, $T_1 \subseteq T_2$. By the definition of $P_{F,T}$, $P_{F_2,T_2} \subseteq P_{F_1,T_1}$. Consequently, $LM(P^h_{F_2,T_2}) \subseteq LM(P^h_{F_1,T_1})$ and, so, $B(F_1) \subseteq B(F_2)$.

(2) Let $T = GL(\overline{F})$. Clearly, $P_{F,T} \subseteq P_T$. Thus, $A(F) = \overline{LM(P^h_T)} \subseteq \overline{LM(P^h_{F,T})} = B(F)$.

(3) We have, $LM(P^h_{T_{wfs}}) = \overline{F_{wfs}}$. It follows that removing from $P^h_{T_{wfs}}$ rules with heads in F_{wfs} and those that contain an atom from F_{wfs} in their bodies does not change the least model. That is,

$$LM(P^h_{F_{wfs},T_{wfs}}) = LM(P^h_{T_{wfs}}).$$

Since, $T_{wfs} = GL(\overline{F_{wfs}})$, $B(F_{wfs}) = \overline{LM(P^h_{F_{wfs},T_{wfs}})}$. Let $F \subseteq F_{wfs}$. Then, by (1), $B(F) \subseteq B(F_{wfs})$. Thus, we have

$$B(F) \subseteq B(F_{wfs}) = \overline{LM(P^h_{F_{wfs},T_{wfs}})} = \overline{LM(P^h_{T_{wfs}})} = F_{wfs}.$$

(4) The least fixpoint of B is given by $lfp(B) = \bigcup B^i(\emptyset)$. By (3), $lfp(B) \subseteq F_{wfs}$. On the other hand, by (1) and (2), $A^i(\emptyset) \subseteq B^i(\emptyset)$. Thus, $F_{wfs} = lfp(A) \subseteq lfp(B)$. It follows that $lfp(B) = F_{wfs}$.

(5) Let $T = GL(\overline{F})$. Since $P_{F,T}$ has no rules with head in F, $LM(P_{F,T}^h) \subseteq \overline{F}$ and, consequently, $F \subseteq B(F)$. Thus, the assertion follows.   □

Theorem 1 allows us to prove the correctness of the following modification of Algorithm 1.

Algorithm 2
> $F := \emptyset$;
>   **repeat**
> $T := true(LM(P \cup \mathbf{not}(F)))$;
> $\Delta F := \overline{F} \setminus LM(P_{F,T}^h)$;
> $F := F \cup \Delta F$;
>   **until** no change in F;
>   **return** T and F.

By Theorem 1, each iteration of the **repeat** loop computes $B(F)$ as the new value for the set F. More formally, the set F just after iteration i, satisfies $F = B^i(\emptyset)$. Thus, when the algorithm terminates, the set F that is returned is the least fixpoint of B. Consequently, by Theorem 1(4), Algorithm 2 is correct.

We will now modify Algorithm 2 to obtain a general template for an alternating-fixpoint algorithm to compute the well-founded semantics. The key idea is to observe that it is enough to compute a subset of ΔF in each iteration and the algorithm will remain correct.

Let us assume that for some operator Δ_w defined for pairs (F, Q), where $F \subseteq At(P)$ and Q is a Horn program such that $At(Q) \subseteq \overline{F}$ (the complement is, as always, evaluated with respect to $At(P)$), we have:

(W1) $\Delta_w(F, Q) \subseteq \overline{F} \setminus LM(Q)$
(W2) $\Delta_w(F, Q) = \emptyset$ if and only if $\overline{F} \setminus LM(Q) = \emptyset$

Let $F \subseteq At(P)$. By the definition of $P_{F,T}$, $At(P_{F,T}^h) \subseteq \overline{F}$. Thus, we define $B_w(F) = F \cup \Delta_w(F, P_{F,T}^h))$, where $T = true(LM(P \cup \mathbf{not}(F)))$. It is clear that for every $F \subseteq At(P)$, $F \subseteq B_w(F) \subseteq B(F)$, the latter inclusion follows from Theorem 1(5). Consequently, for every i,

$$B_w^i(\emptyset) \subseteq B^{i+1}(\emptyset).$$

It follows that $B_w^i(\emptyset) \subseteq lfp(B) = F_{wfs}$. It also follows that there is the first i such that $B_w^i(\emptyset) = B_w^{i+1}(\emptyset)$. Let us denote this set $B_w^i(\emptyset)$ by F_0. Then $F_0 \subseteq F_{wfs}$. In the same time, by condition (W2), $B(F_0) = F_0$. Since F_{wfs} is the least fixpoint of B, $F_{wfs} \subseteq F_0$. It follows that a modification of Algorithm 2 in which line

$$\Delta F := \overline{F} \setminus LM(P_{F,T}^h);$$

is replaced by

$$\Delta F := \Delta_w(F, P_{F,T}^h);$$

correctly computes the well-founded semantics of a program P. Thus, we obtain the following algorithm for computing the well-founded semantics.

Algorithm 3

>$F := \emptyset;$
>**repeat**
>>$T := true(LM(P \cup \mathbf{not}(F)));$
>>$\Delta F := \Delta_w(F, P^h_{F,T});$
>>$F := F \cup \Delta F;$
>**until** no change in F;
>**return** T and F.

We will now refine Algorithm 3. Specifically, we will show that the sets T and F can be computed incrementally.

Let R be a Horn program. We define the *residual* program of R, $res(R)$, to be the Horn program obtained from R by removing all rules of R with the head in $LM(R)$ and by removing from the bodies of the remaining rules those elements that are in $LM(R)$. We have the following technical result.

Lemma 1. *Let R be a Horn program and let M be a set of atoms such that $M \cap head(R) = \emptyset$. Then $LM(R \cup M) = LM(R) \cup LM(res(R) \cup M)$.*

Lemma 1 implies that (we treat here negated literals as new atoms and P as Horn program over the extended alphabet)

$$LM(P \cup \mathbf{not}(F \cup \Delta F)) = LM(P \cup \mathbf{not}(F)) \cup LM(res(P) \cup \mathbf{not}(\Delta F)).$$

Thus, if the set F is expanded by new elements from ΔF, then the new set T can be computed by increasing the old set T by $\Delta T = true(LM(res(P) \cup \mathbf{not}(\Delta F)))$. Important thing to note is that the increment ΔT can be computed on the basis of the residual program and the increment ΔF. Similarly, we have

$$P_{F \cup \Delta F, T \cup \Delta T} = (P_{F,T})_{\Delta F, \Delta T}.$$

Thus, computing $P_{F,T}$ can also be done incrementally on the basis of the program considered in the previous iteration by taking into account most recently computed increments ΔF and ΔT.

This discussion implies that Algorithm 3 can be equivalently restated as follows:

Algorithm 3

1   $T := F := \Delta T := \Delta F := \emptyset;$
2   $R := P;$ (R will be treated as a Horn program *)
3   $Q := P;$
4   **repeat**
5     $\Delta T := true(LM(R \cup \mathbf{not}(\Delta F)));$

6     $R := res(R \cup \mathbf{not}(\Delta F))$;
7     $T := T \cup \Delta T$;
8     $Q := Q_{\Delta F, \Delta T}$;
9     $\Delta F := \Delta_w(F, Q^h)$;
10    $F := F \cup \Delta F$;
11   **until** no change in F;
12   **return** T and F.

We will now estimate the running time of Algorithm 3. Clearly line 1 requires constant time. Setting up appropriate data structures for programs R and Q (lines 2 and 3) takes $O(size(P))$ steps. In each iteration, ΔT is computed and the current program R is replaced by the program $res(R \cup \mathbf{not}(\Delta F))$ (lines 5 and 6). By modifying the algorithm from [7] and assuming that R is already stored in the memory (it is avaliable either as the result of the initialization in the case of the first iteration or as a result of the computation in the previous iteration), both tasks can be accomplished in $O(size(R^o) + |\Delta F| - size(R^n))$ steps. Here R^o denotes the old version of R and R^n denotes the new version of R. Consequently, the total time needed for lines 5 and 6 over all iterations is given by $O(size(P) + |At(P)| - size(R^t)) = O(size(P))$ (where R^t is the program R, when the algorithm terminates). The time needed for all lines 7 is proportional to the number of iterations and is $O(|At(P)|) = O(size(P))$.

Given a logic program Q and sets of atoms ΔT and ΔF, it takes $O(size(Q) - size(Q_{\Delta F, \Delta T}) + |\Delta T| + |\Delta F|)$ steps to compute the program $Q_{\Delta F, \Delta T}$ in line 8. We assume here that Q is already in the memory as a result of the initialization in the case of the first iteration, or as the result of the computation in the previous iteration, otherwise. It follows that the total time over all iterations needed to execute line 8 is $O(size(P) + |At(P)|) = O(size(P))$.

Thus, we obtain that the running time of Algorithm 3 is given by $O(size(P) + m)$, where m is the total time needed to compute $\Delta_w(F, Q)$ over all iterations of the algorithm.

In the standard (Van Gelder's) implementation of Algorithm 3, we compute the whole set $\overline{F} \setminus LM(Q^h)$ as $\Delta_w(F, Q^h)$. In addition, computation is performed in a bottom-up fashion. That is, we first compute the least model of Q^h and then its complement with respect to $\overline{F}$. Such approach requires $O(size(Q^h)) = O(size(P))$ steps per iteration to execute line 9 and leads to $O(|At(P)| \times size(P))$ running-time estimate for the alternating-fixpoint algorithm.

4   Procedure Δ_w

In this section we will focus on the class of programs, $\mathcal{LP}_1$, that is, programs whose rules have no more than one positive atom in their bodies. We describe for programs from this class a particular implementation of a procedure Δ_w and provide an estimate for its running time.

Assume that we have a procedure *false* that, given a Horn program $Q \in \mathcal{LP}_1$, returns a subset of the set $At(Q) \setminus LM(Q)$. Assume also that *false* returns the empty set if and only if $At(Q) = LM(Q)$. For every pair (F, Q), where $F \subseteq At(P)$ and Q is a Horn program such that $At(Q) \subseteq \overline{F}$, we define

$$\Delta_w(F, Q) = (\overline{F} \setminus At(Q)) \cup false(Q).$$

It is easy to see that this operator $\Delta_w(F, Q)$ satisfies conditions (W1) and (W2). Consequently, it can be used in Algorithm 3. Clearly, the procedure Δ_w and its computational properties are determined by the procedure *false*. In the remainder of the paper, we will describe a particular implementation of the procedure *false* and estimate its running time. We will use this estimate to obtain a bound on the running time of the resulting version of Algorithm 3.

A straightforward way to compute the least model of Q and so, to find $At(Q) \setminus LM(Q)$, is "bottom-up". That is, we start with atoms which are heads of rules with empty bodies and use the rules of Q to compute all atoms in $LM(Q)$ by iterating the van Emden-Kowalski operator. An efficient implementation of the process is provided by the Dowling-Gallier algorithm [7].

The approach we follow here in the procedure *false* is "top-down" and gives us, in general, only a part of the set $At(Q) \setminus LM(Q)$. More precisely, for an atom a we proceed "backwards" attempting to construct a proof or to demonstrate that no proof exists. In the process, we either go back to an atom that is the head of a rule with empty body or we show that no proof exists. In the first case, $a \in LM(Q)$. In the latter case, none of the atoms considered while searching for a proof of a are in $LM(Q)$ (because $Q \in \mathcal{LP}_1$ and each rule has at most one antecedent). The problem is that we may find an atom a that does not have a proof only *after* we look at all other atoms first. Thus, in the worst case, to find one new false atom may require time that is proportional to the size of Q.

To improve the time performance, we look for proofs simultaneously for all atoms and grow the proofs "backwards" in a carefully controlled way. This controlled way of looking for proofs for all atoms in which we never let one search to get too much ahead of the other searches is the key idea of our approach and leads to a better performance. We will now provide an informal description of the procedure *false* followed later by a formal specification.

In the procedure, we make use of a new atom, say s, which is not in $At(Q)$. Further, we denote by $head(r)$ the atom in the head of a rule $r \in Q$ and by $tail(r)$ the atom which is either the unique positive atom in the body of r, if such an atom exists, or s otherwise. We call an atom $a \in At(Q)$ *accessible* if there are rules $r_1, ..., r_k$ in Q such that $tail(r_{i+1}) = head(r_i)$, for $i = 1, ..., k-1$, $tail(r_1) = s$ and $head(r_k) = a$. Clearly, the least model $LM(Q)$ of Q is precisely the set of all accessible atoms.

In each step of the algorithm, the set of atoms from $At(Q)$ is partitioned into *potentially false sets* or *pf-sets*, for short. We say that a set $v \subseteq At(Q)$ is a *pf-set* if for each pair of atoms $a, b \in v$ there are rules $r_1, ...r_k$ in Q such that $tail(r_{i+1}) = head(r_i) \in v$, for $i = 1, ..., k-1$, $tail(r_1) = b$ and $head(r_k) = a$. It is clear that if v is a pf-set then either all its elements are accessible (belong to the least model of Q) or none does (they are all false). Clearly, singleton sets consisting of individual atoms in $At(Q)$ are pf-sets. With each pf-set we maintain its *weight*, that is, its cardinality.

Current information about the state of all top-down searches and dependencies among atoms that were discovered so far is maintained in a directed graph $\mathcal{G}$. The vertex set of this graph, say $\mathcal{S}$, consists of $\{s\}$ and of a family of pf-sets forming a partition of the set $At(Q)$. The edges of $\mathcal{G}$ are specified by a *partial* function $pred : \mathcal{S} \to \mathcal{S}$. We write $pred(v) = \textbf{undefined}$ if $pred$ is undefined for v. Now, the set of edges of $\mathcal{G}$ is given by $\{(pred(v), v) : pred(v) \neq \textbf{undefined}\}$. Throughout the algorithm we always have $pred(\{s\}) = \textbf{undefined}$. If both w and v are pf-sets (belong to $\mathcal{S} \setminus \{\{s\}\}$), the existence of the edge (w, v) means that we have already discovered a rule in the original program whose head is in v and whose tail is in w. Thus, if vertices in w are accessible, then so are the vertices in v. Since $pred$ is a partial function, it is easy to see that the connected components of the graph $\mathcal{G}$ are unicyclic graphs or trees rooted in those vertices v for which $pred(v)$ is undefined ($\{s\}$ is one of them). A pf-set that is the root of a tree forming a component of $\mathcal{G}$ is called *active*. If v is an active pf-set then no rule r with $head(r) \in v$ and $tail(r) \notin v$ has been detected so far. Thus, v is a candidate for a set of atoms which does not intersect the least model of Q.

We let active pf-sets grow by gluing them with other pf-sets (or we discard them, if we find that they consist of vertices that belong to the least model of Q). However, we allow to grow only these active pf-sets whose weights (cardinalities) are the least. In each iteration of the algorithm the value of the variable *size* is a lower bound for the cardinalities of active pf-sets. The main loop (lines 6-23) of the algorithm *false* below starts by incrementing *size* followed by a call to procedure $cycle(\mathcal{S}, pred, size, L)$. This procedure scans the graph $\mathcal{G}$ and identifies all its cycles. It then modifies $\mathcal{G}$ by considering each cycle and by gluing its pf-sets into a single pf-set that becomes active. It also computes the weight of each new active pf-set. Finally, it forms a list L of active pf-sets of the cardinality *size*. If no such set is found then we move on to the next iteration of the loop and increment *size* by 1.

For each active pf-set $v \in L$ we consider the tail of each rule with head in v (lines 9-22). If there is a rule r with $head(r) \in v$ and $tail(r) \notin v$ then it is detected (line 15). The value $pred(v)$ is set to this element in $\mathcal{S}$ that contains $tail(r)$ (it may be that this set is $\{s\}$). We also set the variable *success* to **true** (line 16). The pf-set v stops to be active. We move on to the next active pf-set on L.

If such a rule r does not exist then $success = \textbf{false}$ and v is a set of cardinality *size* consisting of atoms which are not in the least model of Q. This set is returned by the procedure *false* (line 21). Hence, for an active pf-set considered in the loop in lines 6-23, either we find a pf-set $pred(v) \in \mathcal{S} \setminus \{v\}$ (and we have to consider the next pf-set on L) or v is returned as a set of atoms of cardinality *size* which are not in the least model of Q (and the procedure *false* terminates). Thus, the procedure *false* is completed if either a nonempty set v of atoms which are not in the least model of Q is found or, after some passes of the loop in lines 6-23, the graph $\mathcal{G}$ has no active pf-sets. In the latter case $\mathcal{G}$ is a tree with the root in $\{s\}$. Thus, $At(Q) = LM(Q)$ and $v = \emptyset$ is returned (line 24).

In the procedure *false*, as formally described below, an input program Q is represented by lists $IN(a)$, $a \in At(Q)$, of all atoms b such that b is the body of some rule with the head a. If there is a rule with the head a and empty body, we insert s into the list $IN(a)$.

We also use an operation *next* on lists and elements. Let l be a list and w be an element, either belonging to l or having a special value **undefined**. Then

$$next(w, l) = \begin{cases} \text{the next element after } w \text{ in } l & \text{if } w \in l \\ \text{the first element in } l & \text{if } w \text{ is } \mathbf{undefined}. \end{cases}$$

The value **undefined** should not be mixed with **nil** which indicates the end of a list.

Finally, we use a procedure $findset(w, \mathcal{S})$ which, for an atom w and a collection $\mathcal{S}$ of disjoint sets, one of which contains w, finds the name of the set in $\mathcal{S}$ containing w (it follows from our assumptions that such a set is unique). Elements of $\mathcal{S}$ are maintained as linked lists. Each element on such a list has a pointer to the head of the list. The head serves as the identifier for the list. When the procedure $findset(w, \mathcal{S})$ is called it returns the head of the list to which w belongs.

```
1    procedure false(Q);
2      S := {{x} : x ∈ At(Q)} ∪ {{s}};
3      for v ∈ S do pred(v) := undefined;
4      for x ∈ At(Q) do {w(x) := undefined; weight(x) := 1};
5      size := 0;
6      while size < |At(Q)| do
7        {size := size + 1;
8        cycle(S, pred, size, L);
9        for all v ∈ L do
10         {success := false;
11         u := next(u, v);
12         while u ≠ nil and not success do
13           w(u) := next(w(u), IN(u));
14           while w(u) ≠ nil and not success do
15             {if findset(w(u), S) ≠ v
16               then {success := true; pred(v) := findset(w(u), S)};
17               else w(u) := next(w(u), IN(u))
18             end while (14)};
19           if not success then u := next(u, v)
20         end while (12)};
21         if not success then return v    (* the procedure terminates *)
22       end for (9)};
23     end while (6)};
24     return v = ∅
25   end false;
```

The following theorem formally establishes two key properties of the procedure *false*.

Theorem 2.   *1. The procedure false returns a set v such that $v \subseteq At(Q) \setminus LM(Q)$.*
2. *false returns the empty set if and only if $At(Q) \setminus LM(Q) = \emptyset$.*

Proof: (1) The statement is trivially true if *false* returns the empty set. Thus assume that the returned set $v \neq \emptyset$. It means that the value of the variable *success* is **false** after all passes of the loop in lines 12-20 for some active pf-set v in the list L. Thus every rule in Q with the head in v has been considered.

Suppose there is a rule r in Q with $head(r) = u \in v$ and $tail(r) = b \notin v$. This rule was considered by the procedure *false* when $u = head(r)$ was a member of some pf-set, say y. Since larger pf-sets are obtained by gluing smaller ones, $y \subseteq v$. While r was being considered, the value of $w(u)$ in the loop in lines 14-18 was b and the value of v was y. Consequently, $findset(b, S) \neq y$ in line 15 because $y \subseteq v$ and $b \notin v$ so $b \notin y$. Hence the value of *success* was set to **true** and $pred(y)$ was defined to be, say, $z = findset(b, S)$ in line 16. The pf-set y stopped to be active. Recall that v is active when the procedure stops. Hence y had to be glued with other pf-sets to obtain v. This is, however, impossible because if y were glued with some other pf-sets to form a larger pf-set x then $pred(y) = z \subseteq x$. Notice that $b \in z \subseteq x \subseteq v$. We have got a contradiction with $b \notin v$.

Hence, there are no rules r in Q with $head(r) \in v$ and $tail(r) \notin v$. Thus no atom in v is accessible so $v \subseteq At(Q) \setminus LM(Q)$.

(2) Suppose *false* returns the empty set and consider the last pass of the loop in lines 6-23, for $size = |At(Q)|$. If the list L is empty then no vertex of $\mathcal{G}$ is an active pf-set. Hence, $\mathcal{G}$ is a tree with the root $\{s\}$. Thus all atoms in $At(Q)$ are accessible and consequently $LM(Q) = At(Q)$.

If the list L is nonempty then it contains one pf-set $v = At(Q)$. The empty set is returned by the procedure *false* so the value of the variable *success* in line 16 is **true** for $v = At(Q)$. It means that for some rule r in Q with $head(r) = u$, $w(u) = tail(r) \notin v = At(Q)$ so $w(u) = s$. Hence, u is accessible and, consequently, all atoms in $At(Q)$ are accessible. That is, we have $At(Q) \setminus LM(Q) = \emptyset$.

The converse of the implication proved above follows immediately from the first part of the theorem.   □

We shall now consider the procedure *cycle* a little bit more carefully. The procedure can be informally written in the following form.

procedure $cycle(S, pred, size, L)$
1. Initialize L to empty.
2. Find all cycles $C_1, C_2, ..., C_p$ in the graph $\mathcal{G}$. Put $\mathcal{C} = \{C_1, C_2, ..., C_p\}$.
3. For every cycle $C = \{v_1, ..., v_q\}$, $C \in \mathcal{C}$, do (i)-(iv).
    (i) set $v_C := v_1 \cup ... \cup v_q$;
    (ii) compute $weight(v_C)$ (sum up the weights of all vertices in C);

(iii) update the function *pred* — for every $i = 1, ..., q$, if $pred(z) = v_i$ (for some $z \in S$) then $pred(z) := v_C$;

(iv) update the set S — $S := (S - \{v_1, ..., v_q\}) \cup \{v_C\}$; (* v_C becomes an active pf-set *)

4. For every vertex of $\mathcal{G}$ that is an active pf-set, if $weight(v) = size$, insert v into the list L.

Since $\mathcal{G}$ is a directed graph whose connected components are either unicyclic graphs or trees, step 2 of the procedure *cycle* can be implemented in $O(|S|)$ time. Since pf-sets are represented as linked lists, with each node on the list pointing to the head of the list, step (i) can be implemented to take $O(|v_C|)$ steps. The time needed for step (ii) is, clearly, $O(|C|)$. Each execution of step (iv) takes also $O(|C|)$. Finally, the running time of each execution of step (iii) is $O(m_C)$, where m_C is the size of the connected component of the graph $\mathcal{G}$ containing C. Thus, an iteration of loop 3 for a cycle $C \in \mathcal{C}$ takes $O(|C| + m_C + |v_C|)$. Clearly, $|C| \leq m_C$. Moreover, $\sum_{C \in \mathcal{C}} m_C \leq |S| - 1 \leq |At(Q)|$ and $\sum_{C \in \mathcal{C}} |v_C| \leq |At(Q)|$ (they are all disjoint subsets of $At(Q)$). Thus, the total time needed for loop 3 is $O(|At(Q)|)$. It is easy to see that the time needed for loop 4 is also $O(|At(Q)|)$. Consequently, the running time of the procedure *cycle* is $O(|At(Q)|)$.

We are now in a position to estimate the running time of the procedure *false*.

Lemma 2. *If the procedure false(Q) returns a nonempty set v, then the running time of false is $O(|v| \times |At(Q)|)$. If false(Q) returns the empty set then its running time is $O(|At(Q)|^2)$.*

Proof: Let $|At(Q)| = n$ and $|v| = k$. As we have already observed the procedure *cycle* runs in time $O(n)$. It is not hard to see that, since we represent all sets occurring in the procedure *false* as linked lists, with each node on a list pointing to the head of the list, the operations: *findset* and *next* require a constant time.

First assume that the output v of the procedure *false* is nonempty. Let us estimate the number of passes of the **while** and **for** loops in the procedure. Clearly, the loop in lines 6-23 is executed k times. Hence the total running time of all calls of the procedure *cycle* is $O(kn)$. The number of passes of the loop in lines 9-22 is not larger than $|L_1| + |L_2| + ... + |L_k|$, where L_i denotes the list L in an iteration i of the loop. Since L_i is a list of disjoint pf-sets of cardinality i, $|L_i| \leq n$, for each $i = 1, 2, ..., k$. Hence the number of passes of the loop in lines 9-22 can be very roughly estimated by kn. The loop in lines 12-20 is executed at most

$$\sum_{i=1}^{k} \sum_{v \in L_i} |v| \leq kn$$

times. This inequality follows from the fact that the sets v in the lists L_i are disjoint subsets of atoms so $\sum_{v \in L_i} |v| \leq n$. The estimation of the number of passes of the loop in lines 14-18 is a little bit more complicated. First notice that in each execution of the loop we check a rule of the program Q and rules are checked only one time. The rules r checked in the loop have either both the head and the tail in some pf-set $v \in S$ or $head(r) \in v$ and $tail(r)$ is in some other pf-set $u \in \mathcal{S}$. In the latter case $pred(v)$ is defined in line 16. The number of executions of line 16 is not larger than the number of passes of the loop in lines 9-22 so it is bounded by kn. When the procedure returns the output, the pf-sets have cardinalities not larger than k. Hence the number of rules with both the head and the tail in the same pf-set that has been checked before the procedure stops is not larger than

$$\sum_{u \in \mathcal{S}} |u|(|u| - 1) \leq (k-1) \sum_{u \in \mathcal{S}} |u| \leq (k-1)n.$$

Thus the number of passes of the loop in lines 14-18 in the whole procedure *false* is less than $2kn$. It follows that if the output v of *false* is nonempty then the running time of *false* is $O(|v| \times |At(Q)|)$.

Now consider the case when the procedure *false* returns the empty set. Clearly the number of passes of the loop in lines 6-23 is n so it takes $O(n^2)$ time for all executions of the procedure *cycle*. Since the rules are checked in the loop in lines 14-18 only one time, the number of passes of this loop is not larger than the number m of rules in Q. Obviously $m \leq n^2$ so the running time of *false* in this case is $O(|At(Q)|^2)$. □

By Lemma 2 and considerations in Section 3 we get an estimation of the running time of Algorithm 3.

Theorem 3. *If P is a program whose rules have at most one positive atom in the body then Algorithm 3 can be implemented such that its running time is $O(|At(P)|^2 + size(P))$.* □

5   Conclusions

The method for computing the well-founded semantics described in the paper is a refinement of the basic alternating-fixpoint algorithm. The key idea is to use a top-down search when identifying atoms that are false. Our method is designed to work with programs whose rules have at most one positive atom in their bodies (class $\mathcal{LP}_1$). Its running time is $O(|At(P)|^2 + size(P))$ (where P is an input program). Thus, our algorithm is an improvement over other known methods to compute the well-founded semantics for programs in the class $\mathcal{LP}_1$. Our algorithm runs in linear time for the class of programs $P \in \mathcal{LP}_1$ for which $size(P) \geq |At(P)|^2$. However, it is not a linear-time algorithm in general. It is an open question whether a linear-time algorithm for computing the well-founded semantics for programs in the class $\mathcal{LP}_1$ exists.

Finally, let us note that the general problem of computing well-founded semantics still remains a challenge. No significant improvement over the alternating-fixpoint algorithm of Van Gelder has been obtained for the class of arbitrary finite propositional logic programs. This paper points to the fact that top-down computation of false atoms may lead to some improvement.

Acknowledgments

This research was supported by the NSF grants CDA-9502645 and IRI-9619233.

References

1. J.J. Alferes, C.V. Damásio, and L.M. Pereira. A logic programming system for nonmonotonic reasoning. *Journal of Automated Reasoning*, 14:93–147, 1995.
2. K. Berman, J. Schlipf, and J.Franco. Computing the well-founded semantics faster. In *Logic Programming and Nonmonotonic Reasoning (Lexington, KY, 1995)*, volume 928 of *Lecture Notes in Computer Science*, pages 113–125, Berlin, 1995. Springer.
3. S. Brass and J. Dix. Characterizations of the disjunctive well-founded semantics: confluent calculi and iterated GCWA. *Journal of Automated Reasoning*, 20(1):143–165, 1998.
4. S. Brass and J. Dix and B. Freitag and U. Zukowski. Transformation-based bottom-up computation of the well-founded model. Manuscript.
5. W. Chen, T. Swift, and D.S. Warren. Efficient top-down computation of queries under the well-founded semantics. *Journal of Logic Programming*, 24(3):161–199, 1995.
6. W. Chen and D.S. Warren. Tabled evaluation with delaying for general logic programs. *Journal of the ACM*, 43(1):20–74, 1996.
7. W.F. Dowling and J.H. Gallier. Linear-time algorithms for testing the satisfiability of propositional Horn formulae. *Journal of Logic Programming*, 1(3):267–284, 1984.
8. M. C. Fitting. Fixpoint semantics for logic programming – a survey. *Theoretical Computer Science*, 1999. To appear.
9. M.C. Fitting. Well-founded semantics, generalized. In *Logic programming (San Diego, CA, 1991)*, MIT Press Series in Logic Programming, pages 71–84, Cambridge, MA, 1991. MIT Press.
10. M. Gelfond and V. Lifschitz. The stable semantics for logic programs. In R. Kowalski and K. Bowen, editors, *Proceedings of the 5th International Symposium on Logic Programming*, pages 1070–1080, Cambridge, MA, 1988. MIT Press.
11. W. Marek and M. Truszczyński. Autoepistemic logic. *Journal of the ACM*, 38(3):588–619, 1991.
12. I. Niemelä and P. Simons. Efficient implementation of the well-founded and stable model semantics. In *Proceedings of JICSLP-96*. MIT Press, 1996.
13. P. Rao, I.V. Ramskrishnan, K. Sagonas, T. Swift, D. S. Warren, and J. Freire. XSB: A system for efficiently computing well-founded semantics. In *Proceedings of LPNMR'97*, pages 430–440. Berlin: Springer-Verlag, 1997. Lecture Notes in Computer Science, 1265.
14. V.S. Subrahmanian, D. Nau, and C. Vago. WFS + branch bound = stable models. *IEEE Transactions on Knowledge and Data Engineering*, 7:362–377, 1995.
15. A. Van Gelder. The alternating fixpoints of logic programs with negation. In *ACM symposium on principles of database systems*, pages 1–10, 1989.
16. A. Van Gelder, K.A. Ross, and J.S. Schlipf. The well-founded semantics for general logic programs. *Journal of the ACM*, 38(3):620–650, 1991.
17. U. Zukowski, S. Brass, and B. Freitag. Improving the alternating fixpoint: the transformation approach. In *Proceedings of LPNMR'97*, pages 40–59. Berlin: Springer-Verlag, 1997. Lecture Notes in Computer Science, 1265.

Computing Equilibrium Models
Using Signed Formulas

David Pearce[1], Inmaculada P. de Guzmán[2], and Agustín Valverde[2]

[1] DFKI, Saarbrücken, Germany
pearce@dfki.de
[2] Dept. of Applied Mathematics, University of Málaga, Spain
{guzman,a_valverde}@ctima.uma.es

Abstract. We discuss equilibrium logic, first presented in Pearce (1997), as a system of nonmonotonic reasoning based on the nonclassical logic N_5 of here-and-there with strong negation. Equilibrium logic is a conservative extension of answer set inference, not only for extended, disjunctive logic programs, but also for significant extensions such as the programs with nested expressions described by Lifschitz, Tang and Turner (forthcoming). It provides a theoretical basis for extending the paradigm of answer set programming beyond current systems such as smodels and dlv. The paper provides proof systems for N_5 and for model-checking in equilibrium logic. The reduction of the latter problem to an unsatisfiability problem of classical logic yields complexity results for the various decision problems concerning equilibrium entailment. The reduction also yields a basis for the practical implementation of an automated reasoning tool.

1 Introduction

Equilibrium logic is a formal system of nonmonotonic reasoning proposed by the first author as a generalisation of inference based on stable models and answer sets [6–8]. While stable models and answer sets are defined for ground (instantiated) *logic programs* whose expressions have a special, restricted syntactic form, equilibrium logic uses an unrestricted propositional language that can therefore be applied also to grounded (predicate logical) theories more general than logic programs. The basic notions and properties of equilibrium logic are discussed in [24, 25]. The present paper is devoted to computational issues, especially the problem of checking efficiently whether a given model of a theory is in equilibrium and whether a given formula is an equilibrium consequence of a theory. We also discuss and characterise the complexity of these tasks.

We approach computational issues using the method of *signing* [20], familiar from the area of automated deduction for many-valued logics. This method translates the problem of deciding the validity of formulas (or entailments) in a many-valued logic to the problem of deciding whether a certain set of *signed* formulas is unsatisfiable. The latter test can then be carried out using standard techniques such as TAS, tableaux, resolution, etc. To our knowledge this paper

J. Lloyd et al. (Eds.): CL 2000, LNAI 1861, pp. 688–702, 2000.

provides the first application of signing to a system of nonmonotonic inference and to the logic on which it is based: the 5-valued logic of here-and-there with strong negation, denoted here by N_5. This application is made possible by using a modification of signed logics called *reduced* signed logics, developed in [11]. In addition, we improve the signing process by using a new technique called *signing-up*.

Since equilibrium inference is a conservative extension of the inference relation associated with stable model semantics, the techniques and results of this paper apply *a fortiori* to stable models for logic programs. There already exist efficient implementations of stable model and answer set semantics, eg [22, 4], using special purpose algorithms tailored to the specific syntax of logic programs. By contrast, the more general theorem proving techniques discussed here apply to the case of full propositional logic and are therefore likely to be of interest to those seeking to extend stable model reasoning beyond the language of logic programs, as for instance the approach of [16] which considers programs with nested expressions. One result that may be of some significance here is that such syntactic extensions do not lead to an increase in the complexity of checking whether a given model is stable (ie. in equilibrium). We hope the methods of this paper may also be of some interest for the field of automated deduction for nonclassical logics; in particular, by illustrating the use of signing in a concrete case (the logic N_5) and by showing how nonmonotonic extensions of many-valued logics may also be amenable to treatment by these methods when suitably extended as here in the form of reduced signed logics.

2   Equilibrium Logic

Equilibrium logic can be viewed, and hence motivated, in different ways. On the one hand it can be seen simply as a general purpose system of nonmonotonic reasoning, based on a notion of negation-by-default. It is currently defined for a propositional language with two kinds of negation, weak and strong, and is therefore also applicable to ground or instantiated theories in a predicate language (without function symbols). Another way to view equilibrium logic is as an extension of stable model or answer set programming. Answer set semantics for extended logic programs was developed already ten years ago [7]. However there has recently been a pronounced revival of interest in answer sets as defining a new programming paradigm.There has been a growing awareness that several well-known types of combinatorial problems have elegant solutions when expressed in the form of answer set programs. In addition, efficient implementations are now available that make computing answer set solutions a viable task. Current implementations, such as dlv, are available for disjunctive as well as normal logic programs and can handle both weak and strong negation [4, 5]. There are also frontends for diagnostic reasoning and for reasoning with inheritance.

There has also been considerable interest in extending the basic language of answer set programs to a more expressive syntax. Already Lifschitz [15] extended the definition of answer set to include languages with integrity constraints and rules with negation-as-failure in their heads. A different but equivalent extension was proposed in [2]. Recently, [9] has treated rules whose bodies may contain conditionals, [27] considers special additional kinds of rules such as (cardinality) constraints, and [16] defines answer sets for programs with nested expressions, that is programs whose formulas comprise implications $\alpha \to \beta$, where α and β may by arbitrary boolean combinations of literals. In equilibrium logic even this last restriction is removed so that all the logical operators may be nested, not only the boolean ones.

We start by giving the original definition of equilibrium logic in terms of Kripke models. Later, for the purposes of computing equilibrium inference, we use an equivalent definition in terms of many-valued matrices.

Equilibrium logic is based on the logic of *here-and-there with strong nega-tion*, which we denote by $\mathbf{N_5}$.[1] We first consider the logic of here-and-there. The language is the propositional language of intuitionistic logic, with formu-las built-up in the usual way using the logical constants: $\wedge, \vee, \to, \neg$, standing respectively for conjunction, disjunction, implication and negation. A *here-and-there* (Kripke) *frame $\mathcal{F}$*, is a pair $\mathcal{F} = \langle W, \leq \rangle$, where W is a set comprising two points (or worlds), 'here' and 'there', denoted by h and t, respectively, and $\leq$ is a partial-ordering on W, such that $h \leq t$. At each point $w \in W$ some primitive propositions (atoms) are verified as *true*, and, once verified at the point h, an atom α remains true at the 'later' point, t. A here-and-there *model $\mathcal{M}$* can there-fore be represented as a frame $\mathcal{F}$ together with an assignment i of sets of atoms to each element of W, such that $i(h) \subseteq i(t)$. An assignment is then extended inductively to all formulas via the following rules:

$\varphi \wedge \psi \in i(w)$ iff $\varphi \in i(w)$ and $\psi \in i(w)$
$\varphi \vee \psi \in i(w)$ iff $\varphi \in i(w)$ or $\psi \in i(w)$
$\varphi \to \psi \in i(w)$ iff for all w' such that $w \leq w'$, $\varphi \in i(w')$ implies $\psi \in i(w')$
$\neg\varphi \in i(w)$ iff for all w' such that $w \leq w'$, $\varphi \notin i(w')$

These are the standard truth-conditions for Kripke models of intuitionistic logic. However they can evidently be simplified in the case of these two-element frames. For instance we see immediately that a negated formula $\neg\varphi$ is true 'here' ($\neg\varphi \in i(h)$) just in case φ is not true 'there' ($\varphi \notin i(t)$).

The logical operator of strong negation adds to intuitionistic logic the in-sight that primitive propositions may not only be constructively *verified* but also constructively *falsified*. The language is accordingly extended by a new, strong negation symbol, '$\sim$', with the interpretation that $\sim\varphi$ is true if φ is con-structively false. A semantics can be obtained through a simple modification of the above Kripke-semantics. As before a model comprises a two element Kripke-frame $\mathcal{F} = \langle W, \leq \rangle$, where $W = \{h, t\}$, together with an assignment i. However i now assigns to each element of W a set of *literals*,[2] such that as before $i(h) \subseteq i(t)$.

---

[1] The symbol 'N' stands for Nelson, the founder of constructive logic with strong negation [21], and '5' expresses that we are dealing with a many-valued extension of Nelson's original logic with five truth-values.

[2] We use the term "literal" to denote an atom or an atom prefixed by strong negation.

An assignment is then extended inductively to all formulas via the previous rules for conjunction, disjunction, implication and (weak) negation together with the following rules governing strongly negated formulas:

$$\sim(\varphi \wedge \psi) \in i(w) \text{ iff } \sim\varphi \in i(w) \text{ or } \sim\psi \in i(w)$$
$$\sim(\varphi \vee \psi) \in i(w) \text{ iff } \sim\varphi \in i(w) \text{ and } \sim\psi \in i(w)$$
$$\sim(\varphi \rightarrow \psi) \in i(w) \text{ iff } \varphi \in i(w) \text{ and } \sim\psi \in i(w)$$
$$\sim\neg\varphi \in i(w) \text{ iff } \sim\sim\varphi \in i(w) \text{ iff } \varphi \in i(w)$$

Weak negation '$\neg$' is definable in $\mathbf{N}_5$ by: $\neg\varphi := \varphi \rightarrow \sim\varphi$. A formula φ is true in a model $\mathcal{M} = \langle W, \leq, i \rangle$ at a point $w \in W$, in symbols $\mathcal{M}, w \models \varphi$, iff $\varphi \in i(w)$. φ is true in a model $\mathcal{M}$, in symbols $\mathcal{M} \models \varphi$, if it is true at both points in $\mathcal{M}$ which is also the case if it is true at h. A formula φ is said to be *valid*, in symbols, $\models \varphi$, if it is true in all models. Logical consequence for $\mathbf{N}_5$ is understood as follows: φ is said to be an $\mathbf{N}_5$-consequence of a set Π of formulas, written $\Pi \models \varphi$, iff for all models $\mathcal{M}$, $\mathcal{M} \models \Pi$ implies $\mathcal{M} \models \varphi$. The logic $\mathbf{N}_5$ can also be presented axiomatically. The above set of valid formulas can be captured via the axioms and rules of intuitionistic logic (see eg. [32]) together with the axiom schemata for strong negation due to Vorob'ev [30, 31], see eg. [32, 26], and in addition the following axiom for here-and-there due to Lukasiewicz [17][3]:

$$(\neg\alpha \rightarrow \beta) \rightarrow (((\beta \rightarrow \alpha) \rightarrow \beta) \rightarrow \beta).$$

$\mathbf{N}_5$ is a conservative extension of the logic of here-and-there[4] in the sense that any formula without strong negation is a theorem of $\mathbf{N}_5$ if and only if it is a theorem of here-and-there. Notice that Nelson's negation '$\sim$' is termed 'strong', since in $\mathbf{N}_5$, $\sim\varphi \rightarrow \neg\varphi$ is a theorem. (See eg. [10, 32]). The derivability relation for $\mathbf{N}_5$ is denoted by $\vdash$. The Kripke semantics is *complete* for $\mathbf{N}_5$ in the sense that for all Π and φ,

Since we are dealing with Kripke frames containing only two points, h and t with $h \leq t$, it is convenient to represent an $\mathbf{N}_5$-model as an ordered pair $\langle H, T \rangle$ of sets of literals, where $H = i(h)$ and $T = i(t)$ under a suitable assignment i. By $h \leq t$, it follows that $H \subseteq T$.

The Kripke semantics for $\mathbf{N}_5$ can be characterised using a many-valued approach, specifically with a five-valued logic where the truth values set is $\mathbf{5} = \{-2, -1, 0, 1, 2\}$. In this approach, the connectives are interpreted in the Nelson algebra:

$$\mathfrak{N} = (\{-2, -1, 0, 1, 2\}, \wedge, \vee, \rightarrow, \neg, \sim)$$

where $\vee = \max$, $\wedge = \min$, $\sim x = -x$,

$$x \rightarrow y = \begin{cases} 2 & \text{if either } x \leq 0 \text{ or } x \leq y \\ y & \text{otherwise} \end{cases} \quad \text{and} \quad \neg x = \begin{cases} 2 & \text{if } x \leq 0 \\ -x & \text{otherwise} \end{cases}$$

---

[3] Smetanich studied the logic of here-and-there in [28] and important results about the logic can also be found in [18].

[4] ie. the logic determined by formulas in the language of intuitionistic logic that are true on all here-and-there frames. This is the greatest logic containing intuitionistic logic and properly contained in classical logic. For more about $\mathbf{N}_5$, see [14].

The relation between Kripke models and many-valued assignments is the following:

$$
\begin{aligned}
\sigma(p) &= \ \ 2 &&\text{iff} && p \in H \\
\sigma(p) &= \ \ 1 &&\text{iff} && p \in T, p \notin H \\
\sigma(p) &= \ \ 0 &&\text{iff} && p \notin T, \sim p \notin T \\
\sigma(p) &= -1 &&\text{iff} && \sim p \in T, \sim p \notin H \\
\sigma(p) &= -2 &&\text{iff} && \sim p \in H
\end{aligned}
$$

This way the many-valued semantics and the Kripke semantics for $\mathbf{N}_5$ are equivalent. In other words, if Π is a set of formulas in $\mathbf{N}_5$ and ψ is a formula, then $\Pi \models \psi$ iff for every assignment σ in $\mathbf{N}_5$, if $\sigma(\varphi) = 2$ for every $\varphi \in \Pi$, then $\sigma(\psi) = 2$

2.1 Equilibrium Models and Equilibrium Inference

Equilibrium models are special kinds of minimal $\mathbf{N}_5$ Kripke models. We first define a partial ordering $\trianglelefteq$ on $\mathbf{N}_5$ models as follows.

Given any two models $\langle H, T \rangle, \langle H', T' \rangle$, we set $\langle H, T \rangle \trianglelefteq \langle H', T' \rangle$ if $T = T'$ and $H \subseteq H'$.

This leads to the following notion of equilibrium: if Π is a set of $\mathbf{N}_5$ formulas and $\langle H, T \rangle$ is a model of Π.

1. $\langle H, T \rangle$ is said to be *total* if $H = T$.
2. $\langle H, T \rangle$ is said to be an *equilibrium* model if it is minimal under $\trianglelefteq$ among models of Π, and it is total.

Using the many-valued semantics we have the following equivalent definitions.

Definition 1. *Let Π be a set of formulas in $\mathbf{N}_5$. The ordering $\sigma_1 \trianglelefteq \sigma_2$ among models σ_1 and σ_2 of Π holds iff for every propositional variable p occurring in Π the following properties hold:*

1. $\sigma_1(p) = 0$ if and only if $\sigma_2(p) = 0$.
2. If $\sigma_1(p) \geq 1$, then $\sigma_1(p) \leq \sigma_2(p)$
3. If $\sigma_1(p) \leq -1$, then $\sigma_1(p) \geq \sigma_2(p)$

Definition 2. *Let $\Pi = \{\varphi_1, \ldots, \varphi_n\}$ be a set of formulas in $\mathbf{N}_5$. A model σ of Π in $\mathbf{N}_5$ is a total model if $\sigma(p) \in \{-2, 0, 2\}$ for every propositional variable p in Π. σ is an equilibrium model if it is total and minimal under the $\trianglelefteq$-ordering.*

Equilibrium logic is the logic determined by the equilibrium models of a theory; we define it formally in terms of a nonmonotonic entailment relation.

Definition 3 (Equilibrium Entailment). *Let $\varphi_1, \ldots, \varphi_n, \varphi$ be formulas in $\mathbf{N}_5$. We define the relation $\hspace{0.1em}\mid\hspace{-0.55em}\sim$ called equilibrium entailment, as follows*

1. If $\Pi = \{\varphi_1, \ldots, \varphi_n\}$ has equilibrium models, then $\varphi_1, \ldots, \varphi_n \mid\hspace{-0.55em}\sim \varphi$ if every equilibrium model of Π is a model of φ in $\mathbf{N}_5$.

2. *If either $n = 0$ or Π has no equilibrium models, then $\varphi_1, \ldots, \varphi_n \mathrel{\vert\!\sim} \varphi$ if $\varphi_1, \ldots, \varphi_n \models \varphi$.*[5]

The process of checking equilibrium entailment, $\Pi \mathrel{\vert\!\sim} \psi$, will be understood as follows:

Step 1. Generate the total models of Π.

Step 2. For every total model of Π, check the equilibrium property. If there are equilibrium models, then go to step 3, else go to step 4.

Step 3. For every equilibrium model of Π, check if it is a model of ψ.

Step 4. If Π doesn't have equilibrium models, just check entailment in $\mathbf{N}_5$.

Part of the interest of equilibrium logic arises from the fact that on a syntactically restricted class of theories it coincides with a well-known nonmonotonic inference relation studied in logic programming, namely that generated by the semantics of *answer sets*. This holds not only for ordinary (extended) logic programs, but also for the generalisation to programs with nested expressions defined in [16].

Theorem 1. *Let Π be a consistent theory having the syntactic shape of a logic program with nested expressions in the sense of [16]. The equilibrium models of Π correspond precisely to the answer sets of Π.*

Proof sketch. Written in usual logical notation, a logic program with nested expressions in the sense of [16] comprises sets of formulas of the form $\alpha \to \beta$, where α, β are arbitrary boolean combinations of literals[6] in the language of $\mathbf{N}_5$. In [16], the authors first define answer sets for programs of this form, and then show, via a series of program transformations, that every such program is (answer set) equivalent to a program whose formulas $\alpha \to \beta$ are such that α is a conjunction of literals and weakly negated literals and β is a disjunction of literals and weakly negated literals. For programs of the latter kind a straightforward extension of the proof of Proposition 10 of [24] shows that answer sets and equilibrium models coincide. Moreover, one may readily verify that the program transformations described in [16] correspond to transformations of formulas that are logically valid in $\mathbf{N}_5$. From this fact the claim follows.

3   Signed Logics

Proof methods for many-valued logic have developed alongside the evolution of the notions of *sign* and *signed formula*. The use of signs and signed formulas allows one to apply classical methods in the analysis of many-valued logics. Forgetting the set of truth-values associated with a given logic, in the metalanguage one may interpret sentences about the many-valued logic as being true-or-false.

---

[5] For the case where a consistent theory has no equilibrium models, entailment can be defined in various different ways. Here we choose a simple option, logical consequence. Another option would be to consider, say, the minimal models, but these choices are not of great issue for the purposes of the present paper.

[6] ie. combinations involving $\wedge, \vee, \neg$.

For example, in a 3-valued logic with truth-values $\{0, 1/2, 1\}$ and with $\{1\}$ as the designated value, the satisfiability of a formula φ can be expressed as: *Is it possible to evaluate φ in $\{1\}$?* In the same way, the unsatisfiability of φ is expressed by: *Is φ always evaluated in $\{0, 1/2\}$?* These questions can be represented by the signed formulas $\{1\}{:}\varphi$ and $\{0,1/2\}{:}\varphi$ which are evaluated on the set $\{0, 1\}$ with the following meaning:

- $\{1\}{:}\varphi$ takes the value 1 when φ is evaluated in $\{1\}$
- $\{0,1/2\}{:}\varphi$ takes the value 1 when φ is evaluated in $\{0, 1/2\}$

In other words, the formulas in a signed logic are constructions of the form $S{:}\varphi$, where S is a set of truth-values of the many-valued logic, called the *sign*, and φ is a formula of that logic. The interpretations that determine the semantics of the signed logic are defined from the interpretations of the many-valued logic as follows:

$$I_\sigma(S{:}\varphi) = 1 \quad \text{if and only if} \quad \sigma(\varphi) \in S$$

The first works to provide a systematic treatment of sets of truth-values as signs were due to Hähnle in [12] and Murray and Rosenthal in [19]. There the notion of *signed formula* is formally introduced. In [12] these tools are used in the framework of truth tables, while in [19] they are used to develop another, nonclausal proof method, that of *disolution*. As a result of these works, the use of signed formulas in the field of automated deduction has been extended, and has led to significant advances in this method.

The notion of *reduced signed logic* was introduced in [11] as a generalisation of previous approaches. It is developed in the general framework of propositional logics, without reference either to an initially given many-valued logic or to a specific algorithm, ie. the definition is completely independent of the particular application at hand. The generalisation consists in introducing a *possible truth values function* to restrict the truth values for each variable. These restrictions can be motivated by the specific application and they can be managed dynamically by the algorithms; for example, in [11] these restrictions are used to improve the efficiency of tableaux methods.

The conversion of a many-valued formula into a signed formula is accomplished via suitable operators called *signing operators*, which are functions between the many-valued logic and the signed logic. Each many-valued logic and each concrete problem requires a specific signing operator. For example, to study the validity of inference in a many-valued logic, the signing operator characterises validity by means of unsatisfiability in the signed logic [29]. In this paper we introduce signing operators to characterise the total and the equilibrium properties of models in $\mathbf{N_5}$.

3.1   Reduced Signed Logics

The formulas in the reduced signed logics are built-up from atomic formulas using the connectives $\wedge$ and $\vee$. The atomic formulas are the ω-*signed literals*: if $\mathbf{n}$ is a finite set of truth-values, $\mathcal{V}$ is the set of propositional variables and

$\omega : \mathcal{V} \to (2^{\mathbf{n}} \smallsetminus \varnothing)$ is a mapping, called the *possible truth-values function*, then the set of ω-*signed literals* is

$$\text{LIT}_\omega = \{S{:}p \mid S \subseteq \omega(p), p \in \mathcal{V}\} \cup \{\bot, \top\}$$

In a literal $\ell = S{:}p$, the set S is called the *sign of* ℓ and p is the *variable of* ℓ. The opposite literal of $S{:}p$ is defined as $\overline{S{:}p} = (\omega(p) \smallsetminus S){:}p$.

The semantics of the *signed logic valued in* $\mathbf{n}$ *by* ω, $\mathbf{S}_\omega$, is defined using the ω-*assignments*. The ω-assignments are mappings from the language into the set $\{0, 1\}$ that interpret $\vee$ as maximum, $\wedge$ as minimum, $\bot$ as falsity, $\top$ as truth and have the following properties:

1. For every p there exists a unique $j \in \omega(p)$ such that $I(\{j\}{:}p) = 1$
2. $I(S{:}p) = 1$ if and only if there exists $j \in S$ such that $I(\{j\}{:}p) = 1$

These conditions arise from the objective for which signed logics were created: the ω-assignment I over $S{:}p$ is 1 if the variable p is assigned a value in S; this value must be unique for every many-valued assignment and thus unique for every ω-assignment.

An important operation in the sequel will be the *reduction* of a signed logic. This operation decreases the possible truth-values set for one or more propositional variables. The reduction will be forced during the application of an algorithm but it can also help us to specify a problem using signed formulas. For instance, in this paper the reductions will be used to describe the equilibrium property in $\mathbf{N}_5$, using this logic. Specifically, we will use two basic reductions: to prohibit a specific value for a given variable, $[p \neq j]$, and to force a specific value for a given variable, $[p = j]$: If ω is a truth-values function, then the possible truth-values functions $\omega[p \neq j]$ and $\omega[p = j]$ are defined as follows:

- $\omega[p \neq j](v) = \omega(v)$ if $v \neq p$ and $\omega[p \neq j](p) = \omega(p) \smallsetminus \{j\}$.
- $\omega[p = j](v) = \omega(v)$ if $v \neq p$ and $\omega[p = j](p) = \{j\}$.

So, if A is a formula in $\mathbf{S}_\omega$, we define the following substitutions:

- $A[p \neq j]$ is a formula in $\mathbf{S}_{\omega[p \neq j]}$ obtained from A by replacing $\{j\}{:}p$ by $\bot$, $\overline{\{j\}{:}p}$ by $\top$ and $S{:}p$ by $(S \smallsetminus \{j\}){:}p$; in addition, the constants are deleted using the 0-1-laws.
- $A[p = j]$ is a formula in $\mathbf{S}_{\omega[p = j]}$ obtained from A by replacing every literal $S{:}p$ with $j \in S$ by $\top$ and every literal $S{:}p$ with $j \notin S$ by $\bot$; in addition, the constants are deleted using the 0-1-laws.

The following result is trivial from the intuitions of the preceding reductions but is important in later sections.

Proposition 1. *Let I be a model of a formula A in $\mathbf{S}_\omega$:*

- *If $I(p) \neq j$, then (the restriction of) I is a model of $A[p \neq j]$ in $\mathbf{S}_{\omega[p \neq j]}$.*
- *If $I(p) = j$, then I is a model of $A[p = j]$ in $\mathbf{S}_{\omega[p = j]}$.*

4 Signability of N_5

As we saw, the application of signed logics in automated deduction for many-valued logics allows us to take a formula in an n-valued logic and construct a signed formula in S_n whose unsatisfiability is equivalent to the validity of the initial formula. Once this transformation is realised, one can apply the various satisfiability tests for signed logics. A special case is created by tableaux algorithms in which one does not carry out an explicit conversion of formulas; rather one uses the conversion rules as expansion rules for the tableaux.

The conversion process described earlier is denoted generically as *signing* and the process of conversion now being considered is called the *signing transformation*. In general, the size of a signed formula obtained by conversion can be different from that of the initial formula. In fact, there are only two possibilities: (i) the size of the signed formula diminishes or grows linearly with respect to the size of the initial formula, or else (ii) it grows exponentially. If it is possible to define a signing transformation with the property (i) for all formulas, then the logic is called *signable*. Several families of signable logics have been described, for example logics with *regular* connectives [13] and the super-family of logics with *ortho-regular* connectives [29].

Here we shall introduce the signing transformation not only for validity but also to generate total models and to check the equilibrium property.

4.1 Signing N_5 for Validity: Signing-Down and Signing-Up

Let S be a set among the following ones: $[\leq j_0] = \{j \in \mathbf{5} \mid j \leq j_0\}$, $[\geq j_0] = \{j \in \mathbf{5} \mid j \geq j_0\}$, for $j_0 \in \mathbf{5}$. We define the operators $(S{:}) : N_5 \to S_5$ as follows:

1. $[\geq j]{:}(\varphi \vee \psi) = [\geq j]{:}\varphi \vee [\geq j]{:}\psi$
2. $[\leq j]{:}(\varphi \vee \psi) = [\leq j]{:}\varphi \wedge [\leq j]{:}\psi$
3. $[\geq j]{:}(\varphi \wedge \psi) = [\geq j]{:}\varphi \wedge [\geq j]{:}\psi$
4. $[\leq j]{:}(\varphi \wedge \psi) = [\leq j]{:}\varphi \vee [\leq j]{:}\psi$
5. $[\geq j]{:}(\sim\varphi) = [\leq -j]{:}\varphi$
6. $[\leq j]{:}(\sim\varphi) = [\geq -j]{:}\varphi$
7. $[\geq j]{:}(\neg\varphi) = [\leq 0]{:}\varphi,\ j \in \{0,1,2\}$
8. $[\geq -1]{:}(\neg\varphi) = [\leq 1]{:}\varphi$
9. $[\leq j]{:}(\neg\varphi) = \{1,2\}{:}\varphi,\ j \in \{-1,0,1\}$

10. $\{-2\}{:}(\neg\varphi) = \{2\}{:}\varphi$
11. $\{2\}{:}(\varphi \to \psi) =$
    $\{-2,-1,0\}{:}\varphi \vee \{2\}{:}\psi \vee (\{-2,-1,0,1\}{:}\varphi \wedge \{1,2\}{:}\psi)$
12. $[\geq j]{:}(\varphi \to \psi) = [\leq 0]{:}\varphi \vee [\geq j]{:}\psi$,
    if $j \in \{-1,0,1\}$.
13. $[\leq j]{:}(\varphi \to \psi) = [\geq 1]{:}\varphi \wedge [\leq j]{:}\psi$,
    if $j \in \{-2,-1,0\}$.
14. $\{-2,-1,0,1\}{:}(\varphi \to \psi) =$
    $(\{1,2\}{:}\varphi \wedge \{-2,-1,0\}{:}\psi) \vee (\{2\}{:}\varphi \wedge \{-2,-1,0,1\}{:}\psi)$

These operators can be used to describe a tableaux prover for the N_5 logic using the approach of [11, 26] and if we apply them to transform the formulas as shown in the following theorem, we can employ other algorithms such as TAS [23, 1] or resolution.

Theorem 2. *1. $\varphi_1, \ldots, \varphi_n \models \psi$ if and only if the following signed formula is unsatisfiable in S_5: $\{2\}{:}\varphi_1 \wedge \cdots \wedge \{2\}{:}\varphi_n \wedge \{-2,-1,0,1\}{:}\psi$*

2. Let $\Pi = \{\varphi_1, \ldots, \varphi_n\}$ be a set of formulas of N_5 and $M_\Pi = \{2\}{:}\varphi_1 \wedge \cdots \wedge \{2\}{:}\varphi_n$, in S_5. Then there is a bijection between the models of Π and the models of M_Π: σ is a model of Π if and only if I_σ is a model of M_Π where $I_\sigma(\{j\}{:}p) = 1$ if and only if $\sigma(p) = j$.

For example, to study the validity of the formula $\varphi = (p \to \neg q) \to (q \to \neg p)$ we use $\{-2,-1,0,1\}{:}((p \to \neg q) \to (q \to \neg p)) =:$

$$((\{-2,-1,0\}{:}p \vee \{-2,-1,0\}{:}q) \wedge \{1,2\}{:}q \wedge \{1,2\}{:}p) \vee ((\{-2,-1,0\}{:}p \vee \{-2,-1,0\}{:}q \vee$$
$$(\{-2,-1,0,1\}{:}p \wedge \{-2,-1,0\}{:}q)) \wedge ((\{1,2\}{:}q \wedge \{1,2\}{:}p) \vee (\{2\}{:}q \wedge \{1,2\}{:}p))))$$

Items 11 and 14 in the definition of the intermediate operator indicate that the logic $\mathbf{N}_5$ is not signable. To improve the definition of intermediate operators we can add more rules to take account of more general schemata of formulas. For example we can replace the rules 11 and 14 by the following:

11a. $\{2\}{:}(\varphi \to \neg\psi) = \{-2,-1,0\}{:}\varphi \vee \{-2,-1,0\}{:}\psi$
11b. $\{2\}{:}(\neg\varphi \to \psi) = \{1,2\}{:}\varphi \vee \{2\}{:}\psi$
11c. $\{2\}{:}(\varphi \to \psi) = \{-2,-1,0\}{:}\varphi \vee \{2\}{:}\psi \vee (\{-2,-1,0,1\}{:}\varphi \wedge \{1,2\}{:}\psi)$
 if $\varphi \neq \neg\varphi'$ and $\psi \neq \neg\psi'$
14a. $\{-2,-1,0,1\}{:}(\neg\varphi \to \psi) = \{-2,-1,0\}{:}\varphi \wedge \{-2,-1,0,1\}{:}\psi$
14b. $\{-2,-1,0,1\}{:}(\varphi \to \neg\psi) = \{1,2\}{:}\varphi \wedge \{1,2\}{:}\psi$
14c. $\{-2,-1,0,1\}{:}(\varphi \to \psi) = (\{1,2\}{:}\varphi \wedge \{-2,-1,0\}{:}\psi) \vee (\{2\}{:}\varphi \wedge \{-2,-1,0,1\}{:}\psi)$
 if $\varphi \neq \neg\varphi'$ and $\psi \neq \neg\psi'$

With this definition, the signed formula for the example above left is:

$$\{-2,-1,0,1\}{:}((p \to \neg q) \to (q \to \neg p)) =$$
$$(((\{-2,-1,0\}{:}p \vee \{-2,-1,0\}{:}q) \wedge \{1,2\}{:}q \wedge \{1,2\}{:}p)) \vee$$
$$\vee ((\{-2,-1,0\}{:}p \vee \{-2,-1,0\}{:}q) \wedge \{1,2\}{:}q \wedge \{1,2\}{:}p)))$$

The improvement obtained with the added rules arises from the fact that a formula of the form $\neg\varphi$ only takes values in the set $\{-2,-1,2\}$. Generalising this line of reasoning, we can once more improve on the definition of the operators, taking account for example of what happens to a formula of type $\varphi \to \psi$ if we know that ψ can only take values in $\{-2,-1,2\}$ but neither φ nor ψ are negated formulas.

To make use of this information we introduce the following notation. Let φ be a formula in $\mathbf{N}_5$ and $S \subset \mathbf{5}$; we write φ_S if every assignment in $\mathbf{N}_5$ evaluates φ on S, ie. φ is S-*tautology*, and there is no S' such that $S' \subset S$ and φ is S'-tautology. For every formula φ, the process called *signing-up* calculates the set S such that φ_S, partially evaluating the function represented by φ in the Nelson algebra (form the variable to the main connective), in contrast to the signing process which passes down the sign from the principal connective until it reaches the variables, *signing-down*. In this way, the original rules 11 and 14 can be replaced by the following:

11a'. $\{2\}{:}(\varphi_{\{-2,-1,2\}} \to \psi_S) = \{-2,-1\}{:}\varphi \vee \{2\}{:}\psi.$
11b'. $\{2\}{:}(\varphi_S \to \psi_{\{-2,-1,2\}}) = \{-2,-1,0\}{:}\varphi \vee \{2\}{:}\psi.$
11c'. $\{2\}{:}(\varphi_S \to \psi_{S'}) = \{-2,-1,0\}{:}\varphi \vee \{2\}{:}\psi \vee (\{-2,-1,0,1\}{:}\varphi \wedge \{1,2\}{:}\psi)$
 if $S \neq \{-2,-1,2\}$ and $S' \neq \{-2,-1,2\}$.

14a'. $\{-2,-1,0,1\}{:}\big(\varphi_{\{-2,-1,2\}} \to \psi_S\big) = \{1,2\}{:}\varphi \wedge \{-2,-1\}{:}\psi.$

14b'. $\{-2,-1,0,1\}{:}\big(\varphi_S \to \psi_{\{-2,-1,2\}}\big) = \{2\}{:}\varphi \wedge \{-2,-1,0,1\}{:}\psi.$

14c'. $\{-2,-1,0,1\}{:}\big(\varphi_S \to \psi_{S'}\big) = \big(\{1,2\}{:}\varphi \wedge \{-2,-1,0\}{:}\psi\big) \vee \big(\{2\}{:}\varphi \wedge \{-2,-1,0,1\}{:}\psi\big)$
   if $S \neq \{-2,-1,2\}$ and $S' \neq \{-2,-1,2\}$.

In the previous example, the size of the formula resulting from the signing is similar to that of the initial formula in $\mathbf{N}_5$

$$\{-2,-1,0,1\}{:}\big((p \to \neg q) \to (q \to \neg p)\big) = \big(\{-2,-1,0\}{:}p \vee \{-2,-1,0\}{:}q\big) \wedge \{1,2\}{:}q \wedge \{1,2\}{:}p$$

4.2   Signing for the Generation of Total Models

Total models evaluate the propositional variables in the set $\mathbf{3} = \{-2,0,2\}$, and therefore we only need to sign over the logic $\mathbf{S}_3$ in order to generate these models. For this we will use the intermediate operators $(S{:})\colon \mathbf{N}_5 \to \mathbf{S}_3$ for the sets S among the following: $[\geq 2] = \{2\}$, $[\geq 0] = \{0,2\}$, $[\leq -2] = \{-2\}$, $[\leq 0] = \{-2,0\}$. The definitions are:

1. $[\geq j]{:}(\varphi \vee \psi) = [\geq j]{:}\varphi \vee [\geq j]{:}\psi$
2. $[\leq j]{:}(\varphi \vee \psi) = [\leq j]{:}\varphi \wedge [\leq j]{:}\psi$
3. $[\geq j]{:}(\varphi \wedge \psi) = [\geq j]{:}\varphi \wedge [\geq j]{:}\psi$
4. $[\leq j]{:}(\varphi \wedge \psi) = [\leq j]{:}\varphi \vee [\leq j]{:}\psi$
5. $[\geq j]{:}(\sim\varphi) = [\leq -j]{:}\varphi$
6. $[\leq j]{:}(\sim\varphi) = [\geq -j]{:}\varphi$
7. $\{2\}{:}(\neg\varphi) = \{0,2\}{:}(\neg\varphi) = \{-2,0\}{:}\varphi$
8. $\{-2\}{:}(\neg\varphi) = \{-2,0\}{:}(\neg\varphi) = \{2\}{:}\varphi$
9. $\{2\}{:}(\varphi \to \psi) = \{-2,0\}{:}\varphi \vee \{2\}{:}\psi$
10. $\{0,2\}{:}(\varphi \to \psi) = \{-2,0\}{:}\varphi \vee \{0,2\}{:}\psi$
11. $\{-2\}{:}(\varphi \to \psi) = \{2\}{:}\varphi \wedge \{-2\}{:}\psi$
12. $\{-2,0\}{:}(\varphi \to \psi) = \{2\}{:}\varphi \wedge \{-2,0\}{:}\psi$

Theorem 3. *Let* $\Pi = \{\varphi_1,\ldots,\varphi_n\}$ *a set of formulas of* $\mathbf{N}_5$ *and let* T_Π *the formula in* $\mathbf{S}_3$ *defined as follows:* $T_\Pi = \{2\}{:}\varphi_1 \wedge \cdots \wedge \{2\}{:}\varphi_n$. *Then there is a bijection between the models of* T_Π *in* $\mathbf{S}_3$ *and the total models of* Π: I *is a model of* T_Π *if and only if* σ_I *is a total model of* Π, *where* $\sigma_I(p) = j$ *if and only if* $I(\{j\}{:}p) = 1$.

The inverse of the bijection in this theorem is defined in a natural way: if σ is a total model of Π, then I_σ is a model of T_Π, where $I_\sigma(\{j\}{:}p) = 1$ if and only if $\sigma(p) = j$. Therefore, we can use any model generator for signed logics applied to $\mathbf{S}_3$ (like tableaux [11] or TAS [23]), and then translate these to total models using the bijection.

4.3   Signing to Check the Equilibrium Property

Given a total model σ of a set of formulas Π we want to decide if this model is in equilibrium, ie. to decide whether it is minimal wrt $\trianglelefteq$ in the set of all models of Π. Then, the question is: is there another model of Π, σ' such that $\sigma' \trianglelefteq \sigma$? Assume that $\{p_1,\ldots,p_m\}$ is the set of propositional variables in Π and:

$$\sigma(p_i) = -2 \text{ if } 1 \leq i \leq k; \quad \sigma(p_i) = 0 \text{ if } k+1 \leq i \leq l; \quad \sigma(p_i) = 2 \text{ if } l+1 \leq i \leq m$$

where $1 \leq k < l < m$. If the model $\sigma' \trianglelefteq \sigma$ exists, then it must verify that:

$$\sigma'(p_i) \leq -1 \text{ if } 1 \leq i \leq k; \ \sigma'(p_i) = 0 \text{ if } k+1 \leq i \leq l; \ \sigma'(p_i) \geq 1 \text{ if } l+1 \leq i \leq m$$

and in addition, $\sigma' \neq \sigma$. Then we are looking for another model of M_Π with these restrictions; that is we are seeking another model for the formula:

$$E_{\Pi,\sigma} = M_\Pi[p_1 \neq 0, p_1 \neq 1, p_1 \neq 2, \ldots, p_k \neq 0, p_k \neq 1, p_k \neq 2,$$
$$p_{k+1} = 0, \ldots, p_l = 0,$$
$$p_{l+1} \neq -2, p_{l+1} \neq -1, p_{l+1} \neq 0, \ldots, p_m \neq -2, p_m \neq -1, p_m \neq 0]$$

By Proposition 1 I_σ is a model of $E_{\Pi,\sigma}$ and thus σ is in equilibrium if and only if I_σ is the unique model of $E_{\Pi,\sigma}$.

Actually, the formula $E_{\Pi,\sigma}$ is a formula in a reduction of $\mathbf{S}_5$ given by the following possible truth-values function: $\omega_\sigma(p) = \{-2, -1\}$, if $\sigma(p) = -2$; $\omega_\sigma(p) = \{0\}$, if $\sigma(p) = 0$; and $\omega_\sigma(p) = \{1, 2\}$, if $\sigma(p) = 2$. Using just its definition, computing Π_σ can be very complicated, however this formula can be obtained with a signing operator over the reduction $\mathbf{S}_{\omega_\sigma}$. To describe this process efficiently, we are going to use the signing-up method introduced earlier, but we need the following property.

Lemma 1. *Let ω be a function such that, for every propositional variable p, either $\omega(p) = \{-2, -1\}$, or $\omega(p) = \{0\}$, or $\omega(p) = \{1, 2\}$. Then, for every formula φ in $\mathbf{N}_\omega$, just one of the following properties holds.*

    a) $\varphi_{\{-2,-1\}}$ b) $\varphi_{\{0\}}$ c) $\varphi_{\{1,2\}}$

Thus, the required intermediate operators are:

1. $S_1:(\varphi_{S_2}) = \bot$, if $S_1 \cap S_2 = \varnothing$
   $S_1:(\varphi_{S_2}) = \top$, if $S_2 \subset S_1$
   $S_1:(\varphi_{S_2}) = (S_1 \cap S_2):\varphi$, otherwise.
2. $\{2\}:(\varphi_{\{1,2\}} \to \psi_{\{1,2\}}) = \{1\}:\varphi \lor \{2\}:\psi$
3. $\{1\}:(\varphi_{\{1,2\}} \to \psi_{\{1,2\}}) = \{2\}:\varphi \land \{1\}:\psi$
4. $\{-2\}:(\varphi_{\{1,2\}} \to \psi_{\{-2,-1\}}) = \{-2\}:\psi$
5. $\{-1\}:(\varphi_{\{1,2\}} \to \psi_{\{-2,-1,0\}}) = \{-1\}:\psi$
6. $\{-2\}:\neg(\varphi_{\{1,2\}}) = \{2\}:\varphi$
7. $\{-1\}:\neg(\varphi_{\{1,2\}}) = \{1\}:\varphi$
8. $\{2\}:\sim(\varphi_{\{-2,-1\}}) = \{-2\}:\varphi$
9. $\{1\}:\sim(\varphi_{\{-2,-1\}}) = \{-1\}:\varphi$

10. $\{-2\}:\sim(\varphi_{\{1,2\}}) = \{2\}:\varphi$
11. $\{-1\}:\sim(\varphi_{\{1,2\}}) = \{1\}:\varphi$
12. $\{2\}:(\varphi_{\{1,2\}} \lor \psi_S) = \{2\}:\varphi \lor \{2\}:\psi_S$
13. $\{1\}:(\varphi_{\{1,2\}} \lor \psi_S) = \{1\}:\varphi \land \{-2,-1,0,1\}:\psi_S$
14. $\{-2\}:(\varphi_{\{-2,-1\}} \lor \psi_{\{-2,-1\}}) =$
    $\{-2\}:\varphi \land \{-2\}:\psi$
15. $\{-1\}:(\varphi_{\{1,2\}} \lor \psi_S) = \{-1\}:\varphi \lor \{-1\}:\psi_S$
16. $\{2\}:(\varphi_{\{1,2\}} \land \psi_{\{1,2\}}) = \{2\}:\varphi \land \{2\}:\psi$
17. $\{1\}:(\varphi_{\{-2,-1\}} \land \psi_{\{-2,-1\}}) = \{1\}:\varphi \lor \{1\}:\psi$
18. $\{-2\}:(\varphi_{\{-2,-1\}} \land \psi_S) = \{-2\}:\varphi \lor \{-2\}:\psi_S$
19. $\{-1\}:(\varphi_{\{-2,-1\}} \land \psi_S) =$
    $\{-1\}:\varphi \land \{-1,0,1,2\}:\psi_S$

Theorem 4. *Let $\Pi = \{\varphi_1, \ldots, \varphi_n\}$ be a set of formulas in $\mathbf{N}_5$, σ a total model of Π and let us consider the signed formula in $\mathbf{S}_{\omega_\sigma}$:*

$$E_{\Pi,\sigma} = \{2\}:\varphi_1 \land \cdots \land \{2\}:\varphi_n$$

Then σ is in equilibrium if and only if I_σ is the unique model of $E_{\Pi,\sigma}$ in $\mathbf{S}_{\omega_\sigma}$.

Example 1. Let us consider the set $\Pi = \{p, q \to r, r \to q\}$; thus, $T_\Pi = \{2\}:p \land (\{-2,0\}:q \lor \{2\}:r) \land (\{-2,0\}:r \lor \{2\}:q)$. The models can be easily obtained by using any model generator for signed formulas. So we obtain the following total models

for Π:

	p	q	r
σ_1	2	2	2

	p	q	r
σ_2	2	0	0

	p	q	r
σ_3	2	0	-2

	p	q	r
σ_4	2	-2	0

	p	q	r
σ_5	2	-2	-2

1. For σ_1: $E_{\Pi,\sigma_1} = \{2\}{:}p \wedge (\{1\}{:}q \vee \{2\}{:}r) \wedge (\{1\}{:}r \vee \{2\}{:}q)$ has a second model, given by: $\tau_1(p) = 2$, $\tau_1(q) = 1$, $\tau_1(r) = 1$; therefore $\tau_1 \trianglelefteq \sigma_1$ and σ_1 is not an equilibrium model.

2. For σ_2: $E_{\Pi,\sigma_2} = \{2\}{:}p$ has a unique model, σ_2, and thus σ_2 is an equilibrium model. Actually, this is the unique equilibrium model of Π.

5 Complexity of Equilibrium Model Generation

The logics $\mathbf{S}_{\omega_\sigma}$ used to check the equilibrium property have the following important properties: if $\sigma(p) = 0$, the signed literals with variable p are logical constants, $\{0\}{:}p \equiv \top$, $\varnothing{:}p \equiv \bot$; if $\sigma(p) = 2$, then $\{1,2\}{:}p \equiv \top$, $\varnothing{:}p \equiv \bot$ and $\{1\}{:}p$ and $\{2\}{:}p$ are opposite literals; if $\sigma(p) = -2$, then $\{-2,-1\}{:}p \equiv \top$, $\varnothing{:}p \equiv \bot$ and $\{-1\}{:}p$ and $\{-2\}{:}p$ are opposite literals. Therefore, the logics $\mathbf{S}_{\omega_\sigma}$ actually form a classical logic. We can define bijections between classical formulas and ω_σ-formulas and between classical assignments and ω_σ-assignments. If $\mathbf{CL}$ denotes classical logic with formulas in negation normal form, the bijection $\Psi \colon \mathbf{S}_{\omega_\sigma} \to \mathbf{CL}$ is defined as follows:

1. $\Psi(\{2\}{:}q) = q$ and $\Psi(\{1\}{:}q) = \neg q$ for every q with $\sigma(q) = 2$.
2. $\Psi(\{-2\}{:}p) = p$ and $\Psi(\{-1\}{:}p) = \neg p$ for every p with $\sigma(p) = 2$.
3. $\Psi(A \vee B) = \Psi(A) \vee \Psi(B)$
4. $\Psi(A \wedge B) = \Psi(A) \wedge \Psi(B)$

The bijection between the sets of assignments, denoted by Ψ, is defined in a natural way: if I is an ω_σ-assignment, $\Psi(I)(p) = 1$ if and only if either $I(\{2\}{:}p) = 1$ or $I(\{-2\}{:}p) = 1$

Therefore, these bijections have the following property: for any ω_σ-formula A and every ω_σ-assignment I, $I(A) = \Psi(I)(\Psi(A))$.

Trivially, we see that: I is a model of a signed formula A in $\mathbf{S}_\omega$ if and only if $\Psi(I)$ is a model of $\Psi(A)$ in classical logic; therefore, A is valid in $\mathbf{S}_\omega$ if and only if $\Psi(A)$ is valid in classical logic. As a consequence we observe that verifying the equilibrium property for a total model can be carried out by means of a satisfiability test for classical logic (although the transformation is not needed for describing an algorithm), and so this problem is also NP-hard.

Actually, the problem of checking the equilibrium property is NP-complete. This fact is also a consequence of the bijection above. From a classical formula we can construct a signed formula with a total model; then using the signing transformation in the reverse direction, we can construct a formula in $\mathbf{N}_5$ with the same total model and the property: the model is in equilibrium if and only if the initial classical formula is satisfiable. Because the described process is polynomial, we have reduced the satisfiability problem in classical logic to the problem of checking the equilibrium property. This yields a proof sketch for the following theorem.

Theorem 5. *The problem of deciding if a model I of a set of formulas is an equilibrium model is NP-complete.*

Because the problem of generating the models of a signed formula is coNP-hard, we obtain the following consequence of this result.

Corollary 1. *(1) The problem of deciding whether a set of formulas has equilibrium models, equilibrium consistency, is Σ_2^P-hard. (2) The decision problem for equilibrium entailment is Π_2^P-hard.*

6   Conclusions

We have presented equilibrium logic as a system of nonmonotonic reasoning based on the nonclassical logic N_5 of here-and-there with strong negation. Equilibrium logic provides a conservative extension of answer set inference, not only for extended, disjunctive logic programs, but also for significant extensions such as the programs with nested expressions described in [16]. The paper provides proof systems for N_5 and for model-checking in equilibrium logic. The reduction of the latter problem to an unsatisfiability problem of classical logic yields complexity results for the various decision problems concerning equilibrium entailment. The reduction also yields a basis for the practical implementation of an automated reasoning tool, which could be based on the TAS methodology developed by the (second and third) authors [1], or, eg. using a system such as QUIP (see [3]) which implements various nonmonotonic formalisms by translating given problems into quantified boolean formulas and applying a QSAT prover to solve the corresponding decision problem. There is currently considerable interest in practical answer set programming and in extending current systems like `smodels` [22] and `dlv` [4] to a richer syntax. Equilibrium logic provides a sound theoretical basis for this, and the method of signed formulas applied here may also yield a basis for practical implementations.

References

1. Aguilera, G, P. de Guzmán, I, Ojeda-Aciego, M and Valverde, A. Reductions for non-clausal theorem proving. *Theoretical Computer Science* (2000). To appear.
2. Alferes, J J, Leite, J A, Pereira, L M, Przymusinska, H, and Przymusinski, T C, Dynamic Logic Programming, in A. Cohn, L. Schubert and S. Shapiro (eds.), *Procs. KR'98*, Morgan Kaufmann,1998.
3. Egly, U, Eiter, T, Tompits, H and Woltran, S, Implementing Default reasoning Using Quantified Boolean Formulae (System Description), in F Bry, U Geske and D Sepiel (eds), *Proc 14. Workshop Logische Programmierung*, GMD Report 90, Jan 2000.
4. Eiter, T, Leone N, Mateis, C, Pfeifer, G and Scarcello, F, A Deductive System for Nonmonotonic Reasoning, in *Proc. LPNMR97*, Springer, 1997.
5. Eiter, T, Leone N, Mateis, C, Pfeifer, G and Scarcello, F, The KR System dlv: Progress Report, Comparisons and Benchmarks, in *Proc. KR98*, Morgan Kaufmann, 1998
6. Gelfond, M, and Lifschitz, V, The Stable Model Semantics for Logic Programs, in K Bowen and R Kowalski (eds), *Proc 5th ICLP*, MIT Press, 1070-1080.

7. Gelfond, M and Lifschitz, V, Logic Programs with Classical Negation, in D Warren and P Szeredi (eds), *Proc ICLP-90*, MIT Press, 1990, 579–597.
8. Gelfond, M, and Lifschitz, V, Classical Negation in Logic Programs and Disjunctive Databases, *New Generation Computing* (1991), 365-387.
9. Greco, S, Leone, N, Scarcello, F, DATALOG with Nested Rules, in *Proc. (LPKR '97)*, Port Jefferson, New York, LNAI 1471, pp. 52-65, Springer, 1998.
10. Gurevich, Y, Intuitionistic Logic with Strong Negation, *Studia Logica* 36 (1977).
11. P. de Guzmán, I., Ojeda-Aciego, M. and Valverde, A. Multiple-Valued Tableaux with Δ-reductions. In *Proc IC-AI'1999*, pp 177–183, Las Vegas, Nevada, USA.
12. Hähnle, R. Towards an efficient tableau proof procedure for multiple-valued logics. In E Börger, H Kleine Büning, M M Richter, and W Schönfeld, eds, *Selected Papers from CSL'90, Heidelberg, Germany*, LNCS 533, pp. 248–260. Springer-Verlag, 1991.
13. Hähnle, R. *Automated Deduction in Multiple-valued Logics*. Oxford UP, 1993.
14. Kracht, M, On Extensions of Intermediate Logics by Strong Negation, *J Philosophical Logic* 27 (1998).
15. Lifschitz,V, Foundations of Logic Programming, in G Brewka (ed), *Principles of Knowledge Representation*, CSLI Publications, 1996.
16. Lifschitz, V, Tang, L R and Turner, H, Nested Expressions in Logic Programs, to appear in *Annals of Mathematics and Artificial Intelligence*.
17. Lukasiewicz, J, Die Logik und das Grundlagenproblem, in *Les Entreties de Zürich sur les Fondaments et la Méthode des Sciences Mathématiques* 6-9, 12 (1938).
18. Maksimova, L, Craig's interpolation theorem and amalgamable varieties, *Doklady Akademii Nauk SSSR*, 237, no. 6, (1977), pp. 1281-1284.
19. Murray, N V and Rosenthal, E. Improving tableau deductions in multiple-valued logics. In *Proc 21st ISMVL*, pp. 230–237, Victoria, May 1991. IEEE Press.
20. Murray, N V and Rosenthal, E. Adapting classical inference techniques to multiple-valued logics using signed formulas. *Fundamenta Informaticae*, 21(3), 1994
21. Nelson, D, Constructible Falsity, *J Symbolic Logic* 14 (1949), 16–26.
22. Niemelä, I and Simons, P, Smodels - an Implementation of the Stable Model and Well-founded Semantics, *Proc LPNMR 97*, Springer, 420-29.
23. Ojeda, M, P. de Guzmán, I, Aguilera, G and Valverde, A. Reducing signed propositional formulas. *Soft Computing*, vol. 2(4):157–166, 1998.
24. Pearce, D, A New Logical Characterisation of Stable Models and Answer Sets, in J Dix, L M Pereira, and T Przymusinski (eds), *Non-monotonic Extensions of Logic Programming. Proc NMELP 96*. Springer, LNAI 1216, 1997.
25. Pearce, D, From Here to There: Stable Negation in Logic Programming, in D Gabbay and H Wansing (eds), *What is Negation?*, Kluwer, 1999.
26. Pearce, D, P. de Guzmán, I, and Valverde, A, A Tableau System for Equilibrium Entailment, Proc TABLEAUX 2000 (To appear).
27. Simons, P, Extending the Stable Model Semantics with more Expressive Rules, in M Gelfond, N Leone and G Pfeifer (eds), *Proc. LPNMR'99*, LNAI 1730, Springer.
28. Smetanich, Ya, S, On Completeness of a Propositional Calculus with an additional Operation of One Variable (in Russian). *Trudy Moscovskogo matrmaticheskogo obshchestva*, 9 (1960), 357-372.
29. Valverde, A. *Δ-Árboles de implicantes e implicados y reducciones de lógicas signadas en ATPs*. PhD thesis, Universidad de Málaga, España, July 1998.
30. Vorob'ev, N N, A Constructive Propositional Calculus with Strong Negation (in Russian), *Doklady Akademii Nauk SSR* 85 (1952), 465–468.
31. Vorob'ev, N N, The Problem of Deducibility in Constructive Propositional Calculus with Strong Negation (in Russian), *Doklady Akademii Nauk SSR* 85 (1952).
32. Wójcicki, R, *Theory of Logical Calculi*, Kluwer, 1988.

Extending Classical Logic
with Inductive Definitions

Marc Denecker

Department of Computer Science, K.U.Leuven,
Celestijnenlaan 200A, B-3001 Heverlee, Belgium.
Phone: +32 16 327555 — Fax: +32 16 327996
marcd@cs.kuleuven.ac.be

Abstract. The goal of this paper is to extend classical logic with a generalized notion of inductive definition supporting positive and negative induction, to investigate the properties of this logic, its relationships to other logics in the area of non-monotonic reasoning, logic programming and deductive databases, and to show its application for knowledge representation by giving a typology of definitional knowledge.

1 Introduction

One of the original ideas underlying the declarative semantics of logic programs with negation as failure was to interpret a logic program as a *definition* of its predicates. This view is underlying both the least model semantics of van Emden and Kowalski [30] and Clark's completion semantics [6]. In [9], the relationship between logic programming and existing formalisations of inductive definitions in mathematical logic is investigated more closely. Standard work on positive or monotone induction was done by Moschovakis [20] and Aczel [1]. As shown in [9], the abstract positive inductive definition logic defined in [1] is formally isomorphic with the formalism of propositional Horn programs under least model semantics.

Not all forms of induction in mathematics are monotone induction. One important application of non-monotone induction is found in the context of inductive definitions in well-founded sets. Perhaps the best-known example of this is the definition of the powers of a non-monotone operator in Tarski's least fixpoint theory of monotone operators [28]. As shown in [9], induction in well-founded sets is in general non-monotone. In the context of mathematical logic, non-monotone forms of induction have been studied in the area of Iterated Inductive Definitions (IID) [11,5]. As argued in [9], the idea underlying such formalisms corresponds to stratification in logic programming. Negative induction appears when the domain of the defined concept(s) can be stratified (possibly in transfinitely many of levels) such that higher level instances of the concept are defined positively or negatively in terms of lower level instances of the predicate. The concept can then be constructed by iterating the principle of positive induction for increasing levels.

J. Lloyd et al. (Eds.): CL 2000, LNAI 1861, pp. 703–717, 2000.
© Springer-Verlag Berlin Heidelberg 2000

As illustrated in [9], encoding even simple inductive definitions in systems of IID requires extremely tedious encoding, which makes these systems rather useless for practical knowledge representation. The main contribution of [9] was to show that the principle of well-founded model in logic programming [31] is a suitable mathematical principle that generalises both monotone and non-monotone induction. The well-founded model is obtained as the least fixpoint of the 3-valued stable operator [23]. The latter operator is a general and robust implementation of the principle of positive induction; negative induction is dealt with by iterating this positive induction operator in a least fixpoint computation.

The study of the role of definitions in knowledge representation has already a long tradition in A.I. As an outcome of a series of investigations to the semantics of semantic networks[1], Brachman and Levesque [4] observed that an important component of expert knowledge is knowledge of the *defining properties* of concepts, and that it is crucial to distinguish between *defining properties* of concepts and *assertional knowledge* on concepts. Description logics are based on this idea, and consist of a Tbox to represent definitional knowledge and an Abox to represent *assertional knowledge*. In the context of non-monotonic reasoning, definitions have received little attention so far. However, Reiter [27] and Amati et al [2] observed that an important method for analysis and computation in common sense knowledge representation is to *compile* non-monotonic theories into first order definitions (i.e. Clark completions). They argue that the advantages of this compilation are that it clarifies the meaning of the original theory and that it yields theories that are better suited for computational purposes. Recently [8] and [29] investigated the use of inductive definitions to represent temporal and causal knowledge.

Consequently, a study of inductive definition could not only lead to a better understanding of the declarative semantics of logic programming but also to a natural and useful knowledge representation logic and a better understanding of the role and contribution of logic programming in the area of knowledge representation. In [9], generalised induction is investigated in the context of an *abstract* infinitary propositional definition logic extending Aczel's positive induction logic. The goal of this paper is to lift this propositional logic to a predicate logic and to show the application of this logic for knowledge representation and for the study of the semantics of logic programming and its extensions.

The structure of the paper is as follows. Section 3 defines an extension of classical logic with generalised inductive definitions, suitable for representing definitions in the context of uncertainty and incomplete knowledge. Section 4 investigates a number of formal properties and methodological guidelines of this logic. In section 5, some of applications of this logic for knowledge representation are sketched and some typology of definitional knowledge is given. Section 6 discusses the relationship with logic programming and its extensions.

Proofs of theorems are omitted due to lack of space.

---

[1] See [24] for a discussion of this topic.

2 An Abstract Logic of Inductive Definitions

In [9], I proposed an extension of Aczel's logic for general monotone and non-monotone inductive definitions. The result is isomorphic with the formalism of infinitary propositional logic programs (with negation) under well-founded semantics. An abstract inductive definition (ID) D in this logic defines a set $Defined(D)$ of symbols, called the set of defined symbols, by a set of rules of the form

$$p \leftarrow B$$

where p is a defined atom and B a set of positive or negative literals. The other atoms are called *open atoms*; their set is denoted $Open(D)$.

In [9] it was argued that Przymusinski's 3-valued extension [22, 23] of Gelfond and Lifschitz' stable model operator [14] is a general and robust implementation of the principle of positive induction, and that its least fixpoint, the well-founded model [31] naturally extends the ideas of Iterated Inductive Definitions and gives the right semantics to generalized inductive definitions.

In general, given an ID D and an interpretation I of the open symbols of D, there is a unique well-founded model extending I. This model will be denoted $\overline{I}^D$. An interpretation M is a model of D iff $M = \overline{M_o}^D$ where M_o is the restriction of M to the open symbols. In general, a model of an inductive definition is a partial (3-valued) interpretation. However, for broad classes of definitions, the well-founded model is known to be total (2-valued).

3 ID-Logic: Classical Logic with Definitions

This section defines a conservative extension of classical logic with definitions. An ID-logic theory T (based on some logical alphabet Σ) consists of a set of classical logic sentences and a set of definitions. A definition D is a pair of a set $Defined(D)$ of predicates and a set $Rules(D)$ of rules of the form:

$$p(\bar{t}) \leftarrow F$$

where $p \in Defined(D)$ and F an arbitrary first order formula based on Σ. Predicates of $Defined(D)$ are called the *defined predicates* of D; other predicates are called *open predicates* of D. A definition defines the defined predicates in terms of the open predicates. More precisely, given some state of the open predicates, the rule set of the definition gives an exhaustive enumeration of the cases in which the defined predicates are true; any defined atom not covered by a rule is defined as false.

A definition will be formally represented as in the example:

$$even, odd :: \left\{ \begin{array}{l} even(0) \leftarrow \\ even(S(x)) \leftarrow odd(x) \\ odd(S(x)) \leftarrow even(x) \end{array} \right\}$$

This is one definition defining two predicates simultaneously.

In ID-logic, definitions are considered as sentences. An ID-logic theory based on Σ consists of sentences and may contain different definitions, even for the same predicates. An Σ-interpretation is a model of an ID-logic theory iff it is a model of all its sentences. So, it suffices to define what is a model of a definition.

The semantics for propositional definitions of section 2 can be lifted quite easily to the predicate case by use of the grounding technique: the technique of reducing a predicate definition to an infinitary propositional definition[2]. In the context of ID-logic, this grounding of a definition is constructed using the domain, the functions and open predicates of some (general non-Herbrand) interpretation I. The intuitive idea is that in the context of the interpretation I, the predicate definition is a shorthand notation for its grounding. The grounding is obtained in three simple steps: instantiation of the free variables in the rules with domain elements of I, evaluation of the compound terms in the head of these ground instantiations and replacement of the formula F in the body of each ground instantiation by *any partial model* of F, i.e. any set of literals of defined predicates that makes F true.

To define the grounding the following terminology is needed. Given an alphabet Σ and a Σ-interpretation I, define the alphabet Σ_I by adding the domain elements of I as constants to Σ[3]. I is naturally extended to Σ_I by defining $I(x) = x$ for each domain element x of I. The evaluation of a ground term t of Σ_I (which may contain domain elements of I) is defined inductively as usual, and is denoted $|t|^I$. Likewise, truth value of a sentence of Σ_I is defined by the usual truth recursion.

Given some partial (3-valued) interpretation I and a definition D, I_o denotes the restriction of I to the constant, functor and open predicate symbols of D. At_I denotes the set of all atoms $p(\overline{d})$ where p is a defined predicate of D and $\overline{d}$ is a tuple of domain elements of I. A ground instance of a rule $p(\overline{t}[\overline{x}]) \leftarrow F[\overline{x}]$ with $\overline{x}$ the tuple of all its free variables, is a rule $p(\overline{t}[\overline{d}]) \leftarrow F[\overline{d}]$ obtained by substituting domain elements $\overline{d}$ for $\overline{x}$.

Note that there is a one-to-one correspondence between partial interpretations extending I_o and *consistent* sets of At_I-literals, i.e. sets that do not contain a pair of complementary literals $p(\overline{d}), \neg p(\overline{d})$. Each partial interpretation J extending I_o defines a unique consistent set S_J of all literals l of At_I that are true in J. Vice versa, each consistent set S defines a unique partial interpretation J_S extending I_o such that $J_S(l) = \mathbf{t}$ iff $l \in S$. Moreover, $J_{S_J} = J$.

Definition 1. *Given an interpretation I, the grounding of a definition D w.r.t. I, denoted I-grounding(D), is the propositional definition defining all atoms of*

---

[2] In [13], an alternative way of defining the well-founded semantics of predicate rules is proposed; it is based on a different treatment of positive and negative occurrences of predicates in the body of rules. I believe both techniques are equivalent but haven't proven this.

[3] Note that Σ_I may be infinite, even non-countable. This is mathematically and philosophically non-problematic because Σ_I is purely used as a semantic device, namely to define the grounding.

At$_I$ and consisting of all rules

$$p(|\bar{t}[\bar{d}]|^I) \leftarrow S_J$$

such that $p(\bar{t}[\bar{d}]) \leftarrow F[\bar{d}]$ is a ground instance of a rule of D and J is a partial model of $F[\bar{d}]$ extending I_o.

Definition 2. *A 3-valued interpretation I is a justified interpretation of D iff S_I is the 3-valued (well-founded) model of the grounding of D w.r.t. I. I is a justified interpretation of a theory T iff it is a justified interpretation of all its definitions and a (3-valued) model of the classical logic sentences of T.*

An interpretation I is a model of a definition D, resp. theory T, iff it is a total (i.e. 2-valued) justified interpretation of D, resp. T.

The above model theory is based on total, general non-Herbrand models. As a consequence, ID-logic is an extension of classical logic. The restriction to total models is not only necessary to get a extension of classical logic, but also because of methodological constraints on the use of definitions, as explained in the next section.

Example 1. The first example shows that different definitions are independent and interact in a monotonic way. Consider the theory consisting of three definitions.

$$\left\{ \begin{array}{l} father :: \{\, father(x,y) \leftarrow parent(x,y) \wedge male(x) \,\} \\ mother :: \{\, mother(x,y) \leftarrow parent(x,y) \wedge female(x) \,\} \\ parent :: \left\{ \begin{array}{l} parent(x,y) \leftarrow father(x,y) \\ parent(x,y) \leftarrow mother(x,y) \end{array} \right\} \end{array} \right\}$$

Note that in the first definition, *father* depends on *parent*, while in the third, *parent* depends on *father*. However, the semantics of a set of definitions is monotonically composed of the semantics of its definitions. Since none of these definitions is recursive, each is equivalent with its completed definition. Consequently, this triple of definitions is equivalent with the FOL theory:

$$\left\{ \begin{array}{l} father(x,y) \leftrightarrow parent(x,y) \wedge male(x) \\ mother(x,y) \leftrightarrow parent(x,y) \wedge female(x) \\ parent(x,y) \leftrightarrow father(x,y) \vee mother(x,y) \end{array} \right\}$$

One can observe that if $male(x) \leftrightarrow \neg female(x)$ holds, then the definition of *parent* is redundant.

Compare this theory with the simultaneous definition obtained by merging the three definitions in one:

$$\left\{ father, mother, parent :: \left\{ \begin{array}{l} father(x,y) \leftarrow parent(x,y) \wedge male(x) \\ mother(x,y) \leftarrow parent(x,y) \wedge female(x) \\ parent(x,y) \leftarrow father(x,y) \\ parent(x,y) \leftarrow mother(x,y) \end{array} \right\} \right\}$$

This new definition is positive recursive. This has the unintended effect that in each model, *father*, *mother* and *parent* are interpreted as the empty relationships.

Example 2. A theory can contain more definitions for the same concept. E.g.

$$\left\{ \begin{array}{l} even :: \left\{ \begin{array}{l} even(0) \\ even(s(x)) \leftarrow \neg even(x) \end{array} \right\} \\ even :: \{ even(0) \leftarrow \neg odd(x) \} \end{array} \right\}$$

In the context of the natural numbers, the first definition defines *even* as the set of even numbers. The second definition defines *even* as the complement of *odd*. Though this theory does not contain a definition for *odd*, it entails that *odd* and *even* are complements, and hence that *odd* is the set of odd numbers.

Definition 3. *A definition is recursive iff a defined predicate appears in the body of a rule. A definition is positive recursive iff all occurrences of the defined predicates in the body of the rules are positive (i.e. occur in the scope of an even number of negations). A simultaneous definition defines more than one predicate. A stratified definition is one in which the defined predicates can be semi-ordered[4] such that each defined predicate occurring positively, resp. negatively, in the body of a rule is less, resp. strictly less, than the predicate in the head.*

A definition hierarchy is a set $\mathcal{D}$ of definitions such that each predicate is defined in at most one definition of $\mathcal{D}$ and $\mathcal{D}$ can be ordered such that each open predicate appearing in a definition is not defined in a later definition.

Below, I define the concept of a well-founded definition. This concept generalizes the principle of definition in a well-founded set.

Definition 4. *A definition D is well-founded in some collection $\mathcal{I}$ of total interpretations of the open predicates of D iff for each $I \in \mathcal{I}$, there exists a well-founded order on the atoms of At_I such that for each ground instance $p(\bar{t}[\bar{d}]) \leftarrow F[\bar{d}]$, the body $F[\bar{d}]$ has the same truth value in all partial interpretations that extend I and are identical on all atoms less than $p(|\bar{t}[\bar{d}]|^I)$.*

The following theorem states an interesting property of well-founded definitions.

Theorem 1. *If D is well-founded in $\mathcal{I}$, then each justified interpretation M of D extending an element I of $\mathcal{I}$ is total (and hence a model) and coincides with the least model of the 3-valued completion of D [12] extending I. M is the unique model of the Clark completion [6] of D extending I.*

Example 3. Consider the definition of even numbers:

$$even :: \left\{ \begin{array}{l} even(0) \leftarrow \\ even(S(x)) \leftarrow \neg even(x) \end{array} \right\}$$

In the context of the natural numbers, this definition is well-founded and the justified interpretation is total. However, in any interpretation where the successor function contains cycles, the justified interpretation is partial.

---

[4] A semi-order is a reflexive, transitive relation.

4   Properties of Definitions

4.1   Well-Defining Definitions

The aim of an inductive definition is to *define* its defined predicates. Therefore, a natural quality requirement is that those justified interpretations that are total in the open predicates, should define truth of all defined predicates, i.e. they should be total in all predicates. As shown by Example 3 the property of having total justified interpretations is context dependent.

Definition 5. *A definition $\mathcal{D}$ is well-defining in a collection $\mathcal{I}$ of total interpretations of its open predicates iff each justified interpretation of $\mathcal{D}$ extending an element of $\mathcal{I}$ is total. Otherwise, $\mathcal{D}$ is called an unfounded definition in $\mathcal{I}$.*

Part of the knowledge representation methodology for representing definitions is to show that each definition in the theory is well-defining in the collection of relevant interpretations of its open predicates. For this purpose, practical mathematical techniques must be developed.

Theorem 2. *Assume that a theory T can be split up in a sequence of theories $T_1, .., T_n$ such that for each i, the predicates with a definition in T_i do not appear in $T_1, .., T_{i-1}$ and for each model I of $T_1 \cup .. \cup T_{i-1}$, the definitions in T_i are well-defining in I.*

Then each justified interpretation of T, total for the subset of predicates without definition in T, is total.

Some syntactic properties that guarantee that a definition is well-defining in every context are well-known from the logic programming literature:

- non-recursive definitions
- positive recursive definitions
- stratified definitions

Other properties guarantee well-defining definitions in some specific context. Inductive definitions corresponding to acyclic [3] or locally stratified logic programs [21] are well-defining in the context of Herbrand interpretations. It follows from theorem 1 that a well-founded definition in context $\mathcal{I}$ is also well-defining in $\mathcal{I}$.

A syntactical criterion that guarantees well-foundedness and hence well-defining-ness is the following.

Definition 6. *Define a relativized definition w.r.t. some strict order $<$ as a definition of a predicate $p(x, \overline{y})$ that consists of rules:*

$$p(x, \overline{t}) \leftarrow F[x]$$

such that each p-atom in F is of the form $p(z, \overline{t}')$ and appears in the scope of a subformula of $F[x]$ of the form $\forall z.z < x \rightarrow G$ or $\exists z.z < x \wedge G$.

Relativized definitions are well-founded when $<$ represents a well-founded order.

Theorem 3. *A relativized definition (w.r.t. to $<$) is well-founded in each interpretation that interprets $<$ as a strict well-founded order.*

Corollary 1. *(of Theorem 1). A relativized definition is well-defining in each interpretation that interprets $<$ as a strict well-founded order.*

4.2 Equivalence of Definitions

In a logic for knowledge representation, there should be a well-understood notion of equivalence. The following example shows that one cannot simply replace bodies of rules by equivalent bodies (w.r.t. 2-valued semantics).

Example 4. The definitions $p :: \{ p \leftarrow \mathbf{t} \}$ and $p :: \{ p \leftarrow p \vee \neg p \}$ have different justified interpretations, respectively the interpretations (represented as literal sets) $\{p\}$ and $\{\}$. Note that their bodies are equivalent w.r.t. 2-valued semantics but not w.r.t. 3-valued semantics.

Some important cases of equivalence preserving rules are sketched below:

- A rule $p(\bar{t}[\bar{x}]) \leftarrow F$ can be replaced by $p(\bar{y}) \leftarrow \exists \bar{x}.\bar{y} = \bar{t}[\bar{x}] \wedge F$.
- In a definition, two rules $p(\bar{t}) \leftarrow F_1$ and $p(\bar{t}) \leftarrow F_2$ can be replaced by one rule $p(\bar{t}) \leftarrow F_1 \vee F_2$. Together with the first rule, it follows that a finite set of rules defining a predicate can always be replaced by one rule. This rule is similar to the Clark completed definition of a predicate.
- The substitution of a sub-formula $F[\bar{x}]$ in the body of a rule of a formula by a formula $G[\bar{x}]$ is equivalence preserving if $F[\bar{x}]$ and $G[\bar{x}]$ are equivalent in 3-valued logic, i.e. if $\forall \bar{x}.F[\bar{x}] \leftrightarrow G[\bar{x}]$ is a tautology in 3-valued logic[5].
- Define the composition of two definitions $Pred_1 :: \{ C_1 \}$ and $Pred_2 :: \{ C_2 \}$ as the definition $Pred_1 \cup Pred_2 :: \{ C_1 \cup C_2 \}$. In general, substituting a pair of definitions by their composition is not equivalence preserving. [32] presents an extensive study of when merging definitions is equivalence preserving in the context of open logic programming, a sub-formalism of the logic defined here. One important example is that a definition hierarchy (Definition 3) is equivalent with its composition. Note that the composition of a definition hierarchy of positive recursive definitions is a stratified definition.

4.3 Monotonicity or Non-monotonicity?

To be able to represent common sense knowledge, *elaboration tolerant* logics are needed; elaboration tolerant logics are necessarily non-monotone [18, 19]. This is the foundational argument for the study of non-monotonic logics.

---

[5] Here the strong Kleene truth table for $\leftrightarrow$ must be used.

On the other hand, monotonicity is important as well. A classical argument in favour of the logical approach to knowledge representation in A.I. is that logic allows for a *modular representation* of knowledge [24]: independent properties of the problem domain can be represented by independent modules (i.e. the axioms) which can be added together to one theory. Obviously though, composing a new theory out of different independent modules should be *modular* , i.e. should preserve the semantics of each module; this property is assured if models of the composition are the models of the independent modules. It is obvious that *modular composition* implies that extension of one module with another is a *monotone* operation.

Non-monotonicity is a necessary condition for elaboration tolerance; monotonicity is a necessary condition for modular representation. How can a logic reconcile these seemingly contradictive requirements? The solution lies in a clean and well-understood distinction between monotone and non-monotone composition and modules. In ID-logic, the distinction is particularly clear:

- Definitions and axioms are monotone modules. Adding a new definition or new axiom to a theory is a monotone operation. This follows trivially from the definition of model.
- Rules in a definition constitute nonmonotone modules. Extending a definition with one or more new rules is in general a non-monotone operation.

4.4   Other Formalizations

The well-founded semantics defines a uniform principle of inductive definition, and gives the correct semantics to a broad class of definitions.

- The well-founded semantics of a non-recursive definition is the semantics of the Clark completion of this definition.
- The well-founded semantics of a well-founded definition in a well-founded order is the semantics of the completion of this inductive definition.
- The well-founded semantics of a positive recursive definition is the least relation (or set of relations) that satisfies the rules. Its semantics can be expressed via circumscription.
- The well-founded semantics of a stratified definition is the semantics of the composition of the positive recursive definitions that constitutes it, and can be expressed via a set of circumscription axioms, one per stratum.

5   Applications of Definitions

Below some applications of ID-logic are given.

Tables.
   The simplest way of defining a concept is by exhaustive enumeration of its elements. A table, as in the context of databases, can naturally be viewed as a definition by exhaustive enumeration. Tables are commonly used to

define concepts, not only in databases but also in common sense knowledge representation, e.g. to define some scenario.

Definitional versus Assertional Knowledge.

As mentioned in the introduction, a major conclusion from the logical analysis of semantic nets in the seventies is that a knowledge representation formalism should support the representation of definitional knowledge and assertional knowledge. The following example recalls the difference and illustrates how to express it in ID-logic.

As an example, take the following definition of an elephant:

$$\{elephant :: \{ elephant(x) \leftarrow animal(x) \wedge grey(x) \wedge has\_trunk(x) \}\}$$

Suppose we knew that *Clyde* is an elephant satisfying this definition. This is assertional knowledge and is represented by adding *elephant(Clyde)* as a FOL axiom. The extended theory entails that *Clyde* is a grey animal with a trunk. Alternatively, suppose that *Clyde* is an elephant but pink (due to a skin disease). To represent this, the definition must be extended with the atomic rule *elephant(Clyde)*. This atomic rule represents a new case of the definition. Additional FOL assertions are needed: *animal(Clyde)*, *pink(Clyde)*, *has_trunk(Clyde)*.

Temporal Reasoning.

In [29], it was shown that Reiter's situation calculus [26] has an equivalent formalization by a set of positive recursive definitions of the fluent predicates and of the effects of actions. Using general inductive definitions (with positive and negative induction), the formalization can be further simplified in ID-logic. Below, I sketch how to do this.

The definition defines all fluent symbols and all causal predicates by simultaneous induction on the poset of situations. I introduce for each fluent f three new predicates: $initially_f$ to represent the initial state of f, and $cause_f$ and $cause_{\neg f}$, representing initiating and terminating causes for f. For each fluent symbol f, the definition contains three cases[6]:

$$f(\overline{x}, S_0) \leftarrow initially_f(\overline{x})$$
$$f(\overline{x}, do(a, s)) \leftarrow cause_f(a, s, \overline{x})$$
$$f(\overline{x}, do(a, s)) \leftarrow f(\overline{x}, s) \wedge \neg cause_{\neg f}(a, s, \overline{x})$$

Note that in contrast to Reiter's situation calculus, this rule set does not contain a rule of the form:

$$\neg f(\overline{x}, do(a, s)) \leftarrow cause_{\neg f}(a, s, \overline{x})$$

However, it is easy to show that the completion of the above 3 rules entails the formula:

$$\neg f(do(a, s)) \leftarrow \neg cause_f(a, s, \overline{x}) \wedge cause_{\neg f}(a, s, \overline{x})$$

---

[6] We assume a many-sorted version of ID-logic, with situation, action and user defined sorts.

which reduces to the causal rule for $\neg f$ if the natural requirement is added that an action cannot cause f and $\neg f$ in the same situation. This requirement is formalised by the clause:

$$\leftarrow cause_{\neg f}(a, s), cause_f(a, s)$$

This illustrates a general methodological principle of using inductive definitions. In an inductive definition, one defines a concept by enumerating the positive cases; given such an enumeration, the closure mechanism of the semantics yields the negative cases.

In addition, per initiating effect of some action represented by an action term $A[\overline{y}]$, there is a case:

$$cause_f(A[\overline{y}], s, \overline{x}) \leftarrow \Psi[\overline{y}, s, \overline{x}]$$

such that the only term in Ψ of the situation sort is s and it appears purely in fluent symbols. Likewise, for each terminating effect there is a case:

$$cause_{\neg f}(A[\overline{y}], s, \overline{x}) \leftarrow \Psi[\overline{y}, s, \overline{x}]$$

Theorem 4. *A definition consisting of the above rules is well-founded in the collection of all interpretations that satisfy the Unique Names Axioms (UNA) axioms [25] and the second order induction axiom for the situation sort[7].*

It follows from theorem 1 that the semantics of this inductive definition coincides with its Clark completion. Note that the completion of this definition is very similar to Reiter's state successor axioms.

The inductive definition representation of situation calculus in ID-logic represents initiating and terminating effects in a case-by-case way. This results in a modular, elaboration tolerant representation of the domain in the sense that one can easily add new cases or drop or refine existing ones. This definition can be further extended with definitions for defined fluents, e.g. the definition of the transitive closure of physical connections in a computer network, in the context in which these physical connections may change:

$$connected(c1, c2, s) \leftarrow physical\_connection(c1, c2, s)$$
$$connected(c1, c2, s) \leftarrow connected(c1, c3, s) \wedge connected(c3, c2, s)$$

Also, similarly as in [29], ramification rules can be added to this theory.

Inductive Definitions as an Approach to Causality.

In [8] we argued that inductive definitions are a suitable formalization of causality. Causality information is an example of constructive information. Effects and forces propagate in a dynamic system through a constructive process in the following sense:

---

[7] The order of the atoms, needed to establish the well-foundedness of the definition is the order generated by the atoms $f(.., do(a, s)) > cause_f(a, s, ..), cause_{\neg f}(a, s, ..) > g(.., s)$, with f, g arbitrary fluents.

- There are no deus ex machina effects. Each effect has a cause; it is caused by a nonempty combination of actions and other effects.
- The causation order among effects is a well-ordering. I.e. there is no pair of effects each of which have caused the other; stronger, there is no infinite descending chain of effects each of which has been caused by the previous one in the chain.

The construction process of an inductive definition formally mimics this physical process of the propagation of the causes and effects. Based on this idea, [8] proposes a general solution to model ramifications. One point of [8] was that effects may easily depend on both presence and absence of other effects. For example, in the case that one latch of a suitcase is open, the effect of opening the second latch produces a derived effect of opening the suitcase, but only if the first latch is not closed simultaneously. As a consequence, if fluents mutually can influence each other, descriptions of ramifications may easily contain positive and negative loops. As shown in [8], the well-founded semantics deals well with these loops.

Induction Axioms; Domain Closure Axiom (DCA).

As a conservative extension of classical logic, ID-logic assumes uncertainty on the domain of discourse (due to the non-Herbrand interpretations). The Domain Closure Axiom (DCA) expresses that the domain of discourse contains only named objects. In [18], McCarthy showed how the DCA can be represented by a combination of circumscription on a set of rules and a FOL assertion. The mapping to ID-logic is straightforward. The set of rules is an inductive definition of a new predicate U; it consists of one case per constant C and per functor f:

$$U :: \left\{ \begin{array}{l} U(C) \leftarrow \\ .. \\ U(f(\overline{x})) \leftarrow U(x_1), .., U(x_n) \end{array} \right\}$$

This defines U as the set of all named objects. The FOL axiom expresses that all objects in the domain are named[8]:

$$\forall x. U(x)$$

The DCA is a generalized induction axiom. In the case of the language of the natural numbers (0 and $S/1$), the above formalization of the DCA is equivalent with Peano's second order induction axiom. The induction axiom for situations as needed in Reiter's situation calculus can be expressed in a similar way.

The semantics of many logics, e.g. logic programming and deductive databases, is based on Herbrand interpretations. This introduces the implicit ontological constraint that all terms in the domain of discourse are named.

---

[8] Note here the distinction between defining knowledge and assertional knowledge. If one would add the FOL assertion as a case to the inductive definition, then U would be defined to be the complete domain of discourse.

This constraint is absent in classical logic and in ID-logic but can be explicitly formalized by the pair of the DCA and the Unique Names Axioms (UNA) [25] or the Clark Equality Theory (CET) [6]. It is easy to show that each model of DCA+UNA is isomorphic with a Herbrand interpretation.

6   Relationship to Logic Programming Extensions

Logic Programming can be embedded in ID-logic in a straightforward way. Some of its extensions can be embedded as well. Abductive logic programming [16] (or open logic programming, as it is called in [7]) can be embedded also in ID-logic. An abductive logic framework is a triple $< A, P, T >$ of a set A of abducible predicates, a set P of rules defining non-abducible predicates and a set T of FOL axioms, called *constraints*. Its embedding in ID-logic is trivial: it is the theory $T \cup \{D_P\}$ where D_P is a definition with $Rules(D) = P$ and with $Defined(D)$ the set of non-abducible predicates. In this embedding, the semantics of an abductive logic program is given by general non-Herbrand well-founded models.

One important implication of this is that the computational techniques developed in Abductive Logic Programming can be used to reason on ID-logic theories. Experiments with the use of abductive solvers for solving satisfiability problems in ID-logic are found in [10].

A question is whether extensions of logic programming with two negations and disjunction [15] have a *natural* embedding in ID-logic. I believe the answer is negative. Extensions with two negations fit in the view of Logic programming as a sub-formalism of autoepistemic logic or default logic. This view is based on various embeddings of Logic Programming in these non-monotone modal logics (for an overview, see [17]). A common feature of these embeddings is that negation as failure literals *not p* are mapped to modal literals (e.g. $\neg Kp$ in autoepistemic logic).

On the other hand, ID-logic has no modal operator and has only one negation symbol. Moreover, its negation symbol is really *objective* negation, similar as in classical logic. Indeed, a close look at the semantics of ID-logic shows that negative literals are evaluated in the context of one interpretation. In contrast, the modal operator of autoepistemic logic and default logic are evaluated with respect to a set of beliefs.

For this reason, in [7] I raised the hypothesis that the autoepistemic and default view on logic programming and the definition view are two fundamentally different declarative interpretations of logic programming. They may lead to different knowledge representation methodologies and different extensions.

Logic programming extensions were introduced to cope with problems of the pure logic programming formalism for knowledge representation. However, the analysis of what these problems are exactly, depends on which view is taken. In the default view, the problem of logic programming was that no definite negative information could be represented; consequently it was natural to introduce strong or classical negation. On the other hand, in the definition view, the problem of pure logic programs is that the semantics assumes that all predicates are defined.

Consequently, it is hard to represent incomplete knowledge. The natural idea here is to introduce open predicates that have no definition, as in ID-logic.

Further analysis of the exact relationship between the inductive definition view and the default or autoepistemic view is needed.

Acknowledgements

This work has benefitted from discussions with many people including Maurice Bruynooghe, Danny Deschreye, Michael Gelfond, Vladimir Lifschitz, Victor Marek, Ray Reiter, Eugenia Ternovskaia, Mirek Truszczynski, Kristof Van Belleghem.

References

1. P. Aczel. An Introduction to Inductive Definitions. In J. Barwise, editor, *Handbook of Mathematical Logic*, pages 739–782. North-Holland Publishing Company, 1977.
2. Gianni Amati, Luigia Carlucci Aiello, and Fiora Pirri. Definability and commonsense reasoning. *Artificial Intelligence Journal*, 93:1 – 30, 1997. Abstract of this paper appeared also in Third Symposium on Logical Formalization of Commonsense Reasoning, Stanford, USA, 96.
3. K.R. Apt and M. Bezem. Acyclic programs. In *Proc. of the International Conference on Logic Programming*, pages 579–597. MIT press, 1990.
4. R. J. Brachman and H.J. Levesque. Competence in Knowledge Representation. In *Proc. of the National Conference on Artificial Intelligence*, pages 189–192, 1982.
5. W. Buchholz, S. Feferman, and W. Pohlers W. Sieg. *Iterated Inductive Definitions and Subsystems of Analysis: Recent Proof-Theoretical Studies*. Springer-Verlag, Lecture Notes in Mathematics 897, 1981.
6. K.L. Clark. Negation as failure. In H. Gallaire and J. Minker, editors, *Logic and Databases*, pages 293–322. Plenum Press, 1978.
7. M. Denecker. A Terminological Interpretation of (Abductive) Logic Programming. In V.W. Marek, A. Nerode, and M. Truszczynski, editors, *International Conference on Logic Programming and Nonmonotonic Reasoning*, Lecture notes in Artificial Intelligence 928, pages 15–29. Springer, 1995.
8. M. Denecker, D. Theseider Dupré, and K. Van Belleghem. An inductive definition approach to ramifications. *Linköping Electronic Articles in Computer and Information Science*, 3(7):1–43, 1998. URL: http://www.ep.liu.se/ea/cis/1998/007/.
9. Marc Denecker. The well-founded semantics is the principle of inductive definition. In J. Dix, L. Fari nas del Cerro, and U. Furbach, editors, *Logics in Artificial Intelligence*, pages 1–16, Schloss Daghstull, October 12-15 1998. Springer-Verlag, Lecture notes in Artificial Intelligence 1489.
10. Marc Denecker and Bert Van Nuffelen. Experiments for integration CLP and abduction. In Krysztof R. Apt, Antonios C. Kakas, Eric Monfroy, and Francesca Rossi, editors, *Workshop on Constraints*, pages 1–15. ERCIM/COMPULOG, October 25-27 1999.
11. S. Feferman. Formal theories for transfinite iterations of generalised inductive definitions and some subsystems of analysis. In A. Kino, J. Myhill, and R.E. Vesley, editors, *Intuitionism and Proof theory*, pages 303–326. North Holland, 1970.

12. M. Fitting. A Kripke-Kleene Semantics for Logic Programs. *Journal of Logic Programming*, 2(4):295–312, 1985.
13. A. Van Gelder. The Alternating Fixpoint of Logic Programs with Negation. *Journal of computer and system sciences*, 47:185–221, 1993.
14. M. Gelfond and V. Lifschitz. The stable model semantics for logic programming. In *Proc. of the International Joint Conference and Symposium on Logic Programming*, pages 1070–1080. IEEE, 1988.
15. M. Gelfond and V. Lifschitz. Classical negation in logic programs and disjunctive databases. *New Generation Computing*, pages 365–387, 1991.
16. A. C. Kakas, R.A. Kowalski, and F. Toni. Abductive Logic Programming. *Journal of Logic and Computation*, 2(6):719–770, 1993.
17. V.W. Marek and M. Truszczyński. *Nonmonotonic Logic Context-Dependent Reasoning*. Springer-Verlag, 1993.
18. J. McCarthy. Circumscription - a form of nonmonotonic reasoning. *Artifical Intelligence*, 13:27–39, 1980.
19. John McCarthy. Elaboration tolerance. In *COMMON SENSE 98, Symposium On Logical Formalizations Of Commonsense Reasoning*, January 1998.
20. Y. N. Moschovakis. *Elementary Induction on Abstract Structures*. North-Holland Publishing Company, Amsterdam- New York, 1974.
21. T.C. Przymusinski. On the semantics of Stratified Databases. In J. Minker, editor, *Foundations of Deductive Databases and Logic Programming*. Morgan Kaufman, 1988.
22. T.C. Przymusinski. Extended Stable Semantics for Normal and Disjunctive Programs. In D.H.D. Warren and P. Szeredi, editors, *Proc. of the seventh international conference on logic programming*, pages 459–477. MIT press, 1990.
23. T.C. Przymusinski. Well founded semantics coincides with three valued Stable Models. *Fundamenta Informaticae*, 13:445–463, 1990.
24. H. Reichgelt. *Knowledge Representation: an AI Perspective*. Ablex Publishing Corporation, 1991.
25. R. Reiter. Equality and domain closure in first-order databases. *JACM*, 27:235–249, 1980.
26. R. Reiter. The Frame Problem in the Situation Calculus: A simple Solution (Sometimes) and a Completeness Result for Goal Regression. In V. Lifschitz, editor, *Artificial Intelligence and Mathematical Theory of Computation: Papers in Honour of John McCarthy*, pages 359–380. Academic Press, 1991.
27. R. Reiter. Nonmonotonic Reasoning: Compiled vs Interpreted Theories. Distributed at the conference of Nonmonotonic Reasoning NMR96 as considerations for the panel discussion, 1996.
28. A. Tarski. Lattice-theoretic fixpoint theorem and its applications. *Pacific journal of Mathematics*, 5:285–309, 1955.
29. E. Ternovskaia. Inductive Definability and the Situation Calculus. In Burkhard Freitag, Hendrik Decker, Michael Kifer, and Andrei Voronkov, editors, *Transactions and Change in Logic Databases*, volume 1472 of *LNCS*. Springer-Verlag, Berlin, 1998.
30. M. van Emden and R.A Kowalski. The semantics of Predicate Logic as a Programming Language. *Journal of the ACM*, 4(4):733–742, 1976.
31. A. Van Gelder, K.A. Ross, and J.S. Schlipf. The Well-Founded Semantics for General Logic Programs. *Journal of the ACM*, 38(3):620–650, 1991.
32. S. Verbaeten, M. Denecker, and D. De Schreye. Compositionality of normal open logic programs. *Journal of Logic Programming*, 41(3):151–183, March 2000.

A Simple Characterization of Extended Abduction

Katsumi Inoue

Department of Electrical and Electronics Engineering
Kobe University
Rokkodai, Nada, Kobe 657-8501, Japan
inoue@eedept.kobe-u.ac.jp

Abstract. To explain positive observations and unexplain negative observations from nonmonotonic background theories, Inoue and Sakama (1995) extended traditional abduction by allowing removal as well as addition of hypotheses. In this paper, we propose a new characterization of extended abduction in which a background theory is written in any logic program possibly containing disjunctions. In this characterization, both removal of hypotheses and anti-explanations can be represented within the framework of traditional abductive logic programming. Using this transformation, updating knowledge bases represented in logic programs as well as restoring consistency for them can also be computed by existing proof procedures for logic programming.

1 Introduction

Abduction is recognized as an important form of reasoning in both AI and logic programming. Since first studied by Peirce, abduction has been defined as an inference to seek explanations, from which, together with the background theory, the given observation is deductively derived. The background theory is usually represented in either classical logic or logic programming. The use of logic programming is often more appropriate to perform abduction in several application domains [17,7]. In this paper, we thus consider *general extended disjunctive programs* [19,15], which belong to the most general class of logic programs. Formally, given a general extended disjunctive program as the background theory, and a literal G as an observation, traditional abduction defines an *explanation* E of G as a set of hypotheses satisfying

1. $K \cup E \models G$,
2. $K \cup E$ is consistent, and
3. E is a set of pre-specified literals and/or rules[1] called *abducibles*.[2]

---

[1] *Abducible rules* are introduced by Poole [22] for hypotheses in the form of first-order clauses and by Inoue [11] for rules in extended logic programs.

[2] Often, there are other conditions to be satisfied by abduced explanations, for example, E being better than any other set E' satisfying the conditions 1–3, according to the given preference criterion.

J. Lloyd et al. (Eds.): CL 2000, LNAI 1861, pp. 718–732, 2000.

Inoue and Sakama [13] extended this traditional abductive framework in two ways as follows.

First extension in [13] is concerned with how to change the theory with abducibles. The issue of *abductive theory change* has to be considered in a dynamic domain. In an evolving world, abductive explanations can be obtained not only by addition of new hypotheses, but also by removal of old hypotheses that become inappropriate. Consider, for example, the extended logic program K_l^0:

$$light \leftarrow switch\text{-}on,$$
$$\neg light \leftarrow switch\text{-}off,$$

where *switch-on* and *switch-off* are abducibles. Given the observed fact *light*, we can abduce *switch-on*, which is then assimilated into our belief K_l^1:

$$K_l^1 = K_l^0 \cup \{switch\text{-}on\}.^3$$

Next, we observe later that $\neg light$ holds. To explain this new observation, we have to remove the old hypothesis *switch-on* and add the new hypothesis *switch-off*, otherwise the theory becomes contradictory. So the new theory K_l^2 becomes:

$$K_l^2 = (K_l^1 \setminus \{switch\text{-}on\}) \cup \{switch\text{-}off\} = K_l^0 \cup \{switch\text{-}off\}.$$

A situation in which removal of hypotheses is necessary can happen even in more static cases. In particular, when a background logic program K is *nonmonotonic*, that is, negation as failure appears in K, contraction of a part of K can lead to a derivation of new literals. For example, consider the well-known bird example:

$$K_b^0 : \quad flies(x) \leftarrow bird(x), not\ ab(x),$$
$$ab(x) \leftarrow broken\text{-}wing(x),$$
$$bird(tweety) \leftarrow ,$$
$$bird(opus) \leftarrow ,$$
$$broken\text{-}wing(tweety) \leftarrow .$$

where *broken-wing* is an abducible predicate. If we observe *flies(tweety)*, the abducible *broken-wing(tweety)* can be removed from K_b^0 to account for the observation. In [13], this kind of extended abduction deals with removal of abducibles by introducing the notion of "negative explanations". Given a background theory K and an observation G, a *negative explanation* N of G is defined as a set of hypotheses satisfying

1. $K \setminus N \models G$,
2. $K \setminus N$ is consistent, and
3. N is a set of abducible literals/rules.

---

[3] Throughout this paper, an abduced literal L is identified with the rule $L \leftarrow$.

An explanation P satisfying $K \cup P \models G$ is then called a *positive explanation*. Usually, both removal and addition are necessary at the same time to explain the observation, as seen in the above example programs K_l^0, K_l^1, K_l^2. Namely, a pair (P, N) is a *(mixed) explanation* of G if

1. $(K \setminus N) \cup P \models G$,[4]
2. $(K \setminus N) \cup P$ is consistent, and
3. P, N are sets of abducible literals/rules.

The second extension in [13] is concerned with types of observations in abduction. Observations are usually seen by observers, but in an evolving world, they may not be observable later. Such an unwanted observation is called a *negative observation*, while the usual one is called a *positive observation*. Then, the notion of "anti-explanations" is introduced to *un*explain negative observations. For example, suppose that an agent with her belief K_b^0 later notices that *opus* does not fly. Since $K_b^0 \models flies(opus)$ holds, we can revise K_b^0 to block the derivation of $flies(opus)$ by assuming $broken\text{-}wing(opus)$:

$$K_b^1 = K_b^0 \cup \{broken\text{-}wing(opus)\}.$$

As in the case of negative explanations, a situation in which anti-explanations are necessary can happen even in a static world. For example, when we have rules:

$$K_s^0 : \quad suspect \leftarrow motivated, \; not \; alibi,$$
$$motivated \leftarrow,$$

in order to prevent one from suspecting a person with a motive, the person must have an alibi. In other words, *alibi* is an anti-explanation of *suspect*. Formally, given a background knowledge base K and a negative observation G, a pair (P, N) of hypotheses is called an *anti-explanation* of G if

1. $(K \setminus N) \cup P \not\models G$,
2. $(K \setminus N) \cup P$ is consistent, and
3. P, N are sets of abducible literals/rules.

Note that the introduction of anti-explanations is necessary for negative observations even in *monotonic* background theories. In fact, negative observations are similar to the concept of *negative examples* in classical inductive learning.

Extended abduction is thus essential to abductive theory revision as well as abduction in nonmonotonic theories. Other applications of extended abduction

---

[4] In the original form of extended abduction [13] and following papers [16, 25], the updated theory is represented as $(K \cup P) \setminus N$ instead of $(K \setminus N) \cup P$. Here, we changed the order of operations by removing the old abducibles N first and then adding the new abducibles P. This new representation is more appropriate to formalize theory revision in terms of contraction, c.f., the Levi identity in the context of [1]. Note that $(K \cup P) \setminus N = (K \setminus N) \cup P$ whenever $P \cap N = \emptyset$.

include *view update* in deductive databases [13], *theory update* [25], *contradiction removal* [13,25], the *system repair* problem with model checking [4], and *inductive logic programming* [24].

One of the major concerns on extended abduction is the question: whether or not extended abduction is reducible to traditional abduction. There are some attempts to establish the relationship between extended abduction and traditional abduction. In [16], *transaction programs* are introduced to compute extended abduction when the background theory is represented in an acyclic normal logic program. In [25], *update programs* are proposed to compute several types of update problems when the background theory is represented in an extended logic program. Both transaction programs and update programs are logic programs specifying changes on abductive hypotheses. However, their computation requires some special treatment for uses of existing proof procedures for logic programming.

In this paper, we provide a new characterization of extended abduction. This new one is attractive for at least the following reasons. First, *the new characterization completely embeds extended abduction to traditional abduction* in a very simple and intuitive way. Second, the proposed translation is applicable to any abductive program in which the background theory is represented in any class of logic programs. Hence, the applicability is larger than any other previously proposed method. Third, any proof procedure for traditional abductive logic programming or any procedure to compute answer sets of logic programs can be used to compute extended abduction. The simplicity of the new translation also contributes to fast computation when extended abduction is applied to various update problems. Note that the fact that extended abduction can easily be embedded in normal abduction never implies that extended abduction is useless; Because extended abduction has a wide range of applications, the importance of the concept of extended abduction remains unchanged.

This paper is organized as follows. Section 2 introduces a theoretical background in this paper, and discusses about previous studies on extended abduction. Section 3 presents a simple characterization of extended abduction, which transforms extended abduction into traditional abduction. Section 4 applies the new characterization of extended abduction to restore consistency for inconsistent logic programs. Section 5 presents related work, and Section 6 concludes the paper. Due to the lack of space, we omit the proofs of theorems in this paper.

2 Extended Abduction

2.1 Definitions

The definition of extended abduction is originally given in autoepistemic logic in [13]. In this paper, we consider a fairly wide subclass of autoepistemic logic which can be represented in logic programming. A knowledge base is represented in a *general extended disjunctive program* (GEDP) [19,15], or simply called a *program*, which consists of rules of the form:

$$L_1; \cdots; L_k; not\, L_{k+1}; \cdots; not\, L_l \leftarrow L_{l+1}, \ldots, L_m, not\, L_{m+1}, \ldots, not\, L_n$$

where each L_i is a literal ($n \geq m \geq l \geq k \geq 0$), and *not* is *negation as failure* (NAF). The left-hand side of the rule is the *head*, and the right-hand side is the *body*. A rule with the empty head is an *integrity constraint*. A rule with variables stands for the set of its ground instances. A GEDP is called an *extended disjunctive program* (EDP) [10] if it contains no NAF in the head of any rule (i.e., $k = l$). An EDP is called an *extended logic program* (ELP) if it contains no disjunction ($l \leq 1$), and an ELP is called a *normal logic program* (NLP) if every L_i is an atom.

The semantics of GEDPs is given by the *answer sets*. The following definition is due to [15]. First, let K be a GEDP without NAF (i.e., $k = l$ and $m = n$) and $S \subseteq \mathcal{L}$, where $\mathcal{L}$ is the set of all ground literals in the language of K. Then, S is an *answer set* of K if S is a minimal set satisfying the conditions:

1. For each ground rule $L_1; \cdots; L_l \leftarrow L_{l+1}, \ldots, L_m$ from K, $\{L_{l+1}, \ldots, L_m\} \subseteq S$ implies $\{L_1, \ldots, L_l\} \cap S \neq \emptyset$;
2. If S contains a pair of complementary literals $L, \neg L$, then $S = \mathcal{L}$.

Second, given *any* GEDP K (with NAF) and $S \subseteq \mathcal{L}$, consider the GEDP (without NAF) K^S obtained as follows: a rule $L_1; \cdots; L_k \leftarrow L_{l+1}, \ldots, L_m$ is in K^S if there is a ground rule of the form

$$L_1; \cdots; L_k; not\, L_{k+1}; \cdots; not\, L_l \leftarrow L_{l+1}, \ldots, L_m, not\, L_{m+1}, \ldots, not\, L_n$$

from K such that $\{L_{k+1}, \ldots, L_l\} \subseteq S$ and $\{L_{m+1}, \ldots, L_n\} \cap S = \emptyset$. Then, S is an *answer set* of K if S is an answer set of K^S. An answer set is *consistent* if it is not $\mathcal{L}$. A GEDP is *consistent* if it has a consistent answer set. An answer set S of K is *minimal* if there is no other answer set S' of K such that $S' \subset S$. Every answer set of any EDP is minimal [10], but the minimality of answer sets no longer holds for GEDPs [19]. For example, the program containing only the rule

$$L; not\, L \leftarrow$$

has two answer sets, $\{L\}$ and $\emptyset$. This type of rules has been used to express the class of abductive programs in terms of GEDPs [15].

The following definition of abductive programs is a generalization of one from [15]. An *abductive program* is a pair $\langle K, \mathcal{A} \rangle$, where K and $\mathcal{A}$ are GEDPs. Each element of $\mathcal{A}$ and its any instance is called an *abducible*. When a rule (resp. literal) is an abducible, it is also called an *abducible rule* (resp. *abducible literal*).

For an abductive program $\langle K, \mathcal{A} \rangle$, we assume that each abducible in $\mathcal{A}$ can be associated with its unique *name* [22, 11]. When an abducible rule $H \leftarrow B$, where H is the head and B is the body (or abducible literal when H is a literal and B is empty), has the name R and free variables $\mathbf{x}$, we often write the rule as $R(\mathbf{x}) = (H \leftarrow B)$. Also, for such a rule $R(\mathbf{x})$ and literals $L_1, \ldots, L_k$, we also write

$$(R(\mathbf{x}) \leftarrow L_1, \ldots, L_k) = (H \leftarrow B, L_1, \ldots, L_k).$$

Now, we give a formal definition for *extended abduction*, which is a slight modification of one from [13, 16, 25]. Let $\langle K, \mathcal{A} \rangle$ be an abductive program.

1. A pair (P, N) is a *scenario for* $\langle K, \mathcal{A} \rangle$ (c.f. [22]) if P, N are sets of instances of elements from $\mathcal{A}$ and $(K \setminus N) \cup P$ is a consistent program.
2. Let G be a ground literal.
   (a) A pair (P, N) is an *explanation of* G *wrt* $\langle K, \mathcal{A} \rangle$ if (P, N) is a scenario for $\langle K, \mathcal{A} \rangle$ such that $(K \setminus N) \cup P \models G$.
   (b) A pair (P, N) is an *anti-explanation of* G *wrt* $\langle K, \mathcal{A} \rangle$ if (P, N) is a scenario for $\langle K, \mathcal{A} \rangle$ such that $(K \setminus N) \cup P \not\models G$.
   (c) An (anti-)explanation (P, N) of G is *minimal* if for any (anti-)explanation (P', N') of G, $P' \subseteq P$ and $N' \subseteq N$ imply $P' = P$ and $N' = N$.

Remark 1. There are two remarks on the definition of extended abduction, which have not been discussed in previous papers.

First, the entailment relation $\models$ is used in the definition. There are two notions for entailment, credulous and skeptical ones. A GEDP K *skeptically entails* a literal L, if L is included in every answer set of P. On the other hand, K *credulously entails* L if L is included in an answer set of P. Similarly, the relation $\not\models$ can also be defined in either credulous or skeptical way. We say (P, N) is a *credulous* (resp. *skeptical*) *(anti-)explanation* if in the above definition $\models$ is defined credulously (resp. skeptically). In this paper, unless otherwise specified, we do not commit ourselves to which definition is used for entailment. In fact, the translation proposed in the next section can be used for both definitions.

Second, when sets S, T of literals/rules contain variables, any set operation $\circ$ is semantically defined on ground programs as $S \circ T = ground(S) \circ ground(T)$, where $ground(S)$ is the ground instances of elements from S. For example, $S \subseteq T$ is defined as $ground(S) \subseteq ground(T)$. For another example, when $p(x) \in K$, $\{p(a)\} \setminus K = \emptyset$ and $K \setminus \{p(a)\} = (K \setminus \{p(x)\}) \cup \{p(y) \mid y \neq a\}$. Here, the set $\{p(y) \mid y \neq a\}$ can also be written in the rule $p(y) \leftarrow y \neq a$. In general, a set $\{R(\mathbf{x}) \mid \mathbf{x} \neq \mathbf{t}_1, \ldots, \mathbf{x} \neq \mathbf{t}_k\}$ can be written as a rule $R(\mathbf{x}) \leftarrow \mathbf{x} \neq \mathbf{t}_1, \ldots, \mathbf{x} \neq \mathbf{t}_k$, where $\mathbf{x}$ and $\mathbf{t}_i$ are tuples of variables and terms, respectively.

Thus, to explain positive observations and unexplain negative observations, extended abduction not only introduces hypotheses to a program but also removes them from it. On the other hand, traditional abduction only introduces hypotheses to explain positive observations. Hence, traditional abduction is a specialization of extended abduction, and is called *normal abduction* hereafter. Formally, a set E is a *scenario for* $\langle K, \mathcal{A} \rangle$ *(under normal abduction)* iff $(E, \emptyset)$ is a scenario for $\langle K, \mathcal{A} \rangle$ (under extended abduction). Also, E is an *explanation of* G *wrt* $\langle K, \mathcal{A} \rangle$ *(under normal abduction)* iff $(E, \emptyset)$ is an explanation of G wrt $\langle K, \mathcal{A} \rangle$ (under extended abduction).

2.2 Previous Characterization of Extended Abduction

There are some previous work on reduction of extended abduction to normal abduction [16, 25]. In [16], *transaction programs* are produced from an abductive program $\langle K, \mathcal{A} \rangle$, in which the background theory K is limited to an acyclic NLP and $\mathcal{A}$ is a set of abducible atoms. A transaction program is a disjunctive logic program, and can provide a declarative specification of update in deductive databases. However, for computing extended abduction, a proof procedure for transaction programs requires an additional task for rewriting literals.

In [25], *update programs* are produced from an abductive program $\langle K, \mathcal{A} \rangle$, in which K is an ELP and $\mathcal{A}$ is a set of abducible literals or rules. An update program is an ELP, and can be used to compute view update, theory update, and inconsistency removal. For computing extended abduction, the only extra task is to select the *U-minimal answer sets* of an update program, where the U-minimality means that update is actually done with minimal change. This method essentially separates the abducibles from the program K, that is, considers $K \setminus \mathcal{A}$, and then reconstructs a consistent theory K' such that (i) K' is the closest to the original program K, and (ii) K' can derive (or cannot derive) the observation. Such a reconstruction is done by the *choice rules* of the form:

$$A \leftarrow not\ A',$$
$$A' \leftarrow not\ A,$$

for every $A \in \mathcal{A}$. Here, the choice A' means that the abducible A is not abduced. The set of choice rules guarantees that every answer set contains complete information on assumed and unassumed hypotheses. Then, the method is computationally weak in that it does not fully take the existence and non-existence of abducibles in the program into account. Then, the minimal change is only realized by selecting the closest one from all the possible scenarios.

Sakama and Inoue [25] also consider another translation of extended abduction into normal abduction. Let $\langle K, \mathcal{A} \rangle$ be an abductive program, and G an observation. For any $P \subseteq \mathcal{A} \setminus K$ and any $N \subseteq \mathcal{A} \cap K$ such that $P \cap N = \emptyset$, it holds that $(K \setminus N) \cup P \models G$ iff $(K \setminus \mathcal{A}) \cup ((K \cap \mathcal{A}) \setminus N) \cup P \models G$. Then, G has an explanation (P, N) wrt $\langle K, \mathcal{A} \rangle$ (under extended abduction) iff G has an explanation $H = ((K \cap \mathcal{A}) \setminus N) \cup P$ wrt $\langle K \setminus \mathcal{A}, \mathcal{A} \rangle$ (under normal abduction). Here, (P, N) can be extracted from H as $P = H \cap (\mathcal{A} \setminus K)$ and $N = (K \cap \mathcal{A}) \setminus H$. Again, this relationship converts $\langle K, \mathcal{A} \rangle$ into $\langle K \setminus \mathcal{A}, \mathcal{A} \rangle$, which separates the abducibles from K and reconstructs a consistent theory that is the closest to K.

In the next section, we show a new translation of extended abduction into normal abduction, which solves the above problems in previous methods.

3   From Extended Abduction to Normal Abduction

We now show that extended abduction is reduced to normal abduction. The proposed reduction method completely embeds extended abduction to normal abduction in a very simple and intuitive way. The proposed translation is applicable to any class of GEDPs, and therefore the applicability is larger than any other previous method. We neither separate the abducibles from the background theory, nor use the choice rules for abducibles. Then, the translated program remains stratified [23] whenever the original background theory is a stratified program. Minimal change with abducibles is realized more naturally without resorting to the search in the space of all scenarios.

3.1 Translation of Explanations

Here, we present a method to translate removal of abducibles from programs to addition of abducibles to programs in order to explain positive observations. The idea is very simple. We give a name to an abducible, but the name can be given in two different ways, according to whether the abducible is to be added or removed. For addition of abducibles, we just give a standard name for them like [11]: for each rule $R(\mathbf{x})$, its name is $add_R(\mathbf{x})$, where $\mathbf{x}$ is the free varaibles appearing in R. For removal of abducibles, we give a name through NAF by $not\ del_R(\mathbf{x})$. Then, deletion of an instance $R(\mathbf{t})$ from the abducibles $R(\mathbf{x})$ is realized by addition of $del_R(\mathbf{t})$ to the program. This simple way of naming through NAF is considered by Satoh [27] to identify the minimal source of inconsistency in a program, but it turns out to be easily accommodated in extended abduction.[5]

Let $\langle K, \mathcal{A} \rangle$ be an abductive program. The translation ν is defined as a mapping from $\langle K, \mathcal{A} \rangle$ to $\nu(K, \mathcal{A}) = \langle K', \mathcal{A}' \rangle$ as follows.

1. For each $R(\mathbf{x}) \in \mathcal{A} \setminus K$,
$$R(\mathbf{x}) \leftarrow add_R(\mathbf{x})$$
is in K';

2. For each $R(\mathbf{x}) \in K \cap \mathcal{A}$,
$$R(\mathbf{x}) \leftarrow not\ del_R(\mathbf{x})$$
is in K';

3. For any $R \in K \setminus \mathcal{A}$, R is in K';

4. $\mathcal{A}'$ is the set of literals of the form $add_R(\mathbf{x})$ and $del_R(\mathbf{x})$.

The translation ν can be simplified in the case of *addition of abducible literals*. In the above 1, if $R(\mathbf{x})$ is an abducible literal in $\mathcal{A} \setminus K$ and there is no rule whose head contains $R(\mathbf{x})$, then we can just put $R(\mathbf{x})$ into $\mathcal{A}'$, instead of introducing $R(\mathbf{x}) \leftarrow add_R(\mathbf{x})$ to K' with the new abducible $add_R(\mathbf{x})$ in $\mathcal{A}'$.

The next theorem establish a 1-1 correspondence between extended abduction and normal abduction wrt the translated program.

Theorem 1. (P, N) is a minimal explanation of G wrt $\langle K, \mathcal{A} \rangle$ under extended abduction iff E is a minimal explanation of G wrt $\nu(K, \mathcal{A})$ under normal abduction, where $P = \{R(\mathbf{t}) \mid add_R(\mathbf{t}) \in E\}$ and $N = \{R(\mathbf{t}) \mid del_R(\mathbf{t}) \in E\}$.

Note that when R has the free variables $\mathbf{x}$, both addition and removal of abducibles are performed at the instance level, that is, variables are always instantiated. In particular, we can remove some set N of instances of a hypothesis. Now, let us consider the case that such explanations are assimilated into the background theory. In the translated abductive theory for normal abduction, suppose that an explanation is obtained as a set:

$$E = \{del_R(\mathbf{t}_1), \ldots, del_R(\mathbf{t}_k), add_{R'}(\mathbf{s}_1), \ldots, add_{R'}(\mathbf{s}_l)\}.$$

---

[5] Satoh recently extended his inconsistency removal method to cover the class of NLPs using a similar naming technique for both addition and removal of abducibles [28].

Then, as explained in Remark on the definition of extended abduction in Section 2.1, the original rule can be replaced with a rule with inequalities in the body. For example, since $N = \{R(\mathbf{t}_1), \ldots, R(\mathbf{t}_k)\}$ is removed from K, the abducible rule $R(\mathbf{x})$ in K is replaced with $R(\mathbf{x}) \leftarrow \mathbf{x} \neq \mathbf{t}_1, \ldots, \mathbf{x} \neq \mathbf{t}_k$. Similarly, since $P = \{R'(\mathbf{s}_1), \ldots, R'(\mathbf{s}_l)\}$ is added to K, a new rule can be represented as $R'(\mathbf{x}) \leftarrow (\mathbf{x} = \mathbf{s}_1; \ldots; \mathbf{x} = \mathbf{s}_l)$.

In [25], removal of abducibles with variables cannot be performed at the instance level, but the abducible itself is removed from the program. Using the above name technique through NAF, we can parameterize hypotheses for removal as well as addition. This is more suitable in extended abduction.

Example 1. Let $\langle K_t^0, \mathcal{A}_t^0 \rangle$ be an abductive program:

$$K_t^0 : \; flies(x) \leftarrow bird(x),$$
$$bird(x) \leftarrow big\_bird(x),$$
$$big\_bird(tweety) \leftarrow , \quad bird(polly) \leftarrow ,$$
$$\mathcal{A}_t^0 : \; flies(x) \leftarrow bird(x),$$
$$\neg flies(x) \leftarrow big\_bird(x).$$

Then, according to the definition of extended abduction, the observation $G_1 = \neg flies(tweety)$ has an explanation (P_1, N_1):

$$(\{\, \neg flies(tweety) \leftarrow big\_bird(tweety)\,\}, \{\, flies(tweety) \leftarrow bird(tweety)\,\}).$$

Now, let us translate extended abduction into normal abduction:

$$K_t^{0'} : \; flies(x) \leftarrow bird(x), \, not\, del_{bf}(x),$$
$$\neg flies(x) \leftarrow big\_bird(x), \, add_{bbnf}(x),$$
$$bird(x) \leftarrow big\_bird(x),$$
$$big\_bird(tweety) \leftarrow , \quad bird(polly) \leftarrow ,$$
$$\mathcal{A}_t^{0'} : \; del_{bf}(x), \; add_{bbnf}(x).$$

Then, the observation $G_1 = \neg flies(tweety)$ has the minimal explanation:

$$E_1 = \{\, del_{bf}(tweety), \, add_{bbnf}(tweety)\,\},$$

which corresponds to the above explanation (P_1, N_1) for extended abduction.

In assimilating this explanation into K_t^0, the new theory becomes

$$K_t^1 : \; flies(x) \leftarrow bird(x), \, x \neq tweety,$$
$$\neg flies(x) \leftarrow big\_bird(x), \, x = tweety,$$
$$bird(x) \leftarrow big\_bird(x),$$
$$big\_bird(tweety) \leftarrow , \quad bird(polly) \leftarrow .$$

On the other hand, a minimal explanation of G_1 is defined as $(P_1', N_1') = (\{\, \neg flies(x) \leftarrow big\_bird(x)\,\}, \{\, flies(x) \leftarrow bird(x)\,\})$ in [25]. Assimilating this explanation into K_t^0 results in the theory that does not contain $flies(x) \leftarrow bird(x)$ any more, so that we lose the information of $flies(polly)$.

3.2 Translation of Anti-explanations

Next, we convert the problem of finding anti-explanations in extended abduction into the problem of finding explanations in normal abduction. To do so, we first translate anti-explanations into explanations within extended abduction as shown by [25]. This can be done for a negative observation G by associating the new rule:

$$G' \leftarrow not\, G,$$

where G' is a new atom. Then, G has an anti-explanation iff G' has an explanation. Strictly speaking, the entailment relation is given as follows.

Theorem 2. Let $\langle K, \mathcal{A} \rangle$ be an abductive program, and G a literal.

1. (P, N) is a *credulous anti-explanation* of G wrt $\langle K, \mathcal{A} \rangle$ (i.e., there is a consistent answer set of $(K \setminus N) \cup P$ in which G is not true) iff (P, N) is a credulous explanation of G' wrt $\langle K \cup \{ G' \leftarrow not\, G \}, \mathcal{A} \rangle$ (i.e., there is a consistent answer set of $(K \cup \{ G' \leftarrow not\, G \} \setminus N) \cup P$ in which G' is true).

2. (P, N) is a *skeptical anti-explanation* of G wrt $\langle K, \mathcal{A} \rangle$ (i.e., (P, N) is a scenario for $\langle K, \mathcal{A} \rangle$ such that G is not true in every consistent answer set of $(K \setminus N) \cup P$) iff (P, N) is a skeptical explanation of G' wrt $\langle K \cup \{ G' \leftarrow not\, G \}, \mathcal{A} \rangle$ (i.e., (P, N) is a scenario for $\langle K \cup \{ G' \leftarrow not\, G \}, \mathcal{A} \rangle$ such that G' is true in every consistent answer set of $(K \setminus N) \cup P$).

Translation of anti-explanations into explanations in normal abduction is now easy as we have shown the translation ν from extended abduction to normal abduction in the previous subsection.

Example 2. Consider the abductive theory $\langle K_t^1, \mathcal{A}_t^1 \rangle$ in Example 1, where $\mathcal{A}_t^0 = \mathcal{A}_t^1$. Suppose that we are now unsure about whether or not *polly* can fly. Then, the minimal anti-explanation of $G_2 = flies(polly)$ is $(P_2, N_2) = (\emptyset, \{ flies(polly) \leftarrow bird(polly) \})$. In assimilating this explanation into K_t^1, the corresponding new rule becomes

$$flies(x) \leftarrow bird(x),\, x \neq tweety,\, x \neq polly.$$

Now, considering the abductive theory $\nu(K_t^1 \cup \{ G_2' \leftarrow not\, G_2 \}, \mathcal{A}_t^1)$, G_2' has the minimal explanation $E_2 = \{ del_{bf}(polly) \}$ under normal abduction, which corresponds to the anti-explanation (P_2, N_2) of G_2 under extended abduction.

3.3 Computing Extended Abduction

We have shown that extended abduction can be reduced to normal abduction. Then, computation of extended abduction can be done using any proof procedure for normal abduction [18, 29, 17, 14]. It is also known that abducibles can be represented in either choice rules [11, 29], disjunctive rules without NAF [26, 6], or disjunctive rules with NAF in heads [15]. Then, according to the class of resultant programs, we can also use procedures to compute answer sets of ELPs [21], EDPs [14, 8, 6], or GEDPs [15].

The computational complexity of extended abduction can also be derived from results for abductive programs by Eiter *et al.* [7] and those for GEDPs and abductive EDPs by Inoue and Sakama [15, 26]. See also some results in [25].

4 Restoring Consistency

In this section, we formalize a method of restoring consistency when a GEDP is inconsistent. Inoue and Sakama [13] consider a general framework for restoring consistency in autoepistemic logic. We consider the logic programming fragment of this framework, and characterize it in normal abduction.

A GEDP may not have a consistent answer set. For example, the program

$$K_c = \{ \neg p \leftarrow , \quad \leftarrow not\, p \}$$

has no answer set. Historically, Doyle resolved such inconsistency by making some disbelieved atoms true through dependency-directed backtracking in Truth Maintenance System. Employing not only expansion but also contraction, a stronger method is proposed for restoring consistency in [13]. Let K and Γ be GEDPs. The theory $r(K) = (K \setminus O) \cup I$, where I, O are sets of instances from elements of Γ, is called a *most coherent theory* of K wrt Γ if

1. $r(K)$ is consistent, and
2. for any pair (I', O') such that $(K \setminus O') \cup I'$ is consistent, $I' \subseteq I$ and $O' \subseteq O$ imply that $I' = I$ and $O' = O$.

Notice that $r(K) = K$ if K is consistent. By definition, each most coherent theory $r(K)$ restores consistency by minimally introducing or removing appropriate rules from Γ. Obviously, most coherent theories can be formalized in extended abduction. That is, $r(K) = (K \setminus O) \cup I$ is a most coherent theory of K wrt Γ iff (I, O) is a scenario for $\langle K, \Gamma \rangle$ such that for any scenario (I', O') for $\langle K, \Gamma \rangle$, $I' \subseteq I$ and $O' \subseteq O$ imply that $I' = I$ and $O' = O$.

There are several ways to determine Γ for restoring consistency. In [13], Γ is set to $\mathcal{L}$. Then, inconsistency of the above K_c can be removed with the scenario $(I, O) = (\{p\}, \{\neg p\})$, which provides the most coherent theory $r(K_c) = \{ p \leftarrow , \quad \leftarrow not\, p \}$. In [25], on the other hand, Γ is set to K. In this case, only contraction is performed to restore consistency, and no new rule nor literal is added. For the above K_c, we then get $r(K_c) = \{ \neg p \leftarrow \}$. Satoh [27] sets Γ as a *part of* K (see also [30]), and again contraction is only allowed.

In any case, we can translate the framework of restoring consistency into normal abduction using the translation ν in Section 3.1.

Theorem 3. Let K and Γ be GEDPs for restoring consistency. Define the abductive program $\langle K', \mathcal{A}' \rangle = \nu(K, \Gamma)$ Then, $r(K) = (K \setminus O) \cup I$ is a most coherent theory of K wrt Γ iff E is a scenario for $\langle K', \mathcal{A}' \rangle$ (under normal abduction) such that no scenario E' for $\langle K', \mathcal{A}' \rangle$ satisfies that $E' \subset E$, and that $I = \{R(\mathbf{t}) \mid add_R(\mathbf{t}) \in E\}$ and $O = \{R(\mathbf{t}) \mid del_R(\mathbf{t}) \in E\}$.

Example 3. (Satoh [27], originally from Borgida [3]) Suppose K_{bs} is an ELP:

$$father(sr, charlie) \leftarrow , \quad age(sr, 14) \leftarrow ,$$
$$\leftarrow father(x, y), age(x, z), z \leq 14,$$
$$\leftarrow father(x, y), age(x, z1), age(y, z2), z1 \leq z2.$$

Let Γ_{bs} be a revisable part of K_{bs}, which consists of the two integrity constraints. Then, $\langle K'_{bs}, \mathcal{A}'_{bs} \rangle = \nu(K_{bs}, \Gamma_{bs})$ is:

$$K'_{bs} : father(sr, charlie) \leftarrow , \quad age(sr, 14) \leftarrow ,$$
$$\leftarrow father(x, y), age(x, z), z \leq 14, \, not \, del_{ic1}(x, y, z),$$
$$\leftarrow father(x, y), age(x, z1), age(y, z2), z1 \leq z2, \, del_{ic2}(x, y, z1, z2),$$
$$\mathcal{A}'_{bs} : del_{ic1}(x, y, z), \quad del_{ic2}(x, y, z1, z2).$$

We have the minimal scenario $\{del_{ic1}(sr, charlie, 14)\}$, which corresponds to the most coherent theory of K_{bs}. Assimilating this change into K_{bs}, the first integrity constraint becomes

$$\leftarrow father(x, y), age(x, z), z \leq 14, \neg(x = sr, y = charlie, z = 14).$$

5   Related Work

Our extended abduction makes an explicit choice of hypotheses that should be removed from the theory. On the other hand, removal of formulas from a theory is implicitly considered by Lobo and Uzcátegui [20] in their abductive change operators, where contraction is done within the standard *revision* operator [1]. When a formula F should be explained from the theory, [20] first contracts $\neg F$ before adding F with abduced hypotheses. Hence, their abductive change operators are not defined as normal abduction.

It is well-known that abduction is used for *view update* in deductive databases. There are two major operations in view update, *insertion* and *deletion*, which are respectively characterized as explanations and anti-explanations in extended abduction [13]. This kind of update can be extended to update with programs called *theory update*, which can be again formalized as extended abduction [25]. Kakas and Mancarella [18] characterize view update through normal abduction, but deletion is defined rather procedurally. They use a top-down abductive procedure for computing view update, which works correctly for locally stratified NLPs. There are also several approaches to formalize update without using abduction. Fernández *et al.* [9] realize database update through construction of minimal models that satisfy an update request. Alferes *et al.* [2] propose a framework of *dynamic logic programming* to realize theory update for a subclass of GEDPs without disjunctions in heads.

There are some work on removing inconsistency in ELPs, e.g., [11, 5, 27, 30]. Inoue [11] resolves inconsistency of an ELP by considering a maximally consistent set of rules from the original program. This is formalized in an abductive framework with the notion of *extension bases*, which corresponds to *extensions* in Poole's default theories [22] rather than abduction. Inoue also considers an abductive framework $\langle K, \mathcal{A} \rangle$ which is used to explain observations. His method gives a name $\delta_R(\mathbf{x})$ to each rule in $\mathcal{A}$, and defines the abducibles as the collection of δ_R atoms. In this kind of abduction, Inoue considers only expansion of a program by formulas. On the other hand, Satoh [27] formalizes a minimal revised program with a new rule in the case that the background knowledge is represented in a Horn program. This can be done by translating a revisable part of Horn clauses into rules with NAF of the form $not\ del_R(\mathbf{x})$ in an NLP, and defines the abducible set as the del_R atoms. Hence, Satoh considers only contraction of formulas from a program. In fact, we do not have to consider expansion in restoring consistency of an inconsistent Horn theory. As discussed in Section 3, the translation method proposed in this paper takes advantage of both translation methods in [11, 27].

Damásio and Pereira [5] remove inconsistency in ELPs with abducible literals under the three-valued well-founded semantics. Removal of abducibles in our extended abduction can be simulated in their abductive system by changing the truth-value of literals from true to false or undefined. In this sense, their abductive framework cannot be defined as normal abduction.

Witteveen and van der Hoek [30] defines a logical framework for *theory recovery* from inconsistent nonmonotonic theories. In their definition, constructing a scenario (P, N) for $\langle K, \mathcal{A} \rangle$ in our extended abduction is classified as a *mixed recovery* approach, in which both expansion and contraction are necessary at the same time. They show that under some conditions, a mixed recovery can be replaced with a successful expansion. Although their formalization is different from ours, their result is related to our transferability of extended abduction into normal abduction in the case of restoring consistency.

6   Concluding Remark

In this paper, we have shown a simple reduction of extended abduction into normal abduction. The new method embeds extended abduction to normal abduction without introducing the source of complexity, and is applicable to abduction with any class of GEDPs. The simplicity of the new translation also contributes to fast computation when extended abduction is applied to various update problems.

Contraction of instances of a rule in our method is based on an associated unique name through NAF in the body of the rule. In a sense, such a rule is weakened by adding an extra condition of the form $not\ del_R(\mathbf{x})$. In fact, this operation is called *specialization* of rules in machine learning. Inoue and Kudoh [12] show a framework for learning default rules in ELPs by specializing general rules with NAF of the form $not\ ab_R(\mathbf{x})$. Hence, there must be a close relationship between removal of rule instances and identification of exceptions of rules. In our method, instances of $del_R(\mathbf{x})$ are collected for rule R to unexplain negative observations or restore consistency. Then, these removed instances can also be seen as *exceptions* to rule R. Often, we would like to generalize such instances and exceptions as

$$ab_{bf}(x) \leftarrow big\_bird(x),$$

which plays the role of a *default cancellation rule*. In this case, instead of assimilating the removed instances into R as

$$flies(x) \leftarrow bird(x),\ x \neq tweety,\ x \neq polly, \ldots ,$$

we can just keep the default rule as

$$flies(x) \leftarrow bird(x), \; not \, ab_{bf}(x),$$

together with default cancellation rules. In this way, knowledge assimilation is performed using both abduction and induction. Formalization and automation of this kind of knowledge evolution is important future work.

Acknowledgements. The author would like to thank Chiaki Sakama for comments on an earlier draft of this paper.

References

1. C. E. Alchourrón, P. Gärdenfors, and D. Makinson. On the logic of theory change: partial meet contraction and revision functions. *Journal of Symbolic Logic*, 50(2):510–530, 1985.
2. J. J. Alferes, J. A. Leite, L. M. Pereira, H. Przymusinska, and T. Przymusinski. Dynamic logic programming. In: *Proceedings of the 6th International Conference on Principles of Knowledge Representation and Reasoning*, pages 98–109, Morgan Kaufmann, 1998.
3. A. Borgida. Language features for flexible handling of exceptions in information systems. *ACM Transactions on Database Systems*, 10:565–603, 1985.
4. F. Buccafurri, T. Eiter, G. Gottlob and L. Leone. Enhancing model checking in verification by AI techniques. *Artificial Intelligence*, 112(1,2):57–104, 1999.
5. C. V. Damásio and L. M. Pereira. Abduction over 3-valued extended logic programs. In: *Proceedings of the 3rd International Conference on Logic Programming and Nonmonotonic Reasoning*, LNAI, 928, pages 29–42, Springer, 1995.
6. T. Eiter, W. Faber, N. Leone, and G. Pfeifer. The diagnosis front-end of the dlv system. *AI Communications*, 12(1,2):99–111, IOS Press, 1999.
7. T. Eiter, G. Gottlob, and N. Leone. Abduction from logic programs: semantics and complexity. *Theoretical Computer Science*, 189(1,2):129–177, 1997.
8. T. Eiter, N. Leone, C. Mateis, G. Pfeifer and F. Scarnello. The KR system dlv: progress report, comparisons and benchmarks. In: *Proceedings of the 6th International Conference on Principles of Knowledge Representation and Reasoning*, pages 406–417, Morgan Kaufmann, 1998.
9. J. Fernández, J. Grant and J. Minker. Model theoretic approach to view updates in deductive databases. *Journal of Automated Reasoning*, 17:171–197, 1996.
10. M. Gelfond and V. Lifschitz. Classical negation in logic programs and disjunctive databases. *New Generation Computing*, 9:365–385, 1991.
11. K. Inoue. Hypothetical reasoning in logic programs. *Journal of Logic Programming*, 18(3):191-227, 1994.
12. K. Inoue and Y. Kudoh. Learning extended logic programs. In: *Proceedings of the 15th International Joint Conference on Artificial Intelligence* (IJCAI-97), pages 176-181, Morgan Kaufmann, 1997.
13. K. Inoue and C. Sakama. Abductive framework for nonmonotonic theory change. In: *Proceedings of the 14th International Joint Conference on Artificial Intelligence* (IJCAI-95), pages 204–210, Morgan Kaufmann, 1995.
14. K. Inoue and C. Sakama. A fixpoint characterization of abductive logic programs. *Journal of Logic Programming*, 27(2):107–136, 1996.

15. K. Inoue and C. Sakama. Negation as failure in the head. *Journal of Logic Programming*, 35(1):39–78, 1998.

16. K. Inoue and C. Sakama. Computing extended abduction through transaction programs. *Annals of Mathematics and Artificial Intelligence*, 25(3,4):339-367, 1999. Shorter version: Specifying transactions for extended abduction. In: *Proceedings of the 6th International Conference on Principles of Knowledge Representation and Reasoning*, pages 394–405, Morgan Kaufmann, 1998.

17. A. C. Kakas, R. A. Kowalski and F. Toni. Abductive logic programming. *Journal of Logic and Computation*, 2:719–770, 1992.

18. A. C. Kakas and P. Mancarella. Database updates through abduction. In: *Proceedings of the 16th International Conference on Very Large Databases*, pages 650–661, Morgan Kaufmann, 1990.

19. V. Lifschitz and T. Y. C. Woo. Answer sets in general nonmonotonic reasoning (preliminary report). In: *Proceedings of the 3rd International Conference on Principles of Knowledge Representation and Reasoning*, pages 603–614, Morgan Kaufmann, 1992.

20. J. Lobo and C. Uzcátegui. Abductive change operators. *Fundamenta Informaticae*, 27:385–412, 1996.

21. I. Niemelä and P. Simons. Efficient implementation of the well-founded and stable model semantics. In: *Proceedings of the Joint International Conference and Symposium on Logic Programming 1996*, pages 289–303, MIT Press, 1996.

22. D. Poole. A logical framework for default reasoning. *Artificial Intelligence*, 36:27–47, 1988.

23. T. C. Przymusinski. On the declarative semantics of deductive databases and logic programs. In: J. Minker, editor, *Foundations of Deductive Databases and Logic Programming*, pages 193–216, Morgan Kaufmann, 1998.

24. C. Sakama. Abductive generalization and specialization. In: P. Flach and A. Kakas, editors. *Abductive and Inductive Reasoning—Essays on their Relation and Integration*, pages 285–300, Kluwer Academic, 2000.

25. C. Sakama and K. Inoue. Updating extended logic programs through abduction. In: *Proceedings of the 5th International Conference on Logic Programming and Nonmonotonic Reasoning*, LNAI, 1730, pages 147-161, Springer, 1999.

26. C. Sakama and K. Inoue. Abductive logic programming and disjunctive logic programming: their relationships and transferability. *Journal of Logic Programming*, 44(1–3):75–100, 2000. Preliminary version: On the equivalence between disjunctive and abductive logic programs. In: *Proceedings of the 11th International Conference on Logic Programming*, pages 489-503, MIT Press, 1994.

27. K. Satoh. Computing minimal revised logical specification by abduction. In: *Proceedings of the International Workshop on Principles of Software Evolution*, pages 177–182, 1998.

28. K. Satoh. Consistency management of normal logic program by top-down abductive proof procedure. In: *Proceedings of the 8th International Workshop on Non-Monotonic Reasoning*, 2000.

29. K. Satoh and K. Iwayama. Computing abduction by using the TMS. In: *Proceedings of the 8th International Conference on Logic Programming*, pages 505–518, MIT Press, 1991.

30. C. Witteveen and W. van der Hoek. Recovery of (non)monotonic theories. *Artificial Intelligence*, 106:139–159, 1998.

A New Equational Foundation
for the Fluent Calculus

Hans-Peter Störr and Michael Thielscher

Artificial Intelligence Institute, Department of Computer Science
Dresden University of Technology, 01062 Dresden, Germany
{haps,mit}@inf.tu-dresden.de

Abstract. A new equational foundation is presented for the Fluent Calculus, an established predicate calculus formalism for reasoning about actions. We discuss limitations of the existing axiomatizations of both equality of states and what it means for a fluent to hold in a state. Our new and conceptually even simpler theory is shown to overcome the restrictions of the existing approach. We prove that the correctness of the Fluent Calculus as a solution to the Frame Problem still holds under the new foundation. Furthermore, we extend our theory by an induction axiom needed for reasoning about integer-valued resources.

Stream: Knowledge Representation and Non-monotonic Reasoning.

1 Introduction

Research in Cognitive Robotics aims at explaining and modeling high-level intelligent agents acting in a complex dynamic world. Among the established predicate calculus formalisms for reasoning about actions, the Fluent Calculus stands out in offering a solution not only to the representational but also the inferential [3] aspect of the fundamental Frame Problem. The basic solution has proven its versatility by allowing extensions regarding a variety of aspects, such as non-deterministic actions, resource-sensitivity, concurrency, ramifications, natural actions in combination with continuous change, sensing actions, and recursive and conditional plans [13, 7, 14, 15]. An implementation of the fluent calculus by means of binary decision diagrams is under way [8].

Central to the Fluent Calculus, which is a many-sorted first-order language, is the representation technique of reification [6]: Terms are used instead of atomic formulas as formal denotations for fluents, i.e., the atomic properties of the world state whose truth-values may change in the course of actions. In the Fluent Calculus these 'atomic' fluent terms are composed to state descriptions by means of a binary function, written as "$\circ$". More precisely, any term of sort *fluent* is also of sort *state*, and if z_1 and z_2 are of sort *state* then so is $z_1 \circ z_2$. For example, if the term $Occupied(x)$ is of sort *fluent*, representing the (temporary) property of a room x to be occupied, and if variable z is of sort *state*, then the term

$$(Occupied(\text{AMT-101}) \circ Occupied(\text{AMT-206})) \circ z \tag{1}$$

J. Lloyd et al. (Eds.): CL 2000, LNAI 1861, pp. 733–746, 2000.
© Springer-Verlag Berlin Heidelberg 2000

describes a world state in which the two rooms AMT-101 and AMT-206 are occupied and in which other fluents z hold.[1]

Based on the concept of state terms, the fundamental Frame Problem is solved in the Fluent Calculus by so-called state update axioms, which specify how the states of the world before and after an action are related [13]: From the Situation Calculus, we adopt the concept of a *situation* as a history of the actions that have been performed [10]. Let the expression $State(s)$ be a denotation of the world state in situation s, let $Do(a,s)$ denote the situation reached after performing action a in situation s, and let the atom $Poss(a,s)$ denote that action a is possible in situation s. Then a state update axiom for an action A with parameters $\boldsymbol{x}$ is of the form,

$$Poss(A(\boldsymbol{x}),s) \supset (\Delta(\boldsymbol{x},s) \supset \Gamma_{A,\Delta}[State(Do(A(\boldsymbol{x}),s)), State(s)]) \qquad (2)$$

where $\Delta(\boldsymbol{x},s)$ is a first-order formula which describes the conditions on $\boldsymbol{x}$ and situation s under which the two states prior and after the action are related in the way specified by $\Gamma_{A,\Delta}$. In the simple case, $\Gamma_{A,\Delta}$ is a mere equational relation between the states:

$$(\exists \boldsymbol{y})\, State(Do(A(\boldsymbol{x}),s)) \circ \vartheta^-(\boldsymbol{x},\boldsymbol{y}) = State(s) \circ \vartheta^+(\boldsymbol{x},\boldsymbol{y}) \qquad (3)$$

where the sub-terms ϑ^- and ϑ^+, which are of sort *state*, contain, respectively, the negative and positive effects of action A under condition Δ.

Consider, for example, the action denoted by $Move(x,y)$ of sending everyone from room x to room y. Suppose that this action has the effect of x no longer being occupied and of room y becoming occupied instead. Suppose further that the action be possible if x is currently occupied and y is not. The following two axioms are a suitable encoding of this specification in the Fluent Calculus:

$$\begin{aligned} Poss(Move(x,y),s) &\supset \\ State(Do(Move(x,y),s)) &\circ Occupied(x) = State(s) \circ Occupied(y) \end{aligned} \qquad (4)$$

$$Poss(Move(x,y),s) \equiv Holds(Occupied(x),s) \wedge \neg Holds(Occupied(y),s) \qquad (5)$$

where $Holds(f,s)$ means that fluent f holds in situation s.

In order that axioms like these entail reasonable conclusions, an axiomatic account of two properties of states is required:

---

[1] A word on the notation: Predicate and function symbols, including constants, start with a capital letter whereas variables are in lower case, sometimes with sub- or superscripts. Free variables in formulas are assumed universally quantified. Throughout the paper, action variables are denoted by the letter a, situation variables by the letter s, fluent variables by the letter f, and state variables by the letter z, all possibly with sub- or superscript. Multisets, i.e. collections, that can contain elements more than once, are written as $\{f_1,\ldots,f_n\}$, and multiset operations are marked by a dot above the operation symbol.

1. What makes two states equal, and what makes them unequal?
2. When does a fluent hold in a state associated to a situation, and when does it not?

An answer to the first question is crucial for solving the representational and inferential Frame Problem by state update axioms whose consequences are equations of the form (3): If a fluent is contained in $State(s)$ and is not among the negative effects $\vartheta^-(\boldsymbol{x}, \boldsymbol{y})$, then the fluent should be contained in $State(Do(A(\boldsymbol{x}), s))$; and if a fluent is not contained in $State(s)$, then it should also not be contained in $State(Do(A(\boldsymbol{x}), s))$ as long as it is not among the positive effects $\vartheta^+(\boldsymbol{x}, \boldsymbol{y})$.[2] An answer to the second question is needed to evaluate both action preconditions and the condition part of state update axioms, and in general to draw any interesting conclusions concerning the values of fluents in situations.

The existing equational foundation of the Fluent Calculus, developed in [9], gives an answer to the two questions based on the equational theory of a commutative monoid along with the notion of unification completeness [12]. In the following section we show the limitations of this approach when it comes to incorporating domain-specific equalities or the definition of functions among domain entities. In Section 3, a new and conceptually simpler equational foundation is developed, which is shown to overcome the restrictions of the existing account. In Section 4, we prove some fundamental properties of the new axiomatization, which in particular ensure that the Fluent Calculus solution to the Frame Problem still is correct under the new foundation. In Section 5, a second-order extension of our theory is presented to enable reasoning about the consumption and production of integer-valued resources. This extension is proved to axiomatically characterize the sort *state* as the finite multisets over the sort *fluent*. We conclude in Section 6.

2 Unification Completeness and Its Limitations

The Fluent Calculus uses classical logic with equality, that is, where the equality relation is assumed to be interpreted as real equality among domain elements. On this basis, the existing equational foundation of the Fluent Calculus consists of the following axioms:

- Equational theory AC1,

$$(z_1 \circ z_2) \circ z_3 = z_1 \circ (z_2 \circ z_3)$$
$$z_1 \circ z_2 = z_2 \circ z_1 \qquad \text{(AC1)}$$
$$z \circ \emptyset = z$$

(where $\emptyset$ is a constant of sort *state*, denoting the empty collection of fluents);
- An AC1-unification complete theory AC1* (details given below).

---

[2] We assume throughout the paper that ϑ^+ and ϑ^- are disjoint and do not contain any fluent more than once.

Theory AC1 essentially says that the order in which the fluent terms occur in repeated applications of ○ is irrelevant, so that, say, $Occupied(\text{AMT-206}) \circ (z \circ Occupied(\text{AMT-101}))$ and (1) denote the very same state. (Justified by the law of associativity, we will omit parentheses in nested applications of ○ in the rest of the paper.) Based on the equational foundation, the notion of fluents holding in states and situations, resp., is defined via two macros which stand for pure equality sentences:

$$Holds(f, z) \stackrel{\text{def}}{=} (\exists z') \, z = f \circ z' \qquad \text{(Holds)}$$
$$Holds(f, s) \stackrel{\text{def}}{=} Holds(f, State(s))$$

That is, a fluent holds in a state or a situation, resp., if it is contained in the respective state terms.

Negating the left and right hand sides of definition (Holds), a fluent f does not hold in a state z if for all z' we have $z \neq f \circ z'$. Deriving inequalities of this kind requires to axiomatize that states not composed of the same fluents are unequal. The AC1-unification complete theory $AC1^*$ serves this purpose [9]. Its definition relies on a complete AC1-unification algorithm, and it comprises an infinite set of axioms which contains the following axiom for any pair of terms t_1, t_2 of sort $state$ and without occurrence of function $State$:

$$t_1 = t_2 \supset \bigvee_{\theta \in \Theta_{\text{AC1}}(t_1, t_2)} \theta_= \qquad (6)$$

where $\Theta_{\text{AC1}}(t_1, t_2)$ is a complete [1] set of AC1-unifiers of t_1, t_2 and where $\theta_=$ is the equational formula $x_1 = r_1 \wedge \ldots \wedge x_n = r_n$ if $\theta = \{x_1/r_1, \ldots, x_n/r_n\}$. In particular, if two terms are not AC1-unifiable, then the disjunction evaluates to falsity, hence the implication simplifies to $t_1 \neq t_2$. Inequalities of state terms can thus be derived from their not being AC1-unifiable.

The rigorousness of unification completeness, however, has the important limitation of making it impossible to add simple domain-specific equalities or to define functions among domain entities.

Observation 1. Consider a Fluent Calculus signature with the two constants AMT-101 and $MainLectureHall$ of the domain sort $room$ and with function $Occupied: room \mapsto fluent$. Then

$$MainLectureHall = \text{AMT-101} \qquad (7)$$

and $AC1^*$ are inconsistent.

Proof. By the standard interpretation of equality and (7) it follows

$$Occupied(MainLectureHall) = Occupied(\text{AMT-101})$$

But the terms $Occupied(MainLectureHall)$ and $Occupied(\text{AMT-101})$ of sort $state$ are not AC1-unifiable; hence, (6) entails

$$Occupied(MainLectureHall) \neq Occupied(\text{AMT-101}) \qquad \square$$

Observation 2. Consider a Fluent Calculus signature with constant AMT-206 of domain sort *room*, constant *Peter* of domain sort *person*, and functions *RoomOf* : *person* $\mapsto$ *room* and *Occupied* : *room* $\mapsto$ *fluent*. Then

$$RoomOf(Peter) = \text{AMT-206} \tag{8}$$

and AC1* are inconsistent.

Proof. As above.   □

The only way of incorporating domain-dependent equalities or definitions of functions without sacrificing the idea of unification completeness is to use an E-unification complete theory instead of simply AC1* where E consists of the axioms AC1 plus all domain-dependent equations. This approach, however, has severe drawbacks: First, the foundational axioms on equality of state terms are domain-dependent so that they need to be adapted to any additional equation or inequality. Second, if the equational theory E is not finitary [1], then the corresponding unification complete theory includes axioms with an infinite number of disjuncts. Finally and most importantly, the definition of an E-unification complete theory appeals to complete sets of E-unifiers so that the existence of such a set for any two terms needs to be proved for any particular domain axiomatization in order that the definition is not rendered meaningless.

The equational foundation for the Fluent Calculus is accompanied by the following foundational axiom, which stipulates non-multiplicity of fluents in state terms that are associated with a situation:

$$State(s) \neq f \circ f \circ z \tag{NonMult}$$

Assuming non-multiplicity instead of stipulating idempotency of $\circ$ is crucial in order not to annul the solution to the Frame Problem offered by state update axioms. To see why, suppose $State(s) = f \circ z$ for some f, s, z, and consider the equation $State(Do(a, s)) \circ f = State(s)$, where f is specified as negative effect. However, neither idempotency of $\circ$ would allow to conclude that f does not occur in $State(Do(a, s))$, nor would this follow without axiom (NonMult).

3   A New Equational Foundation

The limitations of the existing equational foundation for the Fluents Calculus can be overcome by a paradigm shift away from the inference-oriented viewpoint of unification completeness towards a more semantic-oriented view. Intuitively, two state terms shall be equal only if they contain equal fluents. Indeed, a simple, finite first-order axiomatization of this intuition is possible under which the Fluents Calculus solution to the Frame Problem is still valid.[3]

---

[3] In a later section, we will show that it is moreover possible to give a finite but second-order extension of these axioms so as to obtain a characterization of equality of *state* terms precisely up to the ordering of the *fluent* sub-terms—in other words, where in every interpretation the sort *state* is isomorphic to the finite multisets over the sort *fluent*.

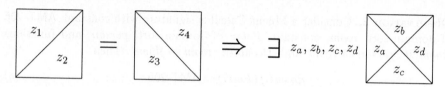

Fig. 1. The Levi axiom: If some state (symbolized by a square) can be partitioned into z_1, z_2 as well as into z_3, z_4, it can be partitioned into z_a, z_b, z_c, z_d such that the same areas denote equal (wrt. (AC1)) parts of the terms.

Definition 1. *The new equational foundation for the Fluent Calculus comprises the following axioms:*

- *Equational theory AC1;*
- *an axiom which specifies that a fluent is an irreducible (wrt. $\circ$) element of state:*

$$z = f \supset z \neq \emptyset \wedge [z = z' \circ z'' \supset z' = \emptyset \vee z'' = \emptyset] \qquad \text{(Irred)}$$

- *the so-called Levi-axiom:[4]*

$$z_1 \circ z_2 = z_3 \circ z_4 \supset (\exists z_a, z_b, z_c, z_d) \begin{pmatrix} z_1 = z_a \circ z_b \wedge z_3 = z_a \circ z_c \wedge \\ z_2 = z_c \circ z_d \wedge z_4 = z_b \circ z_d \end{pmatrix} \qquad \text{(Levi)}$$

Fig. 1 gives a graphical interpretation of this axiom.[5]

These axioms are domain-independent. By EUNA we denote their union along with a set of domain-dependent unique names-axioms UNA.

To demonstrate the gained expressiveness of the new foundation, recall the observations made in Section 2. Suppose given the initial state

$$State(S_0) = Occupied(\text{AMT-206}) \qquad (9)$$

---

[4] The axiom postulated here is proven as a lemma called *Levi's lemma* in trace theory [4]. Since the set of finite multisets with multiset union as an operation is isomorphic to a trace monoid over the same set where all symbols are independent, we turn its role around and postulate this property as an axiom characterizing multisets.

[5] It should be noted that the picture may be a bit misleading: In case z_1, z_2, z_3, z_4 contain multiple occurrences of sub-terms, the states z_a, z_b, z_c, z_d are not necessarily uniquely determined, as the reader may verify with the example $(aoa) \circ (aoa) = ao(aoaoa)$.

along with the axioms $UNA[Occupied]$, $UNA[\text{AMT-101}, \text{AMT-206}]$,[6] and

$$MainLectureHall = \text{AMT-101} \tag{10}$$

Note that this equation does not contradict the axioms of Def. 1, as opposed to the old foundation of the Fluent Calculus (c.f. Observation 1). Suppose further we want to move the current lecture from room AMT-206 to the main lecture hall since the former is too small. This action leads from situation S_0 to $Do(Move(\text{AMT-206}, MainLectureHall), S_0)$. By applying (AC1) and (Irred) to (5) and (9) it follows that $Poss(Move(\text{AMT-206}, MainLectureHall), S_0)$. Thus, from (4) and (9) we conclude that

$$State(Do(Move(\text{AMT-206}, MainLectureHall), S_0)) \circ Occupied(\text{AMT-206}) =$$
$$Occupied(\text{AMT-206}) \circ Occupied(MainLectureHall) \tag{11}$$

While axioms (AC1) and (10) suffice to show that (11) is satisfied by

$$State(Do(Move(\text{AMT-206}, MainLectureHall), S_0)) = Occupied(\text{AMT-101}) \tag{12}$$

our new axioms are needed to *prove* that (12) holds: Applying (10) to (11) we get

$$State(Do(Move(\text{AMT-206}, MainLectureHall), S_0)) \circ Occupied(\text{AMT-206}) =$$
$$Occupied(\text{AMT-206}) \circ Occupied(\text{AMT-101}) \tag{13}$$

According to (Levi) we find z_a, z_b, z_c, z_d such that

$$State(Do(Move(\text{AMT-206}, MainLectureHall), S_0)) = z_a \circ z_b \tag{14}$$
$$Occupied(\text{AMT-206}) = z_c \circ z_d \tag{15}$$
$$Occupied(\text{AMT-206}) = z_a \circ z_c \tag{16}$$
$$Occupied(\text{AMT-101}) = z_b \circ z_d \tag{17}$$

Employing (Irred), we apply case distinction to (15). The case $z_c = \emptyset$ and $z_d = Occupied(\text{AMT-206})$ contradicts equation (17) in view of $UNA[Occupied]$, $UNA[\text{AMT-101}, \text{AMT-206}]$, and (Irred). In case $z_c = Occupied(\text{AMT-206})$ and $z_d = \emptyset$, from (17) and (AC1) it follows that $z_b = Occupied(\text{AMT-101})$; furthermore, from (16) we get $z_a = \emptyset$ according to (Irred). Hence, (15) and (AC1) entail the desired conclusion (12).

The example derivation shows that the new equational foundation successfully handles the domain-dependent equality (10). In a similar fashion we can

---

[6] For domain dependent assumptions of unique names we adopt from [2] the standard notation $UNA[h_1, \ldots, h_n]$ as an abbreviation for the formula

$$\bigwedge_{i \neq j} h_i(x) \neq h_j(y) \wedge \bigwedge_i (h_i(x) = h_i(y) \supset x = y)$$

now introduce functions among domain entities by equations like (8) without producing inconsistency. Admittedly, calculating with pure (Levi) and (Irred) looks rather cumbersome. However, in the next section we will derive two computation rules as logical consequences of our axiomatization, which are of great help when calculating state equations. One of the two rules, for instance, leads directly from (13) to (12).

4 Results

We have seen that our new foundation for the Fluent Calculus allows the incorporation of domain-dependent equations and inequalities. In this section, we prove the crucial result that state update axioms solve the Frame Problem also under the new axioms. More specifically, we prove that the core of a state update axiom, an equation of the form

$$(\exists y)\, State(Do(A(x), s)) \circ \vartheta^-(x, y) = State(s) \circ \vartheta^+(x, y) \tag{18}$$

satisfies the following:

1. All fluents in $\vartheta^+(x, y)$ (the positive effects of the action) do hold in the successor state $State(Do(A(x), s))$;
2. all fluents in $\vartheta^-(x, y)$ (the negative effects of the action) do not hold in the successor state $State(Do(A(x), s))$;
3. all fluents not contained in ϑ^+ or ϑ^- hold in $State(Do(A(x), s))$ if and only if they hold in $State(s)$;
4. the equation is consistent with foundational axiom (NonMult).

The proof is based on two computation rules, the Cancelation Rule and the Distribution Rule. Both are logical consequences of our axiomatization, and they are of great practical value when it comes to calculating with state equations.

Proposition 1. (Cancelation Rule)   *In all models of EUNA we have*

$$f \circ z = f \circ z' \supset z = z' \tag{Cancel}$$

Proof. Assume $f \circ z = f \circ z'$. By (Levi) we find z_a, z_b, z_c, z_d such that

$$f = z_a \circ z_b \ \wedge \ z = z_c \circ z_d \ \wedge \ f = z_a \circ z_c \ \wedge z' = z_b \circ z_d$$

By (Irred) we distinguish two cases:

If $z_a = \emptyset$, then (AC1) implies $f = z_b = z_c$, thus $z = f \circ z_d$ and $z' = f \circ z_d$, and hence by symmetry and transitivity of equality, $z = z'$.

If $z_b = \emptyset$, then $f = z_a$ by (AC1). Applying (Irred) we conclude $f \neq \emptyset$; therefore, $f = z_a \circ z_c$ implies $z_c = \emptyset$, again by (Irred). Hence, $z = \emptyset \circ z_d = z'$. $\square$

The Cancelation Rule allows to cancel out equal *fluent* terms on both sides of a state equation. Note, for instance, that by this rule the rather complicated derivation of (12) from (13) of the preceding section follows directly.

Proposition 2.   (Distribution Rule)   *In all models of EUNA we have*

$$f_1 \neq f_2 \supset f_1 \circ z_1 = f_2 \circ z_2 \supset Holds(f_1, z_2) \tag{Distrib}$$

Proof. Assume $f_1 \neq f_2$ and $f_1 \circ z_1 = f_2 \circ z_2$. Following (Irred) we find z_a, z_b, z_c, z_d such that

$$f_1 = z_a \circ z_b \wedge z_1 = z_c \circ z_d \wedge f_2 = z_a \circ z_c \wedge z_2 = z_b \circ z_d$$

By (Irred) we conclude that either $z_a = \emptyset \wedge z_b = f_1$ or $z_a = f_1 \wedge z_b = \emptyset$. The latter case would imply $f_2 = f_1 \circ z_c$, which contradicts (Irred) given that $f_1 \neq f_2$. Thus, $z_a = \emptyset \wedge z_b = f_1$, hence $z_2 = f_1 \circ z_d$, hence $Holds(f_1, z_2)$.   □

The Distribution Rule in combination with Cancelation allows to rewrite state equations so as to project onto a particular sub-term. A typical application is to rewrite the equation $State(Do(a, s)) \circ f^- = State(s) \circ f^+$ to $(\exists z)(State(s) = f^- \circ z \wedge State(Do(a, s)) \circ f^- = f^- \circ z \circ f^+)$, and then to apply the Cancelation Rule to obtain the projection $(\exists z)(State(Do(a, s)) = z \circ f^+ \wedge State(s) = f^- \circ z)$.

We are now in a position to prove the abovementioned main result. As in [13] we make the following assumption of consistency: State update axioms are designed in such a way that if an equation (18) is entailed, then the positive and negative effects, ϑ^+ and ϑ^-, do not share a fluent, contain no fluent more than once and no fluent is specified as positive effect via ϑ^+ if it holds in $State(s)$ itself. From (NonMult) we furthermore know that no fluent occurs twice in $State(s)$.

Theorem 3. *Consider a set UNA of unique names-axioms and let the terms $\vartheta^- = f_1^- \circ \ldots \circ f_m^-$ and $\vartheta^+ = f_1^+ \circ \ldots \circ f_n^+$ be finite, possibly empty sequences of fluent terms joined together with $\circ$ such that $UNA \models f_i^+ \neq f_-^+$ for all i, j, and $UNA \models f_i^- \neq f_j^-$ as well as $UNA \models f_i^+ \neq f_j^+$ for all $i \neq j$. Then in all models for EUNA we have that*

$$z_1 \circ \vartheta^- = z_2 \circ \vartheta^+ \wedge \bigwedge_{j=1\ldots n} \neg Holds(f_j^+, z_2) \wedge (\forall f) \neg Holds(f \circ f, z_2)^7$$

implies each of the following.

1. $Holds(f_j^+, z_1)$ *(for all $j = 1, \ldots, n$);*
2. $\neg Holds(f_i^-, z_1)$ *(for all $i = 1, \ldots, m$);*
3. $(\forall f)(\neg Holds(f, \vartheta^- \circ \vartheta^+) \supset [Holds(f, z_1) \equiv Holds(f, z_2)]);$
4. $(\forall f) \neg Holds(f \circ f, z_1).$

Proof.

1. Follows from $UNA \models f_i^- \neq f_j^+$ for all f_i^- in ϑ^- by repeated application of the Distribution Rule.

---

[7] where $Holds(\bar{z}, z) \stackrel{\text{def}}{=} (\exists z')\, z = \bar{z} \circ z'$

2. If $z_1 = f_i^- \circ z'$ for some f_i^- in ϑ^- and some z', then

$$f_i^- \circ z' \circ f_1^- \circ \ldots \circ f_i^- \circ \ldots \circ f_m^- = z_2 \circ \vartheta^+ \qquad (19)$$

From $UNA \models f_i^- \neq f_j^+$ for all f_j^+ in ϑ^+ and by n-fold application of the Distribution Rule it follows that $(\exists z'') z_2 = f_i^- \circ z''$; hence, (19) implies, using the Cancelation Rule,

$$(\exists z'') z' \circ f_1^- \circ \ldots \circ f_i^- \circ \ldots \circ f_m^- = z'' \circ \vartheta^+$$

With a similar argument we conclude that $(\exists z''') z'' = f_i^- \circ z'''$; consequently, $(\exists z''') z_2 = f_i^- \circ f_i^- \circ z'''$, which contradicts $(\forall f) \neg Holds(f \circ f, z_2)$.
3. Follows by repeated application of the Distribution Rule.
4. Follows from $(\forall f) \neg Holds(f \circ f, z_2)$ and $\bigwedge_{j=1\ldots n} \neg Holds(f_j^+, z_2)$ with a similar argument as used in the proof of item 2. $\qquad\qquad\square$

5   An Induction Axiom

While our new equational foundation for the Fluent Calculus does not affect the solution to the basic Frame Problem, the axiomatization presented so far is limited when it comes to modeling resources. Generally, the Fluent Calculus offers a very natural way of reasoning about the production and consumption of integer-valued resources, namely, by simply not letting foundational axiom (NonMult) apply to resources. A state may then contain multiple occurrences of a resource. For example, given that wheels (of a certain diameter) and axles (of a certain length) are different things, i.e., $UNA[Wheel, Axle]$, axioms $EUNA$ entail that $Wheel(6'') \circ Wheel(6'') \circ Axle(3.5') \neq Wheel(6'') \circ Axle(3.5') \circ Axle(3.5')$, read: having available two wheels and one axle is different from holding just one wheel but two axles. An example for a state update axiom talking about resources is the following, which specifies the action $Assemble(l, d)$ of assembling a chassis of length l and with two wheels of diameter d:[8]

$$Holds(Axle(l) \circ Wheel(d) \circ Wheel(d), s) \supset$$
$$State(Do(Assemble(l, d), s)) \circ Axle(l) \circ Wheel(d) \circ Wheel(d)$$
$$= State(s) \circ Chassis(l, d)$$

For an adequate treatment of resources, our axiomatization of Section 3 is insufficient because it admits models in which equations like $z \circ f = z$ are true:

Observation 4. $EUNA \cup \{z \circ f = z\}$ is satisfiable.

Proof. We construct a model as follows. Let the domain for sort *state* be the natural numbers $\mathbb{N}$ (incl. 0) augmented by the element ω. The only domain element of sort *fluent* shall be 1. Let $\emptyset$ be interpreted by 0 and $\circ$ by the function

$$\lambda m, n. \begin{cases} m + n & \text{if } m \neq \omega \text{ and } n \neq \omega \\ \omega & \text{otherwise} \end{cases}$$

---

[8] Below, $Holds(\bar{z}, s) \stackrel{\text{def}}{\equiv} (\exists z') State(s) = \bar{z} \circ z'$.

This function is associative, commutative, and has 0 as unit element; hence, (AC1) holds in the model. Furthermore, $1 \neq 0$, and if $1 = m + n$ then either $m = 0$ or $n = 0$; hence, (Irred) holds. Finally, if $n_1 + n_2 = n_3 + n_4$, then (Levi) is satisfied by

$$n_a = \min(n_1, n_3) \qquad n_c = n_2 - n_d$$
$$n_b = n_1 - n_a \qquad n_d = \min(n_2, n_4)$$

in case $n_1 + n_2 \neq \omega$. In case $n_1 + n_2 = n_3 + n_4 = \omega$, let us assume without loss of generality that $n_1 = n_3 = \omega$. If none of n_2, n_4 equals ω, then (Levi) is satisfied by

$$n_a = \omega \qquad n_c = n_2 - n_d$$
$$n_b = \max(0, n_4 - n_2) \qquad n_d = \min(n_2, n_4)$$

else if one and only one of n_2, n_4 equals ω, say n_2, then (Levi) is satisfied by

$$n_a = \omega \ \wedge \ n_b = n_4 \ \wedge \ n_c = \omega \ \wedge \ n_d = 0$$

else if $n_2 = n_4 = \omega$, then (Levi) is satisfied by $n_a = n_b = n_c = n_d = \omega$. Having proved that we have constructed a model for $EUNA$, the claim follows by interpreting z by ω and f by 1, because $\omega + 1 = \omega$. $\qquad\square$

The reader may note that this observation does not contradict the Cancelation Rule, which allows only fluents to be canceled out. The observation is to be contrasted to the old foundation of the Fluent Calculus, where the unification complete theory AC1* includes the axiom $z \circ f \neq z$ since the two terms are not AC1-unifiable.

Observation 4 is unproblematic in the non-resource case, because the equation $State(s) \circ f = State(s)$ *is* unsatisfiable in view of foundational axiom (NonMult).[9] But if we remove the non-multiplicity condition in order to deal with resources, then we need means to prevent such unintended models.

In this section, we introduce two additional axioms through which this problem is solved. Speaking algebraically, we extend $EUNA$ in such a way that in every model $\mathcal{M}$ of that extension we have that the sort $state^{\mathcal{M}}$ is isomorphic to the set of finite multisets over the sort $fluent^{\mathcal{M}}$, where $\emptyset$ represents the empty multiset and $\circ$ the union of multisets. The additional axioms are, first, an induction axiom, which says that the sort $state$ contains exactly the terms which can be constructed by applying $\circ$ to $\emptyset$ and elements of sort $fluent$; and second, an axiom which specifies that $\emptyset$ has no proper divisor:

$$(\forall P) \ [P(\emptyset) \wedge (\forall f, z) \ (P(z) \supset P(f \circ z)) \supset (\forall z) \ P(z)] \qquad \text{(Ind)}$$

$$z \circ z' = \emptyset \supset z = \emptyset \qquad \text{(ZeroDiv)}$$

$EUNA$ augmented by (Ind) and (ZeroDiv) (we call this theory $EUNA^+$) is consistent:

---

[9] Repeated application of the Distribution Rule to $State(s) \circ f = State(s)$ yields $(\exists z) \ State(s) = f \circ f \circ z$.

Proposition 3. *Axioms EUNA $^+$ are satisfiable.*

Proof. We can construct a model for $EUNA^+$ as follows: Let the domain for the sort *fluent* be a set of singleton multisets $\{\{a\} : a \in A\}$, and let the domain for the sort *state* be the set of finite multisets over A. It is easy to verify that (AC1), (Irred), and (ZeroDiv) are true. Furthermore, any instance of (Levi) is satisfied by setting

$$z_a = z_1 \dot{\cap} z_3 \qquad\qquad z_c = z_2 \dot{\setminus} z_d$$
$$z_b = z_1 \dot{\setminus} z_a \qquad\qquad z_d = z_2 \dot{\cap} z_4 .$$

The proof for (Ind) is straightforward by well-founded induction over the set of finite multisets over *fluent* with the ordering relation $\dot{\subset}$. □

In the following, we prove stepwise that for each model of $EUNA^+$, the following function ϱ is an isomorphism. The function is a mapping from finite multisets of fluents onto fluent terms:

$$\varrho\Big(\{ \underbrace{f_1, \ldots, f_1}_{k_1 \text{ times}}, \ldots, \underbrace{f_n, \ldots, f_n}_{k_n \text{ times}} \} \Big) = \emptyset \circ \underbrace{f_1 \circ \cdots \circ f_1}_{k_1 \text{ times}} \circ \cdots \circ \underbrace{f_n \circ \cdots \circ f_n}_{k_n \text{ times}} \qquad (20)$$

Terms which are constructed by applying $\circ$ to $\emptyset$ and terms of sort *fluent*, like the one on the right side of this equation, are called *constructor state terms*.

First, we prove that ϱ is a homomorphism, that is, every equation using $\dot\emptyset$ and $\dot\cup$ which holds between multisets of fluents, also holds after transforming the operands into the Fluent Calculus via ϱ and where $\emptyset$ and $\circ$ replace $\dot\emptyset$ and $\dot\cup$.

Proposition 4. *In every model of* (AC1)*, ϱ is a homomorphism from*

$$\langle \mathcal{M}_{fin}(\text{fluent}); \ \dot\emptyset; \ \dot\cup \rangle$$

into $\langle state; \ \emptyset; \ \circ \rangle$, where $\mathcal{M}_{fin}(\text{fluent})$ is the set of finite multisets over fluent.

The proof is straightforward using the fact that both $\dot\cup$ and $\circ$ are associative and commutative and that $\dot\emptyset$ and $\emptyset$ are the respective unit elements.

Splitting a constructor state term with $\circ$ into two parts, the parts are constructor state terms themselves:

Proposition 5. *In every model of $EUNA \cup \{(ZeroDiv)\}$, for every multiset $\dot{z}$ of fluents we have*

$$\varrho(\dot{z}) = z_1 \circ z_2 \supset (\exists \dot{z}_1, \dot{z}_2) \, [\, z_1 = \varrho(\dot{z}_1) \wedge z_2 = \varrho(\dot{z}_2) \wedge \dot{z} = \dot{z}_1 \dot\cup \dot{z}_2 \,] \qquad (21)$$

Proof. The proof is by induction over the well-founded set of finite multisets with $\dot{\subset}$ as ordering relation. If $\dot{z} = \dot\emptyset$ then (21) is trivially satisfied by $\dot{z}_1 = \dot{z}_2 = \dot\emptyset$ due to (ZeroDiv). If $\dot{z} \neq \dot\emptyset$ then we can find some f and $\dot{z}'$ such that $\dot{z} = \{f\} \dot\cup \dot{z}'$. Assume $\varrho(\dot{z}) = z_1 \circ z_2$, hence $f \circ \varrho(\dot{z}') = z_1 \circ z_2$. We can then apply (Levi) and construct $\dot{z}_1$ and $\dot{z}_2$ using the induction hypothesis for $\dot{z}'$. □

Proposition 5 lays the foundation for proving that ϱ is an injective homomorphism, that is, which maps different multisets onto different elements of *state*:

Proposition 6. *In every model of* $EUNA \cup \{(ZeroDiv)\}$ *we have*

$$\dot{z} \neq \dot{z}' \supset \varrho(\dot{z}) \neq \varrho(\dot{z}') \tag{22}$$

Proof. The proof is by induction over the sum $s = |\dot{z}| + |\dot{z}'|$ of the cardinalities of $\dot{z}$ and $\dot{z}'$. We distinguish three cases. The case of both $\dot{z}$ and $\dot{z}'$ being empty is trivial. If just one of them is empty, say $\dot{z}' = \dot{\emptyset}$, we choose $f \dot{\in} \dot{z}$ and obtain $\varrho(\dot{z}) = f \circ \varrho(\dot{z} \setminus \{f\})$; and by (ZeroDiv) and (Irred) it follows $\varrho(\dot{z}) \neq \emptyset = \varrho(\dot{z}')$, hence (22). In case $\dot{z} \neq \dot{\emptyset} \wedge \dot{z}' \neq \dot{\emptyset}$ we find f, f' such that $f \dot{\in} \dot{z}$ and $f' \dot{\in} \dot{z}'$. Suppose that $\varrho(\dot{z}) = \varrho(\dot{z}')$. Then we can apply (Levi) to $f \circ \varrho(\dot{z} \setminus \{f\}) = f' \circ \varrho(\dot{z}' \setminus \{f'\})$ and prove $\dot{z} = \dot{z}'$ by case distinction and repeated application of (Irred), Proposition 6, and the induction hypothesis.   □

We are almost done. What remains to be shown is that *every* element of *state* corresponds to a finite multiset over *fluent* :

Theorem 5. $EUNA^+$ *specifies that the elements of the sort* state *correspond to multisets of elements of sort* fluent.

Proof. In addition to Proposition 3 we have to prove that ϱ is an isomorphism. Since we know that it is an injective homomorphism (Propositions 4 and 6), it remains to be shown that ϱ is surjective as well, that is, for every element z of *state* there is some $\dot{z}$ such that $\varrho(\dot{z}) = z$. Let P be a monadic relation over *state* such that $P(z)$ holds iff there is some $\dot{z}$ such that $\varrho(\dot{z}) = z$. Then $P(\emptyset)$, and if $P(z)$ then $P(f \circ z)$ holds as well since $f \circ z = \varrho\left(\dot{z} \dot{\cup} \{f\}\right)$. Thus, by (Ind) P holds for all elements of the sort *state*.   □

6   Conclusion

We have presented a new, conceptually simpler equational foundation for the Fluent Calculus which allows for incorporating domain-dependent equations, inequalities, and function definitions. In so doing we have overcome an important limitation of the Fluent Calculus in comparison with the Situation Calculus of [10]. The new axiomatization already proved invaluable for a case study where we have successfully applied the Fluent Calculus to the Traffic World, a complex dynamic domain which has recently been posed as a challenge to the scientific community [11] and which involves actions with ramifications in nondeterministic, concurrent, and continuous domains [5, 14].

We have presented two variants of our new equational foundation. The basic axiomatization of Section 3 has been shown sufficient for guaranteeing that the Frame Problem is still solved by state update axioms. In Section 5, we have presented the extended theory $EUNA^+$, which additionally allows for modeling the concept of resources and by which the sort representing states is made isomorphic to the set of finite multisets of fluents. Theory $EUNA^+$ proved useful as the theoretical foundation for the ongoing implementation of planning with resources in the Fluent Calculus by means of BDDs [8].

References

[1] Franz Baader and Jörg H. Siekmann. Unification theory. In D. M. Gabbay, C. J. Hogger, and J. A. Robinson, editors, *Handbook of Logic in Artificial Intelligence and Logic Programming.* Oxford University Press, 1993.

[2] Andrew B. Baker. A simple solution to the Yale Shooting problem. In R. Brachman, H. J. Levesque, and R. Reiter, editors, *Proceedings of the International Conference on Principles of Knowledge Representation and Reasoning (KR)*, pages 11–20, Toronto, Kanada, 1989. Morgan Kaufmann.

[3] Wolfgang Bibel. Let's plan it deductively! *Artificial Intelligence*, 103(1–2):183–208, 1998.

[4] V. Diekert and G. Rozenberg, editors. *The book of traces.* World Scientific, Singapore etc., 1995.

[5] Andreas Henschel and Michael Thielscher. The LMW traffic world in the fluent calculus, 1999. http://www.ida.liu.se/ext/etai/lmw/TRAFFIC/001.

[6] Steffen Hölldobler and Josef Schneeberger. A new deductive approach to planning. *New Generation Computing*, 8:225–244, 1990.

[7] Steffen Hölldobler and Hans-Peter Störr. Complex plans in the fluent calculus. In S. Hölldobler, editor, *Intellectics and Computational Logic.* Kluwer Academic, 2000.

[8] Steffen Hölldobler and Hans-Peter Störr. Solving the entailment problem in the fluent calculus using binary decision diagrams. In *Proceedings of the First International Conference on Computational Logic (CL)*, 2000. (to appear).

[9] Steffen Hölldobler and Michael Thielscher. Computing change and specificity with equational logic programs. *Annals of Mathematics and Artificial Intelligence*, 14(1):99–133, 1995.

[10] Ray Reiter. The frame problem in the situation calculus: A simple solution (sometimes) and a completeness result for goal regression. In V. Lifschitz, editor, *Artificial Intelligence and Mathematical Theory of Computation*, pages 359–380. Academic Press, 1991.

[11] Erik Sandewall. Logic Modelling Workshop. URL: http://www.ida.liu.se/ext/etai/lmw/, 1999.

[12] John C. Shepherdson. SLDNF-resolution with equality. *Journal of Automated Reasoning*, 8:297–306, 1992.

[13] Michael Thielscher. From Situation Calculus to Fluent Calculus: State update axioms as a solution to the inferential frame problem. *Artificial Intelligence*, 111(1–2):277–299, 1999.

[14] Michael Thielscher. Modeling actions with ramifications in nondeterministic, concurrent, and continuous domains—and a case study. 2000. URL: http://pikas.inf.tu-dresden.de/~mit/publications/conferences/casestudy.ps.

[15] Michael Thielscher. Representing the knowledge of a robot. In A. Cohn, F. Giunchiglia, and B. Selman, editors, *Proceedings of the International Conference on Principles of Knowledge Representation and Reasoning (KR)*, Breckenridge, CO, April 2000. (To appear).

Solving the Entailment Problem in the Fluent Calculus Using Binary Decision Diagrams

Steffen Hölldobler and Hans-Peter Störr

Artificial Intelligence Institute
Department of Computer Science
Dresden University of Technology

Abstract. It is rigorously shown how planning problems encoded as a class of entailment problems in the fluent calculus can be mapped onto satisfiability problems for propositional formulas, which in turn can be mapped to the problem of finding models using binary decision diagrams (BDDs). The mapping is shown to be sound and complete. First experimental results of an implementation are presented and discussed.

1 Introduction

In recent years propositional methods have seen a surprising revival in the field of Intellectics. Greedy satisfiability testing and its variants [17] and the various procedures for answer set computing (e.g. [16, 9]) are just two examples. But only recently researchers have started to investigate whether BDDs may also help to increase the efficiency of algorithms solving typical problems in Intellectics like, for example, planning problems [5, 6, 8]. This comes to a surprise because model checking using BDDs has significantly improved the performance of algorithms and enabled the solution of new classes of problems in areas like formal verification and logic synthesis (see e.g. [3, 4]). Can we adopt this technology for, say, problems occurring in reasoning about situations, actions and causality? Can we enrich these techniques by exploiting the experiences made in the state of the art implementations of propositional logic calculi and systems mentioned at the beginning of this paragraph?

This paper reports on an attempt to find answers for these and related questions in the context of the fluent calculus. The fluent calculus is a formal system for reasoning about situations, actions and causality which admits a well–defined semantics as given in [11] and [20]. In Section 2 a restricted fragment of the fluent calculus is considered, which allows for the specification of planning problems as entailment problems in the spirit of [14]. In Section 3 a transformation is formally defined which maps these entailment problems onto satisfiability problems in propositional logic. The mapping is shown to be sound and complete. Thus, the decidability of the abovementioned fragment of the fluent calculus is established. In Section 4 it is shown how the shortest plan solving the given planning problem can be extracted from the propositional encoding. Finally, in Section 5 first and promising findings of an implementation using BDDs are presented. In

J. Lloyd et al. (Eds.): CL 2000, LNAI 1861, pp. 747–761, 2000.
© Springer-Verlag Berlin Heidelberg 2000

Table 1. Notational conventions.

Symbol	f	$F, G, \ldots$	$\mathcal{F}$	$i, j, \ldots$	z	g	s	t	
Element of	Σ_{Fl}	$\mathcal{L}$	$2^{\mathcal{L}}$	$\mathbb{N}_0$	$\Sigma_{V,St}$	$\Sigma_{V,Fl}$	$\Sigma_{V,Sit}$	constructor state term

this implementation, the propositional logic formulas are represented by reduced and ordered BDDs and techniques from model checking are applied to search for models. A discussion of the achieved results in Section 6 concludes the paper. Due to lack of space most of the proofs had to be omitted. They can be found in detail in [12].

2 Foundations

In this section some notions and notations concerning logics, planning problems, the fluent calculus and binary decision diagrams are presented.

2.1 Logics

Let Σ_V, Σ_F and Σ_P denote disjunct sets of *variables*, *function symbols* and *predicate symbols* respectively. Σ_V is countably infinite, whereas Σ_F and Σ_P are finite. The set of (*first order*) *formulas* is denoted by $\mathcal{L}(\Sigma_V \cup \Sigma_F \cup \Sigma_P)$; we abbreviate this set by $\mathcal{L}$ if the sets Σ_V, Σ_F and Σ_P can be determined from the context. σ denotes a substitution and $X\sigma$ the instance of the syntactic object X under σ.

Table 1 depicts some notational conventions in the sense that, for example, whenever we use z, we implicitly assume $z \in \Sigma_{V,St}$. The sets Σ_{Fl}, $\Sigma_{V,St}$, $\Sigma_{V,Fl}$, $\Sigma_{V,Sit}$ as well as constructor state terms are defined in Section 2.3. All symbols are possibly indexed.

The *entailment problem* $\mathcal{F} \models F$ consists of a set $\mathcal{F}$ of formulas and a formula F and is the question whether $\mathcal{F}$ entails F.

2.2 Planning

In this paper we consider planning problems having the following properties: (i) The set of states is characterized by a set of propositional fluents, i.e., a set of propositional variables, which can take values out of the set $\{\top, \bot\}$ of truth values. (ii) The actions are deterministic and their preconditions as well as effects depend only on the state they are executed in. (iii) The goal of the planning problem is a property which depends solely on the reached state. This class of problems corresponds roughly to the problems from track 1 and 2 of the planning competition held at the 4th International Conference on Artificial Planning Systems (AIPS98). There, planning problems were formulated within a language called PDDL [10]. Unfortunately, PDDL lacks a formal semantics. As shown in [18] this can be rectified by a translation from PDDL into the fluent calculus.

As an example of such a problem consider the so-called GRIPPER class: *A robot equipped with two grippers G_1 and G_2 can move between two rooms A and B. Initially the robot is in room A together with a number of balls $B_1, \ldots, B_n$. The task is to transport these balls into room B.* The problems differ wrt the number of balls and are then called GRIPPER–1, GRIPPER–2.

2.3 The Fluent Calculus

The fluent calculus is a calculus for reasoning about situations, actions and causality. It is based on the idea to consider states as multi–sets of fluents and to represent such states on the term level. The latter is done with the help of a binary function symbol $\circ$, which is associative, commutative and has a constant $\emptyset$ as unit element [11, 19, 20] but is not idempotent. In this paper we consider a restricted version of the calculus as specified in this section.

Formally, the fluent calculus is an order–sorted calculus with sorts ACTION, SIT, FLUENT, and STATE and ordering constraint FLUENT $<$ STATE. The set Σ_V of variables is the union of the disjunct sets $\Sigma_{V,A}$, $\Sigma_{V,Sit}$, $\Sigma_{V,Fl}$ and $\Sigma_{V,St}$, i.e., it consists of a countable set of variables for each sort. The set Σ_F of function symbols is the union $\Sigma_A \cup \Sigma_{Sit} \cup \Sigma_{Fl} \cup \Sigma_{St} \cup \Sigma_O$, where Σ_A is a set of function symbols denoting action names, $\Sigma_{Sit} = \{S_0, do\}$ is the set of function symbols denoting situations, Σ_{Fl} is a set of constant symbols denoting fluent names, $\Sigma_{St} = \{\emptyset, \circ, state\}$ is the set of function symbols denoting states. All sets are mutually disjoint and finite. The mentioned function symbols are sorted as follows:

$$S_0 : \text{SIT} \qquad\qquad\qquad \circ \quad : \text{STATE} \times \text{STATE} \to \text{STATE} \qquad \emptyset : \text{STATE}$$
$$do : \text{ACTION} \times \text{SIT} \to \text{SIT} \qquad state : \text{SIT} \to \text{STATE}$$

The set Σ_P of predicate symbols contains only the equality $=$ with sort STATE $\times$ STATE. The macros *holds* and *set* with sorts FLUENT $\times$ SIT and STATE respectively are often used:

$$holds(f, s) \stackrel{def}{=} (\exists \hat{z})\ state(s) = f \circ \hat{z} \tag{1}$$

$$set(z) \stackrel{def}{=} \neg(\exists f, \hat{z})\ z = f \circ f \circ \hat{z}$$

The language $\mathcal{L}_{FC}$ of the fluent calculus is the set of all well–formed and well–sorted first–order formulas over the given alphabet. State terms of the form $\emptyset \circ f_1 \circ \ldots \circ f_m$, where $f_1, \ldots, f_m \in$ FLUENT, $m \geq 0$, are pairwise distinct, are called *constructor state terms*.

The axioms $\mathcal{F}$ of the fluent calculus considered in this paper are the union $\mathcal{F}_{un} \cup \mathcal{F}_{mset} \cup \mathcal{F}_{S_0} \cup \mathcal{F}_{ms} \cup \mathcal{F}_{su}$.

– $\mathcal{F}_{un}$ is a set of *unique name assumption for fluents* combined with a domain closure axiom for fluents:

$$\mathcal{F}_{un} = \{\neg f_1 = f_2 \mid f_1, f_2 \in \Sigma_{Fl} \text{ and } f_1 \neq f_2\} \cup \{(\forall g) \bigvee_{f \in \Sigma_{Fl}} g = f\} \ .$$

- $\mathcal{F}_{mset}$ is a set of axioms ensuring that the sort STATE denotes finite multisets of fluents[19]. It consists of the following formulas:
  - the standard axioms of equality
  - the axioms AC1 for $\circ$ and $\emptyset$:

$$(\forall z)\ z \circ \emptyset = z$$
$$(\forall z_1,\ z_2)\ z_1 \circ z_2 = z_2 \circ z_1$$
$$(\forall z_1,\ z_2,\ z_3)\ (z_1 \circ z_2) \circ z_3 = z_1 \circ (z_2 \circ z_3)$$

  - an axiom that guarantees that fluents and $\emptyset$ are the only irreducible elements of sort STATE wrt. $\circ$:

$$(\forall z)\ [(\exists g)\ z = g \lor z = \emptyset \leftrightarrow (\forall z', z'')\ z = z' \circ z'' \rightarrow z' = \emptyset \lor z'' = \emptyset]$$

  - a property called Levi's axiom after a lemma used in the theory of trace monoids:

$$(\forall z_1, z_2, z_3, z_4)\ z_1 \circ z_2 = z_3 \circ z_4 \rightarrow (\exists z_a, z_b, z_c, z_d)$$
$$[z_1 = z_a \circ z_b \land z_2 = z_c \circ z_d \land z_3 = z_a \circ z_c \land z_4 = z_b \circ z_d]$$

  - an induction axiom:

$$(\forall P)\ [P(\emptyset) \land (\forall g, z)\ (P(z) \rightarrow P(g \circ z)) \rightarrow (\forall z)\ P(z)]\ .$$

- $\mathcal{F}_{S_0}$ contains a single axiom $\Phi_I(state(s_0))$ of the form $state(s_0) = t$ describing the initial state, where t is a constructor state term.
- $\mathcal{F}_{ms}$ contains an axiom specifying that in each state each fluent may occur at most once:

$$\mathcal{F}_{ms} = \{(\forall s,\ z)\ \neg(\exists g)\ state(s) = g \circ g \circ z\}$$

- $\mathcal{F}_{su}$ is a set of *state update axioms* of the form

$$(\forall) \left[\begin{array}{l} \Delta_p(s) \land \bigwedge_{g \in \vartheta^-} holds(g, s) \land \bigwedge_{g \in \vartheta^+} \neg holds(g, s) \\ \rightarrow state(do(a, s)) \circ \vartheta^- = state(s) \circ \vartheta^+ \end{array} \right], \qquad (2)$$

where ϑ^- and ϑ^+ are constructor state terms denoting the negative and positive direct effects of an action a under condition $\Delta_p(s) \in \mathcal{L}_{FC}$ respectively, $s \in \Sigma_{V,S}$ and $(\forall)$ denotes the universal closure. $\Delta_p(s)$ is a boolean combination of formulas of the form $holds(f, s)$. In the following $\Delta(s)$ will be used to denote the antecedent of (2).

To exemplify $\mathcal{F}_{su}$ and $\mathcal{F}_{S_0}$ consider the GRIPPER class. There are three actions: (i) The robot may *move* from one room to the other. (ii) The robot may *pick* up a ball if it is in the same room as the ball and one of its grippers is empty. (iii) the robot may *drop* a ball if it is carrying one. These actions are specified by the state update axioms:

$$\mathcal{F}_{su} = \{\ holds(at\text{-}robby(r_1), s) \wedge \neg holds(at\text{-}robby(r_2), s)$$
$$\rightarrow state(do(move(r_1, r_2)), s) \circ at\text{-}robby(r_1) = state(s) \circ at\text{-}robby(r_2)\ ,$$

$$holds(at(b, r), s) \wedge holds(at\text{-}robby(r), s) \wedge holds(free(g), s)$$
$$\wedge \neg holds(carry(b, g), s)$$
$$\rightarrow state(do(pick(b, r, g)), s) \circ at(b, r) \circ free(g) = state(s) \circ carry(b, g)\ ,$$

$$holds(carry(b, g), s) \wedge holds(at\text{-}robby(r), s) \wedge \neg holds(at(b, r), s)$$
$$\wedge \neg holds(free(g), s)$$
$$\rightarrow state(do(drop(b, r, g)), s) \circ carry(b, g) = state(s) \circ at(b, r) \circ free(g)\ \}$$

The initial state of a GRIPPER class problem is specified by

$$\mathcal{F}_{S_0} = \{state(S_0) = at(B_1, A) \circ \ldots \circ at(B_n, A) \circ free(G_1) \circ free(G_2) \circ at\text{-}robby(A)\},$$

where n is instantiated to some number, $at(x, y)$ denotes that ball x is in room y, $free(x)$ that gripper x is free and $at\text{-}robby(x)$ that the robot is in room x.

Reasoning problems themselves are specified as entailment problems in the fluent calculus. For the GRIPPER class we obtain the entailment problem

$$\mathcal{F} \models (\exists s)\ holds(at(B_1, B), s) \wedge \ldots \wedge holds(at(B_n, B), s).$$

Expanding abbreviation (1) this can be reformulated as

$$\mathcal{F} \models (\exists s)\ \big[(\exists z)\ state(s) = at(B_1, B) \circ z \wedge \ldots \wedge (\exists z)\ state(s) = at(B_n, B) \circ z\big],$$

which itself is equivalent to

$$\mathcal{F} \models (\exists z)\ \big[(\exists s)\ state(s) = z\ \wedge$$
$$(\exists z')\ z = at(B_1, B) \wedge \ldots \wedge (\exists z')\ z = at(B_n, B) \circ z'\big].$$

In general, reasoning in FC amounts to solving an entailment problem of the form

$$\mathcal{F} \models (\exists z)\big[(\exists s)\ z = state(s) \wedge \varPhi_G(z)\big], \tag{3}$$

where $\varPhi_G(z)$ is a boolean combination of terms of the form $(\exists z') : z = z' \circ f$ for some fluent f. In other words, one is looking for a situation, in which some boolean combination of fluents holds. One should observe that $\varPhi_G(z)$ is independent of $\mathcal{F}_{su} \cup \mathcal{F}_{S_0}$ because it does not contain an expression of sort SIT.

The fluent calculus FC considered in this paper is restricted wrt the general calculus as follows: (i) Only constants are allowed as as fluents. (ii) States are effectively sets of fluents due to $\mathcal{F}_{ms}$. (iii) The initial state is completely specified. (iv) The state update axioms specify only deterministic actions without ramifications or other constraints. The first restriction implies that the set of fluents is finite if Σ_{Fl} is finite. The second restriction implies that there are only finitely many different states uniquely characterized by the set of fluents, which hold in each state, if Σ_{Fl} is finite. As will be shown in this paper these restrictions are sufficient conditions to ensure that the entailment problem (3) in FC is decidable.

2.4 Binary Decision Diagrams

The idea of BDDs is similar to decision trees: a boolean function is represented as a rooted acyclic directed graph. The difference to decision trees is that there is a fixed order of the occurrences of variables in each branch of the diagram, and that isomorphic substructures of the diagram are represented only once.[1] This can lead to exponential savings in space in comparison to representations like decision trees or disjunctive or conjunctive normal form.

Bryant has shown in [2] that, given a fixed variable order, every boolean function is represented by exactly one BDD. Moreover, propositional satisfiability, validity and equivalence problems are decidable over BDDs in linear or constant time. Of course, the complexity of the mentioned problems does not go away: the effort has been moved to the construction of the BDDs. But as Bryant has shown as well, there are efficient algorithms for logical operations, substitutions, restrictions etc. on BDDs, whose cost is in most cases proportional to the size of its operands. BDDs may be used as a theorem prover, i.e., by constructing a BDD corresponding to a logical formula, and checking the BDD for interesting properties, but more often they are used as an implementation tool for algorithms which are semantically based on boolean functions or, equivalently, propositional formulas, or, via the characteristic functions, sets. In the implementation these formulas or sets are always represented as BDDs. The use of BDDs in this paper follows this spirit.

3   Mapping the Fluent Calculus onto Propositional Logic

The envisioned implementation will recursively generate sets of states which are reachable from an initial state by applying actions until one of these states satisfies the goal condition. This two–step behavior is already reflected in (3): The first conjunct expresses the fact that we are looking for a state z such that z is obtained from $state(S_0)$ by applying state update axioms, whereas the second conjunct expresses the fact that in z certain fluents should or should not hold. Starting with the first step and aiming at finding a propositional logic characterization of $\mathcal{F} \models (\exists s)\, z = state(s)$ a relation $\mathbf{T}(z, z')$ is defined which holds iff the state z' is a successor state of z wrt the state update axioms.[2] Moreover, this transformation allows for an encoding of the reasoning process into propositional logic.

One should observe that after expanding the macro *holds* the precondition $\Delta(s)$ of each state update axiom

$$(\forall)\ [\Delta(s) \to state(do(a, s)) \circ \vartheta^- = state(s) \circ \vartheta^+ \in \mathcal{F}_{su}] \tag{4}$$

---

[1] Thus, the BDD is *ordered* and *reduced*, also called ROBDD. These properties are so useful that they are required in almost all BDD applications, so many authors include these properties into the definition of BDDs.

[2] This corresponds to the transition relation in finite state systems.

effectively depends on $state(s)$, and this term contains the only occurrences of terms of sort SIT occurring in the precondition of (4). To explicitly express this dependence we will write $\Delta(state(s))$ instead of $\Delta(s)$. Making use of this notation the expression $\Delta(z)$ denotes the formula Δ, where each occurrence of $state(s)$ has been replaced by z.

For each state update axiom $\phi(a)$ of the form (4) we define

$$\mathbf{T}_{\phi(a)}(z, z') \stackrel{def}{=} \Delta(z) \wedge z' \circ \vartheta^- = z \circ \vartheta^+, \tag{5}$$

and for the set $\mathcal{F}_{su}$ of state update axioms we define

$$\mathbf{T}(z, z') \stackrel{def}{=} \bigvee_{\phi(a) \in \mathcal{F}_{su}} \mathbf{T}_{\phi(a)}(z, z'). \tag{6}$$

This definition is motivated by the following result.

Lemma 1. *Let t and t' be two constructor state terms and $\mathcal{F} \models state(s) = t$. $\mathcal{F} \models state(do(a, s)) = t'$ iff $\mathcal{F}_{un} \cup \mathcal{F}_{mset} \models \mathbf{T}_{\phi(a)}(t, t')$ for some $\phi(a) \in \mathcal{F}_{ua}$.*

A binding of the form z/t, where t is a constructor ground term is called *constructor state binding*. A substitution consisting only of constructor state bindings is called *constructor state substitution*. In the sequel, σ will always denote a constructor state substitution.

The task to encode entailment problems in the fluent calculus into satisfiability problems in propositional logic seems to be impossible on the first glance, because there are infinitely many terms of the sorts SIT and STATE, whereas the set of valuations of a finite propositional program is finite. Fortunately, however, one is primarily interested in logic consequences of the form $(\exists s)\ state(s) = z$ in which the only free variable z is of type STATE. From axiom $\mathcal{F}_{ms}$ one learns that the values for z may contain each fluent at most once. Because there are only finitely many fluents in FC, the set of possible bindings for z is also finite.

More precisely, we want to show that whenever σ is an answer substitution binding z for the entailment problem

$$\mathcal{F} \models ((\exists s)\ [z = state(s) \wedge \Phi_G(z)]),$$

then there exists a propositional valuation $\mathcal{B}_S(\sigma)$ such that $\mathcal{B}_S(\sigma)$ is a model for an appropriately generated propositional logic formula. This formula is obtained by giving an equivalent representation of the entailed formula in terms of $\Phi_I(z)$, $T(z, z')$ and $\Phi_G(z)$ and specifying a mapping $\mathcal{B}$ which maps this representation to a propositional formula.

The basic idea underlying $\mathcal{B}_S$ is as follows. Suppose $\Sigma_{Fl} = \{f_1, \ldots, f_m\}$. Each variable z occurring in a constructor state substitution $\sigma = \{z/t\}$ is represented by m propositional variables $z_{f_1}, \ldots, z_{f_m}$ such that in the propositional valuation $v = \mathcal{B}(\sigma)$ one obtains $v(z_{f_i}) = \top$ iff f_i occurs in t. A formula F is represented by a propositional formula $\mathcal{B}(F)$ such that a ground constructor substitution σ is an answer substitution for $\mathcal{F}_{un} \cup \mathcal{F}_{mset} \models F\sigma$ iff the valuation $\mathcal{B}_S(\sigma)$ fulfills $\mathcal{B}(F)$. We turn now to a formal definition:

Ground Constructor Substitutions: Let z/t be a binding of a constructor state substitution. Then $\mathcal{B}_S(z/t)$ is the valuation v defined by $v(z_f) = \top$ iff f occurs in t, for all $f \in \Sigma_{Fl}$. Let σ be a constructor state substitution. Then

$$\mathcal{B}_S(\sigma) = \bigcup_{z/t \in \sigma} \mathcal{B}_S(z/t).$$

Constructor State Terms: Let $\oplus$ denote the exclusive or. For each $f \in \Sigma_{Fl}$ define: [3]

$$\mathcal{B}_f(\emptyset) = \bot \qquad\qquad \mathcal{B}_f(z) = z_f$$
$$\mathcal{B}_f(f') = \top \text{ iff } f = f' \qquad\qquad \mathcal{B}_f(t_1 \circ t_2) = \mathcal{B}_f(t_1) \oplus \mathcal{B}_f(t_2)$$

Goal Formulas: Recall that each goal formula $\Phi_G(z)$ is a boolean combination of formulas of the form $(\exists z')\ z' = z \circ f$. Define:

$$\mathcal{B}_G((\exists z')\ z = z' \circ f) = z_f, \qquad\qquad \mathcal{B}_G(\neg G) = \neg \mathcal{B}_G(G),$$
$$\mathcal{B}_G(G \wedge H) = \mathcal{B}_G(G) \wedge \mathcal{B}_G(H).$$

F *Formulas:* In the proof of the Theorem 1 $\mathcal{B}$ has to be applied to formulas of the following form. Let $\mathbf{F}$ be the set of formulas defined by (i) $z = t \in \mathbf{F}$ and (ii) if $F(z) \in \mathbf{F}$ and $\mathbf{T}(z, z')$ as defined in (6), then $(\exists z)\ [set(z) \wedge F(z) \wedge \mathbf{T}(z, z)] \in \mathbf{F}$. For this class of formulas define:

$$\mathcal{B}_F(z = t) = \bigwedge_{f \in \mathcal{F}_{Fl}} (z_f \leftrightarrow \mathcal{B}_f(t))$$
$$\mathcal{B}_F((\exists z)\ [set(z) \wedge F(z) \wedge \mathbf{T}(z, z')]) = (\exists (z_f)_{f \in \Sigma_{Fl}})\ [\mathcal{B}_F(F(z)) \wedge \mathcal{B}_T(\mathbf{T}(z, z'))],$$

where

$$\mathcal{B}_T(\mathbf{T}(z, z')) = \bigvee_{\phi(a) \in \mathcal{F}_{su}} \mathcal{B}_T(\mathbf{T}_{\phi(a)}(z, z')),$$
$$\mathcal{B}_T(\mathbf{T}_{\phi(a)}(z, z')) = \mathcal{B}_G(\Delta(z)) \wedge \bigwedge_{f \in \Sigma_{Fl}} (\mathcal{B}_f(z' \circ \vartheta^-) \leftrightarrow \mathcal{B}_f(z \circ \vartheta^+)),$$
$$(\exists (z_f)_{f \in \Sigma_{Fl}}) F = (\exists z_{f_1}) \ldots (\exists z_{f_m}) F \text{ and}$$
$$(\exists z_f) F = F[z_f/\top] \vee F[z_f/\bot]$$

assuming that $\mathcal{B}_T(\mathbf{T}_{\phi(a)}(z, z'))$ is defined as in (5) and $\Sigma_{Fl} = \{f_1, \ldots, f_m\}$. Furthermore, in the last equation F denotes a propositional logic formula and $F[z_f/\top]$ and $F[z_f/\bot]$ denote the formulas obtained from F by replacing all occurrences of z_f in F by $\top$ and $\bot$ respectively.

Initial State. Recall that the initial state is characterized by a formula $\Phi_I(state(s_0))$ with $\Phi_I(z) = (z = t)$.

$$\mathcal{B}_I(z = t) = \bigwedge_{f \text{ occurs in } t} z_f \wedge \bigwedge_{f \text{ does not occur in } t} \neg z_f$$

In the sequel we will omit the index associated with $\mathcal{B}$ if it can be determined from the context to which class of syntactic objects $\mathcal{B}$ is applied.

---

[3] Thus, $\mathcal{B}(\sigma) \models \mathcal{B}_f(t\sigma)$ is true iff fluent f occurs an odd number of times in $t\sigma$.

Lemma 2. *Let F be either $\Phi_I(z)$, $\Phi_G(z)$ or an **F** formula and σ a constructor state substitution such that $F\sigma$ does not contain any free variables. $\mathcal{F}_{un} \cup \mathcal{F}_{mset} \models F\sigma$ iff $\mathcal{B}(\sigma) \models \mathcal{B}(F)$.*

Thus, Lemma 2 provides a way to transform a restricted subset of fluent calculus formulas (which includes $\mathbf{T}(z, z')$) into satisfiability-equivalent propositional formulas. This is the base to transform entailment problems in FC into satisfiability problems in propositional logic. The steps of this transformation are described in the proof of the following theorem.

Theorem 1. *Each entailment problem (3) in FC can be mapped onto a propositional satisfiability problem SAT, such that (3) is solvable iff SAT is solvable.*

Proof. Consider the entailment problem in the fluent calculus:

$$\mathcal{F} \models (\exists z)\big[(\exists s)\; z = state(s) \wedge \Phi_G(z)\big],$$

By $\mathcal{F}_{ms}$ this holds iff there is a constructor state substitution σ such that $\mathcal{F} \models (\exists)\; z\sigma = state(s) \wedge \Phi_G(z\sigma)]$, or, equivalently:

$$\{\sigma \mid \mathcal{F} \models (\exists s)\; z\sigma = state(s) \wedge \Phi_G(z\sigma)\} \neq \emptyset. \tag{7}$$

Because conjunction can be mapped onto set intersection (7) is equivalent to

$$\{\sigma \mid \mathcal{F} \models (\exists s)\; z\sigma = state(s)\} \cap \mathcal{G} \neq \emptyset, \tag{8}$$

where $\mathcal{G} = \{\sigma \mid \mathcal{F}_{mset} \cup \mathcal{F}_{un} \models \Phi_G(z\sigma)\}$. Let m be the number of fluent constants. Because of axiom $\mathcal{F}_{ms}$ there are at most 2^m different states and because preconditions and effects of actions depend only on the current state, the length of the shortest plan can be at most 2^m (such that every state is visited once). Thus (8) is equivalent to

$$\{\sigma \mid \mathcal{F} \models \bigvee_{n=0}^{2^m} (\exists (a_i)_{1 \leq i \leq n})\; z\sigma = state(a_n \ldots a_1 S_0)\} \cap \mathcal{G} \neq \emptyset, \tag{9}$$

where $(a_i)_{1 \leq i \leq n}$ denotes a sequence of actions of length n. Because disjunction can be mapped onto set union (9) is equivalent to

$$\bigcup_{n=0}^{2^m} \mathcal{Z}_n \cap \mathcal{G} \neq \emptyset, \tag{10}$$

where $\quad \mathcal{Z}_n = \{\sigma \mid \mathcal{F} \models (\exists (a_i)_{1 \leq i \leq n})\; z\sigma = state(a_n \ldots a_1 S_0)\}. \tag{11}$

Because $state(S_0)$ depends only on $\mathcal{F}_{S_0} = \{\Phi_I(state(s_0))\}$ and by Lemma 1 equation (11) can be computed recursively by

$$\mathcal{Z}_0 = \{\sigma \mid \mathcal{F}_{mset} \cup \mathcal{F}_{un} \models \Phi_I(z\sigma)\}, \tag{12}$$

$$\mathcal{Z}_n = \{\sigma \mid \mathcal{F}_{mset} \cup \mathcal{F}_{un} \models \mathbf{T}(z\hat{\sigma}, z\sigma), \hat{\sigma} \in \mathcal{Z}_{n-1}\}, \; n > 0. \tag{13}$$

With
$$\mathbf{Z}_0(z) = \Phi_I(z), \tag{14}$$

$$\mathbf{Z}_n(z) = (\exists \hat{z})\; [set(\hat{z}) \wedge \mathbf{Z}_{n-1}(\hat{z}) \wedge \mathbf{T}(\hat{z}, z)], \; n > 0, \tag{15}$$

(12) and (13) can be equivalently combined to

$$\mathcal{Z}_n = \{\sigma \mid \mathcal{F}_{mset} \cup \mathcal{F}_{un} \models \mathbf{Z}_n(z\sigma)\}, n \geq 0. \tag{16}$$

From Lemma 2 we conclude that (16) is equivalent to

$$\mathcal{Z}_n = \{\sigma \mid \mathcal{B}(\sigma) \models \mathcal{B}(\mathbf{Z}_n(z\sigma))\}, n \geq 0. \tag{17}$$

Finally, an application of Lemma 2 to $\mathcal{G}$ guarantees that (10) is equivalent to

$$\bigcup_{n=0}^{2^m} \mathcal{Z}_n \cap \{\sigma \mid \mathcal{B}(\sigma) \models \mathcal{B}(\Phi_G(z\sigma))\} \neq \emptyset, \tag{18}$$

where $\mathcal{Z}_n$ is specified in (17). This, however, is equivalent to the propositional satisfiability problem

$$\left\{\sigma \mid \mathcal{B}(\sigma) \models \left(\bigvee_{n=0}^{2^m} \mathcal{B}(\mathbf{Z}_n)\right) \wedge \mathcal{B}(\Phi_G(z\sigma))\right\} \neq \emptyset,$$

where $\mathbf{Z}_n$ is specified in (14) and (15). □

The following corollary is an immediate consequence of Theorem 1 and the decidability of propositional logic.

Corollary 1. *The entailment problem* (3) *in FC is decidable.*

4   Plan Extraction

In practical applications it is not only relevant whether a sequence of actions (or plan) solving the problem exists, but in most cases one would like to know how such a plan looks like. As it turns out, it is possible to extend the decision procedure presented in the previous section such that a plan can be recovered. Very pleasantly, the extended algorithm returns always the shortest plan.

The main idea for extracting the plan is the following: The sets $\mathcal{Z}_i$ constructed in the proof of Theorem 1 characterize the states reachable from the initial state after i actions. Thus, if $\mathcal{Z}_i \cap \mathcal{G} \neq \emptyset$, i.e., if $\mathcal{Z}_i$ contains a goal state, then there must be a plan of length i. The plan can now be reconstructed step by step by taking a substitution σ (characterizing a state $z\sigma$) from the intersection, computing the intersection of the set of states from which this state may be reached and $\mathcal{Z}_{i-1}$, and repeating this process until eventually the initial state is encountered. Thus, we find a sequence $\sigma_0, \ldots, \sigma_n$ of substitutions representing the states $z\sigma_0, \ldots, z\sigma_n$, where the first one is the initial state specified by $\mathcal{F}_{S_0}$, the last one fulfills the goal $\Phi_G(z\sigma_n)$ and $z\sigma_{i+1}$, $0 \leq i < n$ is reachable from the previous state $z\sigma_i$ by executing an action. The final step is to find actions which transform each $z\sigma_i$ to $z\sigma_{i+1}$ by finding a state update axiom $\phi(a)$ such that $\mathcal{F}_{un} \cup \mathcal{F}_{mset} \models \mathbf{T}_{\phi(a)}(z\sigma_i, z\sigma_{i+1})$.

In the implementation of the algorithm all sets and formulas are represented by in their BDD representation $\mathcal{B}$. Please note that it suffices to compute the sets $(\mathcal{Z}_i)_{i=0,1,\ldots}$ until either a solution is found or it can be determined that all reachable states have been visited (such that the sequence becomes stationary or cyclic).

Algorithm 1. Let $\mathcal{Z}_i$, $i = 0 \leq i \leq 2^m$ be the sets computed by equation (17). If (18) is not fulfilled return "unsolvable", else take the smallest n such that

$$\mathcal{Z}_n \cap \{\sigma \mid \mathcal{B}(\sigma) \models \mathcal{B}(\varPhi_G(z\sigma))\} \neq \emptyset$$

and choose a sequence $\sigma_0, \ldots, \sigma_n$ of substitutions and a sequence $a_1, \ldots, a_n$ of actions such that

$$\sigma_n \in \mathcal{Z}_n \cap \{\sigma \mid \mathcal{B}(\sigma) \models \mathcal{B}(\varPhi_G(z\sigma))\},$$
$$\sigma_{i-1} \in \mathcal{Z}_{i-1} \cap \{\sigma \mid \mathcal{B}(\sigma) \models \mathcal{B}(\mathbf{T}(z, z\sigma_i))\} \text{ and}$$
$$a_i \quad \text{such that} \quad \mathcal{B}(\mathbf{T}_{\phi(a_i)}(z\sigma_{i-1}, z\sigma_i)) = \mathsf{T}$$

Then $s = a_n \ldots a_1 S_0$ corresponds to a shortest plan wrt the goal $\varPhi_G$.

Theorem 2. *Algorithm 1 is correct and complete.*

In other words, the algorithm always proves either that there is no plan or returns a shortest plan solving the problem.

5   An Implementation Using BDDs — First Results

The theoretical results presented in the previous two sections can be applied to use a BDD implementation as the inference engine for solving entailment problems (3) in FC and computing plans. The implementation closely follows the structure of the constructions used in the proofs. Starting from a fluent calculus specification of the entailment problem, the inference engine constructs for each action a the BDD–representations for $\mathcal{B}(\mathbf{T}_{\phi(a)}(z, z'))$, and computes their disjunction $\mathcal{B}(\mathbf{T}(z, z'))$ by (6). The BDDs of the formulas $\mathcal{B}(\mathbf{Z}_i(z))$ are computed iteratively by application of (14) and (15) translated by $\mathcal{B}$. Thus, BDD representations of the sets $\mathcal{Z}_i$ are computed iteratively until either an i is reached such that $\mathcal{Z}_i = \mathcal{Z}_{i+1}$ or $\mathcal{Z}_i \cap \{\sigma \mid \mathcal{B}(\sigma) \models \mathcal{B}(\varPhi_G(z\sigma))\} \neq \emptyset$. Similarly, Algorithm 1 can be implemented using BDDs.

This approach is an implicit[4] breadth first search. In each single step the whole breadth of the search tree in depth i is searched. The sets $\mathcal{Z}_i$ can get quite complex and their BDDs quite large. Even more so, the size of the BDD for $\mathcal{B}(\mathbf{T}(z, z'))$, can quickly become too large to be handled in a graceful manner. Thus, a number of techniques were invented to limit a potential explosion in its size. In the sequel some of these techniques and their effects are sketched using examples from [15].

---

[4] It is called implicit because the calculated sets of states are never explicitly enumerated, but represented as a whole by a BDD, whose size depends more on the structure of the set, than on its actual size.

Variable Order. It is well known that the variable order used in a BDD has a large influence on the size of the BDD. Unfortunately it is still a difficult problem to find even an near optimal variable order.[5] Often, a good variable order is found by empiric knowledge and experimentation. In experiments it has turned out that fluents, which directly influence each other, should be grouped together. We have developed a variable ordering called *sort order*, which employs this idea by grouping fluents by their arguments, since fluents sharing arguments are likely to influence each other. In planning problems that use sorts to restrict the considered argument values for fluents, arguments belonging to large sorts are preferred in this ordering. Due to lack of space a precise definition of this heuristic can not be given here. On some problems this ordering lead to improvements of orders of magnitude in the size of the BDDs if compared to a simple lexicographical ordering, but this depends on the domain of the problem (of course).

Partitioning of the Transition Relation. The maximal size of a BDD is exponential in the number of propositional variables it contains. Thus, the BDD representing $\mathcal{B}(\mathbf{T}(z, z'))$, which contains twice as many propositional variables as the BDDs representing the $\mathcal{Z}_i$, is prone to get very large. A way to reduce this problem is to divide the disjunction $\mathbf{T}(z, z')$ into several parts $\mathbf{T}_1(z, z')$, ..., $\mathbf{T}_n(z, z')$, which correspond to subsets of the state update actions. In experiments, partitioning led to a reduction in the size of the BDDs in most of the tested problems.

On the other hand, such a decrease in the size of the BDDs does not necessarily lead to a decrease in computation time. In each step, the results of applying the parts of the transition relation to the set of states reached so far have to be put together, and this takes time. Nevertheless, partitioning may be useful even if the computation time increases. In the experiments, one problem (MPRIME-X-1) could only be solved after a partitioning of the transition relation; otherwise, the memory exceeded before a solution was found.

Frontier Simplification explores the fact, that the algorithm for solving the entailment problem in the fluent calculus works also if the following two conditions are enforced for all $i \geq 0$: (i) $\mathcal{Z}_i$ represents all states which may be reached by executing i actions, but not by executing less than i actions. (ii) $\mathcal{Z}_i$ does not represent any states which cannot be reached by executing at most i actions. The sets $\mathcal{Z}_i$ can be chosen freely within these limitations. Hence, it is desirable that the algorithm chooses the $\mathcal{Z}_i$ such that their BDD representations are as small as possible. In our experiments, frontier simplification has sometimes lead to moderate improvements both in computation time and memory requirements.

To the end of this section the experimental results on the GRIPPER class are discussed. These problems were quite hard for the systems taking part in the AIPS98 competition. The difficulty is rooted in the combinatorial explosion of

---

[5] The problem to find the optimal variable order is NP-complete.

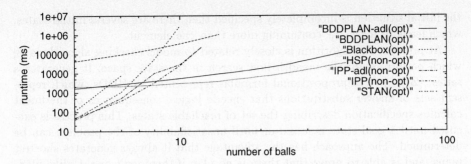

Fig. 1. Runtimes of different planners on GRIPPER class problems (in milliseconds) with different numbers of balls. Planners marked with opt provided optimal (i.e., shortest) plans, planners marked with -adl work on the sorted version of the domains, the others on the STRIPS-version.

alternatives due to the existence of two grippers. In Fig. 1 the runtimes of these planners[6] are compared to our system, BDDPLAN.[7] Only one planner (HSP) was able to solve all of the problems of this class, but it generated only suboptimal plans by using only one of the two grippers, whereas BDDPLAN generates the shortest possible plan by design.

6   Discussion

We have formally specified a mapping from entailment problems in a restricted fluent calculus to satisfiability problems in propositional logic, which is sound and complete, and we have reported some first experimental results of an implementation using BDDs. We are still in the process of investigating how optimization techniques well–known in the area of model checking using BDDs can be adapted such that they increase the efficiency of the implementation.

The mapping is tailored to a specific class of fluent calculus formulas. It seems likely that there is a more general way to translate the formulas of a larger fragment of the fluent calculus while keeping the restriction to propositional fluents, such that we could introduce recent work on the fluent calculus like ramification [20, 21] into the planner without modifying the translation and the proofs. The concept of ramification within the fluent calculus involves a limited use of constructs of second order logic, namely a calculation of the transitive closure of a relation over states, but this does not seem to pose a difficult problem as the set of states is finite and there are algorithms to compute this transitive closure using BDDs [7].

Although the problems considered in this paper admitted only a single initial state (i.e, $\mathcal{Z}_0$ is unitary), the algorithm itself is not restricted to this case. If

---

[6] See http://ftp.cs.yale.edu/pub/mcdermott/aipscomp-results.html.

[7] The runtime of BDDPLAN is measured on a different machine, so it is only accurate up to a constant factor.

the initial situation is incompletely specified then there are several initial states, which leads to a set $\mathcal{Z}_0$ containing more than one element.

At present, our algorithm is closely related to model checking algorithms [3] which perform symbolic breadth first search in the state space. It generates a series $(\mathbf{Z}_i)_{i=0,\dots}$ of propositional formulas represented as BDDs, which represent sets of answer substitutions that encode logical consequences of the fluent calculus specification describing the set of reachable states. This process is executed until a goal state is found or until unsatisfiability of the problem can be determined. The approach has the advantage that it always generates shortest plans, and is able to prove that there is no plan if there isn't one. Unlike planning algorithms based on planning as satisfiability [13] and Graphplan [1] the algorithm presented here is not limited to the generation of polynomial length plans. On the other hand, each time step may take space exponential space, since the maximum size of BDDs is $O(2^n)$ for n propositional variables. However, the experimental results achieved so far indicate that in practice the BDDs are much smaller than the theoretical limit.

Still, the size of the encountered BDDs is the main problem limiting the scalability of the algorithm and is a topic of further research. Since the maximum size of BDDs is exponential in the number of propositional variables, the reduction of this number is a foremost concern. Unlike the approach taken in [6], which explores new possibilities in the generation of plans for non–deterministic domains using BDDs, we can avoid the encoding of the actions with propositional variables in order to reduce the BDD sizes.

The encoding we use at present is "naive" in the sense that each fluent corresponds to a single propositional variable. We assume that the use of domain dependent properties of fluents provides a large space for improvements, as discussed in [8] for the BDD based planning system *Mips*, which is used to explore automated generation of efficient state encodings for STRIPS/ADL/PDDL planning problems and the implementation of heuristic search algorithms with BDDs.

To sum up, our BDD based implementation shows some promising initial results but it is too early to completely evaluate it yet.

Acknowledgment

We benefited from discussions with Sven–Erik Bornscheuer and Enno Sandner.

References

[1] Avrim Blum and Merrick Furst. Fast planning through planning graph analysis. *Artificial Intelligence*, 90:281–300, 1997.

[2] Randal E. Bryant. Graph–based algorithms for boolean function manipulation. *IEEE Transactions on Computers*, 8(C-35):677–691, 1986.

[3] J. Burch, E. Clarke, K. McMillan, and D. Dill. Symbolic model checking: 10^{20} states and beyond. *Information and Computation*, 98(2):142–170, 1992.

[4] J. R. Burch, E. M. Clarke, D. E. Long, K. L. McMillan, and D. L. Dill. Symbolic model checking for sequential circuit verification. *IEEE Transactions on Computer-Aided Design of Integrated Circuits*, 13(4):401–424, April 1994.

[5] A. Cimatti, E. Giunchiglia, F. Giunchiglia, and P. Traverso. "planning via model checking: A decision procedure for ar. In S. Steel and R. Alami, editors, *Proceedings of the Fourth European Conference on Planning (ECP97)*, LNAI 1348 , pages 130–142, Toulouse, France, Sept. 1997. Springer-Verlag.

[6] Alessandro Cimatti, Marco Roveri, and Paolo Traverso. Automatic OBDD-based generation of universal plans on non–deterministic domains. In *Proceedings of the Fifteenth National Conference on Artificial Intelligence (AAAI98)*, Madison, Wisconsin, July 26-30 1998.

[7] E. Clarke, O. Grunberg, and D. Long. Model checking. In *Proceedings of the International Summer School on Deductive Program Design*, Marktoberdorf, 1994.

[8] Stefan Edelkamp and Malte Helmert. Exhibiting knowledge in planning problems to minimize state encoding length. In *ECP'99*, LNAI, pages 135–147, Durham, 1999. Springer.

[9] T. Eiter, N. Leone, C. Mateis, G. Pfeier, and F. Scarnello. The KR system DLV: Progress report, comparisons and benchmarks. In *Proceedings of the 6th International Conference on Principles of Knowledge Representation and Reasoning*, pages 406–417. Morgan Kaufmann Publishers, 1998.

[10] M. Ghallab, A. Howe, C. Knoblock, D. McDermott, A. Ram, M. Veloso, D. Weld, and D. Wilkins. The planning domain definition language. ftp://ftp.cs.yale.edu/pub/mcdermott/software/pddl.tar.gz, march 1998.

[11] S. Hölldobler and J. Schneeberger. A new deductive approach to planning. *New Generation Computing*, 8:225–244, 1990.

[12] S. Hölldobler and H.-P. Störr. Solving the entailment problem in the fluent calculus using binary decision diagrams. Technical Report WV-99-05, AI-Institute, Computer Science Department, Dresden University of Technology, 1999.

[13] Henry Kautz and Bart Selman. Pushing the envelope: Planning, propositional logic, and stochastic search. In *Proceedings of the Thirteenth National Conference on Artificial Intelligence (AAAI-96)*, pages 1194–1201, Portland, Oregon, 1996. AAAI-Press.

[14] J. McCarthy. Situations and actions and causal laws. Stanford Artificial Intelligence Project: Memo 2, 1963.

[15] Drew McDermott. Planning problem repository. ftp://ftp.cs.yale.edu/pub/mcdermott/domains/, 1999.

[16] I. Niemelä and P. Simons. Smodels — an implementation of the well–founded and stable model semantics. In *Proceedings of the 4th International Conderence on Logic Programming and Non–monotonic Reasoning*, pages 420–429, 1997.

[17] B. Selman, H. Levesque, and D. Mitchell. A new method for solving hard satisfiability problems. In *Proceedings of the AAAI National Conference on Artificial Intelligence*, pages 440–446, 1992.

[18] H.-P. Störr. *Planen mit binären Entscheidungsdiagrammen*. PhD thesis, Dresden University of Technology, Department of Computer Science, 2000. (in German; to appear).

[19] H.-P. Störr and M. Thielscher. A new equational foundation for the fluent calculus. In *Proceedings CL 2000*.

[20] Michael Thielscher. Introduction to the Fluent Calculus. *Electronic Transactions on Artificial Intelligence*, 2(3–4):179–192, 1998.

[21] Michael Thielscher. Reasoning about actions: Steady versus stabilizing state constraints. *Artificial Intelligence*, 104:339–355, 1998.

Decidability Results for the
Propositional Fluent Calculus

Helko Lehmann[*] and Michael Leuschel

Department of Electronics and Computer Science
University of Southampton
Highfield, Southampton, SO17 1BJ, UK
{hel99r,mal}@ecs.soton.ac.uk

Abstract. We investigate a small fragment, $\mathcal{FC}_{PL}$, of the fluent calculus. $\mathcal{FC}_{PL}$ can be derived from the fluent calculus by allowing a domain description to contain a finite number of actions and fluents, only. Consequently, it is just powerful enough for specifying certain resource sensitive actions. In this paper, we contribute to the research about the fluent calculus (1) by proving that even in this small fragment the entailment problem for a fairly restricted class of formulas is undecidable. (2) We show decidability of a class of formulas which has interesting applications in resource planning.

We achieve our results by establishing a tight correspondence between models of $\mathcal{FC}_{PL}$–theories and Petri nets. Then, many problems concerning $\mathcal{FC}_{PL}$–theories can be reduced to problems of the well developed Petri net theory. As a consequence of the correspondence on the *structural* level, we also expect strong relationships between more general fluent calculus fragments and more general net classes, e.g. coloured Petri nets or predicate transition systems.

Keywords: Reasoning about Action and Change, Fluent Calculus, Decidability, Petri Nets, Temporal Logics, Model Checking.

Introduction

Arguably, the most widely used computational logic based formalism to reason about action and change is the situation calculus (other approaches are, e.g., the event calculus, action description languages, the features and fluents approach). In the situation calculus a situation of the world is represented by the sequence of actions $a_1, a_2, \ldots, a_k$ that have been performed since the initial situation s_0. Syntactically, a situation is represented by a term $do(a_k, do(a_{k-1}, \ldots, do(a_1, s_0) \ldots))$. There is no explicit representation of what properties hold in any particular situation: this information has to be derived using rules which define which properties are *initiated* and which ones are *terminated* by any particular action a_i.

The fluent calculus ($\mathcal{FC}$) "extends" the situation calculus by adding *explicit state* representations: every situation is assigned a *multi-set* of so called *fluents*. Every action a not only produces a new situation $do(a, \ldots)$ but also modifies

---

[*] The author acknowledges support from the EPSRC under grant no. 99308892

J. Lloyd et al. (Eds.): CL 2000, LNAI 1861, pp. 762–776, 2000.
© Springer-Verlag Berlin Heidelberg 2000

this multi-set of fluents. The latter is implemented using an extended equational theory (EUNA, for extended unique name assumptions [7]) with an associated extended unification (AC1). Syntactically, a multi-set of k fluents is represented as a term of the form $f_1 \circ \ldots \circ f_k$. This allows for a natural encoding of resources (à la linear logic) and it has the advantages that adding and removing fluents to a multi-set M can be very easily expressed using AC1 unification: $Add = M \circ f$ and $Del \circ f = M$.

All this enables the fluent calculus to solve the (representational and inferential) frame problem in a simple and elegant way [6]. The fluent calculus can also more easily handle partial state descriptions and provides a solution to the explanation problem, both of which are harder to come by in (standard logic programming implementations of) the situation calculus.

As in most areas of computer science, decidability issues are very important in the area of reasoning about action and change, but have only recently received increased attention (e.g., [11][14]). Of course, in general the situation as well as the fluent calculus are not decidable. However, when restricting oneself in the situation calculus to a finite set of propositional fluents [14] situations can be seen as finite paths in a finite automaton. For these systems, the validity of wide classes of formulas (e.g., characterized as temporal logics such as CTL*) are known to be decidable ([13]). One might expect that the same restriction to a finite set of propositional fluents applied to the fluent calculus produces a decidable fragment $\mathcal{FC}_{PL}$. In this paper we will show that this is *not* the case!

To prove our result we will first develop a correspondence of this fragment with Petri nets [12], which we prove correct (wrt bisimulation). Based on this, we then show that the validity of formulas expressed in a very restricted subset (CTL_{EF}) of the branching time temporal logic CTL [1] is already undecidable. As a side effect, since Petri nets are strictly more general than finite automata, it follows that $\mathcal{FC}_{PL}$ is strictly more expressive then the restricted situation calculus given in [14]. This result also gives us a new insight about the expressiveness of the fluent calculus compared to the situation calculus.

Furthermore, by reduction to the Petri net reachability problem we prove that questions of the form "Is there an initial situation with property λ_0 and is there a sequence of actions leading from this situation to some final state with property λ_e?" are actually decidable in $\mathcal{FC}_{PL}$. This is interesting, since decision procedures for this type of questions enable for automatic planning of resources.

Finally, the translation of $\mathcal{FC}_{PL}$ to Petri nets also sets the foundation for translating more expressive fragments of the fluent calculus to extended Petri net formalisms, hopefully producing new insights about decidability issues but also pointing at efficient algorithms for certain classes of problems.

In the following section we present the fluent calculus fragment $\mathcal{FC}_{PL}$. In Section 2 we show how certain $\mathcal{FC}_{PL}$–formulas can be characterized by formulas of the temporal logic CTL_{EF}. In Section 3 we develop the correspondence between models of $\mathcal{FC}_{PL}$ theories and Petri nets. We show the undecidability of the entailment relation of $\mathcal{FC}_{PL}$ in Section 4 and the decidability of an interesting class of CTL_{EF} formulas in Section 5.

1   Specifying Systems in the Fluent Calculus

Formally, the propositional fluent calculus $\mathcal{FC}_{PL}$ can be defined as follows (in contrast to the full fluent calculus, fluents and actions have no parameters):

Definition 1. *An $\mathcal{FC}_{PL}$ signature $\Sigma = (SORT, \preceq, FUN, REL)$ is defined as:*

SORT: $S, St, A, F;\ F \preceq St;$
FUN: $1^\circ :\to St;\ \circ : St \times St \to St;\ state : S \to St;$
        $s0 :\to S;\ do : A \times S \to S;$
        $f_1 :\to F; \ldots;\ f_k :\to F;\ (k \in \mathbb{N}\ and\ k \geq 1)$
        $a_1 :\to A; \ldots;\ a_l :\to A;\ (l \in \mathbb{N}\ and\ l \geq 1)$
REL: $<: S \times S;\ Equality\ (=_S\ ,\ =_{St}\ ,\ =_{Action})$

The language of an $\mathcal{FC}_{PL}$ signature Σ is defined as the order–sorted[1] first order language wrt Σ and variable declarations of the form $(x : X)$ where x is a name and X a sort of Σ. By $T_X(Y)$ we denote the terms[2] of sort X wrt Σ and variables Y. $V(t)$ represents the set of variables occurring in a term t.

Objects of sort F are called *fluents* and represent atomic *states* of the world. They can be combined using the binary function $\circ$ to form more complex states of the sort St. Objects of type S are called *situations*; as in the situation calculus they are represented by terms of the form $do(a_k, do(a_{k-1}, \ldots, do(a_1, s_0) \ldots))$ but they are associated an explicit representation of the state via the function *state*. Note that, due to the restriction of fluent terms to finitely many atomic propositions $f_1, \ldots, f_k$, it is not possible to specify an arbitrary natural number as a fluent. However, it is possible to specify a natural number as a term of sort St (e.g., $f \circ (f \circ f)$ might represent 3).

A *domain description* $\mathcal{D}$ for an $\mathcal{FC}_{PL}$–signature Σ contains a certain set of axioms, described in the following.

$\mathcal{D}$ always contains at least the standard equality axioms (reflexivity, symmetry, transitivity, substitutivity) for the sorts of Σ and, the following equational theory which defines a commutative monoid

$$\forall(x, y, z : St).\ (x \circ y) \circ z =_{St} x \circ (y \circ z)$$
$$\forall(x, y : St).\ x \circ y =_{St} y \circ x$$
$$\forall(x : St).\ x \circ 1^\circ =_{St} x$$

This commutative monoid defines the common basis for all fluent calculi, i.e. the way state representations can be combined to form new state representations using the function $\circ$. To be able to infer inequality of terms, every domain description contains a set of axioms, called *Extended Unique Name Assumptions* These assumptions ensure (AC1-) unification completeness[3], see [7].

For convenience, we introduce the following additional shortcut

$$Holds(g, s) \overset{\text{def}}{=} \exists(z : St).\ g \circ z =_{St} state(s)$$

---

[1] The ordering $F \preceq St$ states, that in all models, the sort St contains the sort F.
[2] We omit Σ, since it will be always clear from the context.
[3] This is required since we use inequality in formulas describing temporal properties.

where $g \in St$ and $s \in S$. $Holds(g, s)$ can be understood as the statement "At least the resources described by g are available in situation s".

We associate with every action a in $\mathcal{D}$ three states $St_a^-, St_a^+, St_a^= \in T_{St}(\emptyset)$. Intuitively, the fluents in St_a^- will be removed after executing a while the fluents in St_a^+ will be added. Additionally, to be able to execute the action a in a situation s, it must contain at least the fluents in $St_a^=$ (as well as those in St_a^-). To encode the latter requirement, we define $Poss(a, s)$ as the formula $Holds(St_a^- \circ St_a^=, s)$.

Furthermore, each domain description contains axioms defining a causal ordering over situations (where $s_1 \leq s_2$ is used as a shortcut for $s_1 < s_2 \lor s_1 =_S s_2$):

$$\forall(s_1, s_2 : S), (a : A). (s_1 < do(a, s_2) \leftrightarrow (s_1 \leq s_2 \land Poss(a, s_2)))$$
$$\forall(s_1, s_2 : S). (s_1 < s_2 \to \neg(s_2 < s_1))$$

In fluent calculi, the effect of executing an action is completely described by so called *state update axioms*[4]. For $\mathcal{FC}_{PL}$ the state update axioms in a domain description $\mathcal{D}$ contain exactly one formula of the following form per action a:

$$\forall(s : S). (Poss(a, s) \to state(do(a, s)) \circ St_a^- =_{St} state(s) \circ St_a^+)$$

Note, the condition part of a state update axiom can not depend on a negative statement. Hence, tests for zero like $\neg Holds(f, s)$ with $f \in F$, are not expressible[5]. Also note that the right-hand side may not contain disjunctions, i.e., $\mathcal{FC}_{PL}$ is deterministic.

In the following, we write f^n for a term $f \circ \ldots \circ f$ consisting of n copies of fluent f. Furthermore, let the mapping $|g, f| : St \times F \to \mathbb{N}$ represent the number of occurrences of a fluent f in the state g.

Example 1. ($\mathcal{FC}_{PL}$ domain Description) Consider a $\mathcal{FC}_{PL}$ signature Σ_E containing the fluents f, g, h and the actions a, b, c. Let $Poss(a, s) \overset{\text{def}}{=} Holds(h^3 \circ f^2, s)$, $Poss(b, s) \overset{\text{def}}{=} Holds(g, s)$, $Poss(c, s) \overset{\text{def}}{=} Holds(f^2, s)$ and let $\mathcal{D}_E$ be a domain description to Σ_E that contains the following state update axioms:

$$\forall(s : S). (Poss(a, s) \to state(do(a, s)) \circ h^3 \circ f =_{St} state(s) \circ g)$$
$$\forall(s : S). (Poss(b, s) \to state(do(b, s)) \circ g =_{St} state(s) \circ f)$$
$$\forall(s : S). (Poss(c, s) \to state(do(c, s)) \circ f^2 =_{St} state(s) \circ g \circ h)$$

$\square$

Throughout the paper, we refer to the state update axioms of a domain description $\mathcal{D}$ by $\text{SUA}_{\mathcal{D}}$. The state update axiom describing a particular action $a \in A$ is denoted by $\text{SUA}_{\mathcal{D}}^a$.

To give a semantics to a $\mathcal{FC}_{PL}$ domain description we consider (as usual in fluent calculi) Herbrand–E–models (i.e. Herbrand–models where the equality relation satisfies the equational theory E; see, e.g., [15]). Note that, because $\mathcal{FC}_{PL}$ uses classical negation, we do not always have a least Herbrand model; we therefore consider them all. A formula ϕ of the language of Σ is *valid* (*satisfiable*) in $\mathcal{D}$ iff ϕ is true in all Herbrand–E–models (in at least one Herbrand–E–model)

---

[4] We do not consider extensions to solve the ramification and qualification problems.

[5] Consequently, it is impossible to encode full counter machines in state update axioms.

of $\mathcal{D}$. In general, a formula ϕ is *entailed* by a set Ψ of formulas iff ϕ is true in all models of Ψ. In particular, ϕ is *entailed* by $\mathcal{D}$ iff ϕ is true in all Herbrand–E–models of the axioms of $\mathcal{D}$.

2   Temporal Properties

Many properties of dynamic systems are most easily expressed as formulas in some temporal logic formalism (such as LTL, CTL, CTL^*, or the (modal) μ-calculus). In the *model checking* approach the goal is to verify such temporal formulas for particular dynamic systems.[6] The semantics of these formulas is given wrt specific classes of dynamic systems – most commonly labelled transition systems (graphs where transitions carry action labels), Kripke structures (graphs where nodes are labelled by propositions) or a combination of the two. In this paper we adopt the latter approach, resulting in the following definition of an L–valued transition system as a mathematical representation of the possible behaviours of a dynamic system.

Definition 2. *A tuple* $\Theta = (Z, \rightarrow, T, \alpha)$ *is called L–valued transition system if Z is a non–empty set of states, T is a non–empty set of transitions and $\rightarrow$ is a family of relations such that for each $t \in T$, $\overset{t}{\rightarrow} \in \rightarrow$ and $\overset{t}{\rightarrow} \subseteq Z \times Z$. α is a mapping $L \times Z \rightarrow \{T, F\}$ where L is a non–empty set called* propositions.

A path *in* Θ *is defined as a sequence* $z_0 z_1 z_2 \ldots$ *of states such that* $z_i \overset{t_i}{\rightarrow} z_{i+1}$ *and* $t_i \in T$ *for all* $i \in \mathbb{N}$. *A L–valued transition system is called* rooted *if there is* $z_0 \in Z$ *such that to every* $z \in Z$ *exists a path* $z_0 z_1 \ldots z \ldots$. *Then, z_0 is called* root *of* Θ.

The transition system $K(\mathcal{M})$ that is associated with a particular model $\mathcal{M}$ of an $\mathcal{FC}_{PL}$ domain description $\mathcal{D}$ can be defined as follows. Let $\rightarrow_{\mathcal{M}}$ be the set of relations $\overset{a}{\rightarrow}_{\mathcal{M}}$ where $(s, do_{\mathcal{M}}(a, s)) \in \overset{a}{\rightarrow}_{\mathcal{M}}$ iff $s <_{\mathcal{M}} do_{\mathcal{M}}(a, s)$ for $s \in S_{\mathcal{M}}$.[7] Also, for $g \in St_{\mathcal{M}}$ and $s \in S_{\mathcal{M}}$ let $\alpha_{\mathcal{M}}(Holds(g), s) = T$ iff $\mathcal{M} \models Holds(g, s)$. Clearly, the structure $K(\mathcal{M}) \overset{def}{=} (S_{\mathcal{M}}, \overset{a}{\rightarrow}_{\mathcal{M}}, A_{\mathcal{M}}, \alpha_{\mathcal{M}})$ is an $L_{\mathcal{M}}$–valued transition system, where $L_{\mathcal{M}} = \{Holds(g) \mid g \in St_{\mathcal{M}}\}$.

Example 2. (cont'd) Consider the model $\mathcal{M}_1$ of $\mathcal{D}_E$ with $\mathcal{M}_1 \models state(s0) =_{St} h^3 \circ f^2$. We can depict (parts of) the associated L–valued transition system as follows:

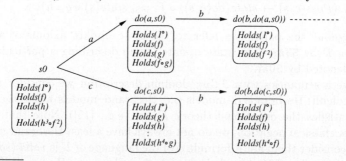

[6] Another approach considers dynamic systems to be defined by temporal formulas.

[7] Equally, we can define $(s, do_{\mathcal{M}}(a, s)) \in \overset{a}{\rightarrow}_{\mathcal{M}}$ iff $\mathcal{M} \models Poss(a, s)$ without considering the definition of $<$.

Having given a transition system semantics to $\mathcal{FC}_{PL}$, we can study the validity of temporal logic formulas, e.g., with the purpose of verification using model checking. To examine the decidability of checking temporal properties of $\mathcal{FC}_{PL}$, we will focus on properties which can be characterized as CTL_{EF}–formulas. CTL_{EF} is a small fragment[8] of the logic CTL [1] (in [2] a very similar logic to CTL_{EF} is called UB^-). CTL_{EF} is particularly interesting since all CTL_{EF} formulas characterize first order $\mathcal{FC}_{PL}$ formulas[9]. Furthermore, as we will show, many interesting properties of systems in the area of Reasoning about action and change can be easily expressed in CTL_{EF}.

Definition 3 (CTL_{EF}). *Formulas of CTL_{EF} are built from* T *and atomic propositions of L recursively using the classical connectives $\neg$ and $\wedge$ as well as the temporal connectives X and EF: if ϕ and ψ are formulas then so are $X(a)\phi$, for all a of some set A, and $EF\phi$.*

The semantics of CTL_{EF} is defined wrt an L–valued transition system K and a state z of K:

$$K, z \models \mathbf{T}$$
$$K, z \models l \quad \text{iff} \quad \alpha(l, z) = \mathbf{T} \text{ and } l \in L$$
$$K, z \models \neg\phi \quad \text{iff} \quad K, z \not\models \phi$$
$$K, z \models \phi \wedge \psi \quad \text{iff} \quad K, z \models \phi \text{ and } K, z \models \psi$$
$$K, z \models X(a)\phi \quad \text{iff} \quad \text{there is some } z' \text{ such that } z \overset{a}{\to} z' \text{ and } K, z' \models \phi$$
$$K, z \models EF\phi \quad \text{iff} \quad \text{there is a path } z_1, z_2, \ldots \text{ with } z = z_1 \text{ and there exists a } z_i \geq 1 \text{ on this path such that } K, z_i \models \phi$$

ϕ is called *valid* iff for all L–valued transition systems K and all states z of K, $K, z \models \phi$ (denoted by $\models \phi$). ϕ is said to be *satisfiable* iff for some L–valued transition system K and for some state z of K, $K, z \models \phi$.

As we can associate a transition system $K(\mathcal{M})$ with every model of $\mathcal{FC}_{PL}$, the semantics of CTL_{EF}–formulas for $\mathcal{FC}_{PL}$ descriptions is clear. We can, however, also encode CTL_{EF}–formulas directly as formulas within $\mathcal{FC}_{PL}$. This ensures that all problems stated in CTL_{EF} actually have a counterpart within $\mathcal{FC}_{PL}$ and can be assigned a meaning using the semantics of $\mathcal{FC}_{PL}$. The translation will also be vital to establish the undecidability result for $\mathcal{FC}_{PL}$ later on.

Definition 4 (Embedding CTL_{EF} into $\mathcal{FC}_{PL}$). *We define Φ, mapping CTL_{EF} formulas and terms of sort situation to $\mathcal{FC}_{PL}$ formulas as follows. Atomic propositions of CTL_{EF} are translated as follows:*
$$\Phi(\mathbf{T}, s) \overset{def}{=} \mathbf{T} \quad \text{and} \quad \Phi(Holds(g), s) \overset{def}{=} Holds(g, s) \text{ for } g \in T_{St}(\emptyset).$$
The classical logical connectives are translated in a canonical way:
$$\Phi(\neg\lambda, s) \overset{def}{=} \neg\Phi(\lambda, s) \quad \text{and} \quad \Phi(\lambda_1 \wedge \lambda_2, s) \overset{def}{=} \Phi(\lambda_1, s) \wedge \Phi(\lambda_2, s)$$
and the temporal operators can be embedded as follows
$$\Phi(X(a)\lambda, s) \overset{def}{=} Poss(a, s) \wedge \Phi(\lambda, do(a, s))$$
$$\Phi(EF\lambda, s) \overset{def}{=} \exists(s' : S).\, (s' \geq s \wedge \Phi(\lambda, s'))$$

---

[8] In contrast to CTL, it does not support the operators EG, EU.

[9] Many other temporal logics allow the expression of properties, which are not first-order definable.

The following proposition establishes soundness of this translation (wrt the semantics of CTL_{EF} on $K(\mathcal{M})$). We do not give a proof here; details can be found in [8].

Proposition 1. *The CTL_{EF}–formula λ is valid for the set of L–valued transition systems specified by a domain description to a $\mathcal{FC}_{PL}$–scheme iff $\forall(s : S).\Phi(\lambda, s)$ is valid in the corresponding domain description $\mathcal{D}$. λ is satisfiable iff $\exists(s : S).\Phi(\lambda, s)$ is satisfiable in $\mathcal{D}$.*

For convenience, we define a temporal operator $AG\phi \stackrel{\text{def}}{=} \neg EF\neg\phi$ and the usual derived logical connectors $\rightarrow$, $\vee$, $\leftrightarrow$. From the definitions follow the corresponding translations to $\mathcal{FC}_{PL}$.

Planning Problem: Assume, an agent knows certain properties (λ_0) of its current situation and it tries to reach a situation with certain goal properties (λ_e) by executing certain actions. Then, answering the following question is crucial: "Is there an initial situation with property λ_0 and is there a sequence of actions leading from this situation to some situation with property λ_e?". This question can be easily expressed as the CTL_{EF}–formula $\lambda_0 \wedge EF\lambda_e$. If this formula is not satisfiable, the agent must give up pursuing his goal. In Section 5 we will prove that this type of question *can* be decided if λ_0, λ_e are restricted to (arbitrary) atomic propositions. Note however, that CTL_{EF} is not powerful enough to express questions like "Do all action sequences executed in a situation with property λ_0 eventually lead to a situation with property λ_e".

To compare transition systems we use the notion of strong bisimulation (see, e.g. [10]). Strong bisimulation is of particular importance in this paper, since the validity of any formula of the modal μ–calculus (and thus CTL and CTL_{EF}) is invariant under strong bisimulation, i.e. proving a property for one system is sufficient to establish it for all strongly bisimilar[10] systems.

Definition 5 (Bisimulation). *Let $\Theta_1 = (Z_1, \{\stackrel{t}{\rightarrow}_1| \ t \in T_1\}, T_1, \alpha_1)$, $\Theta_2 = (Z_2, \{\stackrel{t}{\rightarrow}_2| \ t \in T_2\}, T_2, \alpha_2)$ be L_1–valued and, respectively, L_2–valued transition systems. Let Φ be a relation $\Phi \subseteq Z_1 \times Z_2$. Φ is called bisimulation if there exist mappings $\Psi_1 : L_1 \rightarrow L_2$ and $\Psi_2 : L_2 \rightarrow L_1$ such that $(z_1, z_2) \in \Phi$ implies*

1. *for all $l \in L_1$, $\alpha_1(l, z_1) = \mathbf{T}$ iff $\alpha_2(\Psi_1(l), z_2) = \mathbf{T}$,*
2. *for all $l \in L_2$, $\alpha_2(l, z_2) = \mathbf{T}$ iff $\alpha_1(\Psi_2(l), z_1) = \mathbf{T}$,*
3. *with $z_1 \stackrel{t_1}{\rightarrow}_1 z_1'$, exists $z_2 \stackrel{t_1}{\rightarrow}_2 z_2'$ such that $(z_1', z_2') \in \Phi$*
4. *with $z_2 \stackrel{t_2}{\rightarrow}_2 z_2'$, exists $z_1 \stackrel{t_2}{\rightarrow}_1 z_1'$ such that $(z_1', z_2') \in \Phi$*

$z_1 \in Z_1$ and $z_2 \in Z_2$ are called *bisimilar*, written $z_1 \sim z_2$, if there is a bisimulation Φ such that $(z_1, z_2) \in \Phi$. Θ_1 and Θ_2 are called *bisimilar* if there is a bisimulation Φ such that for all $z_1 \in Z_1$ exists $z_2 \in Z_2$ such that $z_1 \sim z_2$ and for all $z_2 \in Z_2$ exists $z_1 \in Z_1$ such that $z_1 \sim z_2$. Note, that for rooted transition systems it is sufficient to show the existence of a bisimulation for the root states.

---

[10] Since all bisimulations considered here are strong, we omit the word "strong". Bisimulations which take atomic propositions into account are often called *zig–zags*. Furthermore, we extend the common definition slightly, by allowing also mappings Ψ_1, Ψ_2 between atomic propositions.

3   Fluent Calculi and Petri Nets

Petri nets are widely used to model concurrent and possibly infinite state systems. Here we give a short definition and show how Petri nets are related to models of domain descriptions in $\mathcal{FC}_{PL}$.

Definition 6. *A tuple* $\mathcal{P} = (P, T, E, W, m_0)$ *is called* Petri net *if*

1. *P and T are non-empty finite disjoint sets of vertices, elements of P are called* places *and elements of T are called* transitions. *$E \subseteq (P \times T) \cup (T \times P)$ is a set of* edges.
2. *$W : E \to \mathbb{N}^+$, which is called* weight function.
3. *A mapping $m : P \to \mathbb{N}$ is called* marking. *m_0 is a marking and is called* initial marking. *The set $\mathbb{N}^P$ of vectors is understood as the set of all markings.*

For each transition $t \in T$ we define vectors $t^-, t^+, \delta t \in \mathbb{N}^P$, such that $t^-(p) = W(p, t)$, $t^+(p) = W(t, p)$ and $\delta t(p) = t^+(p) - t^-(p)$ for all $p \in P$. Let m_1 and m_2 be two markings, then $m_1 \leq m_2 \overset{\text{def}}{=} \forall (p : P). m_1(p) \leq m_2(p)$. A transition $t \in T$ is called *enabled* iff $t^- \leq m$. If an enabled transition t is *fired*, for the new marking m' of the Petri net $\mathcal{P}$ holds $m' = m + \delta t$ and it is denoted by $m \overset{t}{\to} m'$. The set of all markings which are reachable from m is denoted by $\Re(m)$:

$$\Re(m) = \{m' \mid m \overset{t_1}{\to} \ldots \overset{t_n}{\to} m' \text{ for some } n \in \mathbb{N} \text{ and } t_i \in T \text{ for all } 0 \leq i \leq n\}$$

For all $m, n \in \mathbb{N}^P$ we define $\alpha(m, n) = \mathbf{T}$ iff $m \leq n$. Then, it is easy to see that the tuple $K(\mathcal{P}) = (\Re(m_0), \to, T, \alpha)$, where $\to \overset{\text{def}}{=} \{\overset{t}{\to} \mid t \in T\}$, is a $\mathbb{N}^P$-labelled transition system.

Now we are ready to define a mapping from models $\mathcal{M}$ of domain descriptions $\mathcal{D}$ to Petri nets. Basically, fluents are mapped to places and actions are mapped to transitions. However, the weight function has to reflect both, conditions and (positive and negative) effects of the execution of actions.

Definition 7 ($\mathcal{FC}_{PL} \to$ **Petri Nets**). *Let $\mathcal{D}$ be a domain description in $\mathcal{FC}_{PL}$ and let $\mathcal{M}$ be a model of $\mathcal{D}$. Then, by $\mathcal{P}(\mathcal{D}, \mathcal{M})$ we define a mapping of $\mathcal{M}$ and $\mathcal{D}$ to a Petri net (P, T, E, W, m_0):*

1. $P = F_{\mathcal{M}}$, $T = \{a \mid \text{SUA}_{\mathcal{D}}^a \in \text{SUA}_{\mathcal{D}} \wedge a \in A_{\mathcal{M}}\}$,
2. *let $F(g)$ denote the set of all fluents occurring in $g \in St_{\mathcal{M}}$ and let for each $\text{SUA}_{\mathcal{D}}^a \in \text{SUA}_{\mathcal{D}}$, $a \in A_{\mathcal{M}}$. Then we define with the help of $F_a^- = F(St_a^-)$, $F_a^+ = F(St_a^+)$, $F_a^h = F(St_a^=)$ the edges of the Petri net:*

$$E = \{(F_a^- \cup F_a^h) \times a \mid \text{SUA}_{\mathcal{D}}^a \in \text{SUA}_{\mathcal{D}}\} \cup \{a \times (F_a^h \cup F_a^+) \mid \text{SUA}_{\mathcal{D}}^a \in \text{SUA}_{\mathcal{D}}\}$$

3. *for each $(f, a) \in E$, $W((f, a)) = |St_a^-, f| + |St_a^=, f|$, and for each $(f, a) \in E$, $W((f, a)) = |St_a^+, f| + |St_a^=, f|$.*

For each $g \in St_{\mathcal{M}}$ a marking $m_{\mathcal{M}}(g) : St_{\mathcal{M}} \to \mathbb{N}^P$ is defined as follows:

$$m_{\mathcal{M}}(g) = \{f \to n \mid f \in F_{\mathcal{M}} \wedge n = |g, f|\}$$

Accordingly, for each $s \in S_{\mathcal{M}}$ a marking $m_{\mathcal{M}}(s) : S_{\mathcal{M}} \to \mathbb{N}^P$ is defined as $m_{\mathcal{M}}(s) = m_{\mathcal{M}}(state_{\mathcal{M}}(s))$. In particular, the initial marking m_0 is given by $m_{\mathcal{M}}(s0_{\mathcal{M}})$.

Example 3. (cont'd) The following Petri net corresponds to $\mathcal{M}_1$ of $\mathcal{D}_E$:

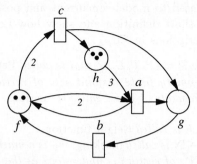

□

The following theorem establishes correctness of the above mapping, thereby enabling the reduction of many problems concerning models of $\mathcal{FC}_{PL}$–descriptions to problems of Petri net theory!

Theorem 1. *Let $K(\mathcal{M})$ be an $L_\mathcal{M}$–valued transition system where $\mathcal{M}$ is a model of a domain description $\mathcal{D}$ in $\mathcal{FC}_{PL}$. Let $\mathcal{P} = (P, T, E, W, m_0) = \mathcal{P}(\mathcal{D}, \mathcal{M})$ be the corresponding Petri net. Then $K(\mathcal{M})$ and $K(\mathcal{P})$ are bisimilar.*

Proof. Let's consider the mappings $\Psi_\mathcal{M} : L_\mathcal{M} \to \mathbb{N}^P$ and $\Psi_\mathcal{P} : \mathbb{N}^P \to L_\mathcal{M}$ between propositions of $K(\mathcal{M})$ and $K(\mathcal{P})$:

$$\Psi_\mathcal{M}(Holds(g)) \stackrel{\text{def}}{=} m_\mathcal{M}(g), \qquad \Psi_\mathcal{P}(m) \stackrel{\text{def}}{=} Holds(f_1^{m(f_1)} \circ f_2^{m(f_2)} \circ \ldots \circ f_k^{m(f_k)})$$

where $\{f_1, f_2, \ldots, f_k\} = P$, $Holds(g) \in L_\mathcal{M}$ and $m \in \mathbb{N}^P$. Since we consider Herbrand–E–models only, the situation $s0_\mathcal{M}$ exists in every $\mathcal{M}$ and is predecessor (wrt $\leq_\mathcal{M}$) of all other $s \in S_\mathcal{M}$, hence $K(\mathcal{M})$ is a rooted transition system. Since $K(\mathcal{P}(\mathcal{D}, \mathcal{M}))$ is rooted as well (in $m_0(s0_\mathcal{M})$), it suffices to show the existence of a bisimulation Φ with $(s0_\mathcal{M}, m_0(s0_\mathcal{M})) \in \Phi$ and the consistency of the mappings $\Psi_\mathcal{P}$ and $\Psi_\mathcal{M}$.

First, we show that for every situation $s \in S_\mathcal{M}$, $\alpha_\mathcal{M}(Holds(g), s)$ with $g \in St_\mathcal{M}$ is true iff $\alpha(\Psi_\mathcal{M}(Holds(g)), m_\mathcal{M}(s))$ is true. From the equational theory for the sort $St_\mathcal{M}$, which must be fulfilled in every model of $\mathcal{D}$, follows that $\mathcal{M} \models Holds(g, s)$ iff for all $g' \in St_\mathcal{M}$, such that $|g', f| = |g, f|$ for all $f \in F_\mathcal{M}$, $\mathcal{M} \models Holds(g', s)$. Furthermore, from the definition of $Holds(g, s)$ follows that $\mathcal{M} \models Holds(g, s)$ iff $|g, f| \leq |state_\mathcal{M}(s), f|$ for all $f \in F_\mathcal{M}$. From the definition of the corresponding Petri net follows $(m_\mathcal{M}(s))(f) = |state_\mathcal{M}(s), f|$ for all $f \in F_\mathcal{M}$ and for markings m' with $m' = \Psi_\mathcal{M}(Holds(g)) = m_\mathcal{M}(g)$ holds $m'(f) = |g, f|$ for all $f \in F_\mathcal{M}$. Hence, $\mathcal{M} \models Holds(g, s)$ iff $\Psi_\mathcal{M}(Holds(g)) \leq m_\mathcal{M}(s)$, i.e. (per definition of $\alpha_\mathcal{M}$ and α) $\alpha_\mathcal{M}(Holds(g), s)$ is true iff $\alpha(\Psi_\mathcal{M}(Holds(g)), m_\mathcal{M}(s))$ is true.

Similarly, for every $m \in \Re(m_0)$ and every $m' : P \to \mathbb{N}$, $\alpha(m', m)$ is true iff $\alpha(\Psi_\mathcal{P}(m'), s)$ is true where $s \in S_\mathcal{M}$ and $m = m_\mathcal{M}(s)$. This follows from the definition of $\Psi_\mathcal{P}$ and the fact that every $s \in S_\mathcal{M}$ with $m = m_\mathcal{M}(s)$ fulfills $|state_\mathcal{M}(s), p| = m(p)$ for all $p \in P$: $\Psi_\mathcal{P}(m') = Holds(p_1^{m'(p_1)} \circ p_2^{m'(p_2)} \circ \ldots \circ p_k^{m'(p_k)}) = Holds(g)$, $\alpha_\mathcal{M}(Holds(g), s)$ is true for $s \in S_\mathcal{M}$ iff $|g, p| \leq |state_\mathcal{M}(s), p|$ for all $p \in F_\mathcal{M}$.

Now let $(s, m) \in \Phi \subseteq S_\mathcal{M} \times \Re(m_0)$ such that $m_\mathcal{M}(s) = m$. We prove that, for every action $a \in A_\mathcal{M}$ and $s \xrightarrow{a}_\mathcal{M} s'$, there exists a marking m' such that $m_\mathcal{M}(s') = m'$ and $m \xrightarrow{a} m'$. From the state update axioms follows for $s' = do_\mathcal{M}(a, s)$ that $\mathcal{M} \models state(do(a, s)) \circ St_a^- =_{St} state(s) \circ St_a^+$ (since $\mathcal{M} \models Holds(St_a^- \circ St_a^=, s)$ if $s \xrightarrow{a}_\mathcal{M} s'$). From the above arguments follows $\mathcal{M} \models Holds(St_a^- \circ St_a^=, s)$ iff $|St_a^-, p| + |St_a^=, p| \leq m(p)$ for all $p \in P$. From the definition of P we conclude that there is a transition $a \in T$ such that $W(p, a) = |St_a^-, p| + |St_a^=, p|$. Hence, a is enabled in $m_{\mathcal{M}}(s)$ iff $\mathcal{M} \models Holds(St_a^- \circ St_a^=, s)$. Furthermore, according to the state update axiom for $a \in A$ for all $f \in F_{\mathcal{M}}$: $|state_{\mathcal{M}}(do_{\mathcal{M}}(a, s)), f| = |state_{\mathcal{M}}(s), f| - |St_a^-, f| + |St_a^+, f|$. If the transition a is fired in P, $m \xrightarrow{a} m'$, then for m' and all $f \in F_{\mathcal{M}}$ holds

$$m'_{\mathcal{M}}(f) = m_{\mathcal{M}}(f) - |St_a^-, f| - |St_a^=, f|) + |St_a^+, f| + |St_a^=, f|$$
$$= m_{\mathcal{M}}(f) - |St_a^-, f| + |St_a^+, f| = |state_{\mathcal{M}}(s'), f|$$

Analogously, for every transition $t \in T$ and $m \xrightarrow{t} m'$, there exists $s' \in S_{\mathcal{M}}$ and $a \in A_{\mathcal{M}}$ such that $m_{\mathcal{M}}(s') = m'$ and $s' = do_{\mathcal{M}}(a, s)$. This follows from the one–to–one mapping of $T_A(\emptyset)$ to T and from the above bidirectional correspondences. Since, for $(s0_{\mathcal{M}}, m_0)$ holds $m_{\mathcal{M}}(s0_{\mathcal{M}}) = m_0$ (see definition), it follows by induction that $s0_{\mathcal{M}} \sim m_0$.   □

This theorem will be applied in Section 5 to reduce satisfiability of $\lambda_0 \wedge EF\lambda_e$ to the (decidable) reachability problem in Petri nets.

However, the question arises whether we can establish a similar correspondence in the opposite direction, i.e. we want to show that for every Petri net, there exists a corresponding model of a domain description in $\mathcal{FC}_{PL}$. To this end, we use the following mapping. Note that in this mapping we do not hardwire the initial marking m_0 of a Petri net; this will enable us to examine richer classes of problems later on.

Definition 8 (Petri Nets $\rightarrow \mathcal{FC}_{PL}$). *Let $\mathcal{P} = (P, T, E, W, m_0)$ be a Petri net. Then by $\mathcal{D}(\mathcal{P})$ a mapping from a Petri net $\mathcal{P}$ to a domain description $\mathcal{D}$ is defined as follows:*

1. *The signature of $\mathcal{D}$ is given by a $\mathcal{FC}_{PL}$ signature where the constants of sort A and F are given by FUN: $\{(p :\to F) \mid p \in P\}$, $\{(t :\to A) \mid t \in T\}$*
2. *Let for each transition t*
$$St_t^= = p_1^{\max(0, W(t,p_1) - W(p_1,t))} \circ \ldots \circ p_k^{\max(0, W(t,p_k) - W(p_k,t))}$$
$$St_t^+ = p_1^{W(t,p_1) - \max(0, W(t,p_1) - W(p_1,t))} \circ \ldots \circ p_k^{W(t,p_k) - \max(0, W(t,p_k) - W(p_k,t))}$$
$$St_t^- = p_1^{W(p_1,t) - \max(0, W(t,p_1) - W(p_1,t))} \circ \ldots \circ p_k^{W(p_k,t) - \max(0, W(t,p_k) - W(p_k,t))}$$
for $\{p_1, \ldots, p_k\} = P$. With $Poss(t, s) = Holds(St_t^- \circ St_t^=, s)$ for every $t \in T$, $SUA_{\mathcal{D}}$ consists of axioms

$$\forall(s : S). (Poss(t, s) \to state(do(t, s)) \circ St_t^- =_{St} state(s) \circ St_t^+)$$

Furthermore, for every domain description $\mathcal{D}$, we assume the domain independent axioms described in Section 1.

The following theorem establishes correctness of the above embedding of Petri nets into $\mathcal{FC}_{PL}$ and it will be the main tool to prove the undecidability of the $\mathcal{FC}_{PL}$ entailment problem in Section 4. (The reason why the theorem does not hold for all models of $\mathcal{D}$ is that the fluent calculus encoding does not contain the initial marking of the Petri net. However, as evident from the proof, the particular model $\mathcal{M}$ can be easily isolated.)

Theorem 2. *For every Petri net $\mathcal{P} = (P, T, E, W, m_0)$, there exists a domain description $\mathcal{D}$ in $\mathcal{FC}_{PL}$ and a model $\mathcal{M}$ of $\mathcal{D}$, such that the $L_{\mathcal{M}}$-valued transition system $K(\mathcal{M})$ and $K(\mathcal{P})$ are bisimilar.*

Proof. We consider the Herbrand–E–models defined by the marking m_0:
$\mathcal{M} \models state(s0) =_{St} p_1^{m_0(p_1)} \circ \ldots \circ p_k^{m_0(p_k)}$ where $P = \{p_1, \ldots, p_k\}$. Furthermore, the mappings $\Psi_\mathcal{M}$ and $\Psi_\mathcal{P}$ describe the mappings between labels of $K(\mathcal{M})$ and $K(\mathcal{P})$.
Now let $(s, m) \in \Phi \subseteq S_\mathcal{M} \times \Re(m_0)$ such that $s \in S_\mathcal{M}(m)$ where $S_\mathcal{M}(m)$ denotes the set of all situations s such that $m_\mathcal{M}(s) = m$. We prove that for every transition $t \in T$ and $m \xrightarrow{t} m'$, there exists a situation s' such that $m_\mathcal{M}(s') = m'$ and $s \xrightarrow{t}_\mathcal{M} s'$ for all $s \in S_\mathcal{M}(m)$. From the definition of $\mathcal{P}$ follows for the marking m', if $m \xrightarrow{t} m'$,

$$m'(p) = m(p) + t^+(p) - t^-(p) = m(p) + W(t, p) - W(p, t)$$

for all $p \in P$, since $t^-(p) = W(p, t) \leq m(p)$ for all $p \in P$.
From the definition of $Holds(g, s)$ follows that $\mathcal{M} \models Holds(g, s)$ with $g \in St_\mathcal{M}$ iff $|g, p| \leq m_\mathcal{M}(s)(p)$ for all $p \in P$. From the definition of $\mathcal{D}$ we conclude that there is a state update axiom $\text{SUA}_\mathcal{D}^t$ with $t \in T_A(\emptyset)$:

$$\forall(s : S).\, (Holds(St_t^- \circ St_t^=, s) \to state(do(t, s)) \circ St_t^- =_{St} state(s) \circ St_t^+)$$

where, in every model of $\mathcal{D}$,

$$St_t^- \circ St_t^= =_{St} p_1^{W(t,p_1) - \max(0, W(t,p_1) - W(p_1,t))} \circ \ldots \circ p_k^{W(t,p_k) - \max(0, W(t,g_k) - W(g_k,t))}$$
$$\circ p_1^{\max(0, W(t,p_1) - W(p_1,t))} \circ \ldots \circ p_k^{\max(0, W(t,g_k) - W(g_k,t))}$$
$$=_{St} p_1^{W(p_1,t)} \circ \ldots \circ p_k^{W(p_k,t)}.$$

Hence, $\mathcal{M} \models Holds(p_1^{W(p_1,t)} \circ \ldots \circ p_k^{W(p_k,t)}, s)$ iff t is enabled in m.
If t is fired, according to the state update axiom for t, for all $p \in F_\mathcal{M}$:

$$|state_\mathcal{M}(do_\mathcal{M}(t, s)), p|$$
$$= |state_\mathcal{M}(s), p| - |St_t^-, p| + |St_t^+, p|$$
$$= |state_\mathcal{M}(s), p| - (W(p, t) - \max(0, W(t, p) - W(p, t)))$$
$$+ W(t, p) - \max(0, W(t, p) - W(p, t)))$$
$$= |state_\mathcal{M}(s), p| + W(t, p) - W(p, t)$$

Analogously, for every action $a \in A_\mathcal{M}$ and $s \xrightarrow{a}_\mathcal{M} s'$, there exists $m' \in \Re(m_0)$ and $t \in T$ such that $m_\mathcal{M}(s') = m'$ and $m \xrightarrow{t} m'$. This follows from the one–to–one mapping of T to $T_A(\emptyset)$ and from the above bidirectional correspondences.
For $(s0_\mathcal{M}, m_0)$ holds $m_\mathcal{M}(s0_\mathcal{M}) = m_0$. By induction follows $s0_\mathcal{M} \sim m_0$. □

As a consequence of this theorem, $\mathcal{FC}_{PL}$ is strictly more expressive than the restricted situation calculus in [14]. For the class of transition systems defined by finite automata is strictly contained in the class defined by Petri nets.

4　Undecidability of CTL_{EF} in $\mathcal{FC}_{PL}$

It is well known (e.g., [13]) that the modal μ–calculus cannot distinguish between strongly bisimilar transition systems, i.e. all formulas that are valid for one transition system are also valid in all bisimilar systems. This allows us to prove the following theorem with the help of Petri net theory.

Theorem 3. *There is a domain description $\mathcal{D}$ in $\mathcal{FC}_{PL}$ and a CTL_{EF}–formula, such that the question whether this CTL_{EF}–formula is satisfiable by $\mathcal{D}$, is undecidable.*

Proof. In [3] with a correction in [4] the undecidability of the model checking problem of the following formula has been shown for Petri nets $\mathcal{P} = (P, T, E, W, m_0)$:

$$\pi = AG(X(t_{AB})\text{T} \to X(t_{AB})EF\, \text{Dead})$$

where $t_{AB} \in T$, $\text{Dead} = \bigwedge_{t \in T} \neg X(t)\text{T}$.

The model checking problem for a Petri net $\mathcal{P} = (P, T, E, W, m_0)$ is defined as the problem to decide whether the associated transition system $K(\mathcal{P})$ with the initial marking m_0 satisfies a formula ϕ. Hence, to prove the claim, it is sufficient to show that there is a domain description $\mathcal{D}$ and a formula π' such that a model $\mathcal{M}$ of $\mathcal{D}$ satisfies π' iff $K(\mathcal{P})$ satisfies π in m_0.

It is easy to see that an initial marking m can be completely characterized as the set of all markings n with $m \leq n \wedge \neg(\overline{m} \leq n)$ where we define $\overline{m}$ as $\overline{m}(p) = m(p) + 1$ for all $p \in P$. I.e., if $\mathcal{P} = (P, T, E, W, m_0)$ and $\mathcal{P}' = (P, T, E, W, m'_0)$ are two Petri nets and both associated transition systems satisfy $m \leq n \wedge \neg(\overline{m} \leq n)$ in m_0 and m'_0, respectively, it follows $m_0 = m'_0 = m$ and $\mathcal{P}$ and $\mathcal{P}'$ are equivalent.

Assume, that $\mathcal{D}(\mathcal{P})$ is the domain description which corresponds to the Petri net constructed in [4]. Then a model $\mathcal{M}$ satisfies

$$\pi' = Holds(g) \wedge \neg Holds(\overline{g}) \wedge$$
$$AG(X(t_{AB})\mathrm{T} \to X(t_{AB})EF \bigwedge_{t \in T} \neg Holds(St_t^= \circ St_t^-))$$

where $Holds(g) = \Psi_\mathcal{P}(m)$ and $Holds(\overline{g}) = \Psi_\mathcal{P}(\overline{m})$ for some $g, \overline{g} \in T_{St}(\emptyset)$, in situation $s_\mathcal{M}$ iff there is a model $\mathcal{M}'$ of $\mathcal{D}(\mathcal{P})$ such that $s0_{\mathcal{M}'}$ satisfies π' (note, that any two L–labelled transition systems for $\mathcal{D}(\mathcal{P})$ rooted in $s_\mathcal{M}$ and $s0_{\mathcal{M}'}$, respectively, where $|state_{\mathcal{M}'}(s0_{\mathcal{M}'}), f| = |state_\mathcal{M}(s_\mathcal{M}), f|$ for all $f \in T_F(\emptyset)$ are isomorphic). The transition system $K(\mathcal{M}')$ is bisimilar to $K(\mathcal{P})$, hence it satisfies π' iff $K(\mathcal{P})$ satisfies π. $\qquad\square$

Corollary 1. *There is a domain description $\mathcal{D}$ in $\mathcal{FC}_{PL}$ and a first order formula, such that the question whether this first order formula is entailed by $\mathcal{D}$, is undecidable.*

Proof. This follows easily from the fact, that for the above Petri net

$$\pi'' = (Holds(g) \wedge \neg Holds(\overline{g})) \to$$
$$AG(X(t_{AB})\mathrm{T} \to X(t_{AB})EF \bigwedge_{t \in T} \neg Holds(St_t^= \circ St_t^-))$$

is entailed by $\mathcal{D}$ iff π' is satisfied by $\mathcal{D}$ (due to the isomorphism mentioned in the previous proof). $\qquad\square$

Note, that the property described by the formula π'' in the above proof can be characterized as follows: "Whenever a certain action a is executable, after the execution of a, it is possible to reach a terminal state". Such propositions could, e.g., be of interest if the resource management of an operating system has to be verified. Furthermore, we can imagine a train entering a fail–safe mode. We might want to know, whether the train, after entering this mode, cannot change certain parameters anymore, e.g. increasing of speed is impossible. The undecidability of the entailment problem restricts the possibility of automated verification of such properties.

5 Decidable Properties in $\mathcal{FC}_{PL}$

Despite of these undecidable problems, important classes of CTL_{EF}–formulas can be decided. To simplify the presentation of the remaining results of this paper we define the set Λ_{Holds} containing all formulas of the form: $Holds(g^p) \wedge \neg Holds(g^n)$ where $g^p, g^n \in T_{St}(\emptyset)$.

Theorem 4. *Let $\mathcal{D}$ be an arbitrary domain description in $\mathcal{FC}_{PL}$. Then, the satisfiability of any formula of the form $\pi = \lambda_0 \wedge EF\lambda_e$ where $\lambda_0, \lambda_e \in \Lambda_{Holds}$ is decidable.*

Proof. We construct $\mathcal{D}'$ and a finite set of formulas Π', such that $\mathcal{D}'$ satisfies some formula $\pi' \in \Pi'$ iff $\mathcal{D}$ satisfies π. Then, we show that the question whether $\mathcal{D}'$ satisfies π' is decidable by reduction to the Petri net reachability problem which is known to be decidable ([9]).

Consider g_0^p, g_0^n to be the terms g^p, g^n of λ_0 and g_e^p, g_e^n to be the terms g^p, g^n of λ_e, respectively.

We define $F_0^n = \{f \mid f \in T_F(\emptyset) \wedge |g_0^n, f| = 0\}$ and $F_e^n = \{f \mid f \in T_F(\emptyset) \wedge |g_e^n, f| = 0\}$. These sets contain those fluents which can appear arbitrary often in the initial state described by λ_0 and in the final state described by λ_e. Now, we introduce a new signature Σ' containing the signature Σ of $\mathcal{D}$ and additionally, two sets, $A_0 = \{a_0^f \mid f \in F_0^n\}$ and $A_e = \{a_e^f \mid f \in F_e^n\}$, of new constants of type A. We augment the domain description $\mathcal{D}$ by the following state update axioms and call the resulting domain description $\mathcal{D}'$:

$\forall(s : S). \mathbf{T} \rightarrow state(do(a_0^f, s)) =_{St} state(s) \circ f$ for each $f \in F_0^n$, and
$\forall(s : S). Holds(f, s) \rightarrow f \circ state(do(a_e^f, s)) =_{St} state(s)$ for each $f \in F_e^n$.

We call the first set of state update axioms (those for F_0^n) SUA$_0$ and the second set of state update axioms (those for F_e^n) SUA$_e$. Now, let Π' be the set of formulas

$$Holds(g_0') \wedge \neg Holds(\overline{g_0'}) \wedge EF(Holds(g_e') \wedge \neg Holds(\overline{g_e'}))$$

for all $g_0', g_e' \in T_{St}(\emptyset)$ with $|g_0^n, f| > |g_0', f| \geq |g_0^p, f|$ for all $f \in T_F(\emptyset)$ where $f \notin F_0^n$ and $|g_0', f| = |g_0^p, f|$ for all $f \in F_0^n$, and $|g_e^n, f| > |g_e', f| \geq |g_e^p, f|$ for all $f \in T_F(\emptyset)$ where $f \notin F_e^n$ and $|g_e', f| = |g_e^p, f|$ for all $f \in F_e^n$.

Since every $\overline{g}$ contains each fluent at least once (see definition in proof to theorem 3), it follows that the set of all g' such that $\forall(z : St). g' \circ z \neq_{St} \overline{g}$ is finite, hence Π' is finite. Now, we show that whenever $\mathcal{D}$ satisfies π there is a $\pi' \in \Pi'$ such that $\mathcal{D}'$ satisfies π'. Assume, $\mathcal{D}$ satisfies π, i.e. there is a model $\mathcal{M}$ and a sequence of situations $s_0 s_1 \ldots s_n$ in $K(\mathcal{M})$ such that λ_0 is true in s_0 and λ_f is true in s_n. Since we did not remove any state update axioms it suffices to show, that there is a $\pi' \in \Pi'$, with the corresponding λ_0, λ_e denoted as $\lambda_0^{\pi'}$ and $\lambda_e^{\pi'}$, and a model $\mathcal{M}'$ of $\mathcal{D}'$ such that

1. there is a situation s_0' with $s_{-m}' \overset{a_{-m}}{\rightarrow} s_{-m}' \overset{a_{-m+1}}{\rightarrow} \ldots \overset{a_{-2}}{\rightarrow} s_{-1}' \overset{a_{-1}}{\rightarrow} s_0'$ such that $\lambda_0^{\pi'}$ holds in s_{-m}' and $|state_{\mathcal{M}}(s_0), f| = |state_{\mathcal{M}'}(s_0'), f|$ for all $f \in T_F(\emptyset)$, and

2. there is a situation s_{n+k}' with $s_n' \overset{a_n}{\rightarrow} s_{n+1}' \overset{a_{n+1}}{\rightarrow} \ldots \overset{a_{n+k-2}}{\rightarrow} s_{n+k-1}' \overset{a_{n+k-1}}{\rightarrow} s_{n+k}'$ such that $\lambda_e^{\pi'}$ holds in s_{n+k}' and $|state_{\mathcal{M}}(s_n), f| = |state_{\mathcal{M}'}(s_n'), f|$ for all $f \in T_F(\emptyset)$.

Assume, there is a situation s_0 fulfilling λ_0 and for a situation $s_{-m}' \in S_{\mathcal{M}'}$ for some model $\mathcal{M}'$ of $\mathcal{D}'$ the number n_f of each fluent f occurring in $state(s_{-m}')$ is given by $|g_0^p, f| \leq n_f < |g_0^n, f|$ if f occurs in g_0^n, and $|g_0^p, f| \leq n_f < |g_0^p, f| + 1$ otherwise (clearly, such a model exists if a model $\mathcal{M}$ exists). Then a situation $s_0' \in S_{\mathcal{M}'}$ such that $|state_{\mathcal{M}}(s_0), f| = |state_{\mathcal{M}'}(s_0'), f|$ for all fluents f can be reached by a finite number of transitions defined by axioms of SUA$_0$ (describing the actions $a_{-1}, \ldots, a_{-m}$). Similarly assume, there is a situation s_n fulfilling λ_e and for a situation $s_{n+k}' \in S_{\mathcal{M}'}$ for some model $\mathcal{M}'$ of $\mathcal{D}'$ the number n_f of each fluent f in $state(s_{n+k}')$ is given by $|g_e^p, f| \leq n_f < |g_e^n, f|$ if f occurs in g_e^n, and $|g_e^p, f| \leq n_f < |g_e^p, f| + 1$ otherwise (again, the $\mathcal{M}'$ exists if there is a model $\mathcal{M}$). Then a situation $s_n' \in S_{\mathcal{M}'}$ such that $|state_{\mathcal{M}}(s_n), f| = |state_{\mathcal{M}'}(s_n'), f|$ for all fluents f leads by a finite number of transitions defined by axioms of SUA$_e$ (describing actions $a_n, \ldots, a_{n+k-1}$) to the situation s_{n+k}'. According to construction of Π', there is a $\pi' \in \Pi'$ such that $\lambda_0^{\pi'}$ and $\lambda_e^{\pi'}$ determine the number of fluents correspondingly.

As a second step, we prove that whenever there is a $\pi' \in \Pi'$ such that $\mathcal{D}'$ satisfies π', $\mathcal{D}$ satisfies π. Suppose, that there is a model $\mathcal{M}'$ and a situation $s_{n+k}' =$

$do(a_{n+k-1}, do(a_{n+k-1}, \ldots, do(a_{-m}, s'_{-m}) \ldots))$ in $\mathcal{M}'$ such that $\lambda_0^{\pi'}$ is true in s'_{-m}, $\lambda_e^{\pi'}$ is true in s'_{n+k} and to determine $state_{\mathcal{M}'}(s'_{n+k})$, m denotes the number of transitions which are described by axioms SUA_0, k denotes the number of transitions which are described by axiom of SUA_e and n denotes the number of transitions which are described by all remaining state update axioms. Then, the following propositions hold:

1. There is a situation $s''_0 \in S_{\mathcal{M}'}$ such that $s''_{-m} \overset{a'_{-m}}{\to} s''_{-m} \overset{a'_{-m+1}}{\to} \ldots \overset{a'_{-2}}{\to} s''_{-1} \overset{a'_{-1}}{\to} s''_0$ where $a'_{-1}, \ldots a'_{-m}$ represent exactly those actions in s'_{n+k} with descriptions in SUA_0 and $\mathcal{M}' \models state(s''_{-m}) =_{St} state(s'_{-m})$. This is due to the fact, that an application of an axiom of SUA_0 strictly increases the number of some fluent, only. Hence, applications of axioms which were possible in situations containing smaller amounts of this fluent, are still possible after increasing the number. Furthermore, clearly, λ_0 is true in all such s''_0.

2. There is a situation $s''_n \in S_{\mathcal{M}'}$ such that $s''_n \overset{a'_n}{\to} s''_{n+1} \overset{a'_{n+1}}{\to} \ldots \overset{a'_{n+k-2}}{\to} s''_{n+k-1} \overset{a'_{n+k-1}}{\to} s''_{n+k}$ where $a'_n, \ldots a'_{n+k}$ represent exactly those actions in s'_{n+k} with descriptions in SUA_e and s''_n with $s''_0 \overset{a'_0}{\to} s''_1 \overset{a'_1}{\to} \ldots \overset{a'_{n-2}}{\to} s''_{n-1} \overset{a'_{n-1}}{\to} s''_n$ where $a'_0, \ldots, a'_{n-1}$ represent exactly those actions in s'_{n+k} with descriptions in SUA in the same order as they appear in s'_{n+k}. This is due to the fact, that an application of an axiom of SUA_e strictly decreases the number of some fluent, only. Hence, applications of axioms which were possible in situations containing greater amounts of this fluent, are still possible before decreasing the number. Note, that $\mathcal{M}' \models state(s''_{n+k}) =_{St} state(s'_{n+k})$ and clearly, λ_e is true in all such s''_n.

Since, $s''_0 \overset{a'_0}{\to} s''_1 \overset{a'_1}{\to} \ldots \overset{a'_{n-2}}{\to} s''_{n-1} \overset{a'_{n-1}}{\to} s''_n$ contains only actions of $\mathcal{D}$ and any pair s''_n and s''_0 fulfills λ_0 and λ_e, respectively, there is a model $\mathcal{M}$ of $\mathcal{D}$ and $s_0 \in S_{\mathcal{M}}$ and $s_n \in S_{\mathcal{M}}$ such that $|state_{\mathcal{M}}(s_0), f| = |state_{\mathcal{M}'}(s''_0), f|$ and $|state_{\mathcal{M}}(s_n), f| = |state_{\mathcal{M}'}(s''_n), f|$ for all fluents f and $s_0 \overset{a'_0}{\to} s_1 \overset{a'_1}{\to} \ldots \overset{a'_{n-2}}{\to} s_{n-1} \overset{a'_{n-1}}{\to} s_n$.

Finally, for every model $\mathcal{M}'$ of $\mathcal{D}'$ which satisfies some $\pi' \in \Pi'$ there is a model $\mathcal{M}''$ where π' is satisfied in $s0_{\mathcal{M}''}$. Hence, there exists a Petri net where $\mathcal{P}(\mathcal{D}', \mathcal{M}'') = (P, T, E, W, m_0)$ such that $\Psi_{\mathcal{M}''}(Holds(g'_0)) \leq m_0 < \Psi_{\mathcal{M}''}(Holds(g'_0))$ (i.e. $m_0 = m_{\mathcal{M}''}(g'_0)$). The formula π' is true in $\mathcal{M}''$ iff there is a sequence of actions $a_0, \ldots, a_{n-1}$ with $n \in \mathbb{N}$ such that $\lambda_e^{\pi'}$ holds in $s_n \in S_{\mathcal{M}''}$ with $s0_{\mathcal{M}''} \overset{a'_0}{\to} s_1 \overset{a'_1}{\to} \ldots \overset{a'_{n-2}}{\to} s_{n-1} \overset{a'_{n-1}}{\to} s_n$. Due to bisimilarity, such an action sequence exists iff there is a corresponding transition sequence in $\mathcal{P}$ such that $m_0 \overset{t_0}{\to} m_1 \overset{t_1}{\to} \ldots \overset{t_{n-1}}{\to} m_e$ and $\Psi_{\mathcal{M}''}(Holds(g'_e)) \leq m_e < \Psi_{\mathcal{M}''}(Holds(\overline{g'_e}))$ (i.e. $m_e = m_{\mathcal{M}''}(g'_e)$). The latter problem is called the *reachability problem* for Petri nets and is known to be decidable, [9]. □

Note, that the algorithm to decide Petri net reachability problems also allows the computation of an appropriate transition sequence.

Conclusions

In this paper we have shown a tight correspondence between models of a restricted fluent calculus, $\mathcal{FC}_{PL}$, and Petri nets. $\mathcal{FC}_{PL}$ is particular interesting since it can be seen as a minimal "core" of the fluent calculus. With the help of the relation to Petri net theory we were able to prove the undecidability of the entailment relation of a fairly restricted class of formulas of $\mathcal{FC}_{PL}$ characterized by the temporal logic CTL_{EF}. This is in contrast to similarly restricted situation calculi where entailment is decidable for a much larger class of temporal formulas [14]. However, as we have shown, some interesting non–trivial properties of systems specified in $\mathcal{FC}_{PL}$ can be automatically verified as well. Both results illustrate that the approach of applying Petri net theory to investigate properties of fluent calculi is very fruitful. Furthermore, the established relationship enables for applications of many efficient Petri net algorithms which exist for particular Petri nets and system properties, e.g. deciding coverability using the minimal coverability graph [5].

In the future, we plan to investigate the relation between other fragments of the fluent calculus and other net classes. E.g., due to the correspondence at the "core"–level, we expect relationships between less restrictive fluent calculi then $\mathcal{FC}_{PL}$ and Higher–Order Petri nets, e.g. coloured Petri nets and Predicate/Transition nets.

References

1. E. Allen Emerson and A. Prasad Sistla. Deciding full branching time logic. *Information and Control*, 61(3):175–201, June 1984.
2. E. Allen Emerson and J. Srinivasan. Branching time temporal logic. In J. W. de Bakker, W.-P. de Roever, and G. Rozenberg, editors, *Linear Time, Branching Time and Partial Order in Logics and Models for Concurrency*, number 354 in Lecture Notes in Computer Science, pages 123–172, Berlin-Heidelberg-New York, 1988. Springer.
3. Javier Esparza. On the decidability of model checking for several mu-calculi and petri nets. In *CAAP: Colloquium on Trees in Algebra and Programming*. LNCS 787, Springer-Verlag, 1994.
4. Javier Esparza. Decidability of model checking for infinite-state concurrent systems. *Acta Informatica*, 34(2):85–107, 1997.
5. A. Finkel. The minimal coverability graph for Petri nets. *Lecture Notes in Computer Science*, 674:210–243, 1993.
6. S. Hölldobler and J. Schneeberger. A new deductive approach to planning. *New Generation Computing*, 8:225–244, 1990.
7. S. Hölldobler and M. Thielscher. Computing change and specificity with equational logic programs. *Annals of Mathematics and Artificial Intelligence*, 14:99–133, 1995.
8. H. Lehmann. Embedding CTL* into fluent calculi. Technical report, University of Southampton, 1999.
9. Ernst W. Mayr. An algorithm for the general Petri net reachability problem. *SIAM Journal on Computing*, 13(3):441–460, 1984.
10. R. Milner. *Communication and Concurrency*. International Series in Computer Science. Prentice Hall, 1989. SU Fisher Research 511/24.
11. F. Pirri and R. Reiter. Some contributions to the metatheory of the situation calculus. *Journal of the ACM*, 46(3):325–361, May 1999.
12. Wolfgang Reisig. *Petri Nets - An Introduction*. Springer Verlag, 1982.
13. C. Stirling. *Handbook of Logic in Computer Science 2*, chapter Modal and Temporal Logics, pages 477–563. Oxford University Press, 1992.
14. E. Ternovskaia. Automata theory for reasoning about actions. In T. Dean, editor, *Proceedings of IJCAI*. Morgan Kaufmann, August 1999.
15. M. Thielscher. *Automatisiertes Schliessen ueber Kausalbeziehungen mit SLDENF-Resolution*. PhD thesis, Darmstadt University of Technology, 1994.

A Meta-logical Semantics for Features and Fluents Based on Compositional Operators over Normal Logic Programs

Vincenzo Pallotta

Theoretical Computer Science Laboratory (LITH)
Swiss Federal Institute of Technology - Lausanne
IN-F Ecublens 1015 Lausanne
Tel. +41-21-6935297,   Fax. +41-21-6935278
Vincenzo.Pallotta@epfl.ch

Abstract *Features & Fluents* is a logical framework proposed by Erik Sandewall for reasoning about action and change by means of a logical language called *discrete fluent logic* (DFL). In this paper we extend the Sandewall's framework for dealing with continuous time and we introduce a knowledge representation language based on a Horn-like fragment of DFL which we called *fluent logic programming*. A meta-logical semantics is described as the proof-theoretical counterpart of FLP in alternative to the Sandewall original *encapsulated semantics*. This semantics makes use of composition operators over general logic programs and can be also considered as an attempt of providing a basis for an effective implementation of a proof-system for a meaningful fragment of the *Features & Fluents* temporal logic.

1   Introduction

We focus on the logical framework *Features & Fluents* (F&F) [23] for describing and reasoning about action and change. *Features & Fluent* is essentially a logical framework for doing qualitative temporal reasoning about qualitative scenario descriptions: the *chronicles*. It also represents a *systematic framework* in which chronicles have been classified into a taxonomy in which epistemological and ontological assumptions are used to asses adequacy of proposed computational reasoning techniques.

1.1   Motivations

Our goal is to show how it is possible to use *logic programming* (LP) to provide a meta-logical semantics to a meaningful fragment of its underlying language *temporal feature logic* (TFL) that we called *Fluent Logic Programming* (FLP).

J. Lloyd et al. (Eds.): CL 2000, LNAI 1861, pp. 777–791, 2000.

The meta-logical semantics is defined by composing a suitable meta-representation of each FLP-statements with an inference engine which encodes its intended semantics. Another important issue is the treatment of non-determinism by means of parametric composition of partial FLP-theories (e.g. their meta-representation) which have been previously and separately generated. This approach is alternative to abduction which has been widely used in Event Calculus [9,26] and recently in Feature & Fluents [6]. From a logical point of view the two methods are equivalent since they can be shown being sound and complete with respect to the underlying semantics which provides an operational way for building intended models. The two approaches differ from a computational perspective since the computational overhead for computing and selecting models by abduction is factorized and performed only once. A proof procedure for abductive logic programming like the one proposed by Esghi and Kowalski in [11] would instead require all the time the generation of the possible models induced by the non-determinism and their successive selection by integrity constraints. We argued that in certain conditions it is possible to perform this step in advance generating a collection of partial theories corresponding to the non-deterministic part of the chronicle which can be composed to deterministic part when proving a certain goal. It is almost always the case that integrity constraints will greatly reduce the set of possible models. Furthermore, using this technique, inconsistent chronicles can be statically recognized.

2   Backgrounds

In order to keep this paper self contained, in this preliminary section we informally provide some little backgrounds about techniques we will use in the rest of the paper.

2.1   Feature and Fluents

This concise and informal introduction aims to give just an intuition about the underlying ideas of *Features & Fluents*. In the rest of the paper we will make use of the following concepts without directly referring to their original meaning even if a strong relation may be apparent. F&F makes use of the following syntactic categories for representing *scenario description* (e.g. *chronicles*):

Features. A *feature* f is a first order term which denotes a property of a class of objects that constitute a scenario (e.g. $color(traffic\_light\_\#1)$), that is a function from the object domain $\mathcal{O}$ to the set of feature values $\mathcal{V}$. The features domain is denoted by $\mathcal{F}$ and for each $f \in \mathcal{F}$, $\mathcal{V}(f)$ denotes the *codomain* of f. $\mathcal{V}(f)$ is thus the set of all possible values for the feature f (e.g. $\mathcal{V}(color(X)) = \{red, yellow, green\}$).

Fluents. A *fluent* $[t]f$ is a first order term which represents a function from time-points to corresponding feature values, and it can be thought of as the trace over time of a particular feature (e.g. $[3]color(traffic\_light\_\#1)$).

Actions. An *action* occurrence $[s, t]a$ happens over an interval of time $[s, t]$ through the intervention of an agent and the action designators domain is denoted by $\mathcal{E}$ (e.g. $[2, 3]switch(traffic\_light\_\#1)$).

At the semantic level, the models of chronicles are represented by *histories*, which are (possibly partial) functions of type $R : \mathcal{T} \times \mathcal{F} \rightarrow \mathcal{V}$ where $\mathcal{T}$ is the time domain, $\mathcal{F}$ is the features domain and $\mathcal{V}$ is the feature-values domain. The set of histories is denoted by $\mathcal{H}$. If a specific feature f is chosen, then the resulting function of time $R(f) : \mathcal{T} \rightarrow \mathcal{V}$ is a *fluent*. Similarly, if a specific time-point t is chosen, then the function obtained $R(t) : \mathcal{F} \rightarrow \mathcal{V}$ is a *state*. The set of *partial states* (e.g. partial functions of type $\mathcal{F} \rightarrow \mathcal{V}$) is denoted by $\mathcal{R}$.

Underlying Semantics. In order to build the intended models of a chronicle (i.e. the possible histories) Sandewall introduces the notion of *underlying semantics* as a game between two players: an *Ego* (e.g. the agent) and a *World* (e.g. the environment). The Ego-World interaction incrementally updates a structure called *finite development* which keeps track of all action occurrences and feature changes over an interval of time $[0, s]$. Let $\mathcal{J}$ be the domain of all possible finite developments. Then we can formally define the Ego **K** and the World **W** as mappings (or transformations) from $\mathcal{J}$ to $\mathcal{J}$ with the special properties that **K** preserves the interval $[0, s]$ over which the development is defined, and **W** extends $[0, s]$ to $[0, s']$ where $s < s'$. Since the *finite history* R (e.g. a history restricted to the closed interval $[0, s]$) is the main information contained in a finite development J, we do not consider here the whole structure J as in the original Sandewall's work[1]. The way a finite history R is gradually extended by an Ego-World game is specified by a system of rules coded by a so called *underlying semantics*. We propose here an adapted version of the Sandewall's *encapsulated semantics* as our underlying semantics, that is a pair $\langle$**Infl, Rstat**$\rangle$ which specifies how the World has to extend the history when an action is carried out by the Ego. The function **Infl** $: \mathcal{E} \times \mathcal{R} \rightarrow 2^{\mathcal{F}}$ specifies a set of features which are influenced by a particular action executed in a particular state. **Rstat** $: \mathcal{E} \times \mathcal{R} \rightarrow 2^{\mathcal{R}}$ specifies a set of states resulting from the successful execution of an action (e.g. action pre-conditions are fulfilled in the given state). Given a state $R(s)$ where $s \in \mathcal{T}$ and an action instance $[s, t]a$, where $a \in \mathcal{E}$, invoked by the Ego then a resulting state r_j is non-deterministically chosen from **Rstat**$(E, R(s)) = \{r_1, \ldots, r_k\}$. The new history R' is obtained from the previous one, R, in the following way:

---

[1] Formally a development J is defined as a 5-tuple $\langle \mathcal{B}, M, R, \mathcal{A}, C \rangle$ where $\mathcal{B}$ is the set of breakpoints (e.g. time-points where persistence is broken), M is an interpretation of constant symbols, R is a finite history, $\mathcal{A}$ is the past action set (e.g. actions performed until the last breakpoint) and C is the set of not yet terminated actions. This structure accounts for a more general notion of scenario. For all details refer to [23].

- $\forall \tau \in (0, s] : R'(\tau) = R(\tau)$
- $f \notin \mathbf{Infl}(a, R(s)) \Rightarrow \forall \tau \in (s, t] : R'(f, \tau) = R(f, \tau)$
- $f \in \mathbf{Infl}(a, R(s)) \Rightarrow (R'(f, t) = r_j(f) \wedge \forall \tau \in (s, t) : R'(f, \tau) = \perp$

Note that the resulting history R' is undefined (e.g. denoted by the symbol $\perp$) for influenced features in $\mathbf{Infl}(a, R(s))$ during the interval (s, t). Any Ego-World game is started in a state denoted by $R(0)$ which contains the initial, possibly partial, knowledge about values of involved features. The above *encapsulated semantics* defines the class $\mathcal{K}\text{-}\mathbf{ReA}^2$ of scenarios descriptions in the Sandewall's taxonomy.

2.2   Logic Programming

The language of logic programs with negation (i.e. general logic programs) will be used here as meta-language for representing FLP-chronicles. FLP is considered the object language which can be mapped into a meta-representation by means of syntactic transformations. We will show how to exploit an existing standard proof procedure for general logic programs to build a proof system for FLP. We assume the reader to be familiar with classical theory of logic programming languages (e.g. logical, fix-point and SLD procedural semantics). More details can be found in [1,14].

General Logic Programs. The underlying language of general (or normal) logic programs is a first order language of terms. Constants and functions are denoted by small letters while variables are capital letters. Terms are constructed in the usual way as in the corresponding first order language. Atoms have the form $p(t_1, \ldots t_n)$, where each t_i is a term and p is a predicate symbol of arity n. A *rule* (or *general clause*) is a statement of the form: $L_0 \leftarrow L_1, \ldots, L_m$ where each L_i is a literal, that is either an atom A_i or its negation *not* A_i for each $i = 1, \ldots, m$ and $m \geq 0$, while $L_0 = A_0$ (e.g. the head of a rule cannot be negated). In the case of $m = 0$ we have unary clauses or *facts*. A literal of the form *not* A is called *negative*. A set of rules is called *general logic program*. General logic programs without any negative literal are called *definite (or positive) logic programs* and their rules are called *definite Horn clauses*. Rules and terms with no variables are called *ground*. A formula Q of the form: $L_1, \ldots, L_n$ with literals L_i is called *query*. A query $L_1, \ldots, L_n$ denotes the formula $\exists \overline{X} : L_1 \wedge \ldots \wedge L_n$ where $\overline{X} = X_1, \ldots, X_k$ is the set of free variables occurring in the query. The set of all constant, function and predicate symbols used in a program P is referred as the *language of* P (e.g. $\mathcal{L}(P)$).

---

[2] The class $\mathcal{K}\text{-}\mathbf{ReA}$ is the extension of the $\mathcal{K}\text{-}\mathbf{IeA}$ class treated in *F&F* for dealing with continuous time. The ontological designator $\mathbf{ReA}$ denotes inertial scenarios with sequentially executed actions whose alternatives are completely and uniquely specified by theirs preconditions and results. The sub-specialty e stands for "encapsulated actions" [18]. A larger class $\mathcal{K}\text{-}\mathbf{RACi}$ (e.g. with indipendent concurrent actions) has been formally defined by Brandano in [6].

Negation in Logic Programming. In the classical formulation of semantics for negation in logic programming we make use of the *Closed World Assumption*, where we can assume as false everything that is not a logical consequence of what is explicitly said to be true. This kind of assumption induces a form of non-monotonic reasoning since if the truth of A depends on the absence of information about the truth of B, just adding the knowledge that B is true, we cannot infer that A is still true. We will make use of the following concept:

- The *Clark's negation as finite failure* [8], where $notQ$ is entailed by a program P if every SLD derivation for the query Q finitely fails.
- The *Clark's completion* of a general logic program $comp(P)$.

We consider here an extension of the SLD decision procedure for dealing with negation as a finite failure: the SLDNF procedure. This procedure has been shown to be sound and complete with respect to a 3-valued logical semantics modeled on the Clark completion and suitable for a meaningful subclass of general logic programs (e.g. the *allowed* programs[3]). All the backgrounds required about negation in logic programming can be found in [2].

Composing General Logic Programs. This section briefly summarizes the main results proposed in [7] about a compositional semantics for *general logic program expressions*. Expressions make use of composition operators and they induce an *algebra* of general logic programs. We focus here only on the *union* operator. Operators are defined syntactically by the following transformation τ which maps general logic programs expressions into plain general logic programs:

$$\tau(P) = P \qquad if\ P\ is\ a\ general\ logic\ program$$
$$\tau(E \cup F) = \{A \leftarrow \overline{L} \mid (A \leftarrow \overline{L}) \in \tau(E) \vee (A \leftarrow \overline{L}) \in \tau(F)\}$$

The union of two logic programs is just the union of their clauses.

The Fitting 3-valued semantics [13] for general logic programs can be extended to general program expressions in the following manner: If $\Phi_p(I) = (J^+, J^-)$, then let be

$$\Phi_P^+(I) = J^+$$
$$\Phi_P^-(I) = J^-.$$

Moreover , if J is an Herbrand interpretation, then the *extension* of J with respect to HB_P (e.g. the Herbrand base of P) is given by:

$$Ext(J) = \{p(\bar{t}) \mid p(\bar{t}) \in HB_P \wedge \exists \bar{u} : p(\bar{u}) \in J\}$$

---

[3] A query $\leftarrow \overline{L} \equiv \leftarrow L_1, \ldots, L_n$ is *allowed* if each variable occurs in positive literals. A clause $A \leftarrow \overline{L}$ is *allowed* if $\leftarrow (not\ A, \overline{L})$ is allowed. A program is *allowed* if all its clauses are allowed.

Let E_1, E_2 be two general logic program expressions and let I be a 3-valued interpretation. Then for the case of the union operator we define:

$$\Phi_{E_1 \cup E_2}(I) = ((\Phi_{E_1}^+(I) \cup \Phi_{E_2}^+(I)), (\Phi_{E_1}^-(I) \cap \Phi_{E_2}^-(I)))$$

The above definition defines a compositional semantics for general logic program expressions. Furthermore in [7] the following results have been shown:

- Let E be a general logic program expression, then for any 3-valued Herbrand interpretation I: $\Phi_E(I) = \Phi_{\tau(E)}(I)$.
- Let E be a program expression over allowed general logic programs, then $\tau(E)$ is an allowed general logic program.

Combining these results with the soundness and completeness theorems of SLDNF proof procedure with respect to the 3-valued Fitting semantics and Clark completion (see [2]), we have that if E is a program expression over allowed general logic programs and $\overline{L}$ is a allowed query, then:

- $\exists m < \omega \; : \; \Phi_E^m(\emptyset) \models_3 \overline{L} \quad \Leftrightarrow \quad \exists m < \omega \; : \; \Phi_{\tau(E)}^m(\emptyset) \models_3 \overline{L} \quad \Leftrightarrow$
  $comp(\tau(E)) \models_3 \overline{L}$
- ϑ is a computed answer substitution such that $\tau(E) \vdash_{SLDNF} \overline{L}\vartheta \quad \Leftrightarrow$
  $comp(\tau(E)) \models_3 \forall \overline{L}\vartheta$
- $\exists n < \omega : \Phi_E^n \models_3 L \quad \Leftrightarrow \quad \exists \vartheta : \tau(E) \vdash_{SLDNF} L\vartheta$.

2.3 Event Calculus

The *event calculus* (EC) [17,22] is a logic programming based formalism capable of dealing with events occurring within time periods and with properties of objects which can persist or change over time. EC is based on the following ontologies or domains: the temporal domain $\mathcal{T}$ is an algebraic structure with a linear order relation $<$ and equality, the properties or features domain $\mathcal{F}$ and the action tokens or events domain $\mathcal{E}$. A *scenario description* is presented by defining the following predicates: *happens* : $\mathcal{E} \times \mathcal{T}$ specifies the occurrence of an event at a certain time-point, *initiates* : $\mathcal{E} \times \mathcal{F}$ and *terminates* : $\mathcal{E} \times \mathcal{F}$ specify the effects of the successful execution of a certain action, *holdsat* : $\mathcal{F} \times \mathcal{T}$ specifies the truth value of a property at a given time-point. The core inference engine is based on the definition of the following rules and relies on the interpretation of negation as finite failure [8]:

$$holdsat(F, T) \leftarrow happens(E, T_1), \qquad clipped(T_1, F, T_2) \leftarrow happens(E, T),$$
$$initiates(E, F), \qquad\qquad\qquad terminates(E, F),$$
$$T_1 < T, \qquad\qquad\qquad\qquad T_1 \leq T, T < T_2.$$
$$not\; clipped(T_1, F, T).$$

In the above definition some epistemological and ontological assumptions are made. In our opinion the most remarkable are the following: (i) only instantaneous actions, (ii) absence of explicit non-determinism, (iii) no partial knowledge and no temporal post-diction. However there are some successful attempts in order to overcome these problems like in [15,25]. An extended version of EC will be used as the basis of the meta-logical semantics for FLP that allows the treatment of non-instantaneous actions.

3 Fluent Logic Programming

Fluent logic programming (FLP) is a slightly modified fragment of Sandewall's TFL. Since we want this language to be effectively implemented, a natural choice is to turn the original full first order predicate calculus language into a *Horn clause-like* one.

Definition 1. *An FLP-chronicle Υ is a collection of statements of the following categories:*

- **Law** *action laws are statement of the two possible forms:*
  - *Deterministic action*

$$[S,T]a \Rrightarrow (f_1 = v_1, \ldots, f_n = v_n) \Rightarrow f := v$$

  - *Non-deterministic action*

$$[S,T]a \Rrightarrow (f_1 = v_1, \ldots, f_n = v_n) \Rightarrow f := [w_1, \ldots, w_k]$$

- **Scd** *action occurrences, are statements of the form:* $[s,t]a$
- **Obs** *observations are statements of the form:* $[t]f = v$

where $a \in \mathcal{E}$, $f, f_1, \ldots, f_n \in \mathcal{F}$, $v, v_1, \ldots, v_n, w_1, \ldots, w_k \in \mathcal{V}$, $s, t \in \mathcal{T}$ and S, T are variables ranging on $\mathcal{T}$.

We have used the meta-symbols a for denoting an action instance, $f, f_1, f_2, \ldots$ for denoting feature names, $v, v_1, \ldots, v_m$ and $w_1, \ldots w_k$ for denoting feature values and s, t for temporal constants in the time structure $\mathcal{T}$. Actions, features and feature values are first order terms while the time structure $\mathcal{T}$ is essentially $(\mathbb{R}^+, \leq)$. We use the symbol $\mathcal{F}_\Upsilon$ for denoting the set of the feature names occurring in the chronicle Υ. As usual capital case is used for logic programming variables. We can partition each FLP-chronicle Υ into three subsets of statements (e.g. $\Upsilon = \mathbf{Law} \cup \mathbf{Scd} \cup \mathbf{Obs}$) according with their syntactical categories. The intuitive reading is that given an instance of an action $[s,t]a$ in **Scd**, the action a is performed during the time interval $[s,t]$. The actions laws in **Law** represent the pre-conditions and the effects of action occurrence. Pre-conditions are expressed as a conjunction of equalities to be checked at the starting time-point of the action duration interval. Effects are expressed as assignments (e.g. using the symbol ":=") of one or more feature values to a feature[4]. If there exists an action law in **Law** whose head (on the left of the symbol "$\Rrightarrow$") unifies with an

---

[4] We will consider the := operator as a syntactic constructor.

action occurrence, we can simply replace it with the body of the action law (on the right of the symbol "$\Rightarrow$"), substituting the variables with the terms occurring in the action occurrence. This step can be expressed by the following rule:

$$\frac{[s,t]act(t_1,\ldots t_n) \in \mathbf{Scd},\ [S,T]act(X_1,\ldots,X_n) \Rightarrow (Pre \Rightarrow Post) \in \mathbf{Law}}{(Pre \Rightarrow Post)\theta \in \mathbf{Law[Scd]}}$$

where $\theta = [s/S, t/T, t_1/X_1, \ldots, t_1/X_n]$ is a set of variable substitutions.

Applying this "unfolding" step to each action in **Scd** we obtain an expanded version of the original chronicle where **Law** and **Scd** are merged in a new set of statements called **Law[Scd]**. Each action instance $[s,t]a$ is then rewritten according to the matching action law in the form:

$$[s,t](f_1 = v_1, \ldots, f_n = v_n) \Rightarrow f := v$$

or in the non-deterministic case:

$$[s,t](f_1 = v_1, \ldots, f_n = v_n) \Rightarrow f := [w_1, \ldots, w_k].$$

According to the encapsulated semantics, the value of the affected feature is undefined during the period of time in which an action is executed. The set of observation statements **Obs** is used to assert constraints to the scenario description. It is assumed that the dynamical part of the chronicle (i.e. **Law** and **Scd**) is consistent with the observations (e.g. epistemological designator $\mathcal{K}$ in the class $\mathcal{K}$-**ReA**). Furthermore a feature cannot be observed having more than one feature value at the same time. Epistemological assumptions provide a general way of defining the chronicles well-formedness. Using the following definition it is always possible to provide an encapsulated semantics for each FLP-chronicles thus characterizing the operational behavior of the corresponding Ego-World game.

Definition 2 (FLP Encapsulated Semantics).

Let $\Upsilon = \mathbf{Law} \cup \mathbf{Scd} \cup \mathbf{Obs}$ be a FLP-chronicle. The encapsulated semantics for Υ is characterized by the pair $\langle \mathbf{Infl}, \mathbf{Rstat} \rangle$ such that for each action occurrence $[s,t]a \in \mathbf{Scd}$ and its corresponding law instance: $[s,t](f_1 = v_1, \ldots, f_n = v_n) \Rightarrow f := [w_1, \ldots, w_k] \in \mathbf{Law[Scd]}$, if R is a history such that $\forall i \in \{1, \ldots, n\}$: $R(s, f_i) = v_i$ then $f \in \mathbf{Infl}(a, R(s))$ and $\forall j \in \{1, \ldots, k\}$: $\exists! r_j \in \mathbf{Rstat}(a, R(s))$ such that $r_j(f) = w_j$.

This definition extends a similar definition of the encapsulated semantics for the class $\mathcal{K}$-**IeA** proposed in [23]. Observe that any initial state $R(0)$ must satisfy the constraint that for each $f \in \mathcal{F}_\Upsilon$ such that $[0]f := v \in \mathbf{Obs}$ there exists a unique value v such that $R(0, f) = v$.

3.1   Non-deterministic Chronicles

The set of possible histories for a chronicle Υ represents the set of its *intended models* and it is denoted by $\Sigma_{\mathcal{K}-\mathbf{ReA}}(\Upsilon)$ if the chronicle Υ belongs to the $\mathcal{K}$-**ReA** class in the Sandewall's taxonomy. A *deterministic chronicle* has only one intended model (e.g. its complete history) while *non-deterministic chronicles*, may have multiple intended models (e.g. deterministic histories consistent with observations). Rather than using the encapsulated semantics to generate the set of intended models, we can suitably transform our FLP-chronicle in order to use a simpler deterministic resulting state function (e.g. **Rstat** $: \mathcal{E} \times \mathcal{R} \rightarrow \mathcal{R}$). The intended model set $\Sigma^{FLP}_{\mathcal{K}-\mathbf{ReA}}(\Upsilon)$ is thus generated by a set of deterministic histories. Each deterministic history is obtained by composing the original FLP-chronicle with a partial deterministic FLP-theory (which contains only action law's instances) taken from a set called *hypothetical theories set* $Hyp(\Upsilon)$. $Hyp(\Upsilon)$ contains deterministic FLP-theories build as a combination of features assignments taken from each occurring non-deterministic actions. In this fashion, incomplete knowledge about the initial state can be modeled as a special case of non-determinism: a dummy instantaneous non-deterministic action with no pre-conditions is executed at time-point 0, assigning all possible values to each feature for which there is no initial knowledge (e.g. no initial observations). More formally the *hypothetical theories set* is characterized by the following definition:

Definition 3 (Hypothetical Theories Set).

Given a FLP-chronicle $\Upsilon = \mathbf{Law} \cup \mathbf{Scd} \cup \mathbf{Obs}$ *let be*

$$\mathbf{InitScd} = \{[0,0]initially(f) \mid f \in \mathcal{F}_\Upsilon \wedge [0]f = v \notin \mathbf{Obs}\}$$

$$\mathbf{InitLaw} = \{[s,t]initially(f) \Rightarrow f := [w_1, \ldots, w_n] \mid$$
$$f \in \mathcal{F}_\Upsilon$$
$$\wedge [0]f = v \notin \mathbf{Obs}$$
$$\wedge \{w_1, \ldots, w_n\} = \mathcal{V}(f)\}$$

and let the expansion of the statements in **InitScd** *w.r.t.* **InitLaw** *be:*

$$\mathbf{InitLaw[InitScd]} = \{[0,0]f := [w_1, \ldots w_n] \mid f \in \mathcal{F}_\Upsilon \wedge$$
$$\wedge [0]f = v \notin \mathbf{Obs}$$
$$\wedge \{w_1, \ldots, w_n\} = \mathcal{V}(f)\}.$$

The hypothetical theories set *is defined by:*

$$Hyp(\Upsilon) = \{\{[s_1, t_1]Pre_1 \Rightarrow f_1 := w_1, \ldots, [s_n, t_n]Pre_n \Rightarrow f_n := w_n\} \mid$$
$$\forall i = 1, \ldots, n :$$
$$[s_i, t_i]Pre_i \Rightarrow f_i := [v_1, \ldots, v_{k_i}] \in \mathbf{Law[Scd]} \cup \mathbf{InitLaw[InitScd]}$$
$$\wedge \bigvee_{j=1}^{k_i} w_i = v_j\}$$

where Pre_i *denotes an action pre-condition of the form* $f_1^i = v_1^i, \ldots, f_{n_i}^i = v_{n_i}^i$.

$Hyp(\Upsilon)$ must be further restricted to those hypotheses which are consistent with the observations made after the initial time-point and it is obtained by keeping only those theories which generate histories containing all the triples $\langle f, v, t \rangle$

corresponding to each non-initial observation $[t]f = v$ in **Obs**[5] (i.e. such that $t > 0$):

Definition 4. *Let by $\overline{\Upsilon}$ be the FLP-chronicle obtained by Υ by removing all non-deterministic action laws from* **Law** *and all non-deterministic action occurrences from* **Scd***, then*

$$Hyp(\Upsilon)\,|_{\mathbf{Obs}} = \{hyp \in Hyp(\Upsilon)|\,\forall f, v, t > 0 :$$
$$([t]f = v \in \mathbf{Obs} \Rightarrow \exists R \in \Sigma_{\mathcal{K}-\mathbf{ReA}}(\overline{\Upsilon} \setminus \mathbf{Obs} \cup hyp) : R(f,t) = v\}$$

The intended model set for a FLP-chronicle Υ is defined as:

$$\Sigma_{\mathcal{K}-\mathbf{ReA}}^{FLP}(\Upsilon) = \Sigma_{\mathcal{K}-\mathbf{ReA}}(\overline{\Upsilon}) \cup \bigcup_{h \in Hyp(\Upsilon)|_{\mathbf{Obs}}} \Sigma_{\mathcal{K}-\mathbf{ReA}}(\overline{\Upsilon} \setminus \mathbf{Obs} \cup hyp)$$

As it can be easily observed, an implementation for the above approach needs a suitable way of composing logical theories in order to generate systematically exactly all the intended models of a non-deterministic FLP-chronicle. It is worthwhile to remark that this solution may seem like an immensely complex alternative to the way in which open theories are usually dealt with in logic programming: on the open predicates just give an integrity constraint providing all possible hypotheses in disjunction. Even simpler: just define something to be open (e.g. abducible predicates) and let abductive procedures propose some consistent closures of the theory. A solution of this kind as been adopted in [6]. On the other hand we argued that equivalent answers can be computed more efficiently using a pre-compiled set of consistent hypothesis rather than computing them every time they are needed in the query processing. However an abductive semantics for FLP is currently under investigation (see [19]).

4   Meta-logical Semantics for FLP

In our investigation summarized in [18] we also provide a transformational meta-logical implementation of FLP, where FLP-theories are transformed into *normal logic programs*. The meta-representation of Υ is denoted by $\pi(\Upsilon)$. Furthermore we add a core inference engine Λ which can be thought as an extension of the *event calculus* inference engine. Instantaneous events have been replaced by extended duration actions and properties have been generalized by features and considered as being their particular case (i.e. boolean valued features). The meta-level representation of the chronicle Υ, completed by Λ, is composed with each element of the meta-representation of *hypothetical theory set* $\pi(Hyp(\Upsilon)|_{\mathbf{Obs}})$. The use of the compositional operator $\cup$ is crucial here since it allows to compose one hypothetical theory at a time with the meta-representation of the chronicle.

---

[5] More details in [18,21]

4.1 Meta-logical Representation of FLP-Chronicles

We provide here the meta representation of a FLP-chronicle together with a mapping for each object-level FLP-statement:

Observations

$$\pi([0]f = v) = initially(f, v).$$

Deterministic Action Laws

$$\pi([S, T]action \Rightarrow (f_1 = v_1, \ldots, f_n = v_n) \Rightarrow f := v)) =$$

$$change(f, v, T) \leftarrow occurs(S, T, action),$$
$$success(f, S, T, action).$$
$$success(f, S, T, action) \leftarrow holds(f_1, v_1, S),$$
$$\vdots$$
$$holds(f_n, v_n, S).$$

Non-deterministic Action Laws

$$\pi([S, T])action \Rightarrow (f_1 = v_1, \ldots, f_n = v_n) \Rightarrow f := [w_1, \ldots, w_k])) =$$

$$success(f, S, T, action) \leftarrow holds(f_1, v_1, S),$$
$$\vdots$$
$$holds(f_n, v_n, S).$$

Action Instance

$$\pi([s, t]action) = occurs(s, t, action).$$

Core Inference Rules

$$\Lambda \equiv change(F, V, 0) \leftarrow initially(F, V).$$
$$holds(F, V, Tau) \leftarrow change(F, V, Tau).$$
$$holds(F, V, Tau) \leftarrow$$
$$\qquad not\ occluded(F, Tau),$$
$$\qquad change(F, V, T_1),$$
$$\qquad T_1 < Tau,$$
$$\qquad not\ clipped(F, T_1, Tau).$$
$$occluded(F, Tau) \leftarrow$$
$$\qquad occurs(S, T, A),$$
$$\qquad success(F, S, T, A),$$
$$\qquad S < Tau, Tau \leq T.$$
$$clipped(F, S, Tau) \leftarrow$$
$$\qquad occurs(S_1, T_1, A),$$
$$\qquad success(F, S_1, T_1, A)$$
$$\qquad S \leq S_1, T_1 < Tau.$$

The predicate *occluded*[6] is true for the feature f at a time-point τ if there is an action $[s, t]a$ influencing f which *occurs* in an interval $[s, t]$ that contains τ. The *success* of its execution depends on its pre-conditions. A feature f is *clipped* in sub-interval $[t, \tau]$ if there exists a successfully executed action influencing f during a sub-interval $[s', t') \subseteq [t, \tau]$. We can check whether an action influences a feature f by verifying that there exists an action instance changing its value at a given time-point. This leads to the definition of the predicate *change*. The four possible situations in which we can ask for deducing a value for a feature f at a certain time-point τ are graphically represented in the following diagram:

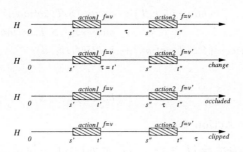

In the first line (from above) at the time-point τ the conditions:

$$\neg occluded(f, \tau) \wedge change(f, v, t') \wedge \neg clipped(f, t', \tau) \wedge t' < \tau$$

holds. In the remaining lines hold respectively $change(f, v, \tau)$, $occluded(f, \tau)$ and $clipped(f, t', \tau)$.

Hypothetical Theories

$$\pi(Hyp(\Upsilon)) = \{$$
$$\{change(f_1, v_1, t_1) \leftarrow success(f_1, s_1, t_1, act_1),$$

$$\vdots \qquad \vdots$$

$$change(f_n, v_n, t_n) \leftarrow success(f_n, s_n, t_n, act_n)\}$$
$$\mid \{[s_1, t_1]Pre_1 \Rightarrow f_1 := w_1, \dots, [s_n, t_n]Pre_n \Rightarrow f_n := w_n\} \in Hyp(\Upsilon)\}$$

Constrained Hypothetical Theories

$$\pi(Hyp(\Upsilon)|_{\mathbf{Obs}}) =$$
$$\{hyp \in \pi(Hyp(\Upsilon)) \mid$$
$$\forall[t]f = v \in \mathbf{Obs}:$$
$$\exists n < \omega : \Phi^n_{\tau(\pi(\Upsilon) \cup \Lambda \cup hyp)} \models_3 holds(f, v, t)\}.$$

---

[6] The term *occluded* has been introduced by Sandewall in the *Features & Fluent* terminology meaning that the value of a fluent is unknown at a given time-point (i.e. is changing during the execution of an action).

4.2   Soundness and Completeness

In [18] we show that using the above meta-representation for FLP-chronicles we obtain proof-theoretically exactly all the intended models (histories) computed by means of the Sandewall's *encapsulated semantics*. In order to prove it, we propose an alternative fix-point semantics which is based on a so called *inertia immediate consequence operator*. This operator is defined over a cpo of well-formed histories and produces as its fix-point exactly the same intended models captured operationally by the Sandewall's *encapsulated semantics*. The following theorem provides a sound theoretical foundation for our meta-logical implementation of a proof-procedure for FLP.

Theorem 1. *Let* $\Upsilon = \mathbf{Law} \cup \mathbf{Scd} \cup \mathbf{Obs}$ *be a FLP-chronicle,* $\pi(\Upsilon)$ *be its meta-level representation, then*

$$\exists R \in \Sigma^{FLP}_{\mathcal{K}-\mathbf{ReA}}(\Upsilon) : R(f,t) = v \Leftrightarrow \exists n < \omega : \Phi_{\tau(\pi(\Upsilon) \cup \Lambda)} \models_3 holds(f,v,t) \vee$$
$$\exists hyp \in \pi(Hyp(\Upsilon)|_{\mathbf{Obs}}) :$$
$$\exists n < \omega : \Phi^n_{\tau(\pi(\Upsilon) \cup \Lambda \cup hyp)} \models_3 holds(f,v,t).$$
$$\Leftrightarrow \tau(\pi(\Upsilon) \cup \Lambda) \vdash_{SLDNF} holds(f,v,t) \vee$$
$$\exists hyp \in \pi(Hyp(\Upsilon)|_{\mathbf{Obs}}) :$$
$$\tau(\pi(\Upsilon) \cup \Lambda \cup hyp) \vdash_{SLDNF} holds(f,v,\tau).$$

Proof. in [18]. It easy to check that our programs are allowed. Furthermore the proof uses an intermediate results which is based on a fix-point semantics for FLP. This fix-point semantics has been shown to be equivalent to the *encapsulated semantics* and it is the model theoretic counterpart of the above meta-logical semantics. More details about the fix-point semantics can be found in [21,20].

5   Conclusions

In this paper we presented a meta-logical semantics for FLP-chronicles belonging to the class $\mathcal{K} - \mathbf{ReA}$ of scenario descriptions in the Sandewall's F&F taxonomy. On the one hand the meta-logical semantics provides the basis for an effective implementation of a proof-system for FLP. On the other hand, it leads to an integration of non-monotonic temporal reasoning and logic programming towards an effective knowledge representation language.

To be more precise, we were dealing only with *ground* scenarios (i.e. the $\mathcal{K}g - \mathbf{ReA}$ class), where we do not allow the use of any global variable and partially specified action instances where variables appear in the duration interval. However we proposed an *abductive semantics* that solves scenarios with non-ground temporal components. Even if we did not provide completeness results, it seems reasonably adequate for treating this kind of problem. We have also implemented an abductive procedure starting from the well-known work of

Esghi-Kowalski [11] and extended it with a restricted and "ad-hoc" tailored form of constructive negation [10]. By combining it with constraint solving capabilities the system will abduce temporal constraints for the duration of a partially specified action instance. Preliminary results are available in [19]. Further extensions will make use of more powerful implementation strategies, like for instance abductive constraint logic programming [16].

The meta-logical semantics can be also extended to cover the full class $\mathcal{K} - \mathbf{RA}$ [7] and for dealing with continuous changes (i.e. *trajectories*) in a way similar to that proposed by [24]. The hypothetical theories method applies also to this case. A first prototype of this system has been successfully implemented in SICStus PROLOG and described in [18] and makes use of a meta-interpreter for general logic program expressions.

Among possible future and related works we envision that reasoning about action and change, and FLP in particular, can be fruitfully applied to computational natural language semantics as an alternative approach to epistemic actions [4] in the context of the View-Finder system for managing reasoning about agents mutual beliefs [3]. Moreover we are also investigating on temporal modeling of multimedia applications [12] and reasoning about properties of logical reactive systems [5]. We consider the results obtained so far quite encouraging and, we think this method will provide a sound basis of future developments for suitably dealing with these possible applications.

References

1. Krzysztof R. Apt. Logic Programming. In J. van Leeuwen, editor, *Handbook of Theoretical Computer Science*, volume B. Elsevier, 1990.
2. Krzysztof R. Apt and Roland N. Bol. Logic programming and negation: A survey. *The Journal of Logic Programming*, 19 & 20:9–72, May 1994.
3. A. Ballim and Y. Wilks. *Artificial Believers*. Lawrence Erlbaum Associates, Hillsdale, New Jersey, 1991.
4. Alexandru Baltag. A logic of epistemic actions. In W. Van der Hoek, J.J. Meyer, and C. Witteveen, editors, *Workshop on Foundations and applications of collective agent based systems (CABS)*, Utrecht, August 1999. ESSLLI99.
5. J.J. Blanc, Rachid Echahed, and Wendelin Serwe. Towards reactive functional logic programming languages. In Herbert Kuchen, editor, *Proc. of 8th Workshop on Functional and Logic Programming*, 1998.
6. Sergio Brandano. A logic-based calculus of fluents. Technical Report TR-98-01, Dipartimento di Informatica, January 12 1998. Sun, 25 Jan 1998 18:08:16 GMT.
7. A. Brogi, S. Contiero, and F. Turini. Programming by Combining General Logic Programs. Technical Report 97-02, Department of Computer Science, University of Pisa, 1997.

---

[7] the full class $\mathcal{K} - \mathbf{RA}$ is obtained relaxing the hypothesis that changes of features happens randomly during the duration of the affecting actions. This is denoted by the ontological designator e. In the most general case it is possible to provide a number of functions (e.g. in case of non-deterministic functions), called *trajectories*, to specify the (possibly continuous) changes of feature values during the action duration period. Trajectory semantics for $\mathcal{K} - \mathbf{RA}$ can be found in [6].

8. K. L. Clark. Negation as failure. In H. Gallaire and J. Minker, editors, *Logic and Data Bases*, pages 293–322. Plenum Press, New York, 1978.

9. M. Denecker, L. Missiaen, and M. Bruynooghe. Temporal reasoning with abductive event calculus. In Bernd Neumann, editor, *Proceedings of the 10th European Conference on Artificial Intelligence*, pages 384–388, Vienna, Austria, August 1992. John Wiley & Sons, Ltd.

10. K.J. Dryllerakis. Residual SLDNF in CLP languages. Technical report, Logic Programming Group Imperial College, 1995.

11. K. Eshghi and R. Kowalski. Abduction compared with negation by failure. In G. Levi and M. Martelli, editors, *Proceedings of the 6th International Conference and 5th Symposium on Logic Programming*, pages 234–254. MIT Press, 1989.

12. Nastaran Fatemi and Philippe Mulhem. A conceptual graph approach for video data representation and retrieval. In M. Berthold, editor, *Proceedings of third symposium on Intelligent Data Analysis IDA'99*. Lecture Notes in Computer Science, 1999.

13. Melvin C. Fitting. A Kripke-Kleene semantics for logic programming. *Journal of Logic Programming*, 4:295–312, 1985.

14. P. M. Hill and J. Gallagher. Meta-programming in logic progamming. In D. M. Gabbay, C. J. Hogger, and J. A. Robinson, editors, *Handbook of Logic in Artificial Intelligence and Logic Programming*, volume 5, pages 421–498. Oxford University Press, 1998.

15. A. Kakas and R. Miller. A simple declarative language for describing narratives with actions. *The Journal of Logic Programming*, 1997.

16. A. Kakas and C. Mourlas. Aclp: Flexible solutions to complex problems. In *Proceedings of Logic Programming and Non-monotonic Reasoning conference LPNMR97*, 1997.

17. R. Kowalski and M. Sergot. A logic based calculus of events. *New Generation Computing*, 4:67–95, 1986.

18. Vincenzo Pallotta. Integrazione della programmazione logica e della logica dei fluenti. Master's thesis, Universitá di Pisa, december 1997. http://lithwww.epfl.ch/~pallotta/tesi.ps.gz.

19. Vincenzo Pallotta. An abductive semantics for fluent logic programming. http://lithwww.epfl.ch/~pallotta/abductive_flp.ps.gz, september 1999.

20. Vincenzo Pallotta. Reasoning about fluents in logic programming. In Rachid Echahed, editor, *Proocedings of 8th International Workshop on Functional and Logic Programming*, volume RR 1021-I- of *Raport de Recherche*, pages 75–91, Grenoble, June 1999. CNRS-INPG, Laboratoire LEIBNIZ - Institute IMAG.

21. Vincenzo Pallotta and Franco Turini. Towards a fluent logic programming. Technical Report TR-98-03, Dipartimento di Informatica, March 9 1998. Wed, 11 Mar 1998 09:26:54 GMT.

22. Fariba Sadri and Robert A. Kowalski. Variants of the event calculus. In Leon Sterling, editor, *Proceedings of the 12th International Conference on Logic Programming*, pages 67–82, Cambridge, June 13–18 1995. MIT Press.

23. E. Sandewall. *Features and Fluents*. Oxford Press, 1994.

24. M. Shanahan. Representing continuous change in the Event Calculus. In *Proceedings of the 9th European Conference on Artificial Intelligence*, page 598, 1990.

25. M.P. Shanahan. *Solving the Frame Problem*. MIT Press, 1997.

26. Murray Shanahan. Prediction is deduction but explanation is abduction. In N. S. Sridharan, editor, *Proceedings of the 11th International Joint Conference on Artificial Intelligence*, pages 1055–1060, Detroit, MI, USA, August 1989. Morgan Kaufmann.

Default Reasoning with Specificity

Phan Minh Dũng[1] and Tran Cao Son[2*]

[1] Department of Computer Science and Information Management
School of Advanced Technology, Asian Institute of Technology
PO Box 2754, Bangkok 10501, Thailand
dung@cs.ait.ac.th
[2] Knowledge Systems Laboratory, Computer Science Department
Stanford University, Stanford, CA 94305, USA
tson@ksl.stanford.edu

Abstract. We present a new approach to reasoning with specificity which subsumes inheritance reasoning[1]. The new approach differs from other approaches in the literature in the way priority between defaults is handled. Here, it is context sensitive rather than context independent as in other approaches. We show that any context independent handling of priorities between defaults as advocated in the literature until now is not sufficient to capture general defeasible inheritance reasoning. We propose a simple and novel argumentation semantics for reasoning with specificity taking the context-dependency of the priorities between defaults into account. Since the proposed argumentation semantics is a form of stable semantics of nonmonotonic reasoning, it inherits a common problem of the latter where it is not always defined for every default theory. We identify the class of stratified default theories which is large enough to accommodate acyclic and consistent inheritance networks and for which the argumentation semantics is always defined. We also prove that the argumentation semantics satisfies the basic properties of a nonmonotonic consequence relation such as deduction, reduction, conditioning, and cumulativity for stratified default theories.

1   Introduction

Reasoning with specificity constitutes an inseparable part of default reasoning as specificity is an important source for conflict resolution in human's commonsense reasoning. In fact, the famous example of whether penguins fly because they are birds [23] in default reasoning is an example of reasoning with specificity. Reasoning with specificity also constitutes a difficult problem which has been studied extensively in the literature [1, 5, 7, 14, 16, 29, 30, 32, 39].

Formally a default theory T could be defined as a pair (E, K) where E is a set of evidence or facts representing what we call the concrete context of T, and

---

* This work was carried out while the author was a student at the University of Texas at El Paso.

[1] In this paper, we consider the graph based, off-path approach to inheritance reasoning [17, 18, 38, 42, 40, 41].

J. Lloyd et al. (Eds.): CL 2000, LNAI 1861, pp. 792–806, 2000.
© Springer-Verlag Berlin Heidelberg 2000

$K = (D, B)$ constitutes the domain knowledge consisting of a set of default rules D and a first order theory B representing the background knowledge. In the literature [1, 5, 7, 14, 16, 29] the principle of reasoning with specificity is "enforced" by first determining a set of priority orders between defaults in D using the information given by the domain knowledge K. Based on these priorities between defaults and following some sensible and intuitive criteria, the semantics of T is then defined either model-theoretically by selecting a subset of the set of all models of $E \cup B$ as the set of preferred models of T or proof-theoretically by selecting certain extensions as preferred extensions. The problem of these approaches is that their obtained semantics is rather weak: *they do not capture general defeasible inheritance reasoning*. There are many intuitive examples of reasoning with specificity (see below) that can not be handled in these approaches. The reason is that the priorities between defaults are defined independent of the context.

Priority orders are strict partial orders [2] between defaults in D. Let PO_K be the set of all these priority orders. For each priority order $\alpha \in PO_K$, where $(d, d') \in \alpha$ means that d is of lower priority than d', a priority order $<_\alpha$ between the sets of defaults in D is defined where $S <_\alpha S'$ means that S is preferred to S'. There are many ways to define $<_\alpha$ [1, 5, 7, 14, 16, 29, 32]. But whatever the definition of $<_\alpha$ is, $<_\alpha$ has to satisfy the following property.

Let d, d' be two defaults in D such that $(d, d') \in \alpha$. Then $\{d'\} <_\alpha \{d\}$.

$<_\alpha$ can be extended into an partial order between models of $E \cup B$ as follows:

$$M <_\alpha M' \text{ iff } D_M <_\alpha D_{M'}$$

where D_M is the set of all defaults in D which are satisfiable in M whereas a default $p \to q$ is said to be satisfiable in M iff the material implication $p \Rightarrow q$ is satisfiable in M.

A model M of $E \cup B$ is defined as a preferred model of T if there exists a partial order α in PO_K such that M is minimal with respect to $<_\alpha$. We then say that a formula β is defeasibly derived from T if β holds in each preferred model of T.

In a previous paper [11], we formally proved that any preferential semantics based on $<_\alpha$ can not account in full for defeasible inheritance reasoning. We include below this proof for the self-containment of the paper.

Example 1. Let us consider the inheritance network representing the normative sentences: (i) "normally, students are not married", (ii) "normally, adults are married", and (iii) "normally, students are young adults", and the subclass relation "young adults are adults."

The inheritance network represented this information is drawn in following picture[3] where the links $s \not\to m$, $a \to m$, and $s \to y$ represent the sentences

---

[2] Strict partial orders are transitive, irreflexive and antisymmetric relations

[3] *Throughout the paper, solid lines and dotted lines represent strict rules and default rules, respectively.*

(i), (ii), and (iii) respectively, and the strict link $y \Rightarrow a$ represents the subclass relation.

This defeasible inheritance network represents the domain knowledge (B, D) with $B = \{y \Rightarrow a\}$, and $D = \{d_1 :\ a \to m,\ d_2 :\ s \to \neg m,\ d_3 :\ s \to y\}$.

Consider now the marital status of a young adult who is also a student. This problem is represented by the default theory $T = (E, B, D)$ with $E = \{s, y, a\}$. The desirable semantics here is represented by the model $M = \{s, y, a, \neg m\}$. To deliver this semantics, all priority-based approaches in the literature [1, 5, 7, 16, 29] assigns default 1 a lower priority than default 2.

Let us consider now the marital status of another student who is an adult but not a young one. Let $T' = (E', B, D)$ with $E' = \{s, \neg y, a\}$. Now, since y does not hold, default 2 can not be considered more specific than default 1. Hence, it is intuitive to expect that neither m nor $\neg m$ should be concluded in this case. This is also the result sanctioned by all semantics of defeasible inheritance networks [17, 18, 38, 42, 40, 41]. In any priority-based system employing the same priorities between defaults with respect to E' as with respect to E, we have $M = \{\neg m, s, \neg y, a\} <_\alpha M' = \{m, s, \neg y, a\}$ since $D_M = \{2\} <_\alpha D'_M = \{1\}$ (due to $(1, 2) \in \alpha$). That means priority-based approaches in the literature conclude $\neg m$ given (E', K) which is not the intuitive result we expect.

To produce a correct semantics, 1 should have lower priority than 2 only in the context $\{s, y, a\}$ where the considered student is young (i.e. default 3 can be applied). In other words, the priority order under the context $\{s, \neg y, a\}$ is different than the priority order under the context $\{s, y, a\}$. In general, the example shows that *specificity cannot be treated independently from the context in which it is defined*.   □

Argumentation has been recognized lately as an important and natural approach to nonmonotonic reasoning [6, 9, 14, 31, 33, 34, 39, 46]. It has been shown in [9] that many major nonmonotonic logics [22, 23, 25, 28, 35] represent in fact different forms of a simple system of argumentation reasoning. Based on the results in [9], a simple logic-based argumentation system has been developed in [6] which captures well-known nonmonotonic logics like autoepistemic logics, Reiter's default logics and logic programming as special cases. In [14] argumentation has been employed to give a proof procedure for conditional logics. In [39], an argumentation system for reasoning with specificity has been developed. Like the proposals based on context-independent priorities, this system is rather weak. It can not deal with many intuitive examples and also fails to capture inheritance reasoning. It does not satisfy many basic properties of defeasible reasoning like the cumulativity. But despite these shortcomings, work like [39] suggests that argumentation offers a natural and intuitive framework for dealing with specificity. As we will show in this paper, argumentation indeed provides a simple and intuitive framework for reasoning with specificity.

In this paper, we extend the approach to reasoning with specificity in [11] to allow *more general propositional default theories*, i.e., we consider default theories with *non-empty background knowledge*. In the process, we simplify the notion of *more specific relation*. We propose a simple and novel argumentation semantics for reasoning with specificity taking the context-dependency of the priorities between defaults into account (Section 2). We then identify a large class of stratified default theories for which the argumentation semantics is always defined (Section 3). We prove that the argumentation semantics satisfies the basic properties of a nonmonotonic consequence relation such as deduction, reduction, conditioning, and cumulativity for stratified default theories (Section 3). We conclude with a discussion about reasoning with specificity in Section 4.

2   A General Framework

We assume a first order language $\mathcal{L}$ that is finite but large enough to contain all constants, function and predicate symbols of interest. The set of ground literals of $\mathcal{L}$ is denoted by $lit(\mathcal{L})$. Literals of $\mathcal{L}$ will be called hereafter simply as literals (or $\mathcal{L}$-literals) for short. Following the literature, a default theory is defined as follows:

Definition 1. *A default theory T is a triple (E, B, D) where*
   (i) E is a set of ground literals representing the evidences of the theory;
   (ii) B is a set of ground clauses;
   (iii) D is a set of defaults of the form $l_1 \wedge \ldots \wedge l_n \to l_0$ where l_i's are ground literals; and
   (iv) $E \cup B$ is a consistent first order theory.

Notice that in the above definition, we use $\to$ to denote a default implication. The material implication is represented by the $\Rightarrow$ symbol. Intuitively, $a \to b$ means that "typically, if a holds then b holds" while $a \Rightarrow b$ means that "whenever a holds then b holds." It is worth noting that default theories considered in [11] do not contain ground clauses, i.e., $B = \emptyset$.

For a default $d \equiv l_1 \wedge \ldots \wedge l_n \to l_0$, we denote $l_1 \wedge \ldots \wedge l_n$ and l_0 by $bd(d)$ and $hd(d)$ respectively.

In the following, we often use clauses and defaults with variables as a shorthand for the sets of their ground instantiations.

Example 2. Consider the famous penguin and bird example:

We have that $B = \{p \Rightarrow b\}$ (penguins are birds) and D consisting of two defaults $p \rightarrow \neg f$ (normally, penguins do not fly) and $b \rightarrow f$ (normally, birds fly)[4].

The question is to determine whether penguins fly. This problem is represented by the default theory $T = (E, B, D)$ where $E = \{p\}$. □

We next define the notion of *defeasible derivation*.

Definition 2. *Let $T = (E, B, D)$ be a default theory and l be a ground literal.*

● *A sequence of defaults $d_1, \ldots, d_n$ $(n \geq 0)$ is said to be a defeasible derivation of l if following conditions are satisfied:*

1. *$n = 0$ and $E \cup B \vdash l$ where the relation $\vdash$ represents the first-order consequence relation, or*
2. *(a) $E \cup B \vdash bd(d_1)$; and*
   (b) for $1 \leq i < n$: $E \cup B \cup \{hd(d_1), \ldots, hd(d_i)\} \vdash bd(d_{i+1})$; and
   (c) $E \cup B \cup \{hd(d_1), \ldots, hd(d_n)\} \vdash l$.

● *We say l is a* possible consequence *of E with respect to B and a set of defaults $K \subseteq D$, denoted by $E \cup B \vdash_K l$, if there exists a defeasible derivation $d_1, \ldots, d_n$ of l such that for all $1 \leq i \leq n$, $d_i \in K$.* □

For a set of literals L we write $E \cup B \vdash_K L$ iff $\forall l \in L : E \cup B \vdash_K l$.

We write $E \cup B \vdash_K \perp$[5] iff there is an atom a such that both $E \cup B \vdash_K a$ and $E \cup B \vdash_K \neg a$ hold.

For the default theory from example 1, it is easy to check that $E \cup B \vdash_{\{s \rightarrow \neg m\}} \neg m$ and $E \cup B \vdash_{\{s \rightarrow y, a \rightarrow m\}} m$. Hence $E \cup B \vdash_D \perp$.

A set of defaults K is said to be *consistent in T* if $E \cup B \not\vdash_K \perp$. K is *inconsistent* if it is not consistent [6].

The "More Specific" Relation

We now define the notion of "more specific" between defaults generalizing the specificity principle of Touretzky in inheritance reasoning. Consider for example the network from the example 1, it is clear that being a student is normally a specific case of being a young adult. Since being a young adult is always a specific case of being an adult, it follows that being a student is a specific case of being an adult if the respective individual is a young adult. This stipulates us to say that the default $s \rightarrow \neg m$ (students are normally not married) is more specific than the default $a \rightarrow m$ (adults are normally married) provided that the default $s \rightarrow y$ (students are normally young adults) can be applied. Similarly, in example 2, since being a penguin is always a specific case of being a bird, we can conclude that the default $p \rightarrow \neg f$ (penguins don't fly) is always more specific than $b \rightarrow f$ (birds fly).

[4] On the other hand, we have to change $p \Rightarrow b$ to $p \rightarrow b$ if we were to use the notion of default theories in [11].

[5] Throughout the paper, we use $\top$ and $\perp$ to denote *True* and *False* respectively.

[6] If there is no possibility for misunderstanding, we often simply say consistent instead of consistent in T

Definition 3. *Let d_1, d_2 be two defaults in D. We say that d_1 is more specific than d_2 with respect to a set of defaults $K \subseteq D$, denoted by $d_1 \prec_K d_2$, if*

1. *$B \cup \{hd(d_1), hd(d_2)\}$ is inconsistent;*
2. *$bd(d_1) \cup B \vdash_K bd(d_2)$; and*
3. *$bd(d_1) \cup B \nvdash_K \perp$.*

In the above definition (1) guarantees that a priority is defined between two defaults only if they are conflicted, (2) ensures that being $bd(d_1)$ is a special case of being $bd(d_2)$ provided that the defaults in K can be applied, and (3) guarantees that K is a sensible set of defaults. *We could say that this is a generalization of Touretzky's specificity principle to general propositional default theories.* In [11], the more specific relation is defined based on the notion of minimal conflict set, which in turn is defined based on the notion of defeasible derivation. As it can be seen, the above definition is much simpler than that was proposed in [11]. Besides, it allows us to deal with default theories with nonempty background knowledge.

If $K = \emptyset$ we say that d_1 is *strictly more specific* than d_2 and write $d_1 < d_2$ instead of $d_1 \prec_\emptyset d_2$.

Example 3. In example 1, $d_2 \prec_{\{d_3\}} d_1$ holds, i.e. d_2 is more specific than d_1 if d_3 is applied. In the context $E = \{s, y, a\}$, d_3 can be applied, and hence d_2 is more specific than d_1 in the context E. But in the context $E' = \{s, \neg y, a\}$, d_3 can not be applied, and hence, d_2 is not more specific than d_1 in E'.

In example 2, it is obvious that $d_2 < d_1$, i.e. d_2 is always more specific than d_1. □

We note that in general the more specific relation is not a strict partial order. For example, in the theory $(\emptyset, \emptyset, \{d_1 : p \to b, d_2 : p \to \neg b\})$, we have that $d_1 < d_2$ and $d_2 < d_1$. Furthermore, it is not always transitive. In the default theory $(\emptyset, \{p \Rightarrow q, q \Rightarrow r\}, \{d_1 : p \to b, d_2 : q \to \neg b, d_3 : r \to b\})$, we have that $d_1 < d_2$ and $d_2 < d_3$ but $d_1 \not< d_3$.

Stable Semantics of Default Reasoning with Specificity

The semantics of a default theory is defined by determining which defaults can be applied to draw new conclusions from the evidences. For example, the semantics of the network in example 1 is defined by determining that the defaults which could be applied are 2 and 3.

In the following, we will see that an argumentation-theoretic notion of attack between a set of defaults K and a default d lies at the heart of the semantics of reasoning with specificity.

Suppose that $K \subseteq D$ is a set of defaults we can apply. Further let d be a default such that $E \cup B \vdash_K \neg hd(d)$. It is obvious that d should not be applied together with K. In this case, we say that K *attacks d by conflict*.

For illustration of attack by conflict, consider the default theory T in example 1. Let $K = \{d_3, d_2\}$. Since $E \cup B \vdash_K \neg m$, K attacks d_1 by conflict. Similarly, $K' = \{d_3, d_1\}$ attacks d_2 by conflict because $E \cup B \vdash_{K'} m$.

The other case where d should not be applied together with K is where it is less specific than some default with respect to K. Formally, this means that if there exists $d' \in D$ such that $d' \prec_K d$ and $E \cup B \vdash_K bd(d')$ then d should not be applied together with the defaults in K. In this case we say that K *attacks* d *by specificity*.

For illustration of attack by specificity, consider again the default theory T in example 1. Let $K = \{d_3\}$. Because $d_2 \prec_{\{d_3\}} d_1$ and $E \cup B \vdash_{\{d_3\}} bd(d_2)$, K attacks d_1 by specificity.

The following definition summarize what we have just discussed:

Definition 4. *Let* $T = (E, B, D)$ *be a default theory. A set of defaults* K *is said to attack a default* d *in* T [7] *if following conditions are satisfied:*

1. *(Attack by Conflict)* $E \cup B \vdash_K \neg hd(d)$; *or*
2. *(Attack by Specificity) There exists* $d' \in D$ *such that* $d' \prec_K d$ *and* $E \cup B \vdash_K bd(d')$.

Note that there is a distinct difference between attack by conflict and inconsistency. It is possible that though K is consistent and $K \cup \{d\}$ is inconsistent but K does not attack d by conflict. It is also possible that K attacks some default d by conflict though $K \cup \{d\}$ is consistent. The "Nixon diamond" example illustrates these points.

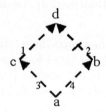

Let $E = \{a\}$, $B = \emptyset$, and $D = \{d_1 : c \to d, d_2 : b \to \neg d, d_3 : a \to c, d_4 : a \to b\}$. Though $K = \{d_1, d_2, d_4\}$ is consistent and $K \cup \{d_3\}$ is inconsistent, K does not attack d_3 by conflict. Further, though $K' = \{d_2, d_4\}$ attacks d_1 by conflict, $K = K' \cup \{d_1\}$ is consistent.

It is obvious that if K attacks d then every superset of K attacks d. K is said to attack some set $H \subseteq D$ if K attacks some default in H. K is said to *attack itself* if K attacks K.

Now we can give a precise definition of what constitutes the semantics of a default theory with specificity.

Definition 5. *Let* $T = (E,B,D)$ *be a default theory. A set of defaults* S *is called an extension of* T *if* S *does not attack itself and attacks every default not belonging to it.*

---

[7] *if there is no possibility for misunderstanding then* T *often is not mentioned*

Definition 6. *Let $T = (E,B,D)$ be a default theory. Let l be a ground literal. We say T entails l, denoted by $T \hspace{1pt}\vdash\hspace{-6pt}\sim\hspace{1pt} l$, if for every extension S of T, $E \cup B \vdash_S l$.*

Because the defeasible consequence relation $\vdash_K$ subsumes the first order consequence relation (definition 2), it is obvious that an inconsistent set of defaults attacks every default. Therefore it is clear that an extension is always consistent.

Example 4. Consider the theory in example 2. We have that $d_2 < d_1$, i.e., d_2 is strictly more specific than d_1. This can be used to prove that $\{d_2\}$ is the unique extension of T. Therefore $T \hspace{1pt}\vdash\hspace{-6pt}\sim\hspace{1pt} \neg f$. □

Example 5. 1. Consider the theory T in example 1. Let $H = \{d_3, d_2\}$. Because $\{s, y, a\} \cup B \vdash_H \neg m$, H attacks d_1 by conflict. Furthermore, since $\{s, y, a\} \cup B \hspace{1pt}\not\vdash_H m$ and $\{s, y, a\} \cup B \hspace{1pt}\not\vdash_H \neg y$, H does not attack itself by conflict. Because there is no default which is more specific than d_2 or d_3 with respect to H, H does not attack itself by specificity. Hence H does not attack itself and attacks every default not belonging to it. Therefore H is an extension of T. Let $K = \{d_1, d_3\}$. Because $d_2 \prec_K d_1$ and $\{s, y, a\} \cup B \vdash_K bd(d_2)$, K attacks d_1 by specificity. Hence K is not an extension of T. It should be obvious now that H is the only extension of T. Hence, $T \hspace{1pt}\vdash\hspace{-6pt}\sim\hspace{1pt} \neg m$.
2. Consider the theory T' in example 1. Let $H = \{d_2\}$ and $K = \{d_1\}$. Since $\{s, \neg y, a\} \vdash_H \neg m$ and $\{s, \neg y, a\} \vdash_K m$, and $\{s, \neg y, a\} \vdash_\emptyset \neg y$, H attacks d_1, d_3 by conflict while K attacks d_2, d_3 by conflict. Due to the fact that d_3 can not be applied, there are no defaults d, d' such that $d \prec_H d'$ or $d \prec_K d'$. Hence both H and K do not attack themselves. Thus, both H and K are extensions of T', and so, $T' \hspace{1pt}\not\vdash\hspace{-6pt}\sim\hspace{1pt} \neg m$ and $T' \hspace{1pt}\not\vdash\hspace{-6pt}\sim\hspace{1pt} m$.

□

The definition 5 of an extension of a default theory corresponds to the stable semantics of argumentation which has been first introduced in [9] and later further studied in [6]. There are also a number of other semantics for argumentation which could be applied to reasoning with specificity. But in this paper we will limit ourselves to the stable semantics.

Existence of Extensions

A well-known problem of stable semantics in nonmonotonic reasoning is that it is not always defined. As our semantics is a form of stable semantics of argumentation, it is expected that the same problem will be encountered in our framework. The following example originated from [7] confirms our expectation.

Example 6 ([7]). Consider $T = (E, \emptyset, D)$ with $E = \{a, b, c\}$ and D consists of the following defaults

$$d_1 : a \wedge q \rightarrow \neg p, d_2 : a \rightarrow p$$
$$d_3 : b \wedge r \rightarrow \neg q, d_4 : b \rightarrow q$$
$$d_5 : c \wedge p \rightarrow \neg r, d_6 : c \rightarrow r$$

It is easy to see that for each $K \subseteq D$, there is no $d \in D$ such that $d \prec_K d_1$ or $d \prec_K d_3$ or $d \prec_K d_5$.

We will prove that T does not have an extension.

Assume the contrary that T has an extension S. We want to prove that $d_1 \notin S$. Assume the contrary that $d_1 \in S$. Since $E \vdash_{\{d_2\}} p$ and S does not attack itself, we conclude that $d_2 \notin S$. This implies that S attacks d_2. There are two cases:

1. S attacks d_2 by conflict. This means that $E \vdash_S \neg p$, which implies that $E \vdash_S q$.
2. S attacks d_2 by specificity. Since the only default in D, that is more specific than d_2, is d_1, S attacks d_2 by specificity implies that $E \vdash_S bd(d_1)$. Thus $E \vdash_S q$.

It follows from the above two cases that $E \vdash_S q$. Therefore S contains d_4. Now, consider the two defaults d_5 and d_6. Since $d_2 \notin S$, $E \nvdash_S bd(d_5)$. Therefore S does not attack d_6 by specificity. Further $E \nvdash_S bd(d_5)$ implies that $E \nvdash_S \neg r$. So, S does not attack d_6 by conflict either. Again, because S is an extension, we have that $d_6 \in S$. However, $E \vdash_{\{d_6\}} bd(d_3)$, which implies that S attacks d_4 by specificity, i.e., S attacks itself. This contradicts the assumption that S is an extension of T. Thus the assumption that $d_1 \in S$ leads to a contradiction. Therefore $d_1 \notin S$.

Similarly, we can prove that $d_3 \notin S$ and $d_5 \notin S$. Since S is a stable extension of T, S attacks d_1. This implies that S must attack d_1 by conflict because there is no default in D which is more specific than d_1. Thus $d_2 \in S$. Similar arguments lead to $d_4 \in S$ and $d_6 \in S$, i.e., $S = \{d_2, d_4, d_6\}$. However, S attacks d_2 by specificity because $d_1 < d_2$ and $E \cup B \vdash_S bd(d_1)$. This means that S attacks itself which contradicts the assumption that S is a stable extension of T. Thus the assumption that there exists an extension leads to a contradiction. Therefore, we can conclude that there exists no extension of T.   □

In the next section we will introduce the class of stratified default theories for which extensions always exist.

3   Stratified Default Theories

The definition of stratified default theories is based on the notion of a *rank function* which is a mapping from the set of ground literals $lit(\mathcal{L}) \cup \{\top, \bot\}$ to the set of nonnegative integers.

Definition 7. *A default theory* $T = (E, B, D)$ *over* $\mathcal{L}$ *is stratified if there exists a rank function of* T, *denoted by rank, satisfying the following conditions:*
   (i) $rank(\top) = rank(\bot) = 0$;
   (ii) for each ground atom l, $rank(l) = rank(\neg l)$;
   (iii) for all literals l and l' occurring in a clause in B, $rank(l) = rank(l')$;
   (iv) for each default $l_1, \ldots, l_m \to l$ in D, $rank(l_i) < rank(l)$, $i = 1, \ldots, m$;

It is not difficult to see that all the default theories in examples 1 and 2 are stratified. We prove that

Theorem 1. *Every stratified default theory has at least one extension.*   □

Notice that stratification does not imply uniqueness of extensions. For example, the default theory $(\{a\}, \emptyset, \{d_1 : c \to d, \; d_2 : b \to \neg d, \; d_3 : a \to c, \; d_4 : a \to b\})$ is stratified and has two extensions $\{d_2, d_4, d_1\}$ and $\{d_2, d_4, d_2\}$.

3.1 General Properties of $\mid\!\sim$

There is a large body of works in the literature [2, 14, 19] on what properties characterize a defeasible consequence relation like $\mid\!\sim$. In general, it is agreed that such a relation should extend the monotonic logical consequence relation. Further, since the intuition of a default rule d is that $bd(d)$ normally implies $hd(d)$, we expect that in the context $E = \{bd(d)\}$, $T \mid\!\sim hd(d)$ holds. Another important property of defeasible consequence relations is related to the adding of proved conclusions to a theory. Intuitively, this means that if $T \mid\!\sim a$ then we expect T and $T + a$ [8] to have the same set of conclusions. Formally, the discussed key properties are given below:

- Deduction: $T \mid\!\sim l$ if $E \cup B \vdash l$;
- Conditioning: If $E = \{bd(d)\}$ for $d \in D$, then $T \mid\!\sim hd(d)$;
- Reduction: If $T \mid\!\sim a$ and $T + a \mid\!\sim b$ then $T \mid\!\sim b$;
- Cumulativity: If $T \mid\!\sim a$ and $T \mid\!\sim b$ then $T + a \mid\!\sim b$;

In the next two theorems, we show that $\mid\!\sim$ satisfies deduction and reduction:

Theorem 2 (Deduction). *Let $T=(E,B,D)$ be an arbitrary default theory. Then, for every $l \in lit(\mathcal{L})$, $E \cup B \vdash l$ implies $T \mid\!\sim l$.*   □

Theorem 3 (Reduction). *Given $T=(E,B,D)$ be an arbitrary default theory and $a, b \in lit(\mathcal{L})$ such that $T \mid\!\sim a$ and $T + a \mid\!\sim b$. Then, $T \mid\!\sim b$.*   □

In general $\mid\!\sim$ does not satisfy cumulativity as the following example shows.

Example 7. Consider the default theory $T = (E, B, D)$

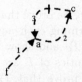

where $E = \{f\}$, $B = \emptyset$, $D = \{d_1 : f \to a, \; d_2 : a \to c, \; d_3 : c \to \neg a\}$ Because the only instance of the more-specific-relation is $d_1 \prec_{\{d_1, d_2\}} d_3$, T has a unique extension $\{d_1, d_2\}$. Hence, $T \mid\!\sim a$ and $T \mid\!\sim c$.

Now consider $T + c$. $T + c$ has two extensions: $\{d_1, d_2\}$ and $\{d_2, d_3\}$. Thus, $T + c \not\mid\!\sim a$. This implies that $\mid\!\sim$ is not cumulative.

---

[8] $T + a$ denotes the default theory $(E \cup \{a\}, B, D)$.

The next theorem proves that stratification is sufficient for cumulativity.

Theorem 4 (Cumulativity). *Let $T = (E, B, D)$ be a stratified default theory and a, b be literals such that $T \hspace{2pt}\vdash\hspace{-6pt}\sim a$, and $T \hspace{2pt}\vdash\hspace{-6pt}\sim b$. Then $T + a \hspace{2pt}\vdash\hspace{-6pt}\sim b$.* ☐

Because stratification does not rule out the coexistence of defaults like $a \to \neg c$, $a \to c$, conditioning does not hold for stratified theories as the next example shows.

Example 8. Let $T = (\{a\}, \emptyset, \{d_1 : a \to \neg c, \ d_2 : a \to c\})$. It is obvious that T is stratified. Because $d_1 < d_2$ and $d_2 < d_1$, both d_1, d_2 are attacked by specificity by the empty set of defaults. Thus the only extension of T is the empty set. Hence, $T \hspace{2pt}\not\vdash\hspace{-6pt}\sim \neg c$, and $T \hspace{2pt}\not\vdash\hspace{-6pt}\sim c$. That means that conditioning is not satisfied.

The coexistence of defaults like $a \to \neg c$, $a \to c$ means that a is normally c and normally not c at the same time which is obviously not sensible. Hence it should not be a surprise that conditioning is not satisfied in such cases. The conditioning property would hold for a default d if in the context of $bd(d)$, d is the most specific default. The following definition formalizes this intuition. For simplicity, we often write $d \prec d'$ if $d \prec_K d'$ for some K. Let $\prec^*$ be the transitive closure of $\prec$.

Definition 8. *A default theory $T = (E,B,D)$ is said to be* conditioning-sensible *if for every default d the following conditions are satisfied:*
(i) $d \not\prec^* d$;
(ii) For every set $K \subseteq D$ such that $bd(d) \cup B \vdash_{K \cup \{d\}} \bot$ and $bd(d) \cup B \not\vdash_K \bot$, there exist $d' \in K$ such that $d \prec_K d'$.

Theorem 5. *Let $T = (E, B, D)$ be a conditioning-sensible default theory, d be a default in D, and $E = bd(d)$. Then $T \hspace{2pt}\vdash\hspace{-6pt}\sim hd(d)$.* ☐

It is interesting to note that conditioning-sensibility and stratification are two independent concepts. Default theories like the one in example 7 are conditioning-sensible but not stratified while default theories like that in example 8 are stratified but not conditioning-sensible. Further while example 8 shows that stratification does not imply conditioning, example 7 shows that conditioning-sensibility does not imply cumulativity.

In the full version of this paper, we prove that our approach captures off-path inheritance reasoning by transforming each acyclic and consistent inheritance network Γ into a default theory T_Γ and show that the conclusions sanctioned by the (off-path) credulous semantics of Γ are also the conclusions of $\hspace{2pt}\vdash\hspace{-6pt}\sim$ with respect to T_Γ. Furthermore, we prove that T_Γ is a stratified default theory. Thus, inheritance entailment based on credulous semantics also satisfies the core properties of a defeasible entailment relation.

4   Discussion and Conclusion

Reiter and Criscuolo [36] are among the first to discuss the importance of specificity (or default interaction, in their terminology) in default reasoning. They discussed various situations, in which the interaction between defaults of a normal default theory can be compiled into the original theory to create a new default theory whose semantics yields the intuitive results. It has been recognized relatively early that priorities between defaults can help in dealing with specificity. In prioritized circumscription, first defined by McCarthy [24], a priority order between predicates is added into each circumscription theory. Lifschitz [27] later proved that prioritized circumscription is a special case of parallel circumscription. A similar approach has been taken by Konolige [20] in using autoepistemic logic to reason with specificity. He defined hierarchical autoepistemic theories in which a preference order between sub-theories and a syntactical condition on the sub-theories ensure that higher priority conclusions will be concluded. Brewka [4] - in defining prioritized default logic - also adds a preference order between defaults into a Reiter's default theory and modifies the semantics of default logic in such a way that guarantees that default of higher priority is preferred. Baader and Hollunder [5] develop prioritized default logic to handle specificity in terminological systems. All of the approaches in [4, 5, 24, 27, 20] assume that priorities between defaults are given by the users.

Computing specificity is another important issue in approaches to reasoning with specificity. Work from Poole [32] is an early attempt to extract the preference between defaults from the theory. Poole defines a notion of "more specific" between pairs consisting of a conclusion and an argument supporting this conclusion. Moinard [26] pointed out that Poole's definition yields unnecessary priority, for example, it can arise even in consistent default theories. Simari and Loui [39] noted that Poole's definition does not take into consideration the interaction between arguments. To overcome this problem they combined Poole's approach and Pollock's theory [31] to define an approach that unifies various approaches to argument-based defeasible reasoning. We have discussed the shortcoming of Simari and Loui's system in the introduction.

Touretzky's specificity principle [43] in inheritance reasoning is a major step in reasoning with specificity. Although this principle is generally accepted, different intuitions on *"what does more specific mean?"* leads to numerous approaches to reasoning with specificity. More interestingly, some seem to contradict the others. Detailed discussions about this problem in inheritance reasoning can be found in Touretzky et al. [44, 45]. Moinard [26] showed that Touretzky's approach does not work well for general default theories. He proposed several principles for determining a preference relation based on specificity in default logic but does not discuss how this preference would change the semantics of a default theory. Furthermore, like Poole he does not take into consideration the interaction between arguments either.

Conditional entailment of Geffner and Pearl [14] bridges the extensional and conditional approaches to default reasoning and is the first approach to reasoning with specificity which satisfies the basic properties of a nonmonotonic consequence relation. Because the priority order between assumptions in [14] is context-independent, conditional entailment, however, is too weak (as also noted by Geffner and Pearl) to capture inheritance reasoning. Pearl also discussed how a preference relation between defaults can be established. In System Z [29], Pearl uses consistency check to determine the order of a default. The lower the order of a default is, the higher is its priority. As in Poole's approach, sometimes System Z introduces unwanted priorities.

The idea of compiling specificities into a general nonmonotonic framework is also used in [7, 11] and in this work. Delgrande and Schaub [7] compiled the preference order between defaults (defined using a order similar to a Z-order of [29]) into the original theory and create a Reiter's default theory whose semantics defines the semantics of the original theory. The compilation of the preference order, however, does not take the context into consideration. As a consequence their approach cannot capture inheritance reasoning. In our approach, the compilation of the more specific relation into the original theory is done in such a way that the context will affect the decision process determining which default can be applied.

Our approach to specificity in this paper is a continuation of our own work in [11]. It could be viewed as a kind of a hybrid between the above approaches. For an intuitive semantical foundation of reasoning with specificity, we develop a general framework, but for implementation, we translate our framework into Reiter's default logics. Wang, You and Yang [47] has applied our idea to give a semantics for possibly cyclic inheritance networks.

Even though our work is not directly related to the recent works on prioritized default theories [8, 15, 37] or adding priority into extended logic programming [3], we believe that there is a mutual benefit between the research done in these works and ours. For example, the more specific relation defined here can be used to specify the priorities between defaults in [8] or the preference relation in [15]. Thus, these two approaches can be extended to realize two different modes of reasoning: one with explicit priority ordering and the other with implicit priority ordering. On the other hand, programs such as that in [47] can be extended to compute the more specific relation and hence allows a fully automatic translation from a default theory $T = (E, B, D)$ into its corresponding Reiter's default theory, R_T. The result of [47] also shows that this can be done in polynomial time for defeasible inheritance networks.

Our work also shows that inheritance networks can be modularly translated into equivalent general nonmonotonic formalism such as Reiter's default theory. We want to note that there are other works on formulating inheritance networks using general nonmonotonic formalisms such as [10, 12, 13, 47] or the works listed in [17]. To the best of our knowledge, our work is the first general propositional approach to default reasoning with specificity which is capable of capturing inheritance reasoning in full.

Acknowledgments

We would like to thank the three anonymous reviewers for their valuable comments that help us to improve the paper in many ways.

References

1. Brewka, G.: Adding Priorities and Specificity to Default Logic, Proc. JELIA 94, LNAI 838, Springer Verlag, 247–260.
2. Brewka, G.: Cumulative default logic: In defense of nonmonotonic inference rules, AIJ'50, 183–205.
3. Brewka, G. and Eiter, T.: Preferred Answer Sets for Extended Logic Programs, AIJ'109, (1999) 297–356.
4. Brewka, G.: Reasoning about Priorities in Default Logic, Proc. AAAI'94, Seatle, 1994.
5. Baader, F. and Hollunder, B.: How to prefer more specific defaults in terminological default logic, Proc. IJCAI'93.
6. Bondarenko A., Dung P.M., Kowalski R.A., Toni F.: An abstract, argumentation-theoretic approach to default reasoning, AIJ'93, (1997) 63–101.
7. Delgrande , J.P. and Schaub, T.H.: A General Approach to Specificity in Default Reasoning, Proc. KR'94, (1994) 47–158.
8. Delgrande , J.P. and Schaub, T.H.: Compiling reasoning with and about preferences into default logic, Proc. IJCAI'97, 1997.
9. Dung, P.M.: On the acceptability of arguments and its fundamental role in non-monotonic reasoning and logic programming and N-person game, AIJ'77, 2 (1995) 321–357.
10. Dung, P.M. and Son, T.C.: Nonmonotonic Inheritance , Argumentation, and Logic Programming, Proc. LPNMR'95, (1995) 316–329.
11. Dung, P.M. and Son, T.C.: An Argumentation-theoretic Approach to Default Reasoning with Specificity, Proc. KR'96, (1996) 407–418.
12. Etherington, D.W. and Reiter, R.: On Inheritance Hierarchies With Exceptions, Proc. AAAI'84, (1984) 104–108.
13. Gelfond, M., Przymusińska, H.: Formalization of Inheritance Reasoning in Au-toepistemic Logic, Fundamental Informaticae XIII, 4(1990), 403–445
14. Geffner, H., and Pearl J.: Conditional entailment: bridging two approaches to default reasoning, AIJ'53, (1992) 209–244.
15. Gelfond, M. and Son T.C.: Prioritized Default Theory, LNAI'1471, Proceeding of the Workshop LPKR'97, (1997) 164–223.
16. Geerts, P. and Viemeir, D.: A nonmonotonic reasoning formalism using implicit specificity information, Proc. LPNRM'94, (1994) 380–396.
17. Horty, J.F.: Some direct Theories of Non-monotonic Inheritance in Handbook of Logic and Artificial Intelligence and Logic Programming, D.Gabbay and C. Hogger, Oxford Uni., 1991.
18. Horty, J.F., Thomason, R.H., and Touretzky, D.S.: A skeptical theory of inheritance in non-monotonic semantic networks, AIJ'42, (1987) 311–348.
19. Kraus, S., Lehmann, D., and Magidor, M.: Nonmonotonic Reasoning, Preferential Models and Cumulative Logics, AIJ'44, (1990) 167–207
20. Konolige, K.: Hierarchic Autoepistemic Theories for Nonmonotonic Reasoning, Proc. AAAI'88, (1988) 439–443.
21. Marek, V.M. and Truszczynski, M.: Nonmonotonic Logic, Springer Verlag, 1993.
22. Moore, R.C.: Semantical Considerations on Nonmonotonic Logics, AIJ'25, 75–94.
23. McCarthy, J.: Circumscription - a form of nonmonotonic reasoning , AIJ'13, (1980) 27–39.
24. McCarthy, J.: Applications of Circumscription to Formalizing Commonsense Knowledge, AI, 1984.

25. McDermott, D. and Doyle, J.: Nonmonotonic Logic I, AIJ'13, (1980) 41–72.
26. Moinard, Y.: Preference by Specificity in Default Logic, 1990.
27. Lifschitz, V.: Computing Circumscription, Proc. IJCAI'85, (1985) 121–127.
28. Lloyd, J.W.: Foundations of Logic Programming, Springer Verlag, 1987.
29. Pearl, J.: System Z: A natural ordering of defaults with tractable applications to nonmonotonic reasoning: A survey; Proc. KR-89, (1989) 505–516.
30. Pereira, L. M., Aparicio, J. N., and Alferes, J. J.: Non–monotonic Reasoning with Logic Programming, Journal of Logic Programming 17(2, 3, & 4):227-263. 1993
31. Pollock, J.L.: Defeasible reasoning. Cognitive Science **17** (1987) 481–518.
32. Poole, D.: On the comparison of theories: Preferring the most specific explanation, Proc. IJCAI'85, (1985) 144–147.
33. Prakken, H., and Sartor, G.: A semantics for argument-based systems with weak and strong negation and with explicit priorities. Draft, July 1995. An extended abstract can be found in Proceedings of the 5th International Conf. on AI and Laws, ACM Press, 1995, 1-9.
34. Prakken, H., and Vreeswijk, G.A.W.: Logics for Defeasible Argumentation, To appear in Handbook of Philosophical Logic, D.Gabbay, Oxford University.
35. Reiter R.: A Logic for Default Reasoning, AIJ'13 1-2 (1980), 81-132.
36. Reiter R. and Criscuolo G.: On interacting defaults, in Readings in Nonmonotonic Reasoning, Edited by M. L. Ginsberg, Morgan Kaufmann Publishers, Inc., Los Altos, California (1987) 94–100
37. Rintanen, J.: Lexicographic priorities in default logics, AIJ'106, 2 (1998) 221–265.
38. Sandewall, E.: Nonmonotonic Inference Rules for Multiple Inheritance with Exceptions, Proceedings of the IEEE, Vol. 74, No. 10, October (1986) 1345–1353
39. Simari, G.R. and Loui, R.P.: A mathematical treatment of defeasible reasoning and its implementation, Elsevier, AIJ'53, (1992) 125–257.
40. Simonet, G. and Ducournau R.: On Stein's paper: resolving ambiguity in nonmonotonic inheritance hierarchies, AIJ'71, 1 (1994) 183–193.
41. Simonet, G.: On Sandewall's paper: Nonmonotonic inference rules for multiple inheritance with exceptions, AIJ'86, 2 (1996) 359–374.
42. Stein, L.A.: Resolving ambiguity in non-monotonic inheritance hierarchies, AIJ'55, 259–310.
43. Touretzky, D. S.: The mathematics of Inheritance Systems, Morgan Kaufmann Pub., Inc., Los Altos, CA, 1986.
44. Touretzky, D. S., Horty, J.F., and Thomason, R.H.: A clash of Intuition: The current state of Non-monotonic Multiple Inheritance Systems, Proc. IJCAI'87, (1987) 476–482
45. Touretzky, D. S., Horty, J.F., and Thomason, R.H.: A skeptic's Menagerie: Conflictors, Preemptors, Reinstaters, and zombies in nonmonotonic Inheritance, Proc. IJCAI'91, (1991) 478–483
46. Vreeswijk, G.A.W.: The feasibility of defeat in defeasible reasoning, KR'91.
47. Wang, X., You, J.H., and Yuan, L.Y.: A default interpretation of defeasible network, Proc. IJCAI'97, 1997.

Planning under Incomplete Knowledge

Thomas Eiter, Wolfgang Faber, Nicola Leone*, Gerald Pfeifer, and Axel Polleres

Institut für Informationssysteme, TU Wien
A-1040 Wien, Austria
{eiter,faber}@kr.tuwien.ac.at
{leone,pfeifer,polleres}@dbai.tuwien.ac.at

Abstract. We propose a new logic-based planning language, called $\mathcal{K}$. Transitions between states of knowledge can be described in $\mathcal{K}$, and the language is well suited for planning under incomplete knowledge. Nonetheless, $\mathcal{K}$ also supports the representation of transitions between states of the world (i.e., states of complete knowledge) as a special case, proving to be very flexible. A planning system supporting $\mathcal{K}$ is implemented on top of the disjunctive logic programming system DLV. This novel system allows for solving hard planning problems, including secure planning under incomplete initial states, which cannot be solved at all by other logic-based planning systems such as traditional satisfiability planners.

1 Introduction

The need for modeling the behavior of robots in a formal way led to the definition of logic-based languages for reasoning about actions and action planning, such as [24, 8, 15, 10, 34, 11, 19, 12, 14]. These languages allow us to specify planning problems of the form "find a sequence of actions that leads from a given initial state to a given goal state."

A state is characterized by the truth values of a number of fluents, describing relevant properties of the domain of discourse. An action is applicable only if some precondition (formula over the fluents) is true in the current state, and its execution changes the current state by modifying the truth values of some fluents. Most of these languages are based on extensions of classical logics and describe transitions among *possible states of the world* (where every fluent must necessarily be either true or false). However, robots usually don't have a *complete* view of the world. Even if their knowledge is incomplete (a number of fluents may be unknown, e.g., whether a door in front of the robot is open), they must take decisions, execute actions, and reason on the basis of their (incomplete) information at hand. For example, if it is not known whether a door is open, the robot might do a sensing action, or decide to push back.

In this paper, we propose a new language, $\mathcal{K}$, for planning under incomplete knowledge. We name it $\mathcal{K}$ to emphasize that it describes transitions among *states of knowledge* rather than among states of the world. Nonetheless, the language is very flexible, and is capable of modeling transitions among states of the world (i.e., states of complete knowledge) and reason about them as a particular case (see below). Compared to similar planning languages, $\mathcal{K}$ is closer in spirit to answer set semantics [7] than to classical

---

* Please address correspondence to this author.

J. Lloyd et al. (Eds.): CL 2000, LNAI 1861, pp. 807–821, 2000.

logics. It allows the use of default negation, exploiting the power of answer sets to deal with incomplete knowledge. We have implemented $\mathcal{K}$ on top of the DLV system [4, 5], and provide a powerful planning system (available on the web), which is ready-to-use for experiments.

initial: goal:

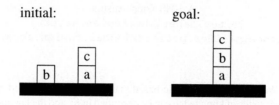

Fig. 1. A blocks world example.

Overview of $\mathcal{K}$

The main features of the language $\mathcal{K}$ (formally defined in Section 2) and our planning system are briefly summarized as follows. We occasionally refer to well-known planning problems in the blocks world, which require to turn one configuration of blocks into another (see Figure 1).

Type Declarations. They specify the ranges of the arguments of fluents and actions. For instance,

```
move(B,L) requires block(B), location(L).
```

specifies the types for the arguments of action *move*. The literals after "requires" (block(B), location(L)) must be positive literals of the static background knowledge, given by a normal (or-free) stratified logic program.

Causation Rules. A (causation) rule, which is main construct of $\mathcal{K}$, is syntactically similar to a rule of the language $\mathcal{C}$ [11, 19, 18] and has the form:

```
caused f if B after A.
```

Intuitively, the above rule says: if B is known to be true in the current state and A is known to be true in the previous state, then f is known to be true in the current state as well. Both the if part and the after part are allowed to be empty (which means that they are true).

Default Negation. not can appear in the bodies of the rules. It allows for natural modeling of inertial properties, default properties, and dealing with incomplete knowledge in general, like in logic programming with answer set semantics. Strong negation ("¬," written in programs as -) is allowed as well. Several shortcuts are defined for $\mathcal{K}$, e.g.

$$\texttt{inertial on(X,Y).}$$

informally states that on(X, Y) holds at the current state if on(X, Y) held at the previous state unless −on(X, Y) is explicitly known to hold. Furthermore,

$$\texttt{default -on(X,Y).}$$

states that -on(X, Y) is assumed, unless on(X, Y) is known to hold (as it has been explicitly entailed by some causation rule).

Executability of Actions. This can be expressed in a direct way: For instance,

```
executable move(X,Y) if not occupied(X), not occupied(Y),
                        X≠Y.
```

states that (block) X can be moved on (location) Y if both X and Y are clear and X ≠ Y. Multiple executable statements for the same action are allowed. A statement with empty body

$$\texttt{executable move(X,Y).}$$

says that move is always executable, provided that the type restrictions on X and Y are respected (and no inconsistency arises from the execution). Execution of an action A under condition B is forbidden by

$$\texttt{nonexecutable A if B.}$$

In case of conflicts, nonexecutable A overrides executable A.

Initial State Constraints. In general, a rule expresses a state constraint that must be fulfilled in all states. An *initial state constraint* (which is preceded by the keyword initially:), must be satisfied only in the initial state. For example,

$$\texttt{initially: caused false if block(B), not supported(B).}$$

enforces the fluent supported to be true on every block at the initial state; the constraint is irrelevant for all subsequent states. Initial state constraints may profitably reduce computation effort: If we are guaranteed that the actions preserve a property, say P, then it is sufficient to check the validity of P only on the initial state for ensuring it holds in any state.

Parallel Execution of Actions. Simultaneous execution of a number of actions is allowed in $\mathcal{K}$. This can be prohibited by the statement

$$\texttt{noConcurrency.}$$

which enforces the execution of at most one action at a time.

Handling of Complete and Incomplete Knowledge. The language allows one also to represent transitions between possible states of the world (which can be seen as states of complete knowledge). First of all, we can easily check that the knowledge on a fluent, say f, is complete, using a rule

```
caused false if not f, not -f.
```

Moreover, we can "totalize" the knowledge of a fluent by declaring

```
total f.
```

which means that, unless a truth value for f can be derived, the cases where f resp. -f is true will be both considered.

Goals and Plans. A goal is a conjunction of ground literals, and a plan for a goal is a sequence of (in general, sets of) actions whose execution leads from an initial state to a state where all literals in the goal are true. In $\mathcal{K}$, the goal is followed by a question mark and by the number of allowed steps in a plan. For instance,

```
on(c,b), on(b,a) ? (3)
```

asks to find a plan of length 3 for the goal of Figure 1.

Secure Plans. A key feature of $\mathcal{K}$ is the command

```
securePlan.
```

by which we ask the system to compute only *secure* plans (a secure plan is often called *conformant* in the literature). Informally, a plan is secure if it is applicable starting at any legal initial state, and enforces, regardless of how the state evolves, the goal. Using this feature, we can also model *possible-worlds planning with an incomplete initial state*, where the initial world is known only partially, and we look for a plan reaching the desired goal from every possible world according to the initial state.

Contribution of the Work

The main contributions of the paper are the following:

- We introduce the planning language $\mathcal{K}$ and provide a declarative model theoretic semantics for it.
- We illustrate the knowledge modeling features of the language by encoding some classical planning problems in $\mathcal{K}$.
- We analyze the computational complexity of language $\mathcal{K}$ in the propositional case. Deciding the existence of an optimistic plan achieving the goal in a fixed number of steps is NP-complete. If the plan should be secure, the problem is obviously harder, because it allows us to encode also planning under incomplete initial states as in [1]. The problem is then Σ_2^P-complete in general, but only mildly harder than NP if concurrent actions are not allowed. On the other hand, deciding existence of a secure plan of variable (arbitrary) length is NEXPTIME-complete, and thus not polynomially reducible to planning in STRIPS-like systems [6] which are PSPACE-complete [2].

An implementation of $\mathcal{K}$ exists as a frontend to the DLV system [4]. This frontend applies a $\mathcal{K}$ evaluator on top of the DLV system, using an efficient translation from $\mathcal{K}$ to disjunctive logic programming.

DLV (including the $\mathcal{K}$ frontend) can be freely retrieved from http://www.dbai.tuwien.ac.at/proj/dlv/.
To the best of our knowledge, this is the first declarative LP-based planning system which allows to solve Σ_2^P-hard planning problems, like planning under incomplete initial states.

For space limitations, we omit some technical material here. Further details can be obtained from the web page mentioned above.

2   Language $\mathcal{K}$

2.1   Syntax

Actions, Fluents, and Types. Let σ^{act}, σ^{fl}, and σ^{typ} be disjoint sets of action, fluent and type names, respectively. These names are effectively predicate symbols with associated arity (≥ 0). Here, $\sigma^{fl} \cup \sigma^{act}$ are used to describe *dynamic knowledge*, whereas σ^{typ} is used to describe *static background knowledge*.

Furthermore, let σ^{con} and σ^{var} be the disjoint sets of constant and variable symbols, respectively.[1]

Given $p \in \sigma^{act}$ (resp. σ^{fl}, σ^{typ}), an action (resp. fluent, type) atom is defined as $p(t_1, \ldots, t_n)$, where n is the arity of p and $t_1, \ldots, t_n \in \sigma^{con} \cup \sigma^{var}$. An action (resp. fluent, type) literal is an action (resp. fluent, type) atom, which is possibly preceded by the true negation symbol "$\neg$". A literal (or any other syntactic object) is *ground* if it does not contain variables.

For any literal l, let $\neg.l$ denote its complement, i.e. $\neg l$ if l is an atom and a if $l = \neg a$. Similarly, for a set L of literals, $\neg.L = \{\neg.l \mid l \in L\}$. A set L of literals is *consistent*, if $L \cap \neg.L = \emptyset$. Furthermore, L^+ (resp., L^-) denotes the set of positive (resp., negative) literals in L.

The set of all action (resp. fluent, type) literals is denoted as $\mathcal{L}_{act}$ (resp. $\mathcal{L}_{fl}$, $\mathcal{L}_{typ}$). Furthermore, let then $\mathcal{L}_{fl,typ} = \mathcal{L}_{fl} \cup \mathcal{L}_{typ}$; $\mathcal{L}_{dyn} = \mathcal{L}_{fl} \cup \mathcal{L}_{act}^+$ (*dyn* stands for *dynamic literals*); and $\mathcal{L} = \mathcal{L}_{fl,typ} \cup \mathcal{L}_{act}^+$.[2]

Action/Fluent Declarations. All actions and fluents have to be declared using an *action* (resp. *fluent*) *declaration* of the form:

$$p(X_1, \ldots, X_n) \text{ requires } t_1, \ldots, t_m \tag{1}$$

where $p \in \mathcal{L}_{act}^+$ (resp. $p \in \mathcal{L}_{fl}^+$), $X_1, \ldots, X_n \in \sigma^{var}$, $t_1, \ldots, t_m \in \mathcal{L}_{typ}$, n is the arity of p, and all X_i occur also in $t_1, \ldots t_n$ and $m \geq 0$. If $m = 0$, the requires part may be skipped.

---

[1] Following logic programming conventions, in this paper constant and variable symbols are denoted as strings starting with a lower or upper case character, respectively.

[2] Note that in this definition only positive action literals are allowed.

Causation Rules. Causation rules are used to define static and dynamic dependencies. *Causation rules* (*rules*, for short) are of the form

$$\text{caused } f \text{ if } b_1, \ldots, b_k, \text{not } b_{k+1}, \ldots, \text{not } b_l \\ \text{after } a_1, \ldots, a_m, \text{not } a_{m+1}, \ldots, \text{not } a_n \tag{2}$$

where $f \in \mathcal{L} \cup \{\texttt{false}\}$, $b_1, \ldots, b_l \in \mathcal{L}_{fl,typ}$, $a_1, \ldots, a_n \in \mathcal{L}$, $l \geq k \geq 0$, and $n \geq m \geq 0$. Rules where $n = 0$ are referred to as *static rules*, all other rules as *dynamic rules*. When $l = 0$, the if part can be omitted; likewise, if $n = 0$, the after part can be skipped. If both $l = n = 0$, also caused is optional. Given a causation rule r, let $h(r) = \{f\}, post^+(r) = \{b_1, \ldots, b_k\}, post^-(r) = \{b_{k+1}, \ldots, b_l\}, pre^+(r) = \{a_1, \ldots, a_m\}, pre^-(r) = \{a_{m+1}, \ldots, a_n\}, lit(r) = \{f, b_1, \ldots, b_l, a_1, \ldots, a_n\}$.

Initial State Constraints. While the scope of general static rules is over all knowledge states, it is often useful to specify rules only for the initial states. *Initial state constraints* are static rules of the form (2) preceded by the keyword initially. For an initial state constraint ic. $h(ic)$, $post^+(ic)$, $post^-(ic)$, $pre^+(ic)$, and $pre^-(ic)$ are defined as for its rule part.

Conditional Executability. $\mathcal{K}$ allows STRIPS-style [6] conditional execution of actions. A difference is that $\mathcal{K}$ allows several alternative executability conditions for an action which are beyond the repertoire of standard STRIPS. An *executability condition* is an expression of the form

$$\text{executable } a \text{ if } b_1, \ldots, b_m, \text{not } b_{m+1}, \ldots, \text{not } b_n \tag{3}$$

where $a \in \mathcal{L}_{act}^+$ and $b_1, \ldots, b_n \in \mathcal{L}$, and $n \geq m \geq 0$. If $n = 0$, the if part is usually skipped, expressing unconditional executability. Given an executability condition e, let $h(e) = \{a\}$, $post^+(e) = post^-(e) = \emptyset, pre^+(e) = \{b_1, \ldots, b_m\}$, $pre^-(e) = \{b_{m+1}, \ldots, b_n\}$, and $lit(e) = \{a, b_1, \ldots, b_n\}$.

Safety Restriction. In $\mathcal{K}$, all rules (including initial state constraints) and executability conditions have to satisfy the following syntactic restriction, which is similar to the notion of safety in logic programs [35]. All variables in a default negated type literal must also occur in some literal which is not a default negated type literal.

Thus, safety is required only for variables appearing in default negated type literals, while it is not required at all for variables appearing in fluent and action literals. The reason is that the range of the latter variables is implicitly restricted by the respective type declaration.

Action Descriptions, Planning Domains, Planning Problems. An *action description* is a pair $\langle D, R \rangle$ where D is a finite set of action and fluent declarations and R is a finite set of safe executability conditions, safe causation rules, and safe initial state constraints.

A *planning domain* is a pair $PD = \langle \Pi, AD \rangle$, where Π is a normal stratified datalog program (referred to as *background knowledge*) that is safe (in the standard LP sense), and AD is an action description. PD is *positive*, if no default negation occurs in AD.

A *query* is of the form

$$g_1, \ldots, g_m, \text{not } g_{m+1}, \ldots, \text{not } g_n ? \ (i) \tag{4}$$

where $g_1, \ldots, g_n \in \mathcal{L}_{fl}$ are variable-free, and $i \geq 0, n \geq m \geq 0$.

A *planning problem* $\langle PD, q \rangle$ is a pair of a planning domain PD and a query q.

2.2   Semantics

First we will define the legal instantiations of a planning problem. This is similar to the grounding of a logic program—the difference is that only correctly typed fluent and action literals are generated.

Instantiation. Let substitutions and their application to syntactic objects be defined as usual (assignments of constants to variables). We first define the notion of legal action (resp. fluent) instantiations:

Let $PD = \langle \Pi, \langle D, R \rangle \rangle$ be a planning domain, and let M be the (unique) answer set of Π. Then, $\theta(p(X_1, \ldots, X_n))$ is a *legal action* (resp. *fluent*) *instantiation* for an action (resp. fluent) declaration $d \in D$ of the form (1), if θ is a substitution defined over all $X_1, \ldots, X_n$ such that $\{\theta(t_1), \ldots, \theta(t_m)\} \subseteq M$. By $\mathcal{L}_{PD}$ we denote the set of all legal action and fluent instantiations.

Based on the above definition of action and fluents instantiations, we define the instantiation of a planning domain, $PD\!\downarrow$, as follows:

$$PD\!\downarrow = \bigcup_{r \in R} \bigcup_{\theta \in \Theta_r} \{\theta(r)\},$$

where Θ_r is the set of all substitutions θ defined over all variables in r, such that $lit(\theta(r)) \cap \mathcal{L}_{dyn} \subseteq \mathcal{L}_{PD}$ and $(post^+(\theta(r)) \cup pre^+(\theta(r))) \cap \mathcal{L}_{typ} \subseteq M$ hold. In other words, actions and fluents must agree with their declarations and positive type literals must agree with the background knowledge.

$PD\!\downarrow$ has a ground action description, in which all fluent and action literals agree with their declarations and all type literals agree with the background knowledge.

States and Transitions. In analogy to the definition of stable models and answer sets [7], we will first define the semantics for positive (i.e., default negation-free) planning problems. Subsequently we define a reduction from general planning problems to positive ones.

A consistent set of ground fluent literals is called *state*. A tuple $t = \langle s, A, s' \rangle$ where s, s' are states and A is a set of action atoms is called a *state transition*.

In what follows, let PD be a planning domain, whose instantiation is $PD\!\downarrow = \langle \Pi, \langle D, R \rangle \rangle$, and M is the unique answer set of Π.

A state s_0 is called *legal initial state* for a positive PD iff for each initial state constraint $c \in R$, $h(c)$ is in s_0 if $post^+(c) \subseteq s_0 \cup M$ holds and s_0 is minimal under this condition.

For a positive PD and a state s, a set $A \subseteq \mathcal{L}_{act}^+$ is called *executable action set* w.r.t. s iff for each $a \in A$ there exists an executability condition $e \in R$ such that $h(e) = \{a\}$, $pre^+(e) \cap \mathcal{L}_{fl,typ} \subseteq s \cup M$, and $pre^+(e) \cap \mathcal{L}_{act}^+ \subseteq A$.[3]

For a positive PD and a state transition $t = \langle s, A, s' \rangle$ is called *legal state transition* if A is an executable action set w.r.t. s and s' is the minimal consistent set that satisfies all causation rules w.r.t. $s \cup A$, i.e. for every causation rule $r \in R$, if (i) $post^+(r) \cap \mathcal{L}_{fl} \subseteq s'$, (ii) $pre^+(r) \cap \mathcal{L}_{fl} \subseteq s$, and (iii) $pre^+(r) \cap \mathcal{L}_{act} \subseteq A$ all hold, then $h(r) \neq \{\texttt{false}\}$ and $h(r) \subseteq s'$. Note that we need not consider type literals, as they have already been dealt with in the instantiation step.

The above definitions are now generalized to a PD containing default negation by defining a reduction to a positive planning domain.

For an arbitrary PD and a state transition $t = \langle s, A, s' \rangle$, the *reduction* $PD^t = \langle \Pi, \langle D, R^t \rangle \rangle$ is a planning domain where R^t is obtained from R by deleting those $r \in R$, for which either $post^-(r) \cap (s' \cup M) \neq \emptyset$ or $pre^-(r) \cap (s \cup A \cup M) \neq \emptyset$ holds, and by deleting all $\texttt{not}\ L$ ($L \in \mathcal{L}$) from the remaining $r \in R$. Note that PD^t is positive and ground.

For an arbitrary PD, a state s_0 is called *legal initial state* iff s_0 is a legal initial state for PD^t with $t = \langle \emptyset, \emptyset, s_0 \rangle$.

A is an *executable action set* in PD w.r.t. a state s iff A is executable w.r.t. s in PD^t with $t = \langle s, A, \emptyset \rangle$.

A transition $t = \langle s, A, s' \rangle$ is a *legal state transition* in PD iff it is a legal transition w.r.t PD^t. A sequence of state transitions $T = \langle \langle s_0, A_1, s_1 \rangle, \ldots, \langle s_{n-1}, A_n, s_n \rangle \rangle$, $n \geq 0$, is a *legal transition sequence* for PD, if s_0 is a legal initial state of PD and all $\langle s_{i-1}, A_i, s_i \rangle$, $1 \leq i \leq n$, are legal state transitions of PD. In particular, $T = \langle \rangle$ is empty if $n = 0$.

We say that an arbitrary planning domain PD is *proper* if, given a state s and an action sequence A, the existence of a legal state transition $\langle s, A, s' \rangle$ is polynomially decidable (i.e., we can check efficiently the existence of a successor state s'). A planning problem $\langle PD, q \rangle$ is *proper* if the underlying planning domain PD is proper.

2.3   Plans

Given a planning problem $PP = \langle PD, q \rangle$, where q has form (4), a sequence of action sets $\langle A_1, \ldots, A_i \rangle$, $i \geq 0$, is an *optimistic plan* for PP, if a legal transition sequence $T = \langle \langle s_0, A_1, s_1 \rangle, \ldots, \langle s_{i-1}, A_i, s_i \rangle \rangle$ in PD exists such that T establishes the goal, i.e., $\{g_1, \ldots g_m\} \subseteq s_i$ and $\{g_{m+1}, \ldots, g_n\} \cap s_i = \emptyset$.

However, the existence of an optimistic plan does not guarantee that executing the plan, due to incomplete information and possible alternative transitions, will always lead to the goal. In case of incomplete initial state specification, we must be sure that

---

[3] This is useful to model dependent actions, i.e. actions which depend on the execution of other actions.

the plan is executable and the goal is reached whatever is the legal initial state consistent with the specification.

An optimistic plan $\langle A_1, \ldots, A_n \rangle$ for PP as previously is a *secure plan*, if for every legal initial state s_0 and legal transition sequence $T = \langle \langle s_0, A_1, s_1 \rangle, \ldots, \langle s_{j-1}, A_j, s_j \rangle \rangle$ such that $0 \leq j \leq n$, it holds that (i) if $j = n$ then T establishes the goal, and (ii) if $j < n$, then A_{j+1} is executable in s_j w.r.t. PD, i.e., some legal transition $\langle s_j, A_{j+1}, s_{j+1} \rangle$ exists.

A plan $\langle A_1, \ldots, A_n \rangle$ is called *sequential* (or *non-concurrent*) if $|A_j| \leq 1$, for all $1 \leq j \leq n$.

3   The Planning System DLV$^{\mathcal{K}}$

We have implemented a fully operational prototype supporting the $\mathcal{K}$ language as a frontend on top of the DLV system [4]. This frontend is invoked by the command-line option -FP of DLV. It reads $\mathcal{K}$ files, that is, files as described in the following subsection whose names carry the extension .plan, and optionally also background knowledge in the form of stratified datalog and transforms these into the core language of DLV. The frontend then invokes the DLV kernel and translates possible solutions back into output appropriate for the planning user.

3.1   Programs in DLV$^{\mathcal{K}}$

A $\mathcal{K}$ program, as implemented in DLV$^{\mathcal{K}}$, consists of various (optional) sections that start with a keyword followed by a colon. The overall structure of a $\mathcal{K}$ program is as follows:

```
fluents:     <fluent declarations>
actions:     <action declarations>
always:      <rules>
initially:   <init rules>

             [noConcurrency.]        [securePlan.]
goal:        <query>?(i)
```

where `<fluent declarations>` and `<action declarations>` are sequences of declarations as defined in Section 2.1, and `<rules>` (resp., `<init rules>`) is a sequence of causation rules and executability conditions which apply to any (resp., any initial) state.

By default, DLV$^{\mathcal{K}}$ will look for plans allowing concurrent actions (that is, plans that may contain transitions $\langle s, A, s' \rangle$ with $|A| > 1$). By specifying noConcurrency. the user can ask for sequential plans. In the presence of securePlan. or the command-line option -FPsec, DLV$^{\mathcal{K}}$ will only compute secure plans, as opposed to the default situation where all (optimistic) plans are computed and the user interactively decides whether to check their safety.[4]

---

[4] In the current implementation, some syntactic conditions, ensuring proper planning domains, are required to allow the security check of the plans. Optimistic plans are computed under no restriction.

3.2   Language Enhancements

In planning it is often useful to declare some fluents as inertial, which means that these fluents keep their truth values in a state transition, unless explicitly affected by an action. In the AI literature this has been studied intensively and is referred to as the *frame problem* [24, 31].

To allow for an easy representation of this kind of situation, we have enhanced the language by a shortcut inertial f. which is equivalent to the rule caused f if not $\neg.f$ after f. where f is a fluent literal.

For reasoning under incomplete knowledge we introduce total f. which is a shortcut for caused f if not $\neg f$.   caused $\neg f$ if not f. where f is a positive fluent literal. Such total statements can be defined in the always: and initially: sections of a DLV$^\mathcal{K}$ program, where in the latter case, only the initial state is completed.

Finally, it may be convenient to explicitly forbid executing an action under specific circumstances. To this end, we introduce nonexecutable a if B. where a is an action atom, as a shortcut for caused false after a, B.

4   Knowledge Representation in $\mathcal{K}$

4.1   A Simple Blocks World Instance

Now we are ready to give a short blocks world example. Referring to Figure 1, we want to turn the initial configuration of blocks into the goal state[5] in three steps, where only one move is allowed in each step (i.e., concurrent moves are not permitted).

First of all, the static background knowledge Π consists of the following rules and actions:

```
block(a). block(b). block(c).
location(table).
location(B) :- block(B).
```

This program describes the relevant objects in our planning domain.

The action description for the blocks world needs one action move and two fluents on, and occupied. We first assume that the knowledge on the initial state is complete (we know the location of all blocks) and correctly specified. We will then show how to deal with incorrect or incomplete initial state specifications.

```
fluents:  on(B,L) requires block(B), location(L).
          occupied(B) requires location(B).
actions:  move(B,L) requires block(B), location(L).
always:   executable move(B,L) if not occupied(B),
                                   not occupied(L), B <> L.
          inertial on(B,L).
```

---

[5] This problem illustrates the well known Sussman anomaly [33].

```
              caused occupied(B) if on(B1,B), block(B).
              caused on(B,L) after move(B,L).
              caused -on(B,L1) after move(B,L), on(B,L1), L <> L1.
initially:    on(a,table). on(b,table). on(c,a).

              noConcurrency.
goal:         on(c,b),on(b,a),on(a,table)? (3)
```

Intuitively, the executable rule says that a block B can be moved on location $L \neq B$ if both B and L are clear (note that the table is always clear, as it is not a block). The causation rules for on and -on specify the effect of a move. It is worthwhile noting that the totality of these fluents is not enforced. Both on(x,y) and -on(x,y) may happen to be not true at a given instant of time.

Actually, the rule for -on could be replaced by a rule stating: wherever a block is, it is not anywhere else (caused -on(B,L1) if on(B,L), L <> L1.). This rule would give us a sharper description of the state making fluent on total at every instant of time. Nevertheless, the extra knowledge derived for -on from this rule is useless for our goal, as -on does not appear in the body of any rule, and -on(x,y) is used only to override the inertial property on(x,y) after moving x from y. Thus, we refrain from using the more general rule which would cause a computational overhead (as more inferences are to be done during the computation) without providing relevant benefits.

The execution of this program on DLV$^{\mathcal{K}}$ computes the following:

```
PLAN: move(c,table,0), move(b,a,1), move(c,b,2)
```

Here, the additional argument in a move atom represents the instant of time when the action is executed. Thus, the above plan requires to first move c on the table, then to move b on top of a, and, finally, to move c on b. It is easy to see that this sequence of actions leads to the desired goal.

4.2   Checking Correctness and Completeness of the Initial State

In the previous example, the knowledge on the block locations in the initial state is complete and correctly specified with respect to domain laws. To ensure that an arbitrary given (partial) knowledge state is not flawed, we should check it properly. We should here verify that every block: (i) is on top of a unique location, (ii) does not have more than one block on top of it, and (iii) is supported by the table (i.e., it is either on the table or on a stack of blocks which is on the table) [20]. To this end, we add the declaration:

```
supported(B) requires block(B).
```

And we add the following rules in the initially section:

```
              caused false if on(B,L), on(B,L1), L<>L1.
              caused false if on(B1,B), on(B2,B), block(B), B1<>B2.
              caused supported(B) if on(B,table).
              caused supported(B) if on(B,B1), supported(B1).
              caused false if not supported(B).
```

The resulting $\text{DLV}^{\mathcal{K}}$ program does not compute any plan if the initial state is either incomplete (in the sense that not all block locations are known) or incorrectly specified. Note that, under noConcurrency, the action move preserves the properties (i),(ii), (iii) above; thus, we do not need to check these properties in all states, if concurrent actions are forbidden.

4.3   Reasoning under Incomplete Knowledge

Suppose now that there is a further block d in Figure 1. The exact location if d is unknown, but we know that it is not on top of c.

We look for a plan that works on every possible initial state (i.e., no matter if on(d,b) or on(d,table) holds), and reaches the goal on(a,c), on(c,d), on(d,b), on(b,table) in four steps. We modify the program Π and the goal q by adding (i) -on(d,c) and total on(X,Y) in the initially section, and (ii) the command securePlan. The execution of this program on $\text{DLV}^{\mathcal{K}}$ computes the following:

    PLAN: move(d,table,0), move(d,b,1), move(c,d,2), move(a,c,3)

The plan is clearly valid on all possible initial legal states. Since the effects of all actions are determined, this plan is also secure.

Note that an optimistic 2-step plan exists: move(c,d,0), move(a,c,1), as c could initially be on b. However, this plan is not secure.

5   Complexity of $\mathcal{K}$

We briefly report some results on the computational complexity of planning in $\mathcal{K}$ for the ground (propositional) case (see [1, 2] and references therein for related results). In particular, we consider deciding existence of a (secure) optimistic plan for a planning program $\langle PD, q \rangle$ and checking whether a given optimistic plan for it is secure.

An optimistic plan can be generated nondeterministically, by guessing the transitions $\langle s_{i-1}, A_i, s_i \rangle$ subsequently, starting from some (nondeterministically generated) legal initial state. Since this requires only polynomial workspace and NPSPACE = PSPACE, the problem is in PSPACE. On the other hand, STRIPS, which is PSPACE-complete [2], can be easily reduced to $\mathcal{K}$. If the number of steps in q is fixed, the complexity decreases because altogether there is fixed number of guesses, which have polynomial size.

Theorem 1. *Deciding whether a given proper ground planning problem* $\langle PD, q \rangle$ *has an optimistic plan is PSPACE-complete, and NP-complete if the number of steps in q is fixed.*

Deciding the existence of a secure plan appears to be harder, since it allows us to encode also planning under incomplete initial states. Already recognizing a secure plan is difficult.

Theorem 2. *Given an optimistic plan P and a proper ground planning problem* $\langle PD, q \rangle$, *deciding whether P is secure is* coNP-*complete. Hardness holds even if the number of steps in q is fixed.*

When looking for a secure plan, these complexities combine, even if the number of steps is bounded.

Theorem 3. *Deciding whether a given proper ground planning problem* $\langle PD, q \rangle$ *has a secure plan is* NEXPTIME-*complete in general and* Σ_2^P-*complete, if the number of steps in q is fixed.*

Intuitively, a secure plan can only be built if we know all states reachable after steps $A_1, \ldots, A_i$ so far when the next step A_{i+1} is generated. This requires exponential work space in general. Note that NEXPTIME strictly contains PSPACE, and thus this problem can not be efficiently translated to traditional STRIPS planning. The Σ_2^P-completeness result implies that even if short secure plans can not be efficiently generated by using systems which allow to solve only problems in NP, such as Blackbox [16], CCALC [21], smodels [25], or satisfiability checkers. The hardness relies on the fact that parallel actions are possible. Note that Baral et al. [1] report the related result that deciding in language $\mathcal{A}$ [8] the existence of an, in our terminology, secure sequential plan of polynomially bounded length is Σ_2^P-complete.

Under no concurrency, the complexity remains unaffected in the general case, but is much lower complexity if the plan length is fixed.

Theorem 4. *Deciding whether a given proper ground planning problem* $\langle PD, q \rangle$ *has a secure sequential plan is* NEXPTIME-*complete in general and* D^P-*complete, if the number of steps in q is fixed. (D^P is the conjunction of* NP *and* coNP.)

Informally, the complexity drops to D^P since in the sequential case only polynomially many candidates for secure plans of fixed length exist, which can be generated in polynomial time. A secure plan exists if (i) some legal initial state exists (which is in NP), and (ii) some of the (polynomially many) candidates has the property that it works on every evolution of every initial state. This check is in coNP for a single candidate and thus, as easily seen, also for all simultaneously. Hence, the problem is in D^P. The hardness for D^P implies, however, that the problem is still not efficiently representable in systems with expressiveness limited to NP.

In arbitrary rather than proper planning domains, security checking as in Theorem 2 is Π_2^P-complete, and deciding the existence of a secure plan of fixed length as in Theorems 3 and 4 is Σ_3^P-complete and Π_2^P-complete, respectively. Intuitively, this is due to an additional nested consistency check. In all other cases, the complexity is the same.

6   Related Work and Conclusion

Planning under incomplete knowledge has been widely investigated in the AI literature. Most works extend algorithms/systems for classical planning, rather than using deduction techniques for solving planning tasks as proposed in this paper. The systems

Buridan [17], UDTPOP [26], Conformant Graphplan [32], CNLP [27] and CASSAN-DRA [28] fall in this class. In particular, Buridan, UDTPOP, and Conformant Graphplan can solve secure planning (also called conformant planning) like $DLV^{\mathcal{K}}$. On the other hand, the systems CNLP and CASSANDRA deal with conditional planning (where the sequence of actions to be executed depends on dynamic conditions).

More recent works propose the use of automated reasoning techniques for planning under incomplete knowledge. In [30] a technique for encoding conditional planning problems in terms of 2-QBF formulas is proposed. The work in [29] proposes a technique based on regression for solving secure planning problems in the framework of the Situation Calculus, and presents a Prolog implementation of such a technique. In [23], sufficient syntactic conditions ensuring security of every (optimistic) plan are singled out. While sharing their logic-based nature, our work presented in this paper differs considerably from such proposals, since it is based on a different formalism.

Work similar to ours has been independently reported in [9]. In that paper, the author presents a SAT-based procedure for computing secure plans over planning domains specified in the action language $\mathcal{C}$ [11, 19, 18]. The main differences between our paper and [9] are (i) the different action languages used for specifying planning domains ($\mathcal{C}$ vs $\mathcal{K}$; the former is closer to classical logic, while the latter is more "logic programming oriented" by the use default negation); (ii) the different computational engines underlying the two systems (a SAT Checker vs a DLP system), which imply completely different translation techniques for the implementation. Other recent studies on secure planning are reported in [3]. Experimental evaluations and a comparison of the performance of the various systems for secure planning are on the agenda for future work.

Acknowledgments. The authors were supported by FWF (Austrian Science Funds) under the projects P11580-MAT and Z29-INF.

This work has greatly benefited from interesting discussions with and comments of Michael Gelfond, Vladimir Lifschitz, Riccardo Rosati, and Hudson Turner.

References

1. C. Baral, V. Kreinovich, and R. Trejo. Computational complexity of planning and approximate planning in presence of incompleteness. *IJCAI '99*, pp. 948–953.
2. T. Bylander. The Computational Complexity of Propositional STRIPS Planning. *AIJ*, 69:165–204, 1994.
3. A. Cimatti, M. Roveri. Conformant Planning via Model Checking. *Proc. ECP'99*, LNCS, 1999.
4. T. Eiter, N. Leone, C. Mateis, G. Pfeifer, and F. Scarcello. The KR System dlv: Progress Report, Comparisons and Benchmarks. *KR'98*, pp. 406–417.
5. W. Faber, N. Leone, and G. Pfeifer. Pushing Goal Derivation in DLP Computations. *LP-NMR'99*, pp. 177–191.
6. R. E. Fikes and N. J. Nilsson. Strips: A new approach to the application of theorem proving to problem solving. *AIJ*, 2(3-4):189–208, 1971.
7. M. Gelfond and V. Lifschitz. Classical Negation in Logic Programs and Disjunctive Databases. *NGC*, 9:365–385, 1991.
8. M. Gelfond and V. Lifschitz. Representing Action and Change by Logic Programs. *JLP*, 17:301–321, 1993.

9. E. Giunchiglia. Planning as Satisfiability with Expressive Action Languages: Concurrency, Constraints and Nondeterminism. *KR '00*.

10. E. Giunchiglia, G. Neelakantan Kartha, and V. Lifschitz. Representing action: Indeterminacy and ramifications. *AIJ*, 95:409–443, 1997.

11. E. Giunchiglia and V. Lifschitz. An Action Language Based on Causal Explanation: Preliminary Report. *AAAI '98*, pp. 623–630.

12. E. Giunchiglia and V. Lifschitz. Action languages, temporal action logics and the situation calculus. *IJCAI'99 Workshop on Nonmonotonic Reasoning, Action, and Change*.

13. S. Hanks and D. McDermott. Nonmonotonic Logic and Temporal Projection. *AIJ*, 33(3):379–412, 1987.

14. L. Iocchi, D. Nardi, and R. Rosati. Planning with sensing, concurrency, and exogenous events: Logical framework and implementation. *KR'2000*.

15. G. Neelakantan Kartha and V. Lifschitz. Actions with indirect effects. *KR '94*, pp. 341–350.

16. H. Kautz and B. Selman. Unifying SAT-based and Graph-based Planning. *IJCAI '99*, pp. 318–325.

17. N. Kushmerick, S. Hanks and D. Weld. An algorithm for probabilistic planning. *Artificial Intelligence*, 76(1–2), pp. 239–286, 1996.

18. V. Lifschitz and H. Turner. Representing transition systems by logic programs. *LPNMR'99*, pp. 92–106.

19. V. Lifschitz. Action Languages, Answer Sets and Planning. *The Logic Programming Paradigm - A 25-Year Perspective*. Springer, 1999.

20. V. Lifschitz. Answer set planning. *ICLP '99*, pp. 23–37.

21. N. McCain. Using the Causal Calculator with the C Input Language. Unpublished draft, 1999.

22. J. McCarthy. *Formalization of common sense, papers by John McCarthy edited by V. Lifschitz*. Ablex, 1990.

23. N. McCain, H. Turner. Fast Satisfiability Planning with Causal Theories. *KR'98*.

24. J. McCarthy and P.J. Hayes. Some philosophical problems from the standpoint of artificial intelligence. *Machine Intelligence 4*.

25. I. Niemelä. Logic Programs with Stable Model Semantics as a Constraint Programming Paradigm. *AMAI*, 25(3-4):241–273, 1999.

26. M. Peot. Decision-theoretic planning. PhD thesis, Dept. of Engineering and Economic Systems, Stanford University, 1998.

27. M. Peot and D. Smith. Conditional nonlinear planning. In *Proc. of AIPS'92*, pp. 189–197, 1992.

28. L. Pryor and G. Collins. Planning for contingencies: a decision-based approach. *Journal of Artificial Intelligence Research*, 4:287–339, 1996.

29. R. Reiter. Open world planning in the situation calculus. To appear in *Proc. of AAAI 2000*.

30. J. Rintanen. Constructing Conditional Plans by a Theorem-Prover. *Journal of Artificial Intelligence Research*, 10:323–352, 1999.

31. S.J. Russel and P. Norvig. *Artificial Intelligence, A Modern Approach*. Prentice-Hall, Inc., 1995.

32. D. Smith and D. Weld. Conformant Graphplan. In *Proc. of AAAI'98*, 1998.

33. G.J. Sussman. The Virtuous Nature of Bugs. *Readings in Planning*, chapter 3. Morgan Kaufmann, 1990. Originally written 1974.

34. H. Turner. Representing Actions in Logic Programs and Default Theories: A Situation Calculus Approach, *JLP*, 31:245–298, 1997.

35. J. D. Ullman. *Principles of Database and Knowledge Base Systems*, volume 1. Computer Science Press, 1989.

36. M. Veloso. *Nonlinear problem solving using intelligent causal-commitment*. Technical Report CMU-CS-89-210, Carnegie Mellon University, 1989.

Wire Routing and Satisfiability Planning

Esra Erdem, Vladimir Lifschitz, and Martin D.F. Wong

Department of Computer Sciences
University of Texas at Austin
Austin, TX 78712, USA
{esra,vl,wong}@cs.utexas.edu

Abstract. Wire routing is the problem of determining the physical locations of all the wires interconnecting the circuit components on a chip.
Since the wires cannot intersect with each other, they are competing
for limited spaces, thus making routing a difficult combinatorial optimization problem. We present a new approach to wire routing that uses
action languages and satisfiability planning. Its idea is to think of each
path as the trajectory of a robot, and to understand a routing problem
as the problem of planning the actions of several robots whose paths
are required to be disjoint. The new method differs from the algorithms
implemented in the existing routing systems in that it always correctly
determines whether a given problem is solvable, and it produces a solution whenever one exists.

1 Introduction

Very large scale integrated circuits (VLSI), with millions of transistors and wires
on a single silicon chip, are too complex to design without the aid of computers.
Advances in integrated circuit technology will result in more complex chips in the
near future—it is predicted that there will be over 1 billion transistors and wires
on a single chip in about 10 years [13]. As a result, research and development
in computer-aided design (CAD) software is very active in both industry and
academia.

Routing is an important step in CAD for VLSI circuits [7]. It is the problem
of determining the physical locations of all the wires interconnecting the circuit
components (transistors, gates, functional units, etc.) on a chip. Since the wires
cannot intersect with each other (otherwise resulting in short circuits), they
are competing for limited spaces, thus making routing a difficult combinatorial
optimization problem. In practice, the routing problem for the whole VLSI chip
is decomposed into smaller routing problems [7]. The chip is partitioned into an
array of rectangular regions. After determining the connections between adjacent
regions, the routing of all the regions are carried out independently. But even
for an individual region the problem is computationally difficult. VLSI routing
has been shown to be NP-complete [14], and there are many heuristic routing
algorithms in the literature [7].

In this paper, we present a new approach to VLSI routing that uses action
languages [3] and satisfiability planning [5]. All existing routing systems are

J. Lloyd et al. (Eds.): CL 2000, LNAI 1861, pp. 822–836, 2000.
© Springer-Verlag Berlin Heidelberg 2000

based on variations of the sequential maze routing approach using a shortest path algorithm connecting one wire at a time [6, 11]. A major shortcoming of these algorithms is that they cannot guarantee finding a routing solution even when one exists. The new method differs from them in that it is complete: it always correctly determines whether a given routing problem is solvable, and it produces a routing solution whenever one exists.

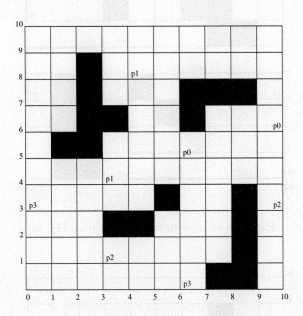

Fig. 1. A routing problem with 4 wires.

Consider, for instance, the routing problem shown in Fig. 1. The wiring space here is a rectangular grid. The goal is to connect 4 pairs of points ("pins")—the two points labeled $p0$, the two points labeled $p1$, and so on—without passing through the obstacles, shown in black. A solution—actually, the solution found by the method proposed in this paper—is given in Fig. 2. If we try to solve this problem by finding first a shortest path between the points labeled $p0$, and then a shortest path between the points labeled $p1$ in the part of the grid that is still available, we will arrive at a partial solution like the one shown in Fig. 3. This partial solution cannot be extended to a complete solution, however, because the points labeled $p2$ cannot be connected without intersecting the first of the two paths selected earlier.

The idea of the new method is to think of each path as the trajectory of a robot moving along the grid lines, and to understand a routing problem as the problem of planning the actions of several robots. In the example above, the problem involves 4 robots. The initial position of Robot 0 is assumed to be $(6,5)$, and its goal is to reach point $(10,6)$ (or the other way around), and similarly for

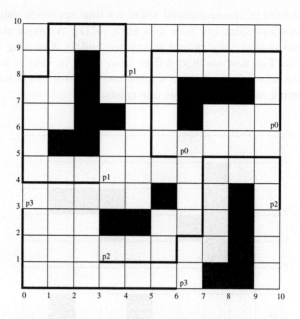

Fig. 2. A solution to the problem from Fig. 1.

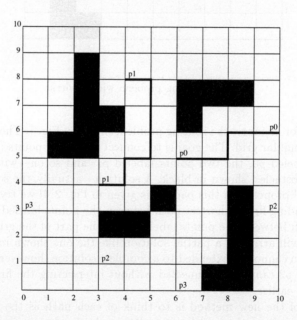

Fig. 3. A partial solution to the problem from Fig. 1. It cannot be extended to a complete solution.

the other robots. The actions that a robot can perform are to move left, right, up or down to the closest grid point, or to do nothing. We describe the effects of these actions in action language C [4].

The action language C is based on the theory of causal explanation proposed in [9]. Therefore, the view of causality adopted in C distinguishes between asserting that a certain fact "holds" and making the stronger assertion that it "is caused" (or "has an explanation").

The language C has propositions of two kinds: *static laws* of the form

$$\textbf{caused } F \textbf{ if } G$$

and *dynamic laws* of the form

$$\textbf{caused } F \textbf{ if } G \textbf{ after } H.$$

Here F and G are formulas whose atomic components represent fluents. The formula H is of a more general kind: in addition to fluents, it is allowed to contain the names of actions. Syntactically, action names are treated as atomic formulas; an assignment of truth values to action names represents the composite action which is executed by performing concurrently all elementary actions whose names are assigned the value *true*.

In the language C,

(i) an expression of the form

$$U \textbf{ causes } F \textbf{ if } G$$

where U is a propositional combination of elementary action names and F, G are propositional combination of fluent names, stands for the dynamic law

$$\textbf{caused } F \textbf{ if } true \textbf{ after } G \wedge U.$$

(ii) an expression of the form

$$\textbf{nonexecutable } U \textbf{ if } F$$

where U is a propositional combination of elementary action names and F is a propositional combination of fluent names, stands for the dynamic law

$$\textbf{caused } false \textbf{ if } true \textbf{ after } F \wedge U.$$

(iii) an expression of the form

$$\textbf{never } F$$

where F is a propositional combination of fluent names, stands for the static law

$$\textbf{caused } false \textbf{ if } F.$$

These and other abbreviations are introduced in [3].

The semantics of $\mathcal{C}$ defines how a set of propositions describes a "transition system"—a directed graph whose vertices are "states" and whose edges are labeled by "actions." A state is characterized by an assignment of truth values to fluent names, and an action is characterized by an assignment of truth values to action names. See [4] for details.

We use the Causal Calculator[1] (CCALC) to find a plan for the planning problem that corresponds to a wire routing problem. The Causal Calculator uses literal completion [9] to reduce a planning problem described in $\mathcal{C}$ to the problem of finding a satisfying interpretation for a set of propositional formulas, and then passes on these formulas to a satisfiability solver, such as RELSAT [1].

In the next two sections we provide a more detailed description of the new method as it applies to the problem above. Then we show that our approach can handle various kinds of additional routing constraints which ensure that a circuit meets its performance specification: constraints on the lengths of the wires, essential because signal delay through a wire is proportional to its length (Sections 4 and 5), and spacing constraints between the wires, related to the problem of avoiding signal interferences (Section 6).

2   Input and Output of CCALC

As discussed in the introduction, for each pair of points that need to be connected we imagine a robot that travels between these points. The position of Robot N is described by the propositional fluents at_x(N,XC) ("the x-coordinate of N is XC") and at_y(N,YC). We also use the expression at(N,XC,YC) that is expanded into the conjunction of these fluents by the CCALC macro expansion mechanism. The actions affecting the position of Robot N are denoted by expressions of the form move(N,D), where D is one of the directions left, right, down, up.

To express that the robots' paths don't loop and don't intersect each other, we use the propositional fluent occupied(N,XC,YC)—"point (XC,YC) has been visited by Robot N." Initially, this fluent is true only if (XC,YC) is the initial position of Robot N. The set of true fluents of this form becomes larger as robots move to new positions.

Fig. 4 shows the CCALC input file representing the routing problem from Fig. 1. The **include** directives in the middle of the file refer to two other files: obstacles0.t, describing the shape of the obstacles in this example, and routing.t, describing the effects and the executability of actions in the routing domain. Parts of file routing.t are discussed in the next section. The number of wires and the size of the grid are represented in that file by the macros k, maxX and maxY. Their numeric values are defined in each particular routing problem.

The description of the planning problem consists of a set of given facts and a goal. The symbol 0: at the beginning of every fact tells CCALC that the fact is assumed to hold at time 0 (that is to say, is an initial condition). The first fact

---

[1] http://www.cs.utexas.edu/users/tag/cc.

```
:- macros k -> 3;
          maxX -> 10;
          maxY -> 10.

:- include 'obstacles0.t'.
:- include 'routing.t'.

:- plan
facts::
0: (occupied(N,XC,YC) ->> at(N,XC,YC)),
0: at(0,6,5),
0: at(1,3,4),
0: at(2,3,1),
0: at(3,0,3);
goal::
12..17: (at(0,10,6) && at(1,4,8) && at(2,10,3) && at(3,6,0)).
```

Fig. 4. Input file for the problem from Fig. 1

characterizes the initial value of `occupied(N,XC,YC)`.[2] We could have replaced this conditional by an equivalence, but there is no need to do this, because file `routing.t` declares `occupied(N,XC,YC)` to be a fluent false by default. The other facts give the initial positions of the robots. The symbol `12..17` in the goal instructs CCALC to try first to find a plan of length 12; if there is no such plan then try length 13, and so on, up to 17. In the case of the routing problem, the length of a plan corresponds to the maximum of the lengths of the wires.

Given this input file, CCALC reports that there is no solution of length 12, 13 or 14, and then produces a plan:

```
0.  at_y(0,5)  at_y(1,4)  at_y(2,1)  at_y(3,3)
    at_x(0,6)  at_x(1,3)  at_x(2,3)  at_x(3,0)

ACTIONS: move(0,left) move(1,left) move(2,right) move(3,down)

1.  at_y(0,5)  at_y(1,4)  at_y(2,1)  at_y(3,2)
    at_x(0,5)  at_x(1,2)  at_x(2,4)  at_x(3,0)

ACTIONS: move(0,up) move(1,left) move(2,right)

2.  at_y(0,6)  at_y(1,4)  at_y(2,1)  at_y(3,2)
    at_x(0,5)  at_x(1,1)  at_x(2,5)  at_x(3,0)

ACTIONS: move(0,up) move(1,left) move(2,right) move(3,down)
```

. . . .

---

[2] In CCALC input files, the propositional connectives are denoted by `->>` (implication), `&&` (conjunction), `++` (disjunction) and `-` (negation).

```
ACTIONS: move(0,down) move(1,down)
```

14. `at_y(0,7)  at_y(1,9)  at_y(2,3)  at_y(3,0)`
     `at_x(0,10)  at_x(1,4)  at_x(2,10)  at_x(3,5)`

```
ACTIONS: move(0,down) move(1,down) move(3,right)
```

15. `at_y(0,6)  at_y(1,8)  at_y(2,3)  at_y(3,0)`
     `at_x(0,10)  at_x(1,4)  at_x(2,10)  at_x(3,6)`

This is the solution shown in Fig. 2. RELSAT took 59 seconds to find it. (In our experiments, we used an UltraSPARC that has 124 MB main memory, runs SunOS 5.5.1, and has a 167 MHz CPU.)

3   The Routing Domain

In file `routing.t`,[3] the effect of action `move(N,right)` is described by the proposition

```
move(N,right) causes at_x(N,X)
              if at_x(N,XC) && X is XC+1 && XC < maxX.
```

(the execution of this action when `at_x(N,XC)` holds for some `XC` that is not at the right boundary of the grid makes `at_x(N,XC+1)` true). There is no need to postulate that the y-coordinate of Robot `N` and the coordinates of the other robots remain the same, because the coordinates of robots are declared to be "inertial"—they don't change their values if there is no evidence that they do. There is no need to say that `at_x(N,XC)` becomes false: the action affects this fluent indirectly, because the uniqueness of the x-coordinate of a robot is postulated in `routing.t` in the form

```
caused -at_x(N,XC)  if at_x(N,XC1) && -(XC=XC1).
```

(whatever value the x-coordinate of Robot `N` currently has, there is a cause for it not to have any other value).[4]

When a robot is on the right edge of the grid, it cannot move right:

```
nonexecutable move(N,right) if at_x(N,XC) && XC>=maxX.
```

Similar postulates describe moves in other directions.

We prevent robots from hitting obstacles by postulating

```
never at(N,XC,YC) && blocked(XC,YC).
```

---

[3] File `routing.t` and other files related to wire routing are available on-line at
http://www.cs.utexas.edu/users/tag/ccalc/ccalc.1.23/examples/routing/ .

[4] The solution to the frame problem and ramification problem incorporated in C and CCALC is based on the ideas of [12, 2, 15, 9].

Here `blocked(XC,YC)` is a macro defining the shape of the obstacles.

Fluent `occupied(N,XC,YC)` is characterized by the propositions

```
caused occupied(N,XC,YC) if at(N,XC,YC).
caused occupied(N,XC,YC) after occupied(N,XC,YC).
```

(the set of points visited by Robot N includes its current position and all points it had visited by the previous time instant). Using this fluent, we can say that paths of different robots don't intersect:

```
never occupied(N,XC,YC) && occupied(N1,XC,YC) && (N < N1).
```

and that a robot never visits the same point twice:

```
caused false if at(N,XC,YC) after occupied(N,XC,YC) && -at(N,XC,YC).
```

The last conjunctive term is necessary to allow a robot not to move; without it, all robots would make the same number of moves, and all paths would have equal lengths.

4   Bus Routing

A bus is a set of wires, each connecting a source pin and a sink pin, where the source pins are all adjacent and the sink pins are all adjacent. In bus routing, given several pairs of points on a rectangular grid, we want to find a configuration of a bus such that all wires are of the same length: we want the signal delays through all wires to be equal. The need to express the equality of the lengths is the main special feature of bus routing problems.

A bus routing problem, along with its solution found by CCALC, is displayed in Fig. 5. The input file for this program is shown in Fig. 6. The equality of the lengths of all paths is expressed there by the proposition

```
caused false if at(N,XC,YC) after at(N,XC,YC).
```

The run time of RELSAT in this example is 36 seconds.

In some cases, a bus routing problem has no solution but becomes solvable if we relax the condition on the lengths of wires. For instance, with the configuration of obstacles shown in Fig. 7, it is impossible to connect all pairs of pins by paths of the same length, but there is an "approximate solution" in which the lenghts of wires do not differ by more than 2 (Fig. 8).

To find an "approximate solution" for the problem presented in Fig. 8 using CCALC, we add a constraint telling that robots always move until their goals have been achieved. Then we can instruct CCALC to look for paths whose lengths are between 11 and 13 by replacing the goal in Fig. 6 with

```
((11: at(0,8,4) ++ 12: at(0,8,4) ++ 13: at(0,8,4)) &&
 (11: at(1,8,5) ++ 12: at(1,8,5) ++ 13: at(1,8,5)) &&
 (11: at(2,8,6) ++ 12: at(2,8,6) ++ 13: at(2,8,6))).
```

If the goal is modified in this way (and file `obstacles1.t` is modified to reflect the configuration of obstacles in Fig. 7), CCALC generates the approximate solution shown in Fig. 8. The run time of RELSAT is 36 seconds.

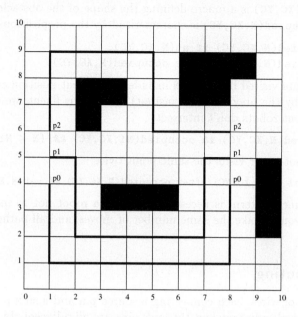

Fig. 5. A bus routing problem. The wires are required to have the same length.

```
:- macros k -> 2;
         maxX -> 10;
         maxY -> 10;
         maxLength -> 15.

:- include 'obstacles1.t'.
:- include 'routing.t'.

% robots always move
caused false if at(N,XC,YC) after at(N,XC,YC).

:- plan
facts::
0: (occupied(N,XC,YC) ->> at(N,XC,YC)),
0: at(0,1,4),
0: at(1,1,5),
0: at(2,1,6);
goal::
12..maxLength: (at(0,8,4) && at(1,8,5) && at(2,8,6)).
```

Fig. 6. Input file for the problem from Fig. 5

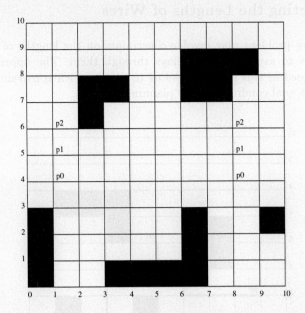

Fig. 7. A bus routing problem that has no precise solution.

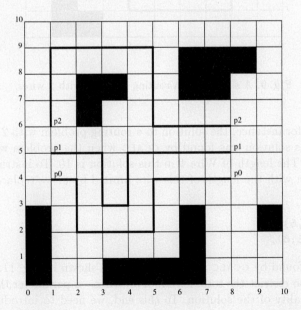

Fig. 8. An approximate solution to the problem from Fig. 7. The differences between the lengths of wires are limited by 2.

5   Restricting the Lengths of Wires

A wire routing problem may involve constraints on the lengths of some of the wires—that is to say, on signal delays through them. The approach to wire routing proposed in this paper allows us to express such constraints by simple changes in the goal condition of the planning problem.

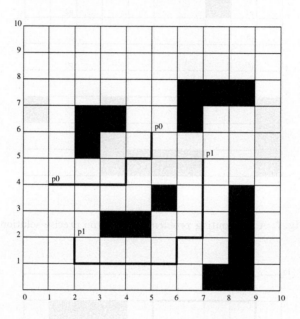

Fig. 9. A solution to a routing problem with 2 wires.

Consider, for instance, the solution to a routing problem with 2 wires shown in Fig. 9. This solution was found by CCALC when the problem was described as in Fig. 10. The length of Wire 1 in this solution is 10. To instruct CCALC to find a solution with the length of this wire limited by 8, we replace the goal in Fig. 10 with

```
8:  at(1,7,5),
10: at(0,5,6).
```

The solution found by CCALC after this change is shown in Fig. 11.

We can also restrict the total length of all wires—a parameter that measures the overall quality of the solution. To this end, we need to introduce auxiliary fluents length(N,L) ("the current length of the path of Robot N equals L"). We assume that initially this length is 0, and postulate that move(N,D) causes it to increase by 1. Then the requirement that the combined length of Wires 0 and 1 be limited by maxTotalLength can be expressed by

```
:- macros k -> 1;
         maxX -> 10;
         maxY -> 10;
         maxLength -> 14.

:- include 'obstacles2.t'.
:- include 'routing.t'.

:- plan
facts::
0: (occupied(N,XC,YC) ->> at(N,XC,YC)),
0: at(0,1,4),
0: at(1,2,2);
goal::
10: (at(0,5,6) && at(1,7,5)).
```

Fig. 10. Input file for the problem from Fig. 9

```
never (\/L0: \/L1: (length(0,L0) && length(1,L1) && L is L0+L1
                                  && L >= maxTotalLength)).
```

The symbol $\backslash/$ represents the existential quantifier (over a finite domain) and is expanded by CCALC into a finite disjunction.

6 Spacing Constraints

We say that two wires in a solution to a routing problem are *adjacent* if a segment of one of them and a segment of the other form two opposite sides of a unit square. In Fig. 2, for instance, Wires 0 and 1 are adjacent, and Wires 2 and 3 are adjacent. In this section we consider the problem of finding a wire routing without adjacent wires. This is a simple spacing constraint, interesting in view of its relation to the problem of avoiding signal interferences.

To describe adjacency, we introduce auxiliary fluents that represent the positions of vertical and horizontal unit segments in the trajectory of every robot. Fluent in_v(N,XC,YC) holds if the part of the trajectory of Robot N constructed so far includes the segment connecting points (XC,YC) and (XC,YC+1). Initially, these fluents are identically false. They are affected by actions move(N,up) and move(N,down) as follows:

```
move(N,up) causes in_v(N,XC,YC) if at(N,XC,YC).
move(N,down) causes in_v(N,XC,Y)
              if at(N,XC,YC) && Y is YC-1 && YC>0.
```

Once such a fluent becomes true, it remains true:

```
caused in_v(N,XC,YC) after in_v(N,XC,YC).
```

Fluents in_h(N,XC,YC) describe the positions of horizontal segments in a similar way.

Using these fluents, we can eliminate adjacent wires by postulating

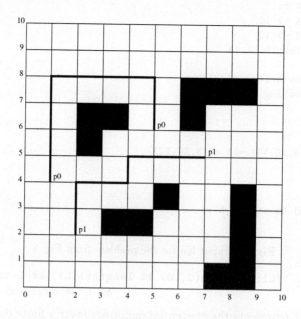

Fig. 11. A solution to the problem from Fig. 9 with the length of Wire 1 limited by 8.

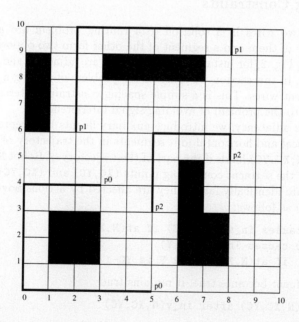

Fig. 12. A solution to a routing problem without adjacent wires.

```
never in_h(N,XC,YC) && in_h(N1,XC,Y)
     && -(N=N1) && Y is YC+1 && YC < maxY.
never in_v(N,XC,YC) && in_v(N1,X,YC)
     && -(N=N1) && X is XC+1 && XC < maxX.
```

Fig. 12 shows a solution to a routing problem, with adjacent wires prohibited, that was generated by CCALC on the basis of such a formalization. In this example, the run time of RELSAT was 156 seconds.

7 Discussion

We showed how satisfiability planning can be applied to wire routing problems of several kinds. Action language $\mathcal{C}$ that we use to describe the effects of actions in the routing domain is much more expressive than older action description languages STRIPS and $\mathcal{A}$ (see [3, Sections 3–6] for references and comparisons). Its expressivity is essential for our purposes.

CCALC transforms planning problems in the routing domains into propositional satisfiability problems, and RELSAT serves as the search engine. In some of our experiments, propositional solver SATO [16] was used instead of RELSAT. On some routing problems it performed much worse than RELSAT, and never much better. In our first example, for instance, RELSAT found a solution after about 1 minute of computation, and SATO did not terminate after 2 hours.

The new approach to wire routing always correctly determines whether a given problem is solvable, and it always produces a solution if it exists. Its other attractive feature is that some enhancements of the basic problem—in which lengths of wires and distances between them come into play—can be easily represented by modifying goals or by adding auxiliary fluents. The CCALC input files for all examples discussed in this paper include the same file routing.t describing the effects and executability of actions in the routing domain. In this sense, our representation method is similar to the work on elaboration tolerance [10] described in [8].

On the negative side, the size of the grid used in our examples is much too small for serious applications. Investigating the applicability of the new routing method to larger problems is a topic for future work.

There are several other possible future directions that we can take. One is to extend the current approach to perform routing on multiple wiring layers. In this paper we only addressed planar routing (i.e., only one layer is available for wiring). Another direction is to consider more complex spacing constraints where adjacent wires are allowed but the total amount of adjacencies between each pair of wires should be bounded. This more general formulation captures the fact that small amount of adjacencies may not produce enough signal interferences to affect circuit performance. Finally, we plan to investigate how to extend our new routing approach to solve the "global routing" problem [7], which is the problem of determining the connections between adjacent regions after an VLSI chip is decomposed into an array of smaller rectangular regions. The global routing problem resembles the routing problem we studied in this paper except that we would allow more than one wire to be placed on a grid edge.

Acknowledgments

We are grateful to Emilio Remolina and Hudson Turner for comments on a draft of this paper. The work of the first two authors was partially supported by the National Science Foundation under Grant No. IIS-9732744. The work of the third author was partially supported by a grant from the Intel Corporation and by the Texas Advanced Research Program under Grant No. 003658288.

References

1. Roberto Bayardo and Robert Schrag. Using CSP look-back techniques to solve real-world SAT instances. In *Proc. IJCAI-97*, pages 203–208, 1997.
2. Hector Geffner. Causal theories for nonmonotonic reasoning. In *Proc. AAAI-90*, pages 524–530. AAAI Press, 1990.
3. Michael Gelfond and Vladimir Lifschitz. Action languages. *Electronic Transactions on AI*, 3, 1998. http://www.ep.liu.se/ea/cis/1998/016.
4. Enrico Giunchiglia and Vladimir Lifschitz. An action language based on causal explanation: Preliminary report. In *Proc. AAAI-98*, pages 623–630. AAAI Press, 1998.
5. Henry Kautz and Bart Selman. Planning as satisfiability. In *Proc. ECAI-92*, pages 359–363, 1992.
6. C. Y. Lee. An algorithm for path connections and its application. *IRE Transactions on Electronic Computers*, EC–10:346–365, 1961.
7. T. Lengauer. *Combinatorial Algorithms for Integrated Circuit Design*. John Wiley & Sons, 1990.
8. Vladimir Lifschitz. Missionaries and cannibals in the causal calculator. In *Principles of Knowledge Representation and Reasoning: Proc. Seventh Int'l Conf.*, pages 85–96, 2000.
9. Norman McCain and Hudson Turner. Causal theories of action and change. In *Proc. AAAI-97*, pages 460–465, 1997.
10. John McCarthy. Elaboration tolerance. In progress, 1999. http://www-formal.stanford.edu/jmc/elaboration.html.
11. T. Ohtsuki. Maze-running and line-search algorithms. In T. Ohtsuki, editor, *Layout Design and Verification*, chapter 3. Elsevier Science Publishers, 1986.
12. Raymond Reiter. A logic for default reasoning. *Artificial Intelligence*, 13:81–132, 1980.
13. Semiconductor Industry Association. The national roadmap for semiconductors, 1997.
14. T. G. Szymanski. Dogleg channel routing is NP-complete. *IEEE Transactions on Computer-Aided Design*, 4(1):31–41, 1985.
15. Hudson Turner. Representing actions in logic programs and default theories: a situation calculus approach. *Journal of Logic Programming*, 31:245–298, 1997.
16. Hantao Zhang. An efficient propositional prover. In *Proc. CADE-97*, 1997.

Including Diagnostic Information in Configuration Models

Tommi Syrjänen*

Helsinki University of Technology, Dept. of Computer Science and Eng.
Laboratory for Theoretical Computer Science
P.O.Box 5400, FIN-02015 HUT, Finland
Tommi.Syrjanen@hut.fi

Abstract. This work presents a new formal model for software configuration. The configuration knowledge is stored in a configuration model
that is specified using a rule-based language. The language has a complete declarative semantics analogous to the stable model semantics for
normal logic programs. In addition, a new method to add diagnostic
information in configuration models is presented. The main idea is to
divide the configuration process into two stages. At the first stage the
user requirements are processed to check whether there exist any suitable
configurations in the configuration model. In the second stage unsatisfiable requirements are diagnosed using a diagnostic model. The diagnostic
model is constructed from the configuration model by adding a new set
of atoms that represent the possible error conditions. The diagnostic output also explains why each problematic component was included in the
configuration. As an example, a subset of the configuration problem for
the Debian GNU/Linux system is formalized using the new rule-based
language. Both configuration and diagnostic models of the problem are
presented. The rule-language is implemented using an existing implementation of the stable model semantics, the Smodels system.

1 Introduction

In a configuration problem, we have a complicated product that consists of
different components, *configuration objects*, that may interact in complex ways.
The collection of objects and relationships between them is called a *configuration
model*. A *configuration* is a set of objects of the configuration model. There may
also be a set of *constraints* imposed on the model that restrict the allowed object
combinations. In a *configuration process*, we are given a configuration model and
a set of *user requirements* and we want to find a configuration that satisfies the
requirements. According to [12] configurations can be divided into three classes:

1. A *valid* configuration satisfies all constraints of the configuration model;
2. A *suitable* configuration is a valid configuration that also satisfies all user
   requirements; and

---

* This work has been supported by the Academy of Finland (project no. 43963) and
Helsinki Graduate School in Computer Science and Engineering (HeCSE).

J. Lloyd et al. (Eds.): CL 2000, LNAI 1861, pp. 837–851, 2000.

3. An *optimal* configuration is a suitable configuration that additionally satisfies some optimality criteria.

Most work that has been done in the configuration management field has focused on finding valid configurations and a recent survey on different configuration methods can be found in [6].

In this work we define a rule-based language RRL that can be used to express configuration knowledge. The RRL language allows the use of variables and it has a declarative semantics that is based on the stable model semantics for normal logic programs [3]. The main advantage of a declarative semantics is implementation-independence. In a configuration system without a well-defined semantics, configurations are defined by the behavior of the configuration tool and if the tool is changed the set of valid configurations of the system may also change. In addition, if there are no suitable configurations at all, we have to explain the user why this is the case. This explanation is difficult to do if the configuration model does not have a well-defined semantics.

One major aim of this work is to closely examine the situation where the user requirements cannot be satisfied. In these cases it is not enough to decide that a suitable configuration does not exist but we also need to give the user a diagnostic explanation that points out the problems. The diagnostic output should have at least the following properties:

1. the diagnosis should identify what components cause the problem;
2. for each component that is a part of the problem, the diagnosis should include an explanation why it was necessary to take it in the configuration; and
3. the diagnosis should be as concise as possible.

The reason for the second property is that the end-user may want to include a pair of components that are not mutually exclusive by themselves but that depend on a pair of conflicting components. If the justification information is not added to the diagnostic model, the user may have a difficult time trying to find out why the configuration system wants to add some seemingly unrelated components in the configuration.

The third property is important when configurations consist of thousands of components. If the diagnosis contains a lot of unessential information, the user will again have a difficult time trying to find the actual problem.

In this work we will take the approach that we will construct two distinct models for the configuration system. A *configuration model* encodes the components and the relationships between them and the diagnostic information is stored in a *diagnostic model*.

During a configuration task, we first try to find a configuration that satisfies the user requirements. If such configuration exists, we can configure the system according to it. Otherwise, we know that we cannot choose the components in such way that the resulting configuration is both valid and satisfies the user requirements and we have to compute a diagnosis. We can do this by constructing an invalid configuration that satisfies all user requirements and explaining why it violates the constraints of the model. This process in illustrated in Figure 1.

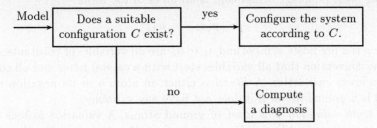

Fig. 1. A conceptual flowchart of a configuration task

The main reason why the two models are separated is simplicity. We find it easier to construct a configuration model when we do not have to worry about adding diagnostic information to it. Similarily, a diagnostic model is easier to construct when we do not have to worry about false alarms that are caused by incompatible optional components. Another reason for separation is efficiency. It seems that the current implementation is more efficient when the models are separated but the results are not conclusive and it is possible that there exists an efficient way to combine the data in one model.

As a practical example, we consider the configuration management problem of the Debian GNU/Linux system [1]. Debian is a distribution of the GNU/Linux operating system and currently with version 2.1 it has over 2500 distinct software packages. A package may interact with several other packages in various ways. A package may depend on functionality provided by another one, two packages may conflict with each other, or a package may recommend that another package is taken into a configuration whenever it is in it. The Debian distribution is an interesting case for configuration management for two main reasons:

1. The relationships between software packages are explicitly described and they are collected in one place. It is possible to generate a configuration model of the system automatically from this information.
2. The large number of software packages makes the configuration management of the Debian system a non-trivial task and if a formal method can handle it well, it can probably also handle other difficult cases.

As it is not possible to model the configuration management of the Debian system completely in this work, we formalize only a small subset of it and concentrate on the diagnostic model. The whole system is modeled in [10] with some preliminary evaluation results.

2   The Rule Language

In this section, we introduce a declarative rule-based formal language RRL which is a subset of the language RL defined in [10]. The language RL is based on a configuration rule language presented in [9].

The basic language component is an *atom* of the form

$$p(a_1, \ldots, a_n) \tag{1}$$

where p is a predicate symbol and a_1 to a_n are all variables or constants. We will use the convention that all variables start with a capital letter and all constants with a lower case letter. A *literal* is either an atom a or its negation $\mathrm{not}\, a$. A literal is a *ground literal* if it does not have any variables.

A *truth valuation* $\mathcal{V}$ is a set of ground atoms. A valuation assigns a truth value to each ground literal. If an atom a is in $\mathcal{V}$, a is *true* in $\mathcal{V}$, otherwise it is *false*. For negative literals the conditions are reversed. If an atom a is in $\mathcal{V}$, the literal $\mathrm{not}\, a$ is *false* in $\mathcal{V}$ and vice versa.

We encode the relationships between atoms using inference *rules* that have two possible forms:

$$h \leftarrow l_1, \ldots, l_n \tag{2}$$
$$\{ h_1, \ldots, h_m \} \leftarrow l_1, \ldots, l_n \tag{3}$$

where the atom h is the rule *head* and the literals $l_1, \ldots, l_n$ form the rule *body*. The rules of the form (2) are called *basic rules* and the rules of the form (3) are called *choice rules*. A basic rule with an empty rule body is called a *fact*. A *ground instance* of a rule is obtained by replacing all variables in it with constants. A RRL *program* is a set of rules.

The intuitive meaning of a basic rule is that if all literals in the rule body are true, the head atom also has to be true. If the body of a choice rule is true, we can include any subset of atoms $h_1, \ldots, h_m$ in our model. Strictly speaking, choice rules are not necessary as they could be replaced by a adding a rule of the form:

$$h_i \leftarrow l_1, \ldots, l_n, \mathrm{not}\, h_i'$$
$$h_i' \leftarrow \mathrm{not}\, h_i \tag{4}$$

for each $1 \leq i \leq m$. However, using choice rules makes programs more compact and the syntax is easy to expand to handle cases where a specific number of atoms $h_1, \ldots, h_m$ has to be true when the body is true [5].

Next we define the formal semantics of RRL. The definition is very similar to the stable model semantics for normal logic programs [3]. The variables are handled by instantiating the rules with all possible constants that are used in the program and computing the stable models of the resulting program.

Definition 1. *The* Herbrand instantiation $\mathbf{HI}(P)$ *of a RRL program P is the set of all ground instances of rules in P that can be constructed using constant symbols in P.*

Example 1. Let $P = \{\mathsf{p}(\mathsf{X}) \leftarrow \mathsf{q}(\mathsf{X}); \mathsf{q}(\mathsf{a}) \leftarrow ; \mathsf{q}(\mathsf{b}) \leftarrow \}$. The program $\mathbf{HI}(P)$ is now

$$\mathbf{HI}(P) = \{ \mathsf{p}(\mathsf{a}) \leftarrow \mathsf{q}(\mathsf{a}); \mathsf{p}(\mathsf{b}) \leftarrow \mathsf{q}(\mathsf{b}); \tag{5}$$
$$\mathsf{q}(\mathsf{a}) \leftarrow ; \mathsf{q}(\mathsf{b}) \leftarrow \}$$

Definition 2. *Given a ground* RRL *program P and a set of atoms M we construct the* reduct P^M *by*

1. *replacing all choice rules*

$$\{ h_1, \ldots, h_m \} \leftarrow l_1, \ldots, l_n \tag{3}$$

with the set

$$\{h_i \leftarrow l_1, \ldots, l_n \mid 1 \leq i \leq m \wedge h_i \in M\} \tag{6}$$

of rules.

2. *removing each rule that has a negative literal* not a *in its body where* $a \in M$; *and*

3. *removing all negative literals from the bodies of the remaining rules.*

Example 2. Let $P = \{\{a\} \leftarrow \text{not } b, \{b\} \leftarrow \text{not } a\}$ and $M_1 = \{a\}$. Now we can construct the reduct

$$P^{M_1} = \{a \leftarrow\} \ .$$

Similarly, if we set $M_2 = \emptyset$, the reduct $P^{M_2} = \emptyset$.

The reduct P^M is a set of Horn clauses so it has a unique minimal model $MM(P^M)$ [11]. If this minimal model coincides with M, we say that M is a *stable model* of P.

Definition 3. *Given a* RRL *program P and a set of atoms M, M is a* stable model *of P if and only if* $M = MM(\mathbf{HI}(P)^M)$.

Example 3. Let $P = \{\{a\} \leftarrow \text{not } b, \{b\} \leftarrow \text{not } a\}$. Now P has three stable models, $M_1 = \{a\}$, $M_2 = \{b\}$, and $M_3 = \emptyset$. As we saw in Example 2, the reduct of P with regards to M_1 is $P^{M_1} = \{a \leftarrow\}$ that has the minimal model $\{a\}$ which coincides to M_1. On the other hand, $M_4 = \{a, b\}$ is a model of P in a propositional sense but it is not a stable model as the reduct $P^{M_4} = \emptyset$ that has an empty minimal model.

Theorem 1. *Given a ground* RRL *program P the question whether there exists a stable model M of P is* NP-*complete.*

Proof. The NP-hardness follows directly from the fact that the problem of existence of a stable model for a normal logic program is NP-complete [4] and all normal logic programs are RRL programs.

If we guess the model M we can construct the reduct P^M in a linear time with respect to the number of literals in rule bodies and the minimal model $MM(P^M)$ can be computed in linear time [2]. This implies that the problem is in NP and thus it is NP-complete.

$$\{ \text{in}(P) \} \leftarrow \text{package}(P), \text{justified}(P)$$
$$\leftarrow \text{in}(P_1), \text{depends}(P_1, P_2), \text{not in}(P_2)$$
$$\leftarrow \text{conflicts}(P_1, P_2), \text{in}(P_1), \text{in}(P_2)$$
$$\leftarrow \text{user-include}(P), \text{not in}(P)$$
$$\leftarrow \text{user-exclude}(P), \text{in}(P)$$
$$\text{justified}(P) \leftarrow \text{user-include}(P)$$
$$\text{justified}(P_2) \leftarrow \text{depends}(P_1, P_2), \text{in}(P_1)$$
$$\text{justified}(P_2) \leftarrow \text{recommends}(P_1, P_2), \text{in}(P_1)$$

Fig. 2. The simplified Debian configuration model CM

3 Configuring a Debian System

In this section we formalize a small subset of the configuration management problem of the Debian GNU/Linux system. In particular, we will formalize only dependency, conflict, and recommendation relations of the system. We will leave out the package version information but we present the outline how it can be included in the model.

A package A *depends on* a package B if A cannot be used at all if B is not installed. A package A *conflicts with* B if A will not operate when B is installed on the system. A package A *recommends* B if B enhances the functionality of A in a significant way. The recommendation relation brings the concept of optionality to the configuration model. If a package recommends another, we can choose to add the recommended package or we can leave it out. The complete formalization of the Debian configuration system is presented in [10].

The Debian configuration model CM is constructed using the RRL language and it can be divided into two parts:

1. a database that stores information about the packages and their relations as facts; and
2. a set of inference rules that construct the valid configurations using the facts stored in the database.

The software packages are modeled as constants in the database. For each package P we add a corresponding constant p to the program. The relations are modeled with predicates, for example, if a package P_1 depends on P_2, the atom depends(P_1, P_2) is added as a fact to the program. The inference rules that form the core of the configuration model are presented in Figure 2.

As a Debian configuration is essentially a set of packages, we will use the predicate in(P) to denote that the package P is chosen to be in the configuration. Thus, valid configurations of a configuration model correspond to the stable models of the RRL program.

The user requirements can be modeled using two predicates user-include(P) and user-exclude(P). A set U of user requirements is a set of facts of the form

$$\text{user-include}(P) \leftarrow \quad \text{and}$$
$$\text{user-exclude}(P) \leftarrow$$

where the atom user-include(P) $\in U$ if the user explicitly selected P to be in the configuration and user-exclude(P) $\in U$ when the user wants to ensure that P is not in the configuration.

Definition 4. *Given a Debian configuration model CM, a set U of user requirements, and a stable model M of $CM \cup U$, a Debian configuration C_M is the set of packages*

$$C_M = \{P \mid \text{in}(P) \in M\} \ . \tag{7}$$

We want the configurations to be compact. They should contain the user selected packages and the packages they depend on and nothing more. Additionally, if a package is recommended by some package in the configuration, it may be included in the configuration but it may also be left out. We encode this principle by using the predicate justified(P) which is true in a stable model if the package P has some reason to be in a configuration.

The basic rule of the configuration model is that a package may be added to a configuration if and only if it can be justified:

$$\{ \ \text{in}(P) \ \} \leftarrow \text{justified}(P), \text{package}(P) \ . \tag{8}$$

The predicate package(P) is added to the rule body to ensure that only available packages may be added to the configuration.

It is an error if a package P_1 is in a configuration but one of its dependencies is not satisfied:

$$\leftarrow \text{in}(P_1), \text{depends}(P_1, P_2), \text{not in}(P_2) \ . \tag{9}$$

We may not have two conflicting packages in one configuration:

$$\leftarrow \text{conflicts}(P_1, P_2), \text{in}(P_1), \text{in}(P_2) \ . \tag{10}$$

If the user made an explicit choice regarding to a package P, the choice must be adhered:

$$\leftarrow \text{user-include}(P), \text{not in}(P) \tag{11}$$
$$\leftarrow \text{user-exclude}(P), \text{in}(P) \ . \tag{12}$$

A package is justified if either the user selected it, some package that has to be in the configuration depends on it, or some included package recommends it.

$$\text{justified}(P) \leftarrow \text{user-include}(P) \tag{13}$$
$$\text{justified}(P_2) \leftarrow \text{depends}(P_1, P_2), \text{in}(P_1) \tag{14}$$
$$\text{justified}(P_2) \leftarrow \text{recommends}(P_1, P_2), \text{in}(P_1) \ . \tag{15}$$

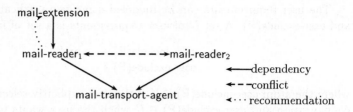

Fig. 3. The relationships between packages in Example 4

As an example we consider a simple system that consists of four different packages. There are two different mail reader packages (mail-reader$_1$ and mail-reader$_2$) that are mutually exclusive and both of them need an installed mail transport agent (mail-transport-agent) package to work correctly. In addition, mail-reader$_1$ recommends an extension package mail-extension that does not work without mail-reader$_1$. The relationships between the packages are shown in Figure 3 and the facts that encode the relationships are presented in Table 1.

Example 4. Suppose that the user selects the mail-reader$_1$ package by adding the atom user-include(mail-reader$_1$) as a fact to the program.

We can conclude by rules (13) and (11) that atoms justified(mail-reader$_1$) and in(mail-reader$_1$) have to be in the stable model of the program. As mail-reader$_1$ has to be in a configuration, we can justify mail-transport-agent by (14) and mail-extension by (15). The last package cannot be justified. We now have two justified packages that we can include in the configuration by the rule (8). The rule (9) forces us to add in(mail-transport-agent) to the model. The only choice we have left is whether to add the mail-extension package or not. Thus, we have two suitable configurations C_1 and C_2.

$$C_1 = \{ \text{ in(mail-reader}_1\text{), in(mail-transport-agent), in(mail-extension) } \}$$
$$C_2 = \{ \text{ in(mail-reader}_1\text{), in(mail-transport-agent) } \}$$

Example 5. Suppose that the user decided to have the mail-extension package and wants to use it with mail-reader$_2$. These requirements are modeled by adding facts user-include(mail-extension) and user-include(mail-reader$_2$) to the program. Now, by (14) the atom in(mail-reader$_1$) has to be in the model which leads to

Table 1. The facts used to encode Example 4.

package(mail-reader$_1$)	depends(mail-reader$_1$, mail-transport-agent)
package(mail-reader$_2$)	depends(mail-reader$_2$, mail-transport-agent)
package(mail-extension)	depends(mail-extension, mail-reader$_1$)
package(mail-transport-agent)	conflicts(mail-reader$_1$, mail-reader$_2$)
recommends(mail-reader$_1$, mail-extension)	

a contradiction with in(mail-reader$_2$) by (10). As a consequence, we do not have any suitable configurations.

The main weakness of the configuration model presented above is that it does not model the version information of the system. This would be unacceptable in real applications so we need to find a way to extend the model. We present here only a brief outline of the extension and the details can be found in [10].

We associate different versions of a package together using the predicate available-version(P, V) that is true when a version V of a package P is present in the configuration model. The predicate in is divided into two cases:

1. An atom in(P, V) is true exactly when a version V of P is chosen to be in the configuration; and
2. An atom in(P) is true when any version of P is in the configuration.

The relationships between packages may be parametrized with version numbers. For example, a package P may depend on Q version V or later. These kinds of dependencies can be modeled using atoms of the form depends(P, Q, Op, V) where Op is the corresponding relational operator. We then add rules that ensure that at least one compatible version of Q is in the configuration when P is in it. These rules may be expressed compactly by extending the language to allow *cardinality literals* of the form:

$$L \leq \{l_1, \ldots, l_n\} \leq U \tag{16}$$

where L and U are integral lower and upper bounds, respectively, and $l_1, \ldots,$ l_n are literals. The intuition of a cardinality literal is that a cardinality literal is satisfied when the number of satisfied literals $l_1, \ldots, l_n$ is between L and U, inclusive. Using cardinality literals the dependency constraint can be expressed as:

$$\begin{aligned}
\leftarrow 0 \leq & \{\text{in}(P_2, V) : \text{available-version}(P_2, V) : V \geq V_2\} \leq 0, \\
& \text{depends}(P_1, P_2, \geq, V_2), \\
& \text{in}(P_1)
\end{aligned} \tag{17}$$

where in(P_2, V) : available-version(P_2, V): V $\geq$ V_2 denotes the set of packages that may potentially satisfy the dependency. This set can be automatically computed during instantiation of the logic program.

4   The Diagnostic Model

We will construct the diagnostic model DM by adding a new set of atoms that represent the potential error conditions and explanations. We modify the constraints in such way that the diagnostic model will always have at least one stable model. The new atoms that are true in a stable model will then identify a set of errors in the requirements and give an explanation why this is the case.

The new atoms can be divided into three classes:

$$\text{in}(P_2) \leftarrow \text{in}(P_1), \text{depends}(P_1, P_2), \text{package}(P_2)$$
$$\text{missing}(P_2) \leftarrow \text{in}(P_1), \text{depends}(P_1, P_2), \text{not package}(P_2)$$
$$\text{in}(P) \leftarrow \text{user-include}(P), \text{package}(P)$$
$$\text{missing}(P) \leftarrow \text{user-include}(P), \text{not package}(P)$$
$$\text{in-conflict}(P_1, P_2) \leftarrow \text{conflicts}(P_1, P_2), \text{in}(P_1), \text{in}(P_2)$$
$$\text{in-conflict}(P, \text{user-exclude}) \leftarrow \text{in}(P), \text{user-exclude}(P)$$
$$\text{needs-reason}(P) \leftarrow \text{missing}(P)$$
$$\text{needs-reason}(P_1) \leftarrow \text{in-conflict}(P_1, P_2), \text{package}(P_1)$$
$$\text{needs-reason}(P_2) \leftarrow \text{in-conflict}(P_1, P_2), \text{package}(P_2)$$
$$\text{needs-reason}(P_1) \leftarrow \text{depends}(P_1, P_2), \text{needs-reason}(P_2), \text{in}(P_1)$$
$$\text{user-selected}(P) \leftarrow \text{needs-reason}(P), \text{user-include}(P)$$
$$\text{needs}(P_1, P_2) \leftarrow \text{needs-reason}(P_2), \text{depends}(P_1, P_2), \text{in}(P_1)$$

Fig. 4. The simplified Debian diagnostic model DM

1. Atoms that denote error conditions. We will use the predicates $\text{missing}(P)$ and $\text{in-conflict}(P_1, P_2)$ for this purpose.
2. Atoms that mark the packages that are in some way part of the problem and thus need an explanation. The predicate $\text{needs-reason}(P)$ is used for this.
3. Atoms that explain why certain packages were taken into the configuration. The predicates $\text{user-selected}(P)$ and $\text{needs}(P_1, P_2)$ are used for this purpose.

Using these predicates we can define a Debian diagnosis formally.

Definition 5. *Given a Debian diagnostic model DM and a set U of user requirements, a diagnosis D is a four-tuple $D = (M, E_M, P_M, R_M)$, where*

1. *M is a stable model of $DM \cup U$;*
2. *E_M is the error set*

$$E_M = \{\text{missing}(P) \in M\} \cup \{\text{in-conflict}(P_1, P_2) \in M\} \; ; \tag{18}$$

3. *P_M is the problem set*

$$P_M = \{P \mid \text{needs-reason}(P) \in M\} \; ; \; and \tag{19}$$

4. *R_M is the explanation set*

$$R_M = \{\text{user-selected}(P) \in M\} \cup \{\text{needs}(P_1, P_2) \in M\} \; . \tag{20}$$

The new program may have more than one diagnosis if there are more than one way to break the constraints. Each diagnosis corresponds to a set of choices that lead to a contradiction. When diagnosing a problem it is often enough to examine only one model. The reason for this is that if all possible choices that we can make lead to a contradiction, it does not matter much what particular set of choices we examine. However, the diagnosis should prefer conflicts over missing packages. The following example shows why this is necessary.

Example 6. Consider the situation where the user wants to have packages A and B in a configuration. The package A needs to have either C or D to work but both C and D conflict with B.

There are three ways to invalidate the constraints. If we add C in the configuration, it is in conflict with B. The same thing happens if we add D. If we leave both out the dependency relation is not satisfied.

The first two cases give us more information than the third one. In both of them we notice the real problem is that including both packages A and B in same configuration leads to a conflict. In the third case we only notice that A does not have its dependencies satisfied but we cannot directly see what caused the problem.

The first modification to the configuration model is that we remove the rule (8) because we want the diagnosis to contain only those packages that have to be in there so that it will be as small as possible. In addition, this ensures that no false alarms are caused by adding unnecessary recommended packages in the configuration.

4.1 Missing Packages

We will use the atom $missing(P)$ to denote that some package in the configuration depends on P but for some reason P is not in the configuration. As we take the approach that we add all necessary packages to a configuration, a package may be missing only if it is not present in the configuration model at all. We replace the rule (9) of the configuration model with the pair of rules

$$in(P_2) \leftarrow in(P_1), depends(P_1, P_2), package(P_2) \qquad (21)$$
$$missing(P_2) \leftarrow in(P_1), depends(P_1, P_2), not\ package(P_2) \ . \qquad (22)$$

The rule (21) ensures that existing packages are added to the model and the rule (22) marks non-existing packages as missing. In addition, it may be the case that a package the user explicitly included in the configuration is not available. To handle this situation we replace the rule (11) with rules

$$in(P) \leftarrow user\text{-}include(P), package(P) \qquad (23)$$
$$missing(P) \leftarrow user\text{-}include(P), not\ package(P) \ . \qquad (24)$$

4.2 Conflicts

We will use the predicate in-conflict to model conflicts. We define the atom $in\text{-}conflict(P_1, P_2)$ to be true exactly when P_1 and P_2 conflict with each other and they both have to be in the configuration.

In the diagnostic model we replace the rule (10) with

$$in\text{-}conflict(P_1, P_2) \leftarrow conflicts(P_1, P_2), in(P_1), in(P_2) \ . \qquad (25)$$

We must also handle the case where the user wants to leave out a package that some other package needs. We will use a special constant user-exclude and the rule

$$\text{in-conflict}(P, \text{user-exclude}) \leftarrow \text{in}(P), \text{user-exclude}(P) \tag{26}$$

to model these cases.

4.3 Justifications

When a package is missing from a configuration or two packages are in conflict, we would like to know why the problematic packages are necessary. In the base case a package is necessary if the user chose it to be in the configuration. A package is also necessary if some mandatory package depends on it.

We will use the predicate needs-reason to mark the atoms that we want to justify. We can find the explanations by first marking the packages that directly cause the problems and then recursively marking all packages that depend on marked packages and are present in the configuration. This can be accomplished with four rules:

$$\text{needs-reason}(P) \leftarrow \text{missing}(P) \tag{27}$$
$$\text{needs-reason}(P_1) \leftarrow \text{in-conflict}(P_1, P_2), \text{package}(P_1) \tag{28}$$
$$\text{needs-reason}(P_2) \leftarrow \text{in-conflict}(P_1, P_2), \text{package}(P_2) \tag{29}$$
$$\text{needs-reason}(P_1) \leftarrow \text{depends}(P_1, P_2), \text{needs-reason}(P_2), \text{in}(P_1) \ . \tag{30}$$

We model the justifications using two predicates, user-selected and needs. The atom user-selected(P) is true when the user chose P to be in the configuration and the atom needs(P_1, P_2) is true if P_2 was included in the configuration because P_1 depends on it. The justifications can be modeled with the following two rules:

$$\text{user-selected}(P) \leftarrow \text{needs-reason}(P), \text{user-include}(P) \tag{31}$$
$$\text{needs}(P_1, P_2) \leftarrow \text{needs-reason}(P_2), \text{depends}(P_1, P_2), \text{in}(P_1) \ . \tag{32}$$

Example 7. Reconsider the situation that was presented in Example 5. By the rule (23) we have to include both atoms in(mail-reader$_2$) and in(mail-extension) in the model and (21) adds atoms in(mail-reader$_1$) and in(mail-transport-agent). By (25) we include the atom in-conflict(mail-reader$_1$, mail-reader$_2$) in the model.

As we have a conflict, we want to find the reason for it. By rules (28) and (29) we know that needs-reason(mail-reader$_1$) and needs-reason(mail-reader$_2$) are in the model. Using the rule (30) we see that we have to find a reason for mail-extension, also.

By using the rule (31), we find explanations user-selected(mail-extension) and user-selected(mail-reader$_2$). We get the justification for the last package by using the rule (32) to find that needs(mail-extension, mail-reader$_2$) has to be in the model. Nothing else has to be included in the model so we now have the full diagnosis:

$$E = \{\text{in-conflict}(\text{mail-reader}_1, \text{mail-reader}_2)\}$$
$$P = \{\text{mail-reader}_1, \text{mail-reader}_2, \text{mail-extension}\}$$
$$R = \{\text{user-selected}(\text{mail-reader}_2), \text{user-selected}(\text{mail-extension}),$$
$$\text{needs}(\text{mail-extension}, \text{mail-reader}_1)\} \ .$$

5   Implementation

The configuration and diagnostic models have been implemented as extended logic programs using the SMODELS system [7, 8] developed in the Laboratory for Theoretical Computer Science in Helsinki University of Technology. The smodels system is available at

http://www.tcs.hut.fi/pub/smodels .

Both the models described in this work and in [10] are available at

http://www.tcs.hut.fi/%7Etssyrjan/configuration/ .

There have been some preliminary tests on the full Debian configuration model and the results are presented in [10]. The model was generated using actual data from Debian version 2.1 with 2260 different packages. The model was tested by generating a random set of user requirements and measuring the time that was used to either find a suitable configuration or a diagnosis. The tests were run on a 233 MHz Intel Pentium II with 128 MB of main memory. The compilation of the model took approximately 13 seconds and after that a valid configuration could be found in about 2 seconds. The results were similar for the diagnostic model.

The models are not yet incorporated into a concrete configuration tool but the test results give hope that it would be possible to use this approach also in practice.

6   Conclusions and Future Work

We presented a method to add diagnostic information to configuration models that are defined using a rule-based language RRL. The approach was to divide the configuration task into two phases. In the first phase we try to find a configuration that satisfies the user requirements. If one is found, the configuration task is completed. Otherwise, in the second phase we diagnose the user requirements trying to find an explanation why they are unsatisfiable.

We generate the diagnostic model by adding a new set of atoms to the configuration model to represent the possible error conditions and modify the rules to ensure the diagnostic model has always at least one stable model whatever the user requirements are. The new atoms that are true in the diagnosis identify a set of errors in the requirements. In addition, the diagnosis also contains explanations that tell for each component that is related to an error the reason why it has to be in the configuration.

We modeled a part of the configuration management problem of the Debian GNU/Linux system using RRL. Both configuration and diagnostic models were constructed. The configuration objects were distinct software packages that may depend on, conflict with, or recommend each other. The models were simplified and the problem of version management was addressed only briefly.

There were two possible error types for user requirements in the Debian configuration model. The first one was that necessary packages might be missing from the configuration. The second one was that two conflicting packages might be in a configuration. We defined the diagnostic model in such way that conflicts were preferred over missing packages because they give more information to the user: if a package is left out because it otherwise would cause a conflict, the user would notice only the absence of the package but the real cause would not be apparent.

The explanations are generated by marking all packages that are missing or in conflict with another one as problematic packages. In addition, all packages that depend on the problematic packages are marked, too. This is done because it is possible that the problems arise because some otherwise unrelated packages depend on conflicting packages.

The full configuration model for the Debian system is presented in [10]. The model has not been incorporated into any existing tool and the next step of this research is to construct a simple back-end that can be used for further testing in real environment. If the results are still promising, the model can be integrated with an existing Debian configuration tool.

References

1. Debian GNU/Linux. Available at: http://www.debian.org.
2. W.F. Dowling and J.H. Gallier. Linear-time algorithms for testing the satisfiability of propositional Horn formulae. *Journal of Logic Programming*, 3:267–284, 1984.
3. M. Gelfond and V. Lifschitz. The stable model semantics for logic programming. In *Proceedings of the 5th International Conference on Logic Programming*, pages 1070–1080, Seattle, USA, August 1988. The MIT Press.
4. W. Marek and M. Truszczyński. Autoepistemic logic. *Journal of the Association for Computing Machinery*, 38:588–619, 1991.
5. Ilkka Niemelä, Patrik Simons, and Timo Soininen. Stable model semantics of weight constraint rules. In *Proceedings of the Fifth Interational Conference on Logic Programming and Nonmonotonic Reasoning*. Springer-Verlag, December 1999.
6. Daniel Sabin and Rainer Weigel. Product configuration frameworks — a survey. *IEEE Intelligent Systems & their applications*, pages 42 – 49, October 1998.
7. P. Simons. Efficient implementation of the stable model semantics for normal logic programs. Research Report 35, Helsinki University of Technology, Helsinki, Finland, September 1995.

8. P. Simons. Extending the stable model semantics with more expressive rules. In *Proceedings of the 5th International Conference on Logic Programming and Nonmonotonic Reasoning*, pages 305–316, El Paso, Texas, USA, December 1999. Springer-Verlag.

9. Timo Soininen and Ilkka Niemelä. Developing a declarative rule language for applications in product configuration. In *Proceedings of the First International Workshop on Practical Aspects of Declarative Languages.* Springer-Verlag, January 1999.

10. T. Syrjänen. A rule-based formal model of software configuration. Research Report A 55, Helsinki University of Technology, Laboratory for Theoretical Computer Science, Helsinki, Finland, December 1999.

11. M.H. van Emden and R.A. Kowalski. The semantics of predicate logic as a programming language. *Journal of the Association for Computing Machinery*, 23:733–742, 1976.

12. B. Wielinga and G. Schreiber. Configuration-design problem solving. *IEEE Expert*, 12 2:49 – 56, March-April 1997.

Comparing the Expressive Powers of Some Syntactically Restricted Classes of Logic Programs

Tomi Janhunen

Helsinki University of Technology
Laboratory for Theoretical Computer Science
P.O.B. 5400, FIN-02015 HUT, Finland

Abstract. This paper studies the expressive powers of classes of logic programs that are obtained by restricting the number of positive literals (atoms) in the bodies of the rules. Three kinds of restrictions are considered, giving rise to the classes of atomic, unary and binary logic programs. The expressive powers of these classes of logic programs are compared by analyzing the existence of polynomial, faithful, and modular (PFM) translation functions between the classes. This analysis leads to a strict ordering of the classes of logic programs. The main result is that binary and unary rules are strictly more expressive than unary and atomic rules, respectively. This is the case even if we consider normal logic programs where negative literals may appear in the bodies of rules. Practical implications of the results are discussed in the context of a particular implementation technique for the stable model semantics of normal logic programs, namely contrapositive reasoning with rules.

1 Introduction

In *logic programming* [20], a simple rule-based language is used for knowledge representation in a declarative fashion (see e.g. [12] for an extensive study and [18] for programming methodology). To enhance the knowledge representation capabilities of logic programs, Clark [2] proposed a form of negation, namely *negation as failure* to prove. Logic programs that involve negation as failure are known as *normal logic programs*. Unfortunately, it turned out that it is difficult to incorporate the negation as failure principle into resolution theorem provers (c.f. SLDNF-resolution in [12]) in a satisfactory way. For example, the order in which rules are considered by the resolution procedure affects the answers to the queries. This feature makes logic programming with negation as failure less declarative and dependent on the implementation of the resolution procedure.

About a decade later, Gelfond and Lifschitz [4] proposed a solution to this problem: the *stable model semantics* for normal logic programs. In this approach, negative literals in rules are interpreted simultaneously which restores the declarative nature of programming with rules. Moreover, the emphasis is more on computing complete models (or answer sets [5]) for logic programs rather than using

J. Lloyd et al. (Eds.): CL 2000, LNAI 1861, pp. 852–866, 2000.

a resolution procedure for query answering. Nowadays, stable model semantics is considered as a constraint programming paradigm of its own [14, 15].

The success of the stable model semantics is much due to implementation techniques that have dramatically improved during the past decade. The basic technique is to use *well-founded models* [21] as approximations in the *branch and bound* approach [19]. However, it is possible to refine well-founded models in order to obtain even tighter approximations. For instance, Niemelä and Simons [16] use additional principles in their implementation (known by the name smodels). One of such principles uses rules contrapositively: assuming that the atom a in the head of a rule $a \leftarrow a_1, \ldots, a_n$ is false in a stable model (being constructed), then one of the atoms in the body $a_1, \ldots, a_n$ must also be false in the model. In particular, this principle becomes effective when $n = 1$ or when $a_2, \ldots, a_n$ are known to be true in the model, for instance. Then the fact that a_1 is false in the model follows immediately and refines the approximation a bit. This suggests that we could facilitate the use of this principle if we could somehow reduce the number of atoms that appear in the bodies of rules. These considerations lead to a fundamental question whether such a reduction is possible in the first place.

This paper answers to this question by analyzing the expressive powers of classes of logic programs that are obtained by limiting the number of positive literals (atoms) in the bodies of rules. Comparisons are based on the existence of polynomial, faithful and modular (PFM) translation functions between these classes. We proceed as follows. We begin in Section 2 by presenting the basic notions of logic programs: syntax and semantics. After this, three central properties of translation functions are distinguished in Section 3 and the comparison method of the paper is explained. PFM translation functions are used in Section 4 to compare the relative expressive powers of the classes of logic programs. Section 5 generalizes the results of previous section to cover normal logic programs, too. Some comparisons with related work are performed in Section 6. Finally, we present our conclusions in Section 7. In particular, the practical implications of our results on contrapositive reasoning with rules are discussed (c.f. the preceding discussion). Guidelines for future work are also sketched.

2 Logic Programs

A *logic program* P is a set of rules of the form

$$a \leftarrow a_1, \ldots, a_n. \tag{1}$$

The atom a is called the *head* of the rule while the atoms $a_1, \ldots, a_n$ form the *body* of the rule. The informal intuition behind the rule (1) is that the head a can be inferred by the rule whenever the atoms $a_1, \ldots, a_n$ in the body of the rule have been inferred. The Herbrand base $\mathrm{Hb}(P)$ of P is the set of atoms that appear in P. In this paper, we restrict to the propositional case and consider only programs that consist of propositional atoms[1].

---

[1] Programs with variables are also covered through Herbrand instantiation.

2.1   Syntactic Restrictions

As a preparation for forthcoming analysis, we distinguish classes of logic programs that are restricted by syntax. A rule of the form (1) is called *atomic,*
unary or *binary,* if $n = 0$, $n \leq 1$ or $n \leq 2$, respectively. Moreover, a rule is
strictly unary if $n = 1$, i.e. it is unary and not atomic. *Strictly* binary rules are
defined analogously, i.e. $n = 2$. We extend these conditions to cover logic programs in the obvious way: a logic program P satisfies any of these five conditions
given that every rule of P satisfies the condition. For instance, a strictly unary
logic program contains only rules of the form a ← b. By these definitions, atomic
programs are unary ones and unary programs are binary ones. This is how we
obtain three classes of logic programs ordered by inclusion: $\mathcal{A} \subseteq \mathcal{U} \subseteq \mathcal{B}$. Outside
these three classes, there are *non-binary* logic programs that contain at least one
rule (1) with $n > 2$. Such programs belong to the class of all logic programs $\mathcal{P}$
which is a superclass of the classes $\mathcal{A}$, $\mathcal{U}$ and $\mathcal{B}$.

2.2   Semantics

We resort to the standard model-theoretic semantics of logic programs that
applies to all programs of $\mathcal{P}$ (see [12] for a complete treatment). An *interpretation*
$I \subseteq \mathrm{Hb}(P)$ of a logic program P determines which atoms of $\mathrm{Hb}(P)$ are true. A
rule a ← $a_1, \ldots, a_n$ of P is satisfied by I if $\{a_1, \ldots, a_n\} \subseteq I$ implies a $\in I$.
An interpretation $M \subseteq \mathrm{Hb}(P)$ is a *model* of P given that every rule of P is
satisfied by M. The semantics of P is determined by the unique minimal model
M of P which is the intersection of all models of P [12]. We let $\mathrm{Mm}(P)$ stand
for this particular model. This semantics coincides with our intuition on rules,
i.e. the minimal model $\mathrm{Mm}(P)$ contains exactly those atoms of $\mathrm{Hb}(P)$ that can
be inferred by using the rules of P recursively. Let us also note the obvious
monotonicity property of minimal models: if $P \subseteq P'$, then $\mathrm{Mm}(P) \subseteq \mathrm{Mm}(P')$.
    The minimal model $\mathrm{Mm}(P)$ can be constructed iteratively as follows [12].
Define an operator T_P for sets of atoms $A \subseteq \mathrm{Hb}(P)$ by setting

$$\mathrm{T}_P(A) = \{a \in \mathrm{Hb}(P) \mid a \leftarrow a_1, \ldots, a_n \in P \text{ and } \{a_1, \ldots, a_n\} \subseteq A\}.$$

The iteration sequence of T_P is defined as follows: $\mathrm{T}_P \uparrow^0 (A) = A$, $\mathrm{T}_P \uparrow^i (A) =$
$\mathrm{T}_P(\mathrm{T}_P \uparrow^{i-1} (A))$ for $i > 0$, and the limit $\mathrm{T}_P \uparrow^\omega (A) = \bigcup_{i < \omega} \mathrm{T}_P \uparrow^i (A)$. It
follows that $\mathrm{Mm}(P) = \mathrm{T}_P \uparrow^\omega (\emptyset) = \mathrm{lfp}(\mathrm{T}_P, \emptyset)$. Note that this fixed point is
reached with a finite number of iterations if P is finite. Moreover, we use the
iterative construction to define the *level* of an atom a $\in \mathrm{Mm}(P)$, denoted by $l(a)$,
which is the least natural number i such that a $\in \mathrm{T}_P \uparrow^i (\emptyset)$.

3   Translations

The author has analyzed the expressive powers of *non-monotonic logics* in a systematic fashion [9, 10] extending previous work by Imielinski [8] and Gottlob [7].
Roughly speaking, the comparison is performed for any pair of non-monotonic

logics by analyzing the existence of certain kinds of translation functions between the logics. As a result of such pairwise comparisons, we have gradually constructed the expressive power hierarchy (EPH) of non-monotonic logics.

In this paper, we propose a similar framework to compare the expressive powers of classes $\mathcal{C}$ of logic programs. Our basic assumptions on any class $\mathcal{C}$ of logic programs are the following. First of all, the class $\mathcal{C}$ is supposed to be *closed under unions*, i.e. given any two programs P and P' from $\mathcal{C}$, then also $P \cup P'$ belongs to $\mathcal{C}$. On the other hand, it is assumed that $\mathcal{C}$ has a semantic operator $\mathrm{Sem}_{\mathcal{C}}$ associated with it. The operator $\mathrm{Sem}_{\mathcal{C}}$ assigns a set of interpretations $I \subseteq \mathrm{Hb}(P)$ to each program P of $\mathcal{C}$. Typically, these interpretations are models of P or *partial models* of P that can be extended to (total) models of P [21]. It is clear that each of the classes $\mathcal{C}$ introduced in Section 2.1 satisfies these criteria: the semantics assigned by the semantic operator is $\mathrm{Sem}_{\mathcal{C}}(P) = \{\mathrm{Mm}(P)\}$.

Let us then list general requirements for a translation function Tr that transforms logic programs P of a class $\mathcal{C}$ into logic programs $\mathrm{Tr}(P)$ of another class $\mathcal{C}'$. The latter class is assumed to be a subclass or a superclass of $\mathcal{C}$. We let $\|P\|$ stand for the *length* of P in symbols.

Definition 1. *Given two classes of logic programs $\mathcal{C}$ and $\mathcal{C}'$ that are closed under unions and the respective semantic operators $\mathrm{Sem}_{\mathcal{C}}$ and $\mathrm{Sem}_{\mathcal{C}'}$, a translation function $\mathrm{Tr} : \mathcal{C} \to \mathcal{C}'$ is*

- **polynomial** *if for all logic programs $P \in \mathcal{C}$, the time required to compute the translation $\mathrm{Tr}(P) \in \mathcal{C}'$ is polynomial in $\|P\|$,*
- **faithful** *if (i) for all logic programs $P \in \mathcal{C}$, the base $\mathrm{Hb}(P) \subseteq \mathrm{Hb}(\mathrm{Tr}(P))$ and (ii) the models/interpretations in $\mathrm{Sem}_{\mathcal{C}}(P)$ and $\mathrm{Sem}_{\mathcal{C}'}(\mathrm{Tr}(P))$ are in a one-to-one correspondence and coincide up to $\mathrm{Hb}(P)$, and*
- **modular** *if (i) for all logic programs $P_1 \in \mathcal{C}$ and $P_2 \in \mathcal{C}$, the translation $\mathrm{Tr}(P_1 \cup P_2) = \mathrm{Tr}(P_1) \cup \mathrm{Tr}(P_2)$ and (ii) $\mathcal{C}' \subset \mathcal{C}$ implies that the translation $\mathrm{Tr}(P') = P'$ for all logic programs $P' \in \mathcal{C}'$.*

A couple of remarks are worthwhile. The faithfulness requirement implies that a translation function Tr may introduce new atoms, but the number of such atoms is clearly bounded by the polynomiality requirement. This is a crucial option (c.f. Theorem 1). Let us also note that if Tr is faithful, then $\mathrm{Sem}_{\mathcal{C}}(P) = \{M \cap \mathrm{Hb}(P) \mid M \in \mathrm{Sem}_{\mathcal{C}'}(\mathrm{Tr}(P))\}$ holds. The intuition behind the modularity condition is as follows. The part (i) enforces locality of Tr, since the translation of a program $P_1 \cup P_2$ is obtained as the union of the translations of the subprograms P_1 and P_2. This implies that programs can be translated rule by rule. The part (ii) handles cases where programs of a class $\mathcal{C}$ are translated into programs in a proper subclass $\mathcal{C}'$ of $\mathcal{C}$. Such a class $\mathcal{C}'$ is typically obtained by restricting the syntax of the rules of the programs in $\mathcal{C}$. In this setting, we require that syntactically restricted rules remain intact in the translation. Note that whenever $\mathcal{C}' \subset \mathcal{C}$ holds, the joint effect of (i) and (ii) is that $\mathrm{Tr}(P' \cup P) = P' \cup \mathrm{Tr}(P)$ holds for all logic programs $P' \in \mathcal{C}'$ and $P \in \mathcal{C}$.

We say that a translation function $\mathrm{Tr} : \mathcal{C} \to \mathcal{C}'$ is PFM if it satisfies all the three criteria. If such a translation function exists, we write $\mathcal{C} \xrightarrow{\text{PFM}} \mathcal{C}'$ and consider

Table 1. Relations used by the Classification Method

Relation	Definition	Explanation
$\mathcal{C} \underset{\text{PFM}}{\Rightarrow} \mathcal{C}'$	$\mathcal{C} \underset{\text{PFM}}{\rightarrow} \mathcal{C}'$ and $\mathcal{C}' \underset{\text{PFM}}{\not\rightarrow} \mathcal{C}$	$\mathcal{C}$ is *less expressive* than $\mathcal{C}'$
$\mathcal{C} \underset{\text{PFM}}{\leftrightarrow} \mathcal{C}'$	$\mathcal{C} \underset{\text{PFM}}{\rightarrow} \mathcal{C}'$ and $\mathcal{C}' \underset{\text{PFM}}{\rightarrow} \mathcal{C}$	$\mathcal{C}$ and $\mathcal{C}'$ are *equally expressive*
$\mathcal{C} \underset{\text{PFM}}{\not\leftrightarrow} \mathcal{C}'$	$\mathcal{C} \underset{\text{PFM}}{\not\rightarrow} \mathcal{C}'$ and $\mathcal{C}' \underset{\text{PFM}}{\not\rightarrow} \mathcal{C}$	$\mathcal{C}$ and $\mathcal{C}'$ are *mutually incomparable*

$\mathcal{C}'$ as expressive as $\mathcal{C}$. In certain cases, we are able to construct a counter-example which shows that a translation function satisfying our criteria does not exist. We use the notation $\mathcal{C} \underset{\text{PFM}}{\not\rightarrow} \mathcal{C}'$ in such cases and we may also drop any of the three letters (referring to the three criteria) given that the corresponding criterion is not needed in the counter-example (note that $\mathcal{C} \underset{\text{FM}}{\not\rightarrow} \mathcal{C}'$ implies $\mathcal{C} \underset{\text{PFM}}{\not\rightarrow} \mathcal{C}'$).

The base relations $\underset{\text{PFM}}{\rightarrow}$ and $\underset{\text{PFM}}{\not\rightarrow}$ among classes of logic programs form the cornerstones of our classification method – giving rise to relations given in Table 1. By these relations, we have accommodated the method proposed for non-monotonic logics [10] to the case of logic programs. The frameworks are analogous, but different. Most importantly, the semantics of a *non-monotonic theory* is determined by a set of *extensions* (propositionally closed theories) while the semantics of a logic program is determined by a set of interpretations/models.

4   Expressive Power Analysis

In this paper, we analyze classes of logic programs $\mathcal{C}'$ that are obtained from other classes $\mathcal{C}$ by restricting the syntax of the rules while the semantics of the programs remains unchanged. This implies directly $\mathcal{C}' \underset{\text{PFM}}{\rightarrow} \mathcal{C}$ by the identity translation, since programs of $\mathcal{C}'$ are also programs of $\mathcal{C}$. By this observation, we obtain the relationships $\mathcal{A} \underset{\text{PFM}}{\rightarrow} \mathcal{U}$, $\mathcal{U} \underset{\text{PFM}}{\rightarrow} \mathcal{B}$ and $\mathcal{B} \underset{\text{PFM}}{\rightarrow} \mathcal{P}$ for free. But it remains open whether these relationships are strict or not.

Let us begin with the relationship of $\mathcal{B}$ and $\mathcal{P}$. Any *non-binary* rule $\mathsf{a} \leftarrow \mathsf{a}_1, \ldots, \mathsf{a}_n$ where $n > 2$ can be rewritten to reduce the number of atoms that appear in the body of the rule. One particular technique is to introduce new atoms $\mathsf{b}_1, \ldots, \mathsf{b}_{n-1}$ and the following binary rules[2]:

$$
\begin{aligned}
&\mathsf{a} \leftarrow \mathsf{a}_1, \mathsf{b}_1 \ ; \\
&\mathsf{b}_1 \leftarrow \mathsf{a}_2, \mathsf{b}_2 \ ; \ \mathsf{b}_2 \leftarrow \mathsf{a}_3, \mathsf{b}_3 \ ; \ \ldots \ ; \ \mathsf{b}_{n-2} \leftarrow \mathsf{a}_{n-1}, \mathsf{b}_{n-1} \ ; \\
&\mathsf{b}_{n-1} \leftarrow \mathsf{a}_n.
\end{aligned}
\tag{2}
$$

Using these binary rules, it is possible to infer a whenever $\mathsf{a}_1, \ldots, \mathsf{a}_n$ are inferable. As a result, any non-binary program P gets translated into a binary one $\text{Tr}_{\text{BIN}}(P)$. Most importantly, this translation satisfies our criteria.

---

[2] We use semicolons to separate program rules.

Theorem 1. $\mathcal{P} \xrightarrow{\text{PFM}} \mathcal{B}$.

Proof sketch. Polynomiality is obvious, since a rule (1) that has $2n + 1$ symbols is translated into n rules having a total of $5n - 1$ symbols. This implies even the linearity of the translation. Modularity follows also easily, since the binary rules of P remain intact. It remains to establish faithfulness.

Let $Q = \text{Tr}_{\text{BIN}}(P)$ so that $\text{Hb}(P) \subseteq \text{Hb}(Q)$, $M = \text{Mm}(P) \subseteq \text{Hb}(P)$ and $N = \text{Mm}(Q) \subseteq \text{Hb}(Q)$. It can be shown that $M = N \cap \text{Hb}(P)$ using induction on i to prove $T_P \uparrow^i (\emptyset) \subseteq N$ and $T_Q \uparrow^i (\emptyset) \cap \text{Hb}(P) \subseteq M$.   □

The next question concerns the strictness of the relationship $\mathcal{U} \xrightarrow{\text{PFM}} \mathcal{B}$. It turns out in the sequel that binary programs cannot be translated into unary ones such that our criteria are met. We need a subsidiary result on unary programs P: if an atom a is included in $\text{Mm}(P)$, then there is a single atomic rule b $\leftarrow$ in P that causes the atom a to be inferable by the rules of P (i.e. to be included in $\text{Mm}(P)$). Note that $\text{Mm}(P) = \emptyset$ for any strictly unary program P.

Lemma 1. *Let $P = P_0 \cup P_1$ be a unary program where P_0 contains the atomic rules of P and P_1 contains the strictly unary rules of P.*

If a $\in \text{Mm}(P_0 \cup P_1)$ and the atomic rule a $\leftarrow$ does not belong to P_0, then there is an atomic rule b $\leftarrow$ in P_0 such that a $\in \text{Mm}(\{b \leftarrow\} \cup P_1)$.

Proof. We use induction on $l(\text{a})$ to prove the claim for an atom a $\in \text{Mm}(P_0 \cup P_1)$ such that a $\leftarrow$ does not belong to P_0. Note that the condition that we impose on a implies that $l(\text{a}) > 0$, since a $\notin T_{P_0 \cup P_1}(\emptyset)$ which is exactly the set of atoms b for which the atomic rule b $\leftarrow$ appears in P_0.

For the base case, assume that $l(\text{a}) = 1$. Then there is a rule a $\leftarrow$ b $\in P_1$ such that b $\in T_{P_0 \cup P_1}(\emptyset)$. It follows that the atomic rule b $\leftarrow$ appears in P_0. It is therefore clear that b $\in T_{\{b \leftarrow\} \cup P_1}(\emptyset)$ and that a $\in \text{Mm}(\{b \leftarrow\} \cup P_1)$.

Then consider the case $l(\text{a}) = i > 1$. Then there is a rule a $\leftarrow$ b $\in P_1$ such that b $\in T_{P_0 \cup P_1} \uparrow^{i-1} (\emptyset)$. Two cases arise. (i) The atomic rule b $\leftarrow$ belongs to P_0. Then a $\in \text{Mm}(\{b \leftarrow\} \cup P_1)$ as in the base case. (ii) Otherwise, the rule b $\leftarrow$ does not belong to P_0. Since $l(\text{b}) < l(\text{a})$, it follows by the inductive hypothesis that there is an atom c such that b $\in \text{Mm}(\{c \leftarrow\} \cup P_1)$. This implies a $\in \text{Mm}(\{c \leftarrow\} \cup P_1)$, because the rule a $\leftarrow$ b $\in P_1$. Consequently, the atomic rule c $\leftarrow$ fulfills the claim of the lemma regarding the atom a.   □

We are ready to establish that $\mathcal{U} \xrightarrow{\text{PFM}} \mathcal{B}$, i.e. unary programs are strictly less expressive than binary ones. The proof below demonstrates how it is impossible to express the conjunctive condition (b and c) in the body of a rule a $\leftarrow$ b, c using only unary rules. In fact, if we attempt to capture this condition in terms of unary rules, the condition turns into a disjunctive one: already b or c alone is sufficient for inferring a (assuming that a does not follow from our translation directly). It is also worth pointing out that our counter-example does not depend on the polynomiality requirement. Consequently, $\mathcal{B} \xrightarrow{\text{FM}} \mathcal{U}$ holds even if we consider arbitrarily large translations of binary programs!

Theorem 2. $\mathcal{B} \not\xrightarrow{\rightarrow}_{FM} \mathcal{U}$.

Proof. Let us assume that there is a faithful and modular translation function Tr_{UN} from binary programs to unary programs. Then consider a strictly binary program $P = \{a \leftarrow b, c\}$. Let us partition $Q = Tr_{UN}(P)$ into a set of atomic rules Q_0 and a set of strictly unary rules Q_1. A case analysis follows.

Consider a set of atomic (and unary) rules $U_1 = \{b \leftarrow ; c \leftarrow\}$. By modularity, the translation $Tr_{UN}(U_1 \cup P) = U_1 \cup Q$. It is clear that $a \in Mm(U_1 \cup P)$ which implies that $a \in Mm(U_1 \cup Q)$ by the faithfulness of the translation. It follows by Lemma 1 that there is an atom d such that the atomic rule $d \leftarrow$ is one of the atomic rules in $U_1 \cup Q_0$ and $a \in Mm(\{d \leftarrow\} \cup Q_1)$. This leaves us three possibilities: (i) the rule $d \leftarrow$ belongs to Q_0, (ii) $d = b$ or (iii) $d = c$.

Then let $U_2 = \{b \leftarrow\}$ so that $Tr_{UN}(U_2 \cup P) = U_2 \cup Q$ holds by modularity. It follows that $a \notin Mm(U_2 \cup P)$ so that also $a \notin Mm(U_2 \cup Q)$ holds by the faithfulness of the translation. This implies that the atomic rule $d \leftarrow$ does not belong to Q_0, since otherwise $a \in Mm(Q)$ and $a \in Mm(U_2 \cup Q)$ follow. Quite similarly, it follows that $d \neq b$, because otherwise $a \in Mm(\{d \leftarrow\} \cup Q_1)$ implies $a \in Mm(U_2 \cup Q)$. Thus $d = c$ is necessarily the case.

Finally, consider $U_3 = \{c \leftarrow\}$ for which $Tr_{UN}(U_3 \cup P) = U_3 \cup Q$ holds by modularity. Then $a \notin Mm(U_3 \cup P)$ holds and $a \notin Mm(U_3 \cup Q)$ follows by the faithfulness of the translation. On the other hand, we know that $a \in Mm(\{c \leftarrow\} \cup Q_1)$ holds by the facts that $a \in Mm(\{d \leftarrow\} \cup Q_1)$ and $d = c$. Since the program $\{c \leftarrow\} \cup Q_1 \subseteq U_3 \cup Q$, we obtain a contradiction $a \in Mm(U_3 \cup Q)$. $\square$

Theorem 3. $\mathcal{U} \not\xrightarrow{\rightarrow}_{FM} \mathcal{A}$.

Proof. Let us assume that there is a faithful and modular translation function Tr_{AT} from unary logic programs to atomic programs. Then consider a strictly unary program $P = \{a \leftarrow b\}$ and the translation $Q = Tr_{AT}(P)$. Let $A = \{b \leftarrow\}$. Since $a \in Mm(A \cup P)$, also $a \in Mm(A \cup Q)$ by the faithfulness and modularity of Tr_{AT}. Since Q is atomic, the rule $a \leftarrow$ must appear in Q.

Note that $Mm(P) = \emptyset$ so that $a \notin Mm(P)$. It follows by the faithfulness and modularity of Tr_{AT} that $a \notin Mm(Q)$. A contradiction, as $a \leftarrow$ appears in Q. $\square$

The last two theorems state that $\mathcal{B} \not\xrightarrow{\rightarrow}_{PFM} \mathcal{U}$ and $\mathcal{U} \not\xrightarrow{\rightarrow}_{PFM} \mathcal{A}$. However, this does not exclude the possibility that polynomial and faithful but *non-modular* translation functions could be devised for these classes. For instance, consider a translation function $Tr_{NM}(P) = \{a \leftarrow | a \in Mm(P)\}$. It is immediately clear that Tr_{NM} is faithful, since $Mm(Tr_{NM}(P)) = Mm(P)$. It is also well known that $Mm(P)$ can be computed in polynomial time (recall the iterative construction given in Section 2.2). Thus Tr_{NM} is also polynomial. To show that Tr_{NM} is non-modular, we use the programs $P = \{a \leftarrow b\}$ and $A = \{b \leftarrow\}$ introduced in the proof of Theorem 3. Now $Tr_{NM}(A \cup P) = \{a \leftarrow ; b \leftarrow\}$, but $Tr_{NM}(A) = \{b \leftarrow\}$ and $Tr_{NM}(P) = \emptyset$, indicating that $Tr_{NM}(A \cup P) \neq Tr_{NM}(A) \cup Tr_{NM}(P)$. Generally speaking, a non-modular translation $Tr(P)$ is often heavily dependent on particular instances of P so that already slight changes to P may alter $Tr(P)$ thoroughly. Consequently, a shortcoming of non-modular translations is that

$$A \underset{\text{PFM}}{\Longrightarrow} \mathcal{U} \underset{\text{PFM}}{\Longrightarrow} \mathcal{B} \underset{\text{PFM}}{\longleftrightarrow} \mathcal{P}$$

Fig. 1. Classes of Logic Programs Ordered by Expressive Power

they do not support updates. This is also clear on the basis of the translation function Tr_{AT} above: consider the effects of deleting A from $\text{Tr}_{NM}(A \cup P)$.

Theorems 1, 2 and 3 establish a strict ordering among the classes of logic programs $\mathcal{A}, \mathcal{U}, \mathcal{B}$ and $\mathcal{P}$ that is summarized in Figure 1.

5   Normal Logic Programs

The next step is to extend our analysis to cover more general classes of logic programs: we let negation (i.e. negative literals) to appear in the bodies of rules. Consequently, the resulting rules are of the form

$$\mathsf{a} \leftarrow \mathsf{a}_1, \ldots, \mathsf{a}_n, \sim\mathsf{b}_1, \ldots, \sim\mathsf{b}_m. \tag{3}$$

where $\mathsf{b}_1, \ldots, \mathsf{b}_m$ are atoms. In the sequel, $\mathsf{a}_1, \ldots, \mathsf{a}_n$ and $\sim\mathsf{b}_1, \ldots, \sim\mathsf{b}_m$ will be called the *positive* and *negative* body literals of the rule (3). Intuitively, this kind of a rule can be used for inferences like the rule (1) given that none of the atoms $\mathsf{b}_1, \ldots, \mathsf{b}_m$ can be inferred. We extend the syntactic restrictions (atomic, unary and binary rules) introduced in Section 2 to cover normal logic programs: negative body literals simply do not count, i.e. they are ignored when rules are classified. For instance, the rule $\mathsf{a} \leftarrow \mathsf{b}, \sim\mathsf{c}$ involving a negative literal $\sim\mathsf{c}$ is strictly unary ($n = 1$) as well as binary ($n \leq 2$). To give another example, the rule $\mathsf{p} \leftarrow \sim\mathsf{p}$ is atomic ($n = 0$). We introduce subscripted symbols $\mathcal{A}_n, \mathcal{U}_n, \mathcal{B}_n$ and $\mathcal{P}_n$ to denote the respective classes of normal logic programs.

The leading semantics for normal logic programs is the *stable model* semantics proposed by Gelfond and Lifschitz [4]. Given a model candidate $M \subseteq \text{Hb}(P)$, a normal logic program P is reduced to a negation-free logic program

$$P^M = \{\mathsf{a} \leftarrow \mathsf{a}_1, \ldots, \mathsf{a}_n \mid \mathsf{a} \leftarrow \mathsf{a}_1, \ldots, \mathsf{a}_n, \sim\mathsf{b}_1, \ldots, \sim\mathsf{b}_m \in P \\ \text{and } M \cap \{\mathsf{b}_1, \ldots, \mathsf{b}_m\} = \emptyset \qquad \}. \tag{4}$$

This is how the negative body literals of all rules of P are simultaneously interpreted with respect to M. Since the reduct P^M is negation-free, it has a straightforward semantics determined by the unique minimal model $\text{Mm}(P^M)$. This suggests that one should accept only *stable models* $M \subseteq \text{Hb}(P)$ of a normal logic program P that satisfy the fixed point condition

$$M = \text{Mm}(P^M). \tag{5}$$

Unfortunately, stable models need not exist for a normal logic program (e.g., $P = \{\mathsf{a} \leftarrow \sim\mathsf{a}\}$) and stable models are not necessarily unique (e.g., the program $P = \{\mathsf{a} \leftarrow \sim\mathsf{b} \; ; \; \mathsf{b} \leftarrow \sim\mathsf{a}\}$ has two stable models $\{\mathsf{a}\}$ and $\{\mathsf{b}\}$). Moreover, negation leads to *non-monotonicity* of reasoning such that conclusions may be retracted (e.g., the programs $P = \{a \leftarrow \sim b\}$ and $P' = P \cup \{b\}$ have unique stable models $\{a\}$ and $\{b\}$, respectively). We will consider the classes of normal logic programs $\mathcal{A}_n$, $\mathcal{U}_n$, $\mathcal{B}_n$ and $\mathcal{P}_n$ under the stable semantics, i.e. $\mathrm{Sem}_{\mathcal{C}_n}(P) = \{M \subseteq \mathrm{Hb}(P) \mid M = \mathrm{Mm}(P^M)\}$ holds for any $\mathcal{C}_n$ and for any $P \in \mathcal{C}_n$.

It is clear that the relations $\mathcal{A}_n \xrightarrow{\mathrm{PFM}} \mathcal{U}_n$, $\mathcal{U}_n \xrightarrow{\mathrm{PFM}} \mathcal{B}_n$ and $\mathcal{B}_n \xrightarrow{\mathrm{PFM}} \mathcal{P}_n$ hold, since the classes involved are obtained by syntactic restrictions that lead to inclusion $\mathcal{A}_n \subseteq \mathcal{U}_n \subseteq \mathcal{B}_n \subseteq \mathcal{P}_n$ in analogy to the monotonic case. From now on, our plan is to generalize Theorems 1, 2 and 3 to the case of normal logic programs. Let us start our considerations with non-binary normal logic programs in $\mathcal{P}_n$.

Theorem 4. $\mathcal{P}_n \xrightarrow{\mathrm{PFM}} \mathcal{B}_n$.

Proof sketch. Let P be a non-binary normal logic program. Then there is at least one rule (3) with $n > 2$. The strategy is to rewrite such rules so that each of the rules (2) is modified by adding the negative body literals $\sim b_1, \ldots, \sim b_m$. Let $Q = \mathrm{Tr_{BIN}}(P)$ be the translation of P obtained by this principle. It is clear that the function $\mathrm{Tr_{BIN}}$ is both polynomial and modular.

Then consider any set of atoms $N \subseteq \mathrm{Hb}(Q)$ and $M = N \cap \mathrm{Hb}(P)$. It is clear that for any binary rule (3) with $n \leq 2$, the rule $a \leftarrow a_1, \ldots, a_n$ belongs to P^M iff it belongs to Q^N. For any non-binary rule (3) with $n > 2$ the rule $a \leftarrow a_1, \ldots, a_n$ belongs to P^M iff the rules (2) belong to Q^N. Thus $\mathrm{Mm}(P^M) = \mathrm{Mm}(Q^N) \cap \mathrm{Hb}(P)$ follows by the technique used in the proof of Theorem 1.

Then it follows easily that if N is a stable model of Q, i.e. $N = \mathrm{Mm}(Q^N)$, then $M = N \cap \mathrm{Hb}(P)$ is a stable model of P, i.e. $M = \mathrm{Mm}(P^M)$. Then consider the case that $M = \mathrm{Mm}(P^M)$. Define N as M augmented with all new atoms b_i (where $0 < i \leq n - 1$) involved in (2) for which P has a corresponding non-binary rule (3) with $n > 2$, the rule $a \leftarrow a_1, \ldots, a_n$ belongs to P^M and $\{a_{i+1}, \ldots, a_n\} \subseteq M$. It follows by the definition of N and the preceding analysis that $N = \mathrm{Mm}(Q^N)$ so that $M = N \cap \mathrm{Hb}(P)$. Moreover, N is the unique stable model of Q satisfying $M = N \cap \mathrm{Hb}(P)$, since the negative literals of Q involve only atoms of $\mathrm{Hb}(P)$ and this makes Q^N unique with respect to M. $\square$

The main result of the paper follows: it is established that binary rules are not expressible in terms of unary rules even if we allow negative body literals.

Theorem 5. $\mathcal{B}_n \xrightarrow{\mathrm{FM}} \mathcal{U}_n$.

Proof. Let us assume that there is a faithful and modular translation function $\mathrm{Tr_{UN}}$ from binary normal logic programs to unary ones. Then consider a strictly binary normal logic program $P = \{a \leftarrow b, c\}$ and the translation $Q = \mathrm{Tr_{UN}}(P)$ which is a unary normal logic program. Let us partition Q into a set of atomic rules Q_0 and a set of strictly unary rules Q_1. Recall that the rules of Q_0 and Q_1 may contain negative body literals and $\mathrm{Hb}(P) \subseteq \mathrm{Hb}(Q)$.

Then consider the sets of rules

$$A_1 = \{b \leftarrow \; ; \; c \leftarrow\}, \; A_2 = \{b \leftarrow\}, \; A_3 = \{c \leftarrow\} \text{ and } U = \{b \leftarrow a \; ; \; c \leftarrow a\}.$$

It follows by the modularity of $\mathrm{Tr_{UN}}$ that $\mathrm{Tr_{UN}}(A_i \cup U \cup P) = A_i \cup U \cup Q$ for all $i \in \{1, 2, 3\}$. Note that $M = \mathrm{Mm}(A_1 \cup U \cup P) = \{a, b, c\}$ is the unique stable model of $A_1 \cup U \cup P$, since $A_1 \cup U \cup P$ does not contain negative literals. Because of the faithfulness of $\mathrm{Tr_{UN}}$, there is a unique stable model N of $A_1 \cup U \cup Q$ such that $M = N \cap \mathrm{Hb}(A_1 \cup U \cup P) = N \cap \{\mathsf{a,b,c}\}$. This implies that $\mathsf{a} \in N$. The reduct $(A_1 \cup U \cup Q)^N = A_1 \cup U \cup Q^N = A_1 \cup U \cup Q_0{}^N \cup Q_1{}^N$ and $N = \mathrm{Mm}(A_1 \cup U \cup Q^N)$. By Lemma 1 there is an atomic rule $\mathsf{d} \leftarrow$ in $A_1 \cup Q_0{}^N$ such that $\mathsf{a} \in \mathrm{Mm}(\{\mathsf{d} \leftarrow\} \cup U \cup Q^N)$. Three cases arise: $\mathsf{d} \leftarrow$ belongs to the atomic part $Q_0{}^N$ of the reduct, $\mathsf{d} = \mathsf{b}$ or $\mathsf{d} = \mathsf{c}$. It follows that (i) $\mathsf{a} \in \mathrm{Mm}(U \cup Q^N)$, (ii) $\mathsf{a} \in \mathrm{Mm}(A_2 \cup U \cup Q^N)$ or (iii) $\mathsf{a} \in \mathrm{Mm}(A_3 \cup U \cup Q^N)$. Since (i) implies both (ii) and (iii), we may conclude that (ii) or (iii) holds.

Recall that U contains the rules $\mathsf{b} \leftarrow \mathsf{a}$ and $\mathsf{c} \leftarrow \mathsf{a}$. Since (ii) or (iii) holds, it follows that $\mathsf{c} \in \mathrm{Mm}(A_2 \cup U \cup Q^N)$ or $\mathsf{b} \in \mathrm{Mm}(A_3 \cup U \cup Q^N)$. Consequently, we have that $\mathrm{Mm}(A_2 \cup U \cup Q^N) = \mathrm{Mm}(A_1 \cup U \cup Q^N)$ or $\mathrm{Mm}(A_3 \cup U \cup Q^N) = \mathrm{Mm}(A_1 \cup U \cup Q^N)$. Thus N is a stable model of $A_2 \cup U \cup Q$ or a stable model of $A_3 \cup U \cup Q$. Note also that $\mathsf{a} \in N$ holds in both cases by (ii) and (iii).

On the other hand, the unique stable models of $A_2 \cup U \cup P$ and $A_3 \cup U \cup P$ are $M_2 = \mathrm{Mm}(A_2 \cup U \cup P) = \{\mathsf{b}\}$ and $M_3 = \mathrm{Mm}(A_3 \cup U \cup P) = \{\mathsf{c}\}$, respectively. Then $\mathsf{a} \notin M_2$ and $\mathsf{a} \notin M_3$ hold, indicating that $\mathrm{Tr_{UN}}$ is not faithful. $\qquad\square$

It remains to explore the strictness of the relationship $\mathcal{A}_\mathrm{n} \overrightarrow{\ \mathrm{PFM}\ } \mathcal{U}_\mathrm{n}$. In the presence of negation, it is *almost* possible to obtain a translation from unary programs to atomic ones. This is demonstrated by the following example.

Example 1. Consider a normal logic program $P = \{\mathsf{a} \leftarrow \mathsf{b} \ ; \ \mathsf{b} \leftarrow \mathsf{c}\}$ and a translation of P into an atomic normal logic program $\mathrm{Tr_{AT}}(P) =$

$$\{\mathsf{a} \leftarrow \mathord{\sim}\mathsf{b'} \ ; \ \mathsf{b} \leftarrow \mathord{\sim}\mathsf{c'} \ ; \ \mathsf{a'} \leftarrow \mathord{\sim}\mathsf{a} \ ; \ \mathsf{b'} \leftarrow \mathord{\sim}\mathsf{b} \ ; \ \mathsf{c'} \leftarrow \mathord{\sim}\mathsf{c}\}$$

where the new atoms $\mathsf{a'}$ $\mathsf{b'}$ and $\mathsf{c'}$ mean that a, b and c are false, respectively. The first two rules of $\mathrm{Tr_{AT}}(P)$ express the rules of P using a kind of double negation while the last three rules of $\mathrm{Tr_{AT}}(P)$ encode the standard closed world assumption [17]. These programs exhibit the following stable models.

A	Stable models of $A \cup P$	Stable models of $A \cup \mathrm{Tr_{AT}}(P)$
$\emptyset$	$\emptyset$	$\{\mathsf{a',b',c'}\}$
$\{\mathsf{a} \leftarrow\}$	$\{\mathsf{a}\}$	$\{\mathsf{a,b',c'}\}$
$\{\mathsf{b} \leftarrow\}$	$\{\mathsf{a,b}\}$	$\{\mathsf{a,b,c'}\}$
$\{\mathsf{c} \leftarrow\}$	$\{\mathsf{a,b,c}\}$	$\{\mathsf{a,b,c}\}$

By the preceding analysis, the translation $\mathrm{Tr_{AT}}(P)$ seems to capture the essentials of P in a modular and faithful manner. However, severe problems arise if P contains a "loop" that lets one to infer a from a, for instance. The simplest possible example of this kind is $P' = \{\mathsf{a} \leftarrow \mathsf{a}\}$ having a minimal model $\mathrm{Mm}(P) = \emptyset$. Unfortunately, the translation $\mathrm{Tr_{AT}}(P') = \{\mathsf{a} \leftarrow \mathord{\sim}\mathsf{a'} \ ; \ \mathsf{a'} \leftarrow \mathord{\sim}\mathsf{a}\}$ has two stable models $\{\mathsf{a'}\}$ and $\{\mathsf{a}\}$. The former is what we would expect on the basis of our example, but the latter is an anomalous stable model. It is proved in the following theorem that such anomalous stable models cannot be avoided.

Theorem 6. $\mathcal{U}_n \overset{\not\rightarrow}{\text{PFM}} \mathcal{A}_n$.

Proof. Let us assume that there is a faithful and modular translation function Tr_{AT} from unary normal logic programs to atomic ones. Then consider the unary (normal) logic program $P = \{a \leftarrow b \; ; \; b \leftarrow a\}$ and the translation $Q = \text{Tr}_{\text{AT}}(P)$ which is an atomic normal logic program. We introduce sets of atomic rules $A_1 = \{a \leftarrow\}$, $A_2 = \{b \leftarrow\}$, $A_3 = \{a \leftarrow \; ; \; b \leftarrow\}$. Note that for each $i \in \{1, 2, 3\}$, the program $A_i \cup P$ has a unique stable model $M = \text{Mm}(A_i \cup P) = \{a, b\}$. In addition, the modularity of Tr_{AT} implies that the translation $\text{Tr}_{\text{AT}}(A_i \cup P) = A_i \cup Q$ for all $i \in \{1, 2, 3\}$. Note also that the Gelfond-Lifschitz reduction $(A_i \cup Q)^N = A_i \cup Q^N$ for any $i \in \{1, 2, 3\}$ and $N \subseteq \text{Hb}(A_i \cup Q)$.

Since M is the unique stable model of $A_1 \cup P$, it follows by the faithfulness of Tr_{AT} that the translation $A_1 \cup Q$ has a unique stable model $N_1 = \text{Mm}(A_1 \cup Q^{N_1})$ such that $N_1 \cap \{a, b\} = M$. This implies that $b \leftarrow$ must belong to the reduct Q^{N_1}, since Q^{N_1} is atomic. Thus also $N_1 = \text{Mm}(A_3 \cup Q^{N_1})$ holds, i.e. N_1 is a stable model of $A_3 \cup Q$. Due to symmetry present in the sets of rules P, A_1, A_2 and A_3, we may conclude that there is a stable model $N_2 = \text{Mm}(A_2 \cup Q^{N_2})$ of $A_2 \cup Q$ such that $N_2 \cap \{a, b\} = M$ and the rule $a \leftarrow$ belongs to Q^{N_2}. Thus N_2 is also a stable model of $A_3 \cup Q$.

Since M is the unique stable model of $A_3 \cup P$, it follows by the faithfulness of Tr_{AT} that $A_3 \cup Q$ has a unique stable model $N_3 = \text{Mm}(A_3 \cup Q^{N_3})$ such that $N_3 \cap \{a, b\} = M$. The uniqueness of N_3 implies that $N_1 = N_2 = N_3$. Consequently, the reductions satisfy $Q^{N_1} = Q^{N_2} = Q^{N_3}$. Therefore, the rules $a \leftarrow$ and $b \leftarrow$ belong to Q^{N_3}. It follows that $N_3 = \text{Mm}(Q^{N_3})$, i.e. N_3 is stable model of Q. Recall that N_3 contains a and b. But this contradicts the faithfulness of Tr_{AT}, since $Q = \text{Tr}_{\text{AT}}(P)$ and P has a unique stable model $\text{Mm}(P) = \emptyset$. $\square$

To make our view complete, we address the relationships between the classes of (negation-free) logic programs and normal logic programs in Theorem 7. Note again that $\mathcal{C} \overset{\rightarrow}{\text{PFM}} \mathcal{C}_n$ holds trivially for any of the classes $\mathcal{C}$. The resulting hierarchy of classes of logic programs is illustrated in Figure 2.

Theorem 7. $\mathcal{C}_n \overset{\not\rightarrow}{\text{F}} \mathcal{C}$ *holds for any class* $\mathcal{C}$ *among* $\mathcal{A}$, $\mathcal{U}$, $\mathcal{B}$ *and* $\mathcal{P}$.

Proof. Let us assume that there is a faithful translation function Tr from $\mathcal{C}_n$ to $\mathcal{C}$. Consider a logic program $P = \{a \leftarrow \sim a\}$ which serves as a representative of the class $\mathcal{C}_n$ of normal logic programs. Let Q be the translation $\text{Tr}(P)$ in $\mathcal{C}$. Now P has no stable models, but the translation Q has a unique stable model $\text{Mm}(Q)$, contradicting the faithfulness of Tr. $\square$

6   Related Work

Let us comment on related work at first. *Partial evaluation* techniques have been introduced to unfold rules of programs in a semantics preserving way. A good example in this respect is the approach by Brass and Dix [1]. They propose *equivalence transformations* for normal and *disjunctive* logic programs under the stable semantics. Let us describe these transformations by restricting to the

$$\mathcal{A}_n \quad \xrightarrow{\text{PFM}} \quad \mathcal{U}_n \quad \xrightarrow{\text{PFM}} \quad \mathcal{B}_n \quad \xrightarrow{\text{PFM}} \quad \mathcal{P}_n$$

$$\Updownarrow_{\text{PFM}} \qquad\qquad \Updownarrow_{\text{PFM}} \qquad\qquad \Updownarrow_{\text{PFM}}$$

$$\mathcal{A} \quad \xrightarrow{\text{PFM}} \quad \mathcal{U} \quad \xrightarrow{\text{PFM}} \quad \mathcal{B} \quad \xleftrightarrow{\text{PFM}} \quad \mathcal{P}$$

Fig. 2. Classes of Logic Programs Ordered by Expressiveness

case of normal logic programs. Two of the transformations eliminate tautologies (which are rules (3) with $a = a_i$ for some i) and inapplicable rules (which are rules (3) with $a_i = b_j$ for some i and j). The third transformation evaluates partially a rule (3) of a normal logic program P with respect to a positive body literal a_i in the rule. This means replacing the rule (3) with a rule

$$a \leftarrow a_1, \ldots, a_{i-1}, a_{i+1}, \ldots, a_n, a'_1, \ldots, a'_{n'}, {\sim}b_1, \ldots, {\sim}b_m, {\sim}b'_1, \ldots, {\sim}b'_{m'}$$

for each rule $a_i \leftarrow a'_1, \ldots, a'_{n'}, {\sim}b'_1, \ldots, {\sim}b'_{m'}$ of P having a_i as the head. This is how the positive occurrences of a_i are replaced by its definition. Compared to the goals of this paper, partial evaluation has a quite opposite effect, as it tends to increase the number of positive body literals.

It is also worthwhile to relate our framework with propositional logic. Given a propositional theory S, i.e. a set of propositional clauses of the form

$$a_1 \vee \ldots \vee a_n \vee \neg b_1 \vee \ldots \vee \neg b_m, \tag{6}$$

a model $M \subseteq \mathrm{Hb}(S)$ of S is a set of atoms (considered to be true) such that all clauses of S evaluate to true. The famous satisfiability problem (SAT) [3] is about checking whether a given set of clauses has a model. It is possible to capture the models of a set of clauses S with the stable models of a translation of S into a normal logic program. In fact, we can do this using only atomic rules. The idea is as follows. The rules $a \leftarrow {\sim}a'$ and $a' \leftarrow {\sim}a$ are needed to select the truth value of each atom $a \in \mathrm{Hb}(S)$. Here a' denotes that a is false (in analogy to Example 1). Given just these rules, we obtain all model candidates for S as stable models of the rules and we have to ensure yet that all clauses of the form (6) are satisfied. This is easily accomplished by introducing a rule[3]

$$f \leftarrow {\sim}f, {\sim}a_1, \ldots, {\sim}a_n, {\sim}b'_1, \ldots, {\sim}b'_m$$

where f is a new atom for each clause (6) in S. These kinds of rules exclude model candidates in which some of the clauses is false. On the other hand, it is impossible to translate an atomic normal logic program P into a propositional theory in a faithful (one-to-one correspondence of models such that corresponding models coincide up to $\mathrm{Hb}(P)$) and modular way. To establish this, let us

---

[3] It would be more intuitive to use a rule of the form $f \leftarrow {\sim}f, {\sim}a_1, \ldots, {\sim}a_n, b_1, \ldots, b_m$, which is not atomic and "double negation" is needed in order to make the rule atomic.

assume that there is such a faithful and modular translation function Tr. Then consider atomic normal logic programs $P_1 = \{a \leftarrow \sim a\}$ and $P_2 = \{a \leftarrow\}$. The program P_1 has no stable models while P_2 has a unique stable model $M = \{a\}$. Since Tr is faithful, the translation $\mathrm{Tr}(P_1)$ must be propositionally inconsistent. By the modularity of Tr, the translation $\mathrm{Tr}(P_1 \cup P_2) = \mathrm{Tr}(P_1) \cup \mathrm{Tr}(P_2)$ which is also propositionally inconsistent, i.e. has no models. But this contradicts the faithfulness of Tr, since M is also the unique stable model of $P_1 \cup P_2$. These observations indicate that propositional theories are already strictly less expressive than *atomic* normal logic programs. By Figure 2 and the transitivity of the relation $\overset{\Rightarrow}{\text{PFM}}$, this holds also for unary and binary logic programs.

Our remarks on computational complexity follow. Marek and Truszczyński [13] establish that finding out whether a normal logic program P has a stable model is an NP-complete problem. By the translation sketched above, the problem SAT is reducible in polynomial time to the problem of checking whether an *atomic/unary/binary* normal logic program has a stable model. This indicates that the computational complexity of the latter problem remains NP-hard under the three syntactic restrictions that are imposed on rules in this paper. Thus, in analogy to our previous experience on classifying non-monotonic logics [10], the method based on PFM translation functions yields a more accurate measure of expressive power than the levels of polynomial time hierarchy (PH) do.

7   Discussion and Conclusions

The analysis in Section 4 reveals the main constituents of rule-based reasoning. In the simplest form, we have just atomic rules $a \leftarrow$ stating that the atom in the head is true. Unary rules enrich this setting by allowing chained inferences with rules. In the richest form, we have binary rules that incorporate conjunctive conditions. Moreover, reasoning with non-binary rules is reducible to these primitive forms. By the results of Section 5 we know that this setting is not affected even if normal logic programs are considered. For instance, negation as failure is not sufficient to compensate conjunctive conditions nor chained inferences (c.f. Example 1). Looking back to the hierarchy in Figure 2, the number of positive body literals seems to be a reasonable criterion for syntactic restrictions, because strict differences result in expressive power.

By Theorem 5 it is impossible to rewrite normal logic programs (as long as we expect modularity and faithfulness) such that binary rules are removed. This provides a quite definite answer to the question posed in the introduction. Given that the head atom a of a binary rule $a \leftarrow b, c$ is false in a stable model M and the truth values of b and c are not known, we know that b is false in M or c is false in M. This leads to a case analysis which can be in the worst case at least as expensive as ordinary branching with respect to b (i.e. analyzing separately the cases that b is true in M and b is false in M) or with respect to c. This is illustrated in our final example.

Example 2. Consider a binary normal logic program

$$P = \{a \leftarrow b, c \ ; \ b \leftarrow \sim b_1 \ ; \ b_1 \leftarrow \sim b \ ; \ c \leftarrow \sim c_1 \ ; \ c_1 \leftarrow \sim c\}$$

which has four stable models: $M_1 = \{a, b, c\}$, $M_2 = \{b, c_1\}$, $M_3 = \{b_1, c\}$ and $M_4 = \{b_1, c_1\}$. Suppose we would like to compute the stable models M of P in which a is false. As suggested by the contrapositive interpretation of $a \leftarrow b, c$, one possibility is to branch the search using the conditions that (i) b is false in M and (ii) c is false in M. While analyzing the case (i), we find the stable models M_3 and M_4. On the other hand, the stable models M_2 and M_4 are discovered when (ii) is analyzed. Thus M_4 is encountered twice during the search. Another approach is to branch according to the condition (i) above and the condition that (iii) b is true in M. In the case (iii), the stable model M_2 is found directly.

A similar analysis can also be accomplished using the system smodels [16] for computations. Given P and the command "compute { not a }" the system finds us the three stable models M_2, M_3 and M_4 of P and informs us that the search involved 2 *choice points*. The choice between the cases (i) and (ii) can be simulated by the commands "compute { not a, not b }" and "compute { not a, not c }". Both cases yield an additional choice point so that the total number of choice points becomes 3. The choice between (i) and (iii) is handled similarly. The command "compute { not a, b }" yields the model M_2 without further choice points. Therefore, only 2 choice points are needed if the search space is split using (i) and (iii). This is exactly the number of choice points passed by smodels given the command "compute { not a }". A larger search tree results if branching is based on the conditions (i) and (ii).

To conclude, binary rules tend to block contrapositive inference in practice. This is because it is impossible to get rid of binary rules in a faithful and modular way (Theorem 5) and there is no guarantee that contrapositive reasoning can be accomplished in polynomial time, if cases arising from binary rules are thoroughly analyzed (Example 2). However, we do not claim that contrapositive reasoning is not useful. In particular, it is reasonable to infer that b is false if a is known to be false in the presence of a unary rule $a \leftarrow b$. Nevertheless, binary rules establish a limit how far it is practical to apply contrapositive reasoning.

Finally, let us sketch future work. The current hierarchy in Figure 1 was obtained as a by-product while the possibilities for reducing the number of positive body literals were analyzed. Consequently, the hierarchy does not cover many interesting classes of logic programs. Extensions to the hierarchy should be searched for by analyzing classes of logic programs with richer syntax (see [5, 6]) and different semantics (see [21]). Our recent results on the relationship of partial stable models and total stable models of disjunctive logic programs [11] provide a promising starting point in this respect.

Acknowledgments

The author wishes to thank Mirek Truszczyński for his suggestion to apply techniques from [9] to the research problem addressed in the paper as well as anonymous referees for comments and suggestions for improvements.

References

1. S. Brass and J. Dix. Semantics of (disjunctive) logic programs based on partial evaluation. *Journal of Logic Programming*, 38(3):167–213, 1999.
2. K.L. Clark. Negation as failure. In H. Gallaire and J. Minker, editors, *Logic and Data Bases*, pages 293–322. Plenum Press, New York, 1978.
3. S. A. Cook. The complexity of theorem proving procedures. In *Proceedings of the third Annual ACM Symposium on Theory of Computing*, pages 151–158, 1971.
4. M. Gelfond and V. Lifschitz. The stable model semantics for logic programming. In *Proceedings of the 5th International Conference on Logic Programming*, pages 1070–1080, Seattle, USA, August 1988. The MIT Press.
5. M. Gelfond and V. Lifschitz. Logic programs with classical negation. In *Proceedings of the 7th International Conference on Logic Programming*, pages 579–597, Jerusalem, Israel, June 1990. The MIT Press.
6. M. Gelfond and V. Lifschitz. Classical negation in logic programs and disjunctive databases. *New Generation Computing*, 9:365–385, 1991.
7. G. Gottlob. Translating default logic into standard autoepistemic logic. *Journal of the Association for Computing Machinery*, 42(2):711–740, 1995.
8. T. Imielinski. Results on translating defaults to circumscription. *Artificial Intelligence*, 32:131–146, 1987.
9. T. Janhunen. Classifying semi-normal default logic on the basis of its expressive power. In M. Gelfond, N. Leone, and G. Pfeifer, editors, *Proceedings of the 5th International Conference on Logic Programming and Non-Monotonic Reasoning, LPNMR'99*, pages 19–33, El Paso, Texas, December 1999. Springer. LNAI 1730.
10. T. Janhunen. On the intertranslatability of non-monotonic logics. *Annals of Mathematics in Artificial Intelligence*, 27(1-4):79–128, 1999.
11. T. Janhunen, I. Niemelä, P. Simons, and J.-H. You. Unfolding partiality and disjunctions in stable model semantics. In A.G. Cohn, F. Giunchiglia, and Selman B., editors, *Principles of Knowledge Representation and Reasoning: Proceedings of KR'2000*, pages 411–422, Breckenridge, Colorado, April 2000.
12. J.W. Lloyd. *Foundations of Logic Programming*. Springer-Verlag, Berlin, 1987.
13. W. Marek and M. Truszczyński. Autoepistemic logic. *Journal of the ACM*, 38:588–619, 1991.
14. W. Marek and M. Truszczyński. Stable models and an alternative logic programming paradigm. In *The Logic Programming Paradigm: a 25-Year Perspective*, pages 375–398. Springer-Verlag, 1999.
15. I. Niemelä. Logic programming with stable model semantics as a constraint programming paradigm. *Annals of Mathematics and Artificial Intelligence*, 25(3,4):241–273, 1999.
16. I. Niemelä and P. Simons. Efficient implementation of the well-founded and stable model semantics. In M. Maher, editor, *Proceedings of the Joint International Conference and Symposium on Logic Programming*, pages 289–303, Bonn, Germany, September 1996. The MIT Press.
17. R. Reiter. On closed world data bases. In H. Gallaire and J. Minker, editors, *Logic and Data Bases*, pages 55–76. Plenum Press, New York, 1978.
18. L. Sterling and E. Shapiro. *The Art of Prolog*. MIT Series in logic programming. The MIT Press, London, 1986.
19. V.S. Subrahmanian, D. Nau, and C. Vago. WFS + branch and bound = stable models. *IEEE Transactions on Knowledge and Data Engineering*, 7(3):362–377, 1995.
20. M.H. van Emden and R.A. Kowalski. The semantics of predicate logic as a programming language. *Journal of the ACM*, 23:733–742, 1976.
21. A. Van Gelder, K.A. Ross, and J.S. Schlipf. The well-founded semantics for general logic programs. *Journal of the ACM*, 38(3):620–650, July 1991.

On Complexity of Updates through Integrity Constraints*

Michael Dekhtyar[1], Alexander Dikovsky[2], and Sergey Dudakov[1]

[1] Dept. of CS, Tver State Univ.
33 Zheljabova str. Tver, Russia, 170000
Michael.Dekhtyar@tversu.ru, p000104@tversu.ru
[2] Université de Nantes. IRIN, UPREF, EA No 2157
2, rue de la Houssinière BP 92208, F 44322 Nantes cedex 3, France
Alexandre.Dikovsky@irin.univ-nantes.fr

Abstract. The computational complexity is explored of finding the minimal real change of a database after an update constrained by a logic program. A polynomial time algorithm is discovered which solves this problem for ground IC in partial interpretations. Formulated in a "property" form, even under the premise of fixed database scheme, this problem turns out to be complete in the first three classes of Σ and Π polynomial hierarchies, depending on many factors: type of interpretation (total or partial), presence of variables, use of negation, arity of predicates, etc. Meanwhile, we show that under strong restrictions to negative constraints the problem is solvable in polynomial time. If the database scheme may vary, the complexity grows exponentially.

1 Introduction

Database updates whose impact on database states is specified by systems of IF-THEN rules or by logic programs are in the focus of research till late 80ies. The interest in such updates has quickened in the past few years by the emergence of databases with intelligent update enforcement features (such as triggers), in particular, of active databases ([9,5,18,31,25,28,6]). Initially, the interest in rule based updates was aroused by the need in generalizations of SQL-like declarative update definitions (cf. [1,2]). Subsequently, this field was influenced by investigation of knowledge base updates initiated by [3]. One approach, influenced by [30], regards the result of a theory update as the theory of its updated (revised) models (see [24,26]). Another approach follows the line of [22], where a propositional update formula transforms an initial formula into a new formula. In the first order case both the updated theory, and the update itself are represented by logic programs (see e.g. [4]). Model based updates provide new models (DB states) minimally deviating (in some sense) from the initial ones, sometimes explicitly, sometimes not. An alternative operational approach to updates

---

* This work was sponsored by the Russian Fundamental Studies Foundation (Grants 98-01-00204, 99-01-00374, 00-01-00254).

J. Lloyd et al. (Eds.): CL 2000, LNAI 1861, pp. 867–881, 2000.

is based on derivations in logic programs. For instance, abduction, sometimes combined with SLD or SLDNF, is used for view updates (cf. [21, 10, 19]).

Still another approach to database updates was proposed in [11, 12, 20], and developed in [13, 14]. It applies to databases with integrity constraints (IC), expressed in the form of a logic program. Accomplishing updates in presence of such IC needs subsequent conflict resolution. This approach departs from the premise that IC is not intended for data or knowledge definition. Rather, they specify the conflicts to avoid after updates. So in this approach the use of exclusively "intended" models of IC may lead to the loss of information or to unjustified conflict resolution failures, which is illustrated by the following simple example.

Example 1. *The IC Φ below expresses a typical case of an exception from a general rule. It consists of two clauses. The first one expresses the general rule: "children (proposition* children*) can bathe (*bathe*) when with parents (*parents*)". The other one expresses an exception from this rule: "children cannot bathe while the ebb tide (proposition* ebb*)":*

$$\text{bathe} \leftarrow \text{children}, \text{parents}$$
$$\neg\text{bathe} \leftarrow \text{children}, \text{ebb}.$$

Let us consider a DB state where children cannot bathe because of the ebb. This state is materialized differently in classical and partial databases. In classical databases the absence of a fact means that its negation holds. In a partial database S a fact a *holds if* $a \in S$, $\neg a$ *holds if* $\neg a \in S$ *explicitly, otherwise* a *is unknown.*

Let us consider first the classical databases. This means that we have the DB state $I = \{\text{children}, \text{ebb}\}$. Suppose that the parents arrive, which is expressed as the addition of the fact parents *to I. This positive update causes the conflict with the first rule. The possible solutions are simple but nontrivial. The first solution is to replace* ebb *by* bathe. *The result is the DB state where children's bathing is allowed: $I_1 = \{\text{children}, \text{parents}, \text{bathe}\}$. The other is just to eliminate* children. *The resulting DB state is that where no children's bathing is needed: $I_2 = \{\text{parents}, \text{ebb}\}$.*

Now, let us consider the same update in the case of partial databases. The initial DB is in this case $I = \{\text{children}, \text{ebb}, \neg\text{bathe}\}$. The first solution is then to replace ebb *and* $\neg$bathe *by* bathe, *the resulting DB state being: $I_1 = \{\text{children}, \text{parents}, \text{bathe}\}$. The other solution is again to eliminate* children, *the resulting DB state being this time: $I_2 = \{\text{parents}, \text{ebb}, \neg\text{bathe}\}$.*

This is why after an update all models of IC are considered, where the update is accomplished. However, among these models one should find one minimally deviating from the initial model. A bit more formally, this "enforced update problem (EUP)" is formulated as follows. Given a logic program Φ which formalizes the IC, a correct initial DB state $I \models \Phi$, and an external update Δ which specifies the facts D^+ to be added to I and the facts D^- to be deleted from it, one should find the *minimal real change* $\Psi(I)$ of I, sufficient to accomplish Δ and to restore Φ if and when it is violated (i.e. to guarantee that $D^+ \subseteq \Psi(I), \Psi(I) \cap D^- = \emptyset$, and $\Psi(I) \models \Phi$). So we see that the EUP is a "function" and not a "property" problem. The closest "property" problems are those of existence of EUP-solutions marked by presence/absence of a given fact (**OFIP**), and of presence/absence of a given fact in all EUP-solutions (**PFIP**). In papers [13, 14] these problems were investigated for databases with ground IC and were shown to be untractable in worst case: namely, complete in first two classes of Σ and Π polynomial hierarchies. In contrast with this, in this paper we find a polynomial time algorithm for the EUP itself in the same class of ground IC in partial interpretations. We suspect that there is no such algorithm in total interpretations.

In this paper we investigate the impact of interpretation type and the use of variables in clauses of IC on the complexity of **OFIP** and **PFIP**. We show that for definite ground IC, and positive updates and initial states these problems are solvable in polynomial time in both interpretations. The use of variables in this positive case makes the problems complete respectively in *NP* and *co-NP*. Possibility of deletions makes them complete respectively in *NP* and *co-NP* for ground definite IC, and complete respectively in Σ_2^p and Π_2^p for definite IC with variables. In general they are respectively Σ_2^p-complete and Π_2^p-complete in partial interpretations, and Σ_3^p-complete and Π_3^p-complete in total interpretations. In the case, where the DB signature may vary, the complexity of these problems grows exponentially.

The paper is organized as follows. The next section contains preliminary notions and notation. The problems we consider are formulated in sections 3 (Enforced Update Problem in terms of conservative update operators) and in section 4 (**OFIP** and **PFIP**). Subsection 4.1 contains complexity results for partial interpretations under the premise of fixed signature. Subsection 4.2 contains the results concerning total interpretations under the same premise. In subsection 4.3 the case of varying signature is considered.

2   Preliminaries

We assume that the reader is familiar with the basic concepts and terminology of logic programming and complexity theory (see [23, 8]) .

Language. Let **S** be a 1st order signature with a set of constants **C** and no other function symbols. Sometimes in this paper **S** will be fixed with infinite **C**, sometimes it will be finite and its size will be considered as a parameter of complexity. A *domain* is a finite subset **D** of **C**. For each domain **D** by $\mathbf{A(S, D)}$, $\mathbf{L(S, D)}$, $\mathbf{B(S, D)}$ and $\mathbf{LB(S, D)}$ we denote respectively the sets of all atoms, all literals, all ground atoms, and all ground literals in the signature **S** with constants in **D**. A literal contrary to a literal l is denoted by $\neg.l$. We set $\neg.M = \{\neg.l \mid l \in M\}$.

Logic Programs. Integrity constraints (IC) will be expressed by generalized logic programs in **S** and **D** with explicit negation, i.e. finite sets of clauses of the form $r = (l \leftarrow l_1, ..., l_n)$ where $n \geq 0$ and $l, l_i \in \mathbf{L(S, D)}$, (note that negative literals are possible in the bodies and in the heads of the clauses). For a clause r $head(r)$ denotes its *head*, and $body(r)$ its *body*. We will treat $body(r)$ as a set of literals. **D** being fixed, we consider groundisations of clauses only over **D**. $gr(\Phi)$ will denote the set of all ground instances of clauses in Φ. $\mathbf{IC(S, D)}$

will denote the set of all integrity constraints in the signature $\mathbf{S}$ with constants in $\mathbf{D}$.

Correct DB States. In this paper we consider both kinds of interpretations of ICs, total and partial, over *closed domains*. This means that a certain domain $\mathbf{D}$ is fixed for each problem. A *partial* interpretation (*DB state*) over $\mathbf{D}$ is a finite subset of $\mathbf{LB}(\mathbf{S},\mathbf{D})$. For such an interpretation $I \subseteq \mathbf{LB}(\mathbf{S},\mathbf{D})$ we set $I^+ = I \cap \mathbf{B}(\mathbf{S},\mathbf{D})$ and $I^- = I \cap \neg.\mathbf{B}(\mathbf{S},\mathbf{D})$. I is *consistent* if it contains no contrary pair of literals $l, \neg.l$. Intuitively, in a consistent partial DB state I the atoms in I^+ are regarded as true, the atoms in $\neg.I^-$ are regarded as false, and all others are regarded as unknown. A partial interpretation I is *total* if $I^+ \cup \neg.I^- = \mathbf{B}(\mathbf{S},\mathbf{D})$ and $I^+ \cap \neg.I^- = \emptyset$. Note that total interpretations are completely defined by their positive parts, so we will identify total interpretations with subsets of $\mathbf{B}(\mathbf{S},\mathbf{D})$. Given an IC $\Phi \in \mathbf{IC}(\mathbf{S},\mathbf{D})$ and a DB state I over $\mathbf{D}$, a ground clause $r = (l \leftarrow l_1,...,l_n)$ in $gr(\Phi)$ is *valid* in I (denoted $I \models r$) if $I \models l$ whenever $I \models l_i$ for each $1 \leq i \leq n$. For a partial DB state I and a ground literal l $I \models l$ means $l \in I$. For a total DB state I and a ground atom a $I \models a$ means $a \in I$, and $I \models \neg.a$ means $a \notin I$. I is *a correct DB state* or a *model* of Φ (denoted $I \models \Phi$) if it is consistent (which is always true for total DB states) and every clause in $gr(\Phi)$ is valid in I.

Consequence Closure. Let $\Phi \in \mathbf{IC}(\mathbf{S},\mathbf{D})$. For a partial interpretation I we set $cl_\Phi(I) = \{l | \exists r = (l \leftarrow l_1,...,l_n) \in gr(\Phi) \ (\bigwedge_{i=1}^{n} I \models l_i)\}$. A strong immediate consequence operator is the total operator

$$T_\Phi^{\in}(I) = \begin{cases} cl_\Phi(I) & : & cl_\Phi(I) \text{ is consistent} \\ \mathbf{LB}(\mathbf{S},\mathbf{D}) & : & cl_\Phi(I) \text{ is inconsistent.} \end{cases}$$

Being continuous, $T_\Phi^{\in}$ has the least fixed point $lfp(T_\Phi^{\in}) = \bigcup_{i=0}^{\infty} (T_\Phi^{\in}(\emptyset))^i$. We denote this set by M_Φ^{min}. It is clear that if M_Φ^{min} is consistent, then it is the least (partial) model of Φ. For any partial DB state I we set $M_\Phi^{min}(I) = M_{\Phi \cup I}^{min}$.

Updates. When partial interpretations over $\mathbf{D}$ are considered, an *update* is a pair $\Delta = (D^+, D^-)$ where D^+, D^- are subsets of $\mathbf{LB}(\mathbf{S},\mathbf{D})$. In the case of total interpretations D^+, D^- are subsets of $\mathbf{B}(\mathbf{S},\mathbf{D})$. In both cases $D^+ \cap D^- = \emptyset$. Intuitively, the literals of D^+ are to be added to DB state I, and those of D^- are to be removed from I. We will denote the components D^+ and D^- respectively by Δ^+ and Δ^-. For both kinds of interpretations $\mathbf{UP}(\mathbf{S},\mathbf{D})$ will denote the set of all updates in the signature $\mathbf{S}$ and with constants in $\mathbf{D}$. We say that Δ is *accomplished* in I if $\Delta^+ \subseteq I$ and $\Delta^- \cap I = \emptyset$.

In the sequel we will omit $\mathbf{S},\mathbf{D}$ when it causes no ambiguity. So when $\mathbf{S}$ and $\mathbf{D}$ are subsumed, in the place of $\mathbf{A}(\mathbf{S},\mathbf{D})$, $\mathbf{L}(\mathbf{S},\mathbf{D})$, $\mathbf{B}(\mathbf{S},\mathbf{D})$, $\mathbf{LB}(\mathbf{S},\mathbf{D})$, $\mathbf{UP}(\mathbf{S},\mathbf{D})$ we will use the notation $\mathbf{A}, \mathbf{L}, \mathbf{B}, \mathbf{LB}, \mathbf{UP}$.

3   Conservative Rule Based Updates

In general, an update may contradict constraints. So a reasonable definition of an update operator should either contain a requirement of "compatibility" of an update and constraints, or specify a part of the update "compatible" with the constraints. The requirement of compatibility is easy to formalize.

Definition 1. *For $\Phi \in$ **IC** and $\Delta \in$ **UP** let us denote by $Acc(\Phi, \Delta)$ the set of all models $I \models \Phi$ where Δ is accomplished. An update Δ is* compatible *with an IC Φ if $Acc(\Phi, \Delta) \neq \emptyset$.*

In [11] we propose the following minimal deviation criterion implementing the intention to keep as much initial facts as possible, and then to add possibly fewer new facts:

Definition 2. *Let I, I_1 be two DB states, and K be a class of DB states. We say that I_1 is* minimally deviating *from I with respect to K if $\forall I_2 \in K \ (\neg(I \cap I_1 \subsetneq I \cap I_2) \ \& \ ((I \cap I_1 = I \cap I_2) \rightarrow \neg(I_2 \setminus I \subsetneq I_1 \setminus I)))$.*

In terms of this criterion the *conservative update operators* we consider have been defined in [12] as follows.

Definition 3. *Let Δ be a given update which is compatible with IC Φ. An operator Ψ on the set of DB states is a* conservative update operator *if for each DB state I :*
- *$\Psi(I)$ is a model of Φ,*
- *Δ is accomplished in $\Psi(I)$,*
- *$\Psi(I)$ is minimally deviating from I with respect to $Acc(\Phi, \Delta)$.*

4   Computational Complexity of Conservative Updates

The Enforced Update Problem (EUP) we discuss in the Introduction is the problem of calculation of a conservative update operator Ψ for some given IC, update and input state. So it is a "function" type problem. In order to measure the complexity of conservative updates in a "property" form we use two standard algorithmic problems: *Optimistic* and *Pessimistic Fall-Into-Problem* (**OFIP** and respectively **PFIP**) (cf. [15]).

OFIP: Given some $\Delta \in$ **UP** compatible with $\Phi \in$ **IC**, an initial state I, and a literal $l \in$ **LB**, one should check whether there exists a DB state I_1 such that:
(a) $I_1 \in Acc(\Phi, \Delta)$,
(b) I_1 is minimally deviating from I with respect to $Acc(\Phi, \Delta)$, and
(c) $I_1 \models l$.

PFIP: requires (c) be true **for all** models I_1 satisfying (a),(b).

We denote respectively by **OFIP** and **PFIP** the sets of all solutions (I, Δ, Φ, l) of these problems.

Typical database updates do not change database scheme. In logical terms this corresponds to the situation, where predicate signature **S** is fixed. Under this premise we consider the combined complexity of **OFIP** and **PFIP** with respect to the problem size evaluated as $N = |\mathbf{D}| + |I| + |\Delta| + |\Phi| + |l|$ (| | being the size of constant or literal sets, and of programs in some standard encoding). Signature **S** being fixed, for a given domain **D** the maximal size of a DB state is bounded by a polynomial of the order $O(|\mathbf{D}|^a)$, where a is the maximal arity of predicates in $\mathbf{S}$. When $\mathbf{S}$ is not fixed, its size is included into the problem size.

In this paper we use the following multiparameter reduction scheme which serves for most lower bounds below in the case of a fixed one-predicate signature.

Let $\mathbf{S} = \{s^{(2)}\}$, $\alpha = d_1 \wedge \ldots \wedge d_n$ be a 3-CNF, where in each clause $d_i = (\neg)u_{i1} \vee (\neg)u_{i2} \vee (\neg)u_{i3}$ $(1 \leq i \leq n)$ u_{ij} are propositional variables. Given a set R of boolean variables we form the set of constants $C(\alpha, R) = \{t, f, t_1, t_2, t_3, f_1, f_2, f_3, 1, 2, 3, p_{000}, p_{001}, \ldots, p_{111}, d_1, \ldots, d_n\} \cup \{c_x | x \in R\}$. Informally, d_i encodes the ith clause, t or f fix its value, 1, 2, or 3 fix j in u_{ij}, t_j or f_j fix the value of u_{ij}, $p_{b_1 b_2 b_3}$ fixes boolean values of u_{i1}, u_{i2}, u_{i3}, and c_x is a DB constant for the boolean variable $x \in R$. We construct the following (α, R)-dependent part $J(\alpha, R)$ of initial DB states.

$J(\alpha, R) = J \cup J_\alpha \cup J_R$, where :
$$J = \{s(t, t_j), s(f, f_j) | 1 \leq j \leq 3\} \cup \{s(t_j, j), s(f_j, j) | 1 \leq j \leq 3\} \cup$$
$$\bigcup_{b_1 b_2 b_3} \{\{s(t_j, p_{b_1 b_2 b_3}) \mid b_j = 1\} \cup \{s(f_j, p_{b_1 b_2 b_3}) \mid b_j = 0\}\};$$
$$J_\alpha = \bigcup_{b_1 b_2 b_3} \{s(d_i, p_{b_1 b_2 b_3}) | \text{ if } i\text{-th clause is true on } b_1 b_2 b_3, 1 \leq i \leq 3\}, \text{ and}$$
$$J_R = \{s(t, c_x), s(f, c_x) \mid x \in R\}.$$

Given α and two sets of variables R_1, R_2, $R_1 \cap R_2 = \emptyset$, we construct the set of atoms
$$\varphi(\alpha, R_1, R_2) = \bigcup_{i=1}^{n} \{s(d_i, P_i)\} \cup \beta_1^i(u_{i1}) \cup \beta_2^i(u_{i2}) \cup \beta_3^i(u_{i3}),$$

where
$$\beta_j^i(x) = \begin{cases} \{s(V_x, c_x), s(V_x, W_{ij}), s(W_{ij}, j), s(W_{ij}, P_i)\} & , \quad \text{for } x \in R_1 \\ \{s(V_x, W_{ij}), s(W_{ij}, j), s(W_{ij}, P_i)\} & , \quad \text{for } x \in R_2. \end{cases}$$

P_i, W_{ij}, V_x being object variables. Intuitively, P_i fixes a triple $p_{b_1 b_2 b_3}$ which makes d_i true, the value of W_{ij} fixes a value b_j of u_{ij} in this triple, and finally, V_x fixes a value $(t$ or $f)$ of x. Therefore, $\beta_j^i(x)$ describes the value of the propositional variable x in j-th literal of i-th clause. Notice that both, $J(\alpha, R)$ and $\varphi(\alpha, R_1, R_2)$ contain only positive literals.

The following lemma relates the satisfiability of α to the validity of φ on J.

Lemma 1. *Let $\overline{x}, \overline{y}$ be a partition of the set of variables of a 3-CNF $\alpha(\overline{x}, \overline{y})$. In our construction let $C = C(\alpha, \overline{x})$ and*
$$I = J(\alpha, \emptyset) \cup \bigcup_{x \in \overline{x}} \{s(t, c_x) \mid \sigma(x) = 1\} \cup \{s(f, c_x) \mid \sigma(x) = 0\},$$
for some boolean substitution $\sigma : \overline{x} \to \{0, 1\}$. Then $\alpha(\sigma \overline{x}, \overline{y})$ is satisfiable iff $I \models \varphi(\alpha, \overline{x}, \overline{y}) \circ \tau$, for some object variables substitution τ.

Proof. If α is satisfiable, then there is an extension σ' of σ to $\overline{y}$ such that $\alpha(\sigma' \overline{x}, \sigma' \overline{y})$ is true. Then we set $\tau P_i = p_{\sigma'(u_{i1} u_{i2} u_{i3})}$,
$$\tau V_u = \begin{cases} t & , \quad \text{if } \sigma'(u) = 1, \\ f & , \quad \text{if } \sigma'(u) = 0, \end{cases} \text{ for all } u \in \overline{x} \cup \overline{y},$$
$$\tau W_{ij} = \begin{cases} t_j & , \quad \text{if } \sigma'(u_{ij}) = 1, \\ f_j & , \quad \text{if } \sigma'(u_{ij}) = 0, \end{cases} \text{ for } 1 \leq i \leq n, 1 \leq j \leq 3.$$

It easy to check that $I \models \varphi(\alpha, \overline{x}, \overline{y}) \circ \tau$.

Now, let $\varphi(\alpha, \overline{x}, \overline{y})$ be valid in I under some object variables substitution τ. Then $\tau P_i \in \{p_{000}, p_{001}, ..., p_{111}\}$ since $I \models s(d_i, P_i) \circ \tau$, $\tau W_{ij} \in \{t_j, f_j\}$ since $I \models s(W_{ij}, j) \circ \tau$, and $\tau V_u \in \{t, f\}$ since $I \models s(V_u, W_{ij}) \circ \tau$. We define σ' from τ as follows : $\sigma'(u) = 1$ if $\tau V_u = t$ and $\sigma'(u) = 0$ otherwise. Let us observe that σ' coincides with σ on $\overline{x}$. Indeed, $\varphi(\alpha, \overline{x}, \overline{y})$ contains a fact $s(V_x, c_x)$ valid in I only if $\sigma(x) = \sigma'(x)$, for all $x \in \overline{x}$. As $\varphi(\alpha, \overline{x}, \overline{y})$ contains the facts $s(V_{u_{ij}}, W_{ij})$, $s(W_{ij}, j)$, and $s(W_{ij}, P_i)$, then $\tau P_i = p_{\sigma'(u_{i1}u_{i2}u_{i3})}$. Now, from $I \models s(d_i, P_i) \circ \tau$ it follows that the clause d_i is true under σ', hence $\alpha(\sigma \overline{x}, \sigma' \overline{y})$ is true. $\square$

The complexity of the problems we consider depends on many factors: presence of variables in clauses of IC, use of negation, arity of predicates, etc. The main factor is the interpretation type. It turns out that the same problems are simpler in partial interpretations than in classical total interpretations. For example, in partial interpretations the compatibility problem $Acc(\Phi, \Delta) \neq \emptyset$ for ground IC Φ is resolved in linear time, whereas, it is NP-complete in total interpretations [13] for the same class of IC. As will be shown, in partial interpretations both problems **OFIP** and **PFIP** have a wide spectrum of complexity depending on specific factors, such as presence of negative literals in DB states or in update. The other important factor is groundness of IC. Such basic problem as model checking is resolved in linear time for ground IC in both interpretations. Meanwhile, even for definite IC Φ the problem $MC = \{< I, \Phi > \mid I \models \Phi\}$ is *co-NP*-complete in both interpretations, which follows for example from the respective complexity bounds for conjunctive queries [7].

4.1 Complexity in Partial Interpretations

We begin with several simple observations.

Proposition 1. *For any IC Φ:*
(1) if $M_\Phi^{min}(S)$ is consistent for some set of literals S, then $M_\Phi^{min}(S) \models \Phi$;
(2) if $I \models \Phi$ and $S \subseteq I$, then $M_\Phi^{min}(S) \models \Phi$;
(3) if Φ is compatible with some Δ, then $M_\Phi^{min}(\Delta^+)$ is the least model in $Acc(\Phi, \Delta)$;
(4) if Φ is a definite IC compatible with some positive Δ (i.e., $\Delta^+ \subseteq \mathbf{B}$ and $\Delta^- = \emptyset$), and $I \subseteq \mathbf{B}$, then $M_\Phi^{min}(\Delta^+ \cup I)$ is the only DB state minimally deviating from I with respect to $Acc(\Phi, \Delta)$.

The premise of fixed predicate signature provides important polynomial time algorithms.

Proposition 2. *Let Φ be an IC and S be a set of literals.*
(1) There is an algorithm that constructs $M_\Phi^{min}(S)$ in polynomial time, if Φ is ground.
(2) There is a nondeterministic uniformly (i.e. in all computations) polynomial time algorithm, which constructs $M_\Phi^{min}(S)$ in some its computation, and a subset of $M_\Phi^{min}(S)$ in any its computation.

These propositions lead to the following interesting characterization of the EUP solutions in partial interpretations.

Theorem 1. *Let Φ and Δ be compatible. Then I_1 is minimally deviating from I with respect to $Acc(\Phi, \Delta)$ iff there is a maximal subset $S \subseteq I$ such that*
$$I_1 = M_{\Phi}^{min}(S \cup \Delta^+) \text{ is consistent and } I_1 \cap \Delta^- = \emptyset.$$

The proof of this theorem uses a construction from the following lemma, which is interesting for itself and provides important consequences for ground IC.

Lemma 2. *There is a polynomial time algorithm constructing some DB state $I_1 \in Acc(\Phi, \Delta)$ minimally deviating from I with respect to $Acc(\Phi, \Delta)$, from an initial DB state I, any DB state $I_0 \in Acc(\Phi, \Delta)$, and ground IC Φ compatible with Δ.*

Proof Scheme: Let $I = \{l_1, l_2, \ldots, l_n\}$, Δ, Φ and some DB state $I_0 \in Acc(\Phi, \Delta)$ be given. We define the following sequence of sets S_i, $0 \le i \le n$.

$$S_0 = (I_0 \cap I) \cup D^+ \text{ and } S_{i+1} = \begin{cases} S_i, & \text{if } M_{\Phi}^{min}(S_i \cup \{l_{i+1}\}) \text{ is inconsistent} \\ & \text{or } M_{\Phi}^{min}(S_i \cup \{l_{i+1}\}) \cap D^- \neq \emptyset \\ S_i \cup \{l_{i+1}\}, & \text{otherwise.} \end{cases}$$

Let $I_1 = M_{\Phi}^{min}(S_n)$. By construction and by Proposition 1, $I_1 \in Acc(\Phi, \Delta)$. No literal $l \in I \setminus I_1$ can be added to I_1, because $\{l\} \cup I_1$ is inconsistent or contradicts Δ^-. No literal $l \in I_1 \setminus I$ can be removed from I_1, because it is inferred from S_n, which contains only literals in I or in D^+. Hence, I_1 minimally deviates from I with respect to $Acc(\Phi, \Delta)$. Note that if I_0 minimally deviates from I with respect to $Acc(\Phi, \Delta)$, then $I_1 = I_0$. Clearly, I_1 is constructed in polynomial time. $\square$

Now we can prove Theorem 1:

Proof Scheme: ($\Rightarrow$) Let $S = I_1 \cap I$ and $I_0 = M_{\Phi}^{min}(S \cup \Delta^+)$. Being a subset of I_1, I_0 is consistent. So $I_0 \models \Phi$. By monotonicity of $M_{\Phi}^{min}(X)$, $\Delta^+ \subseteq I_0$ and $\Delta^- \cap I_0 = \emptyset$, so $I_0 \in Acc(\Phi, \Delta)$. For the same reason, $I_0 \cap I = I_1 \cap I = S$. So if there is some $l \in I_1 \setminus I_0$, then I_1 is not minimally deviating from $Acc(\Phi, \Delta)$.
($\Leftarrow$) Being consistent, $I_1 = M_{\Phi}^{min}(S \cup \Delta^+)$ is a model of Φ. So $I_1 \in Acc(\Phi, \Delta)$. Apply the construction of Lemma 1 to so defined I_1 in the role of I_0. The result will coincide with I_1 by construction. Therefore, I_1 is minimally deviating from $Acc(\Phi, \Delta)$. $\square$

If Φ and Δ are compatible, then by Proposition 1, the model $I_0 = M_{\Phi}^{min}(\Delta^+)$ is in $Acc(\Phi, \Delta)$. So together with Proposition 2, this lemma gives a surprising consequence: for ground IC there is a polynomial time computable conservative update operator, i.e. one can find **some** solution of the EUP in polynomial time.

Corollary 1. *There is a polynomial time algorithm constructing some DB state $I_1 \in Acc(\Phi, \Delta)$ minimally deviating from I with respect to $Acc(\Phi, \Delta)$, from an initial DB state I and ground IC Φ compatible with Δ.*

Sure, this doesn't work for **OFIP**, because the given literal l may not fall into this particular solution. Indeed, as it is shown in [14], **OFIP** is a hard problem even for ground IC.

Theorem 2. *[14] Let IC be ground. Then:*
(1) **OFIP** *and* **PFIP** *belong to P in the case where:*
  a) Φ is normal (i.e. there are no negations in the heads of clauses),
  b) Δ is positive, i.e. $\Delta^+ \subseteq \mathbf{B}$ and $\Delta^- = \emptyset$, and
  c) there are no negations in I, i.e. $I \subseteq \mathbf{B}$.
(2) If any of conditions a), b), c) is violated, then **OFIP** *is NP-complete and* **PFIP** *is co-NP-complete.*

Let us analyze the complexity of **OFIP** and **PFIP** for general IC with variables. There is one very special case, where these problems are solvable in polynomial time: that of positive DB states and updates and definite monadic IC. In this case one can construct the consequence closure of polynomial size. Following to Proposition 1 (4), **OFIP** and **PFIP** are equivalent in this case.

Proposition 3. *There is a polynomial time algorithm, which decides whether $(\Delta, \Phi, I, l) \in$* **OFIP** *(same for* **PFIP***) for definite Φ containing only unary predicates, and for positive Δ, I, and l.*

Even the use of a single binary predicate can increase the complexity of both problems, when Δ is positive and Φ is a definite IC with variables. Interestingly, the complexity depends on positivity of l.

Theorem 3. *In the case, where IC are definite, and updates are positive:*
(1) **OFIP** *is NP-complete if l is positive;*
(2) **OFIP** *is co-NP-complete if l is negative;*
both lower bounds are valid even for a one binary predicate signature.

Proof Scheme: *Lower Bound.* In our reduction scheme for a 3-CNF α with variables V we take some new variable a and set $C = C(\alpha, \{a\})$, $\Delta = (J(\alpha, \emptyset), \emptyset)$, $\Phi = \{s(t, c_a) \leftarrow \varphi(\alpha, \emptyset, V)\}$, and $I = \{\neg s(t, c_a)\}$. Then α is satisfiable iff $(I, \Delta, \Phi, s(t, c_a)) \in$ **OFIP**, and iff $(I, \Delta, \Phi, \neg s(t, c_a)) \notin$ **OFIP**. $\square$

Corollary 2. *In the case, where IC are definite, and Δ and I are positive,* **PFIP** *is NP-complete.*

For the same class of IC and of updates, emergence of negative literals in initial DB states increases the complexity of **PFIP**.

Theorem 4. *In the case, where IC are definite, and Δ are positive,* **PFIP** *is Π_2^p-complete.*

Proof Scheme: *Lower Bound.* Let us consider a sentence $\beta = \forall \overline{x} \exists \overline{y} \alpha(\overline{x}, \overline{y})$, where α is 3-CNF. Let a and b be new different variables. Then we set $C = C(\alpha, \overline{x} \cup \{a, b\})$, $I = J(\alpha, \overline{x}) \cup \{\neg s(t, c_a)\}$, and define Φ by:
$s(t, c_a) \leftarrow s(f, c_a), s(t, c_x), s(f, c_x)$, for $x \in \overline{x}$;
$s(t, c_b) \leftarrow s(t, c_a)$;
$s(t, c_b) \leftarrow \{s(f, c_a)\} \cup \varphi(\alpha, \overline{x}, \overline{y})$;
$s(c_1, c_2) \leftarrow$ for all $s(c_1, c_2) \in J(\alpha, \emptyset)$.
Let $\Delta = (\{s(f, c_a)\}, \emptyset)$ and $l = s(t, c_b)$. Then one can prove that $(I, \Delta, \Phi, l) \in$ **PFIP** iff β is true. $\square$

Discarding the constraint of positivity of updates, we still increase the complexity of both problems. As it concerns monadic definite IC, their complexity is as that of ground IC.

Proposition 4. *In the case, where IC are definite and use only unary predicates,* **OFIP** *is NP-complete, and* **PFIP** *is co-NP-complete.*

For definite IC with arbitrary predicates the problems become complete on the second level of polynomial Σ and Π hierarchies.

Theorem 5. *In the case, where IC are definite:*
(1) **OFIP** *is Σ_2^p-complete;*
(2) **PFIP** *is Π_2^p-complete;*
both lower bounds are valid even for a one binary predicate signature.

Proof Scheme: (1) *Lower Bound.* Let $\beta = \exists \overline{x} \forall \overline{y} \neg \alpha(\overline{x}, \overline{y})$ for a 3-CNF α. We set $C = C(\alpha, \overline{x} \cup \{a, b, c, d\} \cup \{b_x \mid x \in \overline{x}\})$, $I = J(\alpha, \overline{x}) \cup \{s(t, c_d), s(t, c_a)\}$, and define Φ by:
$s(t, c_a) \leftarrow s(t, c_x), s(f, c_x)$, for $x \in \overline{x}$;
$s(t, c_{b_x}) \leftarrow s(t, c_c), s(t, c_x)$, and $s(t, c_{b_x}) \leftarrow s(t, c_c), s(f, c_x)$, for $x \in \overline{x}$;
$s(t, c_a) \leftarrow \{s(t, c_d)\} \cup \varphi(\alpha, \overline{x}, \overline{y})$;
$s(t, c_b) \leftarrow s(t, c_d) \cup \bigcup_{x \in \overline{x}} s(t, c_{b_x})$;
$s(c_1, c_2) \leftarrow$ for all $s(c_1, c_2) \in J(\alpha, \emptyset)$.
Finally, let $\Delta = (\{s(t, c_c)\}, \{s(t, c_a)\})$, and $l = s(t, c_b)$.

Note that for any $I_1 \in Acc(\Phi, \Delta)$ at most one of facts $s(t, c_x)$, $s(f, c_x)$ can belong to I_1. If for some x neither $s(t, c_x)$ nor $s(f, c_x)$ is in I_1 then I_1 doesn't contain $s(t, c_b)$.

Now, if formula β is true, then there is a substitution σ such that $\alpha(\sigma \overline{x}, \overline{y})$ is false for all $\overline{y}$. Let us add $s(t, c_x)$ to I_1 if $\sigma(x) = true$ and $s(f, c_x)$ otherwise. Then we have to add to I_1 also all $s(t, c_{b_x})$. As $\alpha(\sigma \overline{x}, \overline{y})$ is false for all $\overline{y}$, $\varphi(\alpha, \overline{x}, \overline{y})$ cannot be true. Hence we add $s(t, c_d)$ and therefore, also $s(t, c_b)$ to I_1.

If β is false, then for every combination of $s(t, c_x)$ and $s(f, c_x)$ there is a substitution such that $\varphi(\alpha, \overline{x}, \overline{y})$ is true. Hence, we should delete $s(t, c_d)$ from I_1. If we don't delete $s(t, c_d)$, then we must delete some other fact. But we can delete only literals of the form $s(Z, c_x)$ where $Z \in \{t, f\}$. So we remove $s(t, c_x)$ and $s(f, c_x)$ for some x, and we cannot obtain $s(t, c_{b_x})$ for this x. In any case, $s(t, c_b)$ cannot be proven, and does not belong to I_1.

(2) *Lower Bound.* Let us consider a sentence $\beta = \forall \overline{x} \exists \overline{y} \alpha(\overline{x}, \overline{y})$, where α is a 3-CNF. Let a and b be some new variables. We construct $C = C(\alpha, \overline{x} \cup \{a, b\})$, $I = J(\alpha, \emptyset)$, and IC Φ with clauses:
$s(t, c_a) \leftarrow s(f, c_a), s(t, c_x), s(f, c_x)$, for $x \in \overline{x}$;
$s(t, c_b) \leftarrow \{s(f, c_a)\} \cup \varphi(\alpha, \overline{x}, \overline{y})$;
$s(c_1, c_2) \leftarrow$ for all $s(c_1, c_2) \in J(\alpha, \emptyset)$.
We set $\Delta = (\{s(f, c_a)\}, \{s(t, c_a)\})$ and $l = s(t, c_b)$. Then $(I, \Delta, \Phi, l) \in$ **PFIP** iff β is true. $\square$

Interestingly enough, the general case in partial interpretations is polynomially reduced to that of definite IC.

Lemma 3. **OFIP** *and* **PFIP** *for general (ground) IC are polynomial time equivalent to the same problems for definite (ground) IC.*

Proof. We consider only the general case. Let (I, Δ, Φ, l) be an instance of **OFIP** (**PFIP**). We add to **S** a new predicate symbol p' for every predicate $p \in$ **S** and replace all occurrences of $\neg p$ in I, Δ, Φ, and l by p'. Then we fix some new ground atom foo and add it to D^-. Finally, we add to Φ the rule $foo \leftarrow p(\overline{X}), p'(\overline{X})$ for each predicate $p \in$ **S** . Let (I', Δ', Φ', l') be the so constructed instance of **OFIP** (**PFIP**). Evidently, all components of this instance except the update Δ' are positive. It is easy to see that $(I, \Delta, \Phi, l) \in$ **OFIP** (**PFIP**) $\Leftrightarrow$ $(I', \Delta', \Phi', l') \in$ **OFIP** (**PFIP**). □

From this lemma and theorem 5 we get

Corollary 3. *In general case:*
(1) **OFIP** *is Σ_2^p-complete;*
(2) **PFIP** *is Π_2^p-complete.*

4.2   Complexity in Total Interpretations

As it was shown in [13], in the case of ground IC the complexity of **OFIP** and **PFIP** is greater for total interpretations than that in partial ones. In fact, **OFIP** and **PFIP** are "co-problems" in total interpretations in the sense that $(I, \Delta, \Phi, l) \in$ **PFIP** iff $(I, \Delta, \Phi, \neg l) \notin$ **OFIP** . So it is enough to establish complexity bounds for one of the problems, e.g. for **OFIP**, if no constraints are imposed on literal l.

Theorem 6. *[13] In the case, where IC are ground:*
(1) both **OFIP** *and* **PFIP** *belong to P, when IC are definite and updates are positive;*
(2) **OFIP** *is NP-complete, when IC are definite;*
(3) in the general case **OFIP** *is Σ_2^p-complete.*

Corollary 4. *In the case, where IC are ground:*
(1) **PFIP** *is co-NP-complete, when IC are definite;*
(2) **PFIP** *is Π_2^p-complete in the general case.*
(3) **OFIP** *(**PFIP**) is Σ_2^p-complete (Π_2^p-complete) when IC are monadic programs with variables.*

As in the case of partial interpretations, for definite IC and positive updates[1] the problems are equivalent and solvable in polynomial time, when IC are monadic, and are hard otherwise.

Proposition 5. *In the case, where IC are definite:*
(1) **OFIP** *and* **PFIP** *are in P, if IC use only unary predicates, and updates are positive;*

---

[1] in total interpretations this means $\Delta^- = \emptyset$.

(2) **OFIP** *and* **PFIP** *are NP-complete (co-NP-complete), if updates are positive and l is positive (negative);*
(3) **OFIP** *is Σ_2^p-complete in general.*

Corollary 5. **PFIP** *is Π_2^p-complete, when IC are definite.*

In the case of general IC **OFIP** and **PFIP** become complete on the third level of polynomial Σ and Π hierarchies.

Theorem 7.
(1) **OFIP** *(***PFIP***) is Σ_3^p-complete (Π_3^p-complete);*
(2) the lower bounds are valid even for a signature consisting of one binary predicate.

Proof Scheme: *Lower Bound.* Let $\beta = \exists \overline{x} \forall \overline{y} \exists \overline{z} \alpha(\overline{x}, \overline{y}, \overline{z})$, where α is a 3-CNF. We construct $C = C(\alpha, \overline{x} \cup \overline{y} \cup \{a, b\})$, $I = J(\alpha, \emptyset)$, and IC Φ with clauses:
$\neg s(t, c_a) \leftarrow s(t, c_x), s(f, c_x)$, for $x \in \overline{x}$;
$\neg s(t, c_a) \leftarrow \neg s(t, c_x), \neg s(f, c_x)$, for $x \in \overline{x}$;
$s(t, c_b) \leftarrow s(t, c_a), s(t, c_y), s(f, c_y)$, for $y \in \overline{y}$;
$s(t, b) \leftarrow s(t, c_a), \neg s(t, c_y), \neg s(f, c_y)$, for $y \in \overline{y}$;
$s(t, c_y) \leftarrow s(t, c_b)$, and $s(f, c_y) \leftarrow s(t, c_b)$, for $y \in \overline{y}$;
$s(t, c_b) \leftarrow \{s(t, c_a)\} \cup \varphi(\alpha, \overline{x} \cup \overline{y}, \overline{z})$.
We set $\Delta = (\{s(t, c_a)\}, \emptyset)$, and $l = s(t, c_b)$.
Then in every I_1 minimally deviating from $Acc(\Phi, \Delta)$ there is exactly one of the facts $s(t, c_x)$, $s(f, c_x)$ for each $x \in \overline{x}$.

Let β be true. Then there is a substitution σ such that $\forall \overline{y} \exists \overline{z} \alpha(\sigma \overline{x}, \overline{y}, \overline{z})$ is true. Let us include $s(t, c_x)$ in I_1 if $\sigma(x) = 1$ and $s(f, c_x)$ otherwise. Then we also must add at least one of $s(t, c_y)$ and $s(f, c_y)$ for all $y \in \overline{y}$. If for some $y \in \overline{y}$ both $s(t, c_y)$ and $s(f, c_y)$ are present, then $s(t, c_b)$ and all $s(t, c_y)$, $s(f, c_y)$ must be present too. Let us denote this DB state by I_1. In order to obtain some I' which is closer to I than I_1 in our deviation order, we should add to I' exactly one of $s(t, c_y)$, $s(f, c_y)$ for each $y \in \overline{y}$, and we should not add $s(t, c_b)$. This, however, is impossible because $\forall \overline{y} \exists \overline{z} \alpha(\sigma \overline{x}, \overline{y}, \overline{z})$ is true.

Let $l \in I_1$ for some I_1 minimally deviating from $Acc(\Phi, \Delta)$. Then I_1 contains $s(t, c_y)$ and $s(f, c_y)$ for all $y \in \overline{y}$. Hence, it is impossible to select exactly one of $s(t, c_y)$ and $s(f, c_y)$ in order that $\varphi(\alpha, \overline{x} \cup \overline{y}, \overline{z})$ would be false for all substitutions. Therefore, the formula $\forall \overline{y} \exists \overline{z} \alpha(\sigma \overline{x}, \overline{y}, \overline{z})$ is true for the substitution $\sigma(x) = 1$ if $s(t, c_x) \in I_1$, and $\sigma(x) = 0$ otherwise. So formula β is true.$\square$

4.3   The Case of Varying Signature

It is no wonder that without the premise of fixed signature the complexity grows exponentially.

Theorem 8. *When the signature varies, then*
(1) both problems **OFIP** *and* **PFIP** *are* **EXPTIME**-*complete for the class of definite IC in partial and in total interpretations;*

(2) both problems **OFIP** *and* **PFIP** *are* **EXPTIME**-*complete in partial interpretations;*
(3) **OFIP** *is* $\Sigma_2^{EXPTIME}$-*complete and* **PFIP** *is* $\Pi_2^{EXPTIME}$-*complete in total interpretations.*

In fact, the lower bound in (1) follows from the exponential time complexity of Datalog [29, 17] and the lower bound in (3) can be derived from the same order lower bound for Disjunctive Datalog [16]. The point (2) follows from (1) using lemma 3.

We summarize our main results in the following tables.

Complexity of **OFIP** with fixed signature

	Partial		Total	
	ground	Non-ground	ground	Non-ground
Positive case	P	$NP/co\text{-}NP$	P	$NP/co\text{-}NP$
Definite IC	NP	Σ_2^P	NP	Σ_2^P
General case	NP	Σ_2^P	Σ_2^P	Σ_3^P

Complexity of **PFIP** with fixed signature

	Partial		Total	
	ground	Non-ground	ground	Non-ground
Positive case	P	$NP/co\text{-}NP$	P	$NP/co\text{-}NP$
Definite IC	$co\text{-}NP$	Π_2^P	$co\text{-}NP$	Π_2^P
General case	$co\text{-}NP$	Π_2^P	Π_2^P	Π_3^P

5   Conclusion

Our analysis shows that in the worst case the "property" aspects of the EUP are very hard even under the fixed signature premise. Nevertheless, the case of ground IC in partial interpretations presents a rare and surprising exclusion, where the EUP problem itself receives a practical polynomial time solution. As it concerns the EUP-solutions marked by presence or absence of a given fact, in quite a practical situation of definite IC they can be found in polynomial time in the absence of negation/deletions in updates. In the general situation some special means should be used in order to optimize complete choice solutions of the EUP. Some methods of this kind are proposed in [11–14].

Acknowledgements

We are grateful to anonymous referees for their useful comments.

References

1. Abiteboul, S.: Updates a new Frontier. In: *Proc. of the Second International Conference on the Theory of Databases, ICDT'88*. LNCS **326** (1988) 1-18.
2. Abiteboul, S., Vianu, V.: Datalog Extensions for Database Queries and Updates. *JCSS*, **43**, n. 1 (1991) 62–124.
3. Alchourón, C.E., Gärdenfors, P., and Makinson, D.: On the logic of theory change: partial meet contraction and revision functions. *J. Symbolic Logic*. **50** (1985) 510-530.
4. Alferes, J.J.,Pereira, L.M.: Update-Programs Can Update Programs. In J.Dix, L.M. Pereira, T.C. Przymusinski, editors: *Second International Workshop, NMELP'96. Selected Papers*. LNCS **1216** (1997) 110-131.
5. Baral, C., Lobo, J.: Formal Characterization of Active Databases. In Pedreschi, D., Zaniolo, C., editors: *Logic in Databases. Intern. Workshop LID'96. Proceedings*. San Milano, Italy. (1996), 175-195.
6. Baralis E., Ceri S., Paraboschi S.: Improved rule analysis by means of triggering and activation graphs. In T.Sellis, editor: *Rules in Database Systems*, LNCS **985** (1995) 165-181.
7. Chandra A., Merlin P. : Optimal implementation of conjunctive queries in relational databases. In: *Ninth ACM Symp. on Theory of Computing*. (1977) 77-90.
8. Dantsin, E., Eiter, T. Gottlob, G., Voronkov, A. : Complexity and Expressiveness of Logic Programming. In : *Proc. 12th Annual IEEE Conf. On Comput. Compl.* (1997), 82–101.
9. Dayal, U., Hanson,E., and Widom, J.: Active database systems. In: W. Kim, editor, *Modern Database Systems*. Addison Wesley (1995) 436-456
10. Decker H.: An extension of SLD by abduction and integrity maintenance for view updating in deductive databases. In: *Proc. of the 1996 International Conference on Logic Programming*. MIT Press, (1996), 157-169.
11. Dekhtyar, M., Dikovsky, A., Spyratos, N.: On Conservative Enforced Updates. In: Dix, J., Furbach, U., Nerode, A., editors: *Proceedings of 4th International Conference, LPNMR'97*. Dagstuhl Castle, Germany, LNCS **1265** (1997) 244-257.
12. Dekhtyar, M., Dikovsky, A., Spyratos, N.: On Logically Justified Updates. In: J. Jaffar, editor: *Proc. of the 1998 Joint International Conference and Symposium on Logic Programming*. MIT Press, (1998), 250-264.
13. Dekhtyar, M., Dikovsky, A., Dudakov, S., Spyratos, N.: Monotone Expansion of Updates in Logical Databases. In: *Proc. of 5th International Conference LPNMR'99*. LNAI **1730** (1999) 132-147.
14. Dekhtyar, M., Dikovsky, A., Dudakov, S., Spyratos, N.: Maximal Expansions of Database Updates. In *Foundations of Information and Knowledge Systems, FoIKS 2000*. LNCS **1762** (2000) 72-87.
15. Eiter, T., Gottlob, G.: On the complexity of propositional knowledge base revision, updates, and counterfactuals. Artificial Intelligence **57** (1992) 227-270.
16. Eiter, T., Gottlob, G., Mannila, H.: Disjunctive datalog. ACM Transactions on Database Systems **22**(3) 364-418.
17. Immerman, N. : Relational queries computable in polynomial time. Information and Conyrol **68** (1986) 86-104.
18. Gottlob, G., Moerkotte, G., Subrahmanian, V.S.: The PARK semantics for active databases. In: *Proceedings of EDBT'96*. Avignon, France (1996).
19. Guessoum A., Lloyd J.W.: Updating knowledge bases. New Generation Computing, **8** (1990), 71-89.

20. Halfeld Ferrari Alves, M., Laurent, D., Spyratos, N., Stamate, D.: Update rules and revision programs. Rapport de Recherche Université de Paris-Sud, Centre d'Orsay, LRI **1010** (12 / 1995).
21. Kakas A.C., Mancarella P.: Database updates through abduction. IN: *Proc. 16th VLBD Conference.* (1990) 650-661.
22. Katsuno, H., Mendelzon, A. O.: Propositional knowledge base revision and minimal change. Artificial Intelligence **52** (1991) 253-294.
23. Lloyd, J.W., Foundations of Logic Programming. Second, Extended Edition. Springer-Verlag. (1993)
24. Marek, V.W., Truszczyński, M.: Revision programming, database updates and integrity constraints. In: *International Conference on Data Base theory, ICDT.* LNCS **893** (1995) 368-382.
25. Picouet, Ph., Vianu, V.: Expressiveness and Complexity of Active Databases. In: Afrati, F., Kolaitis, Ph., editors, *6th Int. Conf. on Database Theory, ICDT'97.* LNCS **1186** (1997) 155-172.
26. Przymusinski, T.C., Turner, H.: Update by Means of Inference Rules. In: V.W.Marek, A.Nerode, M.Truszczyński, editors, *Logic Programming and Non-monotonic Reasoning.* Proc. of the Third Int. Conf. LPNMR'95, Lexington, KY, USA (1995) 166-174.
27. Raschid, L., Lobo, J.: Semantics for Update Rule Programs and Implementation in a Relational Database Management System. ACM Trans. on Database Systems **21** (December 1996) 526-571
28. Schewe, K.-D., Thalheim, B.: Consistency Enforcement in Active Databases. In: Chakravarty, S., Widom, L., editors: *Research Issues in Data Engineering - Active Databases.* Proceedings. Houston, (1994).
29. Vardi, M. : The complexity of relational query languages. In : *ACM Symposium on Theory of Computing (STOC),* San Francisco, (1982) 137-146.
30. Winslet M.: Reasoning about action using a possible models approach. In:*Proc. AAAI'88, v. 1* (1988) 89-93.
31. Zaniolo, C.: Active database rules with transaction-conscious stable-model semantics. In:*Proceedings of Fourth International Conference, DOOD'95.* LNCS **1013** (1995) 55-72

Computational Complexity of Planning Based on Partial Information about the System's Present and Past States

Chitta Baral[1], Le-Chi Tuan[1], Raúl Trejo[2], and Vladik Kreinovich[2]

[1] Dept. of Computer Science & Engineering
Arizona State University, Tempe, AZ 85287-5406, USA
{chitta,lctuan}@asu.edu
[2] Department of Computer Science, University of Texas at El Paso
El Paso, TX 79968, USA
{rtrejo,vladik}@cs.utep.edu

Abstract. Planning is a very important AI problem, and it is also a very time-consuming AI problem. To get an idea of how complex different planning problems are, it is useful to describe the computational complexity of different general planning problems. This complexity has been described for problems in which planning is based on the (complete or partial) information about the *current* state of the system. In real-life planning problems, we can often complement the incompleteness of our *explicit* knowledge about the current state by using the *implicit* knowledge about this state which is contained in the description of the system's *past behavior*. For example, the information about the system's past failures is very important in planning diagnostic and repair. To describe planning which can use the information about the past, a special language $\mathcal{L}$ was developed in 1997 by C. Baral, M. Gelfond and A. Provetti. In this paper, we expand the known results about computational complexity of planning (including our own previous results) to this more general class of planning problems.

1 Introduction

1.1 Planning Problems: Towards a More Realistic Formulation

Planning Problems: Traditional Approach, with Complete Information about the Initial State. Planning is one of the most important AI problems. Traditional AI formulations of this problem mainly cover situations in which we have a (complete or partial) information about the current state of the system, and we must find an appropriate plan (sequence of actions) which would enable us to achieve a certain goal.

Such situations are described, e.g., by the language $\mathcal{A}$ which was proposed in [8].

In this language, we start with a finite set of properties (fluents) $\mathcal{F} = \{f_1, \ldots, f_n\}$ which describe possible properties of a state.

J. Lloyd et al. (Eds.): CL 2000, LNAI 1861, pp. 882–896, 2000.

A *state* is then defined as a finite set of fluents, e.g., $\{\}$ or $\{f_1, f_3\}$. We are assuming that we have a complete knowledge about the initial state: e.g., $\{f_1, f_3\}$ means that in the initial state, properties f_1 and f_3 are true, while all the other properties $f_2, f_4, \ldots$ are false. The properties of the initial state are described by formulas of the type "initially F," where F is a *fluent literal*, i.e., either a fluent f_i or its negation $\neg f_i$.

There is also a finite set $\mathcal{A}$ of possible *actions*. At each moment of time, an agent can execute an action. The results of different actions $a \in \mathcal{A}$ are described by rules of the type "a causes F if $F_1, \ldots, F_m$", where $F, F_1, \ldots, F_m$ are fluent literals. A reasonably straightforward semantics describes how the state changes after an action:

- If before the action a, the literals $F_1, \ldots, F_m$ were true, and the domain description contains a rule according to which a causes F if $F_1, \ldots, F_m$, then this rule is *activated*, and after the execution of action a, F becomes true. Thus, for some fluents f_i, we will conclude f_i and for some other, that $\neg f_i$ holds in the resulting state.
- If for some fluent f_i, no activated rule enables us to conclude that f_i is true or false, this means that the execution of action a does not change the truth of this fluent. Therefore, f_i is true in the resulting state if and only if it is true in the old state. (This case represents *inertia*.)

Formally, a *domain description D* is a finite set of *value propositions* of the type "initially f" (which describe the initial state), and a finite set of *effect propositions* of the type "a causes f if $f_1, \ldots, f_m$" (which describe results of actions). A *state s* is a finite set of fluents. The *initial state s_0* consists of all the fluents f_i for which the corresponding value proposition "initially f_i" is contained in the domain description. (Here we are assuming that we have complete information about the initial situation.) We say that a fluent f_i *holds* in s if $f_i \in s$; otherwise, we say that $\neg f_i$ holds in s.

The *transition function $res(a, s)$* which describes the effect of an action a on a state s is defined as follows:

- we say that an effect proposition "a causes F if $F_1, \ldots, F_m$" is *activated* in a state s if all m fluent literals $F_1, \ldots, F_n$ hold in s;
- we define $V_D^+(a, s)$ as the set of all fluents f_i for which a rule "a causes f_i if $F_1, \ldots, F_m$" is activated in s;
- similarly, we define $V_D^-(A, S)$ as the set of all fluents f_i for which a rule "a causes $\neg f_i$ if $F_1, \ldots, F_m$" is activated in s;
- if $V_D^+(a, s) \cap V_D^-(a, s) \neq \emptyset$, we say that the result of the action a is *undefined*;
- if the result of the action a is not undefined in a state s (i.e., if $V_D^+(a, s) \cap V_D^-(a, s) = \emptyset$), we define $res(a, s) = (s \cup V_D^+(a, s)) \setminus V_D^-(a, s)$.

A *plan α* is a sequence of of actions $\alpha = [a_1, \ldots, a_n]$; the result $res(a_n, res(a_{n-1}, \ldots, res(a_1, s) \ldots))$ of applying these actions to the state s is denoted by $res(\alpha, s)$.

To complete the description of deterministic planning, we must formulate possible *objectives*. In general, as an objective, we can take a complex combination of elementary properties (fluents) which characterize the final state; for example, a typical objective of an assembling manufacture robot is to reach the state of the world in which all manufactured items are fully assembled. To simplify the description of the problem, we can always add this combination as a new fluent; thus, without losing generality, it is sufficient to consider only objectives of the type $f \in \mathcal{F}$.

In these terms, the *planning* problem can be formulated as follows: given a set of fluents $\mathcal{F}$, a goal $f \in \mathcal{F}$, a set of actions $\mathcal{A}$ and a set of rules D describing how these actions affect the state of the world, to find a sequence of actions $\alpha = [a_1, \ldots, a_k]$ that, when executed from the initial state of the world s_0, makes f true. The problem of *plan checking* is, given $\mathcal{F}$, $\mathcal{A}$, a goal, and a sequence of actions α, to check whether the goal becomes true after execution of α in the initial state.

Next Step: Planning in Case of Incomplete Information about the Initial State. The language $\mathcal{A}$ describes allows planning in the situations with *complete* information, when we know exactly which fluents hold in the initial state and which don't. In real life, we often have only *partial* information about the initial state: about some fluents, we know that they are true in the initial state, about some other fluents, we know that they are false in the initial state; and it is also possible that about some fluents, we do not know whether they are initially true or false.

For example, when we want a mobile robot to reach a certain point, we often do not have a complete information about the state of the world; this is especially true in space applications, when the goal of the robot is to explore new environments whose state is initially unknown. When we plan a diagnostic and repair of a complex object, be it a computer, a car, etc., we do not know which parts are functioning correctly and which parts are not – this is exactly what we are trying to find out. In terms of fluents, this means that we do not know the initial values of the fluents which describe the correct functionality of the system's parts.

Such situations can also be easily described by a simple modification of the above language $\mathcal{A}$. Namely, if for some fluent f, neither the statement "initially f", not the statement "initially $\neg f$" are given, we assume that two different initial situations are possible: when f if initially true, and when $\neg f$ is false in the initial state. As a result, instead of a single initial state s_0, we may have several different initial states which are consistent with our knowledge about the system.

In this case, the notion of a successful plan becomes slightly more complex: namely, we say that a plan is *successful* if for every initial state s which is consistent with our knowledge, after we apply the plan α, the desired fluent g holds in the resulting state $res(\alpha, s)$.

Adding Sensing Actions. In real-life planning problems like the above-mentioned problems of robotic motion or system diagnostic, a reasonable plan involves using *sensors* to find the missing information. Even in simple real-life planning situations, it is often necessary to determine the missing information. For example, if we want the door closed, the required action depends on whether the door was initially open (then we close it), or it was already closed (then we do nothing). Therefore, if we do not know whether the door was initially closed or not, we better somehow find it out, and then, depending on the result of this investigation, perform the corresponding action.

To describe such activities, we must include *sensing actions* – e.g., an action *check*$_i$ which checks whether the fluent f_i holds in a given state – to our list of actions, and allow *conditional* plans, i.e., plans in which the next action depends on the result of the previous sensing action.

To describe such actions, the language $\mathcal{A}$ was enriched by rules of the type "*a* **determines** *f*", meaning that after the action *a* is performed, we know whether *f* is true or not. At any given moment of time, we have the actual state *s* of the system (which may be not completely known to the agent), plus a set Σ of all possible states which are consistent with the agent's knowledge; the pair $\langle s, \Sigma \rangle$ is called a *k-state*. A sensing action does not change the actual state *s*, but it does decrease the set Σ.

Since we will now be dealing with incompleteness of information about the real world, we will need to reason with the agent's knowledge about the world. A *k-state* is defined as pair $\langle s, \Sigma \rangle$, where *s* is the *actual* state, and Σ is the set of all possible states where the agent thinks it may be in. Initially, the set Σ_0 consists of all the states *s* for which:

- a fluent f_i is true ($f_i \in s$) if the domain description D contains the proposition "initially f_i";
- a fluent f_i is false ($f_i \notin s$) if the domain description D contains the proposition "initially $\neg f_i$".

If neither the proposition "initially f_i", nor the proposition "initially $\neg f_i$" are in the domain description, then Σ_0 contains some states with f_i true *and* others with f_i false. The actual initial state s_0 can be any state from the set Σ_0. The transition function due to action execution is defined as follows:

- for proper (*non-sensing*) actions, $\langle s, \Sigma \rangle$ is mapped into $\langle res(a, s), res(a, \Sigma) \rangle$, where:
  - $res(a, s)$ is defined as in the case of complete information, and
  - $res(a, \Sigma) = \{res(a, s') \mid s' \in \Sigma\}$.
- for a *sensing* action *a* which senses fluents $f_1, \ldots, f_k$ – i.e., for which sensing propositions "*a* **determines** f_i" belong to the domain D – the actual state *s* remains unchanged while Σ is down to only those states which have the same values of f_i as *s*: $\langle s, \Sigma \rangle \rightarrow \langle s, \Sigma' \rangle$, where

$$\Sigma' = \{s' \in \Sigma \mid \forall i\, (1 \le i \le k \rightarrow (f_i \in s' \leftrightarrow f_i \in s))\}$$

In the presence of sensing, an action plan may no longer be a pre-determined sequence of actions: if one of these actions is sensing, then the next action may depend on the result of that sensing. In general, the choice of a next action may depend on the results of all previous sensing actions. Such an action plan is called a *conditional plan*.

Possibility of Knowledge about the Past. In the situations when we only have a partial information about the current (present) state, the additional information can be deduced from knowing the *history* of the system's behavior. This additional information about the past is extremely important in diagnostic problems: if we know what types of faulty behavior the system exhibited in the past, it helps in diagnostics (sometimes this information about the past is even sufficient for a successful repair, and no additional sensing is necessary). Similarly, when a medical doctor plans a cure, information about past diseases is as important (and sometimes even more important) than the results of different tests ("sensing actions").

Since this additional information is very important in many practical planning problems, it is desirable to include this information into the corresponding AI formalisms.

To describe the use of knowledge about the past in planning problems, in [1, 2], the language $\mathcal{A}$ was extended to a new language $\mathcal{L}$. In this new language, to describe the history of the system, first of all, the current state s_N is separated from the initial state s_0, so we may have statements about what is true at s_0 ("F at s_0") and statements about what is true at s_N ("F at s_N"). In addition, we may have information about other states in the past; to describe this information, language $\mathcal{L}$ allows to use several constants s_i to describe past moments of time, and allows:

− statements of the type "s_1 precedes s_2" which order past moments of time;
− statements of the type "F at s_i" which describe the properties of the system at the past moments of time, and
− statements which describe past actions:
  • "α between s_1, s_2" means that a sequence of actions α was performed at some point between the moments s_1 and s_2, and
  • "α occurs_at s" means that the sequence of actions α was implemented at s.

The semantics of this history description is as follows:

− a *history* is defined as a triple consisting of an initial state s_0, a sequence of actions $\alpha = [a_1, \ldots, a_m]$, and a mapping t which maps each constant s_i from the history description into an integer $t(s_i) \leq m$ (meaning the moment of time when this constant actually happened, so $t(s_0) = 0$ and $t(s_N) = m$); for this history, we have, at moments of time $0, 1, \ldots, m$, states $s(0) = s_0$, $s(1) = res(a_1, s(0))$, $s(2) = res(a_2, s(1))$, etc., and s_i is identified with $s(t(s_i))$;
− we say that the history is *consistent* with the given knowledge if all the statements from this knowledge become true under this interpretation;
− we say that the history is *possible* if it is consistent and *minimal* in the sense that no history with a proper subsequence of α is consistent.

In this more realistic situation, we can also ask about the existence of a plan, i.e., a sequence (or tree) of actions with a feasible execution time which guarantees that for all possible current states, after this plan, the objective $g \in \mathcal{F}$ will be satisfied.

Let us give an example of such a situation. If a lamp is not broken, then, when we switch it on, the light bulb should be switched on. If in the past, we applied the action *turn_on* but the lamp did not go on, this means that the lamp was broken at that time, and, if we know of no repair actions performed in the past, we can therefore conclude that the lamp is still broken. This narrative can be described by the following rules: "*switch_on* causes *lamp_on* if ¬*broken*", "*switch_on* occurs_at s_1", "s_1 precedes s_2", "¬*lamp_on* at s_2". From these rules, we can conclude that the lamp is currently *broken*.

1.2   Computational Complexity of Planning problem: Why It Is Important, What Is Known, and What We Are Planning to Do

It Is Important to Analyze Computational Complexity of Planning Problems. Planning is one of the most important AI problems, but it is also known to be one of the most difficult ones. While often in practical applications, we need the planning problems to be solved within a reasonable time, the actual application of planning algorithms may take an extremely long time. It is therefore desirable to estimate the potential computation time which is necessary to solve different planning problems, i.e., to estimate the *computational complexity* of different classes of planning problems. Even "negative" results, which show that the problem belongs to one of the high-level complexity classes (e.g., that it is **PSPACE**-hard) are potentially useful: first, they prevent researchers from wasting their time on trying to design a general efficient algorithm; second, they enable the researchers to concentrate on either finding a feasible sub-class of the original class of planning problems, or on finding (and/or justifying) an approximate planning algorithm.

Known Computational Complexity Results: In Brief. There have been several results on computational complexity of planning problems. These results mainly cover the situations in which we have a (complete or partial) information about the current state of the system, and we must find an appropriate plan (sequence of actions) which would enable us to achieve a certain goal. As we have mentioned earlier, such situations are described, e.g., by the language $\mathcal{A}$ which was proposed in [8]. The complexity of planning in $\mathcal{A}$ was analyzed in our earlier paper [3].

Ideally, we want to find cases in which the planning problem can be solved by a *feasible* algorithm, i.e., by an algorithm $\mathcal{U}$ whose computational time $t_\mathcal{U}(w)$ on each input w is bounded by a polynomial $p(|w|)$ of the length $|w|$ of the input w: $t_\mathcal{U}(x) \leq p(|w|)$ (this length can be measured bit-wise or symbol-wise). Since, in practice, we are operating in a time-bounded environment, we should worry not only about the time for *computing* the plan, but we should also worry about the time that it takes to actually *implement* the plan. If an action plan consists of a sequence of 2^{2^n} actions, then this plan is not feasible. It is therefore reasonable to restrict ourselves to *feasible* plans, i.e., by plans u whose length m (= number of actions in it) is bounded by a given polynomial $p(|w|)$ of the length $|w|$ of the input w. For each such polynomial p, we can formulate the following *planning problem*: given a domain description D (i.e., the description of the initial state and of possible consequences of different actions) and a goal g (i.e., a fluent which we want to be true), determine whether it is possible to feasibly achieve this goal, i.e., whether there exists a feasible plan α (with $m \leq p(|D|)$) which achieves this goal.

By solving this problem, we do not yet get the desired plan, we only check whether a plan exists. However, intuitively, the complexity of this problem also represents the complexity of actually finding a plan, in the following sense: if we have an algorithm which solves the above planning problem in reasonable time, then we can also find this plan. Indeed, suppose that we are looking for a plan of length $m \leq P_0$, and an algorithm has told us that such a plan exists. Then, to find the first action of the desired plan, we check (by applying the same algorithm), for each action $a \in \mathcal{A}$, whether from the corresponding state $res(a, s)$ the desired goal g can be achieved in $\leq P_0 - 1$ steps. Since a plan of length $\leq P_0$ does exist, there is such an action, and we can take this action as a_1. After this, we repeat the same procedure to find a_2, etc. As a result, we will be able to find a plan of length $\leq P_0$ by applying the algorithm which checks the existence of the plan $\leq P_0 = p(|D|)$ times; so, if the existence-checking algorithm is feasible, the resulting plan-construction algorithm is feasible as well.

General results on computational complexity of planning are given, e.g., in [5, 7, 11]. For the language $\mathcal{A}$, computational complexity of planning was first studied in [10]; the results about the computational complexity of different planning problems in $\mathcal{A}$ are overviewed in [3, 15].

When sensing is allowed, a plan is not a sequence, but rather a *tree*: every sensing action means that we branch into two possible branches (depending on whether the sensed fluent is true or false), and we execute different actions on different branches. Similarly to the case of the linear plan, we are only interested in plans whose execution time is (guaranteed to be) bounded by a given polynomial $p(|D|)$ of the length of the input. (In other words, we require that for every possible branch, the total number of actions on this branch is bounded by $p(|D|)$.)

For such planning situations, the computational complexity was also surveyed in [3].

What We Are Planning to Do. We have mentioned that a more realistic description of a planning problem involves the use of history (information about the past) in planning. In this paper, we answer the following natural question: *How does the addition of history change the computational complexity of different planning problems?*

Comment. In addition to the possibility of describing history, the language $\mathcal{A}$ can also be extended by adding *static causal laws*, which can make the results of an action non-deterministic. This non-determinism may further increase the complexity of the corresponding planning problem; we are planning to analyze this increase in our future work.

Useful Complexity Notions. Most papers on computational complexity of planning problems classify these problems to different levels of the polynomial hierarchy. For precise definitions of the polynomial hierarchy, see, e.g., [12]. Crudely speaking, a decision problem is a problem of deciding whether a given input w satisfies a certain property P (i.e., in set-theoretic terms, whether it belongs to the corresponding set $S = \{w \mid P(w)\}$).

A decision problem belongs to the class **P** if there is a feasible (polynomial-time) algorithm for solving this problem.

A problem belongs to the class **NP** if the checked formula $w \in S$ (equivalently, $P(w)$) can be represented as $\exists u P(u, w)$, where $P(u, w)$ is a feasible property, and the quantifier runs over words of feasible length (i.e., of length limited by some given polynomial of the length of the input). The class **NP** is also denoted by $\Sigma_1 \mathbf{P}$ to indicate that formulas from this class can be defined by adding 1 existential quantifier (hence Σ and 1) to a polynomial predicate (**P**).

A problem belongs to the class **coNP** if the checked formula $w \in S$ (equivalently, $P(w)$) can be represented as $\forall u P(u, w)$, where $P(u, w)$ is a feasible property, and the quantifier runs over words of feasible length (i.e., of length limited by some given polynomial of the length of the input). The class **coNP** is also denoted by $\Pi_1 \mathbf{P}$ to indicate that formulas from this class can be defined by adding 1 universal quantifier (hence Π and 1) to a polynomial predicate (hence **P**).

For every positive integer k, a problem belongs to the class $\Sigma_k \mathbf{P}$ if the checked formula $w \in S$ (equivalently, $P(w)$) can be represented as $\exists u_1 \forall u_2 \ldots P(u_1, u_2, \ldots, u_k, w)$, where $P(u_1, \ldots, u_k, w)$ is a feasible property, and all k quantifiers run over words of feasible length (i.e., of length limited by some given polynomial of the length of the input).

Similarly, for every positive integer k, a problem belongs to the class $\Pi_k \mathbf{P}$ if the checked formula $w \in S$ (equivalently, $P(w)$) can be represented as $\forall u_1 \exists u_2 \ldots P(u_1, u_2, \ldots, u_k, w)$, where $P(u_1, \ldots, u_k, w)$ is a feasible property, and all k quantifiers run over words of feasible length (i.e., of length limited by some given polynomial of the length of the input).

All these classes $\Sigma_k \mathbf{P}$ and $\Pi_k \mathbf{P}$ are subclasses of a larger class **PSPACE** formed by problems which can be solved by a polynomial-*space* algorithm. It is known (see, e.g., [12]) that this class can be equivalently reformulated as a class of problems for which the checked formula $w \in S$ (equivalently, $P(w)$) can be represented as $\forall u_1 \exists u_2 \ldots P(u_1, u_2, \ldots, u_k, w)$, where the number of quantifiers k is bounded by a polynomial of the length of the input, $P(u_1, \ldots, u_k, w)$ is a feasible property, and all k quantifiers run over words of feasible length (i.e., of length limited by some given polynomial of the length of the input).

A problem is called *complete* in a certain class if, crudely speaking, this is the toughest problem in this class (so that any other general problem from this class can be reduced to it by a feasible-time reduction).

It is still not known (2000) whether we can solve any problem from the class **NP** in polynomial time (i.e., in precise terms, whether **NP=P**). However, it is widely believed that we cannot, i.e., that $\mathbf{NP} \neq \mathbf{P}$. It is also believed that to solve a $\mathbf{NP}$-complete or a $\mathbf{coNP}$-complete problem, we need exponential time $\approx 2^n$, and that solving a complete problem from one of the second-level classes $\Sigma_2 \mathbf{P}$ or $\Pi_2 \mathbf{P}$ requires more computation time than solving $\mathbf{NP}$-complete problems (and solving complete problems from the class $\mathbf{PSPACE}$ takes even longer).

2   Results

In accordance with the above text and with [3], we will consider the following four main groups of planning situations:

- complete information about the initial state, no sensing actions allowed;
- possibly incomplete information about the initial state, no sensing actions allowed;
- possibly incomplete information about the initial state, sensing actions allowed;
- possibly incomplete information about the initial state, full sensing (i.e., every fluent can be sensed).

For comparison, we will also mention the results corresponding to the language $\mathcal{A}$, when neither history nor static causal laws are allowed.

2.1   Complexity of Plan Checking

Before we describe the computational complexity of checking the existence of a plan, let us consider a simpler problem: if, through some heuristic method, we have a plan, how can we check that this plan works?

This plan checking problem makes perfect sense only for the case of no sensing: indeed, if sensing actions are possible, then we can have a branching at every step; as a result, the size of the tree can grow exponentially with the plan's execution time, and even if we can check this tree plan in time polynomial in its size, it will still take un-realistically long.

For the language $\mathcal{A}$, the complexity of this problem depends on whether we have complete information of the initial state or not:

Theorem 1. (Language $\mathcal{A}$, No Sensing)

- *For situations with complete information, the plan checking problem is feasible.*
- *For situations with incomplete information, the plan checking problem is coNP-complete.*

Comment. For readers' convenience, all the proofs are placed in the special (last) section.

Theorem 2. (Language $\mathcal{L}$, No Sensing)

- *For situations with complete information about the initial state, the plan checking problem is $\Pi_2\mathbf{P}$-complete.*
- *For situations with incomplete information about the initial state, the plan checking problem is $\Pi_2\mathbf{P}$-complete.*

Comment. The problem remains $\Pi_2\mathbf{P}$-complete even if we only consider situations with two possible actions. If we only have one action, then for complete information, plan checking is feasible; for incomplete information, it is **coNP**-hard.

2.2   Complexity of Planning

Now, we are ready to describe complexity of planning. In the framework of the language $\mathcal{A}$ (i.e., without history), most planning problems turn out to be complete in one of the classes of the polynomial hierarchy; see, e.g., [3]. However, it turns out that when we allow history, i.e., when we move from language $\mathcal{A}$ to the language $\mathcal{L}$, we get a planning problem that does not seem to be complete within any of the classes from the polynomial hierarchy. To describe the complexity of this program, we therefore had to search for appropriate intermediate classes.

In this search, we were guided by the example of intermediate classes which have been already analyzed in complexity theory: namely, the classes belonging to the so-called *Boolean hierarchy* (see, e.g., [6, 12]). This hierarchy started with the discovery of the first such class – the class **DP** [13, 14]. The original description of these classes uses a language which is slightly different from the language that we used to describe the polynomial hierarchy: namely, we described these classes in terms of the corresponding logical formulas, while the standard description of Boolean hierarchy uses oracles or sets. Therefore, before we explain the new intermediate complexity class which turned out just right for planning, let us first reformulate the notion of the Boolean hierarchy in terms of the corresponding logical formulas.

After $\mathbf{NP} = \Sigma_1\mathbf{P}$ and $\mathbf{coNP} = \Pi_1\mathbf{P}$, the next classes in the polynomial hierarchy are $\Sigma_2\mathbf{P}$ and $\Pi_2\mathbf{P}$. In particular, $\Sigma_2\mathbf{P}$ is a class of problems for which the checked formula $P(w)$ can be represented as $\exists u_1 \forall u_2 P(u_1, u_2, w)$ for some feasible property $P(u_1, u_2, w)$. For each given w, to check whether w satisfies the desired property, we must therefore check whether the following formula holds: $\exists u_1 \forall u_2 Q(u_1, u_2)$, where by $Q(u_1, u_2)$, we denoted $P(u_1, u_2, w)$. In the general definition of this class, for each w, $Q(u_1, u_2)$ can be an arbitrary (feasible) binary predicate. Therefore, in order to find a subclass of this general class $\Sigma_2\mathbf{P}$ for which decision problem is easier than in the general case, we must look for predicates which are simpler than the general binary predicates.

Which predicates are simpler than binary? A natural answer is: unary predicates. It is therefore natural to consider the formulas in which $Q(u_1, u_2)$ is actually a unary predicate, i.e., formulas in which $Q(u_1, u_2)$ depends only on one of its variables. In other words, we have either $Q(u_1, u_2) \equiv Q_2(u_1)$ (here, the subscript 2 in Q_2 means that the predicate does not depend on u_2), or $Q(u_1, u_2) \equiv Q_1(u_2)$. Both these classes of "simpler" binary predicates do lead to simpler complexity classes, but these classes are still within the polynomial hierarchy. Indeed:

- the formula $\exists u_1 \forall u_2 Q_2(u_1)$ is equivalent to $\exists u_1 Q_2(u_1)$ and therefore, the corresponding complexity class is exactly $\Sigma_1 \mathbf{P} \ (= \mathbf{NP})$;
- the formula $\exists u_1 \forall u_2 Q_1(u_2)$ is equivalent to $\forall u_2 Q_1(u_2)$ and therefore, the corresponding complexity class is exactly $\Pi_1 \mathbf{P} \ (= \mathbf{coNP})$.

We get non-trivial intermediate classes if we slightly modify the above idea: namely, if instead of restricting ourselves to binary predicates $Q(u_1, u_2)$ which are actually unary, we consider binary predicates which are Boolean combinations of unary predicates.

For example, we can consider the case when $Q(u_1, u_2)$ is a conjunction of two unary predicates, i.e., when $Q(u_1, u_2)$ is equivalent to $Q_1(u_2)\&Q_2(u_1)$. In this case, the formula $\exists u_1 \forall u_2 (Q_1(u_2)\&Q_2(u_1))$ is equivalent to $\exists u_1 Q_2(u_1)\&\forall u_2 Q_1(u_2)$. If we explicitly mention the variable w, we conclude that $w \in S$ is equivalent to $\exists u_1 P_2(u_1, w)\&\forall u_2 P_1(u_2, w)$, i.e., that the set S is equal to the intersection of a set $S_1 = \{w \mid \exists u_1 P_2(u_1, w)\}$ from the class $\mathbf{NP}$ and a set $S_2 = \{w \mid \forall u_2 P_1(u_2, w)\}$ from the class $\mathbf{coNP}$, i.e., equivalently, to the difference $S_1 - (-S_2)$ between two sets S_1 and $-S_2$ (a complement to S_2) from the class $\mathbf{NP}$. Such sets represent the difference class $\mathbf{DP}$, the first complexity class from the Boolean hierarchy. If we allow more complex Boolean combinations of unary predicates, we get other complexity classes from this hierarchy.

For planning, we need a simpler subclass within the class $\Sigma_3 \mathbf{P}$ of all formulas $P(w)$ of the type $\exists u_1 \forall u_2 \exists u_3 P(u_1, u_2, u_3, w)$. Similarly to the above description of the Boolean hierarchy, it is natural to consider the cases when, for every w, the corresponding ternary predicate $P(u_1, u_2, u_3, w)$ (for fixed w) can be represented as a Boolean combination of binary predicates $P_1(u_2, u_3, w)$, $P_2(u_1, u_3, w)$, and $P_3(u_1, u_2, w)$. Let us give a formal definition of such classes.

Definition. *Let $k \geq 1$ be an integer. By a k-marked propositional variable, we mean an expression of the type v^j, where v is a variable and j is an integer from 1 to k. By a k-Boolean expression B, we mean a propositional formula $B(v_1^{j_1}, \ldots, v_m^{j_m})$ in which all variables are k-marked.*

- *For every k-Boolean expression B, by a class $\Sigma_k(B)\mathbf{P}$, we mean the class of all problems for which the checked formula $P(w)$ can be represented as $\exists u_1 \forall u_2 \ldots P(u_1, u_2, \ldots, u_k, w)$, where $P(u_1, \ldots, u_k, w)$ is equal to the result $B(P_1, \ldots, P_m)$ of substituting, into the Boolean expression $B(v_1^{j_1}, \ldots, v_m^{j_m})$, instead of each variable $v_i^{j_i}$, a feasible predicate P_i which does not depend on the variable u_{j_i}.*
- *For every k-Boolean expression B, by a class $\Pi_k(B)\mathbf{P}$, we mean the class of all problems for which the checked formula $P(w)$ can be represented as $\forall u_1 \exists u_2 \ldots P(u_1, u_2, \ldots, u_k, w)$, where $P(u_1, \ldots, u_k, w) = B(P_1, \ldots, P_m)$ and for each i, the corresponding predicate P_i is feasible and does not depend on the variable u_{j_i}.*

For example, the above class **DP** can be represented as $\Sigma_2(v^1 \& v^2)\mathbf{P}$.

Theorem 3. (Language $\mathcal{L}$, No Sensing) *For situations with complete information about the initial state and with no sensing, the computational complexity of planning is* $\Sigma_3(v^1 \vee v^3)\mathbf{P}$*-complete.*

Comments.

- In other words, the corresponding planning problem is complete for the class of all problems in which $P(w)$ is equivalent to $\exists u_1 \forall u_2 \exists u_3 (P_1(u_2, u_3) \vee P_3(u_1, u_2))$.
- The fact that the planning problem is complete for an intermediate complexity class is not surprising: e.g., in [9], it is shown that several planning problems are indeed complete in some classes intermediate between standard classes of polynomial hierarchy.
- The problem remains $\Sigma_3(v^1 \vee v^3)\mathbf{P}$-complete even if we only consider situations with two possible actions. If we only have one action, then for complete information, planning is feasible; for incomplete information, it is **coNP**-hard.
- For $\mathcal{A}$, the corresponding planning problem is **NP**-complete.

Theorem 4. (Language $\mathcal{L}$, No sensing) *For situations with incomplete information about the initial state and with no sensing, the computational complexity of planning is* $\Sigma_3(v^1 \vee v^3)\mathbf{P}$*-complete.*

For $\mathcal{A}$, this problem is $\Sigma_2\mathbf{P}$-complete.

Theorem 5. (Language $\mathcal{L}$, With Sensing) *For situations with incomplete information about the initial state and with sensing, the computational complexity of planning is* **PSPACE***-complete.*

For $\mathcal{A}$, this problem is also **PSPACE**-complete.

Theorem 6. (Language $\mathcal{L}$, Full Sensing) *For situations with incomplete information about the initial state and with full sensing, the computational complexity of planning is* $\Pi_2\mathbf{P}$*-complete.*

For $\mathcal{A}$, this problem is also $\Pi_2\mathbf{P}$-complete.

What do these complexity results mean in practical terms? At first glance, they may sound gloomy: even **NP**-complete problems are extremely difficult to solve, and the most realistic formulations of the planning problem (with sensing) lead to **PSPACE**-complete problems, i.e., problems at the high end of the polynomial hierarchy. However, they do not sound so gloomy if we take into consideration that these results are about the *worst-case* complexity, and the high worst-case complexity of the problem does not mean that we cannot have good algorithm for many (or even for most) practical instances of this problem.

In plain words, no matter how good a feasible planning algorithm may be, there will always be cases when this algorithm will fail. Our goal is therefore, to design feasible algorithms which will succeed on as many practical planning problems as possible.

Even the traditional planning problem, with no sensing and complete information about the initial state, is known to be **NP**-hard; this complexity result does not prevent us from having successful planners which help in solving many practical planning problems. For situations with incomplete information about the initial state, several ideas of approximate planning were proposed in [4]; the corresponding simplified algorithms are much faster than the algorithms for solving the original planning problem (and the complexity of the corresponding approximate planning problem is indeed smaller; see, e.g., [3]) – the downside being, of course, that sometimes, these approximate algorithms fail to find a plan.

It is desirable to extend these (and other) heuristic planning algorithms to situations when some information about the current state comes in the form of the knowledge about the system's past behavior.

3   Proofs

Proof of Theorem 1. Theorem 1 is, in effect, proven in [3].

Proof of Theorem 2: Main Idea. Let us first show that the plan checking problem belongs to the class $\Pi_2\mathbf{P}$. Indeed, a given plan w is successful if it succeeds for every possible history u_1. For every given history u_1, checking whether a given plan w succeeds is feasible; we will denote the corresponding predicate by $S(u_1, w)$. The condition that the history u_1 is possible means that it is consistent and that none of its sub-histories u_2 is consistent. Checking consistency is feasible (we will denote the corresponding predicate by $C(u)$), and checking whether u_2 is a consistent sub-history of the history u_1 is also feasible; we will denote this other predicate by $H(u_1, u_2)$. So, the possibility of a history u_1 can be expressed as $C(u_1)\&\neg\exists u_2 H(u_1, u_2)$, which is equivalent to $\forall u_2(C(u_1)\&\neg H(u_1, u_2))$. Hence, the success of the plan w can be expressed as $\forall u_1(\forall u_2(C(u_1)\&\neg H(u_1, u_2)) \to S(u_1, w))$, i.e., as a formula $\forall u_1 \exists u_2(\neg C(u_1) \vee H(u_1, u_2) \vee S(u_1, w))$ from the class $\Pi_2\mathbf{P}$. So, the plan checking problem indeed belongs to the class $\Pi_2\mathbf{P}$.

To complete the proof, we must prove that the plan checking problem is $\Pi_2\mathbf{P}$-complete. To show it, we prove that the known $\Pi_2\mathbf{P}$-complete problem – namely, the problem of checking, for a given propositional formula F, whether a formula $\forall x_1 \ldots \forall x_m \exists x_{m+1} \ldots \exists x_n \, F(x_1, \ldots, x_n)$ is true – can be reduced to plan checking. It is sufficient to do this reduction for the case when we have a complete information about the initial state; then, it will automatically follow that a more general problem – corresponding to a case when we may only have partial information about the initial state – is also $\Pi_2\mathbf{P}$-complete. This reduction is done similarly to the proofs from [3] (a detailed proof is posted at http://www.cs.utep.edu/vladik/2000/tr00-13.ps.gz).

Proof of Theorems 3 and 4. Let us first show that the corresponding planning problem indeed belongs to the desired class. The existence of a plan means that there exists a plan u_1 such that for every possible history u_2, *either* the history u_2 is consistent with our knowledge and the plan u_1 succeeds on the current state corresponding to u_2 (we will denote this by $S(u_1, u_2)$); *or* the history u_2 is not minimal, i.e., there exists a different history u_3 for which the sequence of actions is a subsequence of the sequence of actions corresponding to u_2, and u_3 is also consistent with our knowledge (we will denote this property by $M(u_2, u_3)$).

Both binary predicates $S(u_1, u_2)$ and $M(u_2, u_3)$ are feasible to check. Therefore, the existence of a plan is equivalent to a formula $\exists u_1 \forall u_2 (S(u_1, u_3) \vee \exists u_3 M(u_2, u_3))$ with feasible predicates S and M, i.e., to the formula $\exists u_1 \forall u_2 \exists u_3 (S(u_1, u_3) \vee M(u_2, u_3))$ of the desired type.

The fact that the planning problem is complete in this class can be shown by a reduction to a propositional formula, a reduction which is similar to the one from the proofs from [3] and the proof of Theorem 2; the only difference is that in addition to the above reduction – which, crudely speaking, simulates, during the period between the initial and the current state, the computation of the propositional expression corresponding to $M(u_2, u_3)$ – we must also, after the current state, simulate the computation of the expression corresponding to the formula $S(u_1, u_3)$.

Proof of Theorem 5. Let us first show that the corresponding planning problem belongs to the class **PSPACE**. Indeed, the existence of a plan means that there exists an action u_1 such that for every possible sensing result (if any) u_2 of this action, there exists a second action u_2, etc., such that for every history h_1 which is consistent with our initial knowledge and with the follow-up measurements, either we get success, or there exists a "sub"-history h_2. Both success and "sub-history"-ness are feasible to check; thus, the existence of a plan is equivalent to a formula of the type $\exists u_1 \forall u_2 \ldots$, i.e., to a formula from the class **PSPACE**.

As we have shown in [3], this problem is **PSPACE**-complete even for $\mathcal{A}$, i.e., when no history is allowed. Thus, a more general problem from this class **PSPACE** should also be **PSPACE**-hard.

Proof of Theorem 6. Let us first show that the corresponding planning problem belongs to the class $\Pi_2\mathbf{P}$. Since we have unlimited sensing abilities, we do not change our planning abilities if, before we start any planning actions, we first sense the values of all the fluents. We may waste some time on unnecessary sensing, but the total execution time of a plan remains feasible if it was originally feasible; therefore, the existence of a feasible plan is equivalent to the existence of a feasible plan which starts with full sensing. The existence of such a plan means that for every consistent history u_1, either there is a plan u_2 which succeeds for the current state corresponding to u_1, or there exists a sub-history u_3 which is also consistent (which makes u_1 impossible). Checking whether a given plan succeeds for a given history is feasible, and checking whether u_3 is a consistent sub-history is also feasible, so the existence of a plan is equivalent to the formula $\forall u_1 (\exists u_2 P_1(u_1, u_2) \vee \exists u_3 P_2(u_1, u_3))$ for some feasible predicates P_1 and P_2. This formula can be reformulated as $\forall u_1 \exists u_2 P(u_1, u_2)$ with $P(u_1, u_2)$ denoting $P_1(u_1, u_2) \vee P_2(u_1, u_2)$. Therefore, the problem belongs to the class $\Pi_2\mathbf{P}$.

As we have shown in [3], this problem is $\Pi_2\mathbf{P}$-complete even for $\mathcal{A}$, i.e., when no history is allowed. Thus, a more general problem from this class $\Pi_2\mathbf{P}$ should also be $\Pi_2\mathbf{P}$-hard.

Acknowledgments

This work was supported in part by NASA under cooperative agreement NCC5-209, by NSF grants No. DUE-9750858 and CDA-9522207, by United Space Alliance, grant No. NAS 9-20000 (PWO C0C67713A6), by the Future Aerospace Science and Technology Program (FAST) Center for Structural Integrity of Aerospace Systems, effort sponsored by the Air Force Office of Scientific Research, Air Force Materiel Command, USAF, under grant number F49620-95-1-0518, and by the National Security Agency under Grant No. MDA904-98-1-0561.

We are thankful to Luc Longpré, to Tran Cao Son, and to the anonymous referees for valuable discussions.

References

1. Baral, C., Gabaldon, A., Provetti, A.: Formalizing Narratives Using Nested Circumscription, AI Journal **104** (1998) 107–164.
2. Baral, C., Gelfond, M., Provetti, A.: Representing Actions: Laws, Observations and Hypotheses, J. of Logic Programming **31** (1997) 201–243.
3. Baral, C., Kreinovich, V., Trejo, R.: Computational Complexity of Planning and Approximate Planning in Presence of Incompleteness, Proc. IJCAI'99 **2** 948–953 (full paper to appear in AI Journal).
4. Baral, C., Son, T.: Approximate reasoning about actions in presence of sensing and incomplete information, Proc. ILPS'97 387–401.
5. Bylander, T.: The Computational Complexity of Propositional STRIPS Planning, AI Journal **69** (1994) 161–204.
6. Cai, J.-Y. et al.: The Boolean Hierarchy I: Structural Properties, SIAM J. on Computing **17** (1988) 1232–1252; Part II: Applications, in **18** (1989) 95–111.
7. Erol, K., Nau, D., Subrahmanian, V. S.: Complexity, Decidability and Undecidability Results for Domain-Independent Planning, AI Journal **76** (1995) 75–88.
8. Gelfond, M., Lifschitz, V.: Representing Actions and Change by Logic Programs, J. of Logic Programming **17** (1993) 301–323.
9. Gottlob, G., Scarcello, F., Sideri, M.: Fixed-Parameter Complexity in AI and Nonmonotonic Reasoning, Proc. LPNMR'99, Springer-Verlag LNAI **1730** (1999) 1–18.
10. Liberatore, P.: The Complexity of the Language $\mathcal{A}$, Electronic Transactions on Artificial Intelligence **1** (1997) 13–28.
11. Littman, M.: Probabilistic Propositional Planning: Representations and Complexity, Proc. AAAI'97 (1997) 748–754.
12. Papadimitriou, C.: Computational Complexity, Addison-Wesley, Reading, MA, 1994.
13. Papadimitriou, C., Wolfe, D.: The complexity of facets resolved, Proc. FOCS'85 (1985) 74–78; also, J. Computer and Systems Sciences **37** (1987) 2–13.
14. Papadimitriou, C., Yannakakis, M.: The complexity of facets (and some facets of complexity), Proc. STOC'82 (1982) 229–234; also, J. Computer and Systems Sciences **34** (1984) 244–259.
15. Rintanen, J.: Constructing Conditional Plans by a Theorem Prover, Journal of AI Research **10** (1999) 323–352.

Smallest Equivalent Sets for Finite Propositional Formula Circumscription

Yves Moinard[1] and Raymond Rolland[2]

[1] IRISA, Campus de Beaulieu, 35042 Rennes-Cedex, France
Tel.: (33) 2 99 84 73 13, moinard@irisa.fr
[2] IRMAR, Campus de Beaulieu, 35042 Rennes-Cedex, France
Tel.: (33) 2 99 28 60 19, Raymond.Rolland@univ-rennes1.fr

Abstract Circumscription uses classical logic in order to modelize rules with exceptions and implicit knowledge. Formula circumscription is known to be easier to use in order to modelize a situation. We describe when two sets of formulas give the same result, when circumscribed. Two kinds of such equivalence are interesting: the ordinary one (two sets give the same circumscription) and the strong one (when completed by any arbitrary set, the two sets give the same circumscription) which corresponds to having the same closure for logical "and" and "or". In this paper, we consider only the finite case, focusing on looking for the smallest possible sets equivalent to a given set, for the two kinds of equivalence. We need to revisit a characterization result of formula circumscription. Then, we are able to describe a way to get all the sets equivalent to a given set, and also a way to get the smallest such sets. These results should help the automatic computation, and also the translation in terms of circumscription of complex situations.

1 Introduction

Circumscription uses classical logic for representing rules with exceptions. It is often better to use the formula version. An important aspect of formula circumscription has almost not been studied: what are exactly the sets of formulas which give rise to the same circumscription. Answering this question should have important consequences on the automatization of circumscription, and on the knowledge representation side. A possible explanation for the lack of studies on the subject is the complexity of the predicate versions of circumscriptions. We answer this problem in the finite propositional case, providing a way to obtain all the sets which give the same circumscription as a given set. We describe also a way to get the smallest sets, in terms of cardinality. The method given is only semi-constructive but, to our knowledge, no previous study exist.

Section 2 introduces ordinary and formula propositional circumscriptions. Section 3 gives two kinds of equivalence between sets of formulas, the strongest of these equivalences corresponds simply to have the same closure for logical "and" and "or". Section 4 gives a few preliminary technical results, including a new study about a known characterization of formula circumscription. Section 5 gives useful indications in order to find the sets of formulas with as few elements as possible, which are "strongly equivalent", as defined in Section 3, to a given set of formulas Φ. Section 6 uses the results of Sections 4 and 5 in order to get the sets of formulas with as few elements as possible which

J. Lloyd et al. (Eds.): CL 2000, LNAI 1861, pp. 897–911, 2000.

are simply "equivalent" to a given set Φ, meaning which give the same circumscription as Φ. Section 7 provides a few examples. In particular the case where we start from an ordinary circumscription f and where we look for the smallest sets of formulas giving a formula circumscription equal to f, is considered there.

2   Propositional Circumscription

L being a propositional logic, $V(\mathbf{L})$ is the set of its propositional symbols. We suppose $V(\mathbf{L})$ finite in this text. As usual, **L** denotes also the set of all the formulas. We allow empty sets in **partitions** of $V(\mathbf{L})$. $Th(\mathcal{T}) = \{\varphi / \mathcal{T} \models \varphi\}$, the set of **theories** is $\mathbf{T} = \{Th(\mathcal{T}) / \mathcal{T} \subseteq \mathbf{L}\}$. Letters φ, ψ denote formulas in **L**. Letters $\mathcal{T}$, and also Φ, Ψ, or X, Y denote subsets of **L**. $\neg\Phi = \{\neg\varphi \ / \ \varphi \in \Phi\}$. Letters μ and ν denote interpretations for **L**. We denote the interpretations by the subset of $V(\mathbf{L})$ that they satisfy: if $V(\mathbf{L}) = \{P, Q, Z\}$ and $\mu = \{P, Z\}$, then $Th(\mu) = Th(P \wedge \neg Q \wedge Z)$. $\mathbf{M} = \mathcal{P}(V(\mathbf{L}))$ denotes the set of all the interpretations for **L**. For any subset $\mathbf{M}'$ of **M**, we note $Th(\mathbf{M}')$ for the set $\{\varphi \in \mathbf{L} / \mu \models \varphi$ for any $\mu \in \mathbf{M}'\}$. This ambiguous meaning of $\models$ and Th is usual in logic. $\mathbf{M}(\mathcal{T})$ denotes the set of the models of $\mathcal{T}$. The term **formula** will also be used for the quotient of this notion by logical equivalence: $\varphi = \psi$ iff $\mathbf{M}(\varphi) = \mathbf{M}(\psi)$.

Definition 2.1. [15] *A* **preference relation** *in* **L** *is a binary relation* $\prec$ *over* **M**. $\mathbf{M}_\prec(\mathcal{T})$ *is the set of the elements* μ *of* $\mathbf{M}(\mathcal{T})$ **minimal** *for* $\prec$: $\mu \in \mathbf{M}(\mathcal{T})$ *and no* $\nu \in \mathbf{M}(\mathcal{T})$ *is such that* $\nu \prec \mu$. *The* **preferential entailment** $f = f_\prec$ *is defined by*
$f_\prec(\mathcal{T}) = Th(\mathbf{M}_\prec(\mathcal{T}))$, *i.e., as* $V(\mathbf{L})$ *is finite,* $\mathbf{M}(f_\prec(\mathcal{T})) = \mathbf{M}_\prec(\mathcal{T})$. $\square$

Lemma 2.1. [immediate] *If* $\prec$ *is irreflexive, then* $f_\prec = f_{\prec'}$ *iff* $\prec = \prec'$. $\square$

Definition 2.2. [9,13,14] $(\mathbf{P}, \mathbf{Q}, \mathbf{Z})$ *is a partition of* $V(\mathbf{L})$. **P** *is the set of the* **circumscribed** *propositional symbols,* **Z** *of the* **variable** *ones,* **Q** *of the* **fixed** *ones.*
    A circumscription is a preferential entailment $CIRC(\mathbf{P}, \mathbf{Q}, \mathbf{Z}) = f_{\prec(\mathbf{P}, \mathbf{Q}, \mathbf{Z})}$ *where* $\prec_{(\mathbf{P}, \mathbf{Q}, \mathbf{Z})}$ *is defined by:* $\mu \prec_{(\mathbf{P}, \mathbf{Q}, \mathbf{Z})} \nu$ *if* $\mathbf{P} \cap \mu \subset \mathbf{P} \cap \nu$ *and* $\mathbf{Q} \cap \mu = \mathbf{Q} \cap \nu$.
    We define also $\mu \preceq_{(\mathbf{P}, \mathbf{Q}, \mathbf{Z})} \nu$ *by* $\mathbf{P} \cap \mu \subseteq \mathbf{P} \cap \nu$ *and* $\mathbf{Q} \cap \mu = \mathbf{Q} \cap \nu$. $\square$

Instead of using a propositional circumscription, it is often more natural and easier to use formula circumscription [9]. Here is the propositional version.

Definition 2.3. $\Phi, \mathcal{T}$ *are subsets of* **L**, *and* $\mathbf{Q}, \mathbf{Z}$ *is a partition of* $V(\mathbf{L})$. *The* **formula circumscription** $CIRCF$ *of the formulas of* Φ, *with* **Q** *fixed, is as follows: We introduce the set* $\mathbf{P} = \{P_\varphi\}_{\varphi \in \Phi}$ *of new propositional symbols.*
    $CIRCF(\Phi; \mathbf{Q}, \mathbf{Z})(\mathcal{T}) = CIRC(\mathbf{P}, \mathbf{Q}, \mathbf{Z})(\mathcal{T} \cup \{\varphi \Leftrightarrow P_\varphi\}_{\varphi \in \Phi}) \cap \mathbf{L}$.
    If **Q** *is empty, we write* $CIRCF(\Phi)$ *for* $CIRCF(\Phi; \emptyset, V(\mathbf{L}))$. $\square$

Remark 2.1. Any ordinary circumscription is a formula circumscription: $CIRC(\mathbf{P}, \mathbf{Q}, \mathbf{Z}) = CIRCF(\mathbf{P}; \mathbf{Q}, \mathbf{Z} \cup \mathbf{P})$. $\square$

We may generally consider only the case where $\mathbf{Q} = \emptyset$:

Proposition 2.1. [5] $CIRCF(\Phi; \mathbf{Q}, \mathbf{Z}) = CIRCF(\Phi \cup \mathbf{Q} \cup \neg\mathbf{Q})$.
    Thus, $CIRC(\mathbf{P}, \mathbf{Q}, \mathbf{Z}) = CIRCF(\mathbf{P} \cup \mathbf{Q} \cup \neg\mathbf{Q})$. $\square$

Definition 2.4. *Let μ, ν be in **M** and Φ be a subset of **L**.*

(a) *We define the set of formulas $\Phi_\mu = \{\varphi \in \Phi \mid \mu \models \varphi\} = Th(\mu) \cap \Phi$.*

(b) *We define two relations in **M**: $\mu \preceq_\Phi \nu$ if $\Phi_\mu \subseteq \Phi_\nu$, and $\mu \prec_\Phi \nu$ if $\Phi_\mu \subset \Phi_\nu$.*

(b') *If $(\mathbf{Q}, \mathbf{Z})$ is a partition of $V(\mathbf{L})$, we define two relations in **M**: $\mu \preceq_{(\Phi;\mathbf{Q},\mathbf{Z})} \nu$ if $\Phi_\mu \subseteq \Phi_\nu$ and $\mathbf{Q}_\mu = \mathbf{Q}_\nu$, and $\mu \prec_{(\Phi;\mathbf{Q},\mathbf{Z})} \nu$ if $\Phi_\mu \subset \Phi_\nu$ and $\mathbf{Q}_\mu = \mathbf{Q}_\nu$.* $\square$

Lemma 2.2. [immediate] 0. $\preceq_{(\Phi;\mathbf{Q},\mathbf{Z})} = \preceq_{\Phi \cup \mathbf{Q} \cup \neg \mathbf{Q}}$ and $\prec_{(\Phi;\mathbf{Q},\mathbf{Z})} = \prec_{\Phi \cup \mathbf{Q} \cup \neg \mathbf{Q}}$.

1a. $\mu \prec_\Phi \nu$ iff $\mu \preceq_\Phi \nu$ and $\nu \npreceq_\Phi \mu$.

1b. $\mu \preceq_\Phi \nu$ iff for any $\varphi \in \Phi$, if $\mu \models \varphi$ then $\nu \models \varphi$.

2. $\{\varphi\}_\mu \subseteq \{\varphi\}$, thus ($\mu \preceq_{\{\varphi\}} \nu$ or $\nu \preceq_{\{\varphi\}} \mu$) and not ($\mu_1 \prec_{\{\varphi\}} \mu_2$ and $\mu_2 \prec_{\{\varphi\}} \mu_3$).

3a. $\mu \preceq_\Phi \nu$ iff for any $\varphi \in \Phi$, $\mu \preceq_{\{\varphi\}} \nu$.

3b. $\mu \prec_\Phi \nu$ iff for any $\varphi \in \Phi$, $\mu \preceq_{\{\varphi\}} \nu$, and there exists $\varphi \in \Phi$ such that $\mu \prec_{\{\varphi\}} \nu$.

4. $\prec_\Phi$ and $\preceq_\Phi$ are transitive, $\prec_\Phi$ is irreflexive while $\preceq_\Phi$ is reflexive. $\square$

Thus, to know the "useful relation" (see Proposition 2.2) $\prec_\Phi$, we need more than each $\prec_{\{\varphi\}}$, we must know all the $\preceq_{\{\varphi\}}$'s, a more precise information.

Proposition 2.2. [folklore] $CIRCF(\Phi) = f_{\prec_\Phi}$, $CIRCF(\Phi; \mathbf{Q}, \mathbf{Z}) = f_{\prec_{(\Phi;\mathbf{Q},\mathbf{Z})}}$. $\square$

3   Equivalences between Sets of Circumscribed Formulas

We examine when two sets Φ and Φ' give the same formula circumscription.

Definition 3.1. *Φ and Φ' are **c-equivalent**, written $\Phi \equiv_c \Phi'$, if $CIRCF(\Phi) = CIRCF(\Phi')$. Φ and Φ' are **strongly equivalent**, written $\Phi \equiv_{sc} \Phi'$, if, for any set Φ'' of formulas, $CIRCF(\Phi \cup \Phi'') = CIRCF(\Phi' \cup \Phi'')$.* $\square$

If $\Phi \equiv_{sc} \Phi'$, then $\Phi \equiv_c \Phi'$. The strong version is useful because, when another rule, or even, as we are in the propositional case, another "individual", is added, this corresponds to an addition of formula(s): e.g. a new bird B_k, when we know that birds B_i generally fly F_i, provokes the addition of a new formula $B_k \wedge \neg F_k$ to be circumscribed. If we have only the standard equivalence, we may then loose this equivalence.

Definition 3.2. *The $\wedge$-**closure** of Φ is the set $\Phi^\wedge = \{\bigwedge_{\varphi \in \Psi} \varphi / \text{ for any finite } \Psi \subseteq \Phi\}$. The $\vee$-**closure** $\Phi^\vee$ is defined similarly. The $\wedge\vee$-**closure** of Φ is the set $\Phi^{\wedge\vee} = (\Phi^\wedge)^\vee$. $\Phi^\wedge$ (resp. $\Phi^\vee$, or $\Phi^{\wedge\vee}$) is called a set **closed** for $\wedge$ (resp. for $\vee$, for $\wedge$ and $\vee$).* $\square$

We get always $\top \in \Phi^\wedge$, $\bot \in \Phi^\vee$ ($\Psi = \emptyset$) and $(\Phi^\wedge)^\vee = (\Phi^\vee)^\wedge$ from distribution.

Definition 3.3. *1. φ is **accessible** for $f = f_\prec$ if $\varphi \in f(\mathcal{T}) - \mathcal{T}$ for some theory $\mathcal{T}$. The set of the formulas **inaccessible** for f is $I_f = I_\prec = \mathbf{L} - \bigcup_{\mathcal{T} \in \mathbf{T}} (f(\mathcal{T}) - \mathcal{T})$.*

*2. The set of the formulas **positive** for $\prec$ is the set $Pos(\prec)$ of the formulas φ such that, if $\mu \models \varphi$ and $\mu \prec \nu$, then $\nu \models \varphi$.*
*If $\prec = \prec_\Phi$ of Definition 2.4, we write $Pos_e(\Phi)$ for the set $Pos(\prec_\Phi)$, called the set of the formulas **positive in Φ, in the extended acception**.*
*If $\prec = \preceq_\Phi$, we write $Pos_m(\Phi)$ for the set $Pos(\preceq_\Phi)$ of the formulas **positive in Φ, in the minimal acception**.* $\square$

One technical role of the inaccessible formulas for circumscriptions is developed in [10]. Also, I_f is the greatest set Ψ such that $f = CIRCF(\Phi) = CIRCF(\Psi)$ (Theorem 3.3-1 below). $Pos(\prec)$ is closed for $\wedge$ and $\vee$ (next proposition, this gives a justification for the name of this set). We need now to remember a few results which are proved elsewhere (see also [11] for details and examples, these results are restricted here to the finite case).

Proposition 3.1. [12, Proposition 3.1]
1. If $\Phi \subseteq \mathbf{L}$, then $\Phi \subseteq Pos_m(\Phi) \subseteq Pos_e(\Phi)$, $\Phi^{\wedge\vee} = Pos_m(\Phi)$ and $Pos_e(\Phi) = I_{\prec_\Phi}$.
2. If $\prec$ is a binary relation in $\mathbf{M}$, then $Pos(\prec)$ is closed for $\wedge$ and $\vee$. $\square$

It is natural to call the formulas in $\Phi^{\wedge\vee}$, "positive in Φ", thus our notation $Pos_m(\Phi)$. There are also good reasons to call the formulas in the generally greater set $Pos_e(\Phi)$, "positive in Φ", in an **extended acception**.

Lemma 3.1. [12, Lemma 3.6] If $\Phi \subseteq \Psi \subseteq \Phi^{\wedge\vee}$, we have $\preceq_\Phi = \preceq_\Psi$, thus a fortiori $\prec_\Phi = \prec_\Psi$, i.e. $CIRCF(\Phi) = CIRCF(\Psi)$. $\square$

Lemma 3.2. [12, Lemma 3.7] $CIRCF(\Phi) = CIRCF(I_{\prec_\Phi}) = CIRCF(Pos_e(\Phi))$. $\square$

Theorem 3.3. [12, Theorem 3.8] *1.* $\Phi \equiv_c \Psi$ iff $\prec_\Phi = \prec_\Psi$ iff $Pos_e(\Phi) = Pos_e(\Psi)$. $\prec_\Phi = \prec_{Pos_e(\Phi)} = \prec_{Pos_m(\Phi)}$ and $Pos_e(\Phi)$ is the greatest (for $\subseteq$) set Ψ satisfying $\Psi \equiv_c \Phi$.

2a. $\Phi \equiv_{sc} \Psi$ iff $\preceq_\Phi = \preceq_\Psi$ iff $\Phi^{\wedge\vee} = \Psi^{\wedge\vee}$. Also $\preceq_\Phi = \preceq_{\Phi^{\wedge\vee}}$, thus $\prec_\Phi = \prec_{\Phi^{\wedge\vee}}$.
2b. $Pos_m(\Phi) = \Phi^{\wedge\vee}$ is the greatest set Ψ satisfying $\Psi \equiv_{sc} \Phi$ (cf Lemma 3.1).

3. $\Phi \cup \{\varphi\} \equiv_c \Phi$ iff $\Phi \cup \{\varphi\} \equiv_{sc} \Phi$ iff $\varphi \in \Phi^{\wedge\vee}$. $\square$

Point 1 provides necessary and sufficient conditions for two sets of formulas to give the same circumscription. Point 2 provides necessary and sufficient conditions for two sets of formulas to give the same circumscription, even when they are augmented in a similar way. One of these conditions is simply having the same $\wedge\vee$-closure. Point 3 provides a case where c-equivalence is identical to strong equivalence: informally, from point 2 and Lemma 2.2-3, when there is c-equivalence and not strong equivalence between a set and one of its subsets, the added formulas oppose each other. This mutual cancellation is impossible when the two sets differ by one formula only.

4   About the Characterization of Formula Circumscription

From theorem 3.3-2a, we know that the smallest sets strongly equivalent to a set Ψ are the smallest sets Φ such that $\Phi^{\wedge\vee} = \Psi$. We also know that all the elements of the set of all the sets of formulas strongly equivalent to a given set Ψ correspond to the same pre-order relation $\preceq_\Psi$. We will study this set, focusing on the smallest sets of formulas belonging to this set. From theorem 3.3-1 (or directly from lemmas 2.1 and 2.2-4 and from the definitions of $CIRCF$ and $\prec_\Psi$), we know that the set of all the sets of formulas which are c-equivalent to Ψ correspond to the same strict order relation $\prec_\Psi$. From the definitions of $\preceq_\Psi$ and $\prec_\Psi$, we get that various large relations $\preceq_\Psi$ can be associated to a given strict relation $\prec_\Psi$, which is the relation defining a given formula circumscription $CIRCF(\Psi)$. This leads us, firstly to make precise the connections between $\prec_\Phi$ and $\preceq_\Phi$, then to revisit the characterization of finite formula circumscription.

Definition 4.1. *Let* $\prec$ *be some binary relation on a set* E. *We denote by* $s_\prec(e)$ *and* $p_\prec(e)$ *respectively the sets* $s_\prec(e) = \{e' \in E/e \prec e'\}$ *and* $p_\prec(e) = \{e' \in E/e' \prec e\}$.

We suppose now that $\prec$ *is a* **strict order** *(irreflexive and transitive relation). We call* **associated with** $\prec$ *any* **pre-order** *(reflexive and transitive) relation* $\preceq$ *on* E *such that we have, for any* e_1, e_2 *in* E: $e_1 \prec e_2$ *iff* $e_1 \preceq e_2$ *and* $e_2 \not\preceq e_1$. **(Assoc)**

We define the following two relations $\preceq_0$ *and* $\preceq_1$ *on* E: $e_1 \preceq_0 e_2$ *if* $e_1 \prec e_2$ *or* $e_1 = e_2$, *and* $e_1 \preceq_1 e_2$ *if* $e_1 \prec e_2$ *or* $(s_\prec(e_1) = s_\prec(e_2)$ *and* $p_\prec(e_1) = p_\prec(e_2))$. $\square$

Lemma 4.1. 1. $\preceq_0$ and $\preceq_1$ are associated with $\prec$ and, if $\preceq$ is associated with $\prec$ we have, for any e_1, e_2 in E: (1) if $e_1 \preceq_0 e_2$ then $e_1 \preceq e_2$, (2) if $e_1 \preceq e_2$ then $e_1 \preceq_1 e_2$.
  2. $\preceq_0$ is the only order relation $\preceq$ satisfying (Assoc).
  3. A pre-order $\preceq$ "between $\preceq_0$ and $\preceq_1$" is not necessarily associated with $\prec$: $\preceq$ is associated with $\prec$ iff its graph is the reunion of the graphs of $\preceq_0$ and of some universal relations restricted to subsets of E over which $\preceq_1$ is the universal relation.

Proof: Point 1: It is obvious that $\preceq_0$ is associated with $\prec$, that each pre-order $\preceq$ associated with $\prec$ satisfies implication (1), that $\preceq_1$ is reflexive and satisfies (Assoc).

$\preceq_1$ is transitive: We suppose $e_1 \preceq_1 e_2$ and $e_2 \preceq_1 e_3$. If $(e_1 \prec e_2$ and $e_2 \prec e_3)$, or $(e_1 \prec e_2$ and $p_\prec(e_2) = p_\prec(e_3))$, or $(s_\prec(e_1) = s_\prec(e_2)$ and $e_2 \prec e_3)$, then $e_1 \prec e_3$. If $s_\prec(e_1) = s_\prec(e_2)$, $p_\prec(e_1) = p_\prec(e_2)$, $s_\prec(e_2) = s_\prec(e_3)$ and $p_\prec(e_2) = p_\prec(e_3)$, then $s_\prec(e_1) = s_\prec(e_3)$ and $p_\prec(e_1) = p_\prec(e_3)$. In any case $e_1 \preceq_1 e_3$.

Implication (2) [1]: We suppose $e_1 \preceq e_2$. By (Assoc) $e_1 \prec e_2$ or $e_2 \preceq e_1$. If $e_1 \prec e_2$, then $e_1 \preceq_1 e_2$, thus we suppose $e_2 \preceq e_1$. If $e \in p_\prec(e_1)$, then $e \preceq e_1$ by (Assoc) and $e \preceq e_2$ by transitivity. Thus we get $e \prec e_2$ or $e_2 \preceq e$ by (Assoc). If $e_2 \preceq e$, we get $e_1 \preceq e$ by transitivity, thus $e \not\preceq e_1$ by (Assoc), a contradiction: we get $e \prec e_2$. Thus $p_\prec(e_1) \subseteq p_\prec(e_2)$. By similar arguments, we get $s_\prec(e_2) \subseteq s_\prec(e_1)$. As our hypothesis is symmetrical in (e_1, e_2), we get $p_\prec(e_1) = p_\prec(e_2)$ and $s_\prec(e_1) = s_\prec(e_2)$: $e_1 \preceq_1 e_2$.

Point 2: Immediate.

Point 3: "only if": $\preceq$ is associated with $\prec$. We suppose $e_1 \preceq e_2$, $e_2 \preceq e_3$, $\cdots$, $e_{n-1} \preceq e_n$, $\overline{e_1 \not\preceq_0 e_2}$, $e_2 \not\preceq_0 e_3$, $\cdots$, $e_{n-1} \not\preceq e_n$. Then $e_i \not\preceq e_{i+i}$ and, by (Assoc), $e_{i+1} \preceq e_i$: $\preceq$ is universal on the set $\{e_1, e_2, \cdots, e_n\}$. By implication (2), $\preceq_1$ is also universal on this set. The result is then immediate.

"if": $\prec$ is a strict order and the graph of $\preceq$ is the union of the graph of $\preceq_0$ and of the graphs of the universal relation on some subsets of E over which the restriction of $\preceq_1$ is universal. (1) $\preceq$ is reflexive (obvious) and transitive: Let e_1, e_2, e_3 be distinct in E such that $e_1 \preceq e_2$ and $e_2 \preceq e_3$. If $e_1 \preceq_0 e_2$ and $e_2 \preceq_0 e_3$, then $e_1 \preceq_0 e_3$. If $e_1 \preceq_0 e_2$ and $e_2 \not\preceq_0 e_3$ then $e_2 \preceq_1 e_3$ and $e_3 \preceq_1 e_2$ thus $p_\prec(e_2) = p_\prec(e_3)$ and $e_1 \prec e_3$. Similarly, if $e_1 \not\preceq_0 e_2$ and $e_2 \preceq_0 e_3$ then $s_\prec(e_1) = s_\prec(e_2)$ and $e_1 \prec e_3$. (2) $\preceq$ satisfies (Assoc): If $e \preceq e'$ and $e' \not\preceq e$, $\preceq$ is not universal on $\{e, e'\}$, thus $e \preceq_0 e'$ and $e \neq e'$, thus $e \prec e'$. Conversely, we suppose $e \prec e'$. Then $e \preceq e'$ and, if $e' \preceq e$, then $\preceq$, thus $\preceq_1$, is universal on $\{e, e'\}$. As $\prec$ is a strict order, $e' \not\prec e$. Thus, from $e' \preceq_1 e$ we get $s_\prec(e) = s_\prec(e')$, a contradiction. Thus, we get $e \preceq e'$ and $e' \not\preceq e$.

The number of all the pre-orders $\preceq$ associated with a given strict order $\prec$ is then $\Pi_{C \in \mathbf{C}} B_{card(C)}$, where B_k is the Bell (or exponential) number of index k and $\mathbf{C}$ is the set of all the maximal subsets C of E (with $card(C) > 1$) on which $\preceq_1$ is universal. $\square$

---

[1] The first author thanks Éric Badouel for this proof.

Theorem 4.2. [6,3,11] *A pre-circumscription f is a formula circumscription iff it is a preferential entailment associated with a strict order $\prec$.*

Proof: Theorem 4.2 has independently appeared at least three times as [6, Theorems 13-14], [3, Theorem 7] and [11, Proposition 5.24-1]). However, in [6,11] the proof relies on the strict relation (i.e. in fact on the large relation $\preceq_0$), and [3] uses any large relation, but without constructive definition. For our purpose, we need to consider large relations and constructive definitions, which is why we provide a new proof.

"only if": Lemma 2.2-4 and Proposition 2.2.

"if": The proof is built on an old result ([8, Lemma 11.8, Theorems 11.6 and 11.9]): any pre-order $\preceq$ on a set E can be put in correspondence with the relation $\supseteq$ on a subset of $\mathcal{P}(E)$: For any e_1, e_2 in E, we have $e_1 \preceq e_2$ iff $s_\prec(e_2) \subseteq s_\prec(e_1)$. **(MN)**

Step 0: Let $\prec$ be a strict order on $\mathbf{M}$ and $\preceq$ be any pre-order associated with $\prec$.

Step 1, first application of (MN): Let us define the formula $\varphi_\prec(\mu)$, for any $\mu \in \mathbf{M}$, and the set of formulas $\Phi_\prec$ by: $\mathbf{M}(\varphi_\prec(\mu)) = s_\prec(\mu)$ and $\Phi_\prec = \{\varphi_\prec(\mu)\}_{\mu \in \mathbf{M}}$.

From (MN) we get $\mu \preceq \nu$ iff $\varphi_\prec(\nu) \models \varphi_\prec(\mu)$. **(MN1)**

Step 2, second application of (MN): Starting from the set $\Phi_\prec$ pre-ordered by $\models$, we define the set of formulas $s_\models(\psi) = \{\psi' \in \Phi_\prec \,/\, \psi \models \psi'\}$. From (MN) we get, for any μ, ν in $\mathbf{M}$: $\varphi_\prec(\mu) \models \varphi_\prec(\nu)$ iff $s_\models(\varphi_\prec(\nu)) \subseteq s_\models(\varphi_\prec(\mu))$. **(MN2)**

We get $\varphi_\prec(\nu) \in s_\models(\varphi_\prec(\mu))$ iff $\varphi_\prec(\mu) \models \varphi_\prec(\nu)$, $\varphi_\prec(\mu) \models \varphi_\prec(\nu)$ iff $\nu \preceq \mu$ from (MN1), and $\nu \preceq \mu$ iff $\mu \in s_\prec(\nu)$ iff $\mu \models \varphi_\prec(\nu)$. Thus, we get $\varphi_\prec(\nu) \in s_\models(\varphi_\prec(\mu))$ iff $\varphi_\prec(\nu) \in Th(\mu)$. This means, for any $\mu \in \mathbf{M}$: $s_\models(\varphi_\prec(\mu)) = Th(\mu) \cap \Phi_\prec$. From (MN1) and (MN2) we get then $\mu \preceq \nu$ iff $Th(\mu) \cap \Phi_\prec \subseteq Th(\nu) \cap \Phi_\prec$, thus $\mu \prec \nu$ iff $Th(\mu) \cap \Phi_\prec \subset Th(\nu) \cap \Phi_\prec$. Thus, from Proposition 2.2, $f = f_\prec = \widehat{CIRCF}(\Phi_\prec)$. $\square$

Step 0 allows many possibilities. If we want to reduce the size of the set $\Phi_\prec$ of formulas to circumscribe, obtained in step 1, we will see why it is good to choose $\preceq_1$ and why the worst possibility is $\preceq_0$, as done in [6,11]. In step 1, with each pre-order $\preceq$, we associate naturally a set of formulas $\Phi_\prec$. In step 2, with each set Φ of formulas, we associate naturally a pre-order $\preceq_\Phi$ and we get $\preceq = \preceq_{\Phi_\prec}$. Remember that Theorem 3.3-2 allows to reduce the size of the set $\Phi_\prec$ of formulas to circumscribe.

5   The Smallest Sets Strongly Equivalent to a Given Set

We need a few definitions, often given in two forms: in terms of subsets of a set E, and in terms of formulas, where $E = \mathbf{M}$ and a formula can be associated with each subset. This is to relate these results to familiar general results about finite sets.

Definition 5.1. *1. (a) The $\cup$-closure of a set $\mathcal{E}$ of subsets of some given set E is the set $\mathcal{E}^\cup$ of the subsets of E which are unions of elements in $\mathcal{E}$: $\mathcal{E}^\cup = \{\bigcup_{E' \in \mathcal{E}'} E' \,/\, \mathcal{E}' \subseteq \mathcal{E}\}$. The $\cap$-closure of $\mathcal{E}$ is defined similarly and the $\cup\cap$-closure of $\mathcal{E}$ is $\mathcal{E}^{\cup\cap} = (\mathcal{E}^\cup)^\cap = (\mathcal{E}^\cap)^\cup$. (b) We define the sets $\mathcal{E}_\cup = \{E' \in \mathcal{E} / E' \notin (\mathcal{E} - \{E'\})^\cup\}$ and similarly $\mathcal{E}_\cap$. (c) For any set $\mathcal{E}$ of subsets of E, we define an $\cup$-basis of $\mathcal{E}$ as any set $\mathcal{E}'$ of subsets of E having the same $\cup$-closure as $\mathcal{E}$ and which has a cardinal minimal with this property. An $\cap$-basis of $\mathcal{E}$ and an $\cup\cap$-basis of $\mathcal{E}$ are defined similarly.*

2. *Replacing "subset" by "formula", $\cup$ by $\wedge$ and $\cap$ by $\vee$, gives respectively: (a) Definition 3.2, (b) the sets $\Phi_\wedge = \{\varphi \in \Phi / \varphi \notin (\Phi - \{\varphi\})^\wedge\}$ and $\Phi_\vee = \{\varphi \in \Phi / \varphi \notin (\Phi - \{\varphi\})^\vee\}$, and (c) the notions of $\wedge$-basis, $\vee$-basis and $\wedge\vee$-basis of a set Φ of formulas.* $\square$

Proposition 5.1. [Obvious] *If E is finite, then any set $\mathcal{E}$ of subsets of E has exactly one $\cup$-basis, which is $\mathcal{E}_\cup$ and one $\cap$-basis, which is $\mathcal{E}_\cap$. Since $\mathbf{M}$ is finite, any set Ψ of formulas in $\mathbf{L}$ has exactly one $\wedge$-basis, which is $\Psi_\wedge$ and one $\vee$-basis, which is $\Psi_\vee$.* $\square$

Definition 5.2.   *1. Let $\mathcal{E}$ be a set of subsets of E and $\preceq$ be a pre-order in E. We define:*
(a) For each $e \in E$, the set $\mathcal{E}_e$ of subsets of $\mathcal{E}$ by $\bar{\mathcal{E}}_e = \{E_i \in \mathcal{E} \ / \ e \in E_i\}$.
(b) Three relations on E: $e_1 \prec_\mathcal{E} e_2$ if $\mathcal{E}_{e_1} \subset \mathcal{E}_{e_2}$, $e_1 \preceq_\mathcal{E} e_2$ if $\mathcal{E}_{e_1} \subseteq \mathcal{E}_{e_2}$, and $e_1 \preceq\succeq_\mathcal{E} e_2$ if $\mathcal{E}_{e_1} = \mathcal{E}_{e_2}$.
(c) The subsets $F_\preceq = \{s_\preceq(e)/e \in E\}$ and $F_\mathcal{E} = F_{\preceq_\mathcal{E}}$ of $\mathcal{P}(E)$.
*(d) A subset E_1 of E is a **filter for** $\preceq$ if, for any $e_1 \in E_1, e \in E$ such that $e_1 \preceq e$, we have $e \in E_1$. We denote by $\mathcal{F}_\preceq$ the set of all the filters for $\preceq$ and by $\mathcal{F}_\mathcal{E}$ the set $\mathcal{F}_{\preceq_\mathcal{E}}$ of the **filters for** $\mathcal{E}$.*
2. Let X be a set of formulas in $\mathbf{L}$ and $\preceq$ be a pre-order in $\mathbf{M}$. We define:
(a)(b) Definition 2.4 (a), and (b) respectively.
(c) The sets of formulas $\Phi_\preceq$, as in "step 1" in the proof of Theorem 4.2, and $\Phi_X = \Phi_{\preceq_X} = \{\varphi_X(\mu) \ / \ \mu \in \mathbf{M}\}$, where $\varphi_X(\mu) = \varphi_{\preceq_X}(\mu)$.
(d) The sets of formulas $\mathbf{F}_\preceq = \{\varphi \in \mathbf{L}/ \text{ if } \mu \in \mathbf{M}(\varphi), \nu \in \mathbf{M} \text{ and } \mu \preceq \nu, \text{ then } \nu \in \mathbf{M}(\varphi)\}$, and $\mathbf{F}_X = \mathbf{F}_{\preceq_X}$. $\square$

By definition, $\perp \notin \Phi_\preceq$, thus $\perp \notin \Phi_X$. We get $f_{\prec_X} = CIRCF(X)$ from Proposition 2.2. Also, $\preceq_\mathcal{E}$ is associated with $\prec_\mathcal{E}$, and $\preceq_X$ with $\prec_X$. We get then:

Lemma 5.1.   1. Let E be some finite set, and $\mathcal{E}, \mathcal{E}_1, \mathcal{E}_2$ be any set of subsets of E.
   (a) $\preceq_{\mathcal{E}_1} = \preceq_{\mathcal{E}_2}$ iff $\mathcal{E}_1^{\cup\cap} = \mathcal{E}_2^{\cup\cap}$. $\mathcal{F}_\mathcal{E} = \mathcal{E}^{\cup\cap}$.
   (b) The set $F_\mathcal{E}$ is the $\cup$-basis of the set $\mathcal{F}_\mathcal{E} = \mathcal{E}^{\cup\cap}$: $F_\mathcal{E} = (\mathcal{E}^{\cup\cap})_\cup$.
   (c) For any pre-order $\preceq$ on E, we get $\preceq_{\mathcal{F}_\preceq} = \preceq_{F_\preceq} = \preceq$ and $\preceq_{\mathcal{F}_\mathcal{E}} = \preceq_{F_\mathcal{E}} = \preceq_\mathcal{E}$.
   2. In terms of formulas, X and Y being sets of formulas in $\mathbf{L}$, we get:
   (a) $\preceq_X = \preceq_Y$ iff $X^{\wedge\vee} = Y^{\wedge\vee}$. $\mathbf{F}_X = X^{\wedge\vee}$.
   (b) The set Φ_X is the $\vee$-basis of the set $\mathbf{F}_X = X^{\wedge\vee}$. The elements of $\Phi_\preceq$ are $\vee$-**irreducible in $\mathbf{F}_\preceq$**: For any $\varphi \in \Phi_\preceq$, it does not exist any non trivial (without any term equal to the result) disjunction of elements of $\mathbf{F}_\preceq$ which is equal to φ.
   (c) For any pre-order $\preceq$ in $\mathbf{M}$ we get $\preceq_{\mathbf{F}_\preceq} = \preceq_{\Phi_\preceq} = \preceq$. Thus, $\preceq_{\mathbf{F}_X} = \preceq_{\Phi_X} = \preceq_X$. $\square$

These results are known in finite set theory and distributive lattice theory (see e.g. [8,2,4]). Point 2a is Theorem 3.3-2, given here again in order to make precise the correspondence with the "set versions" of point 1a. The left most equalities in point 2c come from point 2a, the right most equalities being step 2 in the proof of Theorem 4.2. Thus, only point 1b (or equivalently 2b) remains, and the proof is straightforward.

Here is an immediate consequence of this lemma (given in terms of formulas only):

Proposition 5.2. *The two operations $\preceq_X$ and $\mathbf{F}_\preceq$ define two reciprocal one-to-one mappings between the set of all the sets X of formulas of $\mathbf{L}$ which are closed for $\wedge$ and $\vee$ and the set of all the pre-orders $\preceq$ defined on $\mathbf{M}$.*
The set of all the sets X of formulas of $\mathbf{L}$ which are closed for $\wedge$ and $\vee$, is the set of all the distributive lattices (with $\top$ and $\perp$) which are sublattices of $\mathbf{L}$, where the operations of the lattices are $\wedge$ (meet) and $\vee$ (join). $\square$

This result can also be extracted from the classical literature about distributive lattices (see e.g. [2, Theorem 3 and Corollary 1, p. 59] or more precisely [4, Theorem 8.19 and Subsection 8.20]). However, this literature uses only orders, and not pre-orders ([8] is a notable exception). The formulation given here makes precise the exact correspondence between having the same pre-order relation on **M** and being "strongly equivalent" with respect to formula circumscription in **L**. Let us give here another useful auxiliary result:

Definition 5.3. A **chain of strict entailment** in a set X of formulas is a sequence $(\varphi_i)_{i \in \{0,1,2,\cdots,n\}}$ of elements of X such that $\varphi_i \models \varphi_{i+1}$ and $\varphi_{i+1} \not\models \varphi_i$ for $i \in \{0, 1, 2, \cdots, n - 1\}$. The **length of this chain** is n, and the length $l(X)$ of X is the length of the longest chains of strict entailment in X. $\square$

Lemma 5.2. For any set of formulas X, $l(\mathbf{F}_X)$ is equal to $card(\Phi_X)$.

Notice that $card(\Phi_X)$ is the number of equivalence classes for $\preceq\succeq_X$ in **M**. Thus, $card(\Phi_X) \leq card(\mathbf{M}) = 2^{card(V(\mathbf{L}))}$. One possible easy <u>proof</u> of this lemma uses the fact that Φ_X constitutes an $\vee$-basis of $\mathbf{F}_X$. Also, it is a consequence of the representation theorem ([2, Theorem 3, p. 59], or e.g., [4, Theorem 8.17]) for finite distributive lattices ($\mathbf{F}_X$ is a distributive lattice). $\square$

Definition 5.4. *1. If $\preceq$ is a pre-order in a finite set E, $Fir_\preceq = \{s_\preceq(e)/e \in E, s_\preceq(e) \notin (F_\preceq - \{s_\preceq(e)\})^\cap\}$ denotes the set of the elements of $\bar{F}_\preceq$ which are $\cap$-irreducible in $\bar{F}_\preceq$. If $\bar{\mathcal{E}} \subseteq \mathcal{P}(E)$, we define $Fir_{\mathcal{E}} = Fir_{\preceq_\varepsilon}$.*
*2. If $\preceq$ is a pre-order in **M**, $\Phi ir_\preceq = \{\varphi \in \Phi_\preceq/\varphi \notin (\Phi_\preceq - \{\varphi\})^\wedge\}$ denotes the set of the formulas of $\Phi_\preceq$ which are $\wedge$-irreducible in $\Phi_\preceq$. If $X \subseteq \mathbf{L}$, we define $\Phi ir_X = \Phi ir_{\preceq_X}$. $\square$*

Notice that $\bot \notin \Phi ir_\preceq$ and $\top \notin \Phi ir_\preceq$. The following result is immediate:

Proposition 5.3. *1. For any set $\mathcal{E}$ of subsets of a finite set E, we have $\mathcal{E}^{\cup\cap} = Fir_{\mathcal{E}}^{\cup\cap}$. Thus, a set $\mathcal{B}$ of subsets of a finite set E is an $\cup\cap$-basis of $\mathcal{E}$ iff we have: $\mathcal{B} \subseteq \mathcal{F}_{\mathcal{E}}$, $Fir_{\mathcal{E}} \subseteq \mathcal{B}^\cap$ and $\mathcal{B}$ has the smallest possible cardinal.*
2. For any set of formulas X, $X^{\wedge\vee} = (\Phi ir_X)^{\wedge\vee}$. Thus, Y is an $\wedge\vee$-basis of X iff we have: $Y \subseteq \mathbf{F}_X$, $\Phi ir_X \subseteq Y^\wedge$ and Y has the smallest possible cardinal. $\square$

This result provides a semi-constructive way for getting an $\wedge\vee$-basis of a given set X of formulas (i.e. one of the smallest sets strongly equivalent to X) by splitting this task in two steps. The first step is constructive: getting the set Φir_X. The second step is much easier than the direct search for an $\wedge\vee$-basis because we need only to search for what could be called an $\wedge$-**basis with respect to $\mathbf{F}_X$ of a given set** Φir_X. This non trivial problem concerns in particular a famous result by Sperner (it is, e.g., "Sperner's theorem" in [1, Part 1.2] and "Sperner's lemma" in [2, p. 98-99]).

Definition 5.5. *Let E be some finite set with $card(E) = n$. An **antichain** in E is a set of subsets of E uncomparable for $\subseteq$. A **weak antichain** $\mathcal{E}$ in E is a set of subsets of E which is equal to its $\cup$-basis $\mathcal{E}_\cup$ (i.e., no set in $\mathcal{E}$ is the union of some other sets in $\mathcal{E}$). $A(n)$ and $WA(n)$ denote respectively the maximal number of elements in an antichain and in a weak antichain in E. $\square$*

As any antichain is a weak antichain, we get $WA(n) \geq A(n)$. Sperner's theorem states that $A(n)$ is the central binomial coefficient $(n, \lfloor n/2 \rfloor)$. This result gives, in some cases (case 2 in next proposition), a fully constructive way for getting an $\wedge\vee$-basis Y of a set X of formulas in $\mathbf{L}$. It does not seem that the exact value of $WA(n)$, not given in [16], is known. It is easy to realize that we get $WA(n) \geq WA1(n) = \Sigma_{i=0}^{n-1}(i, \lfloor i/2 \rfloor)$. Kleitman [7] has shown that a better lower bound for $WA(n)$ is $WA2(n)$ defined by $(n, n/2) + (n, n/2 - 1)/n$ for even n and $2(n-1, (n-1)/2) + (n-1, (n-3)/2)/n$ for odd n. $WA2(n)$ is approached by $(1 + 3/(2n))A(n)$ for odd n and by $(1 + 1/(n+2))A(n)$ for even n [7]. For $n \leq 12$, we have $WA2(n) \leq WA1(n)$ (and maybe $WA(n) = WA1(n)$) but for any $n > 12$ we have $WA2(n) > WA1(n)$.

Proposition 5.4. *Let X be some finite set of formulas in $\mathbf{L}$. We are looking for an $\wedge\vee$-basis Y of X (i.e., some set Y with the minimal cardinality k such that $Y \equiv_{sc} X$). Let $\Phi ir_X = \{\varphi_1, \cdots, \varphi_n\}$ be the set introduced in Definition 5.4, with $n = card(\Phi ir_X)$.*

1. *In any case, $k = card(Y)$ must satisfy $WA(k) \geq n$.*
2. *If Φir_X is made of mutually exclusive formulas ($\varphi \models \neg\psi$ for any distinct φ, ψ), $card(Y)$ is the smallest k satisfying $A(k) \geq n$ and it exists a constructive way for finding Y. This case is particular (it means that $\preceq_X$ is an equivalence relation, thus $\prec_X$ is empty), but it may help to solve more general cases. Applying this result to subsets of Φir_X may help to find Y (see Proposition 7.1 and Example 7.3 below).*
3. *If Φir_X is made of a single chain of strict entailment, then $card(Y) = card(\Phi ir_X)$.*

<u>Proof:</u> <u>1.</u> From Proposition 5.3, we know that we want a subset $Y = \{\varphi_1', \cdots, \varphi_k'\}$ of $\mathbf{F}_X$ such that each $\varphi_i \in \Phi ir_X$ is a conjunction of elements of Y: there exists an injective mapping l from Φir_X to a set of subsets of $\{1, \cdots, k\}$ such that we have

$$\varphi_i = \bigwedge_{j \in l(\varphi_i)} \varphi_j', \text{ where } l(\varphi_i) \subseteq \{1, \cdots, k\} \text{ for any } i \in \{1, \cdots, n\}. \tag{1}$$

Since the formulas in Φir_X are $\vee$-irreducible in $\mathbf{F}_X$, thus in Φir_X, $\{l(\varphi_i)\}_{i\in\{1,\cdots,n\}}$ must be a weak antichain in $\{1, \cdots, k\}$ and k satisfies $WA(k) \geq n$. We will see below (condition $(C : \supseteq \leadsto \models)$ in Example 7.1) how to improve this lower bound for k.

   <u>2.</u> Let l be an injective mapping from Φir_X to a set of subsets of $\{1, \cdots, k\}$ and $\{\varphi_j'\}_{j\in\{1,\cdots,k\}}$ be some set of formulas satisfying (1). As the formulas in Φir_X are mutually exclusive, we get $\varphi_i \not\models \varphi_j$ for any i, j distinct in $\{1, \cdots, n\}$. Thus the set $l(\Phi ir_X) = \{\{l(\varphi_i)\}_{i\in\{1,\cdots,n\}}$ must be an antichain in $\{1, \cdots, k\}$ and $A(k) \geq n$. For any k such that $A(k) \geq n$, it exists an injective mapping l from Φir_X to an antichain in $\{1, \cdots, k\}$. Let us choose one such l, and define the formulas φ_j' as follows:

$$\varphi_j' = \bigvee_{j \in l(\varphi_i)} \varphi_i, \text{ for any } j \in \{1, \cdots, k\}. \tag{2}$$

Clearly, $\varphi_j' \in (\Phi ir_X)^\vee \subseteq \mathbf{F}_X$. As the formulas φ_i are mutually exclusive, we get (1). This shows that the smallest k such that $A(k) \geq n$ is the smallest possible k in this case. Moreover, this gives a fully constructive way for finding a set $Y = \{\varphi_j'\}_{j\in\{1,\cdots,k\}}$.

   <u>3.</u> Φir_X is then a possible Y (obvious, also a consequence of Proposition 5.5 below). $\square$

Example 7.1 below shows that we can sometimes do a slightly better job with weak antichains than with antichains. Case 3 shows that in some cases, we can be much above the best possibility given in 1. Propositions 5.3 and 5.4 provide useful tricks which considerably help the search for an $\wedge\vee$-basis (see also the examples given in Section 7 below). Here is another indication about the size of an $\wedge\vee$-basis of X:

Proposition 5.5. *For any set of formulas X, the cardinal of an $\wedge\vee$-basis Y of X is such that we have: $l(\Phi_X) \leq card(Y) \leq card(\Phi ir_X)$.*

Proof From Proposition 5.3 we know that we have $card(Y) \leq card(\Phi ir_X)$: indeed, in the worst case, we can take Φir_X as our $\wedge\vee$-generator of X. $l(\Phi_X) \leq card(Y)$ is straightforward, we get even $l(\Phi_X) < card(Y)$ if $\top \notin \Phi_X$.   □

6   The Smallest Sets c-Equivalent to a Given Set

We consider now a given $CIRCF(X)$, and we look for the smallest (in terms of cardinality) sets Y such that $CIRCF(Y) = CIRCF(X)$.

Lemma 6.1. Let $\mathcal{E}$ be a set of subsets of some finite set E, closed for $\cup$ and $\cap$ (i.e. such that $\mathcal{E} = \mathcal{F}_{\mathcal{E}}$), and let us consider the relations $\preceq=\preceq_{\mathcal{E}}$ and $\preccurlyeq=\preccurlyeq_{\mathcal{E}}$ (Definition 5.2). Let us call $\cup\cap$-**generator of** $\mathcal{E}$ any subset $\mathcal{G}$ of $\mathcal{E}$ such that $\mathcal{G}^{\cup\cap} = \mathcal{E}$. Let e_1 and e_2 be two elements in E not equivalent for $\preccurlyeq\!\!\succcurlyeq$ and satisfying $p_{\prec}(e_1) = p_{\prec}(e_2)$ and $s_{\prec}(e_1) = s_{\prec}(e_2)$ (Definition 4.1). Let us define the relation $\preceq'$ in E as follows: $e \preceq' e'$ if $e \preceq e'$ or $(e \preccurlyeq\!\!\succcurlyeq e_1$ and $e' \preccurlyeq\!\!\succcurlyeq e_2)$. Then $\preceq'$ is a pre-order in E associated with $\prec$, and we define the set $\mathcal{E}' = \mathcal{F}_{\preceq'}$ of all the filters for $\preceq'$ (clearly $\mathcal{E}' \subseteq \mathcal{E}$).

1. Let $\mathcal{G}$ be a $\cup\cap$-generator of $\mathcal{E}$. Let us denote by $\mathcal{G}'$ the set of all the subsets G' of E defined as follows: For any $G \in \mathcal{G}$,
    $$G' = G \cup \{e \in E \;/\; e \preccurlyeq\!\!\succcurlyeq e_2\} \quad \text{if } \{e_1, e_2\} \cap G = \{e_1\}$$
    $$G - \{e \in E \;/\; e \preccurlyeq\!\!\succcurlyeq e_2\} \quad \text{if } \{e_1, e_2\} \cap G = \{e_2\}$$
    $$G \qquad\qquad \text{otherwise, i.e. if } \{e_1, e_2\} \cap G \text{ is } \emptyset \text{ or } \{e_1, e_2\}.$$
    Then $\mathcal{G}'$ is a $\cup\cap$-generator of $\mathcal{E}'$ and $card(\mathcal{G}') \leq card(\mathcal{G})$.
2. Any $\cup\cap$-basis of $\mathcal{E}'$ has at most as many elements as a $\cup\cap$-basis of $\mathcal{E}$.
    Notice that if we start from $\mathcal{G} = F_{\mathcal{E}}$, which is a $\cup\cap$-generator of $\mathcal{E}$, we get as our set $\mathcal{G}'$ the set $\mathcal{G}' = \mathcal{G} - \{s_{\prec}(e_1), s_{\prec}(e_2)\} \cup \{(s_{\prec}(e_1))', (s_{\prec}(e_2))'\}$ where $(s_{\prec}(e_1))' = s_{\prec'}(e_1) = s_{\prec'}(e_2) = s_{\prec}(e_1) \cup s_{\prec}(e_2)$ and $(s_{\prec}(e_2))' = s_{\prec}(e_1) \cap s_{\prec}(e_2)$.

Proof: Point 1: If we define $\preceq_0$ and $\preceq_1$ from $\prec$ as in Definition 4.1, we know, from Lemma 4.1 (points 1 and 3) that $\preceq'$ is asoociated with $\prec$ and that we have, assimilating a relation to its graph: $\preceq_0 \subseteq \preceq \subseteq \preceq' \subseteq \preceq_1$. Let $\mathcal{G}$ and $\mathcal{G}'$ be as above, and let H be some element of $\mathcal{E}'$. Clearly $card(\mathcal{G}') \leq card(\mathcal{G})$. Let us define the set H'' as follows:
$$H'' = H \cup \{e \;/\; e \preccurlyeq\!\!\succcurlyeq e_2\} \quad \text{if } s_{\prec}(e_1) \subseteq H \text{ and } \{e_1, e_2\} \cap H = \emptyset$$
$$H - \{e \;/\; e \preccurlyeq\!\!\succcurlyeq e_2\} \quad \text{if } \{e_1, e_2\} \subseteq H$$
$$H \qquad\qquad \text{otherwise, i.e. if } s_{\prec}(e_1) \not\subseteq H.$$
It is immediate that if $e \in H''$, then $s_{\prec}(e) \subseteq H''$. Thus, $H'' \in \mathcal{E}$. From $\mathcal{G}^{\cup\cap} = \mathcal{E}$, we get $H'' = \bigcup_{i=1}^{I} \bigcap_{j=1}^{J_i} G_{i,j}$ where each $G_{i,j}$ is in $\mathcal{G}$. Now, it is straightforward to check that we get $H = \bigcup_{i=1}^{I} \bigcap_{j=1}^{J_i} G'_{i,j}$, which establishes $H \in \mathcal{G}'^{\cup\cap}$.
Point 2 The first sentence is an immediate consequence of point 1. The particular case where $\mathcal{G} = F_{\mathcal{E}}$ is a mere application of the definitions involved. □

Proposition 6.1. *(See Definition 4.1) If two pre-orders $\preceq$ and $\preceq'$ on E are associated with the same strict order $\prec$ and if the graph of $\preceq$ is included in the graph of $\preceq'$, then a $\cup\cap$-basis of $\mathcal{F}_{\preceq'}$ has at most as many elements as a $\cup\cap$-basis of $\mathcal{F}_{\preceq}$. In particular, any $\cup\cap$-basis of $\mathcal{F}_{\preceq_1}$ has at most as many elements as a $\cup\cap$-basis of $\bar{\mathcal{F}}_{\prec}$, which has itself at most as many elements as a $\cup\cap$-basis of $\mathcal{F}_{\preceq_0}$.*

Proof: From Lemma 4.1-3, there exists pre-orders $\preceq^i$ with $\preceq=\preceq^0$, $\preceq'=\preceq^p$ and, for any $i \in \{1, \cdots, p\}$, there exists two distinct e_1, e_2 in E such that $e_1 \preceq_1 \succeq_1 e_2$ and the graph of $\preceq^i$ is the graph of $\preceq^{i-1}$ plus $\{(e, e_2) \mid e \succeq \succ e_1\}$. Then, Lemma 6.1 gives the general result, and $(\preceq, \preceq') = (\preceq_0, \preceq)$ or $(\preceq, \preceq_1)$ give the results for $\preceq_0$ and $\preceq_1$. $\square$

Theorem 6.2. *Let Ψ be a set of formulas and $\preceq_1$ and $\preceq_0$ be respectively the greatest and the smallest pre-orders associated with $\prec=\prec_\Psi$ (see Lemma 4.1).*

1. *Any $\wedge\vee$-basis Ψ_1 of the set of formulas $\Phi_{\preceq_1}$ is a set of formulas having the smallest possible number of elements such that $\widetilde{CIRCF}(\Psi) = CIRCF(\Psi_1)$.*
2. *The set $\mathbf{F}_{\preceq_0}$ (see Definition 5.2) is the greatest (for $\subseteq$) set of formulas such that $CIRCF(\bar{\Psi}) = CIRCF(\Psi')$. The set of all the sets Ψ' which are c-equivalent to Ψ is the set of the sets Ψ' such that $\preceq_{\Psi'\wedge\vee}$ (i.e. $\preceq_{\Psi'}$) is associated with $\prec$.*

Proof: 1: Lemmas 4.1-1, 5.1-2a and Proposition 6.1.
2: Rewritted from Theorem 3.3: indeed, $\mathbf{F}_{\preceq_0} = Pos_e(\Psi) = I_{CIRCF(\Psi)}$. $\square$

Thus, $\mathbf{F}_{\preceq_1}$ is the "simplest" set Ψ' of formulas closed for $\wedge\vee$, such that $\Psi \equiv_c \Psi'$, for at least three respects: (1) It has the minimal cardinal possible (Lemma 4.1). (2) It has the smallest maximal chain of strict entailment (Lemma 5.2). (3) Any $\wedge\vee$-basis Ψ_1 of $\mathbf{F}_{\preceq_1}$ (i.e. of $\Phi_{\preceq_1}$) is a set with the smallest possible cardinal such that $\Psi \equiv_c \Psi_1$.

7 A Few Examples

When looking for an $\wedge\vee$-basis Y of a set X of formulas as explained in Section 5, we may get a $k = card(Y)$ smaller than the one given by $A(k) \geq n$ (see Proposition 5.4):

Example 7.1. $V(\mathbf{L}) = \{A, B, C\}$, $X = \{A, B, A\wedge C, B\wedge C\}$. We get $\preceq_X$ (Definition 2.4) described as follows: $\mu \preceq_X \nu$ iff $\mu = \nu$ or $\{\mu, \nu\} = \{\emptyset, \{C\}\}$ or $\mu \prec_X \nu$ with $\mu \prec_X \nu$ iff $((\mu \neq \{C\}, \nu \neq \{C\}$ and $\mu \subset \nu)$ or $(\mu = \{C\}$ and $\nu \notin \{\emptyset, \{C\}\}))$.

We get then the following set $\Phi_X = \{\varphi(\mu)\}_{\mu\in\mathcal{P}(V(\mathbf{L}))-\{C\}}$ (Definition 5.2) with: $\varphi(\mu) = \bigwedge_{P\in\mu} P$ (and $\varphi(\{C\}) = \varphi(\emptyset) = \top$). Thus, $\Phi ir_X = X$ (Definition 5.4). The smallest k such that $A(k) \geq 4 = card(\Phi ir_X)$ is $k = 4$, but we can choose $k = 3$. Here is an injective mapping l from Φir_X to a weak antichain in $\{1, 2, 3\}$: $l(A) = \{1\}, l(B) = \{2\}, l(A \wedge C) = \{1,3\}, l(B \wedge C) = \{2,3\}$. As we want to get (1) page 905, l must satisfy, for any φ, ψ in Φir_X: $\varphi \models \psi$ if $l(\psi) \subseteq l(\varphi)$. Let us call $(C :\supseteq\leadsto\models)$ this condition. We define $Y = \{\varphi'_i\}_{i\in\{1,2,3\}}$, as in (2) page 905, getting $\varphi'_1 = A, \varphi'_2 = B, \varphi'_3 = C \wedge (A \vee B)$. Even if l respects $(C :\supseteq\leadsto\models)$, defining φ'_j by (2) does not always imply that we get (1) page 905. However, here (1) is satisfied, thus $CIRCF(X) = CIRCF(Y)$. As $card(Y) = 3$, Y is one of the sets with the smallest cardinality satisfying $Y \equiv_{sc} X$ from Proposition 5.4. As $\preceq_X=\preceq_Y$ is the greatest relation $\preceq_1$ of Definition 4.1, we get that Y is even one of the smallest sets satisfying $Y \equiv_c X$ from Theorem 6.2-1. $\square$

The next example shows how the results given in Sections 5 and 6 allow to find the various sets of formulas describing a given formula circumscription:

Example 7.2. $V(\mathbf{L}) = \{A, B, C\}$. We consider the set $X = \{A \vee B, C \vee (A \wedge B), \neg C \vee (\neg A \wedge \neg B), (A \vee B) \wedge \neg C, A \wedge B \wedge \neg C, A \wedge \neg B \wedge C, \neg A \wedge B \wedge C, A \wedge B \wedge C\}$ and $f = CIRCF(X)$. Here are the relations $\preceq_X$ and $\prec_X$:

$\emptyset \prec_X \mu$ if $\mu \in \mathbf{M} - \{\emptyset\}, \{A\} \prec_X \{A, B\}, \{B\} \prec_X \{A, B\}, \{C\} \prec_X \{A, B\}$.

$\mu \preceq_X \nu$ if $\mu \prec_X \nu$ or $\mu = \nu$ or $\{\mu, \nu\} = \{\{A\}, \{B\}\}$.

Thus, $\Phi_X = \{\varphi(\mu)\}_{\mu \in \mathcal{P}(V(\mathbf{L})) - \{B\}}$ with $\varphi_X(\emptyset) = \top$, $\varphi_X(\{A\}) = (A \vee B) \wedge \neg C$, $\varphi_X(\{C\}) = (A \wedge B \wedge \neg C) \vee (\neg A \wedge \neg B \wedge C)$, $\varphi_X(\{A, B\}) = A \wedge B \wedge \neg C$, $\varphi_X(\{A, C\}) = A \wedge \neg B \wedge C$, $\varphi_X(\{B, C\}) = \neg A \wedge B \wedge C$, $\varphi_X(\{A, B, C\}) = A \wedge B \wedge C$.

Then, $\Phi ir_X = \{\varphi_X(\{A\}), \varphi_X(\{C\}), \varphi_X(\{A, C\}), \varphi_X(\{B, C\}), \varphi_X(\{A, B, C\})\}$.

Even if we are not in case 2 of Proposition 5.4, we are "close enough" to this case and we can apply the constructive method described there. We are looking for a subset Y of $\mathbf{F}_X$, minimal such that $\Phi ir_X \subseteq Y^\wedge$. We must use four elements in $\mathbf{F}_X$: $WA(3) = 4 < 5 = card(\Phi ir_X) \le 7 = WA(4)$. As we have also $A(3) = 3 < 5 \le 6 = A(4)$, we can start from an antichain without bothering with weak antichains. Let us choose the following injective mapping l from Φir_X into an antichain of $\{1, 2, 3, 4\}$: $l(\varphi_X(\{A\})) = \{1, 2\}$, $l(\varphi_X(\{C\})) = \{1, 3\}$, $l(\varphi_X(\{A, C\})) = \{1, 4\}$, $l(\varphi_X(\{B, C\})) = \{2, 3\}$, $l(\varphi_X(\{A, B, C\})) = \{2, 4\}$, which gives, by (2) page 905, $Y_a = \{\varphi_1', \varphi_2', \varphi_3', \varphi_4'\}$ with

$\varphi_1' = \varphi_X(\{A\}) \vee \varphi_X(\{C\}) \vee \varphi_X(\{A, C\}) = (A \vee B \vee C) \wedge (\neg B \vee \neg C)$,
$\varphi_2' = \varphi_X(\{A\}) \vee \varphi_X(\{B, C\}) \vee \varphi_X(\{A, B, C\}) = (A \wedge \neg C) \vee B$,
$\varphi_3' = \varphi_X(\{C\}) \vee \varphi_X(\{B, C\}) = (A \wedge B \wedge \neg C) \vee (\neg A \wedge \neg B \wedge C) \vee (\neg A \wedge B \wedge C)$,
$\varphi_4' = \varphi_X(\{A, C\}) \vee \varphi_X(\{A, B, C\}) = A \wedge C$.

We get a set Y_a of four formulas with $Y_a \equiv_{sc} X$ (thus $f = f_{\prec_X} = CIRCF(Y_a)$) and Proposition 5.4 gives that no set Y_a' with fewer elements exist with $Y_a' \equiv_{sc} X$.

Let us consider now the greatest pre-order $\preceq_1$ associated with $\prec_X$ (Definition 4.1). We get $\mu \preceq_1 \nu$ iff $\mu \prec_X \nu$ or $\mu = \nu$ or $\{\mu, \nu\} \subseteq \{\{A\}, \{B\}, \{C\}\}$ or $\{\mu, \nu\} \subseteq \{\{A, C\}, \{B, C\}, \{A, B, C\}\}$. We get $\Phi_{\preceq_1} = \{\varphi_{\preceq_1}(\mu)\}_{\mu \in \{\langle \emptyset \rangle, \{A\}, \{A, B\}, \{A, C\}\}}$ where $\varphi_{\preceq_1}(\emptyset) = \top$, $\varphi_{\preceq_1}(\{A\}) = ((A \vee B) \wedge \neg C) \vee (\neg A \wedge \neg B \wedge C)$, $\varphi_{\preceq_1}(\{A, B\}) = A \wedge B \wedge \neg C$, $\varphi_{\preceq_1}(\{A, C\}) = (A \vee B) \wedge C$. The set $\Phi ir_{\preceq_1}$ is then $Y_b = \Phi_{\preceq_1} - \{\varphi_{\preceq_1}(\emptyset)\}$, As $WA(2) = 2 < 3 = card(Y_b) \le WA(3) = 4$, Propositions 5.3 and 5.4 state that we need three elements in any subset X' of $\mathbf{F}_{\preceq_1} = (\Phi_{\preceq_1})^\vee$ such that $Y_b \subseteq (X')^\wedge$. Then, Y_b gives an optimal solution. Y_b is thus one of the sets of formulas X' with as few elements as possible such that $f = f_{\prec_X} = CIRCF(X')$. This example shows that choosing the relation $\preceq_1$ instead of $\preceq_X$ (thus a fortiori of $\preceq_0$) allows to get a smaller set of formulas.

From Lemma 4.1-3, we get here $25 = B_3 \times B_3$ pre-orders $\preceq$ associated with $\prec$. $\square$

As a last example, let us apply our results to ordinary circumscription $CIRC(\mathbf{P}, \mathbf{Q}, \mathbf{Z}) = CIRCF(\mathbf{P}; \mathbf{Q}, \mathbf{Z} \cup \mathbf{P}) = CIRCF(\mathbf{P} \cup \mathbf{Q} \cup \neg \mathbf{Q})$. We want to find one of the smallest sets of formulas Ψ where $CIRC(\mathbf{P}, \mathbf{Q}, \mathbf{Z}) = CIRCF(\Psi; \mathbf{Q}, \mathbf{Z} \cup \mathbf{P})$ and we ask the same question for $CIRC(\mathbf{P}, \mathbf{Q}, \mathbf{Z}) = CIRCF(\Psi)$.

For the first problem, we cannot do better than the set $\mathbf{P}$:

Theorem 7.1. *1. $\mathbf{P}$ is one of the sets Ψ with fewer elements such that we have*
$CIRC(\mathbf{P}, \emptyset, \mathbf{Z}) = CIRCF(\Psi; \emptyset, \mathbf{Z} \cup \mathbf{P}) = CIRCF(\Psi)$.

2. $\mathbf{P}$ *is one of the sets* Ψ *with fewer elements such that we have* $CIRC(\mathbf{P}, \mathbf{Q}, \mathbf{Z}) = CIRCF(\Psi; \mathbf{Q}, \mathbf{Z} \cup \mathbf{P})$ *(and it is the simplest such set).*

Sketch of the proof: 1. It is straightforward (not immediate, but automatic) to see that we have, if $X = \mathbf{P}$ is a set of propositional symbols: $l(\Phi_X) = card(\Phi ir_X) = card(X)$. This is an important case where Proposition 5.5 is very precise. Moreover, if we define $\prec = \prec_{(\mathbf{P}, \emptyset, \mathbf{Z})}$ (Definition 2.2) and $\preceq_1$ as in Definition 4.1, we get $\Phi_{\preceq_1} = \{\bigwedge_{P \in \mathbf{P}'} P\}_{\mathbf{P}' \subseteq \mathbf{P}}$ (and $\mathbf{F}_{\preceq_1} = \mathbf{P}^{\wedge \vee}$). Then use Theorem 6.2.

2. Immediate extension of point 1. $\qquad\square$

The second problem is tougher and partially left to any interested reader:

Proposition 7.1. *There exists a set* Ψ *such that we have* $CIRC(\mathbf{P}, \mathbf{Q}, \mathbf{Z}) = CIRCF(\Psi)$ *satisfying* $card(\Psi) = card(\mathbf{P}) + k_{\mathbf{Q}}$ *where* $k_{\mathbf{Q}}$ *is the smallest integer* k *such that the central binomial coefficient* $A(k) = (k, \lfloor k/2 \rfloor)$ *satisfies* $A(k) \geq 2^{card(\mathbf{Q})}$.

Proof: Let $\mathbf{P}, \mathbf{Q}, \mathbf{Z}$ be a partition of $V(\mathbf{L})$ and Φ be the set of formulas $\Phi = \mathbf{P} \cup \mathbf{Q} \cup \neg \mathbf{Q}$. We know that we have $CIRC(\mathbf{P}, \mathbf{Q}, \mathbf{Z}) = CIRCF(\Phi)$. The set of the formulas Φir_Φ contains a subset composed by formulas involving only the symbols of $\mathbf{Q}$. Let us call $\Phi ir(\mathbf{Q})$ this set. This set is the set of the $2^{card(\mathbf{Q})}$ conjunctions of literals involving all the elements of $\mathbf{Q}$. Thus, this set is made of mutually exclusive formulas. The subset $\mathbf{F}(\mathbf{Q})$ of the formulas of $\mathbf{F}_\Phi$ composed by formulas involving only the symbols of $\mathbf{Q}$ is obviously the set $(\mathbf{Q} \cup \neg \mathbf{Q})^{\wedge \vee}$ of all the formulas made in this vocabulary. We use the method of Proposition 5.4 (case 2) for this subset $\Phi ir(\mathbf{Q})$ of Φir_Φ. We choose a set I with $k_{\mathbf{Q}}$ elements and an injective mapping l from $\Phi ir(\mathbf{Q})$ to the set of subsets of I having $\lfloor k/2 \rfloor$ elements. As with (2) page 905, we define the set $\mathbf{B}(\mathbf{Q}) = \{\varphi'(i)\}_{i \in I}$ where $\varphi'(i) = \bigvee_{i \in l(\varphi), \varphi \in \Phi ir(\mathbf{Q})} \varphi$. Then, we get (1) page 905, thus $\mathbf{B}(\mathbf{Q})^{\wedge \vee} = \mathbf{F}(\mathbf{Q})$. As in the proof of case 2 in Proposition 5.4, we cannot do better: $\mathbf{B}(\mathbf{Q})$ is an $\wedge \vee$-basis of $\mathbf{F}(\mathbf{Q})$. Thus, the set $\Psi = \mathbf{P} \cup \mathbf{B}(\mathbf{Q})$ is such that $\Psi^{\wedge \vee} = (\mathbf{P} \cup \mathbf{Q} \cup \neg \mathbf{Q})^{\wedge \vee}$ and we get $CIRC(\mathbf{P}, \mathbf{Q}, \mathbf{Z}) = CIRCF(\Psi)$. $\square$

This proof can easily be extended to prove that this set Ψ is minimal (in cardinality) among the sets Ψ which are unions of subsets of $\mathbf{P}^{\wedge \vee}$ and of subsets of $(\mathbf{Q} \cup \neg \mathbf{Q})^{\wedge \vee}$ and such that we have $CIRC(\mathbf{P}, \mathbf{Q}, \mathbf{Z}) = CIRCF(\Psi)$. However, this does not prove that Ψ is minimal without this condition: we could imagine some tricky subset of $(\mathbf{P} \cup \mathbf{Q} \cup \neg \mathbf{Q})^{\wedge \vee}$ with fewer elements. We tend to think that this choice is optimal:

Conjecture 7.2. *Any set* Ψ *such that* $CIRC(\mathbf{P}, \mathbf{Q}, \mathbf{Z}) = CIRCF(\Psi)$ *has at least* $card(\mathbf{P}) + k_{\mathbf{Q}}$ *elements.* $\square$

Example 7.3. $\mathbf{P} = \{P\}, \{\mathbf{Q}\} = \{Q_1, Q_2, Q_3\}, \mathbf{Z} = \emptyset$.

We get $card(\Phi ir(\mathbf{Q})) = 2^3 = 8$, $card(\mathbf{Q} \cup \neg \mathbf{Q}) = 2 \times 3 = 6$ and $A(5) = (5, 2) = 10 \geq 8$. Thus, the set $\mathbf{B}(\mathbf{Q})$ has 5 elements, which is better than $\mathbf{Q} \cup \neg \mathbf{Q}$. The difference is not negligible, as when $q = card(\mathbf{Q})$ tends to infinity, $\mathbf{Q} \cup \neg \mathbf{Q}$ has $2 \times q$ elements while $k_{\mathbf{Q}} = card(\mathbf{B}(\mathbf{Q}))$ is approximated by $q + \ln(q)$. Here is a possible mapping l, from $\Phi ir(\mathbf{Q})$ to $\mathcal{I}$, a set of subsets of $I = \{1, \cdots, 5\}$ with two elements:

$l(Q_1 \wedge Q_2 \wedge Q_3) = \{1, 2\}, \quad l(Q_1 \wedge Q_2 \wedge \neg Q_3) = \{1, 3\}, \quad l(Q_1 \wedge \neg Q_2 \wedge Q_3) = \{1, 4\},$
$l(Q_1 \wedge \neg Q_2 \wedge \neg Q_3) = \{1, 5\}, \quad l(\neg Q_1 \wedge Q_2 \wedge Q_3) = \{2, 3\}, \quad l(\neg Q_1 \wedge Q_2 \wedge \neg Q_3) = \{2, 4\},$
$l(\neg Q_1 \wedge \neg Q_2 \wedge Q_3) = \{2, 5\}, \quad l(\neg Q_1 \wedge \neg Q_2 \wedge \neg Q_3) = \{3, 4\}.$

We get then $\mathbf{B}(\mathbf{Q}) = \{\varphi'(i)\}_{i \in \{1,\cdots,5\}}$ with:

$\varphi'(1) = Q_1 [= (Q_1 \wedge Q_2 \wedge Q_3) \vee (Q_1 \wedge Q_2 \wedge \neg Q_3) \vee (Q_1 \wedge \neg Q_2 \wedge Q_3) \vee (Q_1 \wedge \neg Q_2 \wedge \neg Q_3)]$,

$\varphi'(2) = (\neg Q_1 \wedge (Q_2 \vee Q_3)) \vee (Q_2 \wedge Q_3) = l^{-1}(\{1,2\}) \vee^{-1}(\{2,3\}) \vee^{-1}(\{2,4\}) \vee^{-1}(\{2,5\})$,

$\varphi'(3) = (Q_1 \wedge Q_2 \wedge \neg Q_3) \vee (\neg Q_1 \wedge Q_2 \wedge Q_3) \vee (\neg Q_1 \wedge \neg Q_2 \wedge \neg Q_3)]$,

$\varphi'(4) = (Q_1 \wedge \neg Q_2 \wedge Q_3) \vee (\neg Q_1 \wedge Q_2 \wedge \neg Q_3) \vee (\neg Q_1 \wedge \neg Q_2 \wedge \neg Q_3)]$,

$\varphi'(5) = \neg Q_2 \wedge \neg (Q_1 \Leftrightarrow Q_3) \quad [= (Q_1 \wedge \neg Q_2 \wedge \neg Q_3) \vee (\neg Q_1 \wedge \neg Q_2 \wedge Q_3)]$.

Thus, we get as our set Ψ (which in this simple case can be proved to have as few elements as possible) the set $\Psi = \{P\} \cup \mathbf{B}(\mathbf{Q})$ with $CIRC(\mathbf{P}, \mathbf{Q}, \mathbf{Z}) = CIRCF(\Psi)$. $\Box$

Even if we gain a significative number of formulas with respect to the obvious set $\Psi = \mathbf{P} \cup \mathbf{Q} \cup \neg \mathbf{Q}$ when $\mathbf{Q}$ is big enough, the formulas involved are more complicated. However, it is interesting to know that the set $\mathbf{P} \cup \mathbf{Q} \cup \neg \mathbf{Q}$ is not optimal in cardinality, when we allow to replace the set $\mathbf{Q} \cup \neg \mathbf{Q}$ by another subset of $(\mathbf{Q} \cup \neg \mathbf{Q})^{\wedge \vee}$. Conjecture 7.2 (not absolutely certain...) states that even if we allow to "break" the set $(\mathbf{Q} \cup \neg \mathbf{Q})^{\wedge \vee}$, i.e. to forget the information that $\mathbf{Q}$ must be fixed, we cannot do better.

8 Conclusion and Perspective

We have described all the sets of formulas Φ which, when circumscribed, give rise to the same result as a given set Ψ. Also, we have described all the sets Φ which, when completed by any arbitrary set Φ', give rise to the same result as a given set Ψ, when completed by Φ'. Our description is syntactical and very simple in the second case ("strong equivalence"). In the first case ("ordinary equivalence"), we have described a method to get all the possible sets. The method is fully constructive if we consider only sets of formulas which are closed for $\wedge$ and $\vee$ (or for $\wedge$ alone, or $\vee$, thanks to the constructive definitions of the $\wedge$-basis and $\vee$-basis). In particular, we have described the unique greatest and the unique smallest (for set inclusion) such sets which are equivalent to a given set. Also, we have described the greatest (unique, it is the same one as the preceding greatest set) set of formulas which is equivalent to a given set, without other condition. The problem of finding the smallest sets (in terms of cardinality, there is no longer uniqueness here) involves the search for one of the smallest sets having the same closure for $\wedge$ and $\vee$ than a given set of formulas. We have described a semi constructive method for finding these sets in all the cases. The method is fully constructive in two particular but instructive cases, which help finding the solution for more general cases. One of these cases is when we start from an ordinary circumscription $CIRC(\mathbf{P}, \mathbf{Q}, \mathbf{Z})$ where the propositional symbols of $\mathbf{P}$ are circumscribed and those of $\mathbf{Q}$ fixed. In this case, we have proved that the natural and well known set of formulas $\mathbf{P} \cup \mathbf{Q} \cup \neg \mathbf{Q}$ is one of the a smallest possible sets of formulas Ψ which keeps unchanged the set $\mathbf{Q} \cup \neg \mathbf{Q}$ of the fixed literals. More surprisingly, we have shown that we can do better if we allow modifications inside the set of the fixed propositions, and conjectured that our proposition is still the best one, if we "forget the fixed propositions" altogether.

As future work, we should extend these results to the infinite propositional case, then to the predicate case.

Let us add a few words about the importance of such a study. Firstly, this is one of the most fundamental questions to ask: when sets of formulas are equivalent for what we do with them. Secondly, this could help the automatic computation, as we could choose the "easiest" equivalent sets in order to make the computation of a given circumscription. Clearly. a lot of work remains in that direction. Thirdly, this could help the modelization by circumscriptions of complex situations. The idea is to associate with each rule a set of formulas to be circumscribed. Then, in order to combine rules, we would combine the sets. For defining such combinations, it is important to know precisely what are these "sets" and the notions of equivalence give the answers.

References

1. Ian Anderson, *Combinatorics of Finite Sets*, Oxford University Press (Oxford Science Publications), Oxford, 1987.
2. Garret Birkhoff, *Lattice Theory*, American Mathematical Society, 1940, 1948, 1967, Reprinted (1984).
3. Tom Costello, 'The expressive power of circumscription', *Artificial Intelligence*, **104**(1–2), 313–329, (September 1998).
4. B.A. Davey and H.A. Priestley, *Introduction to Lattices and Order*, Cambridge University Press, 1990.
5. Johan de Kleer and Kurt Konolige, 'Eliminating the Fixed Predicates from a Circumscription', *Artificial Intelligence*, **39**(3), 391–398, (July 1989).
6. Michael Freund, 'Preferential reasoning in the perspective of Poole default logic', *Artificial Intelligence*, **98**(1, 2), 209–235, (January 1998).
7. Dan J. Kleitman. personal communication, March 2000.
8. H. M. MacNeille, 'Partially ordered sets', *Transactions of the American Mathematical Society*, **42**, 416–460, (1937).
9. John McCarthy, ' Application of circumscription to formalizing common sense knowledge', *Artificial Intelligence*, **28**(1), 89–116, (February 1986).
10. Yves Moinard and Raymond Rolland, 'Circumscriptions from what they cannot do (Preliminary report)', in *Common Sense'98*, pp. 20–41, University of London, London, (January 1998). http://www.ida.liu.se/ext/etai/nj/fcs-98/listing.html.
11. Yves Moinard and Raymond Rolland, 'Propositional circumscriptions', Technical report, INRIA-IRISA, PI 1211, Rennes, France, (October 1998). http://www.irisa.fr/EXTERNE/bibli/pi/1211/1211.html.
12. Yves Moinard and Raymond Rolland, 'Equivalent sets of formulas for circumscriptions', in *ECAI'2000*, ed., Werner Horn, Berlin, (August 2000). Wiley.
13. Donald Perlis and Jack Minker, 'Completeness results for circumscription', *Artificial Intelligence*, **28**(1), 29–42, (February 1986).
14. Ken Satoh, 'A Probabilistic Interpretation for Lazy Nonmonotonic Reasoning', in *AAAI-90*, pp. 659–664. MIT Press, (1990).
15. Y. Shoham. *Reasoning about change*. MIT Press, Cambridge, 1988.
16. N.J.A Sloane. On-Line Encyclopedia of Integer Sequences. Published electronically at http://www.research.att.com/~njas/sequences/ (as of March, 2000).

A Semantics for Persistency in Propositional Dynamic Logic

Jan Broersen[*][1], Roel Wieringa[2], and John-Jules Meyer[3]

[1] Faculty of Mathematics and Computer Science, *Vrije Universiteit*
De Boelelaan 1081a, 1081 HV Amsterdam, The Netherlands
broersen@cs.vu.nl
[2] Faculty of Computer Science, *University of Twente*
P.O. Box 217, 7500 AE Enschede, The Netherlands
roelw@cs.utwente.nl
[3] Intelligent Systems Group, Department of Computer Science, *Universiteit Utrecht*
Padualaan 14, 3584 CH Utrecht, The Netherlands
jj@cs.uu.nl

Abstract. This paper defines a minimal change semantics for PDL, that is based on minimization over a change ordering of labeled Kripke models. The definition of the change ordering has some striking resemblances with the notion of bisimulation. The minimal change semantics for PDL is shown to behave correctly in case of the notorious Yale shooting and stolen car example scenarios.

1 Introduction

Propositional dynamic logic (PDL) is designed to reason about pre- and postcondition properties of actions exhibiting choice ($\cup$), sequence (;), iteration (*), and test (ϕ?). The formalism has applications in many areas, for instance in normative reasoning [4][13], agent-performed reasoning about action [15][17] and epistemic updates [14][20] and planning [21]. In many of the application areas of PDL, the frame problem is encountered. In our formulation the problem reads as follows.

The Frame Problem: when specifying actions declaratively, we do not want to involve ourselves in describing explicitly and exhaustively for each individual action what conditions do *not* change as the result of it.

Solutions to the frame problem require that somehow a concept of 'minimal change' is imposed. Surprisingly many existing approaches that try to deal with the frame problem in modal action logics such as PDL, mostly focus on the representational problem, that is, on the problem how to extend the language such that persistency can be expressed in an easy, intuitive, and economic way. This

---

[*] This work is sponsored by VU-USF as part of the SINS project, and partially supported by the Esprit Working group Aspire, contract nr. 22704

J. Lloyd et al. (Eds.): CL 2000, LNAI 1861, pp. 912–925, 2000.

is even more surprising if we realize that the emphasis in most first-order based approaches [23][22][7][19][2][18] is on the semantics, that is, on the selection of the intuitively intended first-order models of action descriptions. In this paper we aim to fill in this gap, and focus on the semantics of minimal change for PDL. The semantics is based on a minimal change ordering of labeled Kripke structures, the structures that interpret PDL. The change ordering is achieved by turning the notion of semantical equivalence for PDL, *bisimulation*, into an inequivalence by incorporating a subset criterion of changes between states. The main virtues of the resulting non-monotonic semantics for PDL are (1) its generality, dealing with non-determinism, sequence, iteration and test (2) the simplicity of its definition (3) its intuitive appeal, exemplified by its correct behavior in case of the Yale shooting and stolen car scenarios.

In section 2 we first formally introduce PDL. Section 3 discusses some axiomatic approaches to reasoning about persistency, in PDL and in modal action logics in general. In section 4 we present our semantic definition of persistency in full PDL with choice, sequence, iteration and test. We will start with a reformulation of the notion of bisimulation, and proceed by turning this semantical equivalence into an inequivalences that expresses a change-ordering over Kripke models. In section 5 we will test our theory against the Yale shooting and the stolen car scenarios. Section 6 concludes with a discussion.

2 Propositional Dynamic Logic

Given a set $\mathcal{A}$ of action symbols and $a \in \mathcal{A}$, a set $\mathcal{P}$ of proposition symbols and $p \in \mathcal{P}$, a *well formed formula* ϕ of the language $\mathcal{L}(PDL)$ is defined through the following BNF:

$$\phi ::= p \mid \neg\phi \mid \phi \vee \psi \mid \langle \alpha \rangle \phi$$
$$\alpha ::= a \mid \alpha \cup \alpha' \mid \alpha; \alpha' \mid \alpha^* \mid \phi?$$

We will usually refer to propositions $p \in \mathcal{P}$ as *fluents*, emphasiszing that the non-monotonic minimal change semantics for PDL we define in section 4 focuses on the influence of actions on the values of these propositions. We will call α's (*regular*) *actions* or sometimes *programs*. The intended meaning of a PDL formula $\langle \alpha \rangle \phi$ is that it is possible to execute program α and reach a state where ϕ holds. The following definitional extensions are applied: $\phi \wedge \psi \equiv_{def} \neg(\neg\phi \vee \neg\psi)$, $[\alpha]\phi \equiv_{def} \neg\langle\alpha\rangle\neg\phi$, $\phi \rightarrow \psi \equiv_{def} \neg\phi \vee \psi$, $\phi \leftrightarrow \psi \equiv_{def} (\phi \rightarrow \psi) \wedge (\psi \rightarrow \phi)$, $\top \equiv_{def} \phi \vee \neg\phi$ and $\bot \equiv_{def} \neg\top$.

To interpret PDL, we use standard Kripke models whose transitions are parameterized with respect to actions $a \in \mathcal{A}$. We call these *labeled* Kripke structures (LKSs).

Definition 1. *Given a set $\mathcal{A}$ of action symbols and a set $\mathcal{P}$ of proposition symbols, a structure $\mathcal{S} = \langle S, \pi, R_{\mathcal{A}} \rangle$ is defined as:*

- S is a nonempty set of possible states
- R_A is a set of reachability relations $R_a \subseteq S \times S$ with $a \in \mathcal{A}$
- π is a valuation function $\pi : S \to 2^P$ that assigns to each state s a subset of valid propositions

We use the notation $s \overset{a}{\to} s'$ for an a-transition from state s to s' in a structure $\mathcal{S} = (S, \pi, R_A)$. This notation is extensively used in the definitions of orderings of labeled Kripke structures in section 4.

The semantics of PDL is defined by relating the modality $\langle\,.\,\rangle$. to the reachability relation R_α for regular actions α, which in turn is an extension of the reachability relation R_A for atomic actions a.

Definition 2. *Validity* $\mathcal{S}, s \models \phi$ *of a well-formed formula* ϕ *in a state* s *of a structure* $\mathcal{S}$ *is defined by:*

$$
\begin{aligned}
R_\alpha &= R_a, \text{ for } \alpha = a,\ a \in \mathcal{A} \text{ and } R_a \in R_A \\
R_{\alpha \cup \alpha'} &= R_\alpha \cup R_{\alpha'} \\
R_{\alpha;\alpha'} &= R_\alpha \circ R_{\alpha'} \\
R_{\alpha^*} &= (R_\alpha)^* \\
R_{\phi?} &= \{(s,s) \mid \mathcal{S}, s \models \phi\} \\
\mathcal{S}, s &\models p \quad \text{iff } p \in \pi(s) \\
\mathcal{S}, s &\models \neg\phi \quad \text{iff not } \mathcal{S}, s \models \phi \\
\mathcal{S}, s &\models \phi \wedge \psi \quad \text{iff } \mathcal{S}, s \models \phi \text{ and } \mathcal{S}, s \models \psi \\
\mathcal{S}, s &\models \langle\alpha\rangle\phi \quad \text{iff } \exists s' \in S, \text{ such that } s, s' \in R_\alpha \text{ and } \mathcal{S}, s' \models \phi
\end{aligned}
$$

Validity on a structure $\mathcal{S}$ *is defined as validity in all states of the structure. If* ϕ *is valid on a structure* $\mathcal{S}$, *we say that* $\mathcal{S}$ *is a model for* ϕ[1]. *General validity of a formula* ϕ *is defined as validity on all possible structures. A formula* ϕ *entails a formula* ψ *(notation:* $\phi \models \psi$) *if and only if all models for* ϕ *are also models for* ψ.

Alternatively, the semantics of PDL can be defined by using a *trace* semantics for programs: atomic actions are primitive traces, $\alpha \cup \alpha'$ is defined as the union of the traces that interpret α and α', $\alpha;\alpha'$ is defined as concatenation of the traces of α and α', and finally, α^* is defined as the union of all finitely repeated self-concatenations of the traces that interpret α. Then $\langle\alpha\rangle\phi$ is defined as the existence of a trace from the current state to a state where ϕ holds.

The constructs $\alpha;\alpha'$, $\alpha \cup \alpha'$ and $\phi?$, can also be introduced as definitional extensions of PDL [5]: $[\alpha;\alpha']\phi \equiv_{def} [\alpha][\alpha']\phi$, $[\alpha \cup \alpha']\phi \equiv_{def} [\alpha]\phi \wedge [\alpha']\phi$ and $[\phi?]\psi \equiv_{def} \phi \to \psi$. The iteration cannot be introduced as a definitional extension, which shows that the iteration is responsible for the surplus of expressive power of PDL with respect the multi-modal variant of the basic modal logic K, where modalities are just parameterized with respect to atomic actions a.

In PDL, the intended meaning of formulas of the form $\phi \to [\alpha]\psi$, (which is equivalent to $[\phi?;\alpha]\psi$) is that all executions of α from states where ϕ holds lead

---

[1] Note that we have a clear distinction between structures and models: a model is a structure that is valid for a certain formula.

to states where ψ holds. Formulas of this type appear frequently in applications of dynamic logic, for instance when PDL is used for action domain descriptions in planning. The PDL formula $\phi \rightarrow [\alpha]\psi$ is typically used to describe what changes as the result of the execution of α in the context ϕ. The formula states that it is not possible that if ψ does not hold in the context ϕ, it still does not hold after execution of α. But the formula does not say anything about properties that are independent of ψ; these properties may vary freely over the execution. This is usually not what is intended when formulas $\phi \rightarrow [\alpha]\psi$ are written down. Usually the formula is intended to mean:

> ϕ is a condition under which performing α brings about ψ,
> and nothing else.

To express the 'and nothing else'-part of this intended meaning, we need to able to express that properties are persistent. In the next section we will shortly discuss some approaches.

3   Axiomatic Approaches to Persistency in Modal Action Logics

We discuss three types of approaches: (1) non-monotonic approaches that aim at the definition of intended extensions of modal action logic formulas, as in default logic, (2) monotonic approaches that involve a notion of dependency of fluents on action occurrences, and (3) approaches that only focus on representational aspects.

Of course it is possible to express persistency in PDL by defining completions with the help of formulas of the type $l \rightarrow [a]l$, with l a positive or negated propositional constant, and a an atomic action. But since in more general PDL formulas $\phi \rightarrow [\alpha]\psi$, the actions nor the properties that change value are required to be atomic, the question of how to define such completions intuitively and systematically is far from trivial. Furthermore, the number of frame formulas of the form $l \rightarrow [a]l$ that is needed to complement a general action domain description in PDL to impose the intended meaning, is unacceptably high. One approach that attempts to define completions with formulas of the form $l \rightarrow [a]l$ is that by Giordano, Martelli and Schwind [12]. Their method only applies to the fragment of PDL that contains no iteration. But on the other hand they deal with concurrency. Their basic idea is to define extensions of action descriptions by adding formulas $l \rightarrow [\alpha]l$ in such a way that it is not derivable from the resulting completed description that action α *does* change the value of the literal l. This defines extensions of action theories as in default logic. Weaknesses of the approach are the appearance of multiple extensions, and the absence of iteration.

A second type of approach that might be transposable to the PDL context is that of the 'monotonic' solutions as proposed by Reiter [2][18]. The main idea of this approach is to first take stock of all actions in an action description that may influence a certain atomic property. This way the dependency of value changes of fluents on execution of actions is described explicitly. After this process is completed, formulas (successor state axioms) saying that certain formulas are exclusively influenced by certain actions can be added to impose the intended semantics. A PDL approach, based on the same principles was proposed by De Giacomo [6]. If the intended meaning of the formula $\psi \to [\alpha]l$ is that α exclusively changes l, the formulas $\psi \wedge l \to [\sim \alpha]l$ and $\psi \wedge \neg l \to [\sim \alpha]\neg l$ can be used to express that performance of other actions than α leave the value of l unchanged. A crucial element in this representation of persistency properties is the notion of action negation $\sim \alpha$, that is interpreted as 'union of all actions other than α'. De Giacomo does not define a general procedure for addition of formulas of the form $\psi \wedge \neg l \to [\sim \alpha]\neg l$. Furthermore, it is not clear how persistency of fluents *during* execution of α is dealt with. This relates to the stolen car scenario that we discuss in section 5. Castilho, Gasquet and Herzig [10][3] also make use of an explicitation of the dependency of fluents on action occurrences, and use this explicitation to define how formulas of the form $l \to [a]l$ should be added to action descriptions to obtain the intended semantics. Weaknesses of their approach are that they do not consider iteration, and that frame properties are not really economically expressed by using formulas of the form $l \to [a]l$. This relates to the representational frame problem that we discuss next.

The representational frame problem is the problem of how to express persistency properties in an easy, intuitive and economic way. For PDL this was studied by Prendinger [17]. His main contributions are the addition of the following operators to PDL: (1) terminal preservation expressed by $tpress(\phi, \alpha)$, whose meaning is that ϕ holds before and after execution of α, (2) chronological preservation expressed by $cpress(\phi, \alpha)$ whose meaning is that ϕ is preserved *throughout* the execution of α. Prendinger defines the semantics of these constructs together with their axiomatization, and gives soundness and completeness results. But the notions of terminal and chronological preservation as proposed by Prendinger can also be given as definitional extensions.

Definition 3. *Terminal preservation* $tpres(\phi, \alpha)$ *and chronological preservation* $cpres(\phi, \alpha)$ *of* ϕ *over* α, *as a definitional extensions in PDL:*

$$
\begin{aligned}
tpres(\phi, \alpha) &\equiv_{def} \phi \to [\alpha]\phi \\
cpres(\phi, \alpha) &\equiv_{def} tpres(\phi, \alpha) &&\text{for } \alpha \in \mathcal{A} \\
cpres(\phi, \alpha \cup \beta) &\equiv_{def} cpres(\phi, \alpha) \wedge cpres(\phi, \beta) \\
cpres(\phi, \alpha; \beta) &\equiv_{def} cpres(\phi, \alpha) \wedge [\alpha]cpres(\phi, \beta) \\
cpres(\phi, \alpha^*) &\equiv_{def} [\alpha^*]cpres(\phi, \alpha)
\end{aligned}
$$

We omit the proof of our claim that this exactly defines the preservation notions of Prendinger. An implication of the validity of this claim is that the properties $tpress(\phi, \alpha)$ and $cpress(\phi, \alpha)$ do not add expressiveness to PDL, but can be seen as just convenient abbreviations for complex PDL formulas. In this way the preservation constructs contribute to the representational frame problem. Another implication is a refinement of the commonly made claim (e.g. [9]) that in PDL we cannot talk about properties that hold *'along the way'* when executing a program: it is true that we cannot say in PDL for instance *'there is* a possibility to successfully execute α while preserving ϕ along the way', but definition 3 demonstrates that we *can* say '*for all* possible executions of α we preserve ϕ along the way'.

4   A Semantic Definition of Persistency in PDL

In this section we define a non-monotonic minimal change semantics for PDL. A main difficulty to overcome is caused by the fact that actions in PDL are in general sequential. Due to this sequential nature of actions, we will have to define a notion of minimal change that is in a way *distributed* over series of actions that are being performed one after the other. We accomplish this by turning the well known equivalence relation *bisimulation* for PDL into a minimal change ordering of labeled Kripke structures. The definition of bisimulation deals with sequence of actions correctly due to its recursion. This recursion is also responsible for the correct distribution of minimal change over sequential actions in the change ordering we define.

We want to emphasize that the relation with bisimulation is only meaningfull at the structural level of the definitions. What we are not saying, for instance, is that bisimulation is to coarse to distinguish minimal change from non-minimal change in PDL. We just observe that the recursion in the definition of bisumulation, together with the way that it deals with non-determinism, is exactly what is needed in the definition of minimal change for sequential actions too. First we recall the definition of bisimulation [16].

Definition 4. *Let* $\mathcal{S}_1 = (S_1, \pi_1, R_{\mathcal{A}}^1)$ *and* $\mathcal{S}_2 = (S_2, \pi_2, R_{\mathcal{A}}^2)$ *be two LKSs, and let* $s_1 \in S_1$ *and* $s_2 \in S_2$. *Then* $s_1 \sim_{bis} s_2$ *if and only if:*

 - $\pi_1(s_1) = \pi_2(s_2)$
 - $\exists \, s_1 \overrightarrow{a} s_1' \in R_{\mathcal{A}}^1$ *only if* $\exists \, s_2 \overrightarrow{a} s_2' \in R_{\mathcal{A}}^2$, *such that* $s_1' \sim_{bis} s_2'$
 - $\exists \, s_2 \overrightarrow{a} s_2' \in R_{\mathcal{A}}^2$ *only if* $\exists \, s_1 \overrightarrow{a} s_1' \in R_{\mathcal{A}}^1$, *such that* $s_2' \sim_{bis} s_1'$

We want to emphasize two features of the definition of bisimulation: (1) the recursion (2) the way non-determinism of actions is dealt with. The recursion is needed to guarantee semantical equivalence of states under nesting of modalities in modal languages. In PDL modalities may be explicitly nested, but the nesting can also come 'in disguise' through formulas like $[\alpha; \beta]\phi$ which is equivalent to the nested formula $[\alpha][\beta]\phi$. Our notion of minimal-change will also have to deal with nesting of modalities (or equivalently: sequence of actions), which motivates the recursion in the change ordering we define. PDL also deals with non-deterministic choice between actions. In the definition of bisimulation this is reflected by the requirement that an action is possible in one of the states that are compared, *if and only if* the same action is possible in the other state. It is clear that this *should* hold to guarantee semantical equivalence of both states, because otherwise they could simply be distinguished by a formula of the form $\neg\langle a \rangle \top$, where a denotes an action *missing* in one of the states. Our notion of minimal-change will also have to deal with non-determinism. We do not want that the ordering in any way interferes with the *possibility* of execution of actions. Therefore the definition of our change ordering deals with non-determinsim exactly the same way as bisimulation does. Before defining the change ordering, we first extend the notion of bisimulation to complete models. We also anticipate on the definition of the change ordering by defining bisimulation in terms of changes between states. For this we need a notion of difference between states. The next definition defines that the difference between two states is identified with the set of atomic propositions that change value.

Definition 5. *Given a model* $S = (S, \pi, R_\mathcal{A})$*, the difference* $\delta(s_1, s_2)$ *between state* $s_1 \in S$ *and* $s_2 \in S$ *is defined as the set of propositions* $C = (\pi(s_1) \setminus \pi(s_2) \cup (\mathcal{P} \setminus \pi(s_1))) \setminus (\mathcal{P} \setminus \pi(s_2)))$.

Now we extend bisimulation to models, and reformulate it with the help of the notion of difference between states.

Definition 6. *Let* $S_1 = (S_1, \pi_1, R_\mathcal{A}^1)$ *and* $S_2 = (S_2, \pi_2, R_\mathcal{A}^2)$ *be two LKSs, and let* $s_1 \in S_1$ *and* $s_2 \in S_2$*. Then* $s_1 \sim_\delta s_2$ *if and only if:*

- $\exists\, s_1 \overrightarrow{a} s_1' \in R_\mathcal{A}^1$ *only if* $\exists\, s_2 \overrightarrow{a} s_2' \in R_\mathcal{A}^2$*, such that* $\delta(s_1, s_1') = \delta(s_2, s_2')$ *and* $s_1' \sim_\delta s_2'$
- $\exists\, s_2 \overrightarrow{a} s_2' \in R_\mathcal{A}^2$ *only if* $\exists\, s_1 \overrightarrow{a} s_1' \in R_\mathcal{A}^1$*, such that* $\delta(s_2, s_2') = \delta(s_1, s_1')$ *and* $s_2' \sim_\delta s_1'$

And $S_1 \sim_{bis} S_2$ *if and only if:*

- $\exists\, s_1 \in S_1$ *only if* $\exists\, s_2 \in S_2$*, such that* $\pi_1(s_1) = \pi_2(s_2)$ *and* $s_1 \sim_\delta s_2$
- $\exists\, s_2 \in S_2$ *only if* $\exists\, s_1 \in S_1$*, such that* $\pi_2(s_2) = \pi_1(s_1)$ *and* $s_2 \sim_\delta s_1$

Note that the relation $s_1 \sim_\delta s_2$ is *not* equal to the bisimulation relation $s_1 \sim_{bis} s_2$ of definition 4. The relation $s_1 \sim_\delta s_2$ expresses similarity in the *course of changes* during consecutive executions of atomic actions from states s_1 and s_2. We get bisimulation by adding $\pi_1(s_1) = \pi_2(s_2)$, as is done in the second part of the definition. This second part also states that the relation $S_1 \sim_{bis} S_2$ is a *global* bisimulation relation relating all states of S_1 to all states of S_2.

We are now ready to make the turn from semantical equivalence to semantical inequivalence by incorporating minimal change. The only thing we do is replace equality of changes in the above formulation of global bisimulation by a subsetordering of changes.

Definition 7. *Let* $S_1 = (S_1, \pi_1, R_\mathcal{A}^1)$ *and* $S_2 = (S_2, \pi_2, R_\mathcal{A}^2)$ *be two LKSs, and let* $s_1 \in S_1$ *and* $s_2 \in S_2$*. Then* $s_1 \ll_c s_2$ *if and only if:*

- $\exists\, s_1 \overrightarrow{a} s_1' \in R_\mathcal{A}^1$ *only if* $\exists\, s_2 \overrightarrow{a} s_2' \in R_\mathcal{A}^2$*, such that* $\delta(s_1, s_1') \subseteq \delta(s_2, s_2')$ *and* $s_1' \ll_c s_2'$
- $\exists\, s_2 \overrightarrow{a} s_2' \in R_\mathcal{A}^2$ *only if* $\exists\, s_1 \overrightarrow{a} s_1' \in R_\mathcal{A}^1$*, such that* $\delta(s_2, s_2') \supseteq \delta(s_1, s_1')$ *and* $s_2' \gg_c s_1'$

And $S_1 \sqsubseteq_c S_2$ *if and only if:*

- $\exists\, s_1 \in S_1$ *only if* $\exists\, s_2 \in S_2$, *such that* $\pi_1(s_1) = \pi_2(s_2)$ *and* $s_1 \ll_c s_2$
- $\exists\, s_2 \in S_2$ *only if* $\exists\, s_1 \in S_1$, *such that* $\pi_2(s_2) = \pi_1(s_1)$ *and* $s_2 \gg_c s_1$

Intuitively the ordering says that (1) if model S_1 is below or equal to S_2, then for all possibilities in S_1 to do a sequence of actions, there is a possibility in S_2 to do the same sequence of actions, where each individual action in the sequence in S_1 changes *less* than or as much as the corresponding action in the sequence in S_2, and (2) for all possibilities in S_2 to do a sequence of actions, there is a possibility in S_1 to do the same sequence of actions, where each individual action in the sequence in S_2 changes *more* than or as much as the corresponding action in the sequence in S_1. In section 5, where we discuss the stolen car scenario, we show that this definition distributes minimal change over sequence of action correctly. To get an impression of how this ordering deals with non-determinism of actions, in figure 1 we look at some example models of the formula $(\neg a \wedge \neg b \wedge \neg c) \rightarrow [k](a \vee b)$, where k is an *atomic* action.

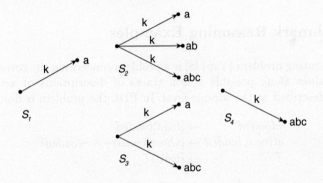

Fig. 1. A comparison of models of $\neg a \wedge \neg b \wedge \neg c \rightarrow [k](a \vee b)$

Clearly all structures in the figure are models of $\neg a \wedge \neg b \wedge \neg c \rightarrow [k](a \vee b)$. Model S_1 is a minimal model under the $\sqsubseteq_c$-ordering, S_2 and S_3 are above S_1 and are indistinguishable from eachother, and S_4 is the model that forms the top of the ordering. Clearly S_1 is not the only minimal model for $\neg a \wedge \neg b \wedge \neg c \rightarrow [k](a \vee b)$ under the $\sqsubseteq_c$-ordering, also the model where action k only makes proposition b true is minimal. And clearly S_2 and S_3 are not the only models that are in between the top model and the minimal models. The figure thus shows only a fragment of the ordering of the models. Metaphorically speaking, going down in the $\sqsubseteq_c$-ordering of models for a PDL-formula ϕ, transitions from certain states look for 'closer' states, that is, states for which it only takes a subset of the current changes to reach them. Of course, they do so under the restriction that they keep satisfying ϕ.

The $\sqsubseteq_c$-ordering is reflexive and transitive, which is to say that it forms a pre-order on LKSs. We define that $S_1 \equiv_c S_2$ if and only if $S_1 \sqsubseteq_c S_2$ and $S_2 \sqsubseteq_c S_1$. The relation $\equiv_c$ defines equivalence classes of models, and we get a partial order by considering the $\sqsubseteq_c$-ordering over these equivalence classes. From definitions

6 and 7 it follows immediately that if two models bisimulate, they cannot be distinguished under the change ordering: $\mathcal{S} \sim_{bis} \mathcal{S}'$ implies $\mathcal{S} \equiv_c \mathcal{S}'$. That the contraposition of this implication does not hold, follows from the above example. It holds that $\mathcal{S}_2 \sqsubseteq_c \mathcal{S}_3$ and $\mathcal{S}_3 \sqsubseteq_c \mathcal{S}_2$. But there is no bisimulation, since the 'middle' transition in $\mathcal{S}_2$ has no equivalent in $\mathcal{S}_3$. But if we restrict ourselves to $\sqsubseteq_c$-minimal models, we do have that two models bisimulate if they cannot be distinguished under the change ordering: $\mathcal{S} \sim_{bis} \mathcal{S}'$ if and only if $\mathcal{S} \equiv_c \mathcal{S}'$. We do not proof this formally here. We only note that this is in agreement with the above example, where $\mathcal{S}_2$ and $\mathcal{S}_3$ are both non-minimal. We now define the non-monotonic minimal change semantics for PDL.

Definition 8. *A PDL formula ϕ preferentially entails ψ under minimal change, notation $\phi \models_c \psi$, if and only if all $\sqsubseteq_c$-minimal models of ϕ are models of ψ.*

In the next section we will demonstrate this minimal change semantics by applying it to the well known Yale shooting and stolen car scenarios.

5   Benchmark Reasoning Examples

The Yale shooting problem (Ysp) [8] is a problem concerning the correct behavior of fluent values along possible action traces of descriptions of actions whose effects are described at the atomic level. In PDL the problem is described as:

$$
\begin{aligned}
\neg loaded &\rightarrow [load]loaded \\
alive \wedge loaded &\rightarrow [shoot](\neg alive \wedge \neg loaded) \\
\top &\rightarrow [wait]\top
\end{aligned}
$$

There are only two fluents in the action description, which implies that minimal models maximally have four states. In each state, each of the actions *load*, *wait* and *shoot* is possible. Figure 2 shows a $\sqsubseteq_c$-minimal model for the Ysp. Transitions with more than one label are used to abbreviate separate transitions relating the same states, and the fluents *loaded* and *alive* are abbreviated to respectively l and a.

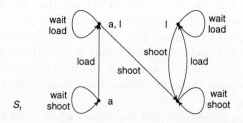

Fig. 2. A minimal Kripke model for the Yale shooting scenario

This is by far not the only minimal model. First of all there are infinitely many models that bisimulate with this model, and where the loops of transitions in certain states are rolled out. As motivated in the previous section all these bisimulating models are minimal under the $\sqsubseteq_c$-ordering. Furthermore, the formulas in our Ysp action description do not extort the possibility of actions in certain situations[2]. Therefore each of the transitions in the above model can be left out to obtain other minimal models. Leaving out transitions in the above model results in minimal models that are not comparable to the above one and to eachother (two models $\mathcal{S}$ and $\mathcal{S}'$ are not comparable if $\mathcal{S} \not\sqsubseteq_c \mathcal{S}'$ and $\mathcal{S}' \not\sqsubseteq_c \mathcal{S}$), since the models will not be equal in the action sequences that are possible. The model of fig 2 is canonical in the sense that minimal models either bisimulate with it or with minimal models that can be formed by leaving out transitions. It is not difficult to perceive that this implies that *all* minimal models satisfy the property: *alive* $\wedge$ ¬*loaded* $\rightarrow$ [*load*; *wait*; *shoot*](¬*alive* $\wedge$ ¬*loaded*).

Most other solutions to the Ysp try to deal with the *trade-off* between the minimizations concerning subsequent actions. The trade-off exists because it is tried to accomplish minimal change of different actions through the minimization of a single abnormality predicate. This results in two extensions for the Ysp scenario: the intended one in which the change of the wait action is none, and that of the shoot action is fatal, and one in which the change in the shoot-action is none and that of the wait-action is, surprisingly, non-empty (the gun becomes unloaded). In our setting, this second extension is just completely non-existent, because the minimal change in the wait action is not 'traded' against minimal change in the shoot action. This means that our semantics does not suffer from the type of problems exemplified by the Yale shooting problem. The solution sketched by Meyer and Doherty [15] behaves well in case of the Ysp for similar reasons. An interesting extension of the Ysp is the one where the *wait*-action is replaced by a *spin*-action that rotates the cylinder of the gun [1]. Our semantics deals with non-determinism in effects of actions, but needs a small extension to deal with this particular type of problems where fluents are explicitly declared *not* to be subject to persistency. We have to constrain the change ordering such that it applies only to changes in fluents that are subject to minimal change. Other propositions are then allowed to change value freely.

In other approaches, the trade-off of minimal change between different actions has elicited answers like *chronological minimization* of changes. This relates to the well-known temporal explanation problem known as 'the stolen car problem' (scp) [11]. The type of problems exemplified by the scp are an important test for our semantics, since they are about the minimal distribution of changes over sequences of actions. In the scp the change concerns the condition that a car becomes stolen. Initially the car is not stolen. Three sequentially performed actions lead from the state where the car is not stolen to the state where it is stolen. In the action description of the scenario, we impose a temporal order on

---

[2] Of course, this is only a choice we made to keep the action description simple. We could also have provided formulas saying for instance that *shoot* is not possible when *loaded* does not hold. Now the action is possible, but has no effect.

the three actions by using formulas of the form $\neg\langle\alpha;\beta\rangle\top$, saying that we cannot execute β immediately after α.

$$\neg\langle wait1; wait3\rangle\top \qquad\qquad \neg\langle wait3; wait2\rangle\top$$
$$\neg\langle wait2; wait1\rangle\top \qquad\qquad \neg\langle wait3; wait1\rangle\top$$
$$\neg stolen \rightarrow [wait1; wait2; wait3]stolen$$

The minimal change semantics also behaves well if we do not force a temporal order on the wait actions. But to be faithfull to the original variant of the problem, we *do* impose the temporal order. The temporal order also makes it simpler to compare the models under the change ordering. And to make the comparison even more simple, in figure 3 we do not compare models globally, but only in a particular point, the starting point of the three subsequent wait actions. To ensure a global comparison of states, many transitions would have to be added, which would obscure the central point of the example.

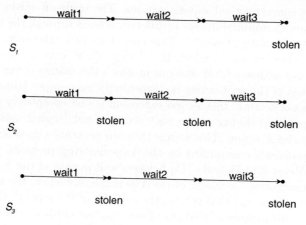

Fig. 3. Models for the stolen car scenario

Model S_1 and S_2 are minimal for the scp action description under the $\sqsubseteq_c$-ordering. That one of the models is not beneath or above the other in the $\sqsubseteq_c$-ordering is easily seen. Both contain the action sequence $wait1, wait2, wait3$. In S_1 the first two of these actions change less than the corresponding ones in S_1, but the third one changes more. So clearly $S_1 \not\sqsubseteq_c S_2$. In S_2 the third action change less than the corresponding one in S_1, but the first two change more. So clearly also $S_2 \not\sqsubseteq_c S_2$. This means that S_1 and S_2 are incomparable. We motivate that nevertheless they are both minimal by comparing them to model S_3. In S_3, after the first wait-action the car is stolen, after the second it has become 'unstolen' mysteriously, and after the third it is stolen again. Clearly here the change from stolen to not stolen is not minimally distributed over the sequence of three actions. If we compare S_1 and S_3, we see that both the first and second wait-action change less, while the third changes as much as the corresponding action in S_3. This means that $S_1 \sqsubseteq_c S_3$ and $S_3 \not\sqsubseteq_c S_1$, meaning that S_1 is beneath S_3 in the ordering. A similar argumentation can be given for the claim that at S_2 is beneath S_3 in the ordering. A third minimal model of the example is of course the one where the stealing takes place during the second wait-action.

6   Discussion

We have defined a non-monotonic minimal change semantics for PDL and we have shown that the semantics behaves well in case of the Yale shooting problem and the stolen car scenario. Our approach contrasts with most other approaches to persistency in modal action logics, for instance with the ones discussed in section 3, in the sense that it is purely semantical. A natural question is whether both types of approaches can be reconciled. But for this to succeed, the axiomatic approaches will have to account for the delicate way in which minimal change is distributed over sequences of actions. Constructs such as $cpress(\phi, \alpha)$ of definition 3 do not help much, because in such examples as the stolen car scenario a construct that defines persistency 'along the way' cannot be used to impose that the change is brought about by either the first, second or third wait action. We know of no axiomatic or proof-theoretic approach that deals with this kind of complexity. However, for nonsequential actions, it might be possible to prove partial soundness and completeness results with respect to for instance the approach by Giordano, Martelli and Schwind [12]. This is a subject for further research. A more fundamental question is whether it is actually possible to define unique completions within PDL that extort the models minimal in the $\sqsubseteq_c$-ordering. It might be the case that this is not possible, and that we need different completions to account for different minimal models.

As observed when we discussed the Yale shooting problem, in some cases (typically in action descriptions consisting of formulas $\psi \rightarrow [\alpha]\phi$ where α is atomic) it is possible to point out a minimal model that is canonical in the sense that all other minimal models either bisimulate with it or with one of the models that can be formed be leaving out certain transitions. We plan to investigate whether these canonical models might be used for model checking.

References

1. C. Baral. Reasoning about actions: non-deterministic effects, constraints and qualification. In *Proceedings of the 14th International Joint Conference on Artificial Intelligence (IJCAI'95)*, pages 2017–2023, 1995.

2. A. Borgida, J. Mylopoulos, and R. Reiter. On the frame problem in procedure specifications. *IEEE Transactions on Software Engineering*, 21:785–798, 1995.

3. Marcos A. Castilho, Olivier Gasquet, and Andreas Herzig. Formalizing action and change in modal logic I: the frame problem. *Journal of Logic and Computation*, 9(5), 1999.

4. F.P.M. Dignum and J.-J.Ch. Meyer. Negations of transactions and their use in the specification of dynamic and deontic integrity constraints. In M.Z. Kwiatkowska,

M.W. Shields, and R.M. Thomas, editors, *Semantics for Concurrency*, pages 61–80. Springer, 1990.

5. K. Fine and G. Schurz. Transfer theorems for stratified multimodal logics. In J. Copeland, editor, *Logic and Reality. Essays in Pure and Applied Logic. In Memory of Arthur Prior*, pages 169–213. Oxford University Press, 1996.

6. Giuseppe De Giacomo and Maurizio Lenzerini. PDL-based framework for reasoning about actions. In *Proceedings of the 4th Congress of the Italian Association for Artificial Intelligence (AI*IA '95)*, Lecture Notes in Artificial Intelligence 992, pages 103–114. Springer-Verlag, 1995.

7. P. Grunwald. Causation and nonmonotonic temporal reasoning. In C. Habel G. Brewka and B. Nebel, editors, *KI-97: Advances in Artificial Intelligence*, pages 159–170. Springer Verlag, Berlin, Germany, 1997. Lecture Notes in Artificial Intelligence no. 1303.

8. S. Hanks and D. Mc Dermott. Default reasoning, nonmonotonic logics, and the frame problem. In *Proceedings of the National Conference on Artificial Intelligence (AAAI86)*, pages 328–333. Morgan Kaufmann Publishers, Inc, 1986.

9. David Harel and Eli Singerman. Computation paths logic: An expressive, yet elementary, process logic (abridged version). In Alberto Marchetti-Spaccamela Pierpaolo Degano, Robert Gorrieri, editor, *Automata, Languages and Programming, 24th International Colloquium, ICALP'97, Bologna, Italy, 7-11 July1997, Proceedings*, pages 408–418. Springer, 1997. Lecture Notes in Computer Science, Vol. 1256.

10. Andreas Herzig and Omar Rifi. Propositional belief base update and minimal change. *Artificial Intelligence Journal*, 115(1):107–138, December 1999.

11. Henry A. Kautz. The logic of persistence. In *Proceedings of the National Conference on Artificial Intelligence (AAAI86)*, pages 401–405. Morgan Kaufmann Publishers, Inc, 1986.

12. Camilla Schwind Laura Giordano, Alberto Martelli. Dealing with concurrent actions in modal action logic. In Henri Prade, editor, *Proceedings ECAI98, 13th European Conference on Artificial Intelligence*, 1998.

13. J. Meyer, W. van der Hoek, and B. van Linder. A logical approach to the dynamics of commitments. *Artificial Intelligence*, 1999.

14. J.-J. Ch. Meyer. Dynamic logic for reasoning about actions and agents. In J. Minker, editor, *Pre-prints Workshop on Logic-Based Artificial Intelligence (LBAI'99, Washington D.C)*, pages 473–484, 1999.

15. John-Jules Ch. Meyer and Patrick Doherty. Preferential action semantics (preliminary report). In J.-J.Ch. Meyer and P.-Y. Schobbens, editors, *Formal Models of Agents*, pages 187–201. Springer, 1999. Lecture Notes in Artificial Intelligence, Vol. 1760.

16. D. Park. Concurrency and automata on infinite sequences. In P. Deussen, editor, *Proceedings 5th GI-Conf. on Theoretical Computer Science*, pages 167–183. Springer, 1981. Lecture Notes in Computer Science, Vol. 104.

17. Helmut Prendinger and Gerhard Schurz. Reasoning about action and change, a dynamic logic approach. *Journal of Logic, Langauge and Information*, 5:209–245, 1996.

18. R. Reiter. The frame problem in the situation calculus: A simple solution (sometimes) and a completeness result for goal regression. In Vladimir Lifschitz, editor, *Artificial Intelligence and Mathematical Theory of Computation: Papers in Honor of John McCarthy*. Academic Press, 1991.

19. Erik Sandewall and Yoav Shoham. Non-monotonic temporal reasoning. In D. M. Gabbay, C. J. Hogger, and J. A. Robinson, editors, *Handbook of Logic in Artificial Intelligence and Logic Programming-Epistemic and Temporal reasoning (Volume 4)*, pages 439–498. Clarendon Press, Oxford, 1994.
20. C. Sierra, J. Godo, R. Lpez de Mntaras, and M. Manzano. Descriptive dynamic logic and its applications to reflective architectures. *Future Generation Computer Systems Journal, Special issue on Reflection and Meta-level AI Architectures*, 12:157–171, 1996.
21. W. Stephan and S. Biundo. A New Logical Framework for Deductive Planning. In *Proceedings IJCAI93*, pages 32–38. Morgan Kaufmann, 1993.
22. Michael Thielscher. Qualified ramifications. In B. Kuipers and B. Webber, editors, *Proceedings of the Fourteenth National Conference on Artificial Intelligence (AAAI)*, Providence, RI, July 1997. MIT Press.
23. Michael Thielscher. From Situation Calculus to Fluent Calculus: State update axioms as a solution to the inferential frame problem. *Artificial Intelligence Journal*, 111(1–2):277–299, 1999.

Applications of Annotated Predicate Calculus to Querying Inconsistent Databases

Marcelo Arenas, Leopoldo Bertossi, and Michael Kifer

[1] P. Universidad Catolica de Chile, Depto. Ciencia de Computacion
Casilla 306, Santiago 22, Chile
{marenas,bertossi}@ing.puc.cl
[2] Department of Computer Science, University at Stony Brook
Stony Brook, NY 11794, USA
kifer@cs.sunysb.edu

Abstract. We consider the problem of specifying and computing consistent answers to queries against databases that do not satisfy given integrity constraints. This is done by simultaneously embedding the database and the integrity constraints, which are mutually inconsistent in classical logic, into a theory in annotated predicate calculus — a logic that allows non trivial reasoning in the presence of inconsistency. In this way, several goals are achieved: (a) A logical specification of the class of all minimal "repairs" of the original database, and the ability to reason about them; (b) The ability to distinguish between consistent and inconsistent information in the database; and (c) The development of computational mechanisms for retrieving consistent query answers, *i.e.*, answers that are not affected by the violation of the integrity constraints.

1 Introduction

Databases that violate stated integrity constraints is an (unfortunate) fact of life for many corporations. They arise due to poor data entry control, due to merges of previously separate databases, due to the incorporation of legacy data, and so on. We call such databases "inconsistent."

Even though the information stored in such a database might be logically inconsistent (and, thus, strictly speaking, *any* tuple should be viewed as a correct query answer), this has not been a deterrent to the use of such databases in practice, because application programmers have been inventing ingenious techniques for salvaging "good" information. Of course, in such situations, what is good information and what is not is in the eyes of beholder, and each concrete case currently requires a custom solution. This situation can be compared to the times before the advent of relational databases, when every database query required a custom solution.

Thus, the problem is: what is the definition of "good information" in an inconsistent database and, once this is settled, what is the meaning of a query in this case. Several proposals to address these problems — both semantically and computationally — are known (*e.g.*, [1]), and we are not going to propose

J. Lloyd et al. (Eds.): CL 2000, LNAI 1861, pp. 926–941, 2000.
© Springer-Verlag Berlin Heidelberg 2000

yet another definition for consistent query answers. Instead, we introduce a new *semantic framework*, based on Annotated Predicate Calculus [9], that leads to a different computational solution and provides a basis for a systematic study of the problem.

Ultimately, our framework leads to the query semantics proposed in [1]. According to [1], a tuple $\bar{t}$ is an answer to the query $Q(\bar{x})$ in a possibly inconsistent database instance r, if $Q(\bar{t})$ holds true in all the "repairs" of the original database, that is in all the databases that satisfy the given constraints and can be obtained from r by means of a "minimal" set of changes (where minimality is measured in terms of a smallest symmetric set difference).

In [1], an algorithm is proposed whereby the original query is modified using the set of integrity constraints (that are violated by the database). The modified query is then posed against the original database (with the integrity constraints ignored). In this way, the explicit integrity checking and computation of all database repairs is avoided.

In this paper, we take a more direct approach. First, since the database is inconsistent with the constraints, it seems natural to embed it into a logic that is better suited for dealing with inconsistency than classical logic. In this paper we use *Annotated Predicate Calculus* (abbr. APC) introduced in [9]. APC is a form of "paraconsistent logic," *i.e.*, logic where inconsistent information does not unravel logical inference and where causes of inconsistency can be reasoned about. APC generalizes a number of earlier proposals [12,11,3] and its various partial generalizations have also been studied in different contexts (*e.g.*, [10]).

The gist of our approach is to embed an inconsistent database theory in APC and then use APC to define database repairs and query answers. This helps understand the results of [1], leads to a more straightforward complexity analysis, and provides a more general algorithm that covers classes of queries not included in [1]. Furthermore, by varying the semi-lattice underlying the host APC theory, it is possible to control how exactly inconsistency is resolved in the original database.

Section 2 formalizes the problem of querying inconsistent databases. Section 3 reviews the basic definitions of Annotated Predicate Calculus, and Section 4 applies this calculus to our problem. In Section 5, we provide a syntactic characterization for database repairs and discuss the associated computational process. Section 6 studies the problem of query evaluation in inconsistent databases and Section 7 concludes the paper.

2   Preliminaries

We assume we have a fixed database schema $P = \{p_1, \ldots, p_n\}$, where $p_1, \ldots, p_n$ are predicates corresponding to the database relations; a fixed, possibly infinite database domain $D = \{c_1, c_2, \ldots\}$; and a fixed set of built-in predicates $B = \{e_1, \ldots, e_m\}$. Each predicate has *arity*, *i.e.*, the number of arguments it takes. An integrity constraint is a closed first-order formula in the language defined by the above components. We also assume a first order language $\mathcal{L} = D \cup P \cup B$ that is based on this schema.

Definition 1. *(Databases and Constraints) A* database instance **DB** *is a finite collection of facts, i.e., of statements of the form* $p(c_1, ..., c_n)$*, where* p *is a predicate in* P *and* $c_1, ..., c_n$ *are constants in* D*.*

An integrity constraint *is a clause of the form*

$$p_1(\bar{T}_1) \vee \cdots \vee p_n(\bar{T}_n) \vee \neg q_1(\bar{S}_1) \vee \cdots \vee \neg q_m(\bar{S}_m)$$

where each p_i *(*$1 \leq i \leq n$*) and* q_j *(*$q \leq j \leq m$*) is a predicate in* $P \cup B$ *and* $\bar{T}_1, ..., \bar{T}_n, \bar{S}_1, ..., \bar{S}_m$ *are tuples (of appropriate arities) of constants or variables. As usual, we assume that all variables in a clause are universally quantified, so the quantifiers are omitted.*

Throughout this paper we assume that both the database instance **DB** and the set of integrity constraints **IC** are consistent when considered in isolation. However, together **DB** $\cup$ **IC** might not be consistent.

Definition 2. *(Sentence Satisfaction) We use* $\models_{DB}$ *to denote the usual notion of formula satisfaction in a database. The subscript* DB *is used to distinguish this relation from other types of implication used in this paper. In other words,*

- **DB** $\models_{DB} p(\bar{c})$*, where* $p \in P$*, iff* $p(\bar{c}) \in$ **DB***;*
- **DB** $\models_{DB} q(\bar{c})$*, where* $q \in B$*, iff* $q(\bar{c})$ *is true;*
- **DB** $\models_{DB} \neg\varphi$ *iff it is not true that* **DB** $\models_{DB} \varphi$*;*
- **DB** $\models_{DB} \phi \wedge \psi$ *iff* **DB** $\models_{DB} \phi$ *and* **DB** $\models_{DB} \psi$*;*
- **DB** $\models_{DB} (\forall X)\phi(X)$ *iff for all* $d \in D$*,* **DB** $\models_{DB} \phi(d)$*;*

and so on. Notice that the domain is fixed, and it is involved in the above definition.

Definition 3. *(IC Satisfaction) A database instance* **DB** *satisfies a set of integrity constraints* **IC** *iff for every* $\varphi \in$ **IC***,* **DB** $\models_{DB} \varphi$*.*

If **DB** *does not satisfy* **IC***, we say that* **DB** *is* inconsistent *with* **IC***. Additionally, we say that a set of integrity constraints is* consistent *if there exists a database instance that satisfies it.*

Next we recall the relevant definitions from [1].

Given two database instances **DB**$_1$ and **DB**$_2$, the *distance* $\Delta(\textbf{DB}_1, \textbf{DB}_2)$ between them is their symmetric difference: $\Delta(\textbf{DB}_1, \textbf{DB}_2) = (\textbf{DB}_1 - \textbf{DB}_2) \cup (\textbf{DB}_2 - \textbf{DB}_1)$. This leads to the following partial order:

$$\textbf{DB}_1 \leq_{\textbf{DB}} \textbf{DB}_2 \quad \text{iff} \quad \Delta(\textbf{DB}, \textbf{DB}_1) \subseteq \Delta(\textbf{DB}, \textbf{DB}_2).$$

That is, $\leq_{\textbf{DB}}$ determines the "closeness" to **DB**. The notion of closeness forms the basis for the concept of a repair of an inconsistent database.

Definition 4. *(Repair) Given database instances* **DB** *and* **DB**′, *we say that* **DB**′ *is a* repair *of* **DB** *with respect to a set of integrity constraints* **IC** *iff* **DB**′ *satisfies* **IC** *and* **DB**′ *is* $\leq_{\textbf{DB}}$-*minimal in the class of database instances that satisfy* **IC**.

Clearly if **DB** is consistent with **IC**, then **DB** is its own repair. Concepts similar to database repair were proposed in the context of database maintenance and belief revision [7,4].

Example 1. (Repairing a Database) Consider a database schema with two unary relations p and q and domain $D = \{a, b, c, \ldots\}$. Let **DB** $= \{p(a), p(b), q(a), q(c)\}$ be a database instance over the domain D and let **IC** $= \{\neg p(x) \lor q(x)\}$ be a set of constraints. This database does not satisfy **IC** because $\neg p(b) \lor q(b)$ is false.

Two repairs are possible. First, we can make $p(b)$ false, obtaining **DB**′ $= \{p(a), q(a), q(c)\}$. Alternatively, we can make $q(b)$ true, obtaining **DB**″ $= \{p(a), p(b), q(a), q(b), q(c)\}$.

Definition 5. *(Consistent Answers) Let* **DB** *be a database instance,* **IC** *be set of integrity constraints and* $Q(\bar{x})$ *be a query. We say that a tuple of constants* $\bar{t}$ *is a* consistent answer *to the query, denoted* **DB** $\models_c Q(\bar{t})$, *if for every repair* **DB**′ *of* **DB**, **DB**′ $\models_{DB} Q(\bar{t})$.

If Q is a closed formula, then true *(respectively,* false*) is a consistent answer to Q, denoted* **DB** $\models_c Q$, *if* **DB**′ $\models_{DB} Q$ *(respectively,* **DB**′ $\not\models_{DB} Q$*) for every repair* **DB**′ *of* **DB**.

3   Annotated Predicate Calculus

Annotated predicate calculus (abbr. APC) [9] is a generalization of annotated logic programs introduced by Blair and Subrahmanian [3]. It was introduced in order to study the problem of "causes of inconsistency" in classical logical theories, which is closely related to the problem of consistent query answers being addressed in our present work. This section briefly surveys the basics of APC used in this paper.

The syntax and the semantics of APC is based on classical logic, except that the classical atomic formulas are annotated with values drawn from a *belief semilattice* (abbr. *BSL*) — an upper semilattice[1] with the following properties:

(i) *BSL* contains at least the following four distinguished elements: **t** (true), **f** (false), ⊤ (contradiction), and ⊥ (unknown);

(ii) For every s ∈ *BSL*, ⊥ ≤ s ≤ ⊤ (≤ is the semilattice ordering);

(iii) lub(**t**, **f**) = ⊤, where lub denotes the least upper bound.

As usual in the lattice theory, lub imposes a partial order on *BSL*: $a \leq b$ iff $b = \text{lub}(a, b)$ and $a < b$ iff $a \leq b$ and a is different from b. Two typical examples of *BSL* (which happen to be complete lattices) are shown in Figure 1. In both

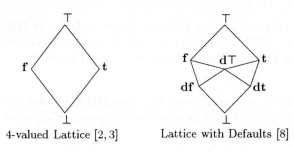

4-valued Lattice [2, 3]   Lattice with Defaults [8]

Fig. 1. Typical Belief Semilattices

of them, the lattice elements are ordered upwards. The specific *BSL* used in this paper is introduced later, in Figure 2.

Thus, the only syntactic difference between APC and classical predicate logic is that the atomic formulas of APC are constructed from the classical atomic formulas by attaching annotation suffixes. For instance, if **s**, **t**, ⊤ are elements of the belief semilattice, then $p(X)$: **s**, q : ⊤, and $r(X, Y, Z)$: **t** all are atomic formulas in APC.

We define only the Herbrand semantics of APC (this is all we need here), and we also assume that the language is free of function symbols (because we are dealing with relational databases in this paper). We thus assume that the *Herbrand universe* is D, the set of all domain constants, and the *Herbrand base*, *HB*, is the set of all ground (*i.e.*, variable-free) atomic formulas of APC.

A *Herbrand interpretation* is any downward-closed subset of *HB*, where a set $I \subseteq HB$ is said to be *downward-closed* iff p : **s** $\in I$ implies that p : **s'** $\in I$ for every **s'** $\in BSL$ such that **s'** $\leq$ **s**. Formula satisfaction can then be defined as follows, where ν is a variable assignment that gives a value in D to every variable:

- $I \models_\nu p$: **s**, where **s** $\in BSL$ and p is a classical atomic formula, if and only if p : **s** $\in I$.
- $I \models_\nu \phi \wedge \psi$ if and only if $I \models_\nu \phi$ and $I \models_\nu \psi$;
- $I \models_\nu \neg\psi$ if and only if not $I \models_\nu \psi$;
- $I \models_\nu (\forall X)\psi(X)$ if and only if $I \models_u \psi$, for *every* u that may differ from v only in its X-value.

It is thus easy to see that the definition of $\models$ looks very much classical. The only difference (which happens to have significant implications) is the syntax of atomic formulas and the requirement that Herbrand interpretations must be downward-closed. The implication $a \longleftarrow b$ is also defined classically, as $a \vee \neg b$.

It turns out that whether or not APC has a complete proof theory depends on which semilattice is used. It is shown in [9] that for a very large and natural class of semilattices (which includes all finite semilattices), APC has a sound and complete proof theory.

---

[1] That is, the least upper bound, $\mathtt{lub}(a, b)$, is defined for every pair of elements $a, b \in BSL$.

The reason why APC is useful in analyzing inconsistent logical theories is because classical theories can be embedded in APC in various ways. The most useful types of embeddings are those where theories that are inconsistent in classical logic become consistent in APC. It then becomes possible to reason about the embedded theories and gain insight into the original inconsistent theory.

The two embeddings defined in [9] are called *epistemic* and *ontological*. Under the epistemic embedding, a (classically inconsistent) set of formulas such as $\mathbf{S} = \{p(1),\ \neg p(1),\ q(2)\}$ is embedded in APC as $\mathbf{S}^e = \{p(1) : \mathbf{t},\ p(1) : \mathbf{f},\ q(2) : \mathbf{t}\}$ and under the ontological embedding it is embedded as $\mathbf{S}^o = \{p(1) : \mathbf{t},\ \neg p(1) : \mathbf{t},\ q(2) : \mathbf{t}\}$.[2] In the second case, the embedded theory is still inconsistent in APC, but in the first case it does have a model: the downward closure of $\{p(1) : \top,\ q(2) : \mathbf{t}\}$. In this model, $p(1)$ is annotated with $\top$, which signifies that its truth value is "inconsistent." In contrast, the truth value of $q(2)$ is $\mathbf{t}$. More precisely, while both $q(2)$ and $\neg q(2)$ follow from $\mathbf{S}$ in classical logic, because $\mathbf{S}$ is inconsistent, only $q(2) : \mathbf{t}$ (but not $q(2) : \mathbf{f}$!) is implied by $\mathbf{S}^e$. Thus, $q(2)$ can be seen as a consistent answer to the query $? - q(X)$ with respect to the inconsistent database $\mathbf{S}$.

In [9], epistemic embedding has been shown to be a suitable tool for analyzing inconsistent classical theories. However, this embedding does not adequately capture the inherent lack of symmetry present in our setting, where inconsistency arises due to the incompatibility of two distinct sets of formulas (the database and the constraints) and only one of these sets (the database) is allowed to change to restore consistency. To deal with this problem, we develop a new type of embedding into APC. It uses a 10-valued lattice depicted in Figure 2, and is akin to the epistemic embedding of [9], but it also has certain features of the ontological embedding.

The above simple examples illustrate one important property of APC: a set of formulas, $\mathbf{S}$, might be *ontologically consistent* in the sense that it might have a model, but it might be *epistemically inconsistent* (abbr. *e-inconsistent*) in the sense that $\mathbf{S} \models p : \top$ for some p, *i.e.*, $\mathbf{S}$ contains at least one inconsistent fact. Moreover, $\mathbf{S}$ can be e-consistent (*i.e.*, it might not imply $p : \top$ for any p), but each of its models in APC might contain an inconsistent fact nonetheless (this fact must then be different in each model, if $\mathbf{S}$ is e-consistent).

It was demonstrated in [9] that ordering models of APC theories according to the amount of inconsistency they contain can be useful for studying the problem of recovering from inconsistency. To illustrate this order, consider $\mathbf{S} = \{p : \mathbf{t},\ p : \mathbf{f} \vee q : \mathbf{t},\ p : \mathbf{f} \vee q : \mathbf{f}\}$ and some of its models:

$\mathcal{M}_1$, where $p : \top$ and $q : \top$ are true;
$\mathcal{M}_2$, where $p : \top$ and $q : \bot$ are true;
$\mathcal{M}_3$, where $p : \mathbf{t}$ and $q : \top$ are true.

Among these models, both $\mathcal{M}_2$ and $\mathcal{M}_3$ contain strictly less inconsistent information than $\mathcal{M}_1$ does. In addition, $\mathcal{M}_2$ and $\mathcal{M}_3$ contain incomparable amounts

---

[2] $\neg p : \mathbf{v}$ is to be always read as $\neg(p : \mathbf{v})$.

of information, and they are both "minimal" with respect to the amount of inconsistent information that they have. This leads to the following definition.

Definition 6. *(E-Consistency Order)   Given $\Delta \subseteq BSL$, a semantic struc-ture I_1 is more (or equally) e-consistent than I_2 with respect to Δ (denoted $I_2 \leq_\Delta I_1$) if and only if for every atom $p(t_1, \ldots, t_k)$ and $\lambda \in \Delta$, whenever $I_1 \models p(t_1, \ldots, t_k) : \lambda$ then also $I_2 \models p(t_1, \ldots, t_k) : \lambda$.*

I is most e-consistent *in a class of semantic structures with respect to Δ, if no semantic structure in this class is strictly more e-consistent with respect to Δ than I (i.e., for every J in the class, $I \leq_\Delta J$ implies $J \leq_\Delta I$).*

4   Embedding Databases in APC

One way to find reliable answers to a query over an inconsistent database is to find an algorithm that implements the definition of consistent answers. While this approach has been successfully used in [1], it is desirable to see it as part of a bigger picture, because consistent query answers were defined at the meta-level, without an independent logical justification. A more general framework might (and does, as we shall see) help study the problem both semantically and algorithmically.

Our new approach is to embed inconsistent databases into APC and study the ways to eliminate inconsistency there. A similar problem was considered in [9] and we are going to adapt some key ideas from that work. In particular, we will define an embedding, $\mathcal{T}$, such that the repairs of the original database are precisely the models (in the APC sense) of the embedded database. This embedding is described below.

First, we define a special 10-valued lattice, $\mathcal{L}^{\mathbf{db}}$, which defines the truth values appropriate for our problem. The lattice is shown in Figure 2. The values $\perp$, $\top$, $\mathbf{t}$ and $\mathbf{f}$ signify undefinedness, inconsistency, truth, and falsehood, as usual. The other six truth values are explained below.

Informally, values $\mathbf{t_c}$ and $\mathbf{f_c}$ signify the truth values as they should be for the purpose of constraint satisfaction. The values $\mathbf{t_d}$ and $\mathbf{f_d}$ are the truth values as they should be according to the database **DB**. Finally, $\mathbf{t_a}$ and $\mathbf{f_a}$ are the *advisory* truth values. Advisory truth values are intended as keepers of the information that helps resolve conflicts between constraints and the database.

Notice that $\mathtt{lub}(\mathbf{f_d}, \mathbf{t_c})$ is $\mathbf{t_a}$ and $\mathtt{lub}(\mathbf{t_d}, \mathbf{f_c})$ is $\mathbf{f_a}$. This means that in case of a conflict between the constraints and the database the advise is to change the truth value of the corresponding fact to the one prescribed by the constraints. Intuitively, the facts that are assigned the advisory truth values are the ones that are to be removed or added to the database in order to satisfy the constraints. The gist of our approach is in finding an embedding of **DB** and **IC** into APC to take advantage of the above truth values.

Embedding the ICs. Given a set of integrity constraints **IC**, we define a new theory, $\mathcal{T}(\mathbf{IC})$, which contains three kinds of formulas:

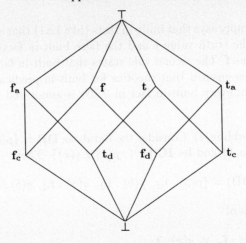

Fig. 2. The lattice $\mathcal{L}^{db}$ with *constraints values*, *database values* and *advisory values*.

1. For every constraint in **IC**:

$$p_1(\bar{T}_1) \quad \vee \quad \cdots \quad \vee \quad p_n(\bar{T}_n) \quad \vee \quad \neg q_1(\bar{S}_1) \quad \vee \quad \cdots \quad \vee \quad \neg q_m(\bar{S}_m),$$

$\mathcal{T}(\mathbf{IC})$ has the following formula:

$$p_1(\bar{T}_1) : \mathbf{t_c} \vee \cdots \vee p_n(\bar{T}_n) : \mathbf{t_c} \vee q_1(\bar{S}_1) : \mathbf{f_c} \vee \cdots \vee q_m(\bar{S}_m) : \mathbf{f_c}.$$

In other words, positive literals are embedded using the "constraint-true" truth value, $\mathbf{t_c}$, and negative literals are embedded using the "constraint-false" truth value $\mathbf{f_c}$.

2. For every predicate symbol $p \in P$, the following formulas are in $\mathcal{T}(\mathbf{IC})$:

$$p(\bar{x}) : \mathbf{t_c} \vee p(\bar{x}) : \mathbf{f_c}, \quad \neg \, p(\bar{x}) : \mathbf{t_c} \vee \neg \, p(\bar{x}) : \mathbf{f_c}.$$

Intuitively, this says that every embedded literal must be either constraint-true or constraint-false (and not both).

Embedding Database Facts. $\mathcal{T}(\mathbf{DB})$, the embedding of the database facts into APC is defined as follows:

1. For every fact $p(\bar{a})$, where $p \in P$: if $p(\bar{a}) \in \mathbf{DB}$, then $p(\bar{a}) : \mathbf{t_d} \in \mathcal{T}(\mathbf{DB})$; if $p(\bar{a}) \notin \mathbf{DB}$, then $p(\bar{a}) : \mathbf{f_d} \in \mathcal{T}(\mathbf{DB})$.

Embedding Built-In Predicates. $\mathcal{T}(\mathcal{B})$, the result of embedding of the built-in predicates into APC is defined as follows:

1. For every built-in fact $p(\bar{a})$, where $p \in B$, the fact $p(\bar{a}) : \mathbf{t}$ is in $\mathcal{T}(\mathcal{B})$ iff $p(\bar{a})$ is true. Otherwise, if $p(\bar{a})$ is false then $p(\bar{a}) : \mathbf{f} \in \mathcal{T}(\mathcal{B})$.

2. $\neg \, p(\bar{x}) : \top \in \mathcal{T}(\mathcal{B})$, for every built-in $p \in B$.

The former rule simply says that built-in facts (like 1=1) that are true in classical sense must have the truth value **t** and the false built-in facts (*e.g.*, 2=3) must have the truth value **f**. The second rule states that built-in facts cannot be both true and false. This ensures that theories for built-in predicates are embedded in 2-valued fashion: every built-in fact in $\mathcal{T}(\mathcal{B})$ is annotated with either **t** or **f**, but not both.

Example 2. (Embedding, I) Consider the database $\mathbf{DB} = \{p(a), p(b), q(a)\}$ over the domain $D = \{a, b\}$ and let **IC** be $\{\neg p(x) \vee q(x)\}$. Then

$$\mathcal{T}(\mathbf{DB}) = \{p(a) : \mathbf{t_d},\ p(b) : \mathbf{t_d},\ q(a) : \mathbf{t_d},\ q(b) : \mathbf{f_d}\}$$

and $\mathcal{T}(\mathbf{IC})$ consists of:

$$p(x) : \mathbf{f_c} \vee q(x) : \mathbf{t_c},$$
$$p(x) : \mathbf{t_c} \vee p(x) : \mathbf{f_c},\ \neg\, p(x) : \mathbf{t_c} \vee \neg\, p(x) : \mathbf{f_c},$$
$$q(x) : \mathbf{t_c} \vee q(x) : \mathbf{f_c},\ \neg\, q(x) : \mathbf{t_c} \vee \neg\, q(x) : \mathbf{f_c}$$

Example 3. (Embedding, II) Let $\mathbf{DB} = \{p(a, a), p(a, b), p(b, a)\}$, $D = \{a, b\}$, and let **IC** be $\{\neg p(x, y) \vee \neg p(x, z) \vee y = z\}$. It is easy to see that this constraint represents the functional dependency $p.1 \rightarrow p.2$. Since this constraint involves the built-in "=", the rules for embedding the built-ins apply.

In this case, $\mathcal{T}(\mathbf{DB}) = \{p(a, a) : \mathbf{t_d},\ p(a, b) : \mathbf{t_d},\ p(b, a) : \mathbf{t_d},\ p(b, b) : \mathbf{f_d}\}$ and $\mathcal{T}(\mathbf{IC})$ is:

$$p(x, y) : \mathbf{f_c} \vee p(x, z) : \mathbf{f_c} \vee y = z : \mathbf{t_c},$$
$$p(x, y) : \mathbf{t_c} \vee p(x, y) : \mathbf{f_c},\ \neg\, p(x, y) : \mathbf{t_c} \vee \neg\, p(x, y) : \mathbf{f_c}.$$

The embedded theory $\mathcal{T}(\mathcal{B})$ for the built-in predicate "=" is: $(a = a) : \mathbf{t}$, $(b = b) : \mathbf{t}$, $(a = b) : \mathbf{f}$, $(b = a) : \mathbf{f}$, $\neg\, (x = y) : \top$. ☐

Finally, we define $\mathcal{T}(\mathbf{DB}, \mathbf{IC})$ as $\mathcal{T}(\mathbf{DB}) \cup \mathcal{T}(\mathbf{IC}) \cup \mathcal{T}(\mathcal{B})$. We can now state the following properties that confirm our intuition about the intended meanings of the truth values in $\mathcal{L}^{\mathbf{db}}$.

Lemma 1. *If $\mathcal{M}$ is a model of $\mathcal{T}(\mathbf{DB}, \mathbf{IC})$, then for every predicate $p \in P$ and a fact $p(\bar{a})$, the following is true:*

1. $\mathcal{M} \models \neg\, p(\bar{a}) : \top.$
2. $\mathcal{M} \models p(\bar{a}) : \mathbf{t} \vee p(\bar{a}) : \mathbf{f} \vee p(\bar{a}) : \mathbf{t_a} \vee p(\bar{a}) : \mathbf{f_a}.$ ☐

The first part of the lemma says that even if the initial database **DB** is inconsistent with constraints **IC**, every model of our embedded theory is *epistemically consistent* in the sense of [9], *i.e.*, no fact of the form $p(\bar{a}) : \top$ is true in any such model.[3] The second part says that any fact is either true, or false, or it has

---

[3] Note that an APC theory *can* entail $p(\bar{a}) : \top$ and be consistent in the sense that it can have a model. However, such a model must contain $p(\bar{a}) : \top$, which makes it epistemically inconsistent.

an advisory value of true or false. This indicates that database repairs can be constructed out of these embeddings by converting the advisory truth values to the corresponding values **t** and **f**. This idea is explored next.

Given a pair of database instances $\mathbf{DB}_1$ and $\mathbf{DB}_2$ over the same domain, we construct the Herbrand structure $\mathcal{M}(\mathbf{DB}_1, \mathbf{DB}_2) = \langle D, I_P, I_B \rangle$, where D is the domain of the database and I_P, I_B are the interpretations for the predicates and the built-ins, respectively. I_P is defined as follows:

$$
I_P(p(\bar{a})) = \begin{cases}
\mathbf{t} & p(\bar{a}) \in \mathbf{DB}_1,\ p(\bar{a}) \in \mathbf{DB}_2 \\
\mathbf{f} & p(\bar{a}) \notin \mathbf{DB}_1,\ p(\bar{a}) \notin \mathbf{DB}_2 \\
\mathbf{f_a} & p(\bar{a}) \in \mathbf{DB}_1,\ p(\bar{a}) \notin \mathbf{DB}_2 \\
\mathbf{t_a} & p(\bar{a}) \notin \mathbf{DB}_1,\ p(\bar{a}) \in \mathbf{DB}_2
\end{cases} \tag{1}
$$

The interpretation I_B is defined as expected: if q is a built-in, then $I_P(q(\bar{a})) = \mathbf{t}$ iff $q(\bar{a})$ is true in classical logic, and $I_P(q(\bar{a})) = \mathbf{f}$ iff $q(\bar{a})$ is false.

Notice that $\mathcal{M}(\mathbf{DB}_1, \mathbf{DB}_2)$ is not symmetric. The intent is to use these structures as the basis for construction of database repairs. In fact, when $\mathbf{DB}_1$ is inconsistent and $\mathbf{DB}_2$ is a repair, I_P shows how the advisory truth values are to be changed to obtain a repair.

Lemma 2. *Given two database instances $\mathbf{DB}$ and $\mathbf{DB}'$, if $\mathbf{DB}' \models_{DB} \mathbf{IC}$, then $\mathcal{M}(\mathbf{DB}, \mathbf{DB}') \models \mathcal{T}(\mathbf{DB}, \mathbf{IC})$.* ☐

The implication of this lemma is that whenever **IC** is consistent, then the theory $\mathcal{T}(\mathbf{DB}, \mathbf{IC})$ is also consistent in APC. Since in this paper we are always dealing with consistent sets of integrity constraints, we conclude that $\mathcal{T}(\mathbf{DB}, \mathbf{IC})$ is always a consistent APC theory.

We will now show how to generate repairs out of the models of $\mathcal{T}(\mathbf{DB}, \mathbf{IC})$. Given a model $\mathcal{M}$ of $\mathcal{T}(\mathbf{DB}, \mathbf{IC})$, we define $\mathbf{DB}_{\mathcal{M}}$ as:

$$
\{p(\bar{a}) \mid p \in P \text{ and } \mathcal{M} \models\ p(\bar{a}) : \mathbf{t} \vee p(\bar{a}) : \mathbf{t_a}\}. \tag{2}
$$

Note that $\mathbf{DB}_{\mathcal{M}}$ can be an infinite set of facts (but finite when $\mathcal{M}$ corresponds to a database instance).

Lemma 3. *If $\mathcal{M}$ is a model of $\mathcal{T}(\mathbf{DB}, \mathbf{IC})$ such that $\mathbf{DB}_{\mathcal{M}}$ is finite, then $\mathbf{DB}_{\mathcal{M}} \models_{DB} \mathbf{IC}$.*

Proposition 1. *Let $\mathcal{M}$ be a model of $\mathcal{T}(\mathbf{DB}, \mathbf{IC})$. If $\mathcal{M}$ is most e-consistent with respect to $\Delta = \{\mathbf{t_a}, \mathbf{f_a}, \top\}$ (see Definition 6) among the models of $\mathcal{T}(\mathbf{DB}, \mathbf{IC})$ and $\mathbf{DB}_{\mathcal{M}}$ is finite, then $\mathbf{DB}_{\mathcal{M}}$ is a repair of $\mathbf{DB}$ with respect to $\mathbf{IC}$.*

Proposition 2. *If $\mathbf{DB}'$ is a repair of $\mathbf{DB}$ with respect to the set of integrity constraints $\mathbf{IC}$, then $\mathcal{M}(\mathbf{DB}, \mathbf{DB}')$ is most e-consistent with respect to $\Delta = \{\mathbf{t_a}, \mathbf{f_a}, \top\}$ among the models of $\mathcal{T}(\mathbf{DB}, \mathbf{IC})$.*

Example 4. (Repairs as Most e-Consistent Models)   Consider a database instance $\mathbf{DB} = \{p(a)\}$ over the domain $D = \{a\}$ and a set of integrity constraints $\mathbf{IC} = \{\neg p(x) \vee q(x), \ \neg q(x) \vee r(x)\}$. In this case $\mathcal{T}(\mathbf{DB}) = \{p(a) : \mathbf{t_d}, \ q(a) : \mathbf{f_d}, \ r(a) : \mathbf{f_d}\}$, and $\mathcal{T}(\mathbf{IC})$ is

$$p(x) : \mathbf{f_c} \vee q(x) : \mathbf{t_c}, \quad q(x) : \mathbf{f_c} \vee r(x) : \mathbf{t_c},$$
$$p(x) : \mathbf{t_c} \vee p(x) : \mathbf{f_c}, \quad \neg p(x) : \mathbf{t_c} \vee \neg p(x) : \mathbf{f_c},$$
$$q(x) : \mathbf{t_c} \vee q(x) : \mathbf{f_c}, \quad \neg q(x) : \mathbf{t_c} \vee \neg q(x) : \mathbf{f_c},$$
$$r(x) : \mathbf{t_c} \vee r(x) : \mathbf{f_c}, \quad \neg r(x) : \mathbf{t_c} \vee \neg r(x) : \mathbf{f_c}$$

This theory has four models, depicted in the following table:

	$p(a)$	$q(a)$	$r(a)$
$\mathcal{M}_1$	t	$\mathbf{t_a}$	$\mathbf{t_a}$
$\mathcal{M}_2$	$\mathbf{f_a}$	f	f
$\mathcal{M}_3$	$\mathbf{f_a}$	f	$\mathbf{t_a}$
$\mathcal{M}_4$	$\mathbf{f_a}$	$\mathbf{t_a}$	$\mathbf{t_a}$

It is easy to verify that $\mathcal{M}_1$ and $\mathcal{M}_2$ are the most e-consistent models with respect to $\Delta = \{\mathbf{t_a}, \mathbf{f_a}, \top\}$ among the models in the table and the database instance $\mathbf{DB}_{\mathcal{M}_1} = \{p(a), q(a), r(a)\}$ and $\mathbf{DB}_{\mathcal{M}_2} = \emptyset$ are exactly the repairs of $\mathbf{DB}$ with respect to $\mathbf{IC}$.

Example 5. (Example 3 Continued)   The embedding of the database described in Example 3 has nine models listed in the following table. The table omits the built-in "$=$", since it has the same interpretation in all models.

	$p(a,a)$	$p(a,b)$	$p(b,a)$	$p(b,b)$
$\mathcal{M}_1$	t	$\mathbf{f_a}$	t	f
$\mathcal{M}_2$	t	$\mathbf{f_a}$	$\mathbf{f_a}$	f
$\mathcal{M}_3$	t	$\mathbf{f_a}$	$\mathbf{f_a}$	$\mathbf{t_a}$
$\mathcal{M}_4$	$\mathbf{f_a}$	t	t	f
$\mathcal{M}_5$	$\mathbf{f_a}$	t	$\mathbf{f_a}$	f
$\mathcal{M}_6$	$\mathbf{f_a}$	t	$\mathbf{f_a}$	$\mathbf{t_a}$
$\mathcal{M}_7$	$\mathbf{f_a}$	$\mathbf{f_a}$	t	f
$\mathcal{M}_8$	$\mathbf{f_a}$	$\mathbf{f_a}$	$\mathbf{f_a}$	f
$\mathcal{M}_9$	$\mathbf{f_a}$	$\mathbf{f_a}$	$\mathbf{f_a}$	$\mathbf{t_a}$

It is easy to see that $\mathcal{M}_1$ and $\mathcal{M}_4$ are the most e-consistent models with respect to $\Delta = \{\mathbf{t_a}, \mathbf{f_a}, \top\}$ among the models in the table, and the database instances $\mathbf{DB}_{\mathcal{M}_1} = \{p(a,a), \ p(b,a)\}$, and $\mathbf{DB}_{\mathcal{M}_4} = \{p(a,b), \ p(b,a)\}$ are exactly the repairs of $\mathbf{DB}$ with respect to $\mathbf{IC}$.

5   Repairing Inconsistent Databases

To construct all possible repairs of a database, $\mathbf{DB}$, that is inconsistent with the integrity constraints $\mathbf{IC}$, we need to find the set of all ground clauses of the form

$$\mathbf{p}_1 : ?_\mathbf{a} \vee \cdots \vee \mathbf{p}_n : ?_\mathbf{a}, \tag{3}$$

that are implied by $\mathcal{T}(\mathbf{DB}, \mathbf{IC})$, where each $?_\mathbf{a}$ is either $\mathbf{t_a}$ or $\mathbf{f_a}$. Such clauses are called *a-clauses*, for advisory clauses.[4]

A-clauses are important because one of the disjuncts of such a clause must be true in each model of $\mathcal{T}(\mathbf{DB}, \mathbf{IC})$. Suppose that, say, $\mathbf{p} : ?_\mathbf{a}$ is true in some model I. This means that the truth value of $\mathbf{p}$ with respect to the database is exactly the opposite of what is required in order for I to satisfy the constraints. This observation can be used to construct a repair of the database by reversing the truth value of $\mathbf{p}$ with respect to the database. We explore this idea next.

Constructing Database Repairs. Let $\mathcal{T}^\mathbf{a}(\mathbf{DB}, \mathbf{IC})$ be the set of all *minimal a-clauses* that are implied by $\mathcal{T}(\mathbf{DB}, \mathbf{IC})$. "Minimal" here means that no disjunct can be removed from any clause in $\mathcal{T}^\mathbf{a}(\mathbf{DB}, \mathbf{IC})$ and still have the clause implied by $\mathcal{T}(\mathbf{DB}, \mathbf{IC})$.

In general, this can be an infinite set, but in most practical cases this set is finite. Conditions for finiteness of $\mathcal{T}^\mathbf{a}(\mathbf{DB}, \mathbf{IC})$ are given in Section 5.1. If $\mathcal{T}^\mathbf{a}(\mathbf{DB}, \mathbf{IC})$ is finite, it can be represented as the following set of clauses:

$$C_1 = \mathbf{p}_{1,1} : \mathbf{a}_{1,1} \vee \cdots \vee \mathbf{p}_{1,n_1} : \mathbf{a}_{1,n_1}$$
$$\cdot \qquad \cdot \qquad \cdot$$
$$C_k = \mathbf{p}_{k,1} : \mathbf{a}_{k,1} \vee \cdots \vee \mathbf{p}_{k,n_k} : \mathbf{a}_{k,n_k}$$

Here, the $\mathbf{p}_{i,j} : \mathbf{a}_{i,j}$ are ground positive literals and their annotations, $\mathbf{a}_{i,j}$, are always of the form $\mathbf{t_a}$ or $\mathbf{f_a}$.

It can be shown that all *a-clauses* can be generated using the APC resolution inference rule [9] between $\mathcal{T}(\mathbf{IC})$, $\mathcal{T}(\mathbf{DB})$, and $\mathcal{T}(\mathcal{B})$. It can be also shown that all *a*-clauses generated in this way are ground and do not contain built-in predicates.

Given $\mathcal{T}^\mathbf{a}(\mathbf{DB}, \mathbf{IC})$ as above, a *repair signature* is a set of APC literals that contains at least one literal from each clause C_i and is minimal in the sense that no proper subset has a literal from each C_i. In other words, a repair signature is a minimal hitting set of the family of clauses $C_1, \ldots, C_k$ [6].

Notice that if the clauses C_i do not share literals, then each repair signature contains exactly k literals and every literal appearing in a clause C_i belongs to some repair signature.

It follows from the construction of repairs in (2) and from Propositions 1 and 2 that there is a one to one correspondence between repair signatures and repairs of the original database instance $\mathbf{DB}$. Given a repair signature $\mathtt{Repair}$, a repair $\mathbf{DB}'$ can be obtained from $\mathbf{DB}$ by removing the tuples $\mathbf{p}(\bar{t})$, if $\mathbf{p}(\bar{t}) : \mathbf{f_a} \in \mathtt{Repair}$, and inserting the tuples $\mathbf{p}(\bar{t})$, if $\mathbf{p}(\bar{t}) : \mathbf{t_a} \in \mathtt{Repair}$. It can be shown that it is not possible for any fact, $\mathbf{p}$, to occur in $\mathcal{T}^\mathbf{a}(\mathbf{DB}, \mathbf{IC})$ with two different annotations. Therefore, it is not possible that the same fact will be inserted and then removed (or vice versa) while constructing a repair as described here.

---

[4] Here, bold face symbols, *e.g.*, $\mathbf{p}$, denote classical ground atomic formulas.

5.1   Finiteness of $\mathcal{T}^a(\mathbf{DB}, \mathbf{IC})$

We now examine the issue of finiteness of the set $\mathcal{T}^a(\mathbf{DB}, \mathbf{IC})$.

Definition 7. *(Range-Restricted Constraints) An integrity constraint, $p_1(\bar{T}_1) \vee \cdots \vee p_n(\bar{T}_n) \vee \neg q_1(\bar{T}_1') \vee \cdots \vee \neg q_m(\bar{T}_m')$, is range-restricted if and only if every variable in $\bar{T}_i$ ($1 \leq i \leq n$) also occurs in some $\bar{T}_j'$ ($1 \leq j \leq m$). Both p_i and q_j can be built-in predicates.*

A set $\mathbf{IC}$ of constraints is range-restricted *if so is every constraint in $\mathbf{IC}$.*

Lemma 4. *Let $\mathbf{IC}$ be a set of range-restricted constraints over a database $\mathbf{DB}$. Then every a-clause implied by $\mathcal{T}(\mathbf{DB}, \mathbf{IC})$ (i.e., every clause of the form (3)) mentions only the constants in the active domain of $\mathbf{DB}$.*[5]

Corollary 1. *If $\mathbf{IC}$ is range-restricted, then $\mathcal{T}^a(\mathbf{DB}, \mathbf{IC})$ is finite.*

6   Queries to Inconsistent Databases

In general, the number of all repair signatures can be exponential in the size of $\mathcal{T}^a(\mathbf{DB}, \mathbf{IC})$, so using this theory directly is not likely to produce a good query engine. In fact, for the propositional case, [5] shows that the problem of deciding whether a formula holds in all models produced by Winslett's theory of updates [4] is Π_2^P-*complete*. Since, as mentioned before, our repairs are essentially Winslett's updated models, the same result applies to our case.

However, there are cases when complexity is manageable. It is easy to see that if k is the number of clauses in $\mathcal{T}^a(\mathbf{DB}, \mathbf{IC})$ and $n_1, ..., n_k$ are the numbers of disjuncts in $C_1, ..., C_k$, respectively, then the number of repair signatures is $O(n_1 \times \ldots \times n_k)$. Therefore, two factors affect the number of repairs:

1. The number of clauses in $\mathcal{T}^a(\mathbf{DB}, \mathbf{IC})$;
2. The number of disjuncts in each clause in $\mathcal{T}^a(\mathbf{DB}, \mathbf{IC})$.

So, we should look into those types of constraints where either k is bound or all but a bound number of n_i's equal 1.

Other cases when query answering is feasible arise when the set of *a-clauses* $\mathcal{T}^a(\mathbf{DB}, \mathbf{IC})$ is precomputed. Precomputing this set might be practical for read-only databases. In other cases, $\mathcal{T}^a(\mathbf{DB}, \mathbf{IC})$ might be easy to compute because of the special form of constraints (and in this case, the size of $\mathcal{T}^a(\mathbf{DB}, \mathbf{IC})$ turns out to be P-bounded). For instance, suppose $\mathbf{IC}$ consists of range-restricted formulas and is closed under the resolution inference rule (e.g. if $\mathbf{IC}$ is a set of functional dependencies). In this case, a-clauses can be generated by converting each constraint into a query that finds all tuples that violate the constraint. For instance, the constraint $p(\bar{x}) \supset q(\bar{x})$ can be converted into the query $p(\bar{x}) \wedge \neg q(\bar{x})$ (which is the denial form of this constraint). If the tuple $\bar{a}$ is an answer, then one *a-clause* is $p(\bar{a}) : \mathbf{f_a} \vee q(\bar{a}) : \mathbf{t_a}$.

---

[5] The active domain consists of the constants in D that appear in some database table.

Answering Ground Conjunctive Queries. To consistently answer a ground conjunctive query of the form $\mathbf{p}_1 \wedge \ldots \wedge \mathbf{p}_k \wedge \neg\mathbf{q}_1 \wedge \ldots \wedge \neg\mathbf{q}_m$, we need to check the following:

For each $\mathbf{p}_i$: if $\mathbf{p}_i \in \mathbf{DB}$ and $\mathbf{p}_i : \mathbf{f_a}$ is not mentioned in $\mathcal{T}^\mathbf{a}(\mathbf{DB}, \mathbf{IC})$; or if $\mathcal{T}^\mathbf{a}(\mathbf{DB}, \mathbf{IC})$ has a clause of the form $\mathbf{p}_i : \mathbf{t_a}$.

For each $\mathbf{q}_j$: if $\mathbf{q}_j \notin \mathbf{DB}$ and $\mathbf{q}_j : \mathbf{t_a}$ is not mentioned in $\mathcal{T}^\mathbf{a}(\mathbf{DB}, \mathbf{IC})$; or if $\mathcal{T}^\mathbf{a}(\mathbf{DB}, \mathbf{IC})$ has a clause of the form $\mathbf{q}_j : \mathbf{f_a}$.

If all of the above holds, *true* is a consistent answer to the query. Otherwise, the answer is *not true*, meaning that there is at least one repair where our conjunctive query is false. (Note that this is not the same as answering *false* in definition 5).

Non-ground Conjunctive Queries. Let $\mathbf{DB}$ have the relations $p_1, \ldots, p_n$. We construct a new database, $\mathbf{DB}^{O,U}$, with relations $p_1^O, \ldots, p_n^O, p_1^U, \ldots, p_n^U$ (where O and U stand for "original" and "unknown", resp.), as follows:

p_i^O *consists of*: all the tuples such that $p_i(\bar{t}) \in \mathbf{DB}$ and $p_i(\bar{t}) : \mathbf{f_a}$ is not mentioned in $\mathcal{T}^\mathbf{a}(\mathbf{DB}, \mathbf{IC})$ plus the tuples $\bar{t}$ such that $p(\bar{t}) : \mathbf{t_a}$ is a clause in $\mathcal{T}^\mathbf{a}(\mathbf{DB}, \mathbf{IC})$.

p_j^U *consists of*: all the tuples $\bar{t}$ such that $p_j(\bar{t}) : \mathbf{t_a}$ or $p_j(\bar{t}) : \mathbf{f_a}$ appear in a clause in $\mathcal{T}^\mathbf{a}(\mathbf{DB}, \mathbf{IC})$ that has more than one disjunct.

To answer an open conjunctive query, for example, $p(x) \wedge \neg q(x)$, we pose the query $p^O(x) \wedge \neg q^O(x) \wedge \neg q^U(x)$ to $\mathbf{DB}^{O,U}$. This can be done in polynomial time in the database size plus the size of the set of *a-clauses*.

Ground Disjunctive Queries. Sound and complete query evaluation techniques for various types of queries and constraints are developed in [1]. Our present framework extends the results in [1] to include disjunctive queries. We concentrate on ground disjunctive queries of the form

$$\mathbf{p}_1 \vee \cdots \vee \mathbf{p}_k \vee \neg\mathbf{q}_1 \cdots \neg\mathbf{q}_r. \tag{4}$$

First, for each p_i we evaluate the query $\mathbf{p}_i^O$ and for each q_j we evaluate the query $\neg\mathbf{q}_j^O \wedge \neg\mathbf{q}_j^U$ against the database $\mathbf{DB}^{O,U}$. If at least one *true* answer is obtained, the answer to (4) is *true*. Otherwise, if all these queries return *false*, we evaluate the queries of the form $\neg\mathbf{p}_i^O \wedge \neg\mathbf{p}_i^U$ and $\mathbf{q}_j^O$ against $\mathbf{DB}^{O,U}$. For each answer *true*, the corresponding literal is eliminated from (4). Let $\mathbf{p}_{i_1} \vee \cdots \vee \mathbf{p}_{i_s} \vee \neg\mathbf{q}_{j_1} \cdots \neg\mathbf{q}_{j_t}$ be the resulting query. If this query is empty, then the answer to the original query is *false*, i.e., the original query is false in every repair. If the resulting query is not empty, we must check if there is a minimal hitting set for $\mathcal{T}^\mathbf{a}(\mathbf{DB}, \mathbf{IC})$, that contains $\{\neg\mathbf{p}_{i_1}, \ldots, \neg\mathbf{p}_{i_s}, \mathbf{q}_{j_1}, \ldots, \mathbf{q}_{j_t}\}$. If such a hitting set exists, the answer to the original query is *maybe*, meaning that there is at least one repair where the answer is *false*. Otherwise, the answer to the query is *true*.

Therefore, the problem of answering disjunctive queries for a given $\mathcal{T}^\mathbf{a}(\mathbf{DB}, \mathbf{IC})$ is equivalent to the problem of deciding whether a given set can be extended to a minimal hitting set of the family. Since this is an *NP-complete* problem, we have the following result.

Proposition 3. *Suppose that $\mathcal{T}^a(\mathbf{DB}, \mathbf{IC})$ has been precomputed. Then the problem of deciding whether true is a consistent answer to a disjunctive ground query is NP-complete with respect to the size of $\mathbf{DB}$ plus $\mathcal{T}^a(\mathbf{DB}, \mathbf{IC})$.*

7 Conclusions

We presented a new semantic framework, based on Annotated Predicate Calculus [9], for studying the problem of query answering in databases that are inconsistent with integrity constraints. This was done by embedding both the database instance and the integrity constraints into a single theory written in an APC with an appropriate truth values lattice. In this way, we obtain a general logical specification of database repairs and consistent query answers.

With this new framework, we are able to provide a better analysis of the computational complexity of query answering in such environments and to develop a more general query answering mechanism than what was known previously [1]. We also identified certain classes of queries and constraints that have lower complexity, and we are looking into better query evaluation algorithms for these classes.

The development of the specific mechanisms for consistent query answering in the presence of universal ICs, and the extension of our methodology to constraints that contain existential quantifiers (*e.g.*, referential integrity constraints) is left for future work.

Acknowledgements

We would like to thank the anonymous referees for their valuable comments. Work supported by Fondecyt Grants # 1980945, # 1000593; and ECOS/CONICYT Grant C97E05.

References

1. M. Arenas, L. Bertossi, and J. Chomicki. Consistent Query Answers in Inconsistent Databases. In *Proc. ACM Symposium on Principles of Database Systems (ACM PODS'99, Philadelphia)*, pages 68–79, 1999.
2. N. Belnap. A Useful Four-Valued Logic. In M. Dunn and G. Epstein, editors, *Modern Uses of Multi-Valued Logic*, pages 8–37. Reidel Publ. Co., 1977.
3. H.A. Blair and V.S. Subrahmanian. Paraconsistent Logic Programming. *Theoretical Computer Science*, 68:135–154, 1989.
4. T. Chou and M. Winslett. A Model-Based Belief Revision System. *J. Automated Reasoning*, 12:157–208, 1994.
5. T. Eiter and G. Gottlob. On the Complexity of Propositional Knowledge Base Revision, Updates, and Counterfactuals. *J. Artificial Intelligence*, 57(2-3):227–270, 1992.
6. M. Garey and D. Johnson. *Computers and Intractability: A Guide to the Theory of NP-Completeness*. W. H. Freeman and Co., 1979.

7. M. Gertz. *Diagnosis and Repair of Constraint Violations in Database Systems.* PhD thesis, Universität Hannover, 1996.
8. M.L. Ginsberg. Multivalued Logics: A Uniform Approach to Reasoning in Artificial Intelligence. *Computational Intelligence*, 4:265–316, 1988.
9. M. Kifer and E.L. Lozinskii. A Logic for Reasoning with Inconsistency. *Journal of Automated Reasoning*, 9(2):179–215, November 1992.
10. M. Kifer and V.S. Subrahmanian. Theory of Generalized Annotated Logic Programming and its Applications. *Journal of Logic Programming*, 12(4):335–368, April 1992.
11. V.S. Subrahmanian. On the Semantics of Quantitative Logic Programs. In *IEEE Symposium on Logic Programming*, pages 173–182, 1987.
12. M.H. van Emden. Quantitative Deduction and its Fixpoint Theory. *Journal of Logic Programming*, 1(4):37–53, 1986.

Querying Inconsistent Databases: Algorithms and Implementation

Alexander Celle and Leopoldo Bertossi

Pontificia Universidad Católica de Chile
Escuela de Ingeniería
Departamento de Ciencia de Computación
Casilla 360, Santiago 22, Chile
{acelle,bertossi}@puc.cl

Abstract. In this paper, an algorithm for obtaining consistent answers to queries posed to inconsistent relational databases is presented. This is a query rewriting algorithm proven to be sound, terminating and complete for some classes of integrity constraints that extend those previously considered in [1]. Complexity issues are addressed.

The implementation of the algorithm in XSB presented here takes advantage of the functionalities of XSB, as a logic programming language with tabling facilities, and the possibility of coupling it to relational database systems.

1 Introduction

It is usually assumed that data stored in a database is consistent; and not having this consistency is considered a dangerous situation. However, it often happens that this is not the case and the database reaches an inconsistent state in the sense that the database instance does not satisfy a given set of integrity constraints IC. This situation may arise due to several reasons. The initial problem was due to poor design of the database schema itself or a malfunctioning application that made the system reach the inconsistent state.

Nowadays, other sources of inconsistencies have appeared. For example, in a datawarehouse context [4], inconsistencies may appear, among other reasons to integration of different data sources. In particular, in the presence of duplicate information, and to delayed update of the datawarehouse views.

Either case, having a consistent database or not, the information stored in it remains relevant to the user and is potentially useful, as long as the distinction between consistent and inconsistent data can be made, and they can be separated when answering queries.

The common solution for the problem of facing inconsistent data is to repair the database and take it back to a consistent state. However, this approach is very expensive in terms of computing power, complexity and in some cases we might lose potentially relevant data in the process. In addition, a particular user, without control on the database administration, might want to impose his/her particular, soft or hard constraints on the database (or some views). In this case, the database cannot be repaired.

J. Lloyd et al. (Eds.): CL 2000, LNAI 1861, pp. 942–956, 2000.
© Springer-Verlag Berlin Heidelberg 2000

Example 1. Consider the inclusion dependency stating that a purchase must have a corresponding client: $\forall(u, v). \, (Purchase(u, v) \Rightarrow Client(x))$. The following database instance r violates the IC:

Purchase		Client
c	e_1	c
d	e_2	
d	e_1	

When repairing the database we might be tempted to remove all the purchases done by client d which provide us with useful information about a client's behavior, no matter whether he is a valid client or not. □

A promising alternative to restoring consistency is to keep the inconsistent data *in* the database and modify the queries in order to retrieve only consistent information. By using this kind of approach we can still use the inconsistent data for analysis (purchases of customer d in Example 1).

A semantic notion of consistent answer to a query was given in [1]. In essence, a tuple answer $\bar{t}$ is a consistent answer to a query $Q(\bar{x})$ if $Q(\bar{t})$ becomes true in every repair of the inconsistent database instance r that can be obtained by a minimal set of changes on r. Of course, the idea is not to construct all possible minimal repairs and then query; this would impossible or too complex. It is necessary to search for an alternative mechanism.

In this context, an operator T_ω was presented in [1] which does not repair the database but that, given the query $Q(\bar{x})$, computes a modified query $T_\omega(Q)(\bar{x})$ whose answers, when posed to the original database instance r, are consistent in the semantic sense already explained. The operator produces query rewritings that are sound, complete and terminating for interesting syntactic classes of queries and constraints [1]. However, this operator has some drawbacks: it is hard to implement due to its recursive nature and a semantic termination condition.

In this paper we address the problem of designing and implementing an alternative operator inspired by T_ω. The new operator corresponds to an algorithm, called $QUECA$, for "QUEry for Consistent Answers", which, given a first order query[1] Q, generates again a new query $QUECA(Q)$, whose answers in r are consistent with IC, but as opposed to T_ω, it guarantees termination, soundness and completeness for a larger set of integrity constraints.

The implementation is done in XSB [6], a powerful logic programming system, which is provided with useful functionalities for the right implementation and operation of the consistent query answering algorithm.

In Section 2, we will show the most relevant characteristics of the operator T_ω and what makes it difficult to implement. We will also give a description of what we will understand by a database repair, query, integrity constraint and consistent answer. Next, in Section 3 we present the algorithms which generate a query $QUECA(Q)$ for a given first order query Q. In Section 4 the properties of these algorithms are analyzed, namely: scope, runtime complexity, termination, soundness and completeness. In Section 5 we describe issues regarding the implementation done in XSB. Finally, in Section 6 we draw some conclusions and

---

[1] Aggregate queries are being treated in [2].

propose some extensions to the solution presented in this article. Due to space restrictions we do not give proofs of propositions; we leave them for an extended version.

2 Preliminaries

2.1 Basic Notions

We start from a fixed set, IC, of integrity constraints associated to fixed relational database schema. We assume that IC is consistent. A database instance r is consistent if it satisfies IC, that is $r \vDash IC$. Otherwise, we say that r is inconsistent. If r is inconsistent, its repairs are database instances (wrt the same schema and domain) that, each of them, satisfy IC and differ from r by a minimal set of inserted or deleted tuples. A tuple $\bar{t}$ is a *consistent* answer to a query $Q(\bar{x})$ wrt IC, and we denote this with $r \vDash_c Q(\bar{t})$, if for every repair r' of r, $r' \vDash Q(\bar{t})$.

Example 2. Consider a distributors database. $Provider(u, v)$ means that product v is provided by u, and $Receives(u, v)$ that product v is received from provider u. The following ICs state that the products supplied by a provider are received from him (and vice versa), and that a provider supplies only one product.

$$\forall u, v. \ (Provider(u, v) \Rightarrow Receives(u, v)) \ ,$$

$$\forall u, v. \ (Receives(u, v) \Rightarrow Provider(u, v)) \ ,$$

$$\forall u, v, z. \ (Provider(u, v) \wedge Provider(u, z) \Rightarrow v = z) \ .$$

The following database instance r, which violates IC,

Provider		Receives	
a	b	a	b
a	c	a	c
d	e	d	e

has two repairs:

r' : Provider		Receives	
a	c	a	c
d	e	d	e

r'' : Provider		Receives	
a	b	a	b
d	e	d	e

Here, the only consistent answer to the query $Provider(u, v)$? in the database instance r is (d, e): $r \vDash_c Provider(d, e)$.

2.2 The T_ω Operator

The T_ω operator [1] is defined based on a previous residue calculation stage[2] which generates the necessary rules to feed the operator. Generally speaking, it is defined as a collection of operators $T_0 \ldots T_n$ (for some n called *finiteness point*), that were calculated based on the residues generated for that query according to the existing set IC of integrity constraints. The (semantical) *finiteness point* was defined as the step in which further computation (i.e. calculate T_{n+1}) had no practical sense because $T_n \Rightarrow T_{n+1}$. We illustrate the application of this operator by means of an example.

---

[2] See Sections 3 and 3.1 for a description of what residues are and how to obtain them.

Example 3. With the set of integrity constraints of example 2 and with the query $P(u, v)$, we will compute $T_\omega(P(u, v))$, letting P stand for *Provider* and R for *Receives*.

$T_0(P(u, v)) = P(u, v)$.

$T_1(P(u, v)) = P(u, v) \land (R(u, v) \land (\neg P(u, z) \lor v = z))$.

$T_2(P(u, v)) = P(u, v) \land ((R(u, v) \land P(u, v)) \land ((\neg P(u, z) \land \neg R(u, z)) \lor v = z))$.

$T_3(P(u, v)) = P(u, v) \land ((R(u, v) \land P(u, v) \land (R(u, v) \land (\neg P(u, w) \lor v = w))) \land$
$$((\neg P(u, z) \land \neg R(u, z) \land \neg P(u, z)) \lor v = z)) .$$

It seems as if T_3 is very different from T_2, however, if we rewrite them by hand we have

$T_2(P(u, v)) = P(u, v) \land (R(u, v) \land P(u, v) \land ((\neg P(u, z) \lor v = z) \land$
$$(\neg R(u, z) \lor v = z))) .$$

$T_3(P(u, v)) = P(u, v) \land (R(u, v) \land P(u, v) \land ((R(u, v) \lor \neg P(u, w)) \land$
$$(R(u, v) \lor v = w) \land (\neg P(u, z) \lor v = z) \land (\neg R(u, z) \lor v = z) \land$$
$$(\neg P(u, z) \lor v = z))) .$$

We can easily see that $T_2(P(u, v)) \equiv T_3(P(u, v))$, therefore the finiteness point is 2 and the modified query is $T_0(P(u, v)) \land T_1(P(u, v)) \land T_2(P(u, v))$.   □

Although operator T_ω is sound, it lacks a more general completeness result; and when thinking of a possible implementation, the termination issue is critical because the finiteness point can be very complicated to detect, even in simple examples like the one above (or may be an undecidable problem). An initial approach consisted in using Otter [5], but it turned out to be cumbersome and sometimes it did not deliver the expected results. For instance, it was not able to solve the previous example. Furthermore, even if it does work, the *offline* nature of such process makes it unsuitable for a real world implementation where a user should interact directly with the query answering system.

Thus we need to modify the previous approach to improve the results regarding termination, and possibly extending completeness as well.

In consequence, we face the problem of modifying T_ω, providing a new, more practical mechanism, but preserving the nice properties T_ω had in terms of soundness and completeness. We need to add a stronger termination property which makes the new mechanism more likely for implementation. The basic approach involves identifying a stronger syntactical condition to achieve semantically correct results.

2.3   Integrity Constraints

In this paper we will only consider only static first order integrity constraints. As in [1], we will only consider *universal* constraints that can be transformed into a standard format

Definition 1. *An integrity constraint is in standard format if it has the form*

$$\forall(\bigvee_{i=1}^{m} P_i(\bar{x}_i) \vee \bigvee_{i=1}^{n} \neg Q_i(\bar{y}_i) \vee \psi) \ ,$$

where $\forall$ represents the universal closure of the formula, $\bar{x}_i$, $\bar{y}_i$ are tuples of variables, the P_i's and Q_i's are atomic formulas based on the schema predicates that do not contain constants, and ψ is a formula that mentions only built–in predicates.

Notice that in these ICs, constants, if needed, can be pushed into ψ. Also notice that equality is allowed in ψ.

Because of implementation issues we shall negate the ICs in standard format, representing ICs as denials, that is as range restricted goals of the form

$$\leftarrow l_1 \wedge \cdots \wedge l_n \ , \tag{1}$$

where each l_i is a literal and variables are assumed to be universally quantified over the whole formula. We must emphasize the fact that this is just notation, and from now on we shall talk about of ICs assuming they are in denial form in the sense of classical logic and not of logic programming.

We shall note, however, that not all integrity constraints may be transformed into standard format, and therefore are not considered in this article. Such is the case of unsafe ICs [7], as $\forall \bar{x} \exists y. \ (P(\bar{x})) \rightarrow Q(\bar{x}, y)$.

3   Query Generation for Consistent Answers

The whole process of query rewriting for consistent answers relies on the concept of *residues* developed in the context of semantic query optimization [3]. Residues, simply put, show the interaction between an integrity constraint and a literal name[3]. Thus, a literal name which does not appear in any constraint does not have any (non–maximal [3]) residues, i.e. there are no restrictions applied to that literal. Similarly, a literal that appears more than once in an IC or set of ICs, may have several residues, which may or may not be redundant (see Definition 2).

To calculate the residues in a database schema, we will introduce Algorithm 1, which shows how to systematically obtain residues for a given literal name. Because only literal names appearing in an integrity constraint generate (non–maximal) residues, the algorithm will only be applied to them, and not to every relation in r.

Once we have calculated all the residues associated to a literal name appearing in IC, we shall present a second algorithm $QUECA$, that will generate the

---

[3] Literal names denote relations, so different literals may have the same literal name, e.g. $P(u)$ and $P(v)$ have the same literal name P. Literal names may be negative, e.g. $\neg P$, where P is a predicate name; and have an associated arity that further differentiates them (like Prolog convention), so from now on when talking about a literal, say $P(u,v)$, we are really talking about its literal name, $P/2$.

queries for consistent answers on the basis of the residues that have been already computed. We will also show how this algorithm differs from the operator T_ω presented in [1], not only in terms of termination, but in the operation itself and the necessary conditions for sound execution.

3.1   Residue Calculation

The first step in the residue calculation determines for whom they are to be calculated. In our case, it is for every literal name appearing in an integrity constraint. Because of this we must first build a list of ICs and a list of the distinct literal names L_P appearing in IC. This list of integrity constraints L_{IC} will only include the bodies of the ICs(represented in the form (1)). That is, given the set of integrity constraints IC, we build $L_{IC} = \{[l_1 \wedge \ldots \wedge l_n] \mid \forall(\leftarrow l_1 \wedge \ldots \wedge l_n) \in IC\}$. It should be noted that when negating a member of L_{IC} we obtain a clause.

Example 4. Let IC be the following set of integrity constraints taken from Example 2 expressed in the form (1).

$$\leftarrow P(u, v) \wedge \neg R(u, v) \ .$$
$$\leftarrow \neg P(u, v) \wedge R(u, v) \ .$$
$$\leftarrow P(u, v) \wedge P(u, z) \wedge y \neq z \ .$$

From this we would generate $L_{IC} = \{[P(u, v) \wedge \neg R(u, v)], [\neg P(u, v) \wedge R(u, v)],$ $[P(u, v) \wedge P(u, z) \wedge y \neq z]\}$ and $L_P = \{P(u, v), R(u, v), \neg P(u, v), \neg R(u, v)\}$. We should recall that in L_P we have the following literal names: $P/2$, $R/2$, $\neg P/2$ and $\neg R/2$.   □

Next, to calculate the residues coming from $l \in L_P$, and $ic \in L_{IC}$, we use the subsumption algorithm presented in [3]. However, because we are dealing with an implementation, we need a systematical procedure to obtain residues. The method utilized is formalized as Algorithm 1.

Example 5. (Example 4 Continued) Applying Algorithm 1 up to line 13, to $l = P(u, v)$ and every member of L_{IC}, we would obtain one residue for each occurrence of $P/2$: $residue_1(P(u, v)) := R(u, v)$, $residue_2(P(u, v)) := \neg P(u, z) \vee v = z$ and $residue_3(P(u, v)) := \neg P(u, w) \vee w = v$. Here we may find redundant residues (see Definition 2).   □

Finally, a conjunction of all the residues associated to a given $l \in L_P$ is created and denoted by $residues(l)$. In this process, we take care of eliminating redundant residues as we build the conjunction (steps 14–21 in Algorithm 1) in order to reduce complexity in the following phase ($QUECA$).

Definition 2 (Residue Redundancy). *Let $R \wedge \varphi$ be a conjunction of residues associated to a literal l, where R is a clause and φ a conjunction of clauses. We will say R is redundant in $R \wedge \varphi$ if exists a clause $R' \in \varphi$ and a substitution $\sigma : (Var(R')^4 \setminus Var(l)) \rightarrow (Var(R) \setminus Var(l))$, such that $R'\sigma \equiv R$.*

---

[4] Var(X) is the set of all (quantified or unquantified) variables in the expression X.

Algorithm 1 Compute $residues(l)$

Require: Set of integrity constraints in denial form IC.
Ensure: $residues(l)$ is a formula in CNF that contains all the residues associated to a
    literal l.

1: Create list L_{IC} of integrity constraint bodies and a list L_P of distinct literal names
    in L_{IC}.
2: **for all** $l \in L_P$ **do**
3:    $i = 1$
4:    **for all** $ic \in L_{IC}$ **do**
5:       **for** each occurrence of l in ic **do**
6:          delete l from $ic \mapsto \overline{ic}$
7:          negate $\overline{ic}$ {Now $\overline{ic}$ is in clausal form}
8:          $residue_i(l) := \overline{ic}$
9:          $i := i + 1$
10:      **end for**
11:   **end for**
12:   $n(l) := i$ {the number of residues associated to l}
13: **end for**
14: **for all** $l \in L_P$ **do**
15:   $residues(l) := \varnothing$
16:   **for all** $i := 1$ to $n(l)$ **do**
17:     **if** $residue_i(l)$ is not redundant **then**
18:       $residues(l) := residues(l) \wedge residue_i(l)$
19:     **end if**
20:   **end for**
21: **end for**

Note that, in the definition above, if R is redundant in $R \wedge \varphi$, then $R \wedge \varphi$ is logically equivalent to φ. The elimination of redundant residues is based on unification and is done in steps 14–21 of Algorithm 1.

Example 6. (Example 5 Continued) By Definition 2, we have that $residue_3(P(u, v))$ is a redundant residue, because there exists a substitution $\sigma : z \mapsto w$, such that $residue_2(P(u,v))\sigma = residue_3(P(u,v))$. Thus, we have $residues(P(u, v)) = [R(u, v)] \wedge [\neg P(u, z) \vee v = z]$.   □

Note that the definition does not state that it detects *all* redundancies, but only those subject to the sufficient condition presented. For example, if we consider the following residues for $R(x)$: $residue_1(R(x)) = P(x) \vee x > 100$ and $residue_2(R(x)) = P(x) \vee x > 50$. Clearly $residue_1$ includes the information in $residue_2$, so $residue_2$ would be redundant; However, Definition 2 does not detect it. This occurs mainly when ICs are redundant, which can easily be avoided for cases like these. As shown in Example 6, functional dependencies are a common case of ICs which generate redundant residues according to Definition 2. The reason why residue redundancy is not treated further is due to the complexity of implementation, which could be far higher than the performance improvement we could get in the next stage ($QUECA$). Besides, residue redundancy can become such a large subject that it would deviate the central point of attention of this article, which is to build the queries for consistent answers.

Example 7. Finally, by applying Algorithm 1 to the set *IC* presented in Example 4, we would obtain:

$$residues(P(u,v)) = (R(u,v)) \land (\neg P(u,z) \lor v = z) \ ,$$
$$residues(\neg P(u,v)) = (\neg R(u,v)) \ ,$$
$$residues(R(u,v)) = P(u,v) \ ,$$
$$residues(\neg R(u,v)) = \neg P(u,v) \ .$$

3.2   Query Generation (*QUECA*)

Once all the residues have been computed, and given a query Q, we can generate the query, $QUECA(Q)$, which will deliver consistent answers from a consistent or inconsistent database. This query differs from Q only when Q has residues, so $QUECA(Q)$ should be only executed for literal names appearing in *IC*.

Initially the query $QUECA(Q)$ is equal to Q, plus a list of pending residues which are the residues associated to Q calculated by Algorithm 1.[5] These residues are not yet part of the query, they form a list of pending clauses that must be resolved via some condition if they should belong to the query. This condition is, informally, if they add new information to it or not. If they do not, they are discarded; but if they do, they must be added to the query and their residues appended at the end of the residue list. This procedure is iterated until no residues are left to resolve, i.e. either we run out of residues or they have all been discarded. We will see later that the procedure does not always terminate.

Example 8. Consider the following hypothetical pairs of queries and residues:

Query :	1. $S(u)$	Residues :	$S(u)$
	2. $M(u)$		$N(u)$
	3. $P(u,v)$		$\forall z \ (P(u,v) \lor \neg Q(u,z))$.

Clearly in the first case, the residue can be discarded because it adds no new information to the query. However, in the second and third cases the residues must be added to the corresponding query, and their residues to the Pending Residue List. So we would have

Query :	1. $S(u)$	Residues :	$\emptyset$
	2. $M(u) \land N(u)$		$residues(N(u))$
	3. $P(u,v) \land \forall z \ (P(u,v) \lor \neg Q(u,z))$		$residues(P(u,v) \lor \neg Q(u,z))$.

$\square$

This method works when only conjunctions are involved (case 2 in Example 8), because determining if a residue should be part of the query or not is easy. However, most of the residues are clauses (case 3 in Example 8), so we must somehow deal with disjunction.

The way to solve this problem is by keeping conjunctions together, i.e. working in DNF. To do so, when a clausal residue adds new information to a query, we make as many copies of the query as literals in the residue we are adding,

---

[5] The residues are in CNF, we will treat every clause as an element of a list.

and append to each of them exactly one of the literals in the residue. The pending residue list of each of these new copies must then be the existing list plus the residues coming from the newly appended literal. We shall informally call this a split operation. These copies, connected together by disjunctions, would constitute the final query $QUECA(Q)$.

Example 9. (Example 8 Continued) In the third case of the previous example we would then have

Query :   Residues :

3. $E_1 : P(u,v) \land P(u,v)$ $R_1 : residues(P(u,v))$
   $E_2 : P(u,v) \land \neg Q(u,z)$ $R_2 : residues(\neg Q(u,z))$.

So, we have $QUECA(Q) = \forall z(E_1 \lor E_2)$ where E_i is a disjunctionless formula, and $Residues = R_1, R_2$, where each R_i belongs to its corresponding E_i.   □

This clarifies the need for a new notation that will enable us to keep track of the residues involved in building each E. Furthermore, this notation should not only include the literals in E and its associated Pending Residue List, but it should also "remember" the last residue that provoked one of these split operations, in order to avoid inserting a residue whose information was already inserted earlier. For these purposes we define a *Temporary Query Unit* (TQU).

Definition 3. *A temporary query unit, $D : E \bullet R$, consists of a set of clauses D, a conjunction of literals E and a conjunction of residues R.*

Both symbols, : and $\bullet$, are only used to separate D, E and R from each other. D represents the last residues involved in building E and R is the conjunction of residues $\phi_1 \land \cdots \land \phi_n$ yet to be resolved. We shall note that all variables coming from a residue appear universally quantified in D and E(see Example 10). Both symbols have higher precedence that any other connective. In this way, $QUECA(Q)$ can be seen as a disjunction of temporary query units, $\bigvee TQU$, when we reach the point in which $R = \varnothing$ for every TQU.

Example 10. (Example 9 Continued) Using the new notation for the third case we would have:

$QUECA(P(u,v))$:

TQU_1 $[\forall z(P(u,v) \lor \neg Q(u,z))] : P(u,v) \land P(u,v) \bullet residues(P(u,v)) \lor$
TQU_2 $\underbrace{[\forall z(P(u,v) \lor \neg Q(u,z))]}_{D} : \underbrace{P(u,v) \land \forall z \neg Q(u,z)}_{E} \bullet \underbrace{residues(\neg Q(u,z))}_{R}$.

□

The critical step is then determining when a residue should be added to the query and when its information is already in it, i.e. it should be discarded. It is easy to see that when $E \vDash \phi_1$[6] or $D \vDash \phi_1$, then ϕ_1 can be discarded. If either condition is not satisfied, the residue must be included in the query.[7] In example 10, we have from TQU_1 that $D \vDash residues(P(u))$, thus they can be

---

[6] The required condition is that every term in ϕ_1 belongs to E.

[7] We will see that sometimes only part of the residue must be included.

discarded and the iteration would have ended for TQU_1. This is the semantic result we want to obtain via syntactical means. The usual way to attain this is via unification.

In our case we will define a sort of one way unification in which only certain types of variables will be involved: New Variables in a TQU and Free Variables in a Residue.

Definition 4. *A New Variable in a $TQU = D : E \bullet R$ associated to a query Q is a variable that belongs to $newVar(TQU) := Var(E) \smallsetminus Var(Q)$ and is universally quantified.*

Definition 5. *Given a $TQU = D : E \bullet R$, a Free Variable in a Residue $\phi \in R$ is a variable that belongs to $freeVar(\phi) := Var(\phi) \smallsetminus Var(E)$ and is universally quantified.*

Because D in a TQU consists of a recently resolved residue, it also behaves as one and has *Free Variables* in the sense of definition 5. For instance, in example 10, we have $newVar(TQU_2) = \{z\}$ and $freeVar(D_1) = \{z\}$. From these definitions it is clear that we can substitute a *freeVar* for any other variable because they occur nowhere else than in that residue.

We can now formally define the meaning of *the information of a residue already in a TQU.*

Definition 6. *We will say the information of a residue $\phi = l_1 \vee \cdots \vee l_n$ is already in a $TQU = D : E \bullet R$, and will write $\phi \mathrel{\widetilde{\in}} D : E$, whenever there exists a substitution $\sigma : freeVar(\phi) \to newVar(TQU) \cup freeVar(D)$, such that $\phi\sigma \in D$ or for all i, $l_i\sigma \in E$. In case only some $l_i\sigma \in E$, we will say the information of a residues is already partially in a TQU, and we will write $\phi \mathrel{{}_p\widetilde{\in}_\sigma} D : E$.*

Notice that if $freeVar(\phi) = \varnothing$, then σ could be ε (the identity).

Consequently we have that, when verifying whether to add a residue $\phi = l_1 \vee \cdots \vee l_m$ to a query, if $\phi \mathrel{\widetilde{\in}} D : E$, then ϕ is discarded. Otherwise, it must be added to E and one of the mentioned split operations must take place. However, if $\phi \mathrel{\widetilde{\in}_{P,\theta}} D : E$, then we must keep a copy of $D : E \bullet R$; and for all the cases in which $l_i\theta \notin E$, $l_i\theta$ must be appended to a copy E_i of E and its residues must be added at the end of a copy R_i of R.

Example 11. (Example 10 Continued) By using the method presented above the second $P(u, v)$ would not be included in TQU_1, that is

$QUECA(P(u, v))$:

$TQU_1 \quad [P(u, v) \vee \neg Q(u, z)] : P(u, v) \bullet residues(P(u, v)) \ \vee$

$TQU_2 \quad [P(u, v) \vee \neg Q(u, z)] : P(u, v) \wedge \forall z \neg Q(u, z) \bullet residues(\neg Q(u, z))$.   □

The procedure just described is formalized in Algorithm 2.

Example 12. (Example 3 Continued) We will show how Algorithm 2 computes $QUECA(P(u, v))$, which is equivalent to $T_2(P(u, v))$, being 2 the finiteness point.

$$QUECA(P(u,v)) = \varnothing$$
$$TQUs = \varnothing : P(u,v) \bullet (R(u,v)) \wedge (\neg P(u,z) \vee v = z)$$
$$QUECA(P(u,v)) = \varnothing$$
$$TQUs = R(u,v) : P(u,v) \wedge R(u,v) \bullet (\neg P(u,z) \vee v = z) \wedge (P(u,v))$$
$$QUECA(P(u,v)) = \varnothing$$
$$TQUs = [(\neg P(u,z) \vee v = z) : P(u,v) \wedge R(u,v) \wedge \neg P(u,z) \bullet$$
$$(P(u,v)) \wedge (\neg R(u,z))] \vee$$
$$[(\neg P(u,z) \vee v = z) : P(u,v) \wedge R(u,v) \wedge v = z \bullet (P(u,v))]$$
$$QUECA(P(u,v)) = \varnothing$$
$$TQUs = [(\neg P(u,z) \vee v = z) : P(u,v) \wedge R(u,v) \wedge \neg P(u,z) \bullet$$
$$(\neg R(u,z))] \vee$$
$$[(\neg P(u,z) \vee v = z) : P(u,v) \wedge R(u,v) \wedge v = z \bullet (P(u,v))]$$
$$QUECA(P(u,v)) = \varnothing$$
$$TQUs = [\neg R(u,z) : P(u,v) \wedge R(u,v) \wedge \neg P(u,z) \wedge \neg R(u,z) \bullet$$
$$(\neg P(u,z))] \vee$$
$$[(\neg P(u,z) \vee v = z) : P(u,v) \wedge R(u,v) \wedge v = z \bullet (P(u,v))]$$
$$QUECA(P(u,v)) = \varnothing$$
$$TQUs = [\neg R(u,z) : P(u,v) \wedge R(u,v) \wedge \neg P(u,z) \wedge \neg R(u,z) \bullet] \vee$$
$$[(\neg P(u,z) \vee v = z) : P(u,v) \wedge R(u,v) \wedge v = z \bullet (P(u,v))]$$
$$QUECA(P(u,v)) = [P(u,v) \wedge R(u,v) \wedge \neg P(u,z) \wedge \neg R(u,z)]$$
$$TQUs = [(\neg P(u,z) \vee v = z) : P(u,v) \wedge R(u,v) \wedge v = z \bullet (P(u,v))]$$
$$QUECA(P(u,v)) = [P(u,v) \wedge R(u,v) \wedge \neg P(u,z) \wedge \neg R(u,z)]$$
$$TQUs = [(\neg P(u,z) \vee v = z) : P(u,v) \wedge R(u,v) \wedge v = z \bullet]$$
$$QUECA(P(u,v)) = \forall z\, [[P(u,v) \wedge R(u,v) \wedge \neg P(u,z) \wedge \neg R(u,z)] \vee$$
$$[P(u,v) \wedge R(u,v) \wedge v = z]]$$

By rearranging the result by hand, we obtain

$$QUECA(P(u,v)) = P(u,v) \wedge R(u,v) \wedge \forall z\, [(\neg P(u,z) \wedge \neg R(u,z)) \vee v = z]$$
$$QUECA(P(u,v)) = P(u,v) \wedge R(u,v) \wedge \forall z\, [(\neg P(u,z) \vee v = z) \wedge$$
$$(\neg R(u,z) \vee v = z)]$$

and we can see how the constraints get spread towards the related literals, in this case $R/2$, where we can see how the functional dependency of the second argument of $P/2$ has generated a functional dependency for the second argument of $R/2$ due to the nature of IC. This example was shown to be non terminating for T_ω (see Example 3), but is now solved by $QUECA$. □

Algorithm 2 Generate a QUEry for Consistent Answers for a literal l: $QUECA(l)$

Require: Algorithm 1 has been executed.
Ensure: $QUECA(l)$ contains the expected results.
1: $QUECA(l) := \varnothing$
2: $TQUs := \varnothing : l \bullet residues(l)$
3: **while** $TQUs \neq \varnothing$ **do**
4:      select(extract) first TQU from $TQUs \mapsto (D : E \bullet R)$
5:      **if** $R = \varnothing$ **then**
6:          $QUECA(l) := QUECA(l) \vee E$
7:      **else**
8:          select(extract) first residue(clause) from $R \mapsto \phi$ $\{\phi = l_1 \vee \cdots \vee l_m\}$
9:          **if** $\phi \tilde{\in} D : E$ **then**
10:             $TQUs = D : E \bullet R \vee TQUs$
11:         **else**
12:             **if** $\phi \; {}_p\tilde{\in}_\theta \; D : E$ **then**
13:                 $append(D, \phi) \mapsto D_0$
14:                 $E_0 := E$
15:                 $R_0 := R$
16:             **else**
17:                 $\theta = \varepsilon$ (identity)
18:             **end if**
19:             **for all** $i \in [1, m]$ **do**
20:                 **if** $l_i\theta \notin E$ **then**
21:                     $D_i := \phi$
22:                     $E_i := E \wedge l_i\theta$
23:                     $R_i := R \wedge residues(l_i\theta)$
24:                 **else**
25:                     Do nothing
26:                 **end if**
27:             **end for**
28:             $TQUs := \bigvee_{i=0}^{m}(D_i : E_i \bullet R_i) \vee TQUs$
29:         **end if**
30:     **end if**
31: **end while**

In the previous example we can see how the $\bullet$ symbol works as a separator between the residues that have been included in the final query and those that are to be resolved. It graphically shows when a TQU is ready to be included in $QUECA$, this occurs when the $\bullet$ reaches the end of R, put in other words, when no residues are left to be resolved.

4 Properties of $QUECA$

In this section we will show that $QUECA$ algorithm is well behaved for an interesting syntactical class of ICs.

Definition 7. *(a) A binary integrity constraint (BIC) is a denial of the form*
$\forall \, (\leftarrow l_1(\bar{x}_1) \wedge l_2(\bar{x}_2) \wedge \psi(\bar{x}))$, *where l_1 and l_2 are database literals, and ψ is a formula that only contains built-in predicates.*
(b) A set of BICs, IC, is fact-oriented[8] if there is a tuple $\bar{a}$ and a literal name L, such that $IC \models L(\bar{a})$.

Usually ICs are not fact-oriented. As a particular case of BICs, we obtain *unary integrity constraints*, which have just one database literal and possibly a formula with built-in predicates. In the class of binary contraints we find functional dependencies, inclusion dependencies, symmetry constraints, and domain and range constraints. In consequence, we are covering most of the static constraints found in traditional relational databases, excluding (existential) referential ICs, transitivity constraints, and possibly other constraints that might be better expressed as rules or views at the application layer.

The following results apply to the case of a finite set of BICs.

Theorem 1. *The worst case runtime complexity of Algorithm 1 for residue computation is $O(n^2)$, where n represents the number of ICs.*

Theorem 2 (Termination). *Given a set of non fact-oriented binary integrity constraints, Algorithm 2 terminates in a finite number of steps.*

The termination property is based on the fact that by restricting execution to BICs only, residues contain one literal name at most, which in the worst case generates an infinite sequence of single literals. The infiniteness of this sequence is then limited by the condition in line 12 of Algorithm 2 and the fact that we only consider range–restricted ICs (1), conditions which ensure that at a given point, pending residues add no new information to the resulting query, thus being discarded. Notice that this result extends the termination results presented in [1], where semantic termination was only ensured for uniform binary constraints.

Theorem 3. *For non fact-oriented binary ICs, and a literal name L, the worst case runtime complexity of Algorithm 2 running on L is $O(nk^{8n})$, where n represents the number of ICs and k is the maximum number of terms per integrity constraint.*

Although this is not an encouraging result, we will see in Section 5 that this process is done at compile–time, so it should not affect the performance from a user's point of view.

---

[8] Fact-oriented integrity constraints can be seen as a special case of tuple-generating dependencies, *tgd's* [7], in which the body may contain equality. A common fact-oriented constraint is of the form $true \Rightarrow L(a)$.

It is possible to prove that the $QUECA$ algorithm can simulate the iterative application of operator T until the point where $QUECA$ stops. At that point we obtain a corresponding semantical termination point for T. The main difference is that, while T would perform split operations and add residues to the pending list (for the whole set of residues) whenever *at least one* of the residues adds new information to the resulting query, $QUECA$ does this on a per-residue basis. This eliminates residues one by one, thus obtaining a much more efficient query (see the difference between $T_3(P(u,v))$ in Example 3 and $QUECA(P(u,v))$ in Example 12). Having mapped $QUECA$'s execution to that of T, we may take advantage of soundeness and completeness results for T.

Theorem 4 (Soundness). *Let r be a database instance, IC a set of binary integrity constraints and $Q(\bar{x})$ a literal query, such that $r \vDash QUECA(Q(\bar{t}))$. If Q is universal or non-universal and domain independent, then $\bar{t}$ is a consistent answer to Q in r, that is, $r \vDash_c Q(\bar{t})$.*

Theorem 5 (Completeness). *Let r be a database instance and IC a set of non fact-oriented binary integrity constraints, then for every ground literal $l(\bar{t})$, if $r \vDash_c l(\bar{t})$, then $r \vDash QUECA(\bar{t})$.*

All the results above can be easily extended to queries that are conjunctions of literals without existential quantifiers.

5   Implementation

To achieve the objectives of this work we need a common framework for data, rules, queries and integrity constraints, to be able to perform operations on them and elaborate the queries for consistent answers mentioned earlier. Logic Programming languages provide this framework and XSB seems an adequate candidate. Generally speaking we prefer an LP language because the algorithms presented in this article need the ability to perform unifications, substitutions and detecting subsumption. Perhaps what makes XSB a better candidate that other LP languages is, apart from the Relational DMBS interface, Foreign Language interface and the fact it runs on multiple platforms, its *tabling* capabilities that improve its efficiency over other systems that would, for example, have to recalculate the residues every time they are needed by Algorithm 2.

Our system consists of a four modules which provide several predicates that allow the user direct interaction with the system. Upon initialization, the program connects itself to a database previously defined by the user, executes both algorithms presented in this paper and stores their results on XSB's tables. This avoids having to recalculate residues, $QUECAs$ or their equivalent SQL strings, thus practically eliminating the relevance of the exponential runtime complexity of Algorithm 2.

The integrity constraints of the form (1) are read from the file named ics, in which they are written with the following syntax:

```
<- [ ... denials ... ].
```

For instance, to include the ICs corresponding to Example 12, we would modify the file `ics` to contain:

```
<- [p(U,V),~r(U,V)].
<- [~p(U,V),r(U,V)].
<- [p(U,V),p(U,Z),~(V==Z)].
```

Once initialization is over, the user may query directly the database or retrieve one of the computed residues, *QUECAs* or SQL strings. For example, by executing | ?-queca(p(X,Y),Q). we would obtain:

```
Q = and(p(id1,id2),all(u1,and(r(id1,id2),or(and(no(p(id1,u1)),
    no(r(id1,u1))),equal(id2,u1)))))
```

With this method we can answer any query that is free of disjunctions and existential quantifiers. Due to space limitations, further details of the implementation are included in an extended version of this paper.

6   Conclusions

We have shown an algorithm to obtain consistent answers to queries posed to inconsistent databases. This algorithm is proved to be terminating, sound and complete for the class of non fact-oriented binary ICs. The termination results extends those obtained in [1].

We also implemented the algorithm on XSB with a program that interfaces directly to a given RDBMS. The next steps towards an effective application include handling queries and integrity constraints with existential quantifiers. Complete elimination of residue redundancy could be addressed as well.

Acknowledgements

This work has been supported by Fondecyt Grants (# 1980945 and # 1000593). We are grateful to Marcelo Arenas for illuminating conversations.

References

1. M. Arenas, L. Bertossi, and J. Chomicki. Consistent Query Answers in Inconsistent Databases. In *Proceedings ACM Symposium on Principles of Database Systems (ACM PODS '99, Philadelphia)*, pages 68–79. ACM Press, 1999.
2. M. Arenas, L. Bertossi, and J. Chomicki. Aggregation in Inconsistent Databases. In Preparation, 2000.
3. U.S Chakravarthy, John Grant, and Jack Minker. Logic-Based Approach to Semantic Query Optimization. *ACM Transactions on Database Systems*, 15(2):162–207, June 1990.
4. S. Chaudhuri and U. Dayal. An Overview of Data Warehousing and OLAP Technology. *SIGMOD Record*, 26:65–74, March 1997.
5. W.W. McCune. *OTTER 3.0 Reference Manual and Guide*. Argonne National Laboratory, Technical Report ANL-94/6, 1994.
6. K. F. Sagonas, T. Swift, and D. S. Warren. XSB as an Efficient Deductive Database Engine. In *Proceedings of SIGMOD 1994 Conference*, pages 442–453. ACM Press, 1994.
7. J.D. Ullman. *Principles of Database and Knoledge-Base Systems*, volume I. Computer Science Press, Maryland, 1988.

On Verification in Logic Database Languages

Francesco Bonchi[1,2], Fosca Giannotti[1], and Dino Pedreschi[2]

[1] CNUCE - CNR
Via Alfieri 1, 56010 Ghezzano, Pisa - Italy
Giannotti@cnuce.cnr.it
[2] Department of Computer Science, University of Pisa
C.so Italia 40, Pisa - Italy
{bonchi,pedre}@di.unipi.it

Abstract. We consider in this paper an extension of Datalog with mechanisms for non-monotonic and non-deterministic reasoning and a simple form of temporal reasoning, which we refer to as Datalog++. First, we show how with this logic database language is possible to express problems in heterogeneous domains, such as operation research and concurrent programming. Second, we provide a methodology for the verification of Datalog++ programs, based on the declarative semantics, which is able to handle both atemporal and temporal properties.

1 Introduction

The name **Datalog++** is used in this paper to refer to Datalog extended with mechanisms supporting:

- *non-monotonic* reasoning, by means of a form of stratified negation w.r.t. the stage arguments, called *XY-stratification* [17];
- *non-deterministic* reasoning, by means of the non-deterministic **choice** construct [12].
- a limited form of *temporal* reasoning, by means of temporal, or *stage*, arguments of relations, ranging over a discrete temporal domain, in the style of Datalog$_{1S}$ [6];

Datalog++, which is essentially a fragment of $\mathcal{LDL}++$ [2], and is advocated in [18, Chap. 10], revealed a highly expressive language, with applications in diverse areas such as AI planning [4], active databases [16], object databases [11], semistructured information management and Web restructuring [11].

In this paper we study a methodology for the development and the verification of Datalog++ programs. Therefore the goal of this paper is twofold: to highlight the expressiveness of Datalog++ programs by providing some realistic examples in diverse programming areas such as operative research and concurrent programming, and to provide the first steps toward a methodology for the verification of Datalog++ programs.

Research in verification in logic programming has focussed on Prolog-like, top-down languages, and relatively little work has addressed the case of deductive

J. Lloyd et al. (Eds.): CL 2000, LNAI 1861, pp. 957–971, 2000.
© Springer-Verlag Berlin Heidelberg 2000

databases and Datalog-like languages [1]. However, Datalog-like languages have a purely declarative reading that makes reasoning about programs simpler than the Prolog-like case, and several verification methods developed for Prolog-like language can be adopted for Datalog-like languages [7]. In these methods, the task of proving a given logic program correct reduces to the task of showing that certain appropriate models of the programs coincide with the intended meaning of the program itself. Clearly, the notion of *appropriate model* is not defined once and for all, but depends on the particular language, and on its use of negation. We adhere to this view, and adopt the stable model semantics as the starting point of our investigation, as Datalog++ programs are non monotonic and employ a rather general form of negation.

Also, we are interested in using Datalog++ to specify concurrent programs, and therefore we need to reason about dynamic properties, such as safety and progress. Unlike formalisms such as UNITY [5] or other temporal logic approaches [14], which use some specialized logic to deal with dynamic properties, we show how a set of interesting safety and progress properties can be handled within the mentioned model-theoretic approach. In this sense, dynamic properties can be formalized and proved as properties of the stable models of the program under consideration.

2   Datalog++: Nondeterministic, Nonmonotonic Datalog

In this paper, we use the name Datalog++ to refer to the Datalog extended by two mechanisms for non-monotonic and non-deterministic reasoning, both based on a form of negation. The first mechanism is represented by XY-programs originally introduced in [17]. The language of such programs is $Datalog_{1S}^\neg$, which admits negation on body atoms and a unary constructor symbol, used to represent a temporal argument usually called the *stage argument*. A general definition of XY-programs is the following. A set P of rules defining mutually recursive predicates, is an XY-program if it satisfies the following conditions:

1. each recursive predicate has a distinguished stage argument;
2. every recursive rule r is either an X-rule or a Y-rule, where:
   - r is an X-rule when the stage argument in every recursive predicates in r is the same variable,
   - r is a Y-rule when (i) the head of r has a stage argument $J+1$, where J is a variable, (ii) some goal of r has J as its stage argument, and (iii) the remaining recursive goals have either J or $J+1$ as their stage argument.

Intuitively, in the rules of XY-programs, an atom $p(J,\_)$ denotes the extension of relation p at the current stage (present time) J, whereas an atom $p(J+1,\_)$ denotes the extension of relation p at the next stage (future time) $J+1$. By using a different *primed* predicate symbol p' in the $p(J+1,\_)$ atoms, we obtain the so-called primed version of an XY-program. We say that an XY-program is *XY-stratified* if its primed version is a stratified program. Intuitively, if the dependency graph of the primed version has no cycles through negated edges, then it is possible to obtain an ordering on the original rules modulo the stage arguments. As a consequence, an XY-stratified program is also locally stratified, and has therefore a unique perfect model. Such a model can be computed by an iterated fixpoint procedure, which uses the ordering imposed by the primed version of the program: the extension of relations at stage J is computed, before proceeding to stage $J + 1$.

Example 1. The following version of the *seminaive* graph-reachability program, discussed in [17], is an example of (XY-stratified) XY-program, which computes all nodes of a graph g reachable from a given node a:

```
delta(0, a).
delta(s(I), Y) ← delta(I, X), g(X, Y), ¬all(I, Y).
all(I, X) ← delta(I, X).
all(s(I), X) ← all(I, X), delta(s(I), _).
```

Observe the use of negation, which is not stratified in the usual sense (delta and all are mutually recursive), although it is stratified modulo the stage. In the outcome of the seminaive program, all(n, b) means that b is a node reachable from a in graph g. At each stage i, delta(i, c) means that c is a newly reached node, and i is also the length of the shortest path from a to c; using relation delta to propagate the search avoids unnecessary recomputations.

The second mechanism is represented by *choice goals*, that are used to non-deterministically select subsets of answers to queries, which obey a specified functional dependences (FD) constraint.

Example 2 (Spanning Tree). The following program [9] computes the spanning tree starting from the source node a for a graph where an arc from node b to node d is represented by the database fact g(b,d).

```
st0 : st(root, a).
st1 : st(X, Y) ← st(_, X), g(X, Y), Y ≠ a, choice((Y), (X)).
```

Observe that, when an arc st(b,d) is added by the second rule, the choice goal ensures that no st(X,d) can later be added with $X \neq b$. The condition $X \neq a$ must be added explicitly to prevent it from generating an arc leading back to a because there is no choice goal in the first rule to avoid it.

The semantics of Choice construct is based on the *stable model* semantics of Datalog¬ programs, a concept originating from autoepistemic logic, which was applied to the study of negation in Horn clause languages in [8]. To define the notion of a stable model we need to introduce a transformation H which, given an interpretation I, maps a Datalog¬ program P into a positive Datalog program $H(P, I)$:

$$H(P, I) = \{A \leftarrow B_1, \ldots, B_n \mid A \leftarrow B_1, \ldots, B_n, \neg C_1, \ldots, \neg C_m \in ground(P) \land \{C_1, \ldots, C_m\} \cap I = \emptyset\}$$

Next, we define:

$$S_P(I) = T_{H(P,I)} \uparrow \omega$$

Then, M is said to be a *stable model* of P if $S_P(M) = M$. In general, Datalog¬ programs may have zero, one or many stable models. The multiplicity of stable models can be exploited to give a declarative account of non determinism. We can in fact define the *stable version* of a program P, $SV(P)$, to be the program transformation where all the references to the *choice* atom in a rule $r : H \leftarrow B, choice(X,Y)$ are replaced by the atom $chosen_r(X,Y)$, and define the $chosen_r$ predicate with the following rules:

$$chosen_r(X,Y) \leftarrow B, \neg diffchoice_r(X,Y).$$
$$diffchoice_r(X,Y) \leftarrow chosen(X,Y'), Y \neq Y'.$$

The various stable-models of the transformed program $SV(P)$ thus correspond to the choice models of the original program [15]. For instance, the various stable models of the program of example 2 correspond to the various spanning tree for graph **g**. Choice programs can be efficiently executed by enforcing the FD constraints during the bottom-up computation [12]. Overall semantics of Datalog++, efficient implementation and optimizations are presented in [10].

3   Programming with Datalog++

Although conceived as a deductive database language, Datalog++ revealed a highly expressive language with applications in other domains. The goal of this section is to highlight the expressiveness of Datalog++ programs by providing some examples in diverse programming areas, ranging from typical procedural algorithms to operation research and concurrent programming.

3.1   Euclid's Algorithm for the Greatest Common Divisor

Our first example illustrates a general programming paradigm, where stages used to record various steps in the computation, **choice** is used to non-deterministically select actions at each step, and rules for the *frame axioms* or *inertia axioms* are used to establish the content of a new state. This technique provides a general programming paradigm that has been applied to many problems, such as planning problem [4] and array ordering problem [9].

The following program computes according to Euclid's algorithm, the greatest common divisor of a set of integers stored as facts of the form **number(X)** in the database.

```
r0 : candidate_GCD(0, X)      ← number(X).

r1 : aux_GCD(J, X, Y)         ← candidate_GCD(J, X), candidate_GCD(J, Y),
                                X > Y, choice((J), (X, Y)).

r2 : candidate_GCD(J + 1, X)  ← candidate_GCD(J, X), ¬aux_GCD(J, X, Y).

r3 : candidate_GCD(J + 1, Z)  ← aux_GCD(J, X, Y), Z = X − Y.

r4 : GCD(X)                   ← candidate_GCD(J, X), ¬aux_GCD(J, _, _).
```

The first rule initializes the staged `candidate_GCD` predicate: at the beginning (stage 0) all integers in the database are candidate to be the greatest common divisor. The second rule nondeterministically selects a pair of candidate integers with different values. Note the use of `choice` to ensure that, at each stage, only one pair of integers out of all the eligible pairs is selected. The third and the fourth rules realize frame axioms: old candidate integers (excluded the greater integer of the selected pair) are copied into the set of candidate integers for the next stage, while a new value, the difference between the two integers of the selected pair, is added. The last rule, according to Euclid's algorithm, simply asserts that when it is no longer possible to select a pair of candidate integers with different values, i.e. when all the candidate integers have the same value, then greatest common divisor has been found.

The objective of this example is to show how it is possible to express typical procedural algorithms in a declarative way. The program we have written is as simple and efficient as its procedural version is. Also, observe that this program computes the greatest common divisor for any set of integers, independently of its cardinality.

3.2 The Ford-Fulkerson Method for the Maximum-Flow Problem

The next program is another example of a typical procedural algorithm in operation research, it is harder than the previous one, but as we show, Datalog++ is naturally geared to cope with graph algorithms. We first introduce some notation.

A *flow-network* $G = (V, E)$ is a directed graph in which each edge $(u, v) \in E$ has a nonnegative capacity $c(u, v) \geq 0$. If $(u, v) \notin E$ we assume that $c(u, v) = 0$. We distinguish two vertex in a flow network: a *source* s and a *sink* t. For convenience we assume that every vertex lies on some path from the source to the sink. Let $G = (V, E)$ be a flow-network (with an implied capacity function c). Let s be the source of the network, and let t be the sink. A *flow* in G is a real-valued function $f : V \times V \to \mathbb{R}$ that satisfies the following three properties:

Capacity Constraint. For all $u, v \in V$, we require $f(u, v) \leq c(u, v)$.
Skew Symmetry. For all $u, v \in V$, we require $f(u, v) = -f(v, u)$.
Flow Conservation. For all $u \in V - \{s, t\}$, we require $\sum_{v \in V} f(u, v) = 0$.

The quantity $f(u, v)$, which can be positive or negative, is called the net flow from vertex u to vertex v.

The Ford-Fulkerson method solves the maximum-flow problem. This method is iterative. We start with $f(u, v) = 0$ for all $u, v \in V$, giving an initial flow of value 0. At each iteration, we increase the flow value by finding an *augmenting path*, which we can think of as a path from the source s to the sink t along which we can push more flow. We repeat this process until no augmenting path can be found; at that moment the flow has reached its maximum value.

We now show how to realize this algorithm with Datalog++. We are given a directed graph, describing the flow network, whose arcs are stored as facts in the database. For each edge (x, y) with capacity c we have a fact $\texttt{g(x,y,c)}$ in the database. We also have a fact $\texttt{g(y,x,c')}$ where $c' = 0$ in the case that does not exist the edge (y, x). The main predicate is $\texttt{flow(J,X,Y,F)}$, describing the value $\texttt{F}$ of the flow from vertex $\texttt{X}$ to vertex $\texttt{Y}$ at stage $\texttt{J}$. First of all we need a flow initializing rule:

$$\texttt{flow}(0, X, Y, 0) \leftarrow \texttt{g}(X, Y, \_).$$

Then we need a predicate describing the *residual capacity network*, that is the graph on which we search a path from the source to the sink along which we can push more flow with respect to the capacity constraint.

$$\texttt{residual\_network}(J, X, Y, C) \leftarrow \texttt{g}(X, Y, C1), \texttt{flow}(J, X, Y, F),$$
$$C = C1 - F1, C > 0.$$

To the purpose of finding a path from the source to the sink on this graph we use the *spanning tree* program, but each time a new edge is added to the spanning three, its residual capacity is compared to the minimum residual capacity of the edges that lie on that path. Therefore, when we reach the sink we already know the minimum residual capacity on the augmenting path, that is the maximum value of flow we can push along the augmenting path.

$$\texttt{augmenting\_path}(J, X, Y, C) \leftarrow \texttt{residual\_network}(J, X, Y, C),$$
$$X = \texttt{source}, \texttt{choice}((J, Y), (X)).$$

$$\texttt{augmenting\_path}(J, X, Y, C) \leftarrow \texttt{augmenting\_path}(J, \_, X, C),$$
$$\texttt{residual\_network}(J, X, Y, C1),$$
$$Y \neq \texttt{source}, C < C1, \texttt{choice}((J, Y), (X)).$$

$$\texttt{augmenting\_path}(J, X, Y, C) \leftarrow \texttt{augmenting\_path}(J, \_, X, C1),$$
$$\texttt{residual\_network}(J, X, Y, C),$$
$$Y \neq \texttt{source}, C < C1, \texttt{choice}((J, Y), (X)).$$

In this way we compute a spanning tree starting from the source. However what we need is a path from the source to the sink. Therefore we have to spot those edges lying on the augmenting path, i.e. the edges on which we push more flow. To do this we can go backwards from the sink to the source.

$$\texttt{flow\_augmentation}(J, X, \texttt{sink}, C) \leftarrow \texttt{augmenting\_path}(J, X, \texttt{sink}, C).$$

$$\texttt{flow\_augmentation}(J, Y, X, C) \leftarrow \texttt{flow\_augmentation}(J, X, \_, C),$$
$$\texttt{augmenting\_path}(J, Y, X, \_).$$

Finally, we need some rules to update, according to the algorithm, the flow at each new stage and a final rule to detect the maximum flow when it is no longer possible to find an augmenting path.

$$\text{flow}(J+1,X,Y,F) \leftarrow \text{flow}(J,X,Y,F1),\text{flow\_augmentation}(J,X,Y,C),$$
$$F = F1 + C.$$

$$\text{flow}(J+1,X,Y,F) \leftarrow \text{flow}(J,X,Y,F1),\text{flow\_augmentation}(J,Y,X,C),$$
$$F = F1 - C.$$

$$\text{flow}(J+1,X,Y,F) \leftarrow \neg\text{flow\_augmentation}(J,X,Y,\_),$$
$$\neg\text{flow\_augmentation}(J,Y,X,\_).$$

$$\text{max\_flow} \qquad\quad \leftarrow \text{flow}(J,X,Y,F),\neg\text{augmenting\_path}(J,\_,\text{sink},\_).$$

3.3 The Readers-Writers Problem

In this last example we show how Datalog++ is able to specify typical concurrent programming problems. We are given a shared resource and some processes. The processes have access to the resource for read or write operations. Any number of reads can proceed concurrently, but a write cannot be executed concurrently with a read or another write. There is no particular priority policy: at each stage it is nondeterministically selected whether to give priority to read or write operations. A process waiting for the right to execute an operation remains in its wait-state until it gets that right and completes its operation. Finally, we assume that all reads and writes complete in a stage. For each process we have in the database a fact of the form process(X), where X is the name of the process.

```
want_to(want_to_read).        action(reading).
want_to(want_to_write).       action(writing).
```

$$p0 : \text{next\_priority}(0,X) \leftarrow \text{action}(X),\text{choice}((),(X)).$$

$$p1 : \text{aux\_priority}(J,X) \leftarrow \text{next\_priority}(J,\_),\text{action}(X),\text{choice}((J),(X)).$$

$$p2 : \text{next\_priority}(J+1,X) \leftarrow \text{aux\_priority}(J,X).$$

$$s0 : \text{state}(0,K,X) \leftarrow \text{process}(K),\text{want\_to}(X),\text{choice}((K),(X)).$$

$$n0 : \text{next\_state}(J,K,\text{writing}) \leftarrow \text{state}(J,K,\text{want\_to\_write}),$$
$$\text{next\_priority}(J,\text{writing}),$$
$$\text{choice}((J),(K)).$$

$$n1 : \text{next\_state}(J,K,\text{writing}) \leftarrow \text{state}(J,K,\text{want\_to\_write}),$$
$$\text{next\_priority}(J,\text{reading}),$$
$$\neg\text{state}(J,\_,\text{want\_to\_read}),$$
$$\text{choice}((J),(K)).$$

$$n2 : \text{next\_state}(J,K,\text{reading}) \leftarrow \text{state}(J,K,\text{want\_to\_read}),$$
$$\text{next\_priority}(J,\text{reading}).$$

$$n3 : \text{next\_state}(J,K,\text{reading}) \leftarrow \text{state}(J,K,\text{want\_to\_read}),$$
$$\text{next\_priority}(J,\text{writing}),$$
$$\neg\text{state}(J,\_,\text{want\_to\_write}).$$

$$n4 : \text{next\_state}(J,K,X) \qquad \leftarrow \text{state}(J,K,Y),\text{action}(Y),$$
$$\text{want\_to}(X),\text{choice}((J,K),(X)).$$

s1 : state(J + 1, K, X) ← next_state(J, K, X).

s2 : state(J + 1, K, X) ← state(J, K, X), want_to(X),
¬next_state(J, K, _).

The first three rules nondeterministically assign the priority, at each stage, to the read or to the write operations. The rule s0 nondeterministically selects a starting state for each process. When the write operations take priority, the rule n0 gives the right to reach the resource to a process waiting for a write operation. Note the use of **choice** to model *mutual exclusion*: only one process, nondeterministically chosen out of all the waiting-for-writing processes, will be able to write at next stage. When the read operations take priority but there are not any processes waiting for reading, the rule n1 acts just like the rule n0. The rules n2 and n3 correspond respectively to the rule n0 and n1 but for the processes that want to read. Note that in this case we do not need the **choice** because any number of reads can be executed concurrently.

Another example of Datalog++ program in the concurrent programming area is the *Alternating Bit Protocol* in [3].

4   Verification of Datalog++ Programs

The goal of this section is that of suggesting a methodology for the verification of Datalog++ programs. Our methodology is based on the distinction between *atemporal* and *temporal* predicates. In fact, for temporal predicates we prove correctness by showing that their stable models match their intended semantics. On the other hand, to show the correctness of temporal predicates we define and prove some standard properties based on their temporal structure.

Definition 3 (X and Y Predicates). *Let* P *be an XY-program, and let* p *be a predicate of* P. *We call* p *an X-predicate if the rules defining* p *are only X-rules; an Y-predicate if at least one rule defining* p *is a Y-rule.*

We assimilate to X-predicates also the predicates of non-staged programs. Intuitively using X-predicates we can deduce only facts for the present time (actual stage), while using Y-predicates we can deduce facts for the future time (next stage). It is important to note that all the programs of the previous section share a similar structure described in Figure 1 for the Ford-Fulkerson example. In fact, Datalog++ programs usually have a single Y-predicate which performs stage transition, and many X-predicates which prepare such transition.

4.1   Properties of the choice Construct

When **choice** constructs are used in XY-programs we must pay attention to the *choice safety* constraint, which requests the stage argument to appear in the domain of the FD (the right argument of a choice goal). Moreover we restrict the use of **choice** at the X-rules, as we have done in all the programs of the previous

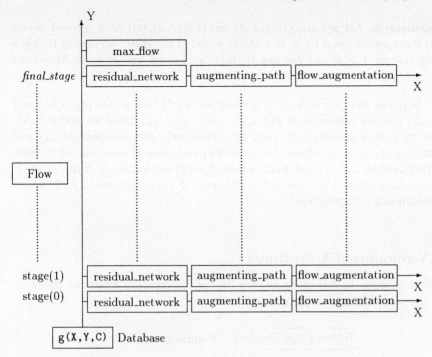

Fig. 1. Structure of the Ford-Fulkerson program

sections. This syntactic restriction, however, does not affect the expressiveness of Datalog++ and makes verification easier.

Now we define a *general choice rule*:

Definition 4 (General choice Rule). *We define a general choice as a rule with the following structure:*

$$p(J, \alpha, \epsilon) \leftarrow q(J, \beta), \mathtt{choice}((J, \delta), (\epsilon)).$$

where Greek letters are sets of variables, $q(J, \beta)$ stands for the conjunction of all the non-choice goals (also the non-staged ones) of the rule, α and δ can be empty sets, $\delta \cap \epsilon = \emptyset$, $\delta, \epsilon \subseteq \beta$.

The stable version of this general choice rule is:

$$\mathtt{sv0} : p(J, \alpha, \epsilon) \qquad\qquad \leftarrow q(J, \beta), \mathtt{chosen}(J, \delta, \epsilon).$$
$$\mathtt{sv1} : \mathtt{chosen}(J, \delta, \epsilon) \qquad \leftarrow q(J, \beta), \neg\mathtt{diffChoice}(J, \delta, \epsilon).$$
$$\mathtt{sv2} : \mathtt{diffChoice}(J, \delta, \epsilon) \leftarrow \mathtt{chosen}(J, \delta, \epsilon'), \epsilon \neq \epsilon'.$$

where ϵ' is derived from ϵ by replacing each $A \in \epsilon$ with a new variable A'.

Following property clarifies what kind of functional dependency is enforced by the choice construct in each stable model.

Proposition 5. *Let* $p(J, \alpha, \epsilon) \leftarrow q(J, \beta), \text{choice}((J, \delta), (\epsilon))$ *be a general choice rule of a program* P, *and let* M *be a stable model of the stable version of* P. *Then for any integer* $J \geq 0$ *and for any* α, *there's at most one atom in* M *ground instance of* $p(J, \alpha, \epsilon)$.

Proof. Suppose that for some $J \geq 0$ there are in M two atoms $p(J, a, \epsilon1)$ and $p(J, a, \epsilon2)$ ground instances of $p(J, a, \epsilon)$, with $\epsilon1 \neq \epsilon2$. Since all stable models are supported models [13], then by clause **sv0**, also $\text{chosen}(J, \delta, \epsilon1)$ and $\text{chosen}(J, \delta, \epsilon1)$ are in M. Hence, by clause **sv1** and since M is supported we have that $\text{diffChoice}(J, \delta, \epsilon1)$ and $\text{diffChoice}(J, \delta, \epsilon2)$ are not in M. Since $\epsilon1 \neq \epsilon2$, it follows from clause **sv2** that either $\text{chosen}(J, \delta, \epsilon1)$ or $\text{chosen}(J, \delta, \epsilon2)$ is not in M which is a contradiction.

□

4.2   Verification of X-Predicates

We are now ready to introduce an overview of the strategy which we follow to prove the correctness of X-predicates.

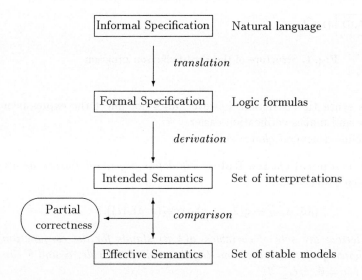

Fig. 2. Our strategy to prove X-predicates partial correctness

We begin by describing in natural language which role in the computation is played by the X-predicate. This description is the *informal specification* of the predicate. The second step consists of translating this description from natural language in a set of logic rules, obtaining the *formal specification*. From this formal specification we derive the *intended semantics* of the predicate. Since the effective semantics of a Datalog++ program is a set of stable models, then, also its intended semantics will be a set of interpretations. Exactly, the set of interpretations which satisfy the logic rules of the formal description.

Definition 6 (Intended Semantics of an X-Predicate). *Let* p *be an X-predicate, and let* S *be a set of logic rules defining the formal specification of* p. *The intended semantics of* p *is the set of interpretations that satisfy each rule in* S.

$$IS(\mathbf{p}) = \{I | I \in B_{\mathbf{p}} \wedge (\forall r \in S.I \models r)\}$$

We can now define *partial correctness* of an X-predicate.

Definition 7 (Partial Correctness of an X-Predicate). *An X-predicate is said to be partially correct with respect to its intended semantics* $IS(\mathbf{p})$ *iff, for each stable model* M *of* p, *there exists an interpretation* $I \in IS(\mathbf{p})$ *such that* M $\subseteq I$.

Example 8 (Partial Correctness of Spanning Tree). Consider the *spanning tree* program of example 2 and assume we wish to prove its correctness. First of all we have to give its informal specification in natural language.

Informal Specification: the st relation is a maximal subset of the g relation. Moreover, st is a tree rooted in a.

Now we have to translate this informal specification in a set of logic formulas. To be a tree means:

$$st(X,Y) \to st(\_,X) \vee Y = a. \tag{1}$$
$$st(X,Y) \to \neg(st(Z,Y) \wedge Z \neq X). \tag{2}$$

To be rooted in a means:

$$st(root,a). \tag{3}$$

To be a maximal subset of g means:

$$st(X,Y) \to g(X,Y) \vee Y = a. \tag{4}$$
$$(g(X,Y) \wedge st(\_,X)) \to st(\_,Y). \tag{5}$$

Intended Semantics: $IS(\mathbf{st}) = \{I | I \subseteq B_{\mathbf{st}} \wedge I \models (1), (2), (3), (4), (5) \}$.
Partial Correctness: Let M be a stable model of st. Then $\exists I \in IS(\mathbf{st})$ such that $M \subseteq I$.

Proof. Property (1) is trivially satisfied by clause st0 and by the definition of model; (2) is satisfied by clause st0, by the goal st(_,X) in the body of clause st1 and since all stable models are supported; (3) is satisfied by the goal Y ≠ a and, for proposition 5, by the choice-goal in the body of clause st1; (4) is satisfied by clause st0, by the goal g(X,Y) in the body of clause st1 and since all stable models are supported; (5) is satisfied because if $(g(X,Y) \wedge st(\_,X))$, then each non-choice goal in the body of clause st1 is satisfied, and then choice has to choose. □

Note how the translation in logic formulas of the informal specification is quite close to the text of the program. This facts hints us a way to exploit the declarative features of Datalog++ programming to give a methodology for program development. Suppose, in fact, we have not yet written the *Spanning tree* program and we wish to develop such program. First we write the informal specification. Then we translate it in logic formulas. At this point the program development become immediate. The logic property (3) trivially gives us the st0 clause. The properties (1) and (4) suggest us the non-choice goal of clause st1. Finally, provided that we recognize in (2) a functional dependence, typically imposed by the choice construct, we obtain the program as we have written before.

4.3 *Safety* and *Progress* Properties for Y-Predicates

For Y-predicates we do not prove partial correctness by reasoning on models, as we have done for X-predicates. We define and prove some standard properties following the approach of UNITY, a computational model with associated a proof system, introduced by Chandy and Misra in [5]. According to Chandy and Misra, we distinguish between *safety* and *progress* properties. We do not define these terms formally. Intuitively safety properties are invariant of the programs, i.e. properties which are satisfied at each stage of the computation. On the other hand, progress properties regard the temporal development of the computation.

We start introducing two kind of safety properties, one characterizing Y-predicates from a semantics point of view, the other one from a quantitative point of view.

The *Meaning* properties express, at each stage, the matching of the role played by the Y-predicate p in the computation with its declarative reading $dr(p)$, i.e. the informal specification.

Definition 9 (Final Stage). *Let* p *be a Y-predicate of a program* P *and* M *a stable model of* P. *If for each stage* $J : 0 \leq J \leq K$ *exists at least one atom of the form* p(J, _) *in* M, *while it does not exist for* $J > K$, *then we say* K *to be the* final_stage *of* p *and we write* $K = final\_stage(p)$. *If such a stage does not exist then* $final\_stage(p) = +\infty$.

Definition 10 (*Meaning*). *A* Meaning *property is the matching of an Y-predicate with its declarative reading. Such a property has the following form:*

$$\forall J : 0 \leq J \leq final\_stage(p), \forall \alpha : db(\alpha) \ . \ p(J, \delta) \equiv dr(p)$$

where α *and* δ *are set of variables such that* $\alpha \subseteq \delta$, *and db is a relation in the database.*

Such kind of properties can be easily proved by induction on the stages as we will show later by providing some examples.

The *HowMany* properties constrain the number of atoms of a given form in every stable model of the program.

Example 11. Recall the program for the *readers-writers problem*. We would like our program to have some desired properties:

1. each process at each stage is in one, and only one, state,
2. two or more write operations can not be executed concurrently,
3. write operations can not be executed concurrently with read operations.

We can express these three properties in terms of number of occurrences of facts of a given form in the stable models:

1. $\forall J, \forall K : process(K) \quad \#\{X|state(J, K, X)\} = 1$
2. $\forall J \quad \#\{K|state(J, K, writing)\} \leq 1$
3. $\forall J \quad \#\{K, W|state(J, K, writing) \wedge state(J, K, reading)\} = 0$

In other words *HowMany* properties are specified using the count aggregate in the stable models or their approximations.

Definition 12 (*HowMany*). *Let $\Pi(J, \kappa, \delta, cost)$ be a logic formula formed only by Y-predicates, where J is the stage argument of the Y-predicates, κ is the set of variables on which we count, δ is the set of all the other variables, cost are he constants. We define* HowMany *property the following expression:*

$$\forall J, K \quad \#\{\kappa|\Pi(J, \kappa, \delta, cost)\} < op > n$$

where n is a nonnegative integer, and $< op > \in \{=, \geq, \leq\}$.

We next define two kinds of progress property, the first one for those programs which reach a fixed point, the second one for those programs that do not terminate (such as the *readers-writers problem*).

Definition 13 (*FixedPoint*). *Let* p *be an Y-predicate. We define* FixedPoint *property the following:*

$$\exists j < +\infty : \quad j = final\_stage(\mathbf{p}).$$

A useful strategy for showing that a Y-predicate always reaches its final_stage is the following: display a function that strictly decreases at each stage and that it's lower bounded, and map the function to the Y-predicate.

Note that in each program of the previous section we have just one Y-predicate which gives the vertical structure to the program and some X-predicate doing the horizontal work. Therefore, if all X-predicates terminate, when we prove that the unique Y-predicate has a finite final_stage, we have that no new atom can be deduced after the final stage, i.e. the computation has reached a fixed point.

The next kind of properties state that the presence of a given fact in a stable model *ensures* that another fact sooner or later will belong to the approximations of stable model.

Definition 14 (*Ensures*). *Let* p *and* q *be Y-predicates of a program* P. *An* Ensures *property is a statement of the form*

$$\forall \alpha, \ \mathbf{p}(J, \alpha) \ \texttt{ensures} \ \exists I > J : \mathbf{q}(I, \beta).$$

Verification of these kind of properties requires a *fairness assumption* which is not treated here due to lack of space. Examples can be found in [3].

4.4   Application of the Methodology

We now apply the methodology introduced to the GCD program. Verification of the Ford-Fulkerson and other programs can be found in [3].

Example 15 (Properties of the GCD Program). Recall the *GCD* program. We wish to prove the following properties:

1. *Meaning:* $\forall J : 0 \leq J \leq final\_stage(\texttt{candidate\_GCD}).\texttt{candidate\_GCD}(\texttt{J}, \texttt{X}) \equiv$ "X is a nonnegative integer which if inserted in the initial set of number doesn't change the GCD."

2. *FixedPoint:* $\exists j < +\infty : j = final\_stage(\texttt{candidate\_GCD})$.

Proof. We prove, by induction on the stages, the *Meaning* property:

Base case (J=0). Trivial. Since only by rule r0 we can deduce facts of the form `candidate_GCD(0,X)`, then X belongs to the initial set of integers.

Induction Step. We can deduce facts of the form `candidate_GCD(n+1,X)` by rules r2 and r3. If `candidate_GCD(n+1,X)` is deduced by the rule r2 then by induction hypothesis X satisfies the property. If `candidate_GCD(n+1,X)` is deduced by the rule r3 then X is the difference between two integers (a,b) such that `candidate_GCD(n,a)` and `candidate_GCD(n,b)`. Since $GCD(a,b) = GCD(a-b,b)$ if $a > b$, and since X = a - b then X satisfies the property.

We now prove that `candidate_GCD` reaches its final stage and thus the program terminates. In fact, at each stage we delete from the set of candidates an integer and we add another integer which is less than the previous one. Therefore, at each stage the sum total of the candidate integers strictly decreases but the sum total is lower bounded. Thus the program terminates. In particular, the program terminates when it is no longer possible to find two candidate_integers with differet values. By the *Meaning* property 1, and since $GCD(a,a) = a$, then, when the program reachs the fixed point we find the GCD of the initial set of integers, as stated by rule r4.

5   Conclusion and Future Work

We briefly presented in this paper a methodology for developing Datalog++ programs and reasoning on their correctness. We believe that Datalog++ is a versatile programming language which supports verification principles, firmly coated in logic. Future research includes a thorough formalization of the verification methodology, as well as the development of tools, automatic or semi-automatic, which support verification of Datalog++ programs.

References

1. K. R. Apt. Program verification and Prolog. In E. Borger, editor, *Specification and Validation methods for Programming languages and systems.* Oxford University press, 1994.
2. N. Arni, K. Ong, S. Tsur, and C. Zaniolo. $\mathcal{LDL}$++: A Second Generation Deductive Databases Systems. Technical report, MCC Corporation, 1993.
3. F. Bonchi. Verification of Datalog++ Programs (in Italian). Master's thesis, Department of Computer Science University of Pisa, 1998.
4. A. Brogi, V. S. Subrahmanian, and C. Zaniolo. The Logic of Totally and Partially Ordered Plans: a Deductive Database Approach. *Annals of Mathematics in Artificial Intelligence*, 19:59–96, 1997.
5. K.M. Chandy and J.Misra. *Parrallel Program Design: A Foundation.* Addison-Wesley, 1988.
6. J. Chomicki. Temporal deductive databases. In A. Tansel, J. Clifford, S. Gadia, S. Jajodia, A. Segev, and R. Snodgrass, editors, *Temporal Databases: Theory, Design and Implementation*, pages 294–320. Benjamin Cummings, 1993.
7. P. Derensart. Proof methods of declarative properties of definite programs. *Theoretical Computer Science*, 118:99–166, 1993.
8. M Gelfond and V. Lifchitz. The Stable Model Semantics for logic programming. In *Proc. of the 5th Int. Conf. on Logic Programming*, pages 1070–1080, 1988.
9. F. Giannotti, S. Greco, D. Saccà, and C. Zaniolo. Programming with non Determinism in Deductive Databases. *Annals of Mathematics in Artificial Intelligence*, 19:97–125, 1997.
10. F. Giannotti, G. Manco, M. Nanni, D. Pedreschi, and F. Turini. Nondeterministic, nonmonotonic logic databases. *To appear in IEEE Transaction on Knowledge and Data Engineering*, 2000.
11. F. Giannotti, G. Manco, and D. Pedreschi. A Deductive Data Model for Representing and Querying Semistructured Data. In *Proc. 5th Int. Conf. on Deductive and Object-Oriented Databases (DOOD97)*, December 1997.
12. F. Giannotti, D. Pedreschi, D. Saccà, and C. Zaniolo. Non-Determinism in Deductive Databases. In *Proc. 2nd Int. Conf. on Deductive and Object-Oriented Databases (DOOD91)*, volume 566 of *Lecture Notes in Computer Science*, pages 129–146, 1991.
13. V. Marek and V.S. Subrahmanian. The relation between stable, supported, default and auto-epistemic semantics for general logic programs. *Theoretical Computer Science*, 103:365–386, 1992.
14. A. Pnueli. The temporal logic of programs. In *Proceedings of the 18 th. IEEE Symposium on Foundations of Computer Science*, pages 44–57, 1977.
15. D. Saccà and C. Zaniolo. Stable Models and Non-determinism in Logic Programs with Negation. In *Proc. of the ACM Symp. on Principles of Database Systems*.
16. C. Zaniolo. Active Database Rules with Transaction Conscious Stable Model Semantics. In *Proc. 4th Int. Conf. on Deductive and Object-Oriented Databases (DOOD95)*, volume 1013 of *Lecture Notes in Computer Science*, pages 55–72, 1995.
17. C. Zaniolo, N. Arni, and K. Ong. Negation and Aggregates in Recursive Rules: The $\mathcal{LDL}$++ Approach. In *Proc. 3rd Int. Conf. on Deductive and Object-Oriented Databases (DOOD93)*, volume 760 of *Lecture Notes in Computer Science*, 1993.
18. C. Zaniolo, S. Ceri, C. Faloutsos, R.T Snodgrass, V.S. Subrahmanian, and R. Zicari. *Advanced Database Systems.* Morgan Kaufman, 1997.

Mining Minimal Non-redundant Association Rules Using Frequent Closed Itemsets

Yves Bastide[1], Nicolas Pasquier[1], Rafik Taouil[1],
Gerd Stumme[1,2], and Lotfi Lakhal[1]

[1] L.I.M.O.S., Université Blaise Pascal – Clermont-Ferrand II
Complexe des Cézeaux, 24 Avenue des Landais, F–63177 Aubière cedex, France
{bastide,pasquier,taouil,lakhal}@libd2.univ-bpclermont.fr
[2] Technische Universität Darmstadt, Fachbereich Mathematik
Schloßgartenstr. 7, D–64289 Darmstadt, Germany
stumme@mathematik.tu-darmstadt.de

Abstract. The problem of the relevance and the usefulness of extracted association rules is of primary importance because, in the majority of cases, real-life databases lead to several thousands association rules with high confidence and among which are many redundancies. Using the closure of the Galois connection, we define two new bases for association rules which union is a generating set for all valid association rules with support and confidence. These bases are characterized using frequent closed itemsets and their generators; they consist of the non-redundant exact and approximate association rules having minimal antecedents and maximal consequents, i.e. the most relevant association rules. Algorithms for extracting these bases are presented and results of experiments carried out on real-life databases show that the proposed bases are useful, and that their generation is not time consuming.

1 Introduction

The purpose of association rule extraction, introduced in [AIS93], is to discover significant relations between binary attributes extracted from databases. An example of association rule extracted from a database of supermarket sales is: "cereals $\wedge$ sugar $\rightarrow$ milk (support 7%, confidence 50%)". This rule states that the customers who buy cereals and sugar also tend to buy milk. The *support* defines the range of the rule, i.e. the proportion of customers who bought the three items among all customers, and the *confidence* defines the precision of the rule, i.e. the proportion of customers who bought milk among those who bought cereals and sugar. An association rule is considered relevant for decision making if it has support and confidence at least equal to some minimal support and confidence thresholds, *minsupport* and *minconfidence*, defined by the user.

The problem of relevance and usefulness of the result is related to the number of extracted association rules – that is in general very large – and to the presence of a huge proportion of redundant rules, i.e. rules conveying the same information, among them. Even though the visualization of a relatively significant number

J. Lloyd et al. (Eds.): CL 2000, LNAI 1861, pp. 972–986, 2000.
© Springer-Verlag Berlin Heidelberg 2000

of rules can be simplified by the use of visualization tools such as the Rule Visualizer system [KMR+94], suppressing redundant association rules requires other solutions. Moreover, as the redundant association rules represent the majority of the extracted rules for several kinds of data, their suppression reduces considerably the number of rules to be managed during the visualization.

Example 1. In order to illustrate the problem of redundant association rules, nine association rules extracted from UCI KDD's archives's dataset MUSH-ROOMS[1] describing the characteristics of 8 416 mushrooms are presented below. These nine rules have identical supports and confidences of 51% and 54% respectively, and the item "free gills" in the antecedent:

1) free gills $\rightarrow$ eatable
2) free gills $\rightarrow$ eatable, partial veil
3) free gills $\rightarrow$ eatable, white veil
4) free gills, white veil $\rightarrow$ eatable
5) free gills, partial veil $\rightarrow$ eatable
6) free gills $\rightarrow$ eatable, partial veil, white veil
7) free gills, partial veil $\rightarrow$ eatable, white veil
8) free gills, white veil $\rightarrow$ eatable, partial veil
9) free gills, partial veil, white veil $\rightarrow$ eatable

Obviously, given rule 6, rules 1 to 5 and 7 to 9 are redundant, since they do not convey any additional information to the user. Rule 6 has minimal antecedent and maximal consequent and it is the most informative among these nine rules. In order to improve the relevance and the usefulness of extracted rules, only rule 6 should be extracted and presented to the user.

Several methods have been proposed in the literature to reduce the number of extracted association rules. Generalized association rules [HF95,SA95] are defined using a taxonomy of the items; they are rules between sets of items that belong to different levels of the taxonomy. The use of statistic measures other than confidence such as conviction, Pearson's correlation or χ^2 test is studied in [BMS97,SBM98]. In [Hec96,PSM94,ST96], the use of deviation measures, i.e. measures of distance between association rules, defined according to their supports and confidences, is proposed. In [BAG99,NLHP98,SVA97], the use of item constraints, that are boolean expressions defined by the user, in order to specify the form of the association rules that will be presented to the user is proposed. The approach proposed in [BG99] is to present to the user rules with maximal antecedents, called A-maximal rules, that are rules for which the population of objects concerned is reduced when an item is added to the antecedent. In [PBTL99c], we adapt the Duquenne-Guigues basis for global implications [DG86,GW99] and the proper basis for partial implications [Lux91] to the association rules framework. It is demonstrated that these bases are minimal with respect to the number of extracted association rules. However, none of these methods allows to generate the non-redundant association rules with minimal antecedents and maximal consequents which we believe are the most relevant and useful from the point of view of the user.

---

[1] ftp://ftp.ics.uci.edu/pub/machine-learning-databases/mushroom/

1.1   Contribution

In the rest of the paper, two kinds of association rules are distinguished:

- Exact association rules whose confidence is equal to 100%, i.e. which are valid for all the objects of the context. These rules are written $l \Rightarrow l'$.
- Approximate association rules whose confidence is lower than 100%, i.e. which are valid for a proportion of objects of the context equal to their confidence. These rules are written $l \rightarrow l'$.

The solution proposed in this paper consists in generating *bases*, or *reduced covers*, for association rules. These bases contain no redundant rule, being thus of smaller size. Our goal is to limit the extraction to the most informative association rules from the point of view of the user.

Using the semantic for the extraction of association rules based on the closure of the Galois connection [PBTL98], the *generic basis for exact association rules* and the *informative basis for approximate association rules* are defined. They are constructed using the frequent closed itemsets and their generators, and they minimize the number of association rules generated while maximizing the quantity and the quality of the information conveyed. They allow for:

1. The generation of only the most informative non-redundant association rules, i.e. of the most useful and relevant rules: those having a minimal antecedent (left-hand side) and a maximal consequent (right-hand side). Thus redundant rules which represent in certain databases the majority of extracted rules, particularly in the case of dense or correlated data for which the total number of valid rules is very large, will be pruned.
2. The presentation to the user of a set of rules covering all the attributes of the database, i.e. containing rules where the union of the antecedents (resp. consequents) is equal to the unions of the antecedents (resp. consequents) of all the association rules valid in the context. This is necessary in order to discover rules that are "surprising" to the user, which constitute important information that it is necessary to consider [Hec96,PSM94,ST96].
3. The extraction of a set of rules without any loss of information, i.e. conveying all the information conveyed by the set of all valid association rules. It is possible to deduce efficiently, without access to the dataset, all valid association rules with their supports and confidences from these bases.

The union of these two bases thus constitutes a small non-redundant generating set for all valid association rules, their supports and their confidences.

In section 2, we recall the semantic for association rules based on the Galois connection. The new bases we propose and algorithms for generating them are defined in section 3. Results of experiments we conducted on real-life datasets are presented in section 4 and section 5 concludes the paper.

2 Semantic for Association Rules Based on the Galois Connection

The association rule extraction is performed from a data mining context, that is a triplet $\mathcal{D} = (\mathcal{O}, \mathcal{I}, \mathcal{R})$, where $\mathcal{O}$ and $\mathcal{I}$ are finite sets of objects and items respectively, and $\mathcal{R} \subseteq \mathcal{O} \times \mathcal{I}$ is a binary relation. Each couple $(o, i) \in \mathcal{R}$ denotes the fact that the object $o \in \mathcal{O}$ is related to the item $i \in \mathcal{I}$.

Example 2. A data mining context $\mathcal{D}$ constituted of six objects (each one identified by its *OID*) and five items is represented in the table 1. This context is used as support for the examples in the rest of the paper.

Table 1. Data mining context $\mathcal{D}$.

OID	Items
1	A C D
2	B C E
3	A B C E
4	B E
5	A B C E
6	B C E

The closure operator γ of the Galois connection [GW99] is the composition of the application ϕ, that associates with $O \subseteq \mathcal{O}$ the items common to all objects $o \in O$, and the application ψ, that associates with an itemset $l \subseteq \mathcal{I}$ the objects related to all items $i \in l$ (the objects "containing" l).

Definition 1 (Frequent Itemsets). *A set of items $l \subseteq \mathcal{I}$ is called an itemset. The support of an itemset l is the percentage of objects in $\mathcal{D}$ containing l: $support(l) = |\psi(l)| / |\mathcal{O}|$. l is a frequent itemset if $support(l) \geq$ minsupport.*

Definition 2 (Association Rules). *An association rule r is an implication between two frequent itemsets $l_1, l_2 \subseteq \mathcal{I}$ of the form $l_1 \to (l_2 \setminus l_1)$ where $l_1 \subset l_2$. The support and the confidence of r are defined as: $support(r) = support(l_2)$ and $confidence(r) = support(l_2) / support(l_1)$.*

The closure operator $\gamma = \phi \circ \psi$ associates with an itemset l the maximal set of items common to all the objects containing l, i.e. the intersection of these objects. Using this closure operator, we define the frequent closed itemsets that constitute a minimal non-redundant generating set for all frequent itemsets and their supports, and thus for all association rules, their supports and their confidences. This property comes from the facts that the support of a frequent itemset is equal to the support of its closure and that the maximal frequent itemsets are maximal frequent closed itemsets [PBTL98].

Definition 3 (Frequent Closed Itemsets). *A frequent itemset $l \subseteq \mathcal{I}$ is a frequent closed itemset iff $\gamma(l) = l$. The smallest (minimal) closed itemset containing an itemset l is $\gamma(l)$, i.e. the closure of l.*

In order to extract the frequent closed itemsets, the Close [PBTL98,PBTL99a] and the A-Close [PBTL99b] algorithms perform a breadth-first search for the *generators* of the frequent closed itemsets in a levelwise manner.

Definition 4 (Generators). *An itemset $g \subseteq \mathcal{I}$ is a (minimal) generator of a closed itemset l iff $\gamma(g) = l$ and $\nexists g' \subseteq \mathcal{I}$ with $g' \subset g$ such that $\gamma(g') = l$. A generator of cardinality k is called a k-generator.*

2.1   Extracting Frequent Closed Itemsets and their Generators with the Close Algorithm

The Close algorithm is an iterative algorithm for the extraction of all frequent closed itemsets. It courses generators of the frequent closed itemsets in a levelwise manner. During the kth iteration of the algorithm, a set FCC_k of candidates is considered. Each element of this set consists of three fields: a candidate k-generator, its closure (which is a candidate closed itemset), and their support (the supports of the generator and its closure being identical). At the end of the kth iteration, the algorithm stores a set FC_k containing the frequent k-generators, their closures which are frequent closed itemsets, and their supports.

The algorithm starts by initializing the set FCC_1 of the candidate 1-generators with the list of the 1-itemsets of the context and then carries out some iterations. During each iteration k:

1. The closures of all k-generators and their supports are computed. This computation is based on the property that the closure of an itemset is equal to the intersection of all the objects in the context containing it. The number of these objects provides the support of the generator. Only one scan of the context is thus necessary to determine the closures and the supports of all the k-generators.
2. All frequent k-generators, which support is greater or equal to *minsupport*, their closures and their supports are inserted in the set FC_k of frequent closed itemsets identified during the iteration k.
3. The set of candidate $(k+1)$-generators (used during the following iteration) is constructed, by joining the frequent k-generators in the set FC_k as follows.
   (a) The candidate $(k+1)$-generators are created by joining the k-generators in FC_k that have the same $k-1$ first items. For instance, the 3-generators {ABC} and {ABD} will be joined in order to create the candidate 4-generator {ABCD}.
   (b) The candidate $(k+1)$-generators that are known to be either infrequent or non-minimal, because one of their subset is either infrequent or non-minimal, are then removed. These generators are identified by the absence of at least one their subsets of size k among the frequent k-generators of FC_k.
   (c) A third phase removes among the remaining generators those which closures were already computed. Such a $(k+1)$-generator g is easily identified since it is included in the closure of a frequent k-generator g' in FC_k: $g' \subset g \subset \gamma(g')$ (i.e. it is not a minimal generator).

The algorithm stops when no new candidate generator can be created. The A-Close algorithm, developed in order to improve the effectiveness of the extraction in the case of slightly correlated data, does not compute the closures of the candidate generators during the iterations, but during an ultimate scan carried out after the end of these iterations.

Example 3. Figure 1 shows the execution of the Close algorithm on the context $\mathcal{D}$ for a minimal support threshold of 2/6. The algorithm carries out two iterations, and thus two dataset scans.

Scan $\mathcal{D}$ $\rightarrow$

FCC_1

Generator	Closed itemset	Support
{A}	{AC}	3/6
{B}	{BE}	5/6
{C}	{C}	5/6
{D}	{ACD}	1/6
{E}	{BE}	5/6

Suppressing infrequent itemsets $\rightarrow$

FC_1

Generator	Closed itemset	Support
{A}	{AC}	3/6
{B}	{BE}	5/6
{C}	{C}	5/6
{E}	{BE}	5/6

Scan $\mathcal{D}$ $\rightarrow$

FCC_2

Generator	Closed itemset	Support
{AB}	{ABCE}	2/6
{AE}	{ABCE}	2/6
{BC}	{BCE}	4/6
{CE}	{BCE}	4/6

Suppressing infrequent itemsets $\rightarrow$

FC_2

Generator	Closed itemset	Support
{AB}	{ABCE}	2/6
{AE}	{ABCE}	2/6
{BC}	{BCE}	4/6
{CE}	{BCE}	4/6

Fig. 1. Extracting frequent closed itemsets from $\mathcal{D}$ with Close for *minsupport* = 2/6.

Experimental results showed that these algorithms are particularly efficient for mining association rules from dense or correlated data that represent an important part of real life databases.

3   Minimal Non-redundant Association Rules

As pointed out in example 1, it is desirable that only the non-redundant association rules with minimal antecedent and maximal consequent, i.e. the most useful and relevant rules, are extracted and presented to the user. Such rules are called *minimal non-redundant association rules*.

Support and confidence indicate the range and the precision of the rule, and thus, must be taken into account for characterizing the redundant association rules. In previous works concerning the reduction of redundant implication rules (functional dependancies), such as the definition of the canonical cover [BB79,Mai80], the notion of non-redundancy considered is related to the inference system using Armstrong axioms [Arm74]. This notion is not to be confused with the notion of non-redundancy we consider here. To our knowledge, such an inference system for association rules, that takes into account supports and confidences of the rules, does not exist. The principle of minimal non-redundant association rules as defined hereafter is to identify the most informative association rules considering the fact that in practice, the user cannot infer all other valid rules from the rules extracted while visualizing them.

An association rule is redundant if it conveys the same information – or less general information – than the information conveyed by another rule of the same usefulness and the same relevance. An association rule $r \in E$ is non-redundant and minimal if there is no other association rule $r' \in E$ having the same support and the same confidence, of which the antecedent is a subset of the antecedent of r and the consequent is a superset of the consequent of r.

Definition 5 (Minimal Non-redundant Association Rules). *An association rule $r : l_1 \rightarrow l_2$ is a minimal non-redundant association rule iff there does not exist an association rule $r' : l'_1 \rightarrow l'_2$ with* support(r) = support(r'), confidence(r) = confidence(r'), $l'_1 \subseteq l_1$ and $l_2 \subseteq l'_2$.

Based on this definition, we characterize the generic basis for exact association rules and the informative basis for approximate association rules, constituted of the minimal non-redundant exact and approximate association rules respectively.

3.1   Generic Basis for Exact Association Rules

The exact association rules, of the form $r : l_1 \Rightarrow (l_2 \setminus l_1)$, are rules between two frequent itemsets l_1 and l_2 whose closures are identical: $\gamma(l_1) = \gamma(l_2)$. Indeed, from $\gamma(l_1) = \gamma(l_2)$ we deduce that $l_1 \subset l_2$ and $support(l_1) = support(l_2)$, and thus $confidence(r) = 1$. Since the maximum itemset among these itemsets (which have same supports) is the itemset $\gamma(l_2)$, all supersets of l_1 that are subsets of $\gamma(l_2)$ have the same support, and the rules between two of these itemsets are exact rules.

Let $G_{\gamma(l_2)}$ be the set of generators of the frequent closed itemset $\gamma(l_2)$. By definition, the minimal itemsets that are supersets of l_1 and are subsets of $\gamma(l_2)$ are the generators $g \in G_{\gamma(l_2)}$. We thus conclude that rules of the form $g \Rightarrow (\gamma(l_2) \setminus g)$ between generators $g \in G_{\gamma(l_2)}$ and the frequent closed itemset $\gamma(l_2)$ are the rules of minimal antecedents and maximal consequents among the rules between the supersets of l_1 and the subsets of $\gamma(l_2)$. The generalization of this property to the set of frequent closed itemsets defines the generic basis consisting of all non-redundant exact association rules with minimal antecedents and maximal consequents, as characterized in definition 5.

Definition 6 (Generic Basis for Exact Association Rules). *Let FC be the set of frequent closed itemsets extracted from the context and, for each frequent closed itemset f, let denote G_f the set of generators of f. The generic basis for exact association rules is:*

$$GB = \{ r : g \Rightarrow (f \setminus g) \mid f \in FC \ \wedge \ g \in G_f \ \wedge \ g \neq f \}.$$

The condition $g \neq f$ ensures that rules of the form $g \Rightarrow \varnothing$ that are non-informative are discarded. The following proposition states that the generic basis does not lead to any loss of information.

Proposition 1. *(i) All valid exact association rules, their supports and their confidences (that are equals to 100%) can be deduced from the rules of the generic basis and theirs supports. (ii) The generic basis for exact association rules contains only minimal non redundant-rules.*

Proof. Let $r : l_1 \Rightarrow (l_2 \setminus l_1)$ be a valid exact association rule between two frequent itemsets with $l_1 \subset l_2$. Since $confidence(r) = 100\%$ we have $support(l_1) = support(l_2)$. Given the property that the support of an itemset is equal to the support of its closure, we deduce that $support(\gamma(l_1)) = support(\gamma(l_2)) \Longrightarrow \gamma(l_1) = \gamma(l_2) = f$. The itemset f is a frequent closed itemset $f \in FC$ and, obviously, there exists a rule $r' : g \Rightarrow (f \setminus g) \in GB$ such that g is a generator of f for which $g \subseteq l_1$ and $g \subset l_2$. We show that the rule r and its support can be deduced from the rule r' and its support. Since $g \subseteq l_1 \subset l_2 \subseteq f$, the rule r can be derived from the rule r'. From $\gamma(l_1) = \gamma(l_2) = f$, we deduce that $support(r) = support(l_2) = support(\gamma(l_2)) = support(f) = support(r')$. $\square$

Algorithm for Constructing the Generic Basis

The pseudo-code of the Gen-GB algorithm for constructing the generic basis for exact association rules using the frequent closed itemsets and their generators is presented in algorithm 1. Each element of a set FC_k consists of three elements: *generator*, *closure* and *support*.

Algorithm 1 Constructing the generic basis with Gen-GB.

Input : sets FC_k of k-groups of frequent k-generators;
Output : set GB of exact association rules of the generic basis;
1) $GB \leftarrow \{\}$
2) **forall** set $FC_k \in FC$ **do begin**
3)   **forall** k-generator $g \in FC_k$ such that $g \neq \gamma(g)$ **do begin**
4) $GB \leftarrow GB \cup \{(r : g \Rightarrow (\gamma(g) \setminus g), \gamma(g).support)\};$
5)   **end**
6) **end**
7) **return** GB;

The algorithm starts by initializing the set GB with the empty set (step 1). Each set FC_k of frequent k-groups is then examined successively (steps 2 to 6). For each k-generator $g \in FC_k$ of the frequent closed itemset $\gamma(g)$ for which g is different from its closure $\gamma(g)$ (steps 3 to 5), the rule $r : g \Rightarrow (\gamma(g) \setminus g)$, whose support is equal to the support of g and $\gamma(g)$, is inserted into GB (step 4). The algorithm returns finally the set GB containing all minimal non-redundant exact association rules between generators and their closures (step 7).

Example 4. The generic basis for exact association rules extracted from the context $\mathcal{D}$ for a minimal support threshold of 2/6 is presented in Table 2. It contains seven rules whereas fourteen exact association rules are valid on the whole.

3.2 Informative Basis for Approximate Association Rules

Each approximate association rule $l_1 \rightarrow (l_2 \setminus l_1)$, is a rule between two frequent itemsets l_1 and l_2 such that the closure of l_1 is a subset of the closure of l_2:

Table 2. Generic basis for exact association rules extracted from $\mathcal{D}$ for *minsupport* = 2/6.

Generator	Closure	Exact rule	Support
{A}	{AC}	A $\Rightarrow$ C	3/6
{B}	{BE}	B $\Rightarrow$ E	5/6
{C}	{C}		
{E}	{BE}	E $\Rightarrow$ B	5/6
{AB}	{ABCE}	AB $\Rightarrow$ CE	2/6
{AE}	{ABCE}	AE $\Rightarrow$ BC	2/6
{BC}	{BCE}	BC $\Rightarrow$ E	4/6
{CE}	{BCE}	CE $\Rightarrow$ B	4/6

$\gamma(l_1) \subset \gamma(l_2)$. The non-redundant approximate association rules with minimal antecedent l_1 and maximal consequent $(l_2 \setminus l_1)$ are deduced from this characterisation.

Let f_1 be the frequent closed itemset which is the closure of l_1, and g_1 a generator of f_1 such as $g_1 \subseteq l_1 \subseteq f_1$. Let f_2 be the frequent closed itemset which is the closure of l_2 and g_2 a generator of f_2 such as $g_2 \subseteq l_2 \subseteq f_2$. The rule $g_1 \Rightarrow (f_2 \setminus g_1)$ between the generator g_1 and the frequent closed itemset f_2 is the minimal non-redundant rule among the rules between an itemset of the interval[2] $[g_1, f_1]$ and an itemset of the interval $[g_2, f_2]$. Indeed, the generator g_1 is the minimal itemset whose closure is f_1, which means that the antecedent g_1 is minimal and that the consequent $(f_2 \setminus g_1)$ is maximal since f_2 is the maximal itemset of the interval $[g_2, f_2]$. The generalization of this property to the set of all rules between two itemsets l_1 and l_2 defines the informative basis which thus consists of all the non-redundant approximate association rules of minimal antecedents and maximal consequents characterized in definition 5.

Definition 7 (Informative Basis for Approximate Association Rules).
Let FC be the set of frequent closed itemsets and let denote G the set of their generators extracted from the context. The informative basis for approximate association rules is:

$$IB = \{r : g \to (f \setminus g) \mid f \in FC \ \wedge \ g \in G \ \wedge \ \gamma(g) \subset f\}.$$

Proposition 2. *(i) All valid approximate association rules, their supports and confidences, can be deduced from the rules of the informative basis, their supports and theirs confidences. (ii) All rules in the informative basis re minimal non-redundant approximate association rules.*

Proof. Let $r : l_1 \to (l_2 \setminus l_1)$ be a valid approximate association rule between two frequent itemsets with $l_1 \subset l_2$. Since $confidence(r) < 1$ we also have $\gamma(l_1) \subset \gamma(l_2)$. For any frequent itemsets l_1 and l_2, there is a generator g_1 such that $g_1 \subset l_1 \subseteq \gamma(l_1) = \gamma(g_1)$ and a generator g_2 such that $g_2 \subset l_2 \subseteq \gamma(l_2) = \gamma(g_2)$. Since $l_1 \subset l_2$, we have $l_1 \subseteq \gamma(g_1) \subset l_2 \subseteq \gamma(g_2)$ and the rule $r' : g_1 \to (\gamma(g_2) \setminus g_1)$ belongs to the informative basis IB. We show that the rule r, its support and its confidence can be deduced from the rule r', its support and its confidence. Since $g_1 \subset l_1 \subseteq \gamma(g_1) \subset g_2 \subset l_2 \subseteq \gamma(g_2)$, the antecedent and the consequent of r can be rebuilt starting from the rule r'. Moreover, we have $\gamma(l_2) =$

---

[2] The interval $[l_1, l_2]$ contains all the supersets of l_1 that are subsets of l_2.

$\gamma(g_2)$ and thus $support(r) = support(l_2) = support(\gamma(g_2)) = support(r')$. Since $g_1 \subset l_1 \subseteq \gamma(g_1)$, we have $support(g_1) = support(l_1)$ and we thus deduce that: $confidence(r) = support(l_2) / support(l_1) = support(\gamma(g_2)) / support(g_1) = confidence(r')$. $\square$

From the definition of the informative basis we deduce the definition of the transitive reduction of the informative basis that is itself a basis for all approximate association rules. We note $l_1 \lessdot l_2$ if the itemset l_1 is an immediate predecessor of the itemset l_2, i.e. $\nexists l_3$ such that $l_1 \subset l_3 \subset l_2$. The transitive rules of the informative basis are of the form $r : g \to (f \setminus g)$ for a frequent closed itemset f and a frequent generator g such that $\gamma(g) \subset f$ and $\gamma(g)$ is not an immediate predecessor of f in FC: $\gamma(g) \not\lessdot f$. The transitive reduction of the informative basis thus contains the rules with the form $r : g \to (f \setminus g)$ for a frequent closed itemset f and a frequent generator g such as $\gamma(g) \lessdot f$.

Definition 8 (Transitive Reduction of the Informative Basis). *Let FC be the set of frequent closed itemsets and let denote G the set of their generators extracted from the context. The transitive reduction of the informative basis for approximate association rules is:*

$$RI = \{r : g \to (f \setminus g) \mid f \in FC \ \wedge \ g \in G \ \wedge \ \gamma(g) \lessdot f\}.$$

Obviously, it is possible to deduce all the association rules of the informative basis with their supports and their confidences, and thus all the valid approximate rules, from the rules of this transitive reduction, their supports and their confidences. This reduction makes it possible to decrease the number of approximate rules extracted by preserving the rules which confidences are the highest (since the transitive rules have confidences lower than the non-transitive rules by construction) without losing any information.

Constructing the Transitive Reduction of the Informative Basis

The pseudo code of the Gen-RI algorithm for constructing the transitive reduction of the informative basis for the approximate association rules using the set of frequent closed itemsets and their generators is presented in algorithm 2. Each element of a set FC_k consists of three fields: *generator*, *closure* and *support*. The algorithm constructs for each generator g considered a set $Succ_g$ containing the frequent closed itemsets that are immediate successors of the closure of g.

The algorithm starts by initializing the set RI with the empty set (step 1). Each set FC_k of frequent k-groups is then examined successively in the increasing order of the values of k (steps 2 to 14). For each k-generator $g \in FC_k$ of the frequent closed itemset $\gamma(g)$ (steps 3 to 18), the set $Succ_g$ of the successors of the closure of $\gamma(g)$ is initialized with the empty set (step 4) and the sets S_j of frequent closed j-itemsets that are supersets of $\gamma(g)$ for $|\gamma(g)| < j \leq \mu^3$ are constructed (steps 5 to 7). The sets S_j are then considered in the ascending order of the values of j (steps 8 to 17). For each itemset $f \in S_j$ that is not

---

[3] We denote μ the size of the longest maximal frequent closed itemsets.

a superset of an immediate successor of $\gamma(g)$ in $Succ_g$ (step 10), f is inserted in $Succ_g$ (step 11) and the confidence of the rule $r : g \rightarrow (f \setminus g)$ is computed (step 12). If the confidence of r is greater or equal to the minimal confidence threshold *minconfidence*, the rule r is inserted in RI (steps 13 to 15). When all the generators of size lower than μ have been considered, the algorithm returns the set RI (step 20).

Algorithm 2 Generating the transitive reduction of the informative basis with Gen-RI.

Input   : sets FC_k of k-groups of frequent k-generators; *minconfidence* threshold;
Output : Transitive reduction of the informative basis RI;

```
1)  RI ← {}
2)  for (k ← 1; k ≤ μ-1; k++) do begin
3)      forall k-generator g ∈ FCₖ do begin
4)          Succ_g ← {};
5)          for (j = |γ(g)|; j ≤ μ; j++) do begin
6)              Sⱼ ← {f ∈ FC | f ⊃ γ(g) ∧ |f| = j};
7)          end
8)          for (j = |γ(g)|; j ≤ μ; j++) do begin
9)              forall frequent closed itemset f ∈ Sⱼ do begin
10)                 if (∄s ∈ Succ_g | s ⊂ f) then do begin
11)                     Succ_g ← Succ_g ∪ f;
12)                     r.confidence ← f.support/g.support;
13)                     if (r.confidence ≥ minconfidence)
14)                     then RI ← RI ∪ {r : g → (f \ g), r.confidence, f.support};
15)                 endif
16)             end
17)         end
18)     end
19) end
20) return RI;
```

Example 5. The transitive reduction of the informative basis for approximate association rules extracted from the context $\mathcal{D}$ for a minimal support threshold of 2/6 and a minimal confidence threshold of 3/6 is presented in Table 3. It contains seven rules, versus ten rules in the informative basis, whereas thirty six approximate association rules are valid on the whole.

4 Experimental Results

We used the four following datasets during these experiments:

- T20I6D100K[4], made up of synthetic data built according to the properties of sales data, which contains 100,000 objects with an average size of 20 items and an average size of the potential maximal frequent itemsets of six items.

---

[4] http://www.almaden.ibm.com/cs/quest/syndata.html

Table 3. Transitive reduction of the informative basis for approximate association rules extracted from $\mathcal{D}$ for *minsupport* $= 2/6$ and *minconfidence* $= 3/6$.

Generator	Closure	Closed superset	Approximate rule	Support	Confidence
{A}	{AC}	{ABCE}	A → BCE	2/6	2/3
{B}	{BE}	{BCE}	B → CE	4/6	4/5
{B}	{BE}	{ABCE}			
{C}	{C}	{AC}	C → A	3/6	3/5
{C}	{C}	{BCE}	C → BE	4/6	4/5
{C}	{C}	{ABCE}			
{E}	{BE}	{BCE}	E → BC	4/6	4/5
{E}	{BE}	{ABCE}			
{AB}	{ABCE}				
{AE}	{ABCE}				
{BC}	{BCE}	{ABCE}	BC → AE	2/6	2/4
{CE}	{BCE}	{ABCE}	CE → AB	2/6	2/4

- MUSHROOMS, that consists of 8,416 objects of an average size of 23 attributes (23 items by objects and 127 items on the whole) describing characteristics of mushrooms.
- C20D10K and C73D10K[5] which are samples of the file Public Use Microdata Samples containing data of the census of Kansas carried out in 1990. They consist of 10,000 objects corresponding to the first 10,000 listed people, each object containing 20 attributes (20 items by objects and 386 items on the whole) for C20D10K and 73 attributes (73 items by objects and 2,178 items on the whole) for C73D10K.

Execution times (not presented here) of the generation of the bases, as for the generation of all valid association rules, are negligible compared to execution times of the frequent (closed) itemsets extraction.

Number of Exact Association Rules Extracted. The total number of valid exact association rules and the number of rules in the generic basis are presented in Table 4. No exact association rule is extracted from T10I4D100K as for this support threshold all the frequent itemsets are frequent closed itemsets: they all have different supports and are thus themselves their unique generator. Consequently, there exists no rule of the form $l_1 \Rightarrow (l_2 \setminus l_1)$ between two frequent itemsets whose closures are identical: $\gamma(l_1) = \gamma(l_2)$ that are the valid exact association rules.

Table 4. Number of exact association rules extracted.

Dataset	Minsupport	Exact rules	Generic basis
T10I4D100K	0.5%	0	0
MUSHROOMS	30%	7,476	543
C20D10K	50%	2,277	457
C73D10K	90%	52,035	1,369

For the three other datasets, made up of dense and correlated data, the total number of valid exact rules varies from more than 2,000 to more than 52,000,

[5] ftp://ftp2.cc.ukans.edu/pub/ippbr/census/pums/pums90ks.zip

which is considerable and makes it difficult to discover interesting relationships. The generic basis represents a significant reduction of the number of extracted rules (by a factor varying from 12 to 50) and since it does not represent any loss of information, it brings a knowledge that is complete, relevant and easily usable from the point of view of the user.

Number of Approximate Association Rules Extracted. The total number of valid approximate association rules and the number of rules in the transitive reduction of the informative basis are presented in Table 5. The total number of valid approximate association rules is for the four datasets very significant since it varies of almost 20,000 rules for T20I6D100K to more than 2,000,000 rules for C73D10K. It is thus essential to reduce the set of extracted rules in order to make it usable by the user. For T20I6D100K, this basis represents a division by a factor of 5 approximately of the number of extracted approximate rules. For MUSHROOMS, C20D10K, and C73D10K, the total number of valid approximate association rules is much more important than for the synthetic data since these data are dense and correlated and thus the number of frequent itemsets is much higher. As a consequence, it is the same for the number of valid approximate rules. The proportion of frequent closed itemsets among the frequent itemsets being weak, the reduction of the informative basis for approximate rules makes it possible to reduce considerably (by a factor varying from 40 to 500) the number of extracted rules.

Table 5. Number of approximate association rules extracted.

Dataset (Minsupport)	Minconfidence	Approximate Rules	Informative basis reduction
T10I4D100K	70%	20,419	4,004
(0.5%)	30%	22,952	4,519
MUSHROOMS	70%	37,671	1,221
(30%)	30%	71,412	1,578
C20D10K	70%	89,601	1,957
(50%)	30%	116,791	1,957
C73D10K	90%	2,053,896	5,718
(90%)	80%	2,053,936	5,718

Comparing rules in the generic basis and the reduction of the informative basis to all valid rules, we checked that these bases do not contain any redundant rules. Considering the example presented in the section 1 concerning the nine approximate rules extracted the dataset MUSHROOMS, only the 6th rule is generated among these nine rules in the bases. Indeed, the itemsets {free gills} and {free gills, eatable, partial veil, white veil} are two frequent closed itemsets of which the first is an immediate predecessor of the second and they are the only frequent closed itemsets of the interval [∅, {free gills, eatable, partial veil, white veil}]. Moreover, the frequent closed itemset {free gills} being itself its unique generator, the rule 6 belongs to the transitive reduction of the informative basis: it is the minimal non-redundant rule among these nine rules.

5 Conclusion

Using the frequent closed itemsets and their generators extracted by the algorithms Close or A-Close, we define the generic basis for exact association rules and the transitive reduction of the informative basis for approximate association rules. The union of these bases provides a non-redundant generating set for all the valid association rules, their supports and their confidences. It contains the minimal non-redundant association rules (of minimal antecedent and maximal consequent) and does not represent any loss of information: from the point of view of the user, these rules are the most useful and the most relevant association rules. All the information conveyed by the set of valid association rules is also conveyed by the union of these two bases. Two algorithms for generating the generic basis and the transitive reduction of the informative basis using the frequent closed itemsets and their generators, are also presented. These bases are also of strong interest for:

- The visualization of the extracted rules since the reduced number of rules in these bases, as well as the distinction of the exact and the approximate rules, facilitate the presentation of the rules to the user. Moreover, the absence of redundant rules in the bases and the generation of the minimal non-redundant rules are of significant interest from the point of view of the user [KMR+94].
- The identification of the minimal non-redundant association rules among the set of valid association rules extracted, using Definition 5. It is thus possible to extend an existing implementation for extracting association rules or to integrate this method in the visualization system in order to present the minimal non-redundant association rules to the user.
- The data analysis and the formal concept analysis since they do not represent any loss of information compared to the set of valid implication rules and are constituted of the most useful and relevant rules. Definition 5 of the minimal non-redundant rules being also valid within the framework of global and partial implication rules between binary sets of attributes, definitions 6 of the generic basis and 7 of the informative basis are also valid for the global and partial implication rules respectively.

Moreover, we think that this approach is complementary with approaches for selecting association rules to be vizualised, such as templates and item constraints, that help the user managing the result.

As pointed out in section 3, up to now, there does not exist any inference system with completeness and soundness properties, for inferring association rules that takes into account supports and confidences of the rules. We think that the definition of such an inference system, equivalent to the Armstrong axioms for implications, constitutes an interesting perspective of future work.

References

[AIS93] R. Agrawal, T. Imielinski, and A. Swami. Mining association rules between sets of items in large databases. *Proc. SIGMOD conf.*, pp 207–216, May 1993.

[AS94] R. Agrawal and R. Srikant. Fast algorithms for mining association rules in large databases. *Proc. VLDB conf.*, pp 478–499, September 1994.

[Arm74] W. W. Armstrong. Dependency structures of data base relationships. *Proc. IFIP congress*, pp 580–583, August 1974.

[BAG99] R. J. Bayardo, R. Agrawal, and D. Gunopulos. Constraint-based rule mining in large, dense databases. *Proc. ICDE conf.*, pp 188–197, March 1999.

[BG99] R. J. Bayardo, and R. Agrawal. Mining the most interesting rules. *Proc. KDD Conference*, pp 145–154, August 1999.

[BB79] C. Beeri, P. A. Bernstein. Computational problems related to the design of normal form relational schemas. *Transactions on Database Systems*, 4(1):30–59, 1979.

[BMS97] S. Brin, R. Motwani, and C. Silverstein. Beyond market baskets: Generalizing association rules to correlation. *Proc. SIGMOD conf.*, pp 265–276, May 1997.

[DG86] V. Duquenne and J.-L. Guigues. Famille minimale d'implications informatives résultant d'un tableau de données binaires. *Mathématiques et Sciences Humaines*, 24(95):5–18, 1986.

[GW99] B. Ganter and R. Wille. *Formal Concept Analysis: Mathematical foundations*. Springer, 1999.

[HF95] J. Han and Y. Fu. Discovery of multiple-level association rules from large databases. *Proc. VLDB conf.*, pp 420–431, September 1995.

[Hec96] D. Heckerman. Bayesian networks for knowledge discovery. *Advances in Knowledge Discovery and Data Mining*, pp 273–305, 1996.

[KMR+94] M. Klemettinen, H. Mannila, P. Ronkainen, H. Toivonen, and A. I. Verkamo. Finding interesting rules from large sets of discovered association rules. *Proc. CIKM conf.*, pp 401–407, November 1994.

[Lux91] M. Luxenburger. Implications partielles dans un contexte. *Mathématiques, Informatique et Sciences Humaines*, 29(113):35–55, 1991.

[Mai80] D. Maier. Minimum covers in relational database model. *Journal of the ACM*, 27(4):664–674, 1980.

[NLHP98] R. T. Ng, V. S. Lakshmanan, J. Han, and A. Pang. Exploratory mining and pruning optimizations of constrained association rules. *Proc. SIGMOD conf.*, pp 13–24, June 1998.

[PBTL98] N. Pasquier, Y. Bastide, R. Taouil, and L. Lakhal. Pruning closed itemset lattices for association rules. *Proc. BDA conf.*, pp 177–196, Octobre 1998.

[PBTL99a] N. Pasquier, Y. Bastide, R. Taouil, and L. Lakhal. Efficient mining of association rules using closed itemset lattices. *Information Systems*, 24(1):25–46, 1999.

[PBTL99b] N. Pasquier, Y. Bastide, R. Taouil, and L. Lakhal. Discovering frequent closed itemsets for association rules. *Proc. ICDT conf.*, LNCS 1540, pp 398–416, January 1999.

[PBTL99c] N. Pasquier, Y. Bastide, R. Taouil, and L. Lakhal. Closed set based discovery of small covers for association rules. *Proc. BDA conf.*, pp 361–381, Octobre 1999.

[PSM94] G. Piatetsky-Shapiro and C. J. Matheus. The interestingness of deviations. *AAAI KDD workshop*, pp 25–36, July 1994.

[ST96] A. Silberschatz and A. Tuzhilin. What makes patterns interesting in knowledge discovery systems. *IEEE Transactions on Knowledge and Data Engineering*, 8(6):970–974, December 1996.

[SBM98] C. Silverstein, S. Brin, and R. Motwani. Beyond market baskets: Generalizing association rules to dependence rules. *Data Mining and Knowledge Discovery*, 2(1):39–68, January 1998.

[SA95] R. Srikant and R. Agrawal. Mining generalized association rules. *Proc. VLDB conf.*, pp 407–419, September 1995.

[SVA97] R. Srikant, Q. Vu, and R. Agrawal. Mining association rules with item constraints. *Proc. KDD conf.*, pp 67–73, August 1997.

Linearly Bounded Reformulations
of Conjunctive Databases
(Extended Abstract)

Rada Chirkova and Michael R. Genesereth

Stanford University, Stanford CA 94305, USA
{rada,genesereth}@cs.stanford.edu

Abstract. *Database reformulation* is the process of rewriting the data and rules of a deductive database in a functionally equivalent manner. We focus on the problem of automatically reformulating a database in a way that reduces query processing time while satisfying strong storage space constraints.

In previous work we have investigated database reformulation for the case of unary databases. In this paper we extend this work to arbitrary arity, while concentrating on databases with conjunctive rules. The main result of the paper is that the database reformulation problem is decidable for conjunctive databases.

1 Introduction

In the life cycle of a database system, there are recurring problems whose solution involves transformations of the database schema and/or queries defined on the schema. Prominent examples are database design, data model translation, schema (de)composition, view materialization, and multidatabase integration. Interestingly, nearly all these problems can be regarded as aspects of the same problem in a theoretical framework that we proceed to describe.

Consider an abstract database transformation problem. Suppose the input to the problem comprises the schema and rules of a deductive database and a set of elementary queries which, together with some algebra, forms a query language on the database. Suppose the objective of database transformation is to build an "optimal" structure of the database with respect to the requirements and constraints that are also provided in the input.

Generally, the transformations of the given database schema and rules need to be performed in such a way that the resulting database satisfies three conditions. First, it should be possible to extract from the transformed database, by means of the input query language, exactly the same information as from the original database. Second, the result should satisfy the input requirements, such as minimizing query processing costs. Finally, the result should satisfy the input constraints; one pervasive constraint is a guarantee of a (low) upper bound on the disk space for storing the transformed database. Notice that since the input

J. Lloyd et al. (Eds.): CL 2000, LNAI 1861, pp. 987–1001, 2000.
© Springer-Verlag Berlin Heidelberg 2000

does not include a specific database instance, all three conditions must hold for *all* instances of the input database and of the transformed database.

We call this problem *database reformulation* and consider logic-based approaches to its solution; a formal definition of the problem is the first contribution of this paper. Database reformulation is the process of rewriting the data and rules of a deductive database in a functionally equivalent manner: it takes as input the schema and rules of a database and a characterization of a query language, and produces as output new schema and rules, as well as a rewriting of (all elementary queries of) the query language in terms of the schema and rules. Notice that database reformulation, unlike query optimization, rewrites multiple rules, thus amortizing over many queries. By specifying various input requirements and constraints, the database reformulation problem translates into any of the database schema/query transformation problems mentioned above.

We focus on database reformulations whose input requirement is to minimize the computational costs of processing the given elementary queries, under strong storage space constraints that guarantee no more than linear increase in database size. In this formulation, the database reformulation framework is most suitable for dealing with the problems of view materialization and multidatabase integration.

This paper treats the base case where all rules in the reformulation input are conjunctive. We show that for such inputs, the database reformulation problem, in the narrow sense described above, is decidable: we describe an algorithm which outputs a solution if there exists at least one satisfactory reformulation of the input. This result is the second contribution of this paper. In previous work we have proposed a solution to the reformulation problem for unary databases; notice that the solution described in this paper works for deductive databases that contain relations of arbitrary arity. Our long-term objective is to extend research in database reformulation to deductive databases whose queries and views are formulated in progressively more general standard query languages (datalog and its extensions), as well as to databases with integrity constraints.

In this extended abstract, all proofs have been omitted. The proof of the main result and additional examples can be found in the appendix.

2   Preliminaries and Terminology

Our representation of the domain includes a set of *relations*; the set of attributes for a relation is called a *relation schema*. A *database schema*, for a given database D, is a collection of relation schemas for all stored relations in D.

A function-free *Horn rule* is an expression of the form

$$p(\bar{X}) \; : - \; p_1(\bar{Y}), \; \dots, \; p_n(\bar{Z}), \tag{1}$$

where p and $p_1, \dots, p_n$ are relation names, and $\bar{X}, \bar{Y}, \dots, \bar{Z}$ are tuples of variables and constants such that any variable appearing in $\bar{X}$ appears also in $\bar{Y} \bigcup \dots \bigcup \bar{Z}$.

A *conjunctive query (view)* is a single non-recursive Horn rule. A *conjunctive query (view) relation* is the relation defined by a conjunctive query (view).

Given a query q, a query q' is called a *rewriting* of q in terms of a set $\mathcal{V}$ of view relations if q and q' are equivalent and q' contains only literals of $\mathcal{V}$, i.e., q' is defined in terms of $\mathcal{V}$. If a query relation $q_\mathcal{V}$ is defined in terms of a set $\mathcal{V}$, and if $\mathcal{R}_\mathcal{V}$ is a set of definitions of view relations in $\mathcal{V}$, an *expansion* $q_{\mathcal{R}_\mathcal{V}}$ of $q_\mathcal{V}$, in terms of $\mathcal{R}_\mathcal{V}$, is a query obtained by replacing, in the body of $q_\mathcal{V}$, every occurrence of a view literal v_i ($v_i \in \mathcal{V}$) by its body in $\mathcal{R}_\mathcal{V}$, with suitable variable renamings.

In this paper we use the notion of a *substitution*, and in this respect generally follow the terminology of [24]. The substitutions we consider are of the form $\{ v_1 \leftarrow t_1, \dots, v_n \leftarrow t_n \}$ where all v_i's are distinct variables, and each t_i is either a variable from among $v_1, v_2, \dots, v_n$ or a constant.

A *containment mapping* [9] from a query q_1 to a query q_2 is a mapping from the variables of q_1 into the variables of q_2, such that every literal in the body of q_1 is mapped to a literal in q_2, and the head of q_1 is mapped into the head of q_2. If both q_1 and q_2 are conjunctive and neither contains built-in predicates, the existence of a containment mapping from q_1 to q_2 is a necessary and sufficient condition for q_1 to contain q_2; this result is called the *containment mapping theorem*.

A conjunctive query q' is a *minimal equivalent* to a conjunctive query q if it has as few subgoals as any query equivalent to q [34]. Both minimization and equivalence of conjunctive queries are shown to be NP-complete in [4, 9].

3   Concept of Database Reformulation

This section gives a definition and a formal specification of the database reformulation problem for the general case where rules are not necessarily conjunctive.

Database reformulation is the process of rewriting the data and rules of a deductive database in a functionally equivalent manner; we use the word "reformulation" both for the process and for its output. We focus on the problem of automatically reformulating a database in a way that reduces the processing time for a prespecified set of queries while satisfying strong storage space constraints. The prespecified set of queries is the set of elementary queries in the input query language; see the Introduction for details.

Let us describe the input and the output of the database reformulation process. Consider a set $\mathcal{P}$ of relation names. Let $\mathcal{S}$ consist of schemas for some relation names in $\mathcal{P}$; $\mathcal{S}$ is the input database schema. Let $\mathcal{R}_\mathcal{S}$ be a set of definitions, in terms of $\mathcal{S}$, for some relations whose names are in $\mathcal{P}$; $\mathcal{R}_\mathcal{S}$ is the set of rules in the input. Let $\mathcal{Q}$ be a set of names of all elementary query relations in the input, such that $\mathcal{Q} \subseteq \mathcal{P}$ and that $\mathcal{R}_\mathcal{S}$ contains definitions of all relations in $\mathcal{Q}$.

Now, let $\mathcal{V}$ consist of schemas for some relation names in $\mathcal{P}$; $\mathcal{V}$ is the output database schema, i.e., the set of schemes of new stored relations which are materialized in the process of database reformulation. Finally, let $\mathcal{R}_\mathcal{V}$ be a set of views defined in terms of $\mathcal{V}$; $\mathcal{R}_\mathcal{V}$ is the set of rules in the output.

Definition 1. *For a given triple* $(\mathcal{S}, \mathcal{R}_\mathcal{S}, \mathcal{Q})$, *a triple* $(\mathcal{V}, \mathcal{R}_\mathcal{V}, \mathcal{Q})$ *is a reformulation of* $(\mathcal{S}, \mathcal{R}_\mathcal{S}, \mathcal{Q})$ *if for each query relation in* $\mathcal{Q}$ *with a definition* $q_\mathcal{S}$ *in* $\mathcal{R}_\mathcal{S}$, $\mathcal{R}_\mathcal{V}$ *contains a rewriting of* $q_\mathcal{S}$.

Let $D_\mathcal{S}$ be an arbitrary database with schema $\mathcal{S}$; let $D_\mathcal{V}$ be a database that consists of the tables for all and only those (materialized, starting from $D_\mathcal{S}$) view relations in $\mathcal{V}$ that are used to define $\mathcal{Q}$. For a fixed database schema $\mathcal{S}$ and for a fixed set of definitions of view relations in $\mathcal{V}$ in terms of $\mathcal{S}$, consider all possible databases $D_\mathcal{S}$ and all corresponding databases $D_\mathcal{V}$, with sizes (in bytes) $|D_\mathcal{S}|$ and $|D_\mathcal{V}|$ respectively.

Definition 2. *A reformulation* $(\mathcal{V}, \mathcal{R}_\mathcal{V}, \mathcal{Q})$ *of an input* $(\mathcal{S}, \mathcal{R}_\mathcal{S}, \mathcal{Q})$ *is linearly bounded with parameter* t, *where* t *is a positive constant, if for all pairs* $(D_\mathcal{S}, D_\mathcal{V})$ *the storage space* $|D_\mathcal{V}|$ *taken up by* $D_\mathcal{V}$ *is no more than linear in both* $|D_\mathcal{S}|$ *and* t:

$$|D_\mathcal{V}| \leq t * |D_\mathcal{S}|. \tag{2}$$

One example of a linear bound is the *no-growth bound*; there, $t = 1$. The no-growth bound may be too restrictive for some applications.

4   Views with Bounded Definition Length

Our objective is to automate the database reformulation process for as general query languages as possible; in other words, we strive to design *reformulation algorithms*. To that end, it is first necessary to understand, for each class of query languages, whether the potentially infinite, for each input, search space of reformulations can be transformed in such a way that it becomes finite but still contains valuable reformulations. One way of making the search space of reformulations more tractable is to restrict the number of view relations that are used to generate rewritings of the input queries.

In this paper we focus on reformulating, in terms of conjunctive views, deductive databases where all rules are conjunctive; in the remainder of the paper we will denote conjunctive queries (views) simply by "queries" ("views"). In the conjunctive case, one might be able to restrict the number of views under consideration by setting an upper bound on the number of subgoals in views. Suppose we could show that in any "good" rewriting of an arbitrary conjunctive input, all participating view relations can be defined by conjunctions of up to a fixed number of subgoals. If this hypothesis were true, the problem of finding all "good" reformulations of the given input would be reduced to the clearly feasible problem of enumerating and combining all "short" views, thereby yielding an *enumeration procedure*. Notice that we do not use the number of subgoals as a cost measure for executing the query.

Consider a database schema $\mathcal{S}$, a set $\mathcal{V}$ of view relations, and a set $\mathcal{R}_\mathcal{V}$ of definitions of relations in $\mathcal{V}$ in terms of $\mathcal{S}$. Consider a query $q_\mathcal{S}$ in terms of $\mathcal{S}$ and a query $q_\mathcal{V}$ in terms of $\mathcal{V}$, with the corresponding expansion $q_{\mathcal{R}_\mathcal{V}}$ in terms of $\mathcal{R}_\mathcal{V}$. For each view literal v_i in the body of $q_\mathcal{V}$ let us denote by r_i the body of v_i in

$q_{\mathcal{R}_V}$. Suppose there is a containment mapping from $q_{\mathcal{R}_V}$ to q_S; such a mapping is called *noninterleaving* if no two r_is in $q_{\mathcal{R}_V}$ map into the same subset of the body of q_S, and if the mapping preserves head variables of all the views involved.

Theorem 1 (Restricted: New Definitions with Fewer Subgoals). *If q_S is minimal, q_S and q_V are equivalent, and there is a noninterleaving containment mapping from $q_{\mathcal{R}_V}$ to q_S, then there exists a set $\mathcal{R}'_V$ of (alternative) definitions of the view relations in V, such that each definition in $\mathcal{R}'_V$ has no more subgoals than q_S.*

Informally, the theorem states that for each view used to define q_V, there exists a "short" definition of the view that has no more subgoals than the original query q_S; thus, in the setting of the theorem, one can apply the enumeration procedure described above to generate all views that can be used in any rewriting of the input query.

Unfortunately, the result stated in Theorem 1 holds in an extremely limited setting and thus is not very useful. It would be desirable to make a similar claim for a more general case. Suppose we could show that if the queries q_S and q_V are equivalent then there exists a set $\mathcal{R}'_V$ of (alternative) definitions of the view relations in V, such that each definition in $\mathcal{R}'_V$ has no more subgoals than q_S. Notice that this formulation is similar to that of Theorem 1, except that we no longer require that q_S be minimal or that there exist a noninterleaving mapping from $q_{\mathcal{R}_V}$ to q_S.

This conjecture, however desirable, is not true: removing the noninterleaving mapping requirement invalidates the claim. Consider a counterexample.

Example 1. Consider a database schema $\mathcal{S}$ that consists of one binary relation schema s, and consider a query q_S:

$$q_S(X, Y) \; :- \; s(X, Y), \; s(Y, X); \tag{3}$$

for a graphic depiction of q_S, see Figure 1.

Consider a set V of two view relations v_1 and v_2 with the following definitions:

$$v_1(X, Y) \; :- \; s(X, Y); \tag{4}$$

$$v_2(Y, X) \; :- \; s(Y, X), \; s(X, Z_1), \; s(Z_1, Z_2), \; \dots \; , \; s(Z_{k-1}, Z_k); \tag{5}$$

let these definitions of v_1 and of v_2 form a set $\mathcal{R}_V$; for a graphic depiction of the views see Figure 2.

q_S

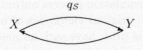

Fig. 1. Graphic depiction of the query for Example 1.

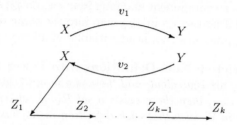

Fig. 2. Graphic depiction of the views for Example 1.

It is easy to show that the query

$$q_\mathcal{V}(X,\ Y)\ :-\ v_1(X,\ Y),\ v_2(Y,\ X) \tag{6}$$

is equivalent to $q_\mathcal{S}$. At the same time, it is not possible to construct a noninterleaving containment mapping from $q_{\mathcal{R}_\mathcal{V}}$ (the expansion of $q_\mathcal{V}$ in terms of $\mathcal{V}$) to $q_\mathcal{S}$.

The number of subgoals of v_2 can be made arbitrarily large by varying the parameter k; it is clear that neither v_1 nor v_2 is redundant in $q_\mathcal{V}$, and therefore no upper bound — one that could be related to the length of $q_\mathcal{S}$ — can be established on the number of subgoals in the definition of v_2.

This example allows us to formulate

Theorem 2 (General: New Definitions with Fewer Subgoals).   *It is not true for all conjunctive queries $q_\mathcal{S}$ and all their rewritings $q_\mathcal{V}$ that each view used in $q_\mathcal{V}$ has an alternative (equivalent) definition which has no more subgoals than $q_\mathcal{S}$.*

The failure of the conjecture formulated above makes one wonder whether it is possible at all to generalize the claim of Theorem 1. Fortunately, the answer is yes: a much more general result is described in the next section.

5   Shorter Views Contained in Longer Views

The main result of the previous section is that it is not possible to rewrite views in an arbitrary formulation of a query, in such a way that each view has no more subgoals than the query itself. However, in this section we show that it is possible to "reformulate" the conjunctive views in an arbitrary rewriting of an arbitrary conjunctive query. This reformulation process outputs views that, although not necessarily equivalent to the original views, constitute an equivalent rewriting of the query and, at the same time, have each no more subgoals than the query itself. Moreover, we show that if, in addition, the input query is linearly bounded with some parameter t (see Definition 2 in Section 3) then the reformulated query is also linearly bounded with the same parameter t.

Example 2. Recall $\mathcal{S}$, $q_{\mathcal{S}}$, $\mathcal{V} = \{ v_1, v_2 \}$, $\mathcal{R}_{\mathcal{V}}$, and $q_{\mathcal{V}}$ introduced in Example 1; we choose $k = 2$ for v_2 which will thus be defined as follows:

$$v_2(Y, X) \; :- \; s(Y, X), \; s(X, Z_1), \; s(Z_1, Z_2). \tag{7}$$

We define a new view relation v_1' (v_2') by applying a substitution to the body of v_1 (v_2). For v_1', consider the trivial substitution applied to the only subgoal $s(X, Y)$ of v_1:

$$v_1'(X, Y) \; :- \; s(X, Y). \tag{8}$$

For v_2', consider a substitution $\{ X \leftarrow X, Y \leftarrow Y, Z_1 \leftarrow Y, Z_2 \leftarrow X \}$ applied to the body of v_2:

$$v_2'(Y, X) \; :- \; s(Y, X), \; s(X, Y). \tag{9}$$

Notice that v_2' is *not* equivalent to v_2.

Now the query $q_{\mathcal{V}'}$:

$$q_{\mathcal{V}'}(X, Y) \; :- \; v_1'(X, Y), \; v_2'(Y, X) \tag{10}$$

is equivalent to both $q_{\mathcal{S}}$ and $q_{\mathcal{V}}$, since the expansion $q_{\mathcal{R}_{\mathcal{V}'}}$ of $q_{\mathcal{V}'}$ is isomorphic to the query $q_{\mathcal{S}}$ (after removing duplicate subgoals). It is easy to see that when $\{ v_1', v_2' \}$ is the schema of the reformulated database (i.e., when both v_1' and v_2' are materialized), the query of interest is computed faster than in databases with schema $\mathcal{S}$, as well as in databases with schema $\mathcal{V}$.

Table 1. Stored relation s and view relations v_2 and v_2' in Example 2.

s		v_2		v_2'	
a	b	a	b	a	b
b	a	b	a	b	a
c	d	c	d	c	d
d	c	d	c	d	c
b	c	b	c		
d	f				

Consider a database instance D with schema $\mathcal{S}$. Suppose the data in the table for s, in that database instance D, is as in Table 1. Table 1 also shows the result of materializing view relations v_2 and v_2' (both v_1 and v_1' are the same as s). Notice that the size of the table for each v_i' is no larger than the size of the table for its corresponding v_i; this is also true for any other database instance with schema $\mathcal{S}$, as will be explained shortly. Thus, if a reformulation that uses the rewriting $q_{\mathcal{V}}$ is linearly bounded with some parameter t, then the reformulation that uses the rewriting $q_{\mathcal{V}'}$ is also guaranteed to be linearly bounded with the same parameter t.

Notice that v_1' is not needed to compute $q_{\mathcal{V}'}$, and thus the reformulation that contains only v_2', in addition to improved computation time, satisfies the no-growth bound compared to the *original* (input) database schema.

In formulating our main result and the reformulation algorithm, we will use the notion of a unifiee of a query:

Definition 3. *Given a query q, a unifiee of q is a query q' such that the body of q' is the result of applying some substitution to some subset of the body of q.*

Consider, as usual, a database schema S and a set V of view relations defined in terms of S. Consider a query q_S defined in terms of S and a query q_V defined in terms of V. In this setting, the following main result holds.

Theorem 3 (Main Result). *If q_S and q_V are equivalent then, for each view literal v_i in q_V, there is a (not necessarily equivalent) view relation v_i' which is a unifiee of q_S, and a query $q_{V'}$ obtained by replacing, in q_V, each v_i with its corresponding v_i', is equivalent to q_V;*
in addition, if both v_i and v_i' are materialized in any database with schema S, then the size of the table for v_i' is no larger than the size of the table for its v_i.

Informally, the theorem states that for any rewriting q_V of a query q_S we can always find an alternative rewriting $q_{V'}$ with two special properties. First, $q_{V'}$ is composed entirely of views with no more subgoals each than in q_S. The second property is that in $q_{V'}$, each v_i' is contained in its corresponding v_i (this becomes clear from the proof of the Theorem — see the appendix); therefore, when the view relations in both rewritings are materialized, the tables for the view relations that define $q_{V'}$ always "fit in" the space required to store the tables for the view relations that define q_V.

Consider again Example 2. By the main result, the table for each v_i' is no larger than the table for its corresponding v_i in any database instance with schema S.

Notice that the theorem is true independently of whether the input query q_S is minimized.

6   A Database Reformulation Algorithm

In this section we describe a database reformulation algorithm for deductive databases where all rules are conjunctive. The algorithm is based on the result described in the previous section: for each space-satisfactory rewriting of a given query there exists another space-satisfactory rewriting, defined in terms of "short" views only, i.e., of those views that have no more subgoals than the query itself. Thus, the idea of the algorithm is, for each input query, to examine all "short" views (obviously there is only a finite number of them) and to construct rewritings of the query by combining such views. The successful rewritings then undergo a storage space check to decide whether they belong to a space-satisfactory reformulation. If such rewritings cannot be found by the algorithm, then, by our results, no rewritings of the query exist.

The reformulation algorithm takes as input a database schema S, a set $\mathcal{R}_S$ of view definitions in terms of S, a set $\mathcal{Q}$ of elementary query relations with definitions in $\mathcal{R}_S$, and the value of parameter t for the linear bound. For each query relation in $\mathcal{Q}$ with definition $q_\mathcal{S}$ in $\mathcal{R}_\mathcal{S}$, the algorithm generates a set of rewritings of $q_\mathcal{S}$ by, first, producing all unifiees of $q_\mathcal{S}$ (see Definition 3 in Section 5) as views and combining the views in conjunctive definitions in all possible ways, and, second, by testing the resulting conjunctions for equivalence with $q_\mathcal{S}$. After all such rewritings of all input queries have been built, the algorithm generates candidate reformulations as all combinations where each candidate reformulation contains one rewriting per input query. Only those candidate reformulation that are linearly bounded for the given value of t, belong in the output of the algorithm.

Theorem 4. *For a given input $(\mathcal{S}, \mathcal{R}_\mathcal{S}, \mathcal{Q})$ and for a given positive number t, the reformulation algorithm outputs only those reformulations $(\mathcal{V}, \mathcal{R}_\mathcal{V}, \mathcal{Q})$ that are linearly bounded with parameter t, and their $\mathcal{R}_\mathcal{V}$ contain only definitions with no more subgoals in each than the number of subgoals in the longest query in $\mathcal{R}_\mathcal{S}$.*

The longest query in $\mathcal{R}_\mathcal{S}$ is the query with the most subgoals. This theorem is true by construction of the algorithm.

Theorem 5. *If, for some input and for some positive number t, the output of the reformulation algorithm is empty then no reformulation of the input in terms of conjunctive views is linearly bounded with parameter t.*

This result follows immediately from Theorem 3 in Section 5.

The reformulation algorithm presented in this section is proof that the database reformulation problem is decidable for conjunctive databases. Notice that the algorithm is, in all probability, too expensive to be used to actually generate reformulations. To see why, it suffices to notice that one of the steps of the algorithm involves testing pairs of conjunctive queries for equivalence, i.e., solving a known NP-complete problem.

7 Related Work

Database schema evolution is an integral part of database design, data model translation, schema (de)composition, and multidatabase integration; fundamental to these problems is the notion of equivalence between database schemata.

The first definition of schema equivalence was proposed in [11]; schema equivalence was studied in [6, 8, 29]. Later, relative information capacity was introduced in [19] as a fundamental theoretical concept which encompasses schema equivalence and dominance. Other work on relative information capacity includes [5, 25, 26]. Tutorial [18] surveys a number of frameworks — relative information capacity among others — for dealing with the issue of semantic heterogeneity arising in database integration.

In practical database systems, database design frequently uses normalization, first introduced in [10] and described in detail in [33]. Papers [7, 20] survey methods and issues in multidatabase integration.

Query transformation is another aspect of database transformation tasks; query rewriting methods complement schema transformation methods in that they are applied to databases that are already operational. Query rewriting is important for query optimization, especially in deductive databases [27] where queries can be complex and the amount of data accessed can be overwhelming. [28] is a survey on implementation techniques and implemented projects in deductive databases.

There is an extensive body of work on theoretical aspects of query rewriting. For an overview of query rewriting methods in datalog and its extensions see [2, 33, 34]. In addition, applications such as data warehousing and multidatabase integration have promoted the study of views in databases. The paper [32] is a survey of containment and rewriting/optimization of queries using views. [1] discusses the complexity of answering queries using materialized views and contains references to major results in the areas of query containment and view materialization. Papers [16, 17, 21, 30] describe approaches to view materialization. [3, 12, 13, 23] treat the problem of using available materialized views for query evaluation. Nearly all results described in the literature concern rewriting of single queries; notice that the database reformulation approach we propose involves simultaneous rewriting of *sets* of queries.

Transformations of database schemas and queries can be considered together as reformulations of logical theories. [31] provides a theoretical foundation for theory reformulations, and [15, 22] contain work on general transformations of logical theories.

Descriptions of basic methods used in this paper can be found, e.g., in [14].

8   Conclusions and Future Work

The first contribution of this paper is that it introduces the notion of database reformulation which is the process of rewriting the data and rules of a deductive database in a functionally equivalent manner. We focus on the problem of automatically reformulating a database in a way that reduces query processing time while satisfying strong storage space constraints.

The second contribution of this paper is a proof that it is decidable to reformulate, using conjunctive views, deductive databases where all rules are conjunctive, in the presence of strong storage space constraints. We have shown that for any space-satisfactory rewriting of a conjunctive query there is a rewriting which is also space-satisfactory and is composed entirely of views that have no more subgoals than the original query. We have described a reformulation algorithm which returns space-satisfactory query rewritings composed of views that have no more subgoals than the longest query in the input. Notice that all the results automatically hold for select-project-join (SPJ) queries in SQL.

There are several directions of future research in database reformulation. A pressing research problem is the issue of update complexity in the reformulated database. On a more long-term scale, it is desirable to develop criteria for comparing different outputs produced by the reformulation algorithm, as well as criteria for choosing the optimal output among the potentially multiple answers. Another challenge is to examine possible interactions between views chosen in support of different queries and to understand how such interactions might influence the quality of a reformulation, in particular its storage space requirements. We also plan to study the complexity of the reformulation problem. Finally, our long-term objective is to extend research in database reformulation to deductive databases whose queries and views are formulated in progressively more general standard query languages, for example include disjunction or negation, as well as to databases with integrity constraints.

Acknowledgements

The authors would like to thank Jeffrey D. Ullman for pointing out the problem of query folding in the first place, which ultimately led to the database reformulation problem. Also we would like to thank Vasilis Vassalos for the reading and extensive discussions of the paper.

References

1. Serge Abiteboul and Oliver Duschka. Complexity of answering queries using materialized views. In *PODS-98*, pages 254–263.
2. Serge Abiteboul, Richard Hull, and Victor Vianu. *Foundations of Databases*. Addison-Wesley, Reading, Mass., 1995.
3. F.N. Afrati, M. Gergatsoulis, and T.G. Kavalieros. Answering queries using materialized views with disjunctions. In *ICDT-99*, pages 435–452.
4. A.V. Aho, Y. Sagiv, and J.D. Ullman. Equivalences among relational expressions. *SIAM J. Comput.*, 8(2):218–246, 1979.
5. J. Albert, Y. Ioannidis, and R. Ramakrishnan. Conjunctive query equivalence of keyed relational schemas. In *PODS-97*, pages 44–50.
6. P. Atzeni, G. Ausiello, C. Batini, and M. Moscarini. Inclusion and equivalence between relational database schemata. *Theoretical Computer Science*, 19:267–285, 1982.
7. C. Batini, M. Lenzerini, and S.B. Navathe. A comparative analysis of methodologies for database schema integration. *ACM Computing Surveys*, 18(4):323–364, 1986.
8. C. Beeri, A.O. Mendelzon, Y. Sagiv, and J.D. Ullman. Equivalence of relational database schemes. *SIAM J. Comput.*, 10(2):352–370, 1981.
9. Ashok K. Chandra and Philip M. Merlin. Optimal implementation of conjunctive queries in relational data bases. In *STOC-77*, pages 77–90.
10. E.F. Codd. A relational model of data for large shared data banks. *Comm. ACM*, 13(6):377–387, June 1970.
11. E.F. Codd. Further normalization of the data base relational model. In R. Rustin, editor, *Database Systems*, pages 33–64. Prentice Hall Inc., Englewood Cliffs, NJ, 1972.
12. Oliver M. Duschka and Michael R. Genesereth. Answering recursive queries using views. In *PODS-97*, pages 109–116.
13. Oliver M. Duschka and Michael R. Genesereth. Query planning with disjunctive sources. In *AAAI-98 Workshop on AI and Information Integration*, 1997.
14. Herbert B. Enderton. *A Mathematical Introduction to Logic*. Academic Press, New York, 1972.

15. Fausto Giunchiglia and Toby Walsh. A theory of abstraction. *Artificial Intelligence*, 57(2-3):323–389, 1992.

16. Himanshu Gupta. Selection of views to materialize in a data warehouse. In *ICDT-97*, pages 98–112.

17. Himanshu Gupta and Inderpal Singh Mumick. Selection of views to materialize under a maintenance cost constraint. In *ICDT-99*, pages 453–470.

18. Richard Hull. Managing semantic heterogeneity in databases: a theoretical perspective. In *PODS-97*, pages 51–61.

19. Richard Hull. Relative information capacity of simple relational database schemata. *SIAM J. Comput.*, 15(3):856–886, August 1986.

20. Won Kim, editor. *Modern Database Systems*. ACM Press, New York, New York, 1995.

21. Yannis Kotidis and Nick Roussopoulos. Dynamat: a dynamic view management system for data warehouses. In *SIGMOD-99*.

22. Alon Y. Levy and P. Pandurang Nayak. A semantic theory of abstractions. In *IJCAI-95*, pages 196–203.

23. A.Y. Levy, A.O. Mendelzon, Y. Sagiv, and D. Srivastava. Answering queries using views. In *PODS-95*, pages 95–104.

24. John Wylie Lloyd. *Foundations of Logic Programming*. Springer-Verlag, 1987.

25. R.J. Miller, Y.E. Ioannidis, and R. Ramakrishnan. The use of information capacity in schema integration and translation. In *VLDB-93*, pages 120–133.

26. R.J. Miller, Y.E. Ioannidis, and R. Ramakrishnan. Schema equivalence in heterogeneous systems: bridging theory and practice. *Information Systems*, 19(1):3–31, 1994.

27. Jack Minker. Logic and databases: a 20 year retrospective. In D. Pedreschi and C. Zaniolo, editors, *Logic in Databases*, pages 3–57. Springer, 1996. (Proceedings of the LID'96 international workshop).

28. Raghu Ramakrishnan and Jeffrey D. Ullman. A survey of deductive database systems. *J. Logic Progr.*, 23(2):125–149, May 1995.

29. J. Rissanen. On equivalences of database schemes. In *PODS-82*, pages 23–26.

30. K.A. Ross, D. Srivastava, and S. Sudarshan. Materialized view maintenance and integrity constraint checking: trading space for time. In *SIGMOD-96*, pages 447–458.

31. Devika Subramanian. *A theory of justified reformulations*. PhD thesis, Stanford University, 1989.

32. Jeffrey D. Ullman. Information integration using logical views. In *ICDT-97*, pages 19–40.

33. Jeffrey D. Ullman. *Principles of Database and Knowledge-Base Systems*, volume I. Computer Science Press, New York, 1988.

34. Jeffrey D. Ullman. *Principles of Database and Knowledge-Base Systems*, volume II. Computer Science Press, New York, 1989.

A   Some Examples and Proofs

A.1   A Recursive Reformulation Example

Here is an example which illustrates the power of database reformulation for a deductive database with recursive rules.

Example 3. Consider the "founding fathers" problem invented by Devika Sub-ramanian [31]. There is just one stored relation in this case: the *father* relation, where $father(X, Y)$ means that X is the father of Y. In addition, there are two views defined as shown below. The (male) *ancestor* relation holds of two people X and Y if X is the father of Y or if there is a third person V who is a child of X and an ancestor of Y. The *samefamily* relation holds of two people if they have a common (male) ancestor.

$$ancestor(X, Y) \; :- \; father(X, Y); \tag{11}$$

$$ancestor(X, Y) \; :- \; father(X, V), \; ancestor(V, Y); \tag{12}$$

$$samefamily(Y, Z) \; :- \; ancestor(X, Y), \; ancestor(X, Z). \tag{13}$$

With the definitions above, determining whether two people are in the same family involves computing all of their ancestors and intersecting the two sets, a fairly expensive operation.

To improve the query processing time, we could materialize the *samefamily* relation. However, the table for that relation, in a database with schema { *father* }, would take up storage space that is, in the worst case, quadratic in the number of people in the database. For large databases, such materialization is impractical.

On the other hand, it is possible to get the same performance gain without any space growth whatsoever. The definitions below show how. We say that a person X is the founding father (*founder*) of the family of person Y if X is an ancestor of Y and there is no person W such that W is the father of X ($\neg$ stands for negation). The *samefamily* relation can then be defined in terms of this new *founder* relation: two people are in the same family if and only if they have the same founding father.

$$hasancestors(X) \; :- \; father(W, X); \tag{14}$$

$$founder(X, Y) \; :- \; ancestor(X, Y), \; \neg \; hasancestors(X); \tag{15}$$

$$samefamily(Y, Z) \; :- \; founder(X, Y), \; founder(X, Z). \tag{16}$$

Using the definitions above, we can materialize the *founder* relation; further-more, if we are interested only in the *samefamily* query we can also dematerialize the *father* relation. With such a reformulation we get the same performance im-provement for our target query as if we did materialize the *samefamily* relation itself. However, the amount of space required for the reformulated database is the same as that required for the input database; in other words, this reformu-lation satisfies the no-growth bound. This reformulation is so good because we have succeeded in defining an equivalence relation (*samefamily*) by choosing a single representative (*founder*) from each equivalence class.

A.2   An Example of Conjunctive Reformulation

Below is a very simple example of database reformulation for a conjunctive deductive database.

Example 4. Suppose in some database there are two stored relations: *parent* and *gender* (either male or female). Suppose the only elementary query of interest is *grandparent* — imagine that we only plan to ask queries about grandfathers or grandmothers. The *grandparent* relation can be defined in terms of the *parent* relation in an obvious way as follows:

$$grandparent\ (X,\ Y)\ :-\ parent\ (X,\ Z),\ parent\ (Z,\ Y). \tag{17}$$

Once we materialize the *grandparent* relation, we can dematerialize the *parent* relation since we are not interested in querying on that relation anyway. As a result, the new database contains only relevant information (relations *gender* and *grandparent*), the processing costs for the queries of interest are minimized, and the reformulation is linearly bounded with $t = 2$.

A.3   Proof of Theorem 3 in Section 5

To prove the theorem, we need the notion of a self-map.

Definition 4. *A containment mapping on a conjunctive query is called a self-map if it maps the query into itself.*

Consider an arbitrary conjunctive query q; consider another query $\tilde{q}$ such that there exist two containment mappings $M_1 : q \rightarrow \tilde{q}$ and $M_2 : \tilde{q} \rightarrow q$, where both M_1 and M_2 preserve head variables of the queries. Consider a composition M of the two mappings; $M : q \rightarrow q$. Notice that M is a self-map by construction.

Then it is easy to show that each such q has the following property:

Lemma 1. *q is equivalent to its image q' under M:*

$$q \equiv q'. \tag{18}$$

We proceed to prove the main result which is formulated as Theorem 3 in Section 5:

Proof (Theorem 3). Let $\mathcal{R}_\mathcal{V}$ be the set of definitions of view relations in $\mathcal{V}$ in terms of $\mathcal{S}$, and let $q_{\mathcal{R}_\mathcal{V}}$ be the (unique and equivalent) expansion of $q_\mathcal{V}$ in terms of $\mathcal{R}_\mathcal{V}$. By transitivity of equivalence, $q_{\mathcal{R}_\mathcal{V}}$ is equivalent to $q_\mathcal{S}$.

From the containment mapping theorem, the equivalence of $q_{\mathcal{R}_\mathcal{V}}$ and of $q_\mathcal{S}$ means that there is a containment mapping $M_{\mathcal{R}\mathcal{S}} : q_{\mathcal{R}_\mathcal{V}} \rightarrow q_\mathcal{S}$ and there is a containment mapping $M_{\mathcal{S}\mathcal{R}} : q_\mathcal{S} \rightarrow q_{\mathcal{R}_\mathcal{V}}$, where both mappings preserve head variables of the queries.

Consider a composition M of $M_{\mathcal{RS}}$ with $M_{\mathcal{SR}}$:

$$M : q_{\mathcal{R}_V} \to q_{\mathcal{R}_V}. \tag{19}$$

By construction, M is a self-map that satisfies the conditions of Lemma 1; therefore, by that lemma, the image $M(q_{\mathcal{R}_V})$ of $q_{\mathcal{R}_V}$ under M is equivalent to $q_{\mathcal{R}_V}$:

$$q_{\mathcal{R}_V} \equiv M(q_{\mathcal{R}_V}). \tag{20}$$

Consider an arbitrary view literal v_i in q_V and the body r_i of the definition of v_i in $q_{\mathcal{R}_V}$. Consider the image r_i' of r_i under M; r_i' is a subset of the body of $M(q_{\mathcal{R}_V})$. Notice that by construction of M, r_i' defines some (at least one — depending on the choice of head variables) unifiee of $q_{\mathcal{S}}$ (see Definition 3 in Section 5).

Let us take r_i' as the body of a definition of some view relation v_i', such that the head variables of v_i' are images, under M, of the head variables of v_i (in r_i).

After we have built a new relation v_i' based on each v_i used in the definition q_V, $M(q_{\mathcal{R}_V})$ can be viewed as an expansion of some conjunctive query $q_{V'}$, where $V' = \bigcup \{v_i'\}$. It is easy to show that $q_{V'}$ exists and is equivalent to $M(q_{\mathcal{R}_V})$; therefore, from transitivity of equivalence, $q_{V'}$ is equivalent to both q_V and to $q_{\mathcal{S}}$.

Consider an arbitary view literal v_i in the body of q_V and its counterpart v_i' in the body of $q_{V'}$. Notice that v_i' is, in fact, constructed as a unifiee of v_i, not of $q_{\mathcal{S}}$, although v_i' is also a unifiee of $q_{\mathcal{S}}$ by properties of the mapping M. Also, by the containment mapping theorem, v_i' is contained in v_i; if M does not preserve head variables of some v_i, we assume that v_i' has the same number of head variables as v_i, only some head variables of v_i' may be unified with each other. Thus we have that in any database instance with schema $\mathcal{S}$, if both v_i and v_i' are materialized, then the table for v_i' takes up at most as much storage space as the table for its corresponding v_i.

MuTACLP: A Language for Declarative GIS Analysis*

Paolo Mancarella, Gianluca Nerbini, Alessandra Raffaetà, and Franco Turini

Dipartimento di Informatica, Università di Pisa
Corso Italia, 40, I-56125 Pisa, Italy
{paolo,nerbini,raffaeta,turini}@di.unipi.it

Abstract. This paper proposes an integration between Geographical
Information System (GIS) technology and constraint logic programming
in order to supply the user with a declarative language that supports
and improves GIS analysis. We present the language MuTACLP, where
spatio-temporal and thematic information can be represented in a uniform way, and the features of constraint logic programming, such as
recursion and constraint handling, can be exploited to perform sophisticated spatio-temporal reasoning. This unifying language seems also
promising to address the key problem of interoperability among different
GISs.
Keywords: Spatio-temporal reasoning, GIS analysis, meta-
programming.

1 Introduction

The manipulation of complex data of very large size, such as spatial and temporal information, and often of very different nature, has become one of the
challenge of todays research [20, 22, 17, 4]. Many applications, such as geographic
information systems (GISs), geometric modeling systems (CAD), and temporal
databases, need the ability of storing and manipulating geometric and temporal
data. Actually, space and time are closely interconnected [15]: much information
which is referenced to space is also referenced to time. Traditional databases
are not able to manage these complex data at a high level of abstraction. Spatial and temporal data differ from conventional data in particular for the fact
that the domains are interpreted and that they often model *infinite* objects. To
fill the gap, many spatial databases and temporal databases have been defined
(e.g., [22, 17, 13, 20, 7]). However, the problem of dealing with correlated spatial
and temporal data has been addressed only recently. The existing models are
not completely satisfactory, especially because they do not provide an explicit
and flexible reasoning mechanism, whereas spatio-temporal information requires
it much more than ordinary data.

In [19] we defined a language, called MuTACLP, where temporal and spatial
information can be represented and handled, and, at the same time, knowledge

---

* This work has been supported by Esprit Working Group 28115 - DeduGIS

J. Lloyd et al. (Eds.): CL 2000, LNAI 1861, pp. 1002–1016, 2000.

can be separated into different theories and combined by means of meta-level composition operations. In particular, the pieces of temporal information are expressed as *temporal annotations* which say at what time(s) the formula to which they are attached is valid. On the other hand, spatial data are represented by using constraints in the style of the constraint databases approaches [14, 3, 13, 12, 8]. The facilities to handle time offered by the language allow one to easily establish spatio-temporal correlations, for instance time-varying areas, or, more generally, moving objects, supporting either discrete or continuous changes.

In this paper, we want to show how MuTACLP can be exploited to integrate GIS technology and constraint logic programming, in order to provide the user with a declarative language which supports and improves GIS analysis at least at the specification level. In fact, one of the frequently stated problems for GISs is that these systems have a complex functionality which is not accessible to non expert end-users. Today GIS user interfaces are not easy to use and require much time to get used to them [22, 9, 18]. Thus a user often knows *what* she/he wants, but does not know *how* to obtain it from the GIS. Moreover, the current GIS analysis approaches are not general and reusable. In fact the analysis is typically based on complex procedural algorithms, and data are built and structured *for the specific application*. We claim that a declarative approach is a better solution for solving this kind of problems at least at the specification level.

In the literature we can find several attempts to exploit the deductive capabilities of logic to *reason* on geographic data [22]. Some approaches go towards the use of artificial intelligence techniques (expert systems), while other approaches express spatial data in an object-oriented style, and add a deductive component to infer knowledge from the spatial objects [1]. Our proposal, based on MuTACLP, relies on the translation of the spatial data stored in a GIS into a logical representation. In this way, all the previously discussed capabilities of MuTACLP can be used to reason on the data contained in a GIS. Having a multi-theory setting is very useful, because often knowledge employed in GIS analysis is fragmented into different sources. For instance, one can get environmental restrictions from the local municipality, the general laws from the government, and the *best place* criteria from the planner. By employing the program composition operations, we can express complex queries on a combination of such analysis criteria. Remarkably, spatial data can be related to temporal information, a great advantage with respect to the current GIS technology where time is almost completely ignored, although recognized as an essential component of geographical information [15, 22]. Furthermore, being based on a uniform representation of data in a common model our approach favors the interoperability among different GISs which is nowadays very difficult to attain [22, 8].

The paper is organized as follows. Section 2 introduces Temporal Annotated Constraint Logic Programming (TACLP) which is the formalism we adopt to describe programs, whereas Section 3 introduces our multi-theory framework, MuTACLP. In Section 4, after presenting the logical representation of GIS data, we show how the classical set-theoretic operations on spatial objects (union, intersection, etc.) can be defined in MuTACLP, and we discuss a logical reconstruction of GIS layers. In Section 5 an example is given to focus on how MuTACLP can support GIS analysis. Finally, Section 6 draws some conclusions.

2   Temporal Annotated Constraint Logic Programming

Temporal Annotated Constraint Logic Programming (TACLP) is a constraint logic programming language where formulae can be annotated with temporal labels and where temporal constraints express relations between these labels. In TACLP, the choice of the temporal ontology is free. In this paper, we consider the subset of TACLP where time points are totally ordered, and sets of time points are convex and non-empty. Moreover only atomic formulae can be annotated and clauses are free of negation. For a more detailed treatment of TACLP we refer the reader to [10]. With an abuse of notation, in the rest of the paper we call TACLP such a subset of the full language.

Time can be discrete or dense. Time points are totally ordered by the relation $\leq$. We denote by D the set of time points, equipped with the usual operations (such as $+$, $-$). We assume that the time-line is left-bounded by 0 and open to the future, with the symbol ∞ used to denote a time point that is later than any other. A *time period* is an interval $[r, s]$ with $0 \leq r \leq s \leq \infty, r, s \in D$ that represents the convex, non-empty set of time points $\{t \mid r \leq t \leq s\}$. Thus the interval $[0, \infty]$ denotes the whole time line.

An *annotated formula* is of the form $A\,\alpha$ where A is an atomic formula and α an annotation. In TACLP there are three kinds of annotations based on time points and time periods. Let t be a time point and let $J = [r, s]$ be a time period. Then

(at) The annotated formula $A\,\text{at}\,t$ means that A holds at time point t.

(th) The annotated formula $A\,\text{th}\,J$ means that A holds *throughout*, i.e., at *every* time point in the time period J. The definition of a th-annotated formula in terms of at is:

$$A\,\text{th}\,J \;\Leftrightarrow\; \forall t\,(t \in J \rightarrow A\,\text{at}\,t).$$

(in) The annotated formula $A\,\text{in}\,J$ means that A holds at *some* time point(s) - but we do not know exactly which - in the time period J. The definition of an in-annotated formula in terms of at is:

$$A\,\text{in}\,J \;\Leftrightarrow\; \exists t\,(t \in J \wedge A\,\text{at}\,t).$$

The in temporal annotation accounts for indefinite temporal information.

The set of annotations is endowed with a partial order relation $\sqsubseteq$ which turns it into a lattice. Given two annotations α and β, the intuition is that $\alpha \sqsubseteq \beta$ if α is "less informative" than β in the sense that for all formulae A, $A\,\beta \Rightarrow A\,\alpha$. More precisely, in addition to Modus Ponens, TACLP has two further inference rules: the rule ($\sqsubseteq$) and the rule ($\sqcup$).

$$\frac{A\,\alpha \qquad \gamma \sqsubseteq \alpha}{A\,\gamma}\;\;rule\;(\sqsubseteq) \qquad\qquad \frac{A\,\alpha \qquad A\,\beta \qquad \gamma = \alpha \sqcup \beta}{A\,\gamma}\;\;rule\;(\sqcup)$$

The rule ($\sqsubseteq$) states that if a formula holds with some annotation, then it also holds with all annotations that are smaller according to the lattice ordering. The rule ($\sqcup$) says that if a formula holds with some annotation and the same formula holds with another annotation then it holds with the least upper bound of the two annotations.

Now, we define the *constraint theory for temporal annotations*. We recall that a constraint theory is a non-empty, consistent first order theory that axiomatizes the meaning of the constraints. First of all, our constraint theory includes an axiomatization of the total order relation $\leq$ on time points D. Then it contains the following axioms defining the partial order on temporal annotations.

$$
\begin{array}{ll}
(\text{at th}) & \text{at } t = \text{th}\,[t, t] \\
(\text{at in}) & \text{at } t = \text{in}\,[t, t] \\
(\text{th } \sqsubseteq) & \text{th}\,[s_1, s_2] \sqsubseteq \text{th}\,[r_1, r_2] \Leftrightarrow r_1 \leq s_1,\, s_1 \leq s_2,\, s_2 \leq r_2 \\
(\text{in } \sqsubseteq) & \text{in}\,[r_1, r_2] \sqsubseteq \text{in}\,[s_1, s_2] \Leftrightarrow r_1 \leq s_1,\, s_1 \leq s_2,\, s_2 \leq r_2
\end{array}
$$

The first two axioms state that $\text{th}\,I$ and $\text{in}\,I$ are equivalent to $\text{at}\,t$ when the time period I consists of a single time point t.[1] Next, if a formula holds at every point of a time period, then it holds at every point in all sub-periods of that period (($\text{th } \sqsubseteq$) axiom). On the other hand, if a formula holds at some points of a time period then it holds at some points in all periods that include this period (($\text{in } \sqsubseteq$) axiom). A consequence of the above axioms is

$$
(\text{in th } \sqsubseteq) \qquad \text{in}\,[s_1, s_2] \sqsubseteq \text{th}\,[r_1, r_2] \Leftrightarrow s_1 \leq r_2, r_1 \leq s_2, s_1 \leq s_2, r_1 \leq r_2
$$

i.e., an atom annotated by in holds in any time period that overlaps with a time period where the atom holds throughout.

Now we axiomatize the least upper bound $\sqcup$ of temporal annotations over time points and time periods. For technical reasons related to the properties of th and in annotations (see [10]) we restrict ourselves to compute the least upper bound between th annotations with overlapping time periods that do not include one another:

$$
(\text{th }\sqcup) \qquad \text{th}\,[s_1, s_2] \sqcup \text{th}\,[r_1, r_2] = \text{th}\,[s_1, r_2] \Leftrightarrow s_1 < r_1, r_1 \leq s_2, s_2 < r_2
$$

We can now define the clausal fragment of TACLP that can be used as an efficient temporal programming language.

Definition 1. *A TACLP clause is of the form:*

$$
A\,\alpha \leftarrow C_1, \ldots, C_n, B_1\,\alpha_1, \ldots, B_m\,\alpha_m \quad (n, m \geq 0)
$$

where A is an atom (not a constraint), α and α_i are (optional) temporal annotations, the C_j's are constraints and the B_i's are atomic formulae. The constraints C_j cannot be annotated. A TACLP program is a finite set of TACLP clauses.

---

[1] Especially in dense time, one may disallow singleton periods and drop the two axioms. This restriction has no effects on the results we are presenting.

3 Multi-theory Temporal Annotated Constraint Logic Programming

In this section we present Multi-theory Temporal Annotated Constraint Logic Programming (MuTACLP), as introduced in [16], a framework where temporal information can be represented and handled, and, at the same time, knowledge can be separated and combined by means of meta-level composition operations. As we will see in the following the use of constraints allows one to represent naturally also spatial and spatio-temporal data.

MuTACLP enriches TACLP with high-level mechanisms for structuring programs and for combining separate temporal knowledge bases. In the style of [6] we provide two operators to combine programs: union $\cup$ and intersection $\cap$. These operations determine a language of program expressions, that may be constructed by starting from a set of *plain* programs, which are TACLP programs, and by repeatedly applying the composition operators. Formally, the language of *program expressions Exp* is defined by the following abstract syntax:

$$Exp ::= Pname \mid Exp \cup Exp \mid Exp \cap Exp$$

where *Pname* is the syntactic category of names of plain programs.

In order to be able to compose programs we add to the constraint theory defined in the previous section the axiomatization of the greatest lower bound $\sqcap$ of two annotations, which is essential in the definition of the intersection operator over program expressions.

$(\mathsf{th}\sqcap)$ $\mathsf{th}\,[s_1, s_2] \sqcap \mathsf{th}\,[r_1, r_2] = \mathsf{th}\,[t_1, t_2] \Leftrightarrow s_1 \le s_2, r_1 \le r_2, t_1 = max\{s_1, r_1\},$
$$t_2 = min\{s_2, r_2\}, t_1 \le t_2$$

$(\mathsf{th}\sqcap')$ $\mathsf{th}\,[s_1, s_2] \sqcap \mathsf{th}\,[r_1, r_2] = \mathsf{in}\,[t_2, t_1] \Leftrightarrow s_1 \le s_2, r_1 \le r_2, t_1 = max\{s_1, r_1\},$
$$t_2 = min\{s_2, r_2\}, t_2 < t_1$$

$(\mathsf{th}\,\mathsf{in}\,\sqcap)$ $\mathsf{th}\,[s_1, s_2] \sqcap \mathsf{in}\,[r_1, r_2] = \mathsf{in}\,[r_1, r_2] \Leftrightarrow s_1 \le r_2, r_1 \le s_2, s_1 \le s_2, r_1 \le r_2$

$(\mathsf{th}\,\mathsf{in}\,\sqcap')$ $\mathsf{th}\,[s_1, s_2] \sqcap \mathsf{in}\,[r_1, r_2] = \mathsf{in}\,[s_2, r_2] \Leftrightarrow s_1 \le s_2, s_2 < r_1, r_1 \le r_2$

$(\mathsf{th}\,\mathsf{in}\,\sqcap'')$ $\mathsf{th}\,[s_1, s_2] \sqcap \mathsf{in}\,[r_1, r_2] = \mathsf{in}\,[r_1, s_1] \Leftrightarrow r_1 \le r_2, r_2 < s_1, s_1 \le s_2$

$(\mathsf{in}\,\sqcap)$ $\mathsf{in}\,[s_1, s_2] \sqcap \mathsf{in}\,[r_1, r_2] = \mathsf{in}\,[t_1, t_2] \Leftrightarrow s_1 \le s_2, r_1 \le r_2, t_1 = min\{s_1, r_1\},$
$$t_2 = max\{s_2, r_2\}$$

Example 1. At 10pm Tom was found dead in his house. The only hint is that the answering machine recorded some messages from 7pm up to 8pm. At a first glance, the doctor said Tom was dead for one to two hours. The detective made a further assumption: Tom did not answer the telephone because he was already dead.

We collect all these hints and assumptions into three programs, HINTS, DOCTOR and DETECTIVE, in order not to mix facts with simple hypotheses that might change during the investigations.

HINTS: *found* at 10*pm*.   *ans-machine* $\mathsf{th}\,[7pm, 8pm]$.

DOCTOR: *dead* $\mathsf{in}\,[T - 2:00, T - 1:00] \leftarrow found$ at T

DETECTIVE: *dead* $\mathsf{in}\,[T_1, T_2] \leftarrow ans\text{-}machine$ $\mathsf{th}\,[T_1, T_2]$

If we combine the hypotheses of the doctor and those of the detective we can extend the period of time in which Tom possibly died. The program expression DOCTOR ∩ DETECTIVE behaves as

$$dead \text{ in } [S_1, S_2] \leftarrow \text{in} \, [T - 2{:}00, T - 1{:}00] \sqcap \text{in} \, [T_1, T_2] = \text{in} \, [S_1, S_2],$$
$$found \text{ at } T,$$
$$ans\text{-}machine \text{ th} \, [T_1, T_2]$$

The constraint $\text{in} \, [T - 2{:}00, T - 1{:}00] \sqcap \text{in} \, [T_1, T_2] = \text{in} \, [S_1, S_2]$ builds the annotation $\text{in} \, [S_1, S_2]$ in which Tom possibly died, and by using axiom $(\text{in} \, \sqcap)$ we know that the resulting interval is $S_1 = min\{T - 2{:}00, T_1\}$ and $S_2 = max\{T - 1{:}00, T_2\}$. In fact, according to the semantics, which is formally presented in the next section, a consequence of the program expression HINTS ∪ (DOCTOR ∩ DETECTIVE) is just $dead \text{ in } [7pm, 9pm]$ since the annotation $\text{in} \, [7pm, 9pm]$ is the greatest lower bound of $\text{in} \, [8pm, 9pm]$ and $\text{in} \, [7pm, 8pm]$.

We next give a first example of how spatial information can be modeled in MuTACLP. In particular we can express spatial relations which are parametric with respect to time, such as moving points or evolving regions.

Example 2. We want to model the area flooded by the water tide, assuming that the front end of the tide is a linear function of time. We can establish such a spatio-temporal correlation as follows

$$floodedarea(X, Y) \text{ at } T \leftarrow 1 \leq Y, Y \leq 10, 3 \leq X, X \leq 10, Y \geq X + 8 - T$$

3.1 Semantics of MuTACLP

In this section we define the operational (top-down) semantics of the language MuTACLP by means of a meta-interpreter. Without loss of generality, we assume all atoms to be annotated with th or in labels. In fact at t annotations can be replaced with th $[t, t]$ by exploiting the (at th) axiom. Moreover, each atom which is not annotated in the object level program is intended to be true throughout the whole temporal domain, and thus can be annotated by th $[0, \infty]$.

The meta-interpreter is obtained by extending the well-known vanilla meta-interpreter for logic programs in order to deal with the annotations and to give meaning to the composition operations. Compositions of programs are realized by combining separate programs at the meta-level, without actually building a new program. The reading of the resulting meta-interpreter is straightforward and, most importantly, the meta-logical definition shows that the multi-theory framework can be expressed from inside constraint logic programming itself.

Following Bowen and Kowalski [5], we employ the two-argument predicate *demo* to represent provability. Namely, $demo(\mathcal{E}, G)$ means that the formula G is provable in the program expression $\mathcal{E}$.

Meta-interpreter. The meta-interpreter is defined by the following clauses.

$$demo(\mathcal{E}, empty). \tag{1}$$

$$demo(\mathcal{E}, (B_1, B_2)) \leftarrow demo(\mathcal{E}, B_1), demo(\mathcal{E}, B_2) \tag{2}$$

$$\begin{aligned} demo(\mathcal{E}, A\,\mathtt{th}\,[T_1, T_2]) \leftarrow & S_1 \leq T_1, T_1 \leq T_2, T_2 \leq S_2, \\ & clause(\mathcal{E}, A\,\mathtt{th}\,[S_1, S_2], B), demo(\mathcal{E}, B) \end{aligned} \tag{3}$$

$$\begin{aligned} demo(\mathcal{E}, A\,\mathtt{th}\,[T_1, T_2]) \leftarrow & S_1 \leq T_1, T_1 < S_2, S_2 < T_2, \\ & clause(\mathcal{E}, A\,\mathtt{th}\,[S_1, S_2], B), demo(\mathcal{E}, B), \\ & demo(\mathcal{E}, A\,\mathtt{th}\,[S_2, T_2]) \end{aligned} \tag{4}$$

$$\begin{aligned} demo(\mathcal{E}, A\,\mathtt{in}\,[T_1, T_2]) \leftarrow & T_1 \leq S_2, S_1 \leq T_2, T_1 \leq T_2, \\ & clause(\mathcal{E}, A\,\mathtt{th}\,[S_1, S_2], B), demo(\mathcal{E}, B) \end{aligned} \tag{5}$$

$$\begin{aligned} demo(\mathcal{E}, A\,\mathtt{in}\,[T_1, T_2]) \leftarrow & T_1 \leq S_1, S_2 \leq T_2, \\ & clause(\mathcal{E}, A\,\mathtt{in}\,[S_1, S_2], B), demo(\mathcal{E}, B) \end{aligned} \tag{6}$$

$$demo(\mathcal{E}, C) \leftarrow constraint(C), C \tag{7}$$

$$clause(\mathcal{E}_1 \cup \mathcal{E}_2, A\,\alpha, B) \leftarrow clause(\mathcal{E}_1, A\,\alpha, B) \tag{8}$$

$$clause(\mathcal{E}_1 \cup \mathcal{E}_2, A\,\alpha, B) \leftarrow clause(\mathcal{E}_2, A\,\alpha, B) \tag{9}$$

$$\begin{aligned} clause(\mathcal{E}_1 \cap \mathcal{E}_2, A\,\gamma, (B_1, B_2)) \leftarrow & clause(\mathcal{E}_1, A\,\alpha, B_1), clause(\mathcal{E}_2, A\,\beta, B_2), \\ & \alpha \sqcap \beta = \gamma \end{aligned} \tag{10}$$

A clause $A\,\alpha \leftarrow B$ of a plain program P is represented at the meta-level by

$$clause(P, A\,\alpha, B) \leftarrow S_1 \leq S_2 \tag{11}$$

where $\alpha = \mathtt{th}\,[S_1, S_2]$ or $\alpha = \mathtt{in}\,[S_1, S_2]$.

Observe that the meta-interpreter implements not only Modus Ponens but also rule ($\sqsubseteq$) and rule ($\sqcup$). Clauses (3), (5) and (6) implement the inference rule ($\sqsubseteq$): the atomic goal to be solved is required to be labelled with an annotation which is smaller than the one labelling the head of the clause used in the resolution step according to axioms ($\mathtt{th}\ \sqsubseteq$), ($\mathtt{in}\,\mathtt{th}\ \sqsubseteq$) and ($\mathtt{in}\ \sqsubseteq$), respectively. Rule ($\sqcup$) is implemented by clause (4). According to the discussion in Section 2, it is applicable only to $\mathtt{th}$ annotations with overlapping time periods which do not include one another. The constraints on temporal variables ensure that the time period $[t_1, t_2]$ is a *new* time period different from $[s_1, s_2]$ and $[s_2, t_2]$ and their subintervals. Clause (7) manages constraints by passing them directly to the constraint solver.

As far as the meta-level definition of the union and intersection operations is concerned, clauses (8) and (9) simply state that a clause $A\,\alpha \leftarrow B$ belongs to the union of two program expressions $\mathcal{E}_1$ and $\mathcal{E}_2$, if it belongs either to $\mathcal{E}_1$ or to $\mathcal{E}_2$. On the other hand, a clause $A\,\alpha \leftarrow B$, belonging to the intersection of two program expressions $\mathcal{E}_1$ and $\mathcal{E}_2$, is built by taking an instance of clause in each program expression $\mathcal{E}_1$ and $\mathcal{E}_2$, such that the head atoms of the two clauses are unifiable. Let such instances of clauses be cl_1 and cl_2. Then B is the conjunction of the bodies of cl_1 and cl_2 and A is the unified atom labelled with the greatest lower bound of the annotations of the heads of cl_1 and cl_2.

As shown in [19] it is also possible to provide MuTACLP with a fixpoint (bottom-up) semantics, based on an immediate consequence operator, and to prove the soundness and completeness of the meta-interpreter with respect to the fixpoint semantics.

4   Declarative GIS Analysis in MuTACLP

Adding a declarative programming layer on top of Geographical Information Systems can permit a better use of them, essentially because a declarative approach is much closer to the natural ways of expressing analysis rules than a procedural approach. First of all, since (constraint) logic programming is essentially a rule-based system, it is possible to build GIS applications with an expert system flavor. Moreover, the multi-theory framework, that provides tools for combining different knowledge components, coded in different programs, seems particularly suited to handle the naturally fragmented knowledge used in GIS analysis.

The approach described in [2] represents a first step for providing the user with a declarative language for GIS analysis. It basically relies on the (enriched) language of program expressions and on the introduction of built-in atoms which can be used to invoke GIS functions. However, this approach still presents some limits such as the inability of directly manipulating the representation of spatial data and the lack of a uniform representation of data. We propose a possible different solution which overcomes these problems. In our proposal the built-in predicates are replaced with an explicit representation of the GIS spatial data in MuTACLP. The main advantage is that we have a declarative language where spatio-temporal and thematic information can be represented in a uniform way and we can exploit the features of constraint logic programming, such as recursion and constraint handling to perform sophisticated spatio-temporal reasoning. Moreover, the use of a unifying language is also promising to support the interoperability among different GISs, which is a topic for future work.

We focus our attention on 2-dimensional spatial objects.

4.1   A Logical Representation of GIS Spatial Data

We propose an automatic translation of the spatial data stored in a GIS into MuTACLP programs, assuming that spatial data are represented according to the Spaghetti Model. Observe that this assumption is reasonable because such a model is very popular and there are also GIS functions that convert data from the Raster Model into the Spaghetti Model and vice versa. Under this hypothesis the translation process consists of two steps:

Step 1. A spatial object is triangulated, and each triangle is represented by a unit clause containing an identifier for the triangle and its three vertexes;

Step 2. By using the implicit representation of a triangle, determined in step 1, i.e., its vertexes, we build a constraint which explicitly defines the set of points belonging to it. A spatial object is then denoted by an expression which represents the union of the triangles which compose the object.

Step 1. In the Spaghetti model, a GIS object is uniquely determined by an identifier, and it has some thematic attributes and a spatial component consisting of a list of points modeling its contour. In the following, we focus on the translation of the spatial component of the object because thematic attributes do not require any particular treatment, and they can be represented by themselves. By using a standard algorithm to triangulate an object we obtain a set of triangles which approximate it. We suppose that if the algorithm returns a triangle with three distinct vertexes, then such points are not all collinear. Now we can define a set of clauses providing the logical representation of the object in the 2-Spaghetti Model.

Definition 2 (2-Spaghetti Model). *An object identified by objId and decomposed into n triangles, with identifiers tId_i and vertexes (x_1^i, y_1^i), (x_2^i, y_2^i), (x_3^i, y_3^i), for $i = 1, \ldots, n$, is represented by the following unit clauses:*

- $n\_tri(objId, n)$.
- $tri(objId, i, tId_i, x_1^i, y_1^i, x_2^i, y_2^i, x_3^i, y_3^i)$.   *for $i = 1, \ldots, n$.*

The first clause states that the object *objId* is composed by n triangles while the predicate *tri* defines the triangles composing the object. A *tri* clause states that the triangle tId_i is the ith triangle of the object *objId* and its vertexes are $x_1^i, y_1^i, x_2^i, y_2^i, x_3^i, y_3^i$. The identifier tId_i is a global (unique) identifier.

Indeed this representation of spatial objects is an intermediate step to obtain a representation based on linear constraints. The second kind of representation has the advantage of giving an explicit characterization of the points which belong to an object (e.g. a polygon is explicitly the infinite set of points it contains versus the implicit definition by means of the sequence of border points). Therefore, it allows us to manipulate spatial objects through standard set operations, such as union, intersection, difference etc.

Step 2. As objects are composed by triangles, we first describe how we can obtain a constraint from the 2-Spaghetti representation of a triangle. We consider a non-degenerate triangle; the translation of points and line segments (degenerate triangles) is similar and it is omitted for space limitation (see [19] for the complete translation). The idea, also exploited by Chomicki and Revesz [8] and by Grumbach et al. [13], is that a triangle, which is the intersection of three half-planes, can be defined as the conjunction of the inequalities defining each half-plane. The predicate *side* expresses the constraint for a half-plane.

$$side(X, Y, X_1, Y_1, X_2, Y_2, X_3, Y_3) \leftarrow (Y_3 - Y_1)(X_2 - X_1) \geq (Y_2 - Y_1)(X_3 - X_1),$$
$$(Y - Y_1)(X_2 - X_1) \geq (Y_2 - Y_1)(X - X_1)$$
$$side(X, Y, X_1, Y_1, X_2, Y_2, X_3, Y_3) \leftarrow (Y_3 - Y_1)(X_2 - X_1) \leq (Y_2 - Y_1)(X_3 - X_1),$$
$$(Y - Y_1)(X_2 - X_1) \leq (Y_2 - Y_1)(X - X_1)$$

The constraint in the clause body is satisfied by the points (X, Y) which are above (or below) the line crossing the points (X_1, Y_1) and (X_2, Y_2) and which are in the same half-plane of (X_3, Y_3).

In order to find the points belonging to a non-degenerate triangle we simply intersect the three half-planes delimited by the lines crossing each couple of the triangle vertexes and including the third one.

$$tri\_con(TrId, X, Y) \leftarrow tri(\_,\_, TrId, X_1, Y_1, X_2, Y_2, X_3, Y_3),$$
$$distinct(X_1, Y_1, X_2, Y_2, X_3, Y_3),$$
$$side(X, Y, X_1, Y_1, X_2, Y_2, X_3, Y_3),$$
$$side(X, Y, X_2, Y_2, X_3, Y_3, X_1, Y_1),$$
$$side(X, Y, X_3, Y_3, X_1, Y_1, X_2, Y_2)$$

where *distinct* is a predicate that checks that the vertexes are all distinct. The resolution of the atom $tri\_con(TrId, X, Y)$ provides the constraint representing all the points of the triangle $TrId$.

Now we can model a spatial object inside our logical framework: an object can be seen as the union of its triangles.

$$obj(ObjId, SpExp) \leftarrow n\_tri(ObjId, N), join(ObjId, N - 1, SpExp)$$
$$join(ObjId, 0, TrId) \leftarrow tri(ObjId, 0, TrId, \_, \_, \_, \_, \_, \_)$$
$$join(ObjId, J, SpExp \oplus TrId) \leftarrow tri(ObjId, J, TrId, \_, \_, \_, \_, \_, \_),$$
$$join(ObjId, J - 1, SpExp)$$

The expression $SpExp$ ($SpExp$ stands for *Spatial Expression*) is a symbolic representation of the object and a means to recover the constraint associated with each triangle composing the object. The intended meaning of $\oplus$ is set-theoretic union and it will be defined formally in the next section.

4.2   Operators on Spatial Objects

In order to manipulate spatial objects we provide the ordinary set-theoretic operations: union $\oplus$, intersection $\otimes$, difference $\setminus$ and complement$^-$. Through these operations we build expressions whose basic components are the triangle identifiers. Formally the set of spatial expressions is defined as follows:

$$SpExp ::= TrId \mid \emptyset \mid SpExp \oplus SpExp \mid SpExp \otimes SpExp \mid SpExp \setminus SpExp \mid SpExp^-$$

where $TrId$ is the syntactic category of triangle identifiers and $\emptyset$ denotes an empty area.

The meaning of such operations is expressed by a set of clauses defining the predicate *belong* which states when a point belongs to a spatial expression.

$$belong(X, Y, TrId) \leftarrow tri\_con(TrId, X, Y)$$
$$belong(X, Y, SpExp_1 \oplus SpExp_2) \leftarrow belong(X, Y, SpExp_1)$$
$$belong(X, Y, SpExp_1 \oplus SpExp_2) \leftarrow belong(X, Y, SpExp_2)$$
$$belong(X, Y, SpExp_1 \otimes SpExp_2) \leftarrow belong(X, Y, SpExp_1), belong(X, Y, SpExp_2)$$
$$belong(X, Y, SpExp_1 \setminus SpExp_2) \leftarrow belong(X, Y, SpExp_1), belong(X, Y, SpExp_2^-)$$
$$belong(X, Y, SpExp^-) \leftarrow complement(X, Y, SpExp)$$

The first clause asserts that a point (x, y) belongs to a triangle $trId$ if it satisfies the constraint representing the triangle (i.e., if $tri\_con(trId, x, y)$ is provable). The definitions of union, intersection and difference are straightforward since they exactly reflect the meaning of the corresponding mathematical operations. The definition of the complement operation is based on the predicate *complement*. To define it, first we provide the representation of the complement of a triangle and then, by exploiting De Morgan laws, we easily obtain a set of clauses for the predicate *complement*. The complement of a non-degenerate triangle is the union of three half-planes which are the complements of the half-planes determined by the predicate *side*. We refer the reader to [19] for a complete definition of such a predicate. It is worth noting that there is no clause for the empty area $\emptyset$ because no point belongs to it.

4.3   Creation of GIS Layers

In a GIS the objects of interest often consist of collections of a quite large number of disjoint areas enjoying a common property, e.g. characterized by the presence of water or where a particular kind of tree grows or with a special kind of ground etc. Such areas form a so-called *layer*. To allow a user to obtain directly these kinds of information, we provide the system with a mechanism (*layer*) that, given a certain property, returns a spatial expression representing the corresponding layer.

To specify that an object $ObId$ enjoys a property $Prop$, we use a unit clause of the form $hasProp(ObId, Prop)$. In order to collect the objects with the same property we define the clause

$$objWithProp(Prop, ListObId) \leftarrow set\_of(ObId, hasProp(ObId, Prop), ListObId)$$

where *set_of* is the Prolog meta-predicate provided to work on sets. In this case, it is used to compute the list of distinct object identifiers which satisfy the goal $hasProp(ObId, Prop)$, that is the list of identifiers of objects which enjoy property $Prop$.

A layer is then represented by a spatial expression, obtained by solving the predicate *layer*

$$layer(Prop, SpExp) \leftarrow objWithProp(Prop, L), extract(L, SpExp)$$
$$extract([], \emptyset).$$
$$extract([ObId], SpExp) \leftarrow obj(ObId, SpExp)$$
$$extract([ObId|L], SpExp \oplus SpE) \leftarrow obj(ObId, SpE), extract(L, SpExp)$$

A layer for the property $Prop$ is denoted by a spatial expression which is the union of the spatial expressions associated with the objects satisfying $Prop$. If no object enjoys the property then the empty area, $\emptyset$, is returned.

It is worth noticing that many definitions, given in this subsection and in the previous ones, are not domain dependent: only n_tri, tri and $hasProp$ are used to represent specific spatial data. Thus we can collect most definitions, provided to handle spatial objects, into a program, called SPACEMOD, which will be combined with the specific theories in all the spatial analyses.

Finally, since the aim of this paper is to improve the GIS analysis ability, the translation process described above does not address the problem of obtaining an efficient representation of objects. To increase the efficiency of our implementation we could use the algorithms proposed in [11] that directly transform a point-based representation into its equivalent constraint representation, but this is left as future work.

5   An Example

In this section we present an application that highlights how analysis criteria can be naturally described in MuTACLP. The application problem we address consists in the analysis of a geographic area, which can be formulated as follows.

> *Find all the zones in a given region that provide a favorable habitat for hares. These animals live in woods, near sources of water, and they eat vegetables, such as lettuce, wild cabbage and turnip. The main predators of hares are foxes, wolves and raptorial birds like eagles. Thus a favorable habitat will be an area rich of water where it is easy to find vegetables and possibly without predators.*

The above description is very general and it refers to the usual behavior of a hare during the year. We can describe the favorable habitat for a hare as follows

HARE-HAB
$$habitat(hares, SpE_1 \otimes SpE_2) \, \text{th} \, [jan, dec] \; \leftarrow \; layer(water, SpE_1),$$
$$layer(vegetable, SpE_2)$$

$$predator(hares, (SpE_1 \oplus SpE_2) \oplus SpE_3) \, \text{th} \, [jan, dec] \leftarrow layer(fox, SpE_1),$$
$$layer(wolf, SpE_2),$$
$$layer(eagle, SpE_3)$$

$$favArea(hares, X, Y) \, \text{th} \, [T_1, T_2] \leftarrow habitat(hares, SpE_1) \, \text{th} \, [T_1, T_2],$$
$$predator(hares, SpE_2) \, \text{th} \, [T_1, T_2],$$
$$belong(X, Y, SpE_1 \setminus SpE_2)$$

The clause for *habitat* states that a zone where hares can live is the intersection of the layer of water and of the layer of vegetables and this holds throughout the year. Since foxes, wolves and eagles are predators of the hare during the entire year we annotate the head of the clause defining *predator* with $\text{th} \, [jan, dec]$. Then a favorable habitat for hares in a certain period $[T_1, T_2]$ is computed by removing from the habitat areas in $[T_1, T_2]$, pieces of land where the predators of hares can be found during that time period.

Figure 1 gives a possible concrete description of the region of interest showing the presence of water, where vegetables grow and the areas where foxes, wolves and eagles live.

The program REG gives the logical description of the region.

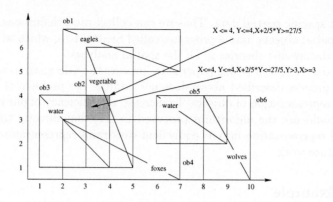

Fig. 1. Favorable habitat

REG

$n\_tri(ob1,2)$.	$tri(ob1,0,tr1,2,7,2,5,7,5)$.	$tri(ob1,1,tr2,2,7,7,5,7,7)$.
$n\_tri(ob2,2)$.	$tri(ob2,0,tr3,3,6,5,1,5,6)$.	$tri(ob2,1,tr4,3,6,3,1,5,1)$.

$\vdots$

$hasProp(ob1, eagle)$.	$hasProp(ob2, vegetable)$.
$hasProp(ob3, water)$.	$hasProp(ob4, fox)$.
$hasProp(ob5, water)$.	$hasProp(ob6, wolf)$.

In our region there are two areas rich of water whereas the layers for vegetables and for the different kinds of predators consist of a single area. To compute the water layer we ask the system

$demo$(REG $\cup$ SPACEMOD, $layer(water, SpE)$)

and the answer is $SpE = ob3 \oplus ob5$. Now to know the favorable habitat in March, we ask the following query

$demo$(HARE-HAB $\cup$ (REG $\cup$ SPACEMOD), $favArea(hares, X, Y)$ th $[mar, mar]$)

The computed favorable habitat, which is painted in grey in Figure 1, is provided by the system returning two solutions to the previous query:

$$X \leq 4, Y \leq 4, X + \tfrac{2}{5} * Y \geq \tfrac{27}{5} \qquad X \leq 4, Y \leq 4, X + \tfrac{2}{5} * Y \leq \tfrac{27}{5}, Y > 3, X \geq 3$$

Indeed we can improve the analysis on the behavior of the hare taking into account how it varies during the year. Let us assume that

during Spring hares like eating corn and in Autumn they feed on also with oil-seeds rich in moisture.

Thus their favorable areas in the cited seasons are more specific: the areas where hares prefer staying should contain respectively corn or oil-seeds, too.

To reflect this more complex behavior of hares we can restrict the program HARE-HAB by using the intersection operation. We define two programs SPRING and AUTUMN which refine the definition of the *favArea* predicate.

Spring
  $habitat(hares, SpE)$ th $[apr, jun]$.
  $predator(hares, SpE)$ th $[apr, jun]$.
  $favArea(hares, X, Y)$ th $[apr, jun]$ ← $layer(corn, SpE), belong(X, Y, SpE)$
Autumn
  $habitat(hares, SpE)$ th $[oct, dec]$.
  $predator(hares, SpE)$ th $[oct, dec]$.
  $favArea(hares, X, Y)$ th $[oct, dec]$ ← $layer(oil\text{-}seed, SpE), belong(X, Y, SpE)$

Spring and Autumn restrict the temporal validity of the definition of *habitat* and *predator*. Thus, when these programs are intersected with a program which contains clauses defining such predicates, those rules holding from April to June or from October to December, respectively, are selected. Moreover, Spring and Autumn add a further constraint both on the temporal validity of *favArea* and on how a favorable zone is computed, i.e., from April to June (resp. from October to December) also *corn* (resp. *oil-seeds*) is required to grow in such an area.

The program expression that captures the season-dependent knowledge is

$$(\text{Hare-Hab} \cap (\text{Spring} \cup \text{Autumn})) \cup$$
$$(\text{Hare-Hab}\Downarrow [jan, mar] \cup \text{Hare-Hab}\Downarrow [jul, sep])$$

where the operator $\Downarrow$ (see [19]) is a derived operator which allows one to restrict the temporal validity of a set of clauses to a time interval.

6 Conclusions

In this paper we have shown how MuTACLP can be used on top of GISs in order to provide users with a more friendly interface for GIS analysis. Although more work is needed to improve the support for spatial data, the examples in the paper highlight that we are already able to perform interesting spatial and spatio-temporal analyses, mainly thanks to the deductive power supplied by the underlying constraint logic programming. By means of recursive predicates we can express the transitive closure of relations, an ability not provided by the traditional approaches in the database field. This ability is very important, for instance, to perform network analysis (see e.g. [19] where it is used to search for connections between objects). More generally, our approach allows one not only to represent data as in constraint databases but also to express rules, an extra feature which makes the difference if we want to use the language as specification and/or analysis language. All these features suggest also the possibility of using MuTACLP in the construction of a software layer, the layer of mediators [21], which allows for the semantic integration of different data sources, and in particular for the semantic interoperability of spatio-temporal knowledge bases, like different geographical information systems.

An interesting direction for future research regards the investigation of some important spatial properties, such as metric properties and topological relations between objects, which, at the moment, are not considered in our framework.

Acknowledgments: We thank Paolo Baldan for his useful comments.

References

1. A.I. Abdelmoty, N.W. Paton, M.H. Williams, A.A.A. Fernandes, M.L. Barja, and A. Dinn. Geographic Data Handling in a Deductive Object-Oriented Database. In *5th International DEXA Conference*, volume 856 of *LNCS*, pages 445–454, 1994.
2. D. Aquilino, P. Asirelli, A. Formuso, C. Renso, and F. Turini. Using MedLan to Integrate Geographical Data. *Journal of Logic Programming*, 43(1):3–14, 2000.
3. A. Belussi, E. Bertino, and B. Catania. An extended algebra for constraint databases. *IEEE TKDE*, 10(5):686–705, 1998.
4. M.H. Böhlen, C.S. Jensen, and M.O. Scholl, editors. *Spatio-Temporal Database Management*, volume 1678 of *LNCS*. Springer Verlag, 1999.
5. K.A. Bowen and R.A. Kowalski. Amalgamating language and metalanguage in logic programming. In *Logic programming*, volume 16 of *APIC studies in data processing*, pages 153–172. Academic Press, 1982.
6. A. Brogi, P. Mancarella, D. Pedreschi, and F. Turini. Modular logic programming. *ACM TOPLAS*, 16(4):1361–1398, July 1994.
7. J. Chomicki. Temporal Query Languages: A Survey. In *Temporal Logic: Proc. of the 1st ICTL'94*, volume 827 of *LNAI*, pages 506–534. Springer Verlag, 1994.
8. J. Chomicki and P.Z. Revesz. Constraint-Based Interoperability of Spatiotemporal Database. *Geoinformatica*, 3(3):211–243, 1999.
9. M. Egenhofer. User interfaces. In *Cognitive Aspects of Human-Computer Interaction for Geographical Information Systems*, pages 1–8. Kluwer Academic, 1995.
10. T. Frühwirth. Temporal Annotated Constraint Logic Programming. *Journal of Symbolic Computation*, 22:555–583, 1996.
11. S. Grumbach, P. Rigaux, M. Scholl, and L. Segoufin. DEDALE, A Spatial Constraint Database. In *Proc. of Intl. Workshop on Database programming Languages*, volume 1369 of *Lecture Notes in Computer Science*, pages 38–59, 1998.
12. S. Grumbach, P. Rigaux, and L. Segoufin. Spatio-Temporal Data Handling with Constraints. In *Proc. of the 6th International Symposium on Advances in GIS*, pages 106–111. ACM Press, 1998.
13. S. Grumbach, P. Rigaux, and L. Segoufin. The DEDALE System for Complex Spatial Queries. In *Proc. of the ACM SIGMOD*, pages 213–224, 1998.
14. P.C. Kanellakis, G.M. Kuper, and P.Z. Revesz. Constraint query languages. *Journal of Computer and System Sciences*, 51(1):26–52, August 1995.
15. G. Langran. *Time in Geographical Information Systems*. Taylor & Francis, 1992.
16. P. Mancarella, A. Raffaetà, and F. Turini. Temporal Annotated Constraint Logic Programming with Multiple Theories. In *10th International DEXA Workshop*, pages 501–508. IEEE Computer Society Press, 1999.
17. Jan Paredaens. Spatial databases, the final frontier. In *Database Theory—ICDT'95*, volume 893 of *LNCS*, pages 14–32. Springer, 1995.
18. Esprit/Essi project no.21580. *Guidelines for best practice in user interface for GIS*. European Commission, 1999.
19. A. Raffaetà. *Spatio-temporal knowledge bases in a constraint logic programming framework with multiple theories*. PhD thesis, Dip. Informatica, Univ. Pisa, 2000.
20. A. Tansel, J. Clifford, S. Gadia, S. Jajodia, A. Segev, and R. Snodgrass editors. *Temporal Databases: Theory, Design, and Implementation*. 1993.
21. G. Wiederhold. Mediators in the Architecture of Future Information Systems. *IEEE Computer*, 25:38–49, March 1992.
22. M. F. Worboys. *GIS - A Computing Perspective*. Taylor & Francis, 1995.

Reasoning about Duplicate Elimination
with Description Logic
(Preliminary Report)

Vitaliy L. Khizder, David Toman, and Grant Weddell

Department of Computer Science
University of Waterloo, Canada

Abstract. Queries commonly perform much better if they manage to avoid duplicate elimination operations in their execution plans. In this paper, we report on a technique that provides a necessary and sufficient condition for removing such operators from object relational conjunctive queries under the standard duplicate semantics. The condition is fully captured as a membership problem in a dialect of description logic called CFD, which is capable of expressing a number of common constraints implicit in object relational database schemas. We also present a PTIME algorithm for arbitrary membership problems in CFD.

1 Introduction

The paper presents a combination of two techniques to provide a very powerful tool for reasoning about duplicate semantics of conjunctive object relational queries, in particular about elimination operations and situations in which these operations can be completely removed. The query language studied in the paper contains many other practical query languages, in particular the conjunctive fragments of SQL92 [13, 17] and OQL [7, 8].

The first technique provides a characterization of situations in which queries can be mowed out of the scope of a duplicate elimination operator: it defines a sufficient and necessary condition in terms of deducing a *uniqueness constraint* in an abstraction of the query. Unlike many other approaches, we show that our technique *completely* characterizes these situations: in the cases the appropriate condition does not hold, we know that the duplicate elimination operator may not be removed.

The second technique is complementary to the first: it defines a dialect of *description logic* called CFD that

- captures usual schema declarations, including the "decidable" part of the SQL IEF (integrity enhancement feature) declarations, and
- has an efficient inference mechanism that runs in PTIME both in the size of the schema and the query.

In addition to the usual integrity constraints, CFD can capture many other *schema declarations*, e.g., inheritance constraints, path functions, etc.

J. Lloyd et al. (Eds.): CL 2000, LNAI 1861, pp. 1017–1032, 2000.

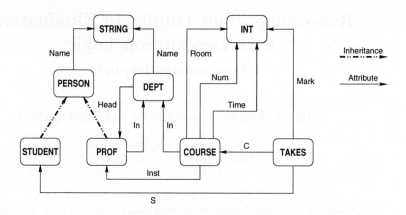

Fig. 1. University Database Schema.

Example 1. We illustrate the approach with an object relational schema for a hypothetical university application illustrated in Figure 1. In particular, consider a request to *"find the unique names of students taking some course taught at the same time as some other course numbered :P2 with an instructor in the department named :P1"*. In SQL-like syntax, the query can be formulated as:

```
select distinct S.Name as Name
from  STUDENT as S, TAKES as T, COURSE as C
where S = T.S and C.Time = T.C.Time and
      C.Inst.In.Name = :P1 and C.Num = :P2
```

The results of this paper enable an efficient rewriting of the query to an equivalent formulation that does not involve any use of a duplicate elimination operation (the removal of the **distinct** keyword in this case):

```
select S.Name as Name
from  STUDENT as S, TAKES as T, COURSE as C
where S = T.S and C.Time = T.C.Time and
      C.Inst.In.Name = :P1 and C.Num = :P2
```

This goal is achieved by describing the integrity constraints that hold in the database schema (Figure 2) and then applying a rewriting rule (Example 10).

1.1 Related Work

Description logics have long been recognized as a valuable tool for conceptual modeling and for the specification of database schemas [2, 6]. More recently, they have found applications in query optimization, in particular for issues relating to deciding view relevance [5]. However, so far as we are aware, such logics have not yet been used to reason about duplicate elimination in query plans.

Conversely, many proposals have utilized *functional dependencies* and *foreign key constraints* to optimize queries, e.g., for predicate movement [16], as a supplement to Magic Set optimization for bag semantics [18], for optimization of joins and semi-joins [19], or for decorelation of complex queries [22], and other more general integrity constraints to optimize queries [12].

This paper links the efforts seeking efficient decision procedures for dialects of description logics [4] with actual techniques used for optimizing queries. The link between these two techniques is non-trivial: conjunctive query subsumption is NP-hard for set semantics [9] and Π_2^p-hard for bag semantics [10], in general. However, using our approach we reduce questions about equivalence of *particular* queries related by common forms of rewrites to subsumption constraints in a dialect of description logic that has an efficient (PTIME) decision procedure.

Both the decision procedure and logic are refinements of earlier versions [4]. In this paper the variety of uniqueness constraints is generalized to include path functional dependencies [24, 23] and the presented decision procedure itself incorporates an optimization for membership tests that involve uniqueness constraints that satisfy a symmetry property.

The rest of the paper is organized as follows: Section 2 defines CFD along with an object relational query language used in the rest of the paper. Section 3 presents the first result: a complete rewriting rule for duplication elimination removal from conjunctive object relational queries with respect to their duplicate semantics. Section 4 presents a complete inference procedure for deducing arbitrary subsumption constraints in CFD. All development is illustrated step-by-step using a running example. The paper concludes with some summary comments and suggestion for several directions of further research.

2 Definitions

This section provides all necessary definitions needed to present the results of the paper. The definitions are followed by examples that illustrate how the individual concepts are used.

2.1 Description Logics and Database Schemas

We begin by defining CFD, a dialect of a description logic that incorporates a constructor for capturing uniqueness constraints. CFD is short for "Classic/FD", the name of an earlier version first defined in [4] in which a simpler form of uniqueness construct is added to an earlier dialect called CLASSIC [3]. CFD has enough expressiveness to capture object relational database schemas including a variety of integrity constraints (cf. Example 3).

Definition 2 (Description Logic CFD). Let C denote primitive concepts and A primitive attributes. The *concept descriptions* are defined by the following

```
PERSON < (Name: STRING),        DEPT < (Name: STRING),
        PERSON(Name -> Id)              (Head: PROF),
                                        DEPT(Name -> Id),
STUDENT < PERSON                        DEPT(Head -> Id)

PROF < PERSON, (In: DEPT)        COURSE < (Num: INT),
                                          (Room: INT),
TAKES < (S: STUDENT),                     (Time: INT),
        (C: COURSE),                      (Inst: PROF),
        (Mark: INT),                      (In: DEPT),
        TAKES(S, C -> Id),                COURSE(Num, In -> Id),
        TAKES(S, C.Time -> C)             COURSE(Room, Time -> Id),
                                          COURSE(Inst.In -> In)
```

Fig. 2. University Database Schema in CFD.

grammar:

$$
\begin{array}{lll}
D :: & ANY & (all\ objects) \\
 & |\ C & (superclass\ construct) \\
 & |\ (\mathsf{Pf} : D) & (typing\ construct) \\
 & |\ C(\mathsf{Pf}_1, \ldots, \mathsf{Pf}_n \rightarrow \mathsf{Pf}) & (uniqueness\ construct;\ n \geq 1) \\
 & |\ \mathsf{Pf}_1 = \mathsf{Pf}_2 & (equational\ construct) \\
 & |\ D_1, D_2 & (conjunction\ construct)
\end{array}
$$

where the *attribute descriptions* Pf are of the form **Id** (identity) or $A.\mathsf{Pf}$ (path composition). The concept descriptions are used to formulate *subsumption constraints* of the form $C < D$.

Intuitively, the *descriptions* describe sets of objects (object id's), the *attributes* (or paths) describe the relationships between objects, and *subsumption constraints* restrict valid instances of the database.

Example 3. The University database schema from Figure 1 is captured using CFD in Figure 2. The constraints introduce primitive classes PERSON, STUDENT, PROF, COURSE, DEPT, TAKES, INT (for integers), and STRING (for strings), and assert that PERSONs have Names (strings), that STUDENTs and PROFs are PERSONs (inheritance constraints); that Name is a key of PERSON (because it determines **Id**—the object id of the person object), and so on. For readability we omit the trailing **Id** in attribute descriptions in our examples.

The semantics of CFD is defined with respect to a possibly infinite collection of entities Dom and a function $(.)^I$. We call the pair $I = (\mathsf{Dom}, (.)^I)$ an *interpretation* or a *database* (these are synonymous in our approach). The second component, $(.)^I$, maps subsumption constraints to truth values, concept descriptions to subsets of Dom, and attribute descriptions to total functions over Dom. There are no further conditions on the interpretation of primitive concepts and attributes. The interpretation of the remaining constructs is constrained as follows:

Definition 4 (Semantics of CFD). Let $\mathcal{C}_C \subseteq \mathsf{Dom}$ be a set for each primitive concept C, and $\mathcal{F}_A : \mathsf{Dom} \to \mathsf{Dom}$ a function on Dom for each attribute A. Then

$$
\begin{aligned}
(ANY)^I &= \mathsf{Dom} \\
(C)^I &= \mathcal{C}_C \\
(\mathsf{Pf} : D)^I &= \{v : (\mathsf{Pf})^I v \in (D)^I\} \\
(C(\mathsf{Pf}_1, \ldots, \mathsf{Pf}_n \to \mathsf{Pf}))^I &= \{v : \forall w \in (C)^I. \\
& \quad (\mathsf{Pf}_i)^I v = (\mathsf{Pf}_i)^I w \Rightarrow (\mathsf{Pf})^I v = (\mathsf{Pf})^I w\} \\
(\mathsf{Pf}_1 = \mathsf{Pf}_2)^I &= \{v : (\mathsf{Pf}_1)^I v = (\mathsf{Pf}_2)^I v\} \\
(D_1, D_2)^I &= (D_1)^I \cap (D_2)^I
\end{aligned}
$$

The meanings of the attribute descriptions **Id** and $A.\mathsf{Pf}$ are defined as $\lambda x.x$ and $\lambda x.(\mathsf{Pf})^I(\mathcal{F}_A \, x)$, respectively. The meaning of a subsumption constraint $C < D$ is defined as $(C)^I \subseteq (D)^I$.

A database schema S is a set of subsumption constraints in CDF. We say that a database I *satisfies* schema S, written $I \models S$, if all subsumption constraints in S are true with respect to $(.)^I$.

Similarly, given subsumption constraint $C < D$, we write $S \models C < D$ to express the condition that $C < D$ is a logical consequence of S, that is $I \models S$ implies $I \models C < D$ for all databases I.

To run in PTIME, the decision procedure presented in Section 4 requires two restrictions on the set S. First, only *regular* path functional dependencies are allowed in S. Description $C(\mathsf{Pf}_1, \ldots, \mathsf{Pf}_n \to \mathsf{Pf})$ is *regular* if Pf (with the possible exception of the last primitive attribute) is a prefix of Pf_i for some $1 \leq i \leq n$ [14]. Second, S may not contain equational constraints. We say that S is *regular* and *equation-free* when it satisfies these conditions. It is easy to verify that the schema in Figure 2 is regular and equation-free.

Relational Databases and Schemas. We have defined databases as pairs of a domain Dom and an interpretation function $(.)^I$. However, it is easy to see that standard SQL table/attribute declarations map to simple subsumption constraints and the databases that satisfy these constraints are equivalent to SQL databases. Consider the declaration

```
CREATE TABLE PERSON(Name char(100))
```

saying that we have a table `PERSON` with a single attribute `NAME`. This is equivalently captured by the subsumption constraint `PERSON < (Name: STRING)`; the function associated with the attribute `Name`, given a person object, returns a string. The SQL IEF (Integrity Enhancement Feature) also allows declaration of *integrity constraints* that must hold on the schema. In this paper we consider the *entity integrity* and the *referential integrity* constraints (the *domain* constraints are captured as above[1]).

---

[1] With the exception of general `CHECK` constraints.

The *entity integrity* (key) constraints are captured in CFD using the uniqueness construct. To declare that `Name` as a key of the `PERSON` table we say `PERSON < PERSON(Name -> Id)` where `Id` is essentially a reference to the object identifier of person (presumed to be unique for each object in the class).

The *referential integrity* constraints in our approach are more limited than in SQL. However, such a restriction is necessary as SQL's referential integrity constraints allow general embedded inclusion dependencies and thus reasoning becomes undecidable [1]. We restrict the referential integrity to unary foreign key constraints (i.e., the target of the dependency must be a key—in our case the object identifier—which reduces to attribute declarations in our model). This restriction leads to efficiently decidable theory (cf. section 4) while capturing a large class of practical schema declarations in SQL.

2.2   Conjunctive Object Relational Queries

We define the core syntax of the conjunctive fragment of object relational queries by the following grammar:

Definition 5 (Object Relational Conjunctive Queries).

$$
\begin{aligned}
Q :: &\; C \text{ as } A && (Primitive\ class) \\
&\mid A.\mathrm{Pf}_1 = B.\mathrm{Pf}_2 && (Equational\ constraint) \\
&\mid \texttt{select } A_1, \dots, A_n\ Q && (Projection) \\
&\mid \texttt{elim } Q && (Duplicate\ elimination) \\
&\mid \texttt{from } Q_1, \dots, Q_k && (Natural\ join)
\end{aligned}
$$

In addition we assume standard *syntactic safety* conditions to be satisfied by the queries[2].

Note that the only *apriori interpreted* operation in the language is equality. All other classes of objects, including built-in classes (relations) are modeled using primitive concepts. Therefore, we have primitive concepts that model all the usual built-in relations, e.g., `LESS` for linear order, `PLUS` for addition, etc.

It is easy to see that the language captures all *conjunctive queries* under duplicate semantics. All other common constructs can be translated to queries formulated in the above fragment and are considered to be mere syntactic sugar. In particular:

Q `where` E `and` $E' \dots$ = `from` $Q, E, E', \dots$
Q `where exists` Q' = `from` $Q, (\texttt{elim select } VQ')$, for V parameters of Q'
`select distinct` VQ = `elim select` VQ

The formal semantics of queries is defined with respect to a database I as follows:

---

[2] For our results to hold we can even allow infinite bags as long as every tuple is duplicated only finitely many times.

Definition 6 (Semantics of Queries). We define the semantic function $[\![.]\!]$ that maps queries to functions from databases I to bags of tuples as follows:

$$[\![C \text{ as } A]\!]I = \{\!\{\langle A : v\rangle : v \in (C)^I\}\!\}$$
$$[\![A.\text{Pf}_1 = B.\text{Pf}_2]\!]I = \{\!\{\langle A : v, B : w\rangle : v, w \in \text{Dom}, (\text{Pf}_1)^I(v) = (\text{Pf}_2)^I(w)\}\!\}$$
$$[\![\text{select } A_1, \ldots, A_n \ Q]\!]I = \{\!\{\langle A_1 : v@A_1, \ldots, A_n : v@A_n\rangle : v \in [\![Q]\!]I\}\!\}$$
$$[\![\text{elim } Q]\!]I = \{v : v \in [\![Q]\!]I\}$$
$$[\![\text{from } Q_1, \ldots, Q_k]\!]I = [\![Q_1]\!]I \bowtie \ldots \bowtie [\![Q_k]\!]I$$

where $\{\!\{\langle A_i : v_i\rangle\}\!\}$ denotes a bag of tuples and $v@A_i$ denotes the value associated with A_i in the tuple v; we require the attribute labels A_i to be the same for each tuple in the bag and for each individual tuple to form a set.

SQL Queries. As in the case of SQL tables mapping directly to primitive concepts, conjunctive queries in SQL (the SELECT-FROM-WHERE blocks) map directly to our object relational query language. The semantics of SQL maps immediately to the semantics presented in Definition 6. The only difference is that, for base tables, SQL retrieves values of all declared attributes in addition to the "tuple id", and thus in equality constraints the already retrieved values are simply compared. (Recall that all path functions in SQL are of the form $A.B$ where A is a tuple variable and B an attribute.)

From this point of view, it is interesting to observe that for SQL queries *tuple identifiers* are never used during query evaluation and therefore do not have to be stored in the database or manipulated by the queries. This approach is similar to introducing *virtual* attributes (record ids) [11, 20].

3   Reasoning about Duplicate Elimination Operators

This section presents the first result: a technique that allows us to remove subqueries (base classes) from the scope of a duplicate elimination operator. The condition of the rewrite rule presents a complete characterization of the situations in which the rewrite is valid.

To simplify the exposition, we first show that every object relational conjunctive query can be written in a *normal form*:

Lemma 7 (Normal Form). Let Q be an arbitrary object relational conjunctive query. Then there is an equivalent query with the form

```
select V
from C₁ as A₁, ..., Cₘ as Aₘ, (elim
                               select W
                               from Cₘ₊₁ as Aₘ₊₁, ..., Cₙ as Aₙ, R)
```

where R is a list of equalities of the form $A_i.\text{Pf}_1 = A_j.\text{Pf}_2$, and V and W sets of attribute names that appear in the signatures of the respective subqueries. Also, we assume that R references $A_{m+1}, \ldots, A_n$ and all attributes in W.

Proof. By induction on the structure of Q using standard equivalence rules.

The normal form yields a set of subsumption constraints in CFD as follows:

Definition 8. Let Q be an object relational conjunctive query in normal form and C_Q a distinguished concept name. We define a set of subsumption constraints

$$S_Q = \{C_Q < (A_1 : C_1), \ldots, C_Q < (A_n : C_n), C_Q < R\}$$

The constraints S_Q mimic the semantics of Q within the description logic. This way, we reduce reasoning about the query Q to reasoning about subsumption constraints in CFD. The ability to reason in CFD allows us to formulate the main result of this section:

Theorem 9 (Duplicate Elimination Reduction). Let S be a database schema. Then for all databases I such that $I \models S$ the query

$$
\begin{aligned}
Q : \; &\texttt{select } V \\
&\texttt{from} \quad C_1 \texttt{ as } A_1, \ldots, C_m \texttt{ as } A_m, (\texttt{elim} \\
&\qquad\quad \texttt{select } W \\
&\qquad\quad \texttt{from } C_{m+1} \texttt{ as } A_{m+1}, \ldots, C_n \texttt{ as } A_n, R)
\end{aligned}
$$

is semantically equivalent to

$$
\begin{aligned}
Q' : \; &\texttt{select } V \\
&\texttt{from} \quad C_1 \texttt{ as } A_1, \ldots, C_{m+1} \texttt{ as } A_{m+1}, (\texttt{elim} \\
&\qquad\quad \texttt{select } W \cup \{A_{m+1}\} \\
&\qquad\quad \texttt{from } C_{m+2} \texttt{ as } A_{m+2}, \ldots, C_n \texttt{ as } A_n, R)
\end{aligned}
$$

if and only if $S \cup S_Q \models C_Q < C_Q(A \cup W \to A_{m+1})$ where $A = \{A_1, \ldots, A_m\}$.

Proof. (sketch)

"$\Rightarrow$": Assume that $S \cup S_Q \not\models C_Q < C_Q(A \cup W \to A_{m+1})$. Then there must be an interpretation I such that $v, w \in (C_Q)^I$ and $\mathcal{F}_{A_i}(v) = \mathcal{F}_{A_i}(w)$ for $A_i \in A \cup W$, but where $\mathcal{F}_{A_{m+1}}(v) \neq \mathcal{F}_{A_{m+1}}(w)$. In addition, v and w satisfy all equational constraints in R. Therefore, using the definition of semantics for the outer **from** clauses of Q and Q' we have

- a single tuple $\langle A_i : \mathcal{F}_{A_i}(v) \rangle$ for Q, but
- at least the two tuples $\langle A_i : \mathcal{F}_{A_i}(v), A_{m+1} : \mathcal{F}_{A_{m+1}}(v) \rangle$
  and $\langle A_i : \mathcal{F}_{A_i}(w), A_{m+1} : \mathcal{F}_{A_{m+1}}(w) \rangle$ for Q';

This fact is preserved by the final duplicate-preserving projection and thus we have $[\![Q]\!]I \neq [\![Q']\!]I$.

"$\Leftarrow$": Conversely, $[\![Q]\!]I \neq [\![Q']\!]I$ is only possible if, similarly to the previous case, the interpretation of Q's outer **from** contains a single tuple while the interpretation of Q' contains two tuples that differ only in the value of A_{m+1}. However, these two tuples can be used to define an interpretation I with exactly two objects in $(C_Q)^I$ that agree on all attributes in $A \cup W$ but disagree on A_{m+1}. As these two objects also satisfy all the other subsumption constraints in S_Q we have $S \cup S_Q \not\models C_Q < C_Q(A \cup W \to A_{m+1})$. $\qquad\square$

The theorem states a sufficient and necessary condition needed to move a conjunct $(C_{m+1}$ as $A_{m+1})$ from the scope of the duplicate elimination operator (elim) into the outer from clause (and vice versa). Let us illustrate this on the query from our introductory Example 1:

Example 10. First, the original query from Example 1 is transformed to the normal form (after replacing syntactic sugar):

```
select :P1, :P2, Name
from elim (
     select :P1, :P2, Name
     from STUDENT as S, TAKES as T, COURSE as C,
          S = T.S, C.Time = T.C.Time, C.Inst.In.Name = :P1,
          C.Num = :P2, Name = S.Name )
```

Note that parameters :P1 and :P2 are converted to "result" attributes on the normalized query (using the standard observation that there is no difference between these). The *query schema* S_Q is defined as follows:

```
CQ < (S: STUDENT), (T: TAKES), (C: COURSE),
     (P1: STRING), (P2: INT), (Name: STRING),
     S = T.S, C.Time = T.C.Time, C.Inst.In.Name = :P1,
     C.Num = :P2, Name = S.Name
```

Now we use our rewriting rule from Theorem 9 to "move" the reference to COURSE out of the scope of the elim operator. The necessary condition is $S \cup S_Q \models$ CQ < CQ(Name,:P1,:P2 -> C); (which is true as we shall see in Section 4). Therefore the query is equivalent to

```
select :P1, :P2, Name
from COURSE as C, elim (
     select C, :P1, :P2, Name
     from STUDENT as S, TAKES as T
          S = T.S, C.Time = T.C.Time, C.Inst.In.Name = :P1,
          C.Num = :P2, Name = S.Name )
```

A sequence of two additional applications of the duplicate elimination rewrite (that check for $S \cup S_Q \models$ CQ < CQ(Name,:P1,:P2,C -> T) to move the TAKES as T subquery and $S \cup S_Q \models$ CQ < CQ(Name,:P1,:P2,C,T -> S) for STUDENT as S) results in the following query:

```
select :P1, :P2, Name
from COURSE as C, TAKES as T, STUDENT as S, elim (
     select C, T, S, :P1, :P2, Name
     from S = T.S, C.Time = T.C.Time, C.Inst.In.Name = :P1,
          C.Num = :P2, Name = S.Name )
```

Note that the set of subsumption constraints S_Q is the same for each of the three steps. In Section 4 we see that the decision procedure can take advantage of this fact and reuse internal data structures to answer the second and third subsumption questions. Using standard simplification that commutes equalities with the duplicate elimination operation we obtain the query we desired in Example 1.

The rewriting rule (Theorem 9) can be integrated with existing query optimizers in two ways:

1. By "moving" an atomic query out of the scope of the `elim` operator (`DISTINCT` and `EXISTS` in SQL), we expand the search space of a join-ordering optimizer. If we manage to move all class references out of the scope of the `elim` operator (as in Example 10), we can completely remove the duplicate elimination operation from the query.
2. Conversely, we can move atomic subqueries into the scope of the `elim` operator. This is especially important in cases where the moved class reference does not contribute values to tuples in the result of the query. In this case the duplicate elimination operation can be replaced with a single index lookup (similarly to processing an `EXISTS` *clause* in SQL).

4   A Decision Procedure for CFD

Our overall algorithm works with *description graphs*, first introduced in [3] and modified in [4] to enable reasoning about simpler forms of uniqueness constraints that resembled (possibly asymmetric) functional dependencies. The algorithm presented here also incorporates an optimization that avoids copying entire description graphs when deducing subsumption by symmetric uniqueness constraints, a property always satisfied when reasoning about duplicate elimination on queries.

Definition 11. A description graph G is a triple (N, E, n) consisting of a set N of nodes, a bag E of directed edges labeled with either primitive attribute names or **Id**, and a distinguished node $n \in N$. Each node $n' \in N$ has three labels: a finite set $\mathsf{DS}(n')$ of concept descriptions, a finite set $\mathsf{PF}(n')$ of attribute descriptions, and a finite set $\mathsf{Fired}(n')$ of subsumption constraints that have already "fired" on n'. (Unless specified otherwise, we will assume that each of the three labels is initially empty for any newly created node.) Elements in E are written as triples (n_1, A, n_2) where n_1 and n_2 are nodes and A is either **Id** or a primitive attribute name.

Intuitively, a description graph may be viewed as a partial database in which nodes correspond to hypothetical or prototypical objects that belong to descriptions in their DS labels, while edges correspond to (some of) their attribute values. Given a database schema S and subsumption constraint $C < D$, the decision procedure constructs this partial database by first creating an initial graph with a single node containing C in its DS label and then invoking a chase-like procedure EXP to create a normalized form for the graph that makes explicit additional constraints that are implicit in S. This normalized form represents a pattern that must always match the structure of *any* C object. The final step of the decision procedure calls a boolean function SUBSUMES to verify that the graph has the properties required by D.

A formal specification of these two procedures is given in the Appendix A. Full proofs of the following theorems are given in [14].

Theorem 12 (Soundness and Completeness). Let S be a regular equation-free database schema and $C_1 < D_1$ and $C_2 < D_2$ arbitrary subsumption constraints for which C_1 does not occur in S. Then

$$S \cup \{C_1 < D_1\} \models C_2 < D_2$$

if and only if

$$\text{SUBSUMES}(D_2, \text{EXP}(G, S \cup \{C_1 < D_1\}), S \cup \{C_1 < D_1\}, C_2, true)$$

where description graph G has the form $(\{n\}, \{\}, n)$ in which $\text{DS}(n) = \{C_2\}$ and $\text{PF}(n) = \text{Fired}(n) = \{\}$.

One of the desirable properties of our decision procedure is the fact that it is incremental; description graphs constructed by earlier invocations of EXP can be reused when the procedure is invoked on a sequence of similar membership problems. For example, a sequence of problems of the form $S \models C < D_i$ can always reuse the graph constructed by the first call to EXP, a circumstance that happens with our example of duplicate elimination (Example 10). Further ways of reusing the work are also possible and are explored in more detail in [14].

Example 13. Figure 3 illustrates the description graph produced by an invocation of SUBSUMES of the form

$$\text{SUBSUMES}(\texttt{CQ(Name,:P1,:P2 -> C)}, \text{EXP}((\{n\}, \{\}, n), S), S, \texttt{CQ}, true)$$

where $\text{DS}(n) = \{\texttt{CQ}\}$ and S consists of the constraints in Figure 1 together with query schema S_Q. Note that only DS labels for nodes are indicated. The nodes are numbered according to the order in which updates E12, E13, E14 of EXP add **Id** to their PF labels. Since in particular the graph "ACCEPTS" attribute description C (note the dashed arc outgoing from the distinguished node), SUBSUMES returns true, thus enabling the first rewrite in Example 10.

Theorem 14 (Complexity). Let S be a regular equation-free database schema with size k, and let $C_1 < D_1$ and $C_2 < D_2$ denote arbitrary subsumption constraints of total size m for which C_1 does not occur in S. Then there is an implementation of EXP and SUBSUMES such that an invocation of the form

$$\text{SUBSUMES}(D_2, \text{EXP}(G, S \cup \{C_1 < D_1\}), S \cup \{C_1 < D_1\}, C_2, true)$$

terminates in $O(mk)$ time if $C_2 < D_2$ has the form $C < C(\text{Pf}_1, \ldots, \text{Pf}_n \to \text{Pf})$, in $O(fm^2k)$ time otherwise (f is the number of uniqueness constructs in D_2).

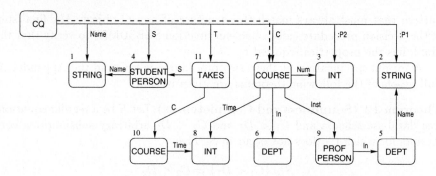

Fig. 3. A description graph for query schema S_Q.

Note that both Theorem 12 and 14 only hold for cases in which database schemas are both regular and equation-free. It is well-known that the membership problem becomes undecidable if equations are allowed in a database schema. If the regularity property is relaxed, the membership problem for CFD becomes DEXPTIME complete [15]. Moreover, regular uniqueness constraints encompass the majority of practical situations (in particular, all of classical functional dependencies and primary keys).

5   Conclusion

The following list summarizes the contributions of the paper.

1. We have defined CFD, a description logic dialect sufficiently expressive to describe object relational database schemas and a wide class of integrity constraints on such schemas.
2. We have devised a rewriting rule for object relational conjunctive queries that completely characterizes situations in which a duplicate elimination operator can be removed from the query. We have shown that a necessary and sufficient condition maps to a question in CFD.
3. We presented an efficient (linear both in size of the schema and the query) procedure that answers the above question.

In addition we have presented a decision procedure for subsumption checking in CFD and discussed the impact of various restrictions we imposed on database schema (or lack of thereof) on the complexity of CFD's decision procedure.

Future work includes several possible directions (presented as conjectures here). Theorem 9 can be straightforwardly modified to handle aggregates in object relational queries (the `elim` operator can be viewed as a degenerate case of the group-by operator). The same theorem can also be easily adapted to handle rewrites that perform various kinds of order optimization, and to discovering *interesting orders* of tables [21]. The addition of disjunction to CFD and/or the query language still leads to a decidable theory, and query rewrites similar to the one presented in this paper are then possible. Moreover, we conjecture that there is a subset of database schemas with amenable computational properties (that includes a limited use of disjunction to capture wider classes of schemas than CFD).

References

1. Serge Abiteboul, Richard Hull, and Victor Vianu. *Foundations of Databases*. Addison-Wesley, 1995.
2. Alexander Borgida. Description logics in data management. *IEEE Transactions on Knowledge and Data Engineering*, 7(5):671–682, 1995.
3. Alexander Borgida and Peter F. Patel-Schneider. A Semantics and Complete Algorithm for Subsumption in the CLASSIC Description Logic. *J. of AI Research*, 1:277–308, 1994.
4. Alexander Borgida and Grant Weddell. Adding uniqueness constraints to description logics (preliminary report). In *International Conference on Deductive and Object-Oriented Databases*, pages 85–102, 1997.
5. Diego Calvanese, Giuseppe De Giacomo, and Maurizio Lenzerini. Answering Queries Using Views in Description Logics. In *6th International Workshop on Knowledge Representation meets Databases (KRDB'99)*, pages 6–10, 1999.
6. Diego Calvanese, Maurizio Lenzerini, and Daniele Nardi. Description logics for conceptual data modelling. In Jan Chomicki and Gunter Saake, editors, *Logics for Databases and Information Systems*, chapter 8. Kluwer, 1998.
7. Rick G. G. Cattell. ODMG-93: A Standard for Object-Oriented DBMSs. In *ACM SIGMOD International Conference on Management of Data*, page 480, 1994.
8. Rick G. G. Cattell, Douglas Barry, Dirk Bartels, Mark Berler, Jeff Eastman, Sophie Gamerman, David Jordan, Adam Springer, Henry Strickland, and Drew Wade. *The Object Database Standard: ODMG 2.0*. Morgan Kaufman, 1997.
9. Ashok K. Chandra and Philip M. Merlin. Optimal implementation of conjunctive queries in relational data bases. In *ACM Symposium on Theory of Computing*, pages 77–90, 1977.
10. Surajit Chaudhuri and Moshe Y. Vardi. Optimization of *real* conjunctive queries. In *ACM Symposium on Principles of Database Systems*, pages 59–70, 1993.
11. Umeshwar Dayal. Of Nests and Trees: A Unified Approach to Processing Queries That Contain Nested Subqueries, Aggregates, and Quantifiers. In *13th International Conference on Very Large Data Bases*, pages 197–208, 1987.
12. Parke Godfrey, John Grant, Jarek Gryz, and Jack Minker. Integrity constraints: Semantics and applications. In Jan Chomicki and Gunter Saake, editors, *Logics for Databases and Information Systems*, chapter 9. Kluwer, 1998.
13. ISO. Database Language SQL. ISO/IEC 9075:1992, International Organization for Standardization, 1992.
14. Vitaliy L. Khizder. *Uniqueness Constraints in Object-Relational Databases and Description Logics*. PhD thesis, University of Waterloo, 1999.
15. Vitaliy L. Khizder, David Toman, and Grant Weddell. On Decidability and Complexity of Description Logics with Uniquwness Constraints. Technical report, Dept. of Computer Science, University of Waterloo, 2000. (submitted).
16. Alon Y. Levy, Inderpal Singh Mumick, and Yehoshua Sagiv. Query Optimization by Predicate Move-Around. In *20th International Conference on Very Large Data Bases*, pages 96–107, 1994.

17. J. Melton and A. R. Simon. *Understanding the new SQL: A Complete Guide.* Morgan Kaufmann Publishers, 1993.
18. Inderpal Singh Mumick, Hamid Pirahesh, and Raghu Ramakrishnan. The Magic of Duplicates and Aggregates. In *16th International Conference on Very Large Data Bases*, pages 264–277, 1990.
19. Glenn N. Paulley and Per-Åke Larson. Exploiting uniqueness in query optimization. In *10th International Conference on Data Engineering*, pages 68–79, 1994.
20. Hamid Pirahesh, Joseph M. Hellerstein, and Waqar Hasan. Extensible/Rule Based Query Rewrite Optimization in Starburst. In *ACM SIGMOD International Conference on Management of Data*, pages 39–48, 1992.
21. Patricia G. Selinger, Morton M. Astrahan, Donald D. Chamberlin, Raymond A. Lorie, and Thomas G. Price. Access Path Selection in a Relational Database Management System. In *ACM SIGMOD International Conference on Management of Data*, pages 23–34, 1979.
22. Praveen Seshadri, Hamid Pirahesh, and T. Y. Cliff Leung. Complex Query Decorrelation. In *12th International Conference on Data Engineering*, pages 450–458, 1996.
23. Martin F. van Bommel and Grant Weddell. Reasoning About Equations and Functional Dependencies on Complex Objects. *IEEE Transactions on Knowledge and Data Engineering*, 6(3):455–469, 1994.
24. Grant Weddell. Reasoning about Functional Dependencies Generalized for Semantic Data Models. *ACM Transactions on Database Systems*, 17(1):32–64, 1992.

A   EXP and SUBSUMES

A specification of procedure EXP and function SUBSUMES are given below in a production system style presumed by the full proofs of Theorems 12 and 14 that can be found in [14]. The actual implementation of these procedures is event driven, and makes use of indices on a given database schema.

Procedure EXP(G, S)

Input: description graph $G = (N, E, n)$; set of subsumption constraints S.

Exhaustively apply the following updates to G in the order presented.

E1. If $e = (n', \mathbf{Id}, n') \in E$, then $E := E - \{e\}$.

E2. If $e = (n', \mathbf{Id}, n) \in E$, then $E := E - \{e\} \cup \{(n, \mathbf{Id}, n')\}^3$.

E3. If $e = (n_1, \mathbf{Id}, n_2) \in E$, then
   (a) $\mathsf{DS}(n_1) := \mathsf{DS}(n_1) \cup \mathsf{DS}(n_2)$.
   (b) $\mathsf{PF}(n_1) := \mathsf{PF}(n_1) \cup \mathsf{PF}(n_2)$.
   (c) $\mathsf{Fired}(n_1) := \mathsf{Fired}(n_1) \cup \mathsf{Fired}(n_2)$.
   (d) For each $e' = (n', A, n_2) \in E$ do $E := E - \{e'\} \cup \{(n', A, n_1)\}$.
   (e) For each $e' = (n_2, A, n') \in E$ do $E := E - \{e'\} \cup \{(n_1, A, n')\}$.
   (f) $E := E - \{e\}; N := N - \{n_2\}$.

E4. If $e_1 = (n_1, A, n_2), e_2 = (n_1, A, n_3) \in E$,
   then $E := E - \{e_2\} \cup \{(n_2, \mathbf{Id}, n_3)\}$.

E5. If $n' \in N$ s.t. $D = (D_1, \ldots, D_n) \in \mathsf{DS}(n')$,
   then $\mathsf{DS}(n') := \mathsf{DS}(n') - \{D\} \cup \{D_1, \ldots, D_n\}$.

---

^{3} Recall that n is the distinguished node in G

E6. If $n_1, n_2 \in N$ s.t. $D = (A.\text{Pf} : D') \in \text{DS}(n_1)$
and $(n_1, A, n_2) \in E$, then
(a) $\text{DS}(n_1) := \text{DS}(n_1) - \{D\}$.
(b) $\text{DS}(n_2) := \text{DS}(n_2) \cup \{(\text{Pf} : D')\}$.

E7. If $n' \in N$ s.t. $D = (A.\text{Pf} : D') \in \text{DS}(n')$
and D' contains an equational constraint,
then invoke $\text{FIND}(n', A.\text{Id}, G)$.

E8. If $n' \in N$ s.t. $D = (\text{Id} : D') \in \text{DS}(n')$,
then $\text{DS}(n') := \text{DS}(n') - \{D\} \cup \{D'\}$.

E9. If $n' \in N$ s.t. $D = (\text{Pf}_1 = \text{Pf}_2) \in \text{DS}(n')$, then
(a) $\text{DS}(n') := \text{DS}(n') - \{D\}$.
(b) Add $(\text{FIND}(n', \text{Pf}_1, G), \text{Id}, \text{FIND}(n', \text{Pf}_2, G))$ to E.

E10. If $n_1, n_2 \in N$ s.t.:
(1) $n_1 \neq n_2$,
(2) there $D = C(\text{Pf}_1, \ldots, \text{Pf}_m \rightarrow \text{Pf}) \in \text{DS}(n_1)$,
(3) $C \in \text{DS}(n_2)$,
(4) for each $1 \leq i \leq m$: $\text{AGREES}(n_1, \text{Pf}_i, n_2, G)$, and
(5) $\neg \text{AGREES}(n_1, \text{Pf}, n_2, G)$,
then add $(\text{FIND}(n_1, \text{Pf}, G), \text{Id}, \text{FIND}(n_2, \text{Pf}, G))$ to E.

E11. If $n' \in N$ s.t. $(C < D) \in S - \text{Fired}(n')$ and $C \in \text{DS}(n')$, then
(a) $\text{Fired}(n') := \text{Fired}(n') \cup \{C < D\}$.
(b) $\text{DS}(n') := \text{DS}(n') \cup \{D\}$.

E12. If $n' \in N$ s.t. $\text{Pf}_1 = A.\text{Pf}_2 \in \text{PF}(n')$, then
(a) $\text{PF}(n') := \text{PF}(n') - \{\text{Pf}_1\}$.
(b) $\text{PF}(\text{FIND}(n', A.\text{Id}, G)) := \{\text{Pf}_2\}$.

E13. If $n' \in N$ s.t.:
(1) $C \in \text{DS}(n')$,
(2) $C(\text{Pf}_1, \ldots, \text{Pf}_m \rightarrow \text{Pf}) \in \text{DS}(n')$,
(3) for each $1 \leq i \leq m$: $\text{ACCEPTS}(n', \text{Pf}_i, G)$, and
(4) $\neg \text{ACCEPTS}(n', \text{Pf}, G)$,
then $\text{PF}(n') := \text{PF}(n') \cup \{\text{Pf}\}$.

E14. If $(n_1, A, n_2) \in E$ s.t. $\text{Id} \in \text{PF}(n_1)$ and $\text{Id} \notin \text{PF}(n_2)$,
then $\text{PF}(n_2) := \text{PF}(n_2) \cup \{\text{Id}\}$.

function SUBSUMES(D, G, S, C, T): Boolean

Input: concept description D; description graph $G = (N, E, n)$; set of subsumption constraints S, primitive concept C and Boolean T.

Branch to the relevant case depending on the form of D.

Case C: Return $C \in \text{DS}(n)$.

Case $(D_1, \ldots, D_m)$:
Return true iff $\text{SUBSUMES}(D_i, G, S, C, T)$ for all $1 \leq i \leq m$.

Case $(\text{Id} : D')$: Return $\text{SUBSUMES}(D', G, S, C, T)$.

Case $(A.\text{Pf} : D')$.
Return $\text{SUBSUMES}((\text{Pf} : D'), \text{EXP}((N, E, \text{FIND}(n, A.\text{Id}, G)), S), S, C, \text{false})$.

Case $\mathsf{Pf}_1 = \mathsf{Pf}_2$:
    (a) $\mathsf{FIND}(n, \mathsf{Pf}_1, G)$, $\mathsf{FIND}(n, \mathsf{Pf}_2, G)$.
    (b) $\mathsf{EXP}(G, S)$.
    (c) Return $\mathsf{FIND}(n, \mathsf{Pf}_1, G) = \mathsf{FIND}(n, \mathsf{Pf}_2, G)$.

Case $C(\mathsf{Pf}_1, ..., \mathsf{Pf}_m \to \mathsf{Pf})$ where T:
    (a) For each $n' \in N : \mathsf{PF}(n') := \{\}$.
    (b) $\mathsf{PF}(n) := \{\mathsf{Pf}_1, ..., \mathsf{Pf}_m\}$.
    (c) Invoke $\mathsf{EXP}((N, E, n), S)$.
    (d) Return $\mathsf{ACCEPTS}(n, \mathsf{Pf}, G)$.

Case $C'(\mathsf{Pf}_1, ..., \mathsf{Pf}_m \to \mathsf{Pf})$ where $C' \neq C$ or $\neg T$:
    (a) Create a copy $G' = (N', E', n')$ of G.
    (b) Add a new node n to N' and a new edge (n, A, n') to E'.
    (c) Add $(B : C')$ to $\mathsf{DS}(n)$.
    (d) For each $1 \leq i \leq m$: add $(A.\mathsf{Pf}_i = B.\mathsf{Pf}_i)$ to $\mathsf{DS}(n)$.
    (e) Invoke $\mathsf{EXP}(G', S)$.
    (f) Return $\mathsf{FIND}(n, A.\mathsf{Pf}, G') = \mathsf{FIND}(n, B.\mathsf{Pf}, G')$.

Case ANY: Return true.

function $\mathsf{FIND}(n, \mathsf{Pf}, G)$: node

Input: description graph $G = (N, E, n'')$; node $n \in N$; attribute description Pf.

Returns the node at the end of the path Pf from a node n in G, potentially creating any missing nodes and edges to ensure such a path exists.

function $\mathsf{AGREES}(n_1, \mathsf{Pf}, n_2, G)$: Boolean

Input: description graph $G = (N, E, n)$; nodes $n_1, n_2 \in N$; attribute description Pf.

Returns true if there is a node $n' \in G$ such that n' is reachable from both n_1 and n_2 by the same prefix of Pf.

function $\mathsf{ACCEPTS}(n_1, \mathsf{Pf}, G)$: Boolean

Input: description graph $G = (N, E, n)$; node $n_1 \in N$; attribute description Pf.

Returns true if **Id** occurs in the PF label of any node on the Pf path starting from node n_1 in G.

A File System Based on Concept Analysis

Sébastien Ferré and Olivier Ridoux

IRISA, Campus Universitaire de Beaulieu, 35042 Rennes cedex
{ferre,ridoux}@irisa.fr

Abstract. We present the design of a file system whose organization is based on Concept Analysis "à la Wille-Ganter". The aim is to combine querying and navigation facilities in one formalism. The file system is supposed to offer a standard interface but the interpretation of common notions like directories is new. The contents of a file system is interpreted as a Formal Context, directories as Formal Concepts, and the sub-directory relation as Formal Concepts inclusion. We present an organization that allows for an efficient implementation of such a Conceptual File System.

1 Introduction: Querying vs. Navigation

Information retrieval includes representation, storage, organization, and access to information. Two information retrieval methods are widely adopted and applied.

The first method is *hierarchical classification*, which is frequently found in computer tools: e.g., file systems, bookmarks, or menus. In this model, searches are done by *navigating* in a classification structure that is built and maintained manually. Navigating implies notions of *place*, being in a place, and going in another place. A notion of *neighborhood* helps specifying the "other place" relatively to the place one is currently in. Many applications require that a place is a place to read from as well as a place to write on. Sometimes, navigation is deemed to be rigid, but this is because it is based on a rigid neighborhood relation: e.g., a tree-like hierarchy. But even a tree can be made more flexible by adding links: e.g., a UNIX-like file system. However, using links opens the door to the problem of dangling links.

The second method is *boolean querying*, often found in information servers such as search engines on the Web (e.g., AltaVista). In this model, searches are done with *queries*, generally expressed in a kind of propositional logic. A recognized difficulty of this model is the necessity of having a good knowledge of the terminology used in the information system, and of having a precise idea of what is searched for.

Then, which search model should be prefered: navigation or querying? In fact, it depends on situations, and it is sometimes needed to use both of them in the same search. Hybrid systems combining hierarchical classification and boolean querying have been proposed in the domain of file systems (FS): e.g.,

J. Lloyd et al. (Eds.): CL 2000, LNAI 1861, pp. 1033–1047, 2000.

— SFS (Semantic File System, [GJSO91]) extends the hierarchical model of usual FSs with virtual directories that correspond to queries. These queries concern file properties that are automatically extracted by *transducers*, and are expressed with valued attributes. So, two organization and storage methods coexist: the standard hierarchy that gives a name to files and virtual directories that enable associative searches on intrinsic file properties. Unfortunately, these two methods cannot be used together in general. In particular, virtual directories are not places to write into.

— HAC (Hierarchy And Content, [GM99]) also uses queries to build directories based on file contents, but these directories are integrated in the hierarchy. This enables to combine hierarchy and content in searches. Users are always allowed to move a file in a directory even if it does not satisfy the query associated to the directory, which results in consistency problems.

The drawback of these hybrid systems is their lack of consistency. Indeed, they have two search models that are not tightly connected, which makes it difficult to switch from one model to the other, and to combine both in the same search. We propose a scheme in which queries are really places to read from and to write into. The scheme is flexible in the sense that the neighborhood relation can be very dense. It incurs no inconsistency or dangling links problem, because the neighborhood relation is managed automatically. Finally, it supports both querying and navigation, and arbitrary combinations of both.

2   Logical Concept Analysis

Formal Concept Analysis (FCA [GW99]) has received attention for its application in many domains such as representing the modular structure of software [Sne98], navigating in software documentation [Lin95], software engineering [KS94], and several applications in Social Sciences. The interest of FCA as a navigation tool in general has also been recognized [GMA93].

Originally, FCA is elaborated using a *Formal Context* that is any relation between a set of objects and a set of attributes. The variety of application domains brings the need for more sophisticated formal contexts than the mere presence/absence of attributes. For instance, many application domains use numerical values (e.g., lengths, prices, ages), and the need to express negation and disjunction is often felt. Several enrichments to the attribute structure have been proposed: e.g., many valued attributes [GW99], and first-order terms [CM98]. However, not a single extended FCA framework covers all the concrete domains, and can pretend covering all the concrete domains to come. We use an extension of FCA that allows for fully abstracting from the object description language [FR99,FR00]. In the rest of this article, we will refer to both the original form of concept analysis, and to its extended form as Logical Concept Analysis (LCA).

2.1   Logical Context and Galois Connection

Definition 1 (Context). *A logical formal context is a triple* $(\mathcal{O}, \mathcal{L}, i)$ *where:*

- $\mathcal{O}$ *is a finite set of objects,*
- $\langle \mathcal{L}; \models \rangle$ *is a lattice of formulas, whose supremum is* $\dot{\vee}$, *and whose infimum is* $\dot{\wedge}$; $\mathcal{L}$ *denotes a logic whose deduction relation is* $\models$, *and whose disjunctive and conjunctive operations are respectively* $\vee$ *and* $\wedge$,
- i *is a mapping from* $\mathcal{O}$ *to* $\mathcal{L}$ *that associates to each object a formula that describes it.*

If $f \models g$ and $g \models f$, f and g are called logically equivalent; we will consider them as different representations of the same equivalence class, and in fact we will consider that elements of $\mathcal{L}$ are the equivalence classes. Given a formal context, one can form a Galois connection between sets of objects (extents) and formulas (intents) with two applications σ and τ.

Definition 2. *Let* $(\mathcal{O}, \mathcal{L}, i)$ *be a logical context,*

$$\sigma : 2^{\mathcal{O}} \to \mathcal{L}, \ \sigma(O) := \bigvee\nolimits_{o \in O} i(o) \quad and \quad \tau : \mathcal{L} \to 2^{\mathcal{O}}, \ \tau(f) := \{o \in \mathcal{O} | i(o) \models f\}$$

Example. The following formal context, K_{ex}, will illustrate the rest of our development on LCA and Conceptual File Systems. It is deliberately small and simple as it is aimed at illustrating theoretic notions. It uses propositional logic. We define context K_{ex} by $(\mathcal{O}_{ex}, \mathcal{P}, i_{ex})$, where $\mathcal{O}_{ex} = \{x, y, z\}$, and where mapping i_{ex} is defined as $\{(x \mapsto a), (y \mapsto b), (z \mapsto c \wedge (a \vee b))\}$.

2.2   Logical Concepts

In this section, we present how formal concepts can be extracted from logical contexts.

Definition 3 (Concept). *In a context* $(\mathcal{O}, \mathcal{L}, i)$, *a concept is a pair* $c = (O, f)$ *where* $O \subseteq \mathcal{O}$, *and* $f \in \mathcal{L}$, *such that* $\sigma(O) \dot{=} f$ *and* $\tau(f) = O$.

The set of objects O *is the concept* extent *(ext(c)), whereas formula* f *is its* intent *(int(c)).*

The set of all concepts that can be built in a context $(\mathcal{O}, \mathcal{L}, i)$ is denoted by $\mathcal{C}(\mathcal{O}, \mathcal{L}, i)$, and is partially ordered by $\leq^c$ defined as follows.

Definition 4. $(O_1, f_1) \leq^c (O_2, f_2) \iff O_1 \subseteq O_2$

This order is compatible with order on intents.

Proposition 1. $(O_1, f_1) \leq^c (O_2, f_2) \iff (f_1 \models f_2)$

Definitions 3 and 4 lead to the following *fundamental theorem.*

Theorem 1. *Let* $(\mathcal{O}, \mathcal{L}, i)$ *be a context, and let* J *be a set of indices. The ordered set* $\langle \mathcal{C}(\mathcal{O}, \mathcal{L}, i); \leq^c \rangle$ *is a finite lattice, whose supremum (least upper bound) and infimum (greatest lower bound) operations are as follows:*

$$\bigvee_{j \in J}^{c} (O_j, f_j) =^c (\tau(\sigma(\bigcup_{j \in J} O_j)), \bigvee_{j \in J} f_j) \quad and \quad \bigwedge_{j \in J}^{c} (O_j, f_j) =^c (\bigcap_{j \in J} O_j, \sigma(\tau(\bigwedge_{j \in J} f_j)))$$

Example. Figure 1.(a) represents the Hasse diagram of the concept lattice of context K_{ex} (introduced in Example 2.1). Concepts are represented by a number and a box containing their extent on the left, and their intent on the right. The higher concepts are placed in the diagram the greater they are for order $\leq^c$. It can be observed that the concept lattice is not isomorphic to the power-set lattice of objects $\langle 2^{\mathcal{O}}; \subseteq \rangle$. E.g., the set of objects $\{x,y\}$ is not the extent of a concept, because $\tau(\sigma(\{x,y\})) = \tau(a \vee b) = \{x,y,z\}$.

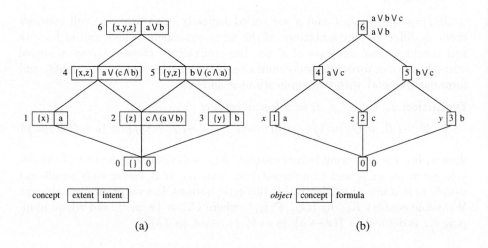

(a)   (b)

Fig. 1. The concept lattice of context K_{ex}, and its labelling.

2.3   Labelling of Concept Lattices

It is possible to label concept lattices with objects and formulas, but in the information system context we are mainly interested in labelling concepts with formulas; formulas are a means for retrieving objects.

Definition 5. *Let* $\mu : \mathcal{L} \to \mathcal{C}(\mathcal{O}, \mathcal{L}, i), \quad \mu(f) := (\tau(f), \sigma(\tau(f)))$

Images of mapping μ are indeed concepts from Definition 3 of concepts, and from properties of applications σ and τ. The next lemma gives interesting properties of the labelling of concept lattices.

Lemma 1. *Let* $(\mathcal{O}, \mathcal{L}, i)$ *be a context, and* $o \in \mathcal{O}, f \in \mathcal{L}, c \in \mathcal{C}(\mathcal{O}, \mathcal{L}, i)$.
(1) $c \leq^c \mu(f) \iff int(c) \models f$ *(2)* μ *is surjective*
(3) $\mu(int(c)) =^c c$ *(4)* $int(\mu(f)) \models f$.

Lemma 1.(1) shows that $\mu(f)$ is the greatest concept whose intent logically entails f; and Lemma 1.(2) establishes that every concept is labelled at least by one formula. Regarding relation between concept intents and concept labels, Lemma 1.(3) shows that every concept is labelled by its intent; and Lemma 1.(4) adds that every formula labelling a concept is logically entailed by the concept intent.

Example. Figure 1.(b) represents the same concept lattice as Figure 1.(a), but it does not associate the same information to concepts. The number of each concept is reused in its box so as to identify it; objects are placed on the left of their labelled concept, and formulas are placed on the right of the concept they label. For instance, concept 1 is labelled by formula a (i.e., $\mu(a) =^c 1$). In this example, we restrict labelling to disjunctive formulas, but every formula labels some context. Note that non-equivalent formulas may label identical concepts: e.g., both formulas $a \vee b$ and $a \vee b \vee c$ label concept 6. Similarly, both formulas c and $c \wedge (a \vee b)$ label concept 2 whose extent is z. This shows that an object can be designated by a formula that is much simpler than its description in the formal context.

Concept lattices support both search models. For navigation, concepts are considered as directories or classes (extent of the concept), and links are realized by generalization/specialization relations between concepts. For querying, concepts are designated/accessed by a query using the labelling function μ, and their extents form the answer. Because concepts serve at the same time as directories and as queries, it is possible to combine both search models in a flexible way. Another advantage is that concept lattices can be automatically built from a context. Therefore, there is no need for a manual maintenance of the information systems. Then, concept lattices appear to be an interesting alternative to usual methods for information retrieving.

3   Informal Specification of a Conceptual Shell

We present a Conceptual File System (CFS) through the use of a Conceptual Shell (CS). Data constitute a formal context $K = (\mathcal{O}, \mathcal{L}, i)$, where i is the mapping that associates to every object a logical description of its properties and features. CS commands are those of the UNIX shell, reinterpreted in the LCA framework as follows: *files* become *objects*, *paths* become *logical formulas*, *directories* become *concepts* or *contextualized formulas*, the *root* becomes concept $\top^c$ or formula $\top$, and the *working directory* becomes a *working concept*. For the rest, commands have essentially the same effects as in a classical shell.

If the Conceptual Shell is instantiated with a logic whose formulas are expressed as conjunctions of names and if the conjunction operator is noted $/$, then formulas can be typed in exactly like classical paths. This Conceptual Shell could be used in the same way as a classical shell but the user would notice that the ordering of names in paths does not matter, that he/she could access a file without giving its whole path, and that answers of `ls` command are larger than expected (offering more navigation paths).

Before specifying CS commands, we introduce terms used in the sequel. Let f be a formula:
— the *concept of f* is the concept associated to f by the labelling mapping μ (see Definition 5), i.e., $\mu(f)$,
— the *extent of f* is in fact the extent of the concept of f; it is also the set of objects whose description satisfies f,

— the *object of f* is the object, if it exists, whose description is *contextually* equivalent to f (it is supposed to be unique to avoid access ambiguities); f serves as a *contextualized description* of this object; an object can thus have several contextualized descriptions (several access paths in a way), and its description is always the most precise of them. Concretely, it is possible to access an object using a formula that is simpler than the actual description of the object in the Formal Context. This can be viewed as implicit completion based on the context.

The following commands are used for navigating and querying in a formal context.

working directory: It is replaced by a stack of formulas corresponding to the *navigation history*. The top of this stack serves as the *working query*, which is noted wq.

pwd: Displays the working query wq.

cd ..:   Pops the navigation history, unless it contains only one element. This command enables to go back in navigation, and replaces the move to the parent directory that is no more possible as the navigation structure is not a tree (this command is in fact similar to command "Back" in Web browsers).

cd *to:*   Let us note $l(to)$ the combination (essentially a conjunction) of *to* with wq. This command pushes $l(to)$ in the navigation history, and "moves" into the concept of $l(to)$. The composition l leaves open the possibility of a notation that distinguishes *relative* formulas, which are combined with wq (e.g., $wq := wq \dot\wedge to$), and *absolute* formulas, which are not combined with wq (e.g., $wq := to$). This implements the "going into some place" part of navigation.

ls *f:*   First, displays the object of $l(f)$, if one exists, and second, displays a list of formulas (preferably simple ones), called *increments*, that enable to refine query $l(f)$ while avoiding to lead to the empty query $\perp^c$, and ensuring that every element of the extent of $l(f)$ is reachable only using increments given by command **ls** (completeness condition). This implements the "looking into a place" part of navigation.

ls -r *f:*   Displays each element of the extent of $l(f)$. This implements querying.

The following commands are used for updating a formal context. They can be used anywhere in conjunction with querying or navigating.

mkfile *f c:*   Creates a new object with contents c and with description $l(f)$.

rm *f:*   Remove the object of $l(f)$, if it exists.

rm -r *f:*   Remove all elements of the extent of $l(f)$.

cp *from to:*   Copies the object of $l(from)$, if it exists, by copying its contents and by "transposing" its description from $l(from)$ to $l(to)$, i.e., by "substracting" $l(from)$ and then by "adding" $l(to)$ (see Section 4.1 for a discussion on the exact meaning of "adding" and "substracting").

cp -r *from to:*   Copies each element of the extent of $l(from)$ by copying its contents and by transposing its description from $l(from)$ to $l(to)$.

mv *from to:*   Move the object of $l(from)$, if it exists, by transposing its description from $l(from)$ to $l(to)$ (identity and contents are kept unchanged).

`mv -r` *from to*:   Move each element of the extent of $l(from)$ by transposing its description from $l(from)$ to $l(to)$ (identity and contents of objects are kept unchanged).

Command `cd` is simple and is essentially useful for handling the working query. Command `ls` deserves more explications. With option `-r` the result is the one that querying systems give to a query: the list of all objects that satisfy the query. Without this option, command `ls` enables navigation, i.e., searching of objects by successive refinements of the working query: an increment x enables to refine the working query wq by $wq \wedge x$.

But a badly chosen refinement $wq \wedge x$ could return as many answers as the previous query (not enough refinement) or no answer at all (too much refinement). So as to avoid these extremes, we must impose the following condition on every increment x for a given working query wq (let us recall that $\tau(f)$ denotes the extent of query f): $\emptyset \subsetneq \tau(wq \wedge x) \subsetneq \tau(wq)$. It can be proved that this condition is equivalent to $\perp^c <^c \mu(wq) \wedge^c \mu(x) <^c \mu(wq)$.

This informal specification shows the relevance of concept lattices to characterize navigation. Moreover, it shows the necessity of these concept lattices because the above condition is not expressible only within logic $\mathcal{L}$. The difficulty is then to find a finite set of increments Inc that satisfies this condition and that is *complete*; i.e., such that for every working query wq and for every object o of the working extent, it exists an increment x in Inc that strictly restricts the working extent while keeping o in the new one. This completeness condition ensures that every object is reachable, only using increments to refine queries. As the conceptual navigation is similar to the classical one (a finite set of increments is used in both cases, increments being formulas in the first case and names in the second case), many facilities offered by classical shells can be applied to our conceptual shell: e.g., name completion, graphical user interface.

In commands resulting in a modification of the context (`mkfile`, `rm`, `cp`, `mv`) the concept lattice is implicitly updated (i.e., formal concepts are used as places one can write into). However, the principle of CS is to provide access to objects by their properties and not through a fixed organization structure, whatever it is. The concept lattice makes no exception: it is interesting for designing and implementing CS, but users need neither know it, nor visualize it explicitly.

4   Formal Specification of a Conceptual Shell

In Section 3, a Conceptual Shell (CS) was presented through its general principles, but was not defined in a precise way. This section aims at giving commands of CS a formal definition based on logic and concept analysis. We begin by describing and defining a set of elementary operations with which CS commands are eventually defined.

4.1   Logical Operations

In CS, objects are described by formulas taken in a logic $\mathcal{L}$. The same formulas are used to express queries (in place of paths). The main logical operation is to compare two formulas in order to know if an object description satisfies a query, i.e., if the object is an answer to the query. The operation that achieves this comparison is the deduction relation $\models$. It establishes a specialization/generalization order on formulas.

In the presentation of CS (cf. Section 3), we talked about "adding" or "substracting" a formula to an object description (in commands cp and mv). "Adding" a formula f to an object description $i(o)$ must be understood as making this object satisfies this formula while keeping its previous properties. Formally, this means that, if we note the "adding" operation by $+$, the following condition has to be true: $i(o) + f \models i(o)$ and $i(o) + f \models f$. The most general formula that satisfies both $i(o)$ and f is $i(o) \dot{\wedge} f$. Then, the "adding" operation is well matched by the conjunction operation $\dot{\wedge}$ of logic $\mathcal{L}$.

"Substracting" a formula f to an object description $i(o)$ consists in generalizing it, which can be understood as the removal of some properties of the object. Formally, if we note the "substracting" operation by $-$, we have $i(o) \models i(o) - f$. Furthermore, "substraction" is combined with "addition" to "transpose" an object from a concept to another: $i'(o) := (i(o) - from) + to$, where $from$ denotes the source of the transposition, and to denotes the target. When such an operation is done on an object, we know from the meaning of CS commands that $i(o) \models from$ (i.e., o is an answer to query $from$). So, in the case where source and target of the transposition are both denoted by formula f, the object description must be kept unchanged, which is formally expressed by $i(o) \models f \implies (i(o) - f) + f \dot{=} i(o)$. Relative complementation is a logical operation that satisfies the two conditions above, and is then a good realization of the "substracting" operation. Relative complement is a weak form of implication, and is defined as follows.

Definition 1. *The* relative complement *is an internal binary operation on $\mathcal{L}$ that is noted $\Leftarrow$, and is defined for all $f, g \in \mathcal{L}$ by $f \Leftarrow g \dot{=} max\{x \in \mathcal{L} | x \dot{\wedge} g \models f\}$.*

As max denotes the greatest element of its argument, not every logic is equiped with a relative complement. Yet, as soon as a logic is equiped with an implication (e.g., the propositional logic), it is equiped with a relative complement, as the later is a weak form of the former.

To summarize, a logic has to be equiped at least with three operations so as to be used in the frame of CS: deduction relation $\models$, and conjunction $\dot{\wedge}$. Relative complement $\Leftarrow$ is necessary for moving and copying objects by "transposition".

4.2   Context Operations

A formal context stores a set of objects $\mathcal{O}$ and their descriptions. We consider that every object o has a contents $c(o)$, and an *extrinsic description* $i_e(o)$ expressed in a logic $\mathcal{L}_e$. From this basic information, we now have to build the mapping i that describes each object. LCA is based on this mapping. First, intrinsic descriptions of objects $i_i(o)$, expressed in a logic $\mathcal{L}_i$, are automatically extracted from the contents of objects through an abstraction function α: $i_i(o) := \alpha(c(o))$.

Then, the whole description of an object is the mere product of its extrinsic and intrinsic decriptions: $i(o) := (i_e(o), i_i(o))$. The logic $\mathcal{L}$ used in LCA framework is therefore the product logic of $\mathcal{L}_e$ and $\mathcal{L}_i$. More precisely, $\mathcal{L}$ is defined as follows:

$$\mathcal{L} := \mathcal{L}_e \times \mathcal{L}_i \qquad (f_e, f_i) {\models} (g_e, g_i) :\Leftrightarrow f_e {\models}_e g_e \wedge f_i {\models}_i g_i$$
$$(f_e, f_i)\, op\, (g_e, g_i) := (f_e\, op_e\, g_e, f_i\, op_i\, g_i), \text{ for } op \text{ in } \{\vee, \wedge, \Leftarrow\}.$$

Moreover, we have the elementary operations new_o and del_o that respectively return a new object and remove a given object, and $extr$ that returns the extrinsic part of a formula.

4.3   Querying and Navigation Operations

Section 3 introduced notions of *extent of a query* and *object of a query*. They correspond to the elementary operations performing querying. The extent of a query q is noted $\tau(q)$ and returns all objects whose description satisfies q. Operation τ is the same as in the Galois connection of LCA (cf. Definition 2).

The object of a query q is noted $t(q)$ and is the object whose description is contextually equivalent to q (i.e., has the same extent):

$$t(q) = o \in \mathcal{O}, \text{ such that } \tau(i(o)) = \tau(q).$$

If there is no such object the query is said *empty* ($\tau(q) = \emptyset$), and if there are several such objects the query is said *ambiguous*.

Navigation is performed by command ls. It returns a set of *increments*, which enable to refine the working query while keeping it non-empty. As already seen in previous section, an increment x of a query q has to satisfy

$$\emptyset \subsetneq \tau(q\dot\wedge x) \subsetneq \tau(q).$$

As $\mathcal{L}$ is a too wide search space, we consider a finite subset X of $\mathcal{L}$ in which increments are selected. The content of X is not strictly determined but it should contain simple formulas (according to the terminology), some often used formulas, and more generally, all formulas that users expect to see in ls responses. X can be finite because terminology and used formulas are. Furthermore, we keep only greatest increments as they correspond to smallest refinement steps. Then, we can now define the set of increments of a query q by

$$Inc(q) := \lceil\{x \in X | \emptyset \subsetneq \tau(q\dot\wedge x) \subsetneq \tau(q)\}\rceil,$$

where $\lceil E \rceil$ denotes the set of greatest elements of E according to the order $\models$.

Because of these seemingly arbitrary selections among possible increments, we can wonder about the completeness of $Inc(q)$. If navigation is seen as a way for finding an object by refining the working query with a sequence of increments, the completeness can be formally expressed by

$$\forall q \in \mathcal{L} : \forall o \in \tau(q) : o \neq t(q) \Rightarrow \exists x \in Inc(q) : o \in \tau(q\dot\wedge x),$$

which means in English: for all working query q and for all object o of its extent, if o is not yet the object of q then it exists an increment that enables to strictly restrict the working extent while keeping o in it. As extents are finite and each increment strictly restricts the working extent, it follows that every navigation terminates and every object can be retrieved through navigation alone (i.e., querying is useful, but not necessary).

We proved that Inc is complete for all contexts if and only if every object description is equivalent to the conjunction of some elements of X.

This characterization leaves some flexibility in the choice of X, because it can be made larger than necessary. This flexibility enables to adjust X in order to make the navigation more progressive and natural.

4.4   Interface Operations

A few elementary operations are defined here to specify interface aspects of CS. For managing the history, we use a stack of queries initialized with one element, the root query $\top$, and equiped with three operations: *push*, *pop*, and *wq* that returns the last pushed query. Beside, we have a function l that combines a formula from a command argument and the history, and a side-effect operation *out* that performs displays.

All elementary operations being defined, CS commands are formally specified in the following table (querying and navigation operations, τ, t, and Inc, are underlined for visibility). Wherever t is used, if it is not defined, the command is aborted and a message warns the user that its query is ambiguous or empty.

CS command	semantics
pwd	$out(wq())$
cd ..	$pop()$
cd *to*	$push(l(to))$
ls f	$out(\underline{t}(l(f))); out(\underline{Inc}(l(f)))$
ls -r f	$out(\underline{\tau}(l(f)))$
mkfile f c	$o := new\_o(); c(o) := c; i_e(o) := extr(l(f))$
rm f	$del\_o(\underline{t}(l(f)))$
rm -r f	forall $o \in \underline{\tau}(l(f))$ do $del\_o(o)$
mv *from to*	$o := \underline{t}(l(from)); i_e(o) := (i_e(o)\Leftarrow extr(l(from)))\dot{\wedge}extr(l(to))$
mv -r *from to*	forall $o \in \underline{\tau}(l(from))$ do $i_e(o) := (i_e(o)\Leftarrow extr(l(from)))\dot{\wedge}extr(l(to))$
cp *from to*	$o := \underline{t}(l(from)); o' := new\_o(); c(o') := c(o);$
	$\quad i_e(o') := (i_e(o)\Leftarrow extr(l(from)))\dot{\wedge}extr(l(to))$
cp -r *from to*	forall $o \in \underline{\tau}(l(from))$ do $\{ o' := new\_o(); c(o') := c(o);$
	$\quad i_e(o') := (i_e(o)\Leftarrow extr(l(from)))\dot{\wedge}extr(l(to)) \}$

5   Algorithms and Complexity

In this section, we present a possible design for data structures and algorithms that implement the elementary operations defined in Section 4. We also discuss about the complexity of these algorithms.

5.1   Data Structures

Contents and extrinsic descriptions, which are the basic information of a context, are stored in arrays indexed by object identifiers. Intrinsic descriptions are extracted from contents by an abstraction function α. As this abstraction can be costly, it is important to cache its results to avoid to redo it at each access (there are well known problems of coherence between contents and intrinsic descriptions, but we do not want to focus on them here). The whole description of an object is then easily composed from its extrinsic and intrinsic ones.

A basic principle in CS is to access objects (and achieve some operations on them) through formulas. Elementary operations τ and t, the most often used ones, consist in finding one or several objects from a formula. There are two extreme solutions for implementing these operations. The first one consists in having no structure at all, and computing these operations, according to their definition, from scratch every time they are used. For $\tau(q)$ (the extent of q), this amounts to computing $i(o) \models q$ for every object o of the system, which must be avoided. The second one consists in representing the whole concept lattice. However, even if concept lattices are finite, their size increases with the richness of the logic used in descriptions and the number of objects, and it quickly becomes unacceptable (exponential in the worst case). Happily, such a representation is not necessary.

> The solution we propose consists in representing only a subdiagram $(F, \prec)$ of the Hasse diagram (i.e., a subgraph that is anti-reflexive and anti-transitive) of the (possibly infinite) formula lattice $\langle \mathcal{L}; \models \rangle$, where F contains $\dot{\top}$ (the root), $i(\mathcal{O})$ (all object descriptions), and a set X of increments (see elementary operation Inc in Section 4.3).

Why use a diagram of formulas rather than a diagram of concepts? Firstly, what is interesting in concepts is their extents (recall that we aim at identifying objects with formulas), and not their intents which can be too complicated to be exploitable. Nevertheless, any formula that labels a concept by μ is a consistent representation of it. Moreover, the extent of every concept is related to each formula labelling it by the application τ, which can be defined without using the notion of concept $(\forall f \in \mathcal{L} : ext(\mu(f)) = \tau(f))$: so, the diagram of formulas is sufficient for retrieving all information relative to extents, and therefore to concepts. Secondly, the diagram of formulas is easier to use than the concept lattice because command parameters are formulas, and not concepts, and easier to maintain because it is stable (it is defined by the logic $\mathcal{L}$, and more precisely by $\models$), whereas the concept lattice evolves according to the context (i.e., every time an object is created, updated or removed). Why choose a subdiagram that is anti-reflexive and anti-transitive? This avoids redundancies and lighten the structure. Furthermore, relation $\models$ can easily be retrieved from $\prec$ (by reflexive and transitive closure). Why F must contain $\dot{\top}$, $i(\mathcal{O})$, and X? $\dot{\top}$ is the root of the diagram and is used as an entry point for diagram traversals. Diagram nodes that are labelled by object descriptions are used to attach corresponding objects on them. X is used by Inc in command ls. Each node in F can be seen as a *view* that records the answers to a query, and $(F, \prec)$ is then a kind of *view hierarchy* that organizes and facilitates access to information.

Example. Assuming objects of context K_{ex} (cf. Example 2.1) have been created in the order x, z, y, Figure 2 draws the diagram of formulas before and after

y is created. Formulas represented in these diagrams are object descriptions (labelled by the object) or increments which are parts of these descriptions, seen as conjunctions. Circles gather formulas that have the same extent, i.e, that label the same concept. In other words, each circle matches a concept in Figure 1.(b). Not all concepts are represented in diagrams, which is a good point considering that there can be an exponential number of concepts in some contexts.

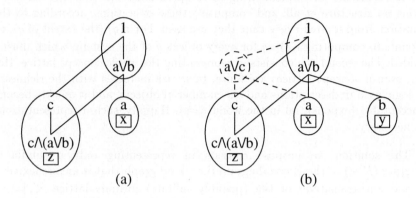

Fig. 2. Hasse diagrams of formulas for K_{ex} with (a) $\mathcal{O} = \{x, z\}$, and (b) $\mathcal{O} = \{x, z, y\}$.

5.2 Algorithms for Operations τ, t, and Inc

We express operations τ, t, and Inc using elementary accesses to the Hasse diagram of formulas: Inf, Inf^*, Sup, Sup^*, obj. The first two are defined for all $f \in F$ by

$$Inf(f) := \{g \in F | g \prec f\} \qquad Inf^*(f) := \{g \in F | g \models f\}.$$

Sup and Sup^* are defined dually, and $obj(f)$ is the object that is attached to f (it exists only if f is an object description). From definitions given in Section 4, we get the following equalities for every $f \in F$:

- $\tau(f) = \{o \in \mathcal{O} | \exists g \in Inf^*(f) : obj(g) = o\}$,
- $t(f) = obj(max_\prec \{g \in Inf^*(f) | obj(g) \text{ is defined}\})$,
- $Inc(f) = \lceil \{x \in X | 0 < |\tau(f) \cap \tau(x)| < |\tau(f)|\} \rceil$.

These equalities show that algorithms for τ, t, and Inc consist in traversing the set Inf^* of some nodes of the diagram of formulas, while performing simple operations (e.g. collect an object, test and set some marks). These algorithms are independant from $\mathcal{L}$ because logical operations are not used here. More precisely, all useful consequences of the deduction relation, $\models$, are cached in the diagram.

Example. In the diagram of Figure 2.(b), the following results can be computed with the above algorithms:

$\tau(a \vee b) = \{x, y, z\}$ $t(a \vee b)$ is undefined $Inc(a \vee b) = \{a, b, c\}$
$\tau(c) = \{z\}$ $t(c) = z$ $Inc(c) = \{\}$.

We see that $a \vee b$ is an ambiguous query because $t(a \vee b)$ is undefined and $\tau(a \vee b)$ is not empty; whereas c identifies the object z, and has an empty set of increments because $\tau(c)$ is a singleton.

5.3   Algorithms for Locating and Inserting Formulas in the Diagram

Some formulas need to be located and inserted in the diagram of formulas F: descriptions of new objects, new increments, and arguments of τ, t and Inc. Thus, we need an algorithm that takes a formula as an argument, inserts it as a node in F, and returns this node. If a formula f is already in F (modulo $\doteq$), it is not inserted as a new node, but the existing node is returned. Inserting a formula f in F consists in computing $Inf(f)$ and $Sup(f)$. We designed an algorithm *insert* based on traversals of $(F, \prec)$ and comparisons between formulas with $\models$ that achieves these computations (by lack of place, we do not detail it here).

Even if we tried to minimize the use of $\models$, whose complexity depends on the chosen logic, algorithm *insert* remains costly and we avoid it as often as possible. Firstly, we observe that in practice the working query is built incrementally as a conjunction of increments. Indeed, the usual navigation paradigm is to alternate commands `ls` and `cd`. Even if a query is used instead of an increment given by `ls`, this query can be inserted as a new increment and then conjuncted to the working query. Secondly, algorithms for τ, t and Inc traverse only Inf^* and not Sup^*; and practice shows that they are the most often applied to the working query: in other cases (e.g, `ls -r f`), the command can be decomposed so that it becomes the case (e.g., `cd f; ls -r .; cd ..`).

These observations lead us to introduce a special node wq for representing the working query. This node is special in the sense that only $Inf(wq)$ is defined ($Sup(wq)$ and $obj(wq)$ are not), and the formula of wq is a conjunction of increments (elements of X). The advantage of this is that we have an algorithm *refine* that refines the working query to $wq \wedge x$ from wq and the node of an increment x by traversing $Inf^*(wq)$ and $Inf^*(x)$ without any call to $\models$. Moreover, if x is already in F in the same syntactic form, it could be located in F in constant time, using a hashtable for example.

Example. From Figure 2, we can see the effect of adding the object y whose description is b, and the effect of refining the working query with formula $a \vee c$ that leads to insert $a \vee c$ in the diagram of formulas (in dotted lines on the figure).

5.4   Discussion about Complexity

In this section, we evaluate the complexity of the algorithms presented above according to the number of objects n and the complexity of $\models$, which we note $O(\models)$. We begin by stating some reasonable assumptions. First, we assume that each object description is the conjunction of a set of formulas whose elements belong to the set of increments X, and whose average size is a constant k. This assumption is rather natural and easily satisfied. Second, we assume that F is somewhat homogeneous, i.e., every increment x has a number of subformulas in F proportionnal to the size of its extent: i.e., the ratio $\frac{|Inf^*(x)|}{|\tau(x)|}$ does not depend on x.

From these assumptions, it comes that the average complexity of τ, t and $refine$ is $k(1 + \frac{n}{|X|})$, and that the average complexity of Inc is $k(n + |X|)$, where $|X|$ is the number of increments.

A good compromise is to give X a size proportional to n. So doing, the average complexity of τ, t and $refine$ is constant, and the one of Inc is linear in n.

For algorithm $insert$, the worst case complexity is $nO(\models)$, which is unavoidable in some situations: for instance, the insertion of a new increment x, that is incomparable to existing ones, leads to compare x with all object descriptions.

The best average complexity of $insert$, theoretically speaking, is $(\ln n)O(\models)$. This optimal complexity is realized under the conditions that, in the diagram of formulas, the height (the greatest path length) is in $(\ln n)$, and the size of Inf is bound.

To put a concrete form on these conditions, let us observe that if F is structured as a tree, it satisfies all conditions we put on the diagram of formulas.

To conclude, although the structure and the management of the diagram of formulas must be further specified to precise how to satisfy the above conditions, we already know that it is possible to implement the CS at a reasonable cost. Moreover, this is valid for any decidable logic and without any restriction to the model presented in section 3.

6   Conclusion and Further Works

We have presented the design of a file system shell in which the designation of objects is made by using formulas via Concept Analysis. In this design, conventional notions such as files and directories are matched by the notions of objects and concepts. The reference to an arbitrary logic may seem to challenge the practicalness of the design, but we have shown that the actual usage of a theorem prover for taking into account the logic is very limited. In fact, deductions can be "cached" in a partially ordered diagram of formulas that does no depend on the formal context. Thus, it needs not be updated when the Formal Context changes. Explicitly managing an evolving Concept Lattice is costly, and we have shown how to avoid it. Only an approximation of the Concept Lattice is actually represented.

This design has been implemented as a high-level generic Conceptual Shell prototype (CS) in which a theorem prover can be plugged in, and as a lower level File System prototype (RFS for relational file system) in which a simple logic (a logic of sets of attributes) is wired in a file system. The prototypes have been tested with different applications: a Vietnamese cookbook (e.g., cd fish_sauce/pineapple) as an example of a small-size consumer oriented application, the management of home directories as an example of a medium-size professional application (we used CS with up to 5000 objects), and a personal organizer.

Further works on the short and medium term is to develop the algorithmic aspects of CFS, improve the navigation facilities, and develop a graphical user interface. Long term further works is to implement it at the level of a file system. This is necessary because not all accesses to objects are done via a shell; many more are done via system commands. So, one must offer the CFS service at this level.

References

[CM98]   L. Chaudron and N. Maille. 1st order logic formal concept analysis: from logic programming to theory. *Computer and Information Science*, 13(3), 1998.

[FR99]   S. Ferré and O. Ridoux. Une généralisation logique de l'analyse de concepts logique. Technical Report RR-3820, Inria, Institut National de Recherche en Informatique et en Automatique, December 1999. An english version is available at http://www.irisa.fr/lande/ferre.

[FR00]   Sébastien Ferré and Olivier Ridoux. A logical generalization of formal concept analysis. In Guy Mineau and Bernhard Ganter, editors, *International Conference on Conceptual Structures*, August 2000. To appear.

[GJSO91] David K. Gifford, Pierre Jouvelot, Mark A. Sheldon, and James W. Jr O'Toole. Semantic file systems. In *Proceedings of 13th ACM Symposium on Operating Systems Principles*, pages 16–25. ACM SIGOPS, October 1991.

[GM99]   Burra Gopal and Udi Manber. Integrating content-based access mechanisms with hierarchical file systems. In *Proceedings of third symposium on Operating Systems Design and Implementation*, pages 265–278. USENIX Association, 1999.

[GMA93]   R. Godin, R. Missaoui, and A. April. Experimental comparison of navigation in a Galois lattice with conventional information retrieval methods. *International Journal of Man-Machine Studies*, 38(5):747–767, 1993.

[GW99]   B. Ganter and R. Wille. *Formal Concept Analysis — Mathematical Foundations*. Springer, 1999.

[KS94]   M. Krone and G. Snelting. On the inference of configuration structures from source code. In *Proceedings of the 16th International Conference on Software Engineering*, pages 49–58. IEEE Computer Society Press, May 1994.

[Lin95]   C. Lindig. Concept-based component retrieval. In *IJCAI95 Workshop on Formal Approaches to the Reuse of Plans, Proofs, and Programs*, 1995.

[Sne98]   G. Snelting. Concept analysis — A new framework for program understanding. *ACM SIGPLAN Notices*, 33(7):1–10, July 1998.

A Semantic Approach for Schema Evolution and Versioning in Object-Oriented Databases

Enrico Franconi[1], Fabio Grandi[2], and Federica Mandreoli[2]

[1] Univ. of Manchester, Dept. of Computer Science, Manchester M13 9PL, UK
franconi@cs.man.ac.uk
[2] Univ. di Bologna, Dip. di Elettronica, Informatica e Sistemistica, Bologna, Italy
{fgrandi, fmandreoli}@deis.unibo.it

Abstract. In this paper a semantic approach for the specification and the management of databases with evolving schemata is introduced. It is shown how a general object-oriented model for schema versioning and evolution can be formalized; how the semantics of schema change operations can be defined; how interesting reasoning tasks can be supported, based on an encoding in description logics.

1 Introduction

The problems of schema evolution and versioning arose in the context of long-lived database applications, where stored data were considered worth surviving changes in the database schema [23]. According to a widely accepted terminology [18], a database supports *schema evolution* if it permits modifications of the schema without the loss of extant data; in addition, it supports *schema versioning* if it allows the querying of all data through user-definable version interfaces. For the sake of brevity, schema evolution can be considered as a special case of schema versioning where only the current schema version is retained. With schema versioning, different schemata can be identified and selected by means of a suitable "coordinate system": symbolic labels are often used in design systems to this purpose, whereas proper time values are the elective choice for temporal applications [13, 14].

In this paper, we present and discuss a formal approach, for the specification and management of schema versioning in a very general object-oriented data model. The adoption of an object-oriented data model is the most common choice in the literature concerning schema evolution, though schema versioning in relational databases [10] has also been studied deeply. The approach is based on:

- the definition of an extended object-oriented model supporting evolving schemata (equipped with all the usually adopted schema changes) for which a semantics is provided;
- the formulation of interesting reasoning tasks, in order to support the design and the management of an evolving schema;

J. Lloyd et al. (Eds.): CL 2000, LNAI 1861, pp. 1048–1062, 2000.

- an encoding, which has been proved correct, as inclusion dependencies in a suitable Description Logic, which can then be used to solve the tasks defined for the schema versioning.

Within such a framework, the main problems connected with schema versioning support will be formally characterised, both from a logical and computational viewpoint, leading to the following enhancements.

- The complexity of schema changes becomes potentially unlimited: in addition to the classical schema change primitives (a well-known comprehensive taxonomy can be found in [3]), our approach enables the definition of complex and articulated schema changes.
- We define different notions of consistency, related to the existence of a legal database for the global schema or for a single schema version, or related to the consistency of single classes within a consistent schema (version). Classification tasks we define include the discovery of implicit inclusion/inheritance relationships between classes ([4]). Decidability and complexity results are available for the above mentioned tasks in our framework; tools based on Description Logics can be used for solving these tasks.
- The process of schema transformation can be formally checked. The provided semantics of the various schema change operations makes it possible to reduce the correctness proof of complex sequences of schema changes to solvable reasoning tasks.

However, our semantic approach has not thoroughly addressed the so-called *change propagation* problem yet, which concerns the effects of schema changes on the underlying data instances. In general, change propagation can be accomplished by populating the new schema version with the results of queries involving extant data connected to previous schema versions. In Section 6, our proposal will be reviewed in the light of previous approaches involving query languages (e.g. [1, 9, 17, 19]), and directions for future developments will also be sketched.

The paper is organised as follows. After a survey of the current status of the field, Section 3 first introduces the object-oriented model for evolving schemata, and then formally defines the relevant reasoning problems supporting the design and the management of an evolving schema. Section 5 introduces a provably correct encoding of the model into a Description Logic, so that theoretical, computational and practical results can be proved. A critical discussion (Sec. 6) about the proposed approach precedes the conclusions (Sec. 7).

2   Related Work

The problems of schema evolution and schema versioning support have been diffusively studied in relational and object-oriented database papers: [23] provides an excellent survey on the main issues concerned. The introduction of schema change facilities in a system involves the solution of two fundamental problems:

the *semantics of change*, which refers to the effects of the change on the schema itself, and the *change propagation*, which refers to the effects on the underlying data instances. The former problem involves the checking and maintenance of schema consistency after changes, whereas the latter involves the consistency of extant data with the modified schema.

In the object-oriented field, two main approaches were followed to ensure consistency in pursuing the "semantics of change" problem. The first approach is based on the adoption of *invariants* and *rules*, and has been used, for instance, in the ORION [3] and O$_2$ [11] systems. The second approach, which was proposed in [22], is based on the introduction of *axioms*. In the former approach, the invariants define the consistency of a schema, and definite rules must be followed to maintain the invariants satisfied after each schema change. In the latter approach, a sound and complete set of axioms (provided with an inference mechanism) formalises the *dynamic schema evolution*, which is the actual management of schema changes in a system in operation. The compliance of the available primitive schema changes with the axioms automatically ensures schema consistency, without need for explicit checking, as incorrect schema versions cannot actually be generated.

For the "change propagation" problem, several solutions have been proposed and implemented in real systems [3, 11, 21]. In most cases, simple *default* mechanisms can be used or user-supplied conversion functions must be defined for non-trivial extant object updates. A notable exception is [19], where a formal notion of logical consistency of the global approach is devised and proved decidable, in the context of a simple object-oriented data model. This work is different from the previous solutions in that there is no automatic reorganisation of the data after the schema update, but only a consistency check of the resulting database.

As far as complex schema changes are concerned, [20] considered sequences of schema change primitives to make up high-level useful changes, solving the propagation to objects problem with simple schema integration techniques. However, with this approach, the consistency of the resulting database is not guaranteed nor checked. In [5], high-level primitives are defined as *well-ordered* sets of primitive schema changes. Consistency of the resulting schema is ensured by the use of invariants' preserving elementary steps and by *ad-hoc* constraints imposed on their application order. In other words, consistency preservation is dependent on an accurate design of high-level schema changes and, thus, still relies on the designer's skills.

3   An Object-Oriented Data Model for Evolving Schemata

The object-oriented model we propose allows for the representation of multiple schema versions. It is based on an expressive version of the "snapshot" – i.e., single-schema – object-oriented model introduced by [1] and further extended and elaborated in its relationships with Description Logics by [7, 8]; in this paper we borrow the notation from [7]. The language embodies the features of the static parts of UML/OMT and ODMG and, therefore, it does not take into account those aspects related to the definition of methods.

The definition of an evolving schema $\mathcal{S}$ is based on a set of class and attribute names ($\mathcal{C}_\mathcal{S}$ and $\mathcal{A}_\mathcal{S}$ respectively) and includes a partially ordered set of schema versions. The initial schema version of $\mathcal{S}$ contains a set of class definitions having one of the following forms:

$$\underline{\text{Class}} \ C \ \underline{\text{is-a}} \ C_1, \ldots, C_h \ \underline{\text{disjoint}} \ C_{h+1}, \ldots, C_k \ \underline{\text{type-is}} \ T.$$
$$\underline{\text{View-class}} \ C \ \underline{\text{is-a}} \ C_1, \ldots, C_h \ \underline{\text{disjoint}} \ C_{h+1}, \ldots, C_k \ \underline{\text{type-is}} \ T.$$

A class definition introduces just necessary conditions regarding the type of the class – this is the standard case in object-oriented data models – while views are defined by means of both necessary and sufficient conditions. The symbol T denotes a type expression built according to the following syntax:

$$
\begin{aligned}
T \rightarrow \ &C \ | \\
&\underline{\text{Union}} \ T_1, \ldots, T_k \ \underline{\text{End}} \ | \quad &\text{(union type)} \\
&\underline{\text{Set-of}} \ [\text{m,n}] \ T \ | \quad &\text{(set type)} \\
&\underline{\text{Record}} \ A_1{:}T_1, \ldots, A_k{:}T_k \ \underline{\text{End}} . \quad &\text{(record type)}
\end{aligned}
$$

where $C \in \mathcal{C}_\mathcal{S}$, $A_i \in \mathcal{A}_\mathcal{S}$, and [m,n] denotes an optional cardinality constraint.

A schema version in $\mathcal{S}$ is defined by the application of a sequence of schema changes to a preceding schema version. The schema change taxonomy is built by combining the model elements which are subject to change with the elementary modifications, add, drop and change, they undergo. In this paper only a basic set of elementary schema change operators will be introduced; it includes the standard ones found in the literature (e.g., [3]); however, it is not difficult to consider the complete set of operators with respect to the constructs of the data model.

$$
\begin{aligned}
M \rightarrow \ &\underline{\text{Add-attribute}} \ C, A, T \ \underline{\text{End}} \ | \\
&\underline{\text{Drop-attribute}} \ C, A \ \underline{\text{End}} \ | \\
&\underline{\text{Change-attr-name}} \ C, A, A' \ \underline{\text{End}} \ | \\
&\underline{\text{Change-attr-type}} \ C, A, T' \ \underline{\text{End}} \ | \\
&\underline{\text{Add-class}} \ C, T \ \underline{\text{End}} \ | \\
&\underline{\text{Drop-class}} \ C \ \underline{\text{End}} \ | \\
&\underline{\text{Change-class-name}} \ C, C' \ \underline{\text{End}} \ | \\
&\underline{\text{Change-class-type}} \ C, T' \ \underline{\text{End}} \ | \\
&\underline{\text{Add-is-a}} \ C, C' \ \underline{\text{End}} \ | \\
&\underline{\text{Drop-is-a}} \ C, C' \ \underline{\text{End}} .
\end{aligned}
$$

In this paper, we omit the definition of a schema version coordinate mechanism and simply reference distinct schema versions by means of different subscripts. Any kind of versioning dimension usually considered in the literature could actually be employed – such as transaction time, valid time and symbolic labels – provided that a suitable mapping between version coordinates and index values is defined.

Definition 1. *An evolving object-oriented schema is a tuple* $\mathcal{S} = (\mathcal{C}_\mathcal{S}, \mathcal{A}_\mathcal{S}, \mathcal{SV}_0,$ $\mathcal{M}_\mathcal{S})$, *where:*

- $\mathcal{C}_\mathcal{S}$ *is a finite set of class names;*
- $\mathcal{A}_\mathcal{S}$ *is a finite set of attribute names;*
- $\mathcal{SV}_0$ *is the initial schema version, which includes class and view definitions for some* $C \in \mathcal{C}_\mathcal{S}$;
- $\mathcal{M}_\mathcal{S}$ *is a set of modifications* $\mathcal{M}_{ij}$, *where* i, j *denote a pair of version coordinates. Each modification is a finite sequence of elementary schema changes.*

The set $\mathcal{M}_\mathcal{S}$ induces a partial order $\mathcal{SV}$ over a finite and discrete set of schema versions with minimal element $\mathcal{SV}_0$. Hence $\mathcal{SV}_0$ precedes every other schema version and the schema version $\mathcal{SV}_j$ represents the outcome of the application of $\mathcal{M}_{ij}$ to $\mathcal{SV}_i$. $\mathcal{S}$ is called *elementary* if every $\mathcal{M}_{ij}$ in $\mathcal{M}_\mathcal{S}$ contains only one elementary modification, and every schema version $\mathcal{SV}_i$ has at most one immediate predecessor. In the following we will consider only elementary evolving schemata.

Let us now introduce the meaning of an evolving object-oriented schema $\mathcal{S}$. Informally, the semantics is given by assigning to each schema version a possible legal database state – i.e., a legal instance of the schema version – conforming to the constraints imposed by the sequence of schema changes starting from the initial schema version.

Formally, an instance $\mathcal{I}$ of $\mathcal{S}$ is a tuple $\mathcal{I} = (\mathcal{O}^\mathcal{I}, \rho^\mathcal{I}, (\mathcal{I}_0, \dots, \mathcal{I}_n))$, consisting of a finite set $\mathcal{O}^\mathcal{I}$ of object identifiers, a function $\rho^\mathcal{I} : \mathcal{O}^\mathcal{I} \mapsto \mathcal{V}_{\mathcal{O}^\mathcal{I}}$ giving a value to object identifiers, and a sequence of version instances $\mathcal{I}_i$, one for each schema version $\mathcal{SV}_i$ in $\mathcal{S}$. The set $\mathcal{V}_{\mathcal{O}^\mathcal{I}}$ of values is defined by induction as the smallest set including the union of $\mathcal{O}^\mathcal{I}$ with all possible "sets" of values and with all possible "records" of values. Although the set $\mathcal{V}_{\mathcal{O}^\mathcal{I}}$ is infinite, we consider for an instance $\mathcal{I}$ the finite set $\mathcal{V}_\mathcal{I}$ of *active values*, which is the subset of $\mathcal{V}_{\mathcal{O}^\mathcal{I}}$ formed by the union of $\mathcal{O}^\mathcal{I}$ and the set of values assigned by $\rho^\mathcal{I}$ ([7]).

A version instance $\mathcal{I}_i = (\pi^{\mathcal{I}_i}, \cdot^{\mathcal{I}_i})$ consists of a total function $\pi^{\mathcal{I}_i} : \mathcal{C}_\mathcal{S} \mapsto 2^{\mathcal{O}^\mathcal{I}}$, giving the set of object identifiers in the extension of each class $C \in \mathcal{C}_\mathcal{S}$ for that version, and of a function $\cdot^{\mathcal{I}_i}$ (the *interpretation* function) mapping type expressions to sets of values, such that the following is satisfied:

$$C^{\mathcal{I}_i} = \pi^{\mathcal{I}_i}(C)$$

$$(\underline{\text{Union}}\ T_1, \dots, T_k\ \underline{\text{End}})^{\mathcal{I}_i} = T_1^{\mathcal{I}_i} \cup \dots \cup T_k^{\mathcal{I}_i}$$

$$(\underline{\text{Set-of}}\ [\text{m,n}]\ T)^{\mathcal{I}_i} = \{\{\!|\ v_1, \dots, v_k\ |\!\}\ |\ m \le k \le n, v_j \in T^{\mathcal{I}_i},$$
$$\text{for } j \in \{1, \dots, k\}\}$$

$$(\underline{\text{Record}}\ A_1{:}T_1, \dots, A_k{:}T_k\ \underline{\text{End}})^{\mathcal{I}_i} = \{[\![A_1 : v_1, \dots, A_k : v_k, \dots, A_h : v_h]\!]\ |$$
$$\text{for some } h \ge k,$$
$$v_j \in T_j^{\mathcal{I}_i}, \text{for } j \in \{1, \dots, k\},$$
$$v_j \in \mathcal{V}_{\mathcal{O}^\mathcal{I}}, \text{for } j \in \{k+1, \dots, h\}\}$$

Add-attribute **C, A, T**	$\pi^{\mathcal{I}_j}(\mathbf{C}) = \pi^{\mathcal{I}_i}(\mathbf{C}) \cap \{o \in \mathcal{O}^{\mathcal{I}} \mid \rho^{\mathcal{I}}(o) = [\dots, \mathbf{A} : v, \dots] \wedge v \in \mathbf{T}^{\mathcal{I}_j}\},$ $\pi^{\mathcal{I}_i}(D) = \pi^{\mathcal{I}_j}(D)$ for all $D \neq \mathbf{C}$
Drop-attribute **C, A**	$\pi^{\mathcal{I}_i}(\mathbf{C}) = \pi^{\mathcal{I}_j}(\mathbf{C}) \cap \{o \in \mathcal{O}^{\mathcal{I}} \mid \rho^{\mathcal{I}}(o) = [\dots, \mathbf{A} : v, \dots]\},$ $\pi^{\mathcal{I}_i}(D) = \pi^{\mathcal{I}_j}(D)$ for all $D \neq \mathbf{C}$
Change-attr-name **C, A, A'**	$\pi^{\mathcal{I}_i}(\mathbf{C}) \cap \{o \in \mathcal{O}^{\mathcal{I}} \mid \rho^{\mathcal{I}}(o) = [\dots, \mathbf{A} : v, \dots]\} =$ $\pi^{\mathcal{I}_j}(\mathbf{C}) \cap \{o \in \mathcal{O}^{\mathcal{I}} \mid \rho^{\mathcal{I}}(o) = [\dots, \mathbf{A'} : v, \dots]\},$ $\pi^{\mathcal{I}_i}(D) = \pi^{\mathcal{I}_j}(D)$ for all $D \neq \mathbf{C}$
Change-attr-type **C, A, T'**	$\pi^{\mathcal{I}_i}(\mathbf{C}) \cap \{o \in \mathcal{O}^{\mathcal{I}} \mid \rho^{\mathcal{I}}(o) = [\dots, \mathbf{A} : v, \dots] \wedge v \in \mathbf{T'}^{\mathcal{I}_j}\} =$ $\pi^{\mathcal{I}_j}(\mathbf{C}) \cap \{o \in \mathcal{O}^{\mathcal{I}} \mid \rho^{\mathcal{I}}(o) = [\dots, \mathbf{A} : v, \dots]\},$ $\pi^{\mathcal{I}_i}(D) = \pi^{\mathcal{I}_j}(D)$ for all $D \neq \mathbf{C}$
Add-class **C, T**	$\pi^{\mathcal{I}_i}(\mathbf{C}) = \emptyset, \quad \rho^{\mathcal{I}}(\pi^{\mathcal{I}_i}(\mathbf{C})) \subseteq \mathbf{T}^{\mathcal{I}_j}, \quad \pi^{\mathcal{I}_i}(D) = \pi^{\mathcal{I}_j}(D)$ for all $D \neq \mathbf{C}$
Drop-class **C**	$\pi^{\mathcal{I}_j}(\mathbf{C}) = \emptyset, \quad \pi^{\mathcal{I}_i}(D) = \pi^{\mathcal{I}_j}(D)$ for all $D \neq \mathbf{C}$
Change-class-name **C, C'**	$\pi^{\mathcal{I}_i}(\mathbf{C}) = \pi^{\mathcal{I}_j}(\mathbf{C'}), \quad \pi^{\mathcal{I}_i}(D) = \pi^{\mathcal{I}_j}(D)$ for all $D \neq \mathbf{C}, \mathbf{C'}$
Change-class-type **C, T'**	$\pi^{\mathcal{I}_j}(\mathbf{C}) = \pi^{\mathcal{I}_i}(\mathbf{C}) \cap \{o \in \mathcal{O}^{\mathcal{I}} \mid \rho^{\mathcal{I}}(o) \in \mathbf{T'}^{\mathcal{I}_j}\},$ $\pi^{\mathcal{I}_i}(D) = \pi^{\mathcal{I}_j}(D)$ for all $D \neq \mathbf{C}$
Add-is-a **C, C'**	$\pi^{\mathcal{I}_j}(\mathbf{C}) = \pi^{\mathcal{I}_i}(\mathbf{C}) \cap \pi^{\mathcal{I}_i}(\mathbf{C'}), \quad \pi^{\mathcal{I}_i}(D) = \pi^{\mathcal{I}_j}(D)$ for all $D \neq \mathbf{C}$
Drop-is-a **C, C'**	$\pi^{\mathcal{I}_i}(\mathbf{C}) = \pi^{\mathcal{I}_j}(\mathbf{C}) \cap \pi^{\mathcal{I}_j}(\mathbf{C'}), \quad \pi^{\mathcal{I}_i}(D) = \pi^{\mathcal{I}_j}(D)$ for all $D \neq \mathbf{C}$

Fig. 1. Semantics of the schema changes.

where an open semantics for records is adopted (called *-interpretation in [1]) in order to give the right semantics to inheritance. In a set constructor if the minimum or the maximum cardinalities are not explicitly specified, they are assumed to be zero and infinite, respectively.

The semantics of schema changes is shown in Fig. 1. For each schema change $\mathcal{M}_{ij}$, it defines a relationship between the instances of the involved schema versions.

A *legal* instance $\mathcal{I}$ of a schema $\mathcal{S}$ should satisfy the constraints imposed by the class definitions in the initial schema version and by the schema changes between schema versions.

Definition 2. *An instance $\mathcal{I}$ of a schema $\mathcal{S}$ is said to be legal if*

- *for each class definition in $\mathcal{SV}_0$*
  Class C is-a $C_1, \dots, C_h$ disjoint $C_{h+1}, \dots, C_k$ type-is T, it holds that:
  $C^{\mathcal{I}_0} \subseteq C_j^{\mathcal{I}_0}$ *for each* $j \in \{1, \dots, h\}$,
  $C^{\mathcal{I}_0} \cap C_j^{\mathcal{I}_0} = \emptyset$ *for each* $j \in \{h+1, \dots, k\}$,
  $\{\rho^{\mathcal{I}}(o) \mid o \in \pi^{\mathcal{I}_0}(C)\} \subseteq T^{\mathcal{I}_0}$;
- *for each view definition in $\mathcal{SV}_0$*
  View-class C is-a $C_1, \dots, C_h$ disjoint $C_{h+1}, \dots, C_k$ type-is T, it holds that:
  $C^{\mathcal{I}_0} \subseteq C_j^{\mathcal{I}_0}$ *for each* $j \in \{1, \dots, h\}$,
  $C^{\mathcal{I}_0} \cap C_j^{\mathcal{I}_0} = \emptyset$ *for each* $j \in \{h+1, \dots, k\}$,
  $\{\rho^{\mathcal{I}}(o) \mid o \in \pi^{\mathcal{I}_0}(C)\} = T^{\mathcal{I}_0}$;
- *for each schema change $\mathcal{M}_{ij}$ in $\mathcal{M}$, the version instances $\mathcal{I}_i$ and $\mathcal{I}_j$ satisfy the equations of the corresponding schema change type at the right hand side of Tab. 1.*

4   Reasoning Problems

According to the semantic definitions given in the previous section, several reasoning problems can be introduced, in order to support the design and the management of an evolving schema.

Definition 3. *Reasoning problems:*

a. *Global/local Schema Consistency: an evolving schema S is globally consistent if it admits a legal instance; a schema version SV_i of S is locally consistent if the evolving schema $S_{\downarrow i}$ – obtained from S by reducing the set of modifications $\mathcal{M}_{S_{\downarrow i}}$ to the linear sequence of schema changes in $\mathcal{M}_S$ which led to the version SV_i from SV_0 – admits a legal instance. In the following, a global reasoning problem refers to S, while a local one refers to $S_{\downarrow i}$.*

b. *Global/local Class Consistency: a class C is globally inconsistent if for every legal instance $\mathcal{I}$ of S and for every version SV_i its extension is empty, i.e., $\forall i. \; \pi^{\mathcal{I}_i}(C) = \emptyset$; a class C is locally inconsistent in the version SV_i if for every legal instance $\mathcal{I}$ of $S_{\downarrow i}$ its extension is empty, i.e., $\pi^{\mathcal{I}_i}(C) = \emptyset$.*

c. *Global/local Disjoint Classes: two classes C, D are globally disjoint if for every legal instance $\mathcal{I}$ of S and for every version SV_i their extensions are disjoint, i.e., $\forall i. \; \pi^{\mathcal{I}_i}(C) \cap \pi^{\mathcal{I}_i}(D) = \emptyset$; two classes C, D are locally disjoint in the version SV_i if for every legal instance $\mathcal{I}$ of $S_{\downarrow i}$ their extensions are disjoint, i.e., $\pi^{\mathcal{I}_i}(C) \cap \pi^{\mathcal{I}_i}(D) = \emptyset$.*

d. *Global/local Class Subsumption: a class D globally subsumes a class C if for every legal instance $\mathcal{I}$ of S and for every version SV_i the extension of C is included in the extension of D, i.e., $\forall i. \; \pi^{\mathcal{I}_i}(C) \subseteq \pi^{\mathcal{I}_i}(D)$; a class D locally subsumes a class C in the version SV_i if for every legal instance $\mathcal{I}$ of $S_{\downarrow i}$ the extension of C is included in the extension of D, i.e., $\pi^{\mathcal{I}_i}(C) \subseteq \pi^{\mathcal{I}_i}(D)$.*

e. *Global/local Class Equivalence: two classes C, D are globally/locally equivalent if C globally/locally subsumes D and viceversa.*

Please note that the classical *subtyping* problem – i.e., finding the explicit representation of the partial order induced on a set of type expressions by the containment between their extensions – is a special case of class subsumption, if we restrict our attention to view definitions.

As to the *change propagation* task, which is one of the fundamental task addressed in the literature (see Sec. 2), it is usually dealt with by populating the classes in the new version with the result of queries over the previous version. The same applies for our framework: a language for the specification of views can be defined for specifying how to populate classes in a version from the previous data. Formally, we require a query language for expressing views providing a mechanism for explicit creation of object identifiers. At present, our approach includes one single data pool and a set of version instances which can be thought as views over the data pool. Therefore we consider update as a *schema augmentation* problem in the sense of [17], where the original logical schema is augmented and the new data may refer to the input data. The result of applying any view to a source data pool may involve OIDs from the source

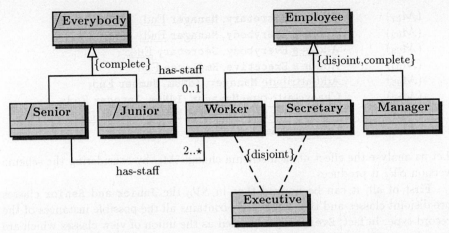

Fig. 2. The Employee initial schema version in UML notation.

besides the new required OIDs to be created. The association between the source OIDs and the target ones should not be destroyed, and only the target data pool will be retained. In Section 6 an alternative approach will be discussed.

Of course, at this point the problem of global consistency of an evolving schema S becomes more complex, since it involves the additional constraints defined by the data conversions: an instance would therefore be legal if it satisfies not only the constraints of Definition 2 but also the constraints specified by the views. Obviously, a schema S involving a schema change for which the corresponding semantics expressed by the equation in Tab. 1 and the associated data conversions are incompatible would never admit a legal instance. In general, the introduction of data conversion views makes all the reasoning problems defined above more complex.

We will try to explain the application of the reasoning problems through an example. Let us consider an evolving schema S describing the employees of a company. The schema includes an initial schema version SV_0 defined as follows:

<u>Class</u> Employee <u>type-is</u> <u>Union</u> Manager, Secretary, Worker <u>End</u>;
<u>Class</u> Manager <u>is-a</u> Employee <u>disjoint</u> Secretary, Worker ;
<u>Class</u> Secretary <u>is-a</u> Employee <u>disjoint</u> Worker ;
<u>Class</u> Worker <u>is-a</u> Employee;
<u>View-class</u> Senior <u>type-is</u> <u>Record</u> has_staff: <u>Set-of</u> [2,n] Worker <u>End</u>;
<u>View-class</u> Junior <u>type-is</u> <u>Record</u> has_staff: <u>Set-of</u> [0,1] Worker <u>End</u>;
<u>Class</u> Executive <u>disjoint</u> Secretary, Worker;
<u>View-class</u> Everybody <u>type-is</u> <u>Union</u> Senior, Junior <u>End</u> <u>End</u>;

Figure 2 shows the UML-like representation induced by the initial schema SV_0; note that classes with names prefixed by a slash represent the views. The evolving schema S includes a set of schema modifications M_S defined as follows:

$(\mathcal{M}_{01})$	Add-is-a Secretary, Manager End;
$(\mathcal{M}_{02})$	Add-is-a Everybody, Manager End;
$(\mathcal{M}_{23})$	Add-is-a Everybody, Secretary End;
$(\mathcal{M}_{04})$	Add-is-a Executive, Employee End;
$(\mathcal{M}_{45})$	Add-attribute Manager, IdNum, Number End;
$(\mathcal{M}_{56})$	Change-attr-type Manager, IdNum, Integer End;
$(\mathcal{M}_{67})$	Change-attr-type Manager, IdNum, String End;
$(\mathcal{M}_{68})$	Drop-class Employee End;

Let us analyse the effect of each schema change $\mathcal{M}_{ij}$ by considering the schema version $\mathcal{SV}_j$ it produces.

First of all, it can be noticed that in $\mathcal{SV}_0$ the Junior and Senior classes are disjoint classes and that Everybody contains all the possible instances of the record type. In fact, Everybody is defined as the union of view classes which are complementary with respect to the record type: any possible record instance is the value of an object belonging either to Senior or Junior.

Secretary is inconsistent in $\mathcal{SV}_1$ since Secretary and Manager are disjoint: its extension is included in the Manager extension only if it is empty (for each version instance $\mathcal{I}_1$, Secretary$^{\mathcal{I}_1} = \emptyset$). Therefore, Secretary is *locally inconsistent*, as it is inconsistent in $\mathcal{SV}_1$ but not in $\mathcal{SV}_0$.

The schema version $\mathcal{SV}_3$ is inconsistent because Secretary and Manager, which are both superclasses of Everybody, are disjoint and the intersection of their extensions is empty: no version instance $\mathcal{I}_3$ exists such that Everybody$^{\mathcal{I}_3} \subseteq \emptyset$. It follows that $\mathcal{S}$ is locally inconsistent with respect to $\mathcal{SV}_3$ and, thus, globally inconsistent (although is locally consistent wrt the other schema versions).

In $\mathcal{SV}_4$, it can be derived that Executive is locally subsumed by Manager, since it is a subclass of Employee disjoint from Secretary and Worker (Manager, Secretary and Worker are a partition of Employee).

The schema version $\mathcal{SV}_5$ exemplifies a case of attribute inheritance. The attribute IdNum which has been added to the Manager class is inherited by the Executive class. This means that *every* legal instance of $\mathcal{S}$ should be such that every instance of Executive in $\mathcal{SV}_5$ has an attribute IdNum of type Number, i.e., Executive$^{\mathcal{I}_5} \subseteq \{o \mid \rho^{\mathcal{I}}(o) = [\![\ldots, \text{IdNum} : v, \ldots]\!] \land v \in \text{Number}^{\mathcal{I}_5}\}$. Of course, there is no restriction on the way classes are related via subsumption, and multiple inheritance is allowed as soon as it does not generate an inconsistency.

The Change-attr-type elementary schema change allows for the modification of the type of an attribute with the proviso that the new type is not incompatible with the old one, like in $\mathcal{M}_{56}$. In fact, the semantics of elementary schema changes as defined in Tab. 1 is based on the assumption that the updated view should coexist with the starting data, since we are in the context of update as *schema augmentation*. If an object changes its value, then its object identifier should change, too. Notice that, for this reason, $\mathcal{M}_{67}$ leads to an inconsistent version if Number and String are defined to be non-empty disjoint classes. Since the only elementary change that can refer to *new* objects is Add-class, in order to specify a schema change involving a restructuring of the data and the creation of new objects – like in the case of the change of the type of an attribute

$$
\begin{aligned}
C, D \rightarrow \quad & A \mid \\
& \top \mid & \top^{\mathcal{I}} &= \Delta^{\mathcal{I}} \\
& \bot \mid & \bot^{\mathcal{I}} &= \emptyset \\
& \neg C \mid & (\neg C)^{\mathcal{I}} &= \Delta^{\mathcal{I}} \setminus C^{\mathcal{I}} \\
& C \sqcap D \mid & (C \sqcap D)^{\mathcal{I}} &= C^{\mathcal{I}} \cap D^{\mathcal{I}} \\
& C \sqcup D \mid & (C \sqcup D)^{\mathcal{I}} &= C^{\mathcal{I}} \cup D^{\mathcal{I}} \\
& \forall R.C \mid & (\forall R.C)^{\mathcal{I}} &= \{ i \in \Delta^{\mathcal{I}} \mid \forall j.\; R^{\mathcal{I}}(i,j) \Rightarrow C^{\mathcal{I}}(j) \} \\
& \exists R.C \mid & (\exists R.C)^{\mathcal{I}} &= \{ i \in \Delta^{\mathcal{I}} \mid \exists j.\; R^{\mathcal{I}}(i,j) \wedge C^{\mathcal{I}}(j) \} \\
& \geq nR.C \mid & (\geq nR.C)^{\mathcal{I}} &= \{ i \in \Delta^{\mathcal{I}} \mid \sharp\{ j \in \Delta^{\mathcal{I}} \mid R^{\mathcal{I}}(i,j) \wedge C^{\mathcal{I}}(j) \} \geq n \} \\
& \leq nR.C & (\leq nR.C)^{\mathcal{I}} &= \{ i \in \Delta^{\mathcal{I}} \mid \sharp\{ j \in \Delta^{\mathcal{I}} \mid R^{\mathcal{I}}(i,j) \wedge C^{\mathcal{I}}(j) \} \leq n \}
\end{aligned}
$$

$$
\begin{aligned}
R, S \rightarrow \quad & P \mid \\
& R^{-} & (R^{-})^{\mathcal{I}} &= \{ (i,j) \in \Delta^{\mathcal{I}} \times \Delta^{\mathcal{I}} \mid R^{\mathcal{I}}(j,i) \}
\end{aligned}
$$

Fig. 3. $\mathcal{ALCQI}$ concept and role expressions and their semantics.

with an incompatible new type – a sequence of Drop-class and Add-class should be specified, together with a data conversion view specifying how the data is converted from one version to the other.

The deletion of the class Employee in $\mathcal{SV}_8$ does not cause any inconsistency in the resulting schema version. In $\mathcal{SV}_8$ the Employee extension is empty and the former Employee subclasses continue to exist (with the constraint that their extensions are subsets of the extension of Employee in $\mathcal{SV}_6$). Notice that, in a classical object model where the class hierarchy is explicitly based on a DAG, the deletion of a non-isolated class would require a restructuring of the DAG itself (e.g. to get rid of dangling edges).

5   Reasoning Using Description Logics

In this section we establish a relationship between the proposed model for evolving schemata and the $\mathcal{ALCQI}$ description logic. To this end, we provide an encoding from an evolving schema into an $\mathcal{ALCQI}$ knowledge base Σ, such that the reasoning problems mentioned in the previous section can be reduced to corresponding description logics reasoning problems, for which extensive theories and well founded and efficient implemented systems exist. The encoding is grounded on the fact that there is a correspondence between the models of the knowledge base and the legal instances of the evolving schema.

We give here only a very brief introduction to the $\mathcal{ALCQI}$ description logic; for a full account, see, e.g., [6]. The basic types of a description logic are *concepts* and *roles*. The syntax rules at the left hand side of Figure 3 define valid concept and role expressions. Concepts are interpreted as sets of individuals—as for unary predicates—and roles as sets of pairs of individuals—as for binary predicates. Formally, an *interpretation* is a pair $\mathcal{I} = (\Delta^{\mathcal{I}}, \cdot^{\mathcal{I}})$ consisting of a set $\Delta^{\mathcal{I}}$ of individuals (the *domain* of $\mathcal{I}$) and a function $\cdot^{\mathcal{I}}$ (the *interpretation function* of $\mathcal{I}$) mapping every concept to a subset of $\Delta^{\mathcal{I}}$ and every role to a subset of $\Delta^{\mathcal{I}} \times \Delta^{\mathcal{I}}$, such that the equations at the right hand side of Figure 3 are satisfied.

A *knowledge base* is a finite set Σ of axioms of the form $C \mathrel{\dot{\sqsubseteq}} D$, involving concept expressions C, D; we write $C \equiv D$ as a shortcut for both $C \mathrel{\dot{\sqsubseteq}} D$ and $D \mathrel{\dot{\sqsubseteq}} C$. An interpretation $\mathcal{I}$ satisfies $C \mathrel{\dot{\sqsubseteq}} D$ if and only if the interpretation of C is included in the interpretation of D, i.e., $C^{\mathcal{I}} \subseteq D^{\mathcal{I}}$; it is said that C is subsumed by D. An interpretation $\mathcal{I}$ is a *model* of a knowledge base Σ iff every axiom of Σ is satisfied by $\mathcal{I}$. If Σ has a model, then it is *satisfiable*. Σ *logically implies* an axiom $C \mathrel{\dot{\sqsubseteq}} D$ (written $\Sigma \models C \mathrel{\dot{\sqsubseteq}} D$) if $C \mathrel{\dot{\sqsubseteq}} D$ is satisfied by every model of Σ. Reasoning in $\mathcal{ALCQI}$ (i.e., deciding knowledge base satisfiability and logical implication) is decidable, and it has been proven to be an EXPTIME-complete problem [6].

As in [7], the encoding of an object-oriented schema in an $\mathcal{ALCQI}$ knowledge base is based on the *reification* of type expressions – i.e., explicit individuals exist to denote values of complex types. We introduce the concept AbstractClass to represent the classes, the concepts RecType, SetType to represent types, the role value to model the association between classes and types, and the role member to specify the type of the elements of a set. In particular, a record is represented as an individual connected by means of (functional) roles – corresponding to attributes – to the fillers of its attributes. The mapping function ψ_i translates type expressions into $\mathcal{ALCQI}$ concepts as follows:

$$\psi_i(\mathrm{C}) = C_i$$
$$\psi_i(\underline{\text{Union}}\ T_1, \ldots, T_k\ \underline{\text{End}}) = \psi_i(T_1) \sqcup \ldots \sqcup \psi_i(T_k)$$
$$\psi_i(\underline{\text{Set-of}}\ [\mathrm{m,n}]\ T) = \mathsf{SetType} \sqcap \forall \mathsf{member}.\psi_i(T) \sqcap$$
$$\geq m\mathsf{member}.\top \sqcap \leq n\mathsf{member}.\top$$
$$\psi_i(\underline{\text{Record}}\ A_1{:}T_1, \ldots, A_k{:}T_k\ \underline{\text{End}}) = \mathsf{RecType} \sqcap \exists A_1.\psi_i(T_1) \sqcap \ldots \sqcap \exists A_k.\psi_i(T_k)$$

The translation function ψ_i is contextualised to the ith schema version, since a class in different schema version may have different extensions, and it is mapped into distinct concepts.

Definition 4. *The $\mathcal{ALCQI}$ knowledge base $\Sigma = \psi(\mathcal{S})$ corresponding to the object-oriented evolving schema $\mathcal{S} = (\mathcal{C_S}, \mathcal{A_S}, \mathcal{SV}_0, \mathcal{M_S})$ is composed by the following axioms:*

- *Axioms on basic types:*
  $$\mathsf{AbstractClass} \sqsubseteq \exists \mathsf{value}.\top \sqcap \leq 1\mathsf{value}.\top$$
  $$\mathsf{RecType} \sqsubseteq \forall \mathsf{value}.\bot$$
  $$\mathsf{SetType} \sqsubseteq \forall \mathsf{value}.\bot \sqcap \neg \mathsf{RecType}$$
- *For each class definition*
  $\underline{\textit{Class}}\ C\ \underline{\textit{is-a}}\ C_1, \ldots, C_h\ \underline{\textit{disjoint}}\ C_{h+1}, \ldots, C_k\ \underline{\textit{type-is}}\ T\ \textit{in}\ \mathcal{SV}_0$:
  $$\psi_0(C) \sqsubseteq \mathsf{AbstractClass} \sqcap \psi_0(C_1) \sqcap \ldots \sqcap \psi_0(C_h) \sqcap \forall \mathsf{value}.\psi_0(T)$$
  $$\psi_0(C) \sqsubseteq \neg \psi_0(C_{h+1}) \sqcap \ldots \sqcap \neg \psi_0(C_k)$$
- *For each view definition*
  $\underline{\textit{View-class}}\ C\ \underline{\textit{is-a}}\ C_1, \ldots, C_h\ \underline{\textit{disjoint}}\ C_{h+1}, \ldots, C_k\ \underline{\textit{type-is}}\ T\ \textit{in}\ \mathcal{SV}_0$:
  $$\psi_0(C) \sqsubseteq \mathsf{AbstractClass} \sqcap \psi_0(C_1) \sqcap \ldots \sqcap \psi_0(C_h)$$
  $$\psi_0(C) \sqsubseteq \neg \psi_0(C_{h+1}) \sqcap \ldots \sqcap \neg \psi_0(C_k)$$
  $$\psi_0(C) \equiv \forall \mathsf{value}.\psi_0(T)$$

Add-attribute **C, A, T**	$\psi_j(\mathbf{C}) \equiv \psi_i(\mathbf{C}) \sqcap \forall \mathsf{value}.(\mathsf{RecType} \sqcap \exists \mathsf{A}.\psi_j(\mathbf{T}))$,
	$\psi_i(D) \equiv \psi_j(D)$ for all $D \neq \mathbf{C}$
Drop-attribute **C, A**	$\psi_i(\mathbf{C}) \equiv \psi_j(\mathbf{C}) \sqcap \forall \mathsf{value}.(\mathsf{RecType} \sqcap \exists \mathsf{A}.\top)$,
	$\psi_i(D) \equiv \psi_j(D)$ for all $D \neq \mathbf{C}$
Change-attr-name **C, A, A′**	$\psi_i(\mathbf{C}) \sqcap \forall \mathsf{value}.(\mathsf{RecType} \sqcap \exists \mathsf{A}.\top) \equiv$
	$\qquad \psi_j(\mathbf{C}) \sqcap \forall \mathsf{value}.(\mathsf{RecType} \sqcap \exists \mathsf{A}'.\top)$,
	$\psi_i(D) \equiv \psi_j(D)$ for all $D \neq \mathbf{C}$
Change-attr-type **C, A, T′**	$\psi_i(\mathbf{C}) \sqcap \forall \mathsf{value}.(\mathsf{RecType} \sqcap \exists \mathsf{A}.\psi_j(\mathbf{T}')) \equiv$
	$\qquad \psi_j(\mathbf{C}) \sqcap \forall \mathsf{value}.(\mathsf{RecType} \sqcap \exists \mathsf{A}.\top)$,
	$\psi_i(D) \equiv \psi_j(D)$ for all $D \neq \mathbf{C}$
Add-class **C, T**	$\psi_i(\mathbf{C}) \equiv \bot$, $\psi_j(\mathbf{C}) \sqsubseteq \mathsf{AbstractClass} \sqcap \forall \mathsf{value}.\psi_j(\mathbf{T})$,
	$\psi_i(D) \equiv \psi_j(D)$ for all $D \neq \mathbf{C}$
Drop-class **C**	$\psi_j(\mathbf{C}) \equiv \bot$, $\psi_i(D) \equiv \psi_j(D)$ for all $D \neq \mathbf{C}$
Change-class-name **C, C′**	$\psi_i(\mathbf{C}) \equiv \psi_j(\mathbf{C}')$, $\psi_i(D) \equiv \psi_j(D)$ for all $D \neq \mathbf{C}, \mathbf{C}'$
Change-class-type **C, T′**	$\psi_j(\mathbf{C}) \equiv \psi_i(\mathbf{C}) \sqcap \forall \mathsf{value}.\psi_j(\mathbf{T}')$,
	$\psi_i(D) \equiv \psi_j(D)$ for all $D \neq \mathbf{C}$
Add-is-a **C, C′**	$\psi_j(\mathbf{C}) \equiv \psi_i(\mathbf{C}) \sqcap \psi_i(\mathbf{C}')$, $\psi_i(D) \equiv \psi_j(D)$ for all $D \neq \mathbf{C}$
Drop-is-a **C, C′**	$\psi_i(\mathbf{C}) \equiv \psi_j(\mathbf{C}) \sqcap \psi_j(\mathbf{C}')$, $\psi_i(D) \equiv \psi_j(D)$ for all $D \neq \mathbf{C}$

Fig. 4. The axioms induced by the schema changes.

- *For each attribute in $\mathcal{A}_S$:*
  $\exists A_i.\top \sqsubseteq \, \leq 1 A_i.\top$
- *For each schema modification $\mathcal{M}_{ij} \in \mathcal{M}_S$ a corresponding axiom from Tab. 4.*

Based on the results of [8], we have proved in [12] that the encoding is correct, in the sense that there is a correspondence between the models of the knowledge base and the legal instances of the evolving schema. The semantic correspondence is exploited to devise a correspondence between reasoning problems at the level of evolving schemata and reasoning problems at the level of the description logic.

Theorem 1. *Given an evolving schema $\mathcal{S}$, the reasoning problems defined in the previous section are all decidable in EXPTIME with a PSPACE lower bound. The reasoning problems can be reduced to corresponding satisfiability problems in the $\mathcal{ALCQI}$ Description Logic.*

Please note that the worst case complexity between PSPACE and EXPTIME does not imply bad practical computational behaviour in the real cases: in fact, a preliminary experimentation with the Description Logic system FaCT [16] shows that reasoning problems in realistic scenarios of evolving schemata are solved very efficiently.

As a final remark, it should be noted that the high expressiveness of the Description Logic constructs can capture an extended version of the presented object-oriented model, at no extra cost with respect to the computational complexity, since the target Description Logic in which the problem is encoded does not change. This includes not only taxonomic relationships, but also arbitrary boolean constructs, inverse attributes, n-ary relationships, and a large class of integrity constraints expressed by means of $\mathcal{ALCQI}$ inclusion dependencies [7]. The last point suggests that axioms modeling schema changes can be freely combined in order to transform a schema in a new one. Some combination can be defined at database level by introducing new non-elementary primitives.

6   Discussion

In this paper we have introduced an approach to schema versioning which considers a (conceptual) schema change as a (logical) schema augmentation, in the sense of [17]. In fact, the sequence of schema versions can be seen as an increasing set of constraints, as defined in Table 1; every elementary schema change introduces new constraints over a vocabulary augmented by the classes for the new version. An update of the schema is also reflected by the introduction of materialised views at the level of the data which specify how to populate the classes of the new version from the data of the previous version. Formally, in our approach the materialised views coexist together with the base data in the same pool of data. In some sense, there is no proper evolution of the objects themselves, since the emphasis is given to the evolution of the schema.

More complex is the case when it is needed that a particular object maintains its identity over different version – i.e., the object evolves by varying its structural properties – and it is requested to have an overview of its evolution over the various versions. This is the case when a query – possibly over more than one conceptual schema – requires an answer about an object from more than one version.

In this case an explicit treatment of the partial order over the schema versions induced by the schema changes is required at the level of the semantics. Formally, this partial order defines some sort of "temporal structure" which leads us to consider the evolving data as a (formal) temporal database with a temporally extended conceptual data model [15, 2]. With such an approach, different formal "timestamps" can be associated with different schema versions: all the objects connected with a schema version are assigned the same timestamp, such that each data pool represents a homogeneous state (snapshot) in the database evolution along the formal time axis[1]. Objects belonging to different versions can be distinguished by means of the object's OID and the timestamp.

In such a framework, the (materialised) views expressing the data conversions can be expressed as temporal queries. In some sense, we can say that such a query language operates in a *schema translation* fashion [9] instead of a schema augmentation, where new data are presumed to be independent of the

---

[1] This case corresponds to the multi-pool solution for temporal schema versioning of snapshot data in the [10] taxonomy.

source data and an explicit mapping between them has to be maintained. Multischema queries can be seen as temporal queries involving in their formulation distinct (formal) timestamps. Moreover, in case (bi)temporal schema versioning is adopted, this "formal" temporal dimension has also interesting and nontrivial connections, which deserve further investigation, with the "real" temporal dimension(s) used for versioning.

7 Conclusions

This paper deals with the support of database schema evolution and versioning by introducing a general framework based on a semantic approach. The reducibility of a general Object- Oriented conceptual model to the proposed framework made it possible to provide a sound foundation for the purposes stated in the Introduction. In particular, the adoption of a Description Logic for the framework specification implies the availability of powerful services (like consistency checking and classification) which can be proved decidable.

References

1. S. Abiteboul and P. Kanellakis. Object identity as a query language primitive. *Journal of the ACM*, 45(5):798–842, 1998. A first version appeared in SIGMOD'89.
2. Alessandro Artale and Enrico Franconi. Temporal ER modeling with description logics. In *Proc. of the International Conference on Conceptual Modeling (ER'99)*. Springer-Verlag, November 1999.
3. J. Banerjee, W. Kim, H.-J. Kim, and H. F. Korth. Semantics and Implementation of Schema Evolution in Object-Oriented Databases. In *Proc. of the ACM-SIGMOD Annual Conference*, pages 311–322, May 1987.
4. S. Bergamaschi and B. Nebel. Automatic Building and Validation of Multiple Inheritance Complex Object Database Schemata. *International Journal of Applied Intelligence*, 4(2):185–204, 1994.
5. P. Brèche. Advanced Principles of Changing Schema of Object Databases. In *Proc. of the 8th Int'l Conf. on Advanced Information Systems Engineering (CAiSE)*, pages 476–495, May 1996.
6. D. Calvanese, G. De Giacomo, M. Lenzerini, and D. Nardi. Reasoning in expressive description logics. In A. Robinson and A. Voronkov, editors, *Handbook of Automated Reasoning*. Elsevier, 2000. To appear.
7. D. Calvanese, M. Lenzerini, and D. Nardi. Description logics for conceptual data modeling. In J. Chomicki and G. Saake, editors, *Logics for Databases and Information Systems*, pages 229–263. Kluwer, 1998.
8. D. Calvanese, M. Lenzerini, and D. Nardi. Unifying class-based representation formalisms. *Journal of Artificial Intelligence Research*, 11:199–240, 1999.
9. Ti-Pin Chang and Richard Hull. Using witness generators to support bi-directional update between object-based databases. In *Proc. of the 1995 ACM SIGACT SIGMOD SIGART Symposium on Principles of Database Systems (PODS'95)*, 1995.
10. C. De Castro, F. Grandi, and M. R. Scalas. Schema Versioning for Multitemporal Relational Databases. *Information Systems*, 22(5):249–290, 1997.

11. F. Ferrandina, T. Meyer, R. Zicari, G. Ferran, and J. Madec. Schema and Database Evolution in the O_2 Object Database System. In *Proc. of the 21st Int'l Conf. on Very Large Databases (VLDB)*, pages 170–181, September 1995.

12. Enrico Franconi, Fabio Grandi, and Federica Mandreoli. A semantic approach for schema evolution and versioning in object-oriented databases. Technical report, Department of Computer Science, University of Manchester, UK, 2000.

13. F. Grandi and F. Mandreoli. ODMG Language Extensions for Generalized Schema Versioning Support. In *Proc. of ECDM'99 Workshop (in conj. with ER)*, November 1999.

14. F. Grandi, F. Mandreoli, and M. R. Scalas. A Generalized Modeling Framework for Schema Versioning Support. In *Proc. of 11th Australasian Database Conference (ADC 2000)*, January 2000.

15. H. Gregersen and C. S. Jensen. Temporal Entity-Relationship Models - A Survey. *IEEE Transaction on Knowledge and Data Engineering*, 11(3):464–497, 1999.

16. I. Horrocks, U. Sattler, and S. Tobies. Practical reasoning for expressive description logics. In *Proc. of the 6th International Conference on Logic for Programming and Automated Reasoning (LPAR'99)*, pages 161–180, 1999.

17. Richard Hull and Masatoshi Yoshikawa. ILOG: Declarative creation and manipulation of object identifiers. In *Proc. of the 16th VLDB Conference*, 1990.

18. C. S. Jensen, J. Clifford, S. K. Gadia, P. Hayes, and S. Jajodia et al. The Consensus Glossary of Temporal Database Concepts - February 1998 Version. In O. Etzion, S. Jajodia, and S. Sripada, editors, *Temporal Databases - Research and Practice*, pages 367–405. Springer-Verlag, 1998. LNCS No. 1399.

19. J-B Lagorce, A. Stockus, and E. Waller. Object-oriented database evolution. In *Proc. of ICDT'97*, 1997.

20. S.-E. Lautemann. A Propagation Mechanism for Populated Schema Versions. In *Proc. of the 13th International Conference on Data Engineering (ICDE)*, pages 67–78, April 1997.

21. D. J. Penney and J. Stein. Class Modification in the GemStone object-oriented DBMS. In *Proc. of the Int'l Conf. on Object-Oriented Programming Systems, Languages, and Applications (OOPSLA)*, pages 111–117, December 1987.

22. R. J. Peters and M. T. Özsu. An Axiomatic Model of Dynamic Schema Evolution in Objectbase Systems. *ACM Transaction on Database Systems*, 22(1):75–114, 1997.

23. J. F. Roddick. A Survey of Schema Versioning Issues for Database Systems. *Information and Software Technology*, 37(7):383–393, 1996.

SLDMagic — The Real Magic
(With Applications to Web Queries)*

Stefan Brass

University of Pittsburgh, Dept. of Information Science and Telecommunications
135 N. Bellefield Ave., Pittsburgh, PA 15260, USA
sbrass@sis.pitt.edu

Abstract. The magic set technique is a standard technique for query evaluation in deductive databases, and its variants are also used in modern commercial database systems like DB2. Numerous improvements of the basic technique have been proposed. However, each of these optimizations makes the transformation more complicated, and combining them in a single system is at least difficult.

In this paper, a new transformation is introduced, which is based on partial evaluation of a bottom-up meta-interpreter for SLD-resolution. In spite of its simplicity, this technique gives us a whole bunch of optimizations for free: For instance, it contains a tail recursion optimization, it transforms non-recursive into non-recursive programs, it can pass arbitary conditions on the parameters to called predicates, and it saves the join necessary to get subquery results back into the calling context. In this way, it helps to integrate many of the previous efforts.

The usefulness of these optimizations is illustrated with example programs querying the World Wide Web.

1   Introduction

Many current developments aim at integrated systems consisting of a programming language and a database management system. For instance, object-oriented database systems combine both functionalities, but also stored procedures and triggers in relational systems go into this direction. Deductive databases offered such an integrated language for a long time. Theoretically, this is very appealing since here a declarative language is also used for the programming part. Declarativity has proven to be very useful in SQL.

Deductive database systems have also become interesting again because they are well suited to process graph-structured data, and the World Wide Web can be seen as a large directed graph of interconnected documents. This view of the WWW is the basis of web query languages, e.g. [KS95,MMM97,HLLS97]. Also, recently proposed data models for semi-structured data and XML [ABS00] as well as the RDF model for Web metadata are graph-structured.

---

* This paper is a completely rewritten and significantly extended version of a paper which appeared in the electronic proceedings of the International Workshop on "Advances in Databases and Information Systems", Moscow, 1996.

J. Lloyd et al. (Eds.): CL 2000, LNAI 1861, pp. 1063–1077, 2000.
© Springer-Verlag Berlin Heidelberg 2000

One of the biggest problems of deductive databases is still the performance, which is quite far behind other integrated DB/PL systems. It is known that "Bottom-Up [evaluation with magic sets] Beats Top-Down for Datalog" [Ull89a]. However, as noted by Ross [Ros91] (see also [Ull89a]), this does not mean that current deductive databases are at least as efficient as Prolog implementations. This is not even true asymptotically (in O-notation). So let us quickly explain the main difference between magic sets and SLD-resolution (which is the basis of Prolog evaluation). Although both are top-down evaluation methods, and in fact equally goal-directed (see, e.g., [Bra95]), there are important differences.

The magic set method treats predicates (views) like procedures, which are called with a set of bindings for the input (bound) arguments. This input relation is the so-called "magic set". They return a relation for all arguments, such that every returned tuple agrees with one input tuple in the bound arguments. So the result is the semijoin of the magic set and the full extension of the predicate. Of course, the trick is to avoid computing this full extension.

For instance, consider a predicate local_link(From_URL, To_URL, Label) which returns links in the web page From_URL refering to a page To_URL on the same server. An invocation with the first argument bound could look as follows:

From_URL	local_link	From_URL	To_URL	Label
`http://x.edu/`	$\longrightarrow$	`http://x.edu/`	`http://x.edu/a`	...
`http://y.edu/`		`http://x.edu/`	`http://x.edu/b`	...
		`http://y.edu/`	`http://y.edu/c`	...

In contrast, SLD-resolution works by repeatedly "unfolding" query literals — it replaces the predicate call by the predicate definition. This is what many relational database systems do with view definitions, but in SLD-resolution this is the only computation mechanism and works also with recursive views. Let local_link be defined as follows:

local_link(From_URL, To_URL, Label) ← link(From_URL, To_URL, Label) ∧
                                       same_server(From_URL, To_URL).

Furthermore, let the query be

local_link('http://www.pitt.edu', URL, Label) ∧
like(Label, '%Inf%Sc%').

SLD-resolution replaces this query by

link('http://www.pitt.edu', URL, Label) ∧
same_server('http://www.pitt.edu', URL) ∧
like(Label, '%Inf%Sc%').

In SLD-resolution, there is no explicit procedure call and return. Instead, we always work on complete continuations of the computation. Even if we should choose to evaluate next the calls to link and same_server, the control passes then immediately to like without entering the rule for local_link again. This is essential for tail recursions. Furthermore, we can choose a different evaluation sequence, for instance evaluate the call to like before the call to same_server. This gives us a much bigger optimization potential than the sideways information passing rule of magic sets, which can only locally reorder the body literals within a rule (or decide not to use all available bindings)[1].

Of course, SLD-resolution also has its problems, the most important being the possibility of non-termination. There are tabulation techniques which avoid this [SSW94], but these are essentially equivalent the magic set method. In this paper, we present a new method to combine advantages of bottom-up evaluation and SLD-resolution. The title says that this is the "real magic", because we believe that it was from the beginning the goal of the magic set transformation to combine bottom-up evaluation with Prolog evaluation (i.e. SLD-resolution).

Deductive databases are normally applied when there are large sets of facts which Prolog implementations cannot handle. While we do SLD-resolution as Prolog, we execute it on a bottom-up machine using set-oriented evaluation techniques. Whereas Prolog always does nested loop joins, we can apply merge-joins or hash-joins. Also, we will see that the SLD-resolution selection function, which is not used in Prolog, can be an important means for query optimization.

Our approach is based on the idea of partially evaluating a meta-interpreter. BRY has done this for the standard magic set technique [Bry90], we only start with another meta-interpreter and do a bit more involved partial evaluation. It is fascinating how many optimizations we get for free based on this idea. Such optimizations are known for the magic set method [MFPR90,Ros91,GM92], but integrating them in a single system is at least hard work.

2   Problems of Magic Set Query Evaluation

Let us consider some examples which demonstrate weak points of the standard magic set technique. We will see that an approach based on SLD-resolution can avoid these problems. Specialized solutions to most of these shortcomings have already been developed. Our contribution is an integrated approach which solves all of these problems (and is actually quite simple).

2.1   Tail Recursions

It is a standard task to find all documents which are reachable from a given document via local links (i.e. links refering to documents on the same server). In order to do this, we first define a predicate for the transitive closure (corresponding to $\longrightarrow^*$ in WebSQL [MMM97]):

local_reachable$(X, Y) \leftarrow$ local_link$(X, Y, \_)$.
local_reachable$(X, Z) \leftarrow$ local_link$(X, Y, \_) \wedge$ local_reachable(Y, Z).

---

[1] "Informally, for a rule of a program, a sip represents a decision about the order in which predicates of the rule will be evaluated, and how values for variables are passed from predicates to other predicates during evaluation." [BR91]

Then we can call this predicate with the given start document, say d_0:

$$\mathsf{local\_reachable}(d_0, D).$$

To keep the example simple, let us consider the following hypertext structure:

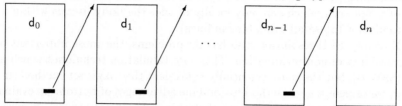

However, the same problem appears when we have additional links, and this path is only a subgraph. Actually, we could have used any reasonable connection of $n + 1$ pages (e.g. a star topology with backlinks).

In order to solve the task, we must only follow the links and output every page we reach. Thus a complexity of $O(n)$ seems reasonable, or $O(n * \log(n))$, if we check for cycles due to backlinks. But if we use the magic set technique in this example, the complexity is at least $O(n^2)$. The reason is that this method explicitly represents the results of subqueries. We start with the call $\mathsf{local\_reachable}(d_0, D)$, but since there is a link to page d_1, we get the recursive call $\mathsf{local\_reachable}(d_1, D)$, and so on, for any page of the chain. For each such subquery, the magic set method computes all matching facts which follow from the original program. So we not only get $\mathsf{local\_reachable}(d_0, d_1), \ldots, \mathsf{local\_reachable}(d_0, d_n)$, but also $\mathsf{local\_reachable}(d_1, d_2)$, and so on. This is a quadratic number of facts, thus the complexity is at least $O(n^2)$, and probably higher due to join computations and duplicate eliminations.

In contrast, Prolog can process this example in linear time, and this can be understood without looking inside Prolog implementations. The tree of goals (queries) created by SLD-resolution for the above program and data (including the rule for $\mathsf{local\_link}$) contains $8n + 5$ nodes, and all nodes have ≤ 3 literals.

However, SLD-resolution will not terminate for cyclic hypertext graphs. But our method of evaluating SLD-resolution bottom-up will compute only a finite number of SLD-goals, and does so in the required time $O(n * \log(n))$. In contrast, previous tabulation methods for making SLD-resolution terminate, such as those used in the XSB-system [SSW94], have the same problem as magic sets: They store proven instances of literals in a table, which is already a quadratic number.

The magic set method with tail-recursion optimization developed in [Ros91] and further analyzed in [RS91,SR93] solves the problem. There are also methods for more specific kinds of tail-recursions [NRSU89,Ull89b,KRS90]. However, our method contains such optimizations, and solves many other problems as well.

Current query languages for the web, semistructured data, and XML typically contain path expressions for following edges in the graph. There are specialized algorithms for evaluating these expressions which of course do not have this problem. While path expressions work well for XML, retrieving a page on the web is an expensive operation, so we might need the full power of Datalog to describe as precisely as possible which links we want to follow.

2.2   Nonrecursive Programs

The following predicate computes pages reachable via at most two local links:

$$\text{reach2}(X, Y) \leftarrow \text{local\_link}(X, Y, \_).$$
$$\text{reach2}(X, Z) \leftarrow \text{local\_link}(X, Y, \_) \wedge \text{local\_link}(Y, Z, \_).$$

The program is non-recursive and should be easy to evaluate. However, if we use the magic set technique for the query $\text{reach2}(d_0, D)$, we get a recursive program. The reason for this problem is that the magic set technique collects all calls to a predicate (with the same "binding pattern") into a single magic predicate. But here, due to the second rule for reach2, the queries for local_link (in the second body literal) depend on solutions for local_link (in the first body literal). And of course, solutions for a predicate always depend conversely on the queries.

In contrast, SLD-resolution treats the two calls to local_link separately, and thus the problem does not occur. Of course, merging calls sometimes can be advantageous, if this helps to avoid recomputations. Therefore our method can be parameterized in such a way that for every body literal either magic sets or SLD-resolution can be chosen.

The methods of [GM92] ensure that non-recursive programs are transformed into non-recursive programs. The basic approach is also to distinguish the two calls. In one of their solutions, they also do some unfolding, and add a "covered subgoal elimination" which we do not (yet) have. Again, the strength of our solution is that it solves different problems at the same time.

2.3   Getting Results Back into the Context of the Caller

Suppose we have a relation my_links(URL, Last_Visited) in which we store our personal collection of most interesting web pages. It is the combination of such local information with a web interface which makes web query languages a useful and powerful tool. Now the following predicate returns those pages which have changed since the time of last visit:

$$\text{has\_changed}(URL) \leftarrow \text{my\_links}(URL, Last\_Visited) \wedge$$
$$\text{doc\_mtime}(URL, Modif) \wedge$$
$$Modif > Last\_Visited.$$

When has_changed is called with URL free, the magic set method will evaluate the body literals in the given sequence. So it first accesses the relation my_links. This gives bindings for the two variables URL and Last_Visited. Let us assume that doc_mtime is also an IDB-predicate:

$$\text{doc\_mtime}(URL, Modif) \leftarrow \text{www\_get}(URL, Title, Modif, Contents).$$

Then a magic set for doc_mtime is constructed by projecting the bindings for URL and Last_Visited on the variable URL. The predicate doc_mtime returns bindings for URL and Modif. But in the context of the calling rule, all three variables URL,

$$\text{my\_links(URL, Last\_Visited)} \land \text{doc\_mtime(URL, Modif)} \land \text{Modif} > \text{Last\_Visited}$$

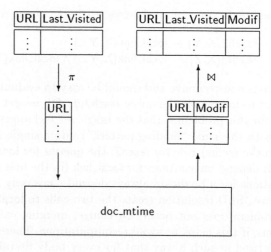

Fig. 1. Projection and Join During Magic Set Evaluation

Last_Visited, and Modif are bound, and all three variables are still needed. Thus, the two relations must be joined on the attribute URL (see Figure 1).

Since a join is expensive, it would have been better not to project the variable Last_Visited away. SLD-resolution always retains the complete bindings for all variables which are still needed: The goals in the SLD tree contain the full continuation of the computation.

Magic sets with supplementary predicates do not solve this problem. This method reduces unnecessary recomputations while evaluating a single rule, but does not change the arguments of the IDB-predicates, as would be required here.

Magic sets could be advantageous to SLD-resolution if e.g. my_links would produce several solutions for a single URL (In the given example, this cannot happen because URL is key). Then the projection could do a duplicate elimination and thereby reduce the input to doc_mtime.

2.4 Passing Conditions on the Parameters to Called Predicates

Suppose that we are again interested in pages from our hotlist which were modified since our last visit, but only from a specific server. Then we use the query

$$\text{has\_changed(URL)} \land \text{on\_server(URL, 'www.sis.pitt.edu')}.$$

Consider now the evaluation of has_changed: While my_links is a locally stored relation, the call to the WWW-interface predicate doc_mtime is very expensive: We have to fetch each page under all URLs stored in my_links, and only later throw out all pages which are not on the given server.

The problem here is that for the magic set technique, the structure of the program in predicates is significant: The "sideways information passing" strategy cannot move literals between predicate boundaries. However, in this case, the optimal sequence would be

$$my\_links(URL, Last\_Visited) \land$$
$$on\_server(URL, 'www.sis.pitt.edu') \land$$
$$doc\_mtime(URL, Modif) \land$$
$$Modif > Last\_Visited.$$

The literals on_server(URL, 'www.sis.pitt.edu') and Modif > Last_Visited are very cheap to evaluate, however, they can only be evaluated after their arguments are bound. And of course, we should try to "fail as early as you can", at least before very expensive literals are evaluated. This corresponds to the classical optimization strategy to push selections as far "down" as possible, and especially evaluate them before expensive joins.

The magic set technique can pass only conditions of the form $X = const$ on the parameters to the called predicates. The rectification transformation [Ull89b] was invented to handle conditions of the form $X = Y$. The technique of [MFPR90] can pass conditions of the form $X < const$. Our method inherits from SLD-resolution the possibility to evaluate arbitrary conditions of the parameters as soon as they become bound. In SLD-resolution this kind of "global optimization" is done by means of the selection function: It decides which literal from the continuation should be evaluated next. In this way, it considerably generalizes the magic set SIP-strategy (at least the reordering part. The SIP-strategy also can decide to use only a subset of the available bindings.)

While we reach the same optimization as [MFPR90], the method of [SR92] has features which would have to be added to our approach. It can move linear arithmetic constraints both from the uses of a predicate into its rules as well as from the definitions towards its uses. Our method breaks up the rule structure so that constraints to be satisfied are visible when we evaluate a predicate. However, it evaluates them only as soon as the become bound, we do not yet check the constraints for consistency. We also do not generate constraints for predicates which would help to detect inconsistencies earlier. On the other hand, our method is not limited to any particular type of constraints. Any predicate which can be evaluated cheaply can act as a constraint.

2.5 Combining Conditions for Index Access

This greater flexibility in the evaluation order is also important for index structures which can evaluate conjunctions of literals. For instance, when we submit a query to a search engine, we should first collect all literals specifying search terms for the same document.

Suppose we have defined a predicate containing the URLs of possible job offers in the Web:

$$job\_offer(URL) \leftarrow keyword('Job\ Opportunity', URL).$$
$$job\_offer(URL) \leftarrow keyword('Free\ Positions', URL).$$

Here the predicate keyword gives access to a search engine. While this particular definition of the predicate job_offer is very naive, such predicates can be used to represent knowledge about searching in the WWW. The possibility to reuse and share such knowledge is an important issue for future web querying systems.

Now suppose that we are interested only in job offers mentioning "Prolog":

$$\text{job\_offer}(\text{URL}) \wedge \text{keyword}('\text{Prolog}', \text{URL}).$$

Then it might be important that when we evaluate the call to job_offer, we already see that there is another call to the predicate keyword. It will certainly be better to combine the search terms, and not to collect first all job offers and then to select those mentioning "Prolog".

In general, index structures often allow to evaluate conjunctions of literals at once. Even a classical B-tree over e.g. the attribute Sal of the relation emp allows us to evaluate a conjunction like $\text{emp}(X, Y, \text{Sal}) \wedge \text{Sal} \geq 1000 \wedge \text{Sal} \leq 1500$ in one shot. However, in the source program, these conditions might not be contained in the same rule. Therefore, good query optimization needs the unfolding power of SLD-resolution.

It is sometimes assumed that standard relational query optimization can be done after the magic-set transformation. In our view, this is an error. The result of the transformation prescribes more or less the evaluation order. So many physical parameters (such as the existence of indexes) must already be taken into account when the transformation is done.

3   The Meta-interpreter

Often, an evaluation method can be explained by presenting an interpreter for it. If this interpreter is written in the language itself, it is called a meta-interpreter. It is a standard exercise in Prolog programming courses to write an interpreter for Prolog in Prolog. However, BRY clarified in [Bry90] that such interpreters depend heavily on the machine model used to execute them. While the standard meta-interpreter runs only on Prolog, BRY developed a meta-interpreter which formalized top-down evaluation, but run itself on a bottom-up machine. He used explicit call and return, and in this way reconstructed the standard magic set transformation. So all we have to do now is to start with a meta-interpreter which describes real SLD-resolution.

3.1   Bottom-Up Execution of SLD-Resolution

We present SLD-goals (nodes of the SLD-tree) by lists of literals which still have to be proven. For instance, the query local_reachable(d_0, D) gives the root node of the SLD-tree:

$$\text{node}\big([\text{local\_reachable}(d_0, D)]\big).$$

The rules of the given program are stored in the form rule(Head, Body), e.g.

$$\text{rule}\big(\text{local\_reachable}(X, Z), [\text{local\_link}(X, Y, \_), \text{local\_reachable}(Y, Z)]\big).$$

Now the SLD-resolution step can be described by means of the following main rule of our meta-interpreter (for simplicity, we have chosen here the "first literal" selection function of Prolog):

$$\text{node}(\text{Child}) \leftarrow$$
$$\text{node}([\text{Lit}|\text{Rest}]) \wedge$$
$$\text{rule}(\text{Lit}, \text{Body}) \wedge$$
$$\text{append}(\text{Body}, \text{Rest}, \text{Child}).$$

Our meta-interpreter will be evaluated bottom-up, so you have to read the rule from right to left: If we insert, e.g., the above node- and rule-facts, we will derive the following node-fact:

$$\text{node}\big([\text{local\_link}(d_0, Y, \_), \text{local\_reachable}(Y, D)]\big).$$

Bottom-up evaluation with non-ground facts does the necessary unification, and renames the variables of the used "facts" before that in order to avoid name clashes. In addition, it treats derived facts as duplicates if they differ only by a variable renaming from known facts. This is important for the termination and can be easily achieved by normalizing variable names (e.g. $X_1, X_2, \ldots$).

There is the small problem that in this way it is difficult to track the binding for the answer variable D. When all literals are proven, we get the empty goal $\text{node}([])$, but the answer substitution is lost. We solve this problem by adding to each derived node-fact the current instance of the query. This will be the first argument of the predicate node, the second argument will be the current goal as above. So instead of the above node-fact we really derive

$$\text{node}\big(\text{local\_reachable}(d_0, D), [\text{local\_link}(d_0, Y, \_), \text{local\_reachable}(Y, D)]\big).$$

This is similar to a rule where the head always remains an instance of the query and we iteratively unfold the body. Since the substitutions are also applied to the first argument, it contains the proven query instance as soon as the goal becomes empty:

$$\text{node}\big(\text{local\_reachable}(d_0, d_2), []\big).$$

The complete meta-interpreter is shown in Figure 2. We assume there that EDB-facts from the database are stored in the predicate db. The distinction between program rules with empty bodies and database facts becomes relevant only later when we do partial evaluation. For simplicity, we assume that the query is a single literal stored in the predicate query. The meta-interpreter can be executed by deductive database systems like CORAL [RSSS94] which allow structured terms and non-ground facts.

Theorem 1 (Relation to SLD-Resolution). *Let the above meta-interpreter be executed on* rule, db, *and* query-*facts corresponding to a program* P, *database* DB, *and query* Q. *Then it computes the goals in the SLD-tree for* $P \cup DB \cup \{\leftarrow Q\}$:

- *For every node* $\mathcal{N}$ *in the SLD-tree with goal* $\leftarrow A_1 \wedge \cdots \wedge A_n$, *there is a fact* $\text{node}\big(Q\theta, [A'_1, \ldots, A'_n]\big)$ *which is derivable from the meta-interpreter and a*

```
/* Initialization (Root Node): */
node(Query, [Query]) ←
    query(Query).

/* SLD-Resolution: */
node(Query, Child) ←
    node(Query, [Lit|Rest]) ∧
    rule(Lit, Body) ∧
    append(Body, Rest, Child).

/* Evaluation of DB-Literal: */
node(Query, Rest) ←
    node(Query, [Lit|Rest]) ∧
    db(Lit).

/* Turn Proven Query into Answer: */
answer(Query) ←
    node(Query, []).
```

Fig. 2. Bottom-Up Meta-Interpreter for SLD-Resolution

variable-renaming σ *such that* $A'_i\sigma = A_i$, $i = 1, \ldots, n$, *and* $Q\theta\sigma$ *is the result of applying to the query all most general unifiers which SLD-resolution used on the way from the root node to* $\mathcal{N}$.

- *And vice versa, every derivable fact corresponds in this way to (at least) one node in the SLD-tree.*

From the soundness and completeness of SLD-resolution, we directly get the following corollary:

Theorem 2 (Soundness and Completeness). *Let the meta-interpreter be executed on* rule, db, *and* query-*facts corresponding to a program* P, *database* DB, *and query* Q.

- *For every derived fact* answer($Q\theta$), *the substitution* θ *is a correct answer substitution.*
- *For every correct answer substitution* θ, *there is a derived fact* answer($Q\theta'$) *and a substitution* σ *with* $\theta = \theta'\sigma$.

3.2 Termination

So our meta-interpreter correctly simulates SLD-resolution. As explained in Section 2, this is advantageous for many applications. But do we get in exchange for these advantages also the problem of possible non-termination? The answer is: Often not. Since we do not compute the nodes themselves, but only the goals attached to them, the termination behaviour is better than that of SLD-resolution. For instance, the rule $p(X) \leftarrow p(X)$ poses no problem at all, since it does not yield new goals. In general, we can guarantee the termination for all tail-recursive Datalog-programs using only finite database predicates. We do not suggest to simulate SLD-resolution for predicates with other kinds of recursions. For such programs, we will later present a combined method which allows to use the "magic set" behaviour (tabulation) for calling some literals.

Definition 1 (Tail-Recursive Program). *A program is at most tail-recursive iff for every rule*

$$A \leftarrow B_1 \wedge \cdots \wedge B_m,$$

the predicates of B_i, $1 \leq i \leq m-1$, do not depend on the predicate of A, i.e. no body literal except possibly the last is recursive.

Note that this class of programs is larger than the class for which the "right recursion optimization" of [Ull89b] is applicable. Most practical programs are covered. The condition ensures that the number of literals in SLD-goals is bounded (assuming the left-to-right selection function).

Theorem 3 (Sufficient Condition for Termination). *Let P be an at most tail-recursive program, DB a database, and Q be a query such that $P \cup DB \cup \{\leftarrow Q\}$ is finite and does not contain structured terms. Then the bottom-up evaluation of the above meta-interpreter terminates, i.e. there are only finitely many facts derivable from it (modulo variable renamings).*

3.3 Adding "Magic Set" Behaviour

Because of the problems with general recursive calls, we might be interested to evaluate such literals with the magic set technique. Also, the strength of magic sets is that every predicate is evaluated only once for the same input values. While often the behaviour of SLD-resolution is better, we sometimes might want to table calls and computed results in order to avoid unnecessary recomputations. Fortunately, it is easy to extend the meta-interpreter in such a way that we can choose for every body literal whether it should be evaluated via SLD-resolution or via magic sets.

Let us enclose body literals intended for magic set evaluation into the special predicate call. Then it suffices to add the two rules in Figure 3 to our meta-interpreter. The idea is that we allow SLD-resolution to call itself recursively for evaluating certain literals (like standard SLD-resolution does for negative literals). So we now construct not a single SLD-tree, but one for each recursive call. This explict call and return is the key to understanding the difference between magic sets and SLD-resolution. One can view the two rules also as describing SLD-resolution with tabulation: The first rule enters a predicate call into a table, and the second rule takes solutions from a table in order to solve this literal.

If all IDB-literals are evaluated in subproofs, we get something very similar to magic sets with supplementary predicates: The query-facts correspond to magic facts, answer-facts correspond to derived IDB-facts, and node-facts correspond to facts of the supplementary predicates.

```
/* Set Up Recursive Call (Derive Magic Fact): */
query(Lit) ←
        node(_, [call(Lit)|_]).

/* Get Result of Recursive Call: */
node(Query, Rest) ←
        node(Query, [call(Lit)|Rest]) ∧
        answer(Lit).
```

Fig. 3. Additional Meta-Interpreter Rules for "Magic Set" Behaviour

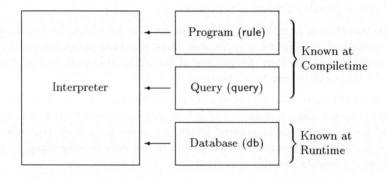

Fig. 4. Inputs of the Meta-Interpreter

4   Partial Evaluation

While the above meta-interpreter can be directly executed (e.g. on CORAL), the use of lists and non-ground facts significantly decreases the performance. It is well known that from an interpreter, one can get a compiler via partial evaluation. Such a compiler will transform a program intended for SLD-evaluation into a program which runs on a bottom-up machine. For BRY's meta-interpreter, it was sufficient to unfold the call to the predicate rule. In our case, partial evaluation becomes a bit more complicated. There are a number of papers which investigate partial evaluation for Prolog (i.e. top-down evaluation), but partial evaluation for bottom-up execution seems to be a new problem.

Our task is to evaluate the meta-interpreter as far as possible, given program and query, but with a yet unknown database (see Figure 4). Especially, we should try to avoid using lists and non-ground facts. This is feasible, since the number of literals in node-facts is bounded as long as the program is at most tail-recursive or other recursions are evaluated via call.

Our main idea is to use conditional facts of the form A ← B to separate what is known at compile-time (A) from what is only at runtime (B). For instance, we might know at compilation time that we can derive facts of the form

$$\mathsf{node}\big(\mathsf{local\_reachable}(\mathsf{d}_0, \mathsf{D}),\ [\mathsf{local\_reachable}(\mathsf{d}, \mathsf{D})]\big).$$

This corresponds to the situation that we have followed links from the start page d_0 to some page d, and therefore any page D reachable from d is also reachable from d_0. Of course, the possible values for d depend on the data, and are not yet known at compile time. So we would encode this knowledge as

$$\mathsf{node}\big(\mathsf{local\_reachable}(\mathsf{d}_0, \mathsf{D}),\ [\mathsf{local\_reachable}(\mathsf{X}, \mathsf{D})]\big) \leftarrow \mathsf{p}(\mathsf{X})$$

where p is a new predicate used for the runtime computations.

Let us now explain the partial evaluation in more detail. Basically, we do a standard bottom-up fixpoint computation, but we work now with conditional facts. So we have a set COND of conditional facts which will increase until a fixpoint is reached. An important invariance is that COND will never contain two different conditional facts with the same predicate p in the body. In this way, we can translate facts produced later at runtime (e.g. $\mathsf{p}(\mathsf{d})$) uniquely back to facts of the original program.

We start with the following facts COND (if we want to partially evaluate our meta-interpreter):

- $\mathsf{db}\big(\mathsf{p}(\mathsf{X}_1, \ldots, \mathsf{X}_n)\big) \leftarrow \mathsf{p}(\mathsf{X}_1, \ldots, \mathsf{X}_n)$ for every EDB-predicate p. Actually, if there are certain small lookup-tables which seldom change, we might be allowed to compile them into our program. In this case we would have a conditional fact $\mathsf{db}\big(\mathsf{p}(\mathsf{c}_1, \ldots, \mathsf{c}_n)\big) \leftarrow \mathsf{true}$ for every row $(\mathsf{c}_1, \ldots, \mathsf{c}_n)$ in the lookup-table.
- $\mathsf{query}(\mathsf{Query}) \leftarrow \mathsf{true}$ for the given query literal Query. If we want to run the query repeatedly with different constants, we can replace them by variables $\mathsf{X}_1, \ldots, \mathsf{X}_n$ and start with $\mathsf{query}(\mathsf{Query}) \leftarrow \mathsf{p}(\mathsf{X}_1, \ldots, \mathsf{X}_n)$ instead. When the constants are known at runtime, we would add the corresponding p-fact.
- $\mathsf{rule}\big(\mathsf{A}, [\mathsf{B}_1, \ldots, \mathsf{B}_m]\big) \leftarrow \mathsf{true}$ for each rule $\mathsf{A} \leftarrow \mathsf{B}_1, \ldots, \mathsf{B}_m$ in the given input program.

In addition we have a set PROG of program rules which are the result of the partial evaluation. The set PROG starts out empty.

Now let $\mathsf{A} \leftarrow \mathsf{B}_1, \ldots, \mathsf{B}_m$ be a rule of our meta-interpreter (or whatever program we want to partially evaluate). We choose conditional facts $\mathsf{B}_i' \leftarrow \mathsf{C}_i$ from COND (but with fresh variables) such that there is an mgu θ of $(\mathsf{B}_1, \ldots, \mathsf{B}_m)$ and $(\mathsf{B}_1', \ldots, \mathsf{B}_m')$. Then the result of the unfolding with respect to the given conditional facts is

$$\mathsf{A}\theta \leftarrow \mathsf{C}_1\theta \wedge \cdots \wedge \mathsf{C}_m\theta.$$

Now the body is already in the right form, but we want to encode also the head via a conditional fact. Let $\mathsf{Y}_1, \ldots, \mathsf{Y}_n$ be those variables which appear in $\mathsf{A}\theta$ and in at least one of the $\mathsf{C}_i\theta$. Then we search COND for a conditional fact of the form $\mathsf{A}\theta \leftarrow \mathsf{p}(\mathsf{Y}_1, \ldots, \mathsf{Y}_n)$ (with any predicate p and the variables possibly renamed). If there is none, we insert this conditional fact with a new predicate p

into COND. Finally, we add the rule $p(Y_1, \ldots, Y_n) \leftarrow C_1\theta \wedge \cdots \wedge C_m\theta$ to PROG. Of course, duplicate elimination is needed here: We normalize the variables in such a way that we do not get two rules in COND or PROG which differ only in a renaming of variables.

Some body literals (like the call to append) can already be evaluated fully at compile-time, so there is no need for a matching fact pattern.

When a fixpoint is reached, PROG is the result of the partial evaluation. Each fact derivable from PROG can be translated back into the syntax of the original program by a unique rule from COND.

In the special case of the meta-interpreter, we can guarantee that partial evaluation terminates under the above conditions (all recursions other than tail-recursions are evaluated via call, the input program contains no structured terms, program and database are finite). We also can handle structured terms at least when we move them into the conditional fact bodies which are evaluated at runtime. More research is needed for deciding which function symbols can in general be evaluated during partial evaluation.

5   Conclusions

SQL-3 contains recursion, and current applications like web queries really need it. The main techniques for evaluating recursion are magic sets (with many variants) and SLD-resolution (used in Prolog). In this paper, we have clarified the differences between these two techniques. We have shown that SLD-resolution is often advantageous, and that SLD-resolution can be evaluated in a set-oriented fashion using database techniques. A first prototype implementation of the transformation is available from http://www2.sis.pitt.edu/~sbrass/sldmagic/.

It seems that for future performance improvements, we have to look more at the internal data structures. Especially, we want to avoid copying variable values. Our goal is to reach the performance of Prolog systems. This also needs a powerful program analysis to avoid duplicate eliminations.

For simplicity, we have considered only negation-free programs. Adding stratified negation is not difficult, although some care has to be taken to make the output stratified. We are currently working on using our ideas from [BD99,ZBF97] to handle general negation.

References

[ABS00]   S. Abiteboul, P. Bunemann, D. Suciu (eds.): *Data on the Web: From Relations to Semistructured Data and XML*. Morgan Kaufmann, 2000.

[BD99]   S. Brass, J. Dix: Semantics of (disjunctive) logic programs based on partial evaluation. *The Journal of Logic Programming 40 (1999)*, 1–46.

[BR91]   C. Beeri, R. Ramakrishnan: On the power of magic. *The Journal of Logic Programming 10 (1991)*, 255–299.

[Bra95]   S. Brass: Magic sets vs. SLD-resolution. In J. Eder, L. A. Kalinichenko (eds.), *Advances in Databases and Information Systems (ADBIS'95)*, 185–203, Springer, 1995.

[Bry90]   F. Bry: Query evaluation in recursive databases: bottom-up and top-down
            reconciled. *Data & Knowledge Engineering 5 (1990)*, 289–312.

[GM92]   A. Gupta, I. S. Mumick: Magic-sets transformation in nonrecursive systems.
            In *Proc. of the Eleventh ACM SIGACT-SIGMOD-SIGART Symposium on
            Principles of Database Systems (PODS'92)*, 354–367, 1992.

[HLLS97]   R. Himmeröder, G. Lausen, B. Ludäscher, C. Schlepphorst: On a declarative
            semantics for web queries. In *Fifth International Conference on Deductive
            and Object-Oriented Databases (DOOD'97)*, 1997.

[KRS90]   D. B. Kemp, K. Ramamohanarao, Z. Somogyi: Right-, left- and multi-linear
            rule transformations that maintain context information. In D. McLeod,
            R. Sacks-Davis, H. Schek (eds.), *Proc. Very Large Data Bases, 16th
            Int. Conf. (VLDB'90)*, 380–391, Morgan Kaufmann Publishers, 1990.

[KS95]   D. Konopnicki, O. Shmueli: W3QS: A query system for the world-wide web.
            In U. Dayal, P. M. D. Gray, S. Nishio (eds.), *Proc. of the 21st Int. Conf. on
            Very Large Data Bases, (VLDB'95)*, 54–65, Morgan Kaufmann, 1995.

[MFPR90]   I. S. Mumick, S. J. Finkelstein, H. Pirahesh, R. Ramakrishnan: Magic
            conditions. In *Proc. of the Ninth ACM SIGACT-SIGMOD-SIGART Sym-
            posium on Principles of Database Systems (PODS'90)*, 314–330, 1990.

[MMM97]   A. O. Mendelzon, G. Mihaila, T. Milo: Querying the world wide web.
            Journal of Digital Libraries 1 (1997), 68–88.

[NRSU89]   J. F. Naughton, R. Ramakrishnan, Y. Sagiv, J. D. Ullman: Efficient evalu-
            ation of right-, left-, and multi-linear rules. In *Proceedings of the 1989 ACM
            SIGMOD International Conference on Management of Data*, 235–242, 1989.

[Ros91]   K. A. Ross: Modular acyclicity and tail recursion in logic programs. In
            *Proc. of the Tenth ACM SIGACT-SIGMOD-SIGART Symp. on Princ. of
            Database Systems (PODS'91)*, 92–101, 1991.

[RS91]   R. Ramakrishnan, S. Sudarshan: Top-down vs. bottom-up revisited. In
            V. Saraswat, K. Ueda (eds.), *Proc. of the 1991 Int. Symposium on Logic
            Programming*, 321–336, MIT Press, 1991.

[RSSS94]   R. Ramakrishnan, D. Srivastava, S. Sudarshan, P. Seshadri: The CORAL
            deductive system. *The VLDB Journal 3 (1994)*, 161–210.

[SR92]   D. Srivastava, R. Ramakrishnan: Pushing constraint selections. In *Proc. of
            the Eleventh ACM SIGACT-SIGMOD-SIGART Symposium on Principles
            of Database Systems (PODS'92)*, 301–315, 1992.

[SR93]   S. Sudarshan, R. Ramakrishnan: Optimizations of bottom-up evaluation
            with non-ground terms. In D. Miller (ed.), *Proceedings of the International
            Logic Programming Symposium (ILPS'93)*, 557–574, MIT Press, 1993.

[SSW94]   K. Sagonas, T. Swift, D. S. Warren: XSB as an efficient deductive database
            engine. In R. T. Snodgrass, M. Winslett (eds.), *Proc. of the 1994 ACM
            SIGMOD Int. Conf. on Management of Data (SIGMOD'94)*, 442–453, 1994.

[Ull89a]   J. D. Ullman: Bottom-up beats top-down for Datalog. In *Proc. of the Eighth
            ACM SIGACT-SIGMOD-SIGART Symposium on Principles of Database
            Systems (PODS'89)*, 140–149, 1989.

[Ull89b]   J. D. Ullman: *Principles of Database and Knowledge-Base Systems, Vol. 2.*
            Computer Science Press, 1989.

[ZBF97]   U. Zukowski, S. Brass, B. Freitag: Improving the alternating fixpoint: The
            transformation approach. In A. Nerode (ed.), *Proc. of the 4th Int. Conf.
            on Logic Programming and Non-Monotonic Reasoning (LPNMR'97)*, 40–59,
            LNAI 1265, Springer, 1997.

FLORA: Implementing an Efficient DOOD System Using a Tabling Logic Engine*

Guizhen Yang and Michael Kifer

Department of Computer Science, SUNY at Stony Brook
Stony Brook, NY 11794, U.S.A.
{guizyang,kifer}@CS.SunySB.EDU

Abstract. This paper reports on the design and implementation of FLORA — a powerful DOOD system that incorporates the features of F-logic, HiLog, and Transaction Logic. FLORA is implemented by translation into XSB, a tabling logic engine that is known for its efficiency and is the only known system that extends the power of Prolog with an equivalent of the Magic Sets style optimization, the well-founded semantics for negation, and many other important features. We discuss the features of XSB that help our effort as well as the areas where it falls short of what is needed. We then describe our solutions and optimization techniques that address these problems and make FLORA much more efficient than other known DOOD systems based on F-logic.

1 Introduction

Deductive object-oriented databases (abbr. DOOD) attracted much attention in early 1990's but difficulties in realizing these ideas and performance problems had dampened the initial enthusiasm. Nevertheless, the second half of the last decade witnessed several experimental systems [33, 19, 2, 23, 16, 26]. They, along with the proliferation of the Web and many recent developments, such as the RDF[1] standard, have fueled renewed interest in DOOD systems; in particular, systems for logic-based processing of object-oriented meta-data [15, 17, 27, 4, 5]. Also, a new field — processing of semistructured data — is emerging to address a specialized segment of the research on DOOD systems [1].

In this paper, we report our work on FLORA, a *practical* DOOD system that has already been successfully used to build a number of sophisticated Web-based information systems, as reported in [13, 18, 25]. By "practical" we mean a DOOD system that has high expressive power, is built on strong theoretical foundations and offers competitive performance and convenient software development environment.

FLORA is based on F-logic [21], HiLog [11], and Transaction Logic [8, 6, 9], which are all incorporated into a single, coherent logic language along the lines

---

* Work supported in part by a grant from New York State through the program for Strategic Partnership for Industrial Resurgence, by XSB, Inc., through the NSF SBIR Award 9960485, and by NSF grant INT9809945.

[1] http://www.w3.org/RDF/

J. Lloyd et al. (Eds.): CL 2000, LNAI 1861, pp. 1078–1093, 2000.

described in [21, 20]. However, rather than developing our own deductive engine for F-logic (such as the ones developed for FLORID [16, 26] or SiLRI [15]), we chose to utilize an existing engine, XSB [28], and implement FLORA through source-level translation to XSB. Apart from the benefits of saving considerable amount of time, our choice of XSB was motivated by the following considerations:

1. XSB augments OLD-resolution [31] with *tabling*, which extends the well-known Magic Sets method [3], thereby offering both goal-driven top-down evaluation and data-driven bottom-up evaluation [30].
2. Mapping of F-logic and HiLog into predicate calculus is well known [21, 11].
3. XSB is known to be an order of magnitude faster than other similar logic systems, such as LDL and CORAL [28].
4. XSB has compile-time optimizations particularly suited for source-level translation, such as specialization [29], unification factoring [14], and trie-based indexing (which permits indexing on multiple arguments of a predicate).

To the best of our knowledge, the first functioning F-logic prototype based on the source-level translation approach was FLIP [24]. FLIP served as the starting point and the inspiration for our own work. Fortunately, there was plenty of work left for us to do, because FLIP's translation was essentially identical to that described in [21] and it was rather naively relying on the ability of XSB to apply the right optimizations. As a result, the implementation of FLIP suffered from a number of serious problems. In particular:

1. As a compiler optimization, XSB's specialization does not apply to many programs obtained from a direct translation of F-logic [21]. This is even more so when HiLog terms (which FLIP did not have) occur in the program.
2. Although fundamental to evaluating F-logic programs, tabling cannot be used without discretion. First, tabling can, in some cases, cause unnecessary overhead. Second, tabling and databases updates do not work well together.
3. FLIP did not have a consistent object model and had limited support for path expressions, functional attributes, and meta-programming.
4. Finally, FLIP did not provide any module system, which basically confined users to a single program file, making serious software development difficult.

In this paper we discuss how these problems are resolved in FLORA. The full paper will present performance results, which compare FLORA with other systems that implement F-logic.

2   Preliminaries

In this section we review the technical foundations of FLORA — F-logic [21], HiLog [11], and Transaction Logic [8, 7] — and describe their naive translation using "wrapper" predicates. This discussion forms the basis for understanding the architecture of FLORA and the optimizations built into it.

2.1   F-Logic

F-logic subsumes predicate calculus while both its syntax and semantics are still defined in object-oriented terms. On the other hand, much of F-logic can be viewed as a syntactic variant of classical logic, which makes implementation through source-level translation possible.

Basic Syntax. F-logic uses Prolog *ground* (*i.e.*, variable-free) terms to represent object identities (abbr., oid's), *e.g.*, john and father(mary). Objects can have scalar (single-valued), multivalued, or Boolean attributes, for instance,

> mary[spouse→john, children→↠{alice, nancy}].
> mary[children→↠{jack}; married].

Here spouse→john says that mary has a scalar attribute spouse, whose value is the oid john; children→↠{alice, nancy} says that the value of the multivalued attribute children is a set that *contains* two oid's: alice and nancy. We emphasize "contains" because sets do not need to be specified all at once. For instance, the second fact above says that mary has one other child, jack. The attribute married in the second fact is Boolean: its value is *true* in the above example.

While some attributes of an object can be specified explicitly as facts, other attributes can be defined using inference rules. For instance, we can derive john[children→↠{alice, nancy, jack}] with the help of the following rule:

$$X[\text{children}→↠\{C\}] :− Y[\text{spouse}→X, \text{children}→↠\{C\}]. \qquad (1)$$

Here we adopt the usual Prolog convention that capitalized symbols denote variables, while symbols beginning with a lower case letter denote constants.

F-logic objects can also have *methods*, *i.e.*, functions that return a value or a set of values when appropriate arguments are provided. For instance,

> john[grade@(cs305,f99)→100, courses@(f99)→↠{cs305, cs306}].

says that john has a scalar method, grade, whose value on the arguments cs305 and f99 is 100, and a multivalued method courses, whose value on the argument f99 is a set of oid's that contains cs305 and cs306. As attributes, methods can also be defined using rules.

One might wonder about the purpose of the "@"-sign in method specification. Indeed, why not write grade(cs305,f99) instead? The purpose is to enable meta-programming without using meta-logic. The "@"-sign trick makes methods into objects so that variables can range over them. For instance, the following rules

$$X[\text{methods}→↠\{M\}] :− X[M@(\_)→\_].$$
$$X[\text{methods}→↠\{M\}] :− X[M@(\_,\_)→\_]. \qquad (2)$$

where the symbol "_" denotes a new unique variable, define a new method, methods, which for any given object collects those of the object's methods that take one or two arguments.

Thus, the "@"-sign is just a syntactic gimmick that permits F-logic to stay within the boundary of first-order logic syntax and avoids having to deal with terms like M(X,Y), where M is a variable. However, there is a better gimmick, HiLog [11], which will be discussed shortly.

Finally, we note that F-logic can specify *class membership* (*e.g.*, john : student), *subclass relationship* (*e.g.*, student :: person), *types* (*e.g.*, person[name⇒string]), and many other things that are peripheral to the subject of this paper.

Translation into Predicate Calculus. A general translation technique, called *flattening*, was described in [21]. It used a small, fixed assortment of *wrapper predicates* to encode different types of specifications. For instance, the scalar attribute specification mary[age→30] is encoded as fd(age,mary,[ ],30) whereas the multivalued method specification john[courses@(f99)→↠{cs305, cs306}] is encoded as mvd(courses,john,[f99],cs305) ∧ mvd(courses,john,[f99],cs306).

However, one problem is that the indexing advantage is lost due to the small number of wrapper predicates used, since most Prolog systems index on predicate names. At first thought, one might think that the problem can be easily avoided if the encoding used method and attribute names as predicates instead of the "faceless" general wrappers. However, this is not the case, because variables are allowed to occur in place of method names, which would make the translated program second-order.

Recursion presents another serious difficulty. The naive translation scheme will most likely produce rules that are highly recursive, due to the small number of wrapper predicates used. For instance, consider the rule (1) presented earlier; its naive translation is as follows:

mvd(children,X,[ ],C) : − fd(spouse,Y,[ ],X), mvd(children,Y,[ ],C).

In general, evaluating such rules using a regular Prolog-style engine will go to infinite loop even if logically there is only a finite number of possible answers. In contrast, such rules present no problems to a tabling logic engine, like XSB, which uses memorization to terminate unnecessary loops in the evaluation.

For completeness, we note that class membership has its own translation, *e.g.*, isa(john,student), and so does the subclass relationship, *e.g.*, subclass(student,person). Type specifications have their own translation as well. In addition, a set of axioms must be added to enforce various properties of F-logic. For instance, we have to ensure that scalar attributes yield at most one value for any given object, that the subclass relationship is transitively closed, and that subclass membership is contained in the superclass membership.

Last but not least, although the non-monotonic part of F-logic— inheritance — cannot be directly translated into predicate calculus, it can still be encoded using Prolog-style rules and computed using XSB's efficient implementation of the *well-founded semantics* for negation [32].

2.2   HiLog

We have seen that one can do certain amount of meta-programming in F-logic, mostly owing to the "@"-sign gimmick. Although the rules in (2) show that all method names can be collected using this trick, it is not easy to collect all method invocations (*i.e.*, methods plus their arguments). Our experience with FLORA 1.0 also shows that it is very convenient to treat both method names *and* method invocations uniformly as objects, because the "@"-sign trick is error-prone: people tend to forget to write down the "@"-sign (in F-logic, grade@(cs305,f99) is different from grade(cs305,f99)).

Fortunately, with the extension of HiLog [11], all these problems disappear. We illustrate HiLog through examples. The simplest yet most unusual one is the definition of the standard Prolog meta-predicate, call: $call(X) :- X$. This means that HiLog does not distinguish between function terms and atomic formulas: the same variable can range over both. Variables can also range over function symbols, as in $X(Y,a)$. A query of the form $?- p(X), X, X(Y,X)$ is well within the boundaries of HiLog. The syntax for HiLog terms also extends that of classical logic. For instance, $g(X)(f(a,X),Y)(b,Y)$ is perfectly fine. Of course, such powerful syntax should be used sparingly, but people have found many important uses for these features (see [11] for some).

Obviously HiLog is a suitable replacement for the "@"-sign gimmick. Now with the HiLog extension, users can write, say,

$$X[methods \twoheadrightarrow \{M\}] :- X[M(\_,\_) \rightarrow \_]$$

instead of the rules shown earlier in (2). Trivial as it might appear, HiLog completely eliminates the need for special meta-syntax used in FLORA 1.0, and reduces the danger of programming mistakes. In addition, the underlying conceptual object model becomes much more consistent. The HiLog extension is implemented in the upcoming FLORA 2.0. Section 4 discusses the techniques that were developed to optimize the translation.

Encoding in Predicate Calculus. It turns out that the semantics of HiLog is inherently first-order and that it can actually be encoded using standard predicate calculus [11]. Although the translation is rather subtle, it is defined with just two recursive transformation functions (we omit steps irrelevant to the main subject): $encode_a$, for translating formulas, and $encode_t$, for translating terms:

1. $encode_t(X) = X$, for each variable X.
2. $encode_t(s) = s$, for each function symbol s.
3. $encode_t(t(t_1,\ldots,t_n)) = apply_{n+1}(encode_t(t), encode_t(t_1),\ldots, encode_t(t_n))$.
4. $encode_a(A) = call(encode_t(A))$, where A is a HiLog atomic formula.
5. $encode_a(A \wedge B) = encode_a(A) \wedge encode_a(B)$.

For instance, $f(a,X)(b,Y) \wedge X(Y) \wedge Z$ is encoded as:

$$apply_3(apply_3(f,a,X),b,Y) \wedge apply_2(X,Y) \wedge call(Z)$$

Note that this naive HiLog encoding uses essentially one wrapper predicate per arity. For a Prolog-style implementation, this poses an even greater challenge than F-logic, since all predicate-level indexing is lost. To overcome this problem, two kinds of compiler optimizations can be used: unification factoring [14] and specialization [29]. They both are source-level transformations aimed at improving predicate-level indexing. These techniques are discussed in Section 4.

2.3   Transaction Logic

An important aspect of an object-oriented language is the ability to update the internal states of objects. In this respect, F-logic is only partly object-oriented, since it is just a query language. To address this problem, [22] introduced techniques based on preserving the history of object states, so different object states can be distinguished through the extra state argument. However, such techniques do not support modular design. For instance, one cannot define more and more complex update transactions using the previously defined subroutines.

In our view, subroutines are fundamental to programming, and any practical proposal for dealing with updates in a logic-based programming language must address this issue. *Transaction Logic* [8, 7, 9] is one such proposal, which provides a comprehensive theory of updates in logic programming. The utility of Transaction Logic has been demonstrated in various applications ranging from database updates, to robot action planning, to reasoning about actions, to workflow analysis, and many more [8, 10, 12].

In FLORA 2.0, F-logic and Transaction Logic are integrated along the lines of the proposal in [20], and the corresponding implementation issues are described in Section 4. In Transaction Logic, both actions (transactions) and queries are represented as predicates. In the context of F-logic, transactions are expressed as object methods. Underlying Transaction Logic are just a few basic ideas:

1. *Execution ≡ Truth.* Execution of an action is tantamount to it being true on a *path*, *i.e.*, a sequence of database states that represent the execution trace.

2. *Elementary Updates.* These are the building blocks for constructing complex transactions. Their behavior can be specified by a separate program (*e.g.*, in the C language) or via a set of axioms. In this paper, we shall use only two types of elementary updates: insert and delete.

3. *Atomicity of Updates.* A transaction should either execute entirely (in which case it is true along the execution path) or not at all. Although common in databases, this behavior is not typical in logic programming, where assert and retract are not backtrackable.

The following program is a FLORA 2.0 adaptation of the block-stacking program from [8]. Here, the action stack is defined as a Boolean method of a robot. The

"#"-sign marks transactional methods that change the database state.

R[#stack(0,X)] :− R:robot.
R[#stack(N,X)] :− R:robot, N > 0,
                     Y[#move(X)], R[#stack(N-1,Y)].
Y[#move(X)]   :− Y:block, Y[clear], X[clear], X[wider(Y)],
                     del(Y[on→Z]), ins(Z[clear]), ins(Y[on→X]), del(X[clear]).

Informally, the program says that to stack a pyramid of N blocks on top of block X, the robot must find a block Y, move it onto X, and then stack N-1 blocks on top of Y. To move Y onto X, both of them must be "clear" (*i.e.*, with no block on top), and X must be wider than Y. If these conditions are satisfied, the database will be updated accordingly (ins and del are elementary insert and delete transactions, respectively).

Note that because of the non-backtrackable nature of Prolog updates, using assert and retract to translate the ins and del transactions in the above program would not work properly. However, backtrackable updates can be implemented efficiently in XSB at the engine level, due to XSB's use of tries — a special data structure for storing dynamic data. Transaction Logic provides semantics to this type of updates.

3   Implementation Issues

3.1   Transactions in a Tabling Environment

As mentioned in Section 2.1, translation from F-logic to predicate calculus requires tabling all the wrapper predicates used for flattening. It turns out, however, that tabling and database updates are fundamentally at odds: tabling has the effect that whenever the same query is repeated, it is not evaluated and instead the previously computed answers are returned. Even a subsumed query does not necessarily need to be evaluated. Its answers can be computed from the answers for the corresponding subsuming query. Obviously, this hurts the semantics of update transactions and other procedures that have side effects. To see the problem, consider the following program:

    :− table p/1.   p(X) :− write(X).

The first time p(a) is called, the system will print out "a" and return the answer yes. However, if p(a) is called the second time, the system will only answer yes without the "side effect" of "a" being printed out.

This problem implies that update transactions in Transaction Logic should *not* be translated using tabled predicates. Moreover, a tabled predicate p should not depend (directly or indirectly) on an update transaction q, since the semantics of such dependency is murky: the first call to p will execute q while subsequent calls might not. Therefore, FLORA must check that regular F-logic methods and attributes do not depend on update transactions. A special syntax is introduced to help FLORA perform proper translation: transactional methods are preceded by a "#"-sign to distinguish them from regular F-logic methods. Primitive update transaction, such as insertion and deletion, also look special:

ins(smith : professor[teach(1999,fall)→cse100])
del(cse200[taught_by(1999,spring)→david])

A more difficult problem arises when a transaction changes the base facts that a tabled predicate depends on. In this case, the changes should propagate to all answers that are already tabled for this predicate. This is similar to the view maintenance problem in databases, but the overhead associated with database view maintenance methods is unacceptable for fast in-memory logic engines. Currently, FLORA takes a rather drastic approach of abolishing all tables and letting subsequent queries rebuild them. However, this problem is not specific to FLORA, and a more efficient solution can be developed at the XSB engine level.

3.2   Problems with Naive Translation of HiLog and F-Logic

Choice Points and Indexing. In Section 2 we described the naive translation from F-logic and HiLog into classical predicate calculus. Such translation, however, cannot be the basis for practical implementation. The first problem is that the naive translation lays down too many choice points in the top-down execution tree and thus causes excessive backtracking. Consider the following program and its encoding using the apply predicate (we consider translation of HiLog, because it illustrates the problem more dramatically):

$$p(X,Y) :- f(X), g(Y). \qquad apply(p,X,Y) :- apply(f,X), apply(g,Y). \qquad (3)$$
$$s(X,Y) :- p(X,Y). \qquad apply(s,X,Y) :- apply(p,X,Y).$$

If apply(p,X,Y) is evaluated, it will unify with all the rules even though its unification with the last rule is bound to fail. In large programs this might cause a serious performance penalty.

Degradation of indexing is another source of performance penalty. Typically, a deductive system indexes on the predicate name plus one of the arguments, *e.g.*, the first. In the naive translation, however, predicate-level indexing is lost, because there are too few predicates used. For instance, in the above example, the translated program has no indexing mechanism corresponding to the first-argument indexing in predicates p and s in the original program.

These problems are not new to logic programming. To tackle them, XSB has developed compiler optimization techniques known as specialization [29] and unification factoring [14], which both perform source-to-source transformation.

Specialization takes place when a goal can only unify with a subset of the candidate rules. By replacing this goal's predicate with a different predicate that can only unify with the heads of *some* of the rules, specialization throws out the unnecessary choice points. For instance, performing specialization on the translated program in (3) yields the following more efficient program, where some occurrences of the predicate apply are replaced with apply_1:

apply(p,X,Y) :- apply(f,X), apply(g,Y).   apply(s,X,Y) :- apply_1(X,Y).
apply_1(a,X) :- apply(f,X), apply(g,Y).

In contrast to specialization, unification factoring is driven by the patterns in rule heads. The idea is to factor out common function symbols to save on unification and achieve better indexing. Consider the following program:

$$p(apply(a),X) :- q(X). \qquad p(apply(b),X) :- r(X).$$

and the query ?- p(apply(X),Y). Here unification for apply has to take place once with each rule head. However, this repeated unification can be avoided if the same goal is executed against the following transformed program:

$$p\_apply(a,X) :- q(X). \qquad p(apply(X),Y) :- p\_apply(X,Y).$$
$$p\_apply(b,X) :- r(X).$$

Because apply is used to encode HiLog terms, common functors, as in the above example, occur very frequently in a translated FLORA program. It turns out that the native XSB unification factoring performs quite well with FLORA-translated programs. XSB specialization, however, exhibits subtle problems.

Double Tabling. The first problem with specialization is tabling. In HiLog translation, it is not very clear how a tabling directive like :−table p/2 should be translated. If FLORA handles this by tabling apply/3, then XSB specialization may cause "double tabling" — a situation where certain predicates are tabled unnecessarily. For instance, consider the following program (which computes transitive closure) and its naive encoding:

$$
\begin{array}{ll}
:- \text{table } p/2. & :- \text{table } apply/3. \\
p(a,b). & apply(p,a,b). \\
p(b,c). & apply(p,b,c). \\
t(X,Y) :- p(X,Y). & apply(t,X,Y) :- apply(p,X,Y). \\
t(X,Y) :- p(X,Z), t(Z,Y). & apply(t,X,Y) :- apply(p,X,Z), apply(t,Z,Y).
\end{array}
\qquad (4)
$$

XSB specialization on the translated program (4) would yield the following:

$$
\begin{array}{ll}
:- \text{table } apply/3. & \\
:- \text{table } apply\_1/2. & :- \text{table } apply\_2/2. \\
apply\_1(a,b). & apply\_2(X,Y) :- apply\_1(X,Y). \\
apply\_1(b,c). & apply\_2(X,Y) :- apply\_1(X,Z), apply\_2(Z,Y). \\
apply(p,a,b). & apply(t,X,Y) :- apply\_1(X,Y). \\
apply(p,b,c). & apply(t,X,Y) :- apply\_1(X,Z), apply\_2(Z,Y).
\end{array}
$$

Being essentially another copy of apply(t,X,Y), tabling the tuples of apply_2(X,Y) is redundant, although this caching is needed to guarantee termination of the specialized program. The size of the compiled code is also considerably larger than the original.

Meta-programming. Yet another problem is due to meta-programming, which tends to produce programs that preclude XSB specialization. To see the crippling effect of meta-rules on XSB specialization, consider the following program and its naive translation:

$$
\begin{array}{ll}
\mathsf{p(a).} & \mathsf{apply(p,a).} \\
\mathsf{p(b).} & \mathsf{apply(p,b).} \\
\mathsf{X(Y):-X=p,\ Y=c.} & \mathsf{apply(X,Y):-X=p,\ Y=c.} \\
\mathsf{t(X):-p(X).} & \mathsf{apply(t,X):-apply(p,X).}
\end{array}
\tag{5}
$$

XSB specialization on the previous translated program (5) looks as follows:

$$
\begin{array}{ll}
\mathsf{apply(p,a).} & \mathsf{apply\_1(p,a).} \\
\mathsf{apply(p,b).} & \mathsf{apply\_1(p,b).} \\
\mathsf{apply(X,Y):-X=p,\ Y=c.} & \mathsf{apply\_1(X,Y):-X=p,\ Y=c.} \\
\mathsf{apply(t,X):-apply\_1(p,X).}
\end{array}
$$

In this program, the predicate apply_1(p,X) still has to unify with all the apply_1 facts and rules. Not only the unification on p is repeated, but indexing on the first argument in the original program is lost as well.

Note that although so far we have been illustrating the XSB specialization problems using HiLog only, F-logic exhibits the same problem. Consider the following F-logic program and its naive translation:

$$
\begin{array}{ll}
\mathsf{obja[atta \rightarrow vala].} & \mathsf{fd(atta,obja,[\ ],vala).} \\
\mathsf{objb[atta \rightarrow valb].} & \mathsf{fd(atta,objb,[\ ],valb).} \\
\mathsf{objc[X \rightarrow Y]:-X=atta,\ Y=valc.} & \mathsf{fd(X,objc,[\ ],Y):-X=atta,\ Y=valc.} \\
\mathsf{O[attb \twoheadrightarrow \{X\}]:-O[atta \rightarrow X].} & \mathsf{mvd(attb,O,[\ ],X):-fd(atta,O,[\ ],X).}
\end{array}
\tag{6}
$$

It is easy to see that the translation is just another version of the previous HiLog program (5) and thus it cripples XSB specialization just as badly.

The next section proposes a new kind of specialization, called *skeleton-based specialization*, which is used in FLORA 2.0 to optimize source-level translation for F-logic and HiLog. The system is designed in such a way that skeleton-based specialization and XSB specialization compliment each other.

4   Solutions

As explained in Section 3, a major problem with the naive translation of F-logic and HiLog is the loss of indexing and while XSB unification factoring performs well for the translated programs, specialization often fails to yield any improvements and, in some cases, it might even cause unnecessary overhead. In this section we propose *skeleton-based specialization*, which supplements the native XSB specialization and fixes the aforesaid problems.

4.1   Skeleton-Based Specialization Algorithm

Definition 1 (Skeleton). *Given a HiLog term* T, *its skeleton* Skel(T) *is an abstract view of the syntactic structure of* T. Skel(T) *is defined as follows:*

1. Skel(T) = T, *if* T *is a constant.*
2. Skel(T) = _, *if* T *is a variable.*
3. Skel(T) = Skel(F)/n, *if* T = F(T$_1$,...,T$_n$).

Example 1 (Skeletons of HiLog Terms).

1. Skel(f) = f
2. Skel(X(a,b)(Y)) = _/2/1
3. Skel(X(f(Y))) = _/1

Input: a FLORA program F consisting of rules (including facts)
Output: an XSB program that encodes F
```
1     HL := {L | L is a literal in a rule head of F};
2     BL := {L | L is a literal in a rule body of F};
3     HS := {Skel(L) | L ∈ HL};
4     BS := {Skel(L) | L ∈ BL};
5     for each skeleton S ∈ HS ∪ BS do seq(S) := a unique integer;
6     for each rule H:−B from the input program F do {
7         H′ := flatten(H,Skel(H));
8         B′ := B;
9         for each literal L ∈ B′ do L := flatten(L,Skel(L));
10        output the rule H′:−B′;
11    }
12    for each literal H ∈ HL do {
13        H′ := naive(H);
14        H″ := flatten(H,Skel(H));
15        output the rule H′:−H″;
16    }
17    for each literal L ∈ BL do
18        for each rule H:−B from the input program F do
19            if L unifies with H with the mgu θ and Skel(L) ≠ Skel(H) then {
20                H′ := flatten(Hθ,Skel(L));
21                B′ := B;
22                for each literal T ∈ B′ do {
23                    S := Tθ;
24                    if Skel(S) ∈ BS
25                        then T := flatten(S,Skel(S));
26                        else T := flatten(S,Skel(T));
27                output the rule H′:−B′;
28            }
```

Fig. 1. Skeleton-Based Specialization Algorithm

The algorithm in Figure 1 describes FLORA skeleton-based specialization. It applies to F-logic and HiLog translation separately, since the set of wrapper predicates used for F-logic translation is disjoint from those wrapper predicates used for HiLog predicates.

First we explain the algorithm in the context of HiLog translation. It takes a FLORA program as input and yields an equivalent program in predicate logic; the algorithm has the following steps:

Skeleton Analysis (Lines 1 – 5). First we collect all the literals in rule heads into the set HL and all the literals in rule bodies into the set BL.[2] Then, the algorithm computes the set of skeletons HS and BS for each literal in HL and BL, respectively. Each unique skeleton in the union of HS and BS is assigned a unique sequence number.

The rest of the algorithm consists of three main tasks: *flattening, trap rule generation*, and *instantiation*.

Flattening (Lines 6 – 11). The purpose of flattening is to eliminate unnecessary wrapper predicates and unification. Let $S = X/n_1/.../n_k$, where X is either "_" or a constant, and L be of the form $T(T_{1n_1},...,T_{n_1n_1})...(T_{1n_k},...,T_{n_kn_k})$. The transformation procedure flatten(L,S) then does the following: Let n be the sequence number assigned to the skeleton S, then the wrapper predicate used to encode the HiLog literal L is apply_n, which is unique across HiLog translation. Next, if X is a constant in $X/n_1/.../n_k$, then so must be T (in Lines 7, 14 and 25 the skeleton argument of flatten is that of the literal argument whereas in Lines 20 and 26 the skeleton either subsumes or is the same as that of the literal) and flatten(L,S) yields $apply\_n(E_{1n_1},...,E_{n_1n_1},...,E_{1n_k},...,E_{n_kn_k})$. Otherwise, X is "_" and T might be any HiLog term, then flatten(L,S) will return $apply\_n(E,E_{1n_1},...,E_{n_1n_1},...,E_{1n_k},...,E_{n_kn_k})$, where E, $E_{ij} = encode_t(T)$, $encode_t(T_{ij})$, respectively, $encode_t$ is the naive encoding of HiLog terms described in Section 2.2. For instance, if the sequence number assigned to the skeleton $f/1/2$ is 2, then flatten(f(Y)(a,Z),f/1/2) will produce apply_2(Y,a,Z). The reason why the functor symbol f can be omitted is because it is already encoded in the sequence number for the skeleton.

Trap Rule Generation (Lines 12 – 16). These steps generate rules to "trap" the naive encoding of literals. The translation outputs a rule whose head is the naive encoding of the original rule-head, while the body is the result of flattening the head. For instance, the trap rule for f(Y)(a,Z):−body is like apply(apply(f,Y),a,Z):−apply_2(Y,a,Z). Trap rule generation is indispensable for inter-module communications in FLORA. Since specialization in principle has no knowledge of other modules, calls referring to other modules have to be encoded using the naive translation. Due to space limits, we will not elaborate on this topic further.

Instantiation (Lines 17 – 28). Even when two literals unify, their encodings might not unify after flattening. For instance, X(Y) and f(a)(Z) unify, but their flattened forms, *e.g.*, apply_1(X,Y) and apply_2(a,Z) (with respect to the skeletons _/1 and f/1/1, respectively), do not unify.

---

[2] Each HiLog literal is assumed to have the functor part and the arity. Propositional constants are treated as 0-ary literals, *e.g.*, p().

Instantiation ensures that unifiability is preserved after specialization. The idea is that if a body literal unifies with the head of a rule, R, using the mgu θ, but the two literals have different skeletons, then a new rule, $R\theta$, must be generated. For instance, consider the following program:

$$g(X):-p(X). \qquad Y(Z):-q(Y,Z).$$

Here $p(X)$ will be flattened as apply_1(X) and $Y(Z)$ as apply_2(Y,Z). Because $p(X)$ unifies with $Y(Z):-q(Y,Z)$, this rule must be instantiated using the substitution Y/p, yielding $p(Z):-q(p,Z)$. Specializing this rule yields apply_1(Z):$-$apply_2(p,Z), which ensures that the semantics of the original program is preserved.

However, rule instantiation might generate body literals with *new* skeletons that have not been seen before in the original program. Thus, instantiation might have to be applied again, using these new body literals. This opens up the possibility of an infinite instantiation process. For instance, in the following program:

$$g(X):-p(X). \qquad Y(Z):-Y(Z)(Z).$$

when the second rule is instantiated with Y/p (the mgu of $p(X)$ and $Y(Z)$), a new rule $p(Z):-p(Z)(Z)$ is generated. The literal $p(Z)(Z)$ has a completely new skeleton: $p/1/1$. If $p(X)(X)$ is flattened with respect to $p/1/1$, the rule $Y(Z):-Y(Z)(Z)$ has to be instantiated with $Y/p(X)$, the mgu of $p(X)(X)$ and $Y(Z)$. Thus yet another new skeleton $p/1/1/1$ will emerge, and so on.

Lines 24 – 26 in the algorithm are designed to ensure termination of the instantiation process. The solution is simple: the quality of specialization is traded in for termination. When a literal with a new skeleton shows up in a newly instantiated rule, its skeleton must extend the skeleton of that literal before instantiation. Thus, we can flatten the instantiated literal with respect to the skeleton of the original literal. Unifiability is also preserved by such translation. For instance, specializing the above example yields the following program (where the trap rules are omitted):

apply_1(X):$-$apply_2(X).   apply_2(X):$-$apply_4(p,X,X).
apply_3(Y,Z):$-$apply_4(Y,Z,Z).   apply_4(Y,Z,Z):$-$apply_4(apply(Y,Z),Z,Z).

4.2   Putting It All Together

For the translated program (4), which computes transitive closure, the result of skeleton-based specialization is as follows:

:$-$table apply_2/2.
apply_1(a,b).   apply_2(X,Y):$-$apply_1(X,Y).
apply_1(b,c).   apply_2(X,Y):$-$apply_1(X,Z), apply_2(Z,Y).

The following program is the result of skeleton-based specialization of the program shown in (5):

apply_1(a).   apply_3(X) : − apply_1(X).
apply_1(b).   apply_1(X) : − p=p, X=c.
apply_2(X,Y) : − X=p, Y=c.

Note that although we illustrate the idea of skeleton-based specialization using HiLog translation, our algorithm applies to F-logic translation as well. In fact, the translation views F-logic literals as just another kind of HiLog literals, which just happen to use different wrapper predicates.

For instance, a slight variation of the naive F-logic translation can convert O[M→V] into the HiLog literal M(O,V) and then further convert it to predicate logic using the wrapper predicate fd instead of apply. Likewise, O[M↠V] can be converted to M(O,V) and then to predicate calculus using mvd as a wrapper. Therefore, skeleton-based specialization can be performed on HiLog and F-logic independently. The only part of the algorithm that needs to be changed is the prefix used to construct the wrappers. For instance, instead of apply_2 we would use fd_2. Thus, the result of applying skeleton-based specialization to the program (6) would be the following (where the trap rules are omitted):

fd_1(obja,vala).   mvd_1(O,X) : − fd_1(O,X).
fd_1(objb,valb).   fd_1(objc,Y) : − atta=atta, Y=valc.
fd_2(X,objc,Y) : − X=atta, Y=valc.

Our experiments show that even for small programs discussed in this section FLORA skeleton-based specialization can speed up programs by a factor of 2.1, whereas XSB native specialization reduces execution time only by a factor of 1.85. A more detailed comparison will be reported in the full version of this paper. Nevertheless, as said earlier, FLORA specialization is not intended to replace XSB specialization. Instead, it is used as a first-line optimization technique. Then the FLORA-translated program is further optimized through the native XSB specialization and unification factoring.

Another observation about FLORA specialization is that better-quality specialization is possible with more detailed skeleton representation. Indeed, considering HiLog terms as trees, we could define skeletons as the abstract view of their structures at some depth level. For example, a two-level skeleton for f(X)(X,a,f(b)) would be f/(_)/(_,a,(f/1)). There is a subtle relationship, though, between the amount of detail preserved in skeletons and the quality of specialized programs. More detailed skeletons normally mean better specialized programs and thus better performance, but longer compilation time and larger program size.

5   Conclusion

This paper discusses techniques for building efficient DOOD systems by translation into lower-level Prolog syntax and utilizing an existing tabling logic engine, such as XSB [28]. The feasibility of our approach has been demonstrated by the F-logic based FLORA system, which delivers very encouraging performance. (Performance results will be included in the full version of this paper.) We also discuss the compiler optimization techniques that were used to achieve this performance; some of them are just native XSB optimizations, while others are designed specifically for FLORA. Due to lack of space we omitted a number of other implementation issues, such as the FLORA module system and performance optimizations related to handling path expressions. Details can be found at http://www.cs.sunysb.edu/~guizyang/papers/floratech.ps.

Acknowledgement

We would like to thank Hasan Davulcu, Kostis Sagonas, C.R. Ramakrishnan, and David S. Warren for their patience in explaining us the intricacies of XSB optimization techniques. We are also grateful to Bertram Ludäscher and the anonymous referees for the very helpful comments.

References

1. S. Abiteboul, P. Buneman, and D. Suciu. *Data on the Web*. Morgan Kaufmann, San Francisco, CA, 2000.
2. M.L. Barja, A.A.A. Fernandes, N.W. Paton, A.H. Williams, A. Dinn, and A.I. Abdelmoty. Design and implementation of ROCK & ROLL: A deductive object-oriented database system. *Information Systems*, 20(3):185–211, 1995.
3. C. Beeri and R. Ramakrishnan. On the power of magic. *Journal of Logic Programming*, 10:255–300, April 1991.
4. T. Berners-Lee. Semantic web road map. http://www.w3.org/DesignIssues/Semantic.html, September 1998.
5. T. Berners-Lee. The semantic toolbox: Building semantics on top of XML-RDF. http://www.w3.org/DesignIssues/Toolbox.html, May 1999.
6. A.J. Bonner and M. Kifer. Transaction logic programming. In *Int'l Conference on Logic Programming*, pages 257–282, Budapest, Hungary, June 1993. MIT Press.
7. A.J. Bonner and M. Kifer. An overview of transaction logic. *Theoretical Computer Science*, 133:205–265, October 1994.
8. A.J. Bonner and M. Kifer. Transaction logic programming (or a logic of declarative and procedural knowledge). Technical Report CSRI-323, University of Toronto, November 1995. http://www.cs.toronto.edu/~bonner/transaction-logic.html.
9. A.J. Bonner and M. Kifer. A logic for programming database transactions. In J. Chomicki and G. Saake, editors, *Logics for Databases and Information Systems*, chapter 5, pages 117–166. Kluwer Academic Publishers, March 1998.
10. A.J. Bonner and M. Kifer. Results on reasoning about updates in transaction logic. In Transactions and Change in Logic, B. Freitag et al.,Springer-Verlag, Berlin LNCS 1472, 1998.
11. W. Chen, M. Kifer, and D.S. Warren. HiLog: A foundation for higher-order logic programming. *Journal of Logic Programming*, 15(3):187–230, February 1993.
12. H. Davulcu, M. Kifer, C.R. Ramakrishnan, and I.V. Ramakrishnan. Logic based modeling and analysis of workflows. In *ACM Symposium on Principles of Database Systems*, pages 25–33, Seattle, Washington, June 1998.
13. H. Davulcu, G. Yang, M. Kifer, and I.V. Ramakrishnan. Design and implementation of the physical layer in webbases: The XRover experience. In *Int'l Conference on Computational Logic (DOOD-2000 Stream)*, July 2000.

14. S. Dawson, C.R. Ramakrishnan, I.V. Ramakrishnan, K. Sagonas, S. Skiena, T. Swift, and D.S. Warren. Unification factoring for efficient evaluation of logic programs. In *ACM Symposium on Principles of Programming Languages*, 1995.

15. S. Decker, D. Brickley, J. Saarela, and J. Angele. A query and inference service for RDF. In *QL'98 - The Query Languages Workshop*, December 1998.

16. J. Frohn, R. Himmeroeder, P.-Th. Kandzia, G. Lausen, and C. Schlepphorst. FLORID – A prototype for F-logic. In *Proc. Intl. Conference on Data Engineering (ICDE, Exhibition Program)*. IEEE Computer Science Press, 1997.

17. R.V. Guha, O. Lassila, E. Miler, and D. Brickley. Enabling inferencing. In *QL'98 - The Query Languages Workshop*, December 1998.

18. A. Gupta, B. Ludäscher, and M. E. Martone. Knowledge-based integration of neuroscience data sources. In *12th Intl. Conference on Scientific and Statistical Database Management (SSDBM)*, Berlin, Germany, July 2000. IEEE Computer Society.

19. M. Jarke, R. Gallersdörfer, M.A. Jeusfeld, M. Staudt, and Stefan Eherer. Concept-Base – A deductive object base for meta data management. *Journal of Intelligent Information Systems*, February 1995.

20. M. Kifer. Deductive and object-oriented data languages: A quest for integration. In *Int'l Conference on Deductive and Object-Oriented Databases*, volume 1013 of *Lecture Notes in Computer Science*, pages 187–212, Singapore, December 1995. Springer-Verlag. Keynote address at the 3d Int'l Conference on Deductive and Object-Oriented databases.

21. M. Kifer, G. Lausen, and J. Wu. Logical foundations of object-oriented and frame-based languages. *Journal of ACM*, 42:741–843, July 1995.

22. G. Lausen and B. Ludäscher. Updates by reasoning about states. In *2-nd International East/West Database Workshop*, Klagenfurt, Austria, September 1994.

23. M. Liu. A deductive object base language. *Information Systems*, 21(5):431–457, 1996.

24. B. Ludäscher. Tour de FLIP. The FLIP manual, 1998.

25. B. Ludäscher, A. Gupta, and M. E. Martone. A mediator system for model-based information integration. In *Int'l Conference on Very Large Data Bases*, Cairo, Egypt, 2000. system demonstration.

26. B. Ludäscher, R. Himmeröder, G. Lausen, W. May, and C. Schlepphorst. Managing semistructured data with FLORID: A deductive object-oriented perspective. *Information Systems*, 23(8):589–613, 1998.

27. Mozilla RDF/Enabling inference. http://www.mozilla.org/rdf/doc/inference.html, 1999.

28. K. Sagonas, T. Swift, and D.S. Warren. XSB as an efficient deductive database engine. In *ACM SIGMOD Conference on Management of Data*, pages 442–453, New York, May 1994. ACM.

29. K. Sagonas and D.S. Warren. Efficient execution of HiLog in WAM-based Prolog implementations. In *Int'l Conference on Logic Programming*, 1995.

30. T. Swift and D. S. Warren. An abstract machine for SLG resolution: Definite programs. In *Int'l Logic Programming Symposium*, Cambridge, MA, November 1994. MIT Press.

31. H. Tamaki and T. Sato. OLD resolution with tabulation. In *Int'l Conference on Logic Programming*, pages 84–98, Cambridge, MA, 1986. MIT Press.

32. A. Van Gelder, K.A. Ross, and J.S. Schlipf. The well-founded semantics for general logic programs. *Journal of ACM*, 38(3):620–650, 1991.

33. K. Yokota and H. Yasukawa. Towards an integrated knowledge-base management system. In *Proceedings of the Int'l Conference on Fifth Generation Computer Systems*, pages 89–109, June 1992.

Design and Implementation of the Physical Layer in WebBases: The XRover* Experience**

Hasan Davulcu[1], Guizhen Yang[2], Michael Kifer[2], and I.V. Ramakrishnan[2]

[1] XSB Inc., Stony Brook Software Incubator
Nassau Hall Suite 115, Stony Brook, NY 11794 USA
hdavulcu@xsb.com
[2] Dept. of Computer Science, SUNY Stony Brook
Stony Brook, NY 11794, USA
{guizyang,kifer,ram}@cs.sunysb.edu

Abstract. Webbases are database systems that enable creation of Web applications that allow end users to shop around for products and services at various Web sites without having to manually browse and fill out forms at each of these sites. In this paper we describe *XRover* which is an implementation of the physical layer of the webbase architecture. This layer is primarily responsible for automatically locating and extracting dynamic data from Web sites, i.e data that can only be obtained by form fill-outs. We discuss our experience in building XRover using FLORA, a deductive object-oriented system.

1 Introduction

The World Wide Web is becoming the dominant medium for information delivery and electronic commerce. The number of users who routinely use the Web to buy goods and services continues to increase at a rapid pace. In response, software robots (called "shopbots") that allow consumers to quickly find out the best prices for comparable goods and services are beginning to emerge. Information about prices and other attributes of products are typically obtained by filling out forms at a vendor's site. Software robots retrieve such information by automatically navigating to relevant sites, locating the correct forms, filling them out and extracting the data of interest from web pages returned as the result.[1] Hence tools that can do automatic form fill-outs and extract relevant information from the data pages returned in response, are becoming very important.

One such enabling technology is a *webbase* [11,3,2,6], which is a database system for managing and querying the dynamic Web content (i.e., data that can

---

* XRover is a registered trademark of XSB Inc.

** Work supported in part by the ARCHIMEDES Contract SP0103-99-C-002 from Defense Logistics Agency, by NSF SBIR Award 9960485, by NSF grants CCR-9711386, EIA-9705998, and INT9809945, and by a SPIR grant from New York State and XSB, Inc.

[1] Jango and mySimon [8] are two examples of such shopbots.

J. Lloyd et al. (Eds.): CL 2000, LNAI 1861, pp. 1094–1105, 2000.
© Springer-Verlag Berlin Heidelberg 2000

only be extracted by filling out multiple forms). Designing webbases is an active area of current database research in view of the rapid proliferation of shopbots. Managing the dynamic Web content encompasses automating several tasks that include specifying and locating the data of interest (e.g. price information) in a Web site and extracting and integrating information from multiple sites into a coherent view.

In [6] we proposed a 3-layer architecture for designing and implementing webbases — an architecture that is akin to the traditional layering of database systems. The most significant difference between a webbase and a database is the absence of the traditional physical layer. The actual data in webbases is the exclusive domain of the Web server, and the only way a webbase can access it is by filing requests to the server, such as following links or filling out forms. Hence, the notion of *virtual physical layer (VPL)* was introduced for the lowest layer in the webbase architecture in order to provide a unifying view of all the data that can be retrieved by filing requests to the server. While the physical layer in databases describes data storage, VPL specifies how to navigate to the various data sources in the Web. In this way, VPL provides *navigation independence* by shielding the user from the complexities associated with retrieving raw data from Web sources and thereby presents a database view of the Web to the upper layers of the webbase architecture, namely the *logical layer* and the *external schema layer*. While these layers are similar to the corresponding upper layers in traditional databases, they have special semantic meaning in webbases. For instance, the logical layer provides *site independence* in the sense that it integrates and reconciles heterogeneous information available from different sites, which is available through VPL in navigation-independent, but nonetheless site-specific form.

We had proposed techniques centered around Transaction F-Logic [10, 9] that facilitate creation of wrappers for the virtual physical layer [6]. Our architecture makes it possible to automate data extraction from web data sources to a much higher degree than was previously possible. But the design and implementation of the VPL itself was left open and is the subject of this paper. Specifically we describe our experience with implementing the XRover using FLORA [14], a deductive object-oriented system that we recently developed.

A Case for Deductive Object-Oriented Design of VPL: The first step in the design process is to develop a suitable data model for HTML pages. Observe that an HTML page is a semistructured data source comprising several elements, each having a tag that identifies the type of the element. For instance, a tag can identify an element as a paragraph, an image, a link, a table, a form, etc. We designed a syntactic *HTML object data model* to represent the elements in a page. In this model we define an object class corresponding to every tag. The HTML page is parsed and its elements are assigned an object class based on their tags.

HTML is a display-oriented mark-up language with only limited structural capabilities. In particular, it provides no machine understandable information to describe the *contents* of a page. Hence, we also need a semantic data model so as to be able to structure the syntactic objects presented in HTML and invoke meaningful operations on them, such as *follow a link object, fill-out a form object*, or *query the value of a certain attribute* (say, in a table). For this purpose, we designed a semantic *navigation object model*, which consists of aggregate objects that draw information from the HTML model and enable automated navigation in Web sites. In database terms, navigation objects are semantic *views* over the purely syntactic HTML objects.

The first step, converting an HTML page into a set of objects, is a relatively simple task. The crux of the VPL is the design of the navigation object model and the *mapping* between the syntactic HTML object model and the semantic navigation object model. One important issue in this design is the *resilience* of that mapping, namely, the ability of the mapping to yield correct navigation objects in the face of variations and changes in the page layout. We propose a deductive rule-based approach for locating and extracting information from objects in Web pages. Such a paradigm lets us efficiently search for objects and their associated attributes with high degree of independence from the page layout.

The rest of this paper is organized as follows: In Section 2 we provide an overview of our approach to the design of the VPL. Section 3 describes the details of the design. Section 4 discusses XRover, our implementation of VPL using FLORA,[2] a recently developed deductive object-oriented system based on F-logic [10]. Our implementation experience is discussed in Section 5.

2   Our Approach

One of the most important tasks that a shopbot must do is to collect information and services from different sites and present it to the customer in an integrated, unified view. In many shopbot sites, most of this extraction happens automatically, by "learning" regular expressions that match the desired information. The learning process is guided by a set of simple heuristics, such as those described in [12]. These techniques work well for a typical consumer site, where information is obtained by filling out a simple keyword-based search form and the result is presented in a simple, structured table. It is much more difficult to deal with sites that cater to business customers where search forms allows complex parametric queries based on multiple attributes, and results are presented in multiple related HTML segments. For instance, Figure 1 shows part of a search result page on the Web site of a large distributor of electronic components.

The page consists of three visible tables (each providing a different kind of information for the electronic part), many more invisible tables, one form to enable purchase, plus a plain text header that provides classification information for the retrieved part. Such complex result pages vary widely from site to site and, to the best of our knowledge, no automatic techniques exist for extracting and integrating such complex information. However, the semantic structure of Web

---

[2] http://xsb.sourceforge.net/flora/

pages can be *mapped* with relative ease with the help of appropriate graphical tools. The purpose of such a tool is to let the user identify (and specify to the system) the objects of interest, such as the relevant tables, forms and links. The physical virtual layer of our webbase system provides the needed infrastructure to support the process of site mapping and complex information extraction.

Mfg. Part Number: 29021
Category: Chemicals & Solder/Threadlockers

Pricing

Order Quantity	Unit Price
1 - 9	16.08
10 - 50	13.16
Call 1-800-PQRSTUV for pricing on other quantities.	

Add Part # 00Z787 to Shopping Cart

[Add] [1   ]

Component Detail

Attribute	Value
Mfg Pt no	29021
Manufacturer	LOCTITE CORP.
Available	38
Description	CHEMICALS & SOLDER~THREADLOCKERS
Price each	16.08
Min Buy	1
Cat 117 Page No.	111
Cat 116 Page No.	162
Buy Mult	1
Cat 115 Page No	160

Additional Information for Threadlockers

Link/ Download	Description	Type	Size (Bytes)
Download	Catalog 116 View	text/html	Not Available
Download	Catalog Detail (117)	text/HTML	Not Available

Fig. 1. A Complex Catalog Search Result Page

The architecture of the VPL is object-oriented and it is implemented using FLORA. The approach has two main components:

1. A general mechanism for locating objects of interest on a page; and
2. An object model for describing aggregate objects in the navigation model. Navigation objects are queried by the higher levels of the webbase.

The first mechanism is based on the *object locator language* (OLL) — a special declarative language that allows the user to specify object location in a flexible way. It is akin to the language of extended path expressions in semistructured query languages [1]. The system includes a FLORA program that acts as an interpreter for this language. Since FLORA implements F-logic, which in itself is a powerful query language for semistructured data, building such an interpreter for OLL is very easy. Thus, when the user points to an HTML object of interest, an OLL expression must be generated in order to arrange for the subsequent retrieval of the object.

The unique aspect of our approach is how these expressions are generated. First, an OLL expression for the desired object is *automatically* created. This expression is fairly simple-minded, as it specifies the location of the object in rather rigid terms. This initial expression is similar to URI's in XML: it provides a sequence of simple navigation commands that direct the search towards the requisite object. However, such expressions are not appropriate for locating Web information, because the location of an object can change due to a page redesign or simply because the page is generated dynamically, by a script. Such changes tend to break Web extraction systems so resilience cannot be achieved by rigid, brittle locator expressions. Thus, at the next stage, we transform the initial OLL expression into an *unambiguous* and *resilient* expression that extracts to the same object. Here "unambiguous" means that the expression identifies just one object; this requirement guards against the possibility of over-generalizing the initial OLL expressions. "Resilience" means that the expression will be able to locate the requisite object under a large class of variations in the page layout. Some of the techniques used to create unambiguous resilient expressions are detailed in [7].

To illustrate the idea, consider the second visible table in Figure 1 (below the "Component Detail" header). This table is actually part of a bigger, invisible table, so the initial OLL expression would be generated as follows:

$$\texttt{table, table.tr, tr.td, td.img, table, table, td,}$$
$$\texttt{table, img, table, text, table, table, form, text, table}$$

The actual initial expression is much more detailed—we skipped many of the intermediate features of the Web page. In this expression, the symbols correspond to HTML objects, the period "." means that the search must nest inside a complex data element, such as a table or a form, and the comma "," signifies horizontal scan accross the siblings in the HTML tree. The above expression tells us that in order to find the second visible table, we have to find the second top-level table in the HTML source, go inside the table (nest), find the second row and then start examining the fields of that row. Having found the second field, which happens to have complex internal structure, we must nest into that structure. Then we must scan this structure horizontally to find an image, skip two tables, find an out-of-place `<td>` element (which happens to be a formatting bug on this page), and then skip a number of images, tables, and text items to locate the table we need.

The problem with this addressing schema is that it is too brittle. It will get us the desired table for a particular instance of the page, but a page generated for a different catalog search request might look slightly different and the above address might then point to a wrong item (or not point anywhere at all). This problem was addressed in [7]. Combining the techniques described in that work with other heuristics, we can create a much more resilient OLL expression:

$$\texttt{*.text[contents} \rightarrow' \texttt{* Component*], table}$$

This expression says that in order to find the desired table, we must find a text object that matches the word "Component" at any level of nesting and then scan horizontally to the first table. This expression is much more resilient to changes in the page contents than the original one, and it stands a much better chance of being able to fetch the right object regardless of the actual search parameters, even in the presence of many types of page layout changes. Not only is the above expression more resilient, but it also can be processed faster using a deductive system, such as FLORA, because we can build an index on the contents attribute of the text class.

The second layer in our architecture, the aggregate navigation objects that unify the information scattered in disparate HTML segments, is essentially a view over the basic HTML model of a Web page. This view is specified using the *page extraction map*, which itself is a set of F-logic objects that use the OLL expressions to tell the system where the individual components of the navigation object are coming from. Page extraction maps are composed together to form a *site map* for the Web site.

The page extraction map object corresponding to the second table in the above example looks as follows:

```
oll(*.text[contents -> '*Component*'],table) : normal_table[
        column_names -> rel_oll( .tr(1) );
        init_row -> 2;
        row(Row) -> rel_oll( .tr(Row) );
        total_rows -> rel_oll( .last )
].

oll(*.text[contents -> '*Component*'],table.tr(1))
: header_row[
        column_name(Column) -> rel_oll( .th(Column).text );
        width -> rel_oll( .last )
].

oll(*.text[contents -> '*Component*'],table.tr(Row))
: data_row[
        column(Column) -> rel_oll( .td(Column).text );
        width -> rel_oll( .last )
].
```

The above specifies that the HTML segment pointed to by

$$*.\text{text}[\text{contents} \to' * Component *'], \text{table}$$

is a *normal_table* in the navigation object model and its header column can be extracted from the segment pointed to by the OLL expression

$$*.\text{text}[\text{contents} \to' * Component *'], \text{table.tr}(1)$$

where $\text{tr}(1)$ means the first row in the table. The rows can be extracted from the segment pointed to by $*.\text{text}[\text{contents} \to '*\text{Component}*']$, $\text{table.tr}(\text{Row})$ where *Row* is a parameter. The second extraction map object is interpreted similarly.

Some of the navigation objects extracted with the help of this extraction map object are as follows:

```
nav_obj3     : normal_table.        nav_obj4     : header_row.
nav_obj3[                           nav_obj4[
   column_names -> nav_obj4;           column_name(1) -> 'Attribute';
   row(1) -> nav_obj5;                 column_name(2) -> 'Value';
   row(2) -> nav_obj6;                 width -> 2
   ...                              ].
   total -> 10
].

nav_obj5     : data_row.            nav_obj6     : data_row.
nav_obj5[                           nav_obj6[
   column(1) -> 'Mfg Pt No';           column(1) -> 'Manufacturer';
   column(2) -> '29021';               column(2) -> 'LOCTITE CORP.';
   width -> 2                          width -> 2
].                                  ].
```

We discuss navigation objects in further detail in subsequent sections.

3   Architecture of the Virtual Physical Layer (VPL)

There are two aspects in VPL implementation:

1. *Site Mapping* which is done *once* per site.
2. *Run-time query processing* driven by the site maps.

We first explain the process of site map construction.

Site Map Construction. The process is shown in Figure 2. XRover begins by using an HTTP library to fetch the Web page. This page is then parsed by an HTML parser that translates the page into a set of F-Logic objects, and for each object its OLL expression is computed. For instance, the following objects describe two consecutive tables in an HTML page:

```
htmlobj3        : table.            htmlobj11    : table.
htmlobj3[                           htmlobj11[
   parent -> htmlobj2;                 parent -> htmlobj2;
   position -> 0;                      position -> 1;
   rows -> htmlobj4;                   rows -> htmlobj12;
   oll -> [table];                     oll -> [table,table];
```

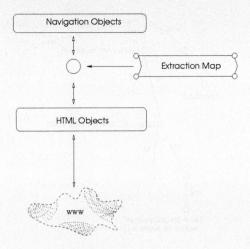

Fig. 2. Site Map Construction

```
    width -> 640;
    border -> 0
].                              ].
```

Next, a page extraction map is created using a graphical editor by drag and drop operations on the HTML object tree, such as the one illustrated in Figure 3. The oll's in the page map are then optimized and made more resilient as described in Section 2. This process is repeated for every page of interest, including those dynamically generated by scripts.

Extraction maps for individual pages are put together to form a *site map*, which encodes all access paths to the data of interest. A site map can be viewed as a labeled directed graph where the nodes represent the extraction map objects, and the labeled edges represent possible actions on the navigation objects (i.e., following a link or filling out a form) that can be executed from that page.

The overall structure of a site-map for an electronics catalog could be as depicted in Figure 4.

The above represents a simple site map with three nodes: **page1**, **page2** and **page3**. There is an edge from **page1** to **page2** labeled **table(2).tr(2).td(2). form(1)** which corresponds to a form invocation. The **items** attribute of the form in the page extraction map would describe its queriable attributes. Also, there is an edge from **page2** to **page3** with the label **table(2).tr(1).td(1).a.action** which represents a link that could be followed to retrieve additional part information such as the information presented in Figure 1.

Runtime Query Processing. The purpose of this sub-system is to automatically extract data in response to user queries. Its overall operation is as depicted in Figure 5. When a user query arrives, the *navigation planner* determines the sequences of pages to be followed using the site maps and navigation objects

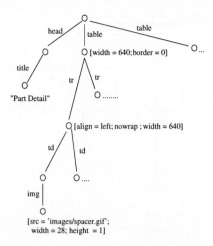

Fig. 3. An HTML parse-tree

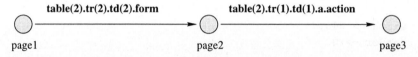

Fig. 4. A simple site map.

that are needed to answer the user's query. It then constructs a *navigation plan* for the query. For example, if the user just requests pricing information for an electronic part then only the pricing table needs to be extracted from the HTML page of Figure 1.

Next, the *navigation plan* is passed to the *plan evaluator* which accesses the actual Web pages. It parses and translates page contents into FLORA HTML objects. From these objects, the *Extractor* module extracts the navigation objects of interest using the page extraction map, and the cycle repeats until the entire query plan evaluation is completed. The resulting navigation objects are returned to the user or to the higher levels of XRover.

4   XRover Implementation: Status and Statistics

XRover was built using FLORA, a deductive object-oriented system implemented through source-to-source translation into XSB [13], which is a fast deductive engine that is based on tabled resolution approach. This technique is known to produce fast executable code and combines the advantages of top-down and bottom-up query processing.

The overall system is about 1,500 lines of FLORA code and it took less than two man months to implement. The average size of a site map is under 100 lines.

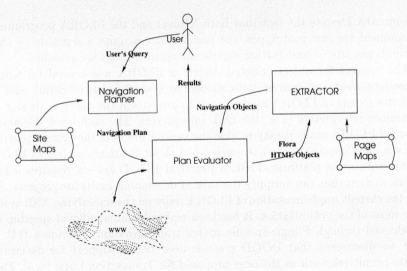

Fig. 5. Run-time query processing.

We also developed a graphical site-mapping tool to facilitate the job of building site maps. Using this tool one can construct the extraction map for a page by dragging and dropping the relevant objects from the HTML parse tree. The site-mapping GUI was written entirely in Java using the Swing library.

Even though both FLORA and XRover are just prototypes, we observed that the system has very acceptable performance. A typical number of XRover accesses per Web site is three pages, and results are returned within 3 seconds. In most cases, the response time is dominated by network delays.

So far we have built two applications with XRover – a direct mail marketing service for a large pharmaceutical company and a electronic parts portal for the U.S. Defense Logistics Agency. In the former we extract names and addresses of potential customers from phone directories posted at the web sites of various medical institutions. The parts portal provides price, availability and technical data of electronic parts from various vendor and OEM catalogs on the Web.

5   Conclusion

We described the object-oriented architecture of the virtual physical layer of XRover, a Web based information system that presents a unified database view over multiple Web sites. The implementation was done using FLORA — a DOOD system based on F-logic. The experience gained during the course of this project is perhaps the most interesting part, because DOOD systems are still rare and there are not that many applications developed with them. As expected, the use of a high-level DOOD language significantly reduced the implementation effort: the entire VPL layer was implemented in less than two man-months. Despite the fact that both XRover and the FLORA programming environment are just prototypes, the performance is quite acceptable — about 3 seconds per site — and further significant optimizations are possible.

The support for object-oriented design in FLORA was crucial for helping us produce clear and concise data models at several levels of detail, and the deductive nature of FLORA made it easy to implement the query evaluator and the various interpreters (e.g., the OLL interpreter). The high-level, declarative nature of FLORA made it easy to glue the various pieces of the system together.

Even more important is what was learned about the shortcomings of FLORA as implementation platform. First, a practical DOOD system requires a good module system that can simplify the task of developing multi-file projects. Second, the current implementation of FLORA relies on the underlying XSB system to do most of the optimization. It has been realized that significant speedup can be achieved through F-logic-specific source transformation techniques [14]. Finally, we discovered that DOOD systems need better support for declarative update primitives, such as the ones proposed for Transaction Logic [4,5]. These features are being added in the upcoming implementation of FLORA 2.0 [14].

Acknowledgement

The authors would like to thank the anonymous referees for their helpful comments.

References

1. S. Abiteboul, P. Buneman, and D. Suciu. *Data on the Web*. Morgan Kaufmann, San Francisco, CA, 2000.
2. J.L. Ambite, N. Ashish, G. Barish, C.A. Knoblock, S. Minton, P.J. Modi, I. Muslea, A. Philpot, and S. Tejada. Ariadne: A system for constructing mediators for internet sources. In *Proc. of SIGMOD*, 1998.
3. P. Atzeni, A. Masci, G. Mecca, P. Merialdo, and E. Tabet. Ulixes: Building relational views over the web. In *Proc. of ICDE*, page 576, 1997.
4. A.J. Bonner and M. Kifer. An overview of transaction logic. *Theoretical Computer Science*, 133:205–265, October 1994.
5. A.J. Bonner and M. Kifer. A logic for programming database transactions. In J. Chomicki and G. Saake, editors, *Logics for Databases and Information Systems*, pages 117–166. Kluwer Academic Publishers, 1998.
6. H. Davulcu, J. Freire, M. Kifer, and I.V. Ramakrishnan. A layered architecture for querying dynamic web content. In *ACM SIGMOD Conference on Management of Data*, June 1999.
7. H. Davulcu, G. Yang, M. Kifer, and I.V. Ramakrishnan. Computational aspects of resilient data extraction from semistructured sources. In *ACM Symposium on Principles of Database Systems*, May 2000.
8. http://www.jango.com. Jango Corporation.
9. M. Kifer. Deductive and object-oriented data languages: A quest for integration. In *Proc. of DOOD*, pages 187–212, 1995.

10. M. Kifer, G. Lausen, and J. Wu. Logical foundations of object-oriented and frame-based languages. *Journal of ACM*, 42:741–843, July 1995.
11. G. Mecca, P. Atzeni, A. Masci, P. Merialdo, and G. Sindoni. The araneus web-base management system. In *Proc. of SIGMOD*, pages 544–546, 1998.
12. M. Perkowitz, R.B. Doorenbos, O. Etzioni, and D.S. Weld. Learning to understand information on the internet: An example-based approach. *Journal of Intelligent Information Systems*, 8(2):133–153, March 1997.
13. K. Sagonas, T. Swift, and D.S. Warren. XSB as an efficient deductive database engine. In *ACM SIGMOD Conference on Management of Data*, pages 442–453, New York, May 1994. ACM.
14. G. Yang and M. Kifer. Implementing an efficient dood system using a tabling logic engine. In *First International Conference on Computational Logic, DOOD-2000 Stream*, July 2000.

A Dynamic Approach to Termination Analysis for Active Database Rules

James Bailey, Alexandra Poulovassilis, and Peter Newson

Department of Computer Science, Birkbeck College, Univ. of London
Malet Street, London WC1E 7HX, UK
{james,ap,pete}@dcs.bbk.ac.uk

Abstract. An important behavioural property for sets of active database rules is that of termination. In current commercial database systems, termination is guaranteed by imposing a fixed upper limit on the number of recursive rule firings that may occur. This can have undesirable effects such as prematurely halting correct executions. We describe a new approach based on a dynamic upper limit to the number of rule firings. This limit reflects knowledge about past rule behaviour on the database and provides a more accurate measure for when the DBMS should terminate rule execution. The approach incurs little cost and can easily be integrated with current techniques for static analysis of active rules.

1 Introduction

Active databases provide the functionality of traditional databases and additionally are capable of reacting automatically to state changes without user intervention. This is achieved by means of Event-Condition-Action (ECA) rules of the form *on* event *if* condition *do* action. One of the problems of using ECA rules is the inherent difficulty of analysing and controlling their behaviour. An important behavioural property is that of *termination*, since when multiple ECA rules have been defined in an active DBMS, possibly by different people at different times, there is the possibility that the rules may trigger each other indefinitely.

The research community has addressed this problem by focusing principally on static analysis of rule sets. The aim here has been to develop methods which can predict whether a set of rules is always guaranteed to terminate [1, 7, 4]. Since the problem is undecidable even for simple rule languages [3], these methods cannot achieve full precision. Also, given the lack of any consensus on what constitutes a "typical" terminating or non-terminating rule set, it is not easy to compare various methods with one another.

These difficulties are recognised by the current SQL3 standard for triggers [12], which does not attempt to prescribe methods for ensuring termination. Thus, commercial database products do not use any static analysis on rule sets, and termination is enforced by imposing a fixed upper limit (hereafter referred to as k or the k *limit*) on the number of recursive rule firings allowed (in Oracle 8, for example, this limit is 64). If k is reached, the actions of all the rules are rolled back. This approach has the limitation that correct sequences of rule firings may

J. Lloyd et al. (Eds.): CL 2000, LNAI 1861, pp. 1106–1120, 2000.

be prematurely halted due to an overly conservative (i.e. too low) choice of k. Conversely, allowing k to be too high can lead to unnecessary rule processing if a non-terminating computation occurs. This wasted effort may be problematic for applications such as real-time systems, where there are hard deadlines on transaction execution time and where minimising work is important.

In this paper, we describe a new approach to termination management based on a *variable* upper limit on the number of recursive rule firings. Before rule execution begins, some analysis is first performed to calculate a "suitable" k limit for that particular execution. This calculation is performed using information about the past execution behaviour of the rules. The aim is that calculating the k limit dynamically will allow rule executions to run for longer if eventual termination can definitely be predicted. This in turn helps with the second difficulty above, which occurs when the k limit is too high. This is because the rule designer can now choose a lower default k limit, more confident in the knowledge that fewer correct rule execution sequences will be aborted.

The paper is structured as follows. Section 2 defines our assumed rule execution semantics. Section 3 describes our method for inferring future rule termination from past rule execution behaviour using incremental inferencing techniques. Section 4 extends the treatment to detect the possibility of future rule non-termination by checking for repeating states. Section 5 discusses the practical usefulness and applicability of our approach, including how it fits within the overall transaction execution, and how it can be applied to analysis of SQL3 triggers. In Section 6 we compare our work with other approaches and in Section 7 we summarise our results and outline directions for future research.

2   Rule Execution Semantics

We assume that active rules are of the form *on* event *if* condition *do* action. The event part is of the form $ins(R)$ or $del(R)$, where R is a relation. The condition part is an SQL query. The action part is a sequence of insertions or deletions of the form $\pm R \leftarrow query$ where R is a relation and *query* an SQL query. In this paper we do not consider UPDATE events as found in SQL3, but the approach described here could easily be extended to cater for these also.

Events occur as transactions execute. A rule is *triggered* when the event specified in its event part occurs. A rule *fires* if it is triggered and its condition part evaluates to true. A rule set is *terminating* if for any initial event and database state, rule processing always terminates. In this paper we will be considering specific execution sequences and are thus interested in whether rule execution terminates from a *given* database state when triggered by a *given* event.

We specify the assumed rule execution semantics as a function, **execRules**. This inputs the current database and an initial schedule of rule actions. It repeatedly pops the first action off the schedule, executes it (by calling **updateDB**), determines which rules have fired as a result (in the `for` loop) and places their actions on the schedule. `execRules` terminates when the schedule is empty [1].

```
function execRules(db:DB,s:Sched):DB;
var  i      : Nat;
     action: Action;
while s != [] do {
    action:= head s;
    s      := tail s;
    db     := updateDB(db,action);
    for i := 1 to NoOfRules do
        if nonEmpty(eval(eventQueries[i],db)) and
           nonEmpty(eval(condQueries[i],db)) then
               s := bind(actions[i],db) ++ s;
}
return(db);
```

Rules are identified by numbers `1..NoOfRules`, in order of increasing priority. A schedule is a list of rule actions waiting execution. We assume the initial update initiating rule execution is itself the action part of one of the rules[2], so the initial schedule passed to `execRules` is a singleton list `[a]` for some action `a`.

A database is a set of pairs of relation names and relation extents. Relations are of three kinds: (i) user-defined ones; (ii) for each user-defined relation R, two *delta* relations, $\triangle R$ and $\triangledown R$; $\triangle R$ ($\triangledown R$) contains tuples inserted into (deleted from) R by the latest action executed; (iii) for each user-defined relation R, two *event* relations, *insEventR* and *delEventR*; *insEventR* (*delEventR*) is non-empty if and only if the latest action executed was an insertion into (deletion from) R.

The types `DB` and `Sched` are defined as follows, where the types `RelName`, `deltaRelName`, `Tuple`, `Query`, `List` and `Set` are self-explanatory:

```
type DB     = Set(RelName,Set(Tuple));
type Action = (DeltaRelName,Query);
type Sched  = List(Action);
```

A number of global variable declarations representing the rules are assumed:

```
var eventQueries:array[1..NoOfRules] of DeltaRelName;
var condQueries :array[1..NoOfRules] of Query;
var actions     :array[1..NoOfRules] of List(Action);
```

`eventQueries` records for each rule the name of the relation which, if it is non-empty, triggers the execution of the rule: if the rule's event part is $ins(R)$ ($del(R)$), this relation will be $\triangle R$ ($\triangledown R$)[3]. `condQueries` represents the condition

---

[1] We use the notation $[x_1, x_2, \ldots]$ for lists, $< x_1, x_2, \ldots >$ for tuples and $[i]$ for indexing array elements. For any list $[x_1, x_2, \ldots]$, *head* $[x_1, x_2, \ldots]$ returns x_1 and *tail* $[x_1, x_2, \ldots]$ returns $[x_2, \ldots]$. $++$ is the list concatenation operator.

[2] If not, then the original rule set can be extended with a new rule whose action part is the initial update and whose event part is not triggered by any rule.

[3] This is **semantic** triggering i.e. rules are triggered if delta relations are non-empty. Later we will also consider **syntactic** triggering where rules are triggered when up-

part of each rule, which is just an SQL query. `actions` is the list of updates constituting the action part of each rule. An insertion $+R \leftarrow query$ is represented by the pair $(\triangle R, query)$ and a deletion $-R \leftarrow query$ by $(\triangledown R, query)$.

`execRules` calls four other functions (which are straightforward and so not given here): `updateDB` applies the first action on the schedule to the database and returns the resulting database (including updated delta and event relations). `eval` evaluates a query with respect to the database and returns a set of tuples. `nonEmpty` tests whether a set is non-empty. `bind` takes a list of rule actions and the current database, and substitutes all occurrences of delta relations in the bodies of the rule actions by their current values in the database.

We have assumed *Immediate* rule coupling mode whereby the actions of a fired rule are placed at the front of the schedule[4]. This is the coupling mode assumed by SQL3. However, our method is also applicable to Deferred coupling mode, or mixtures of coupling modes. For reasons of space we do not consider this issue here, and refer the reader to [5] which discusses a general framework for abstract interpretation of active rule execution.

3   Incremental Inference of Termination Behaviour

Our method for inferring future rule termination behaviour is specified below as a function, INC, which performs an incremental inferencing of future rule behaviour using knowledge about past behaviour:

```
function INC(deltaVals:array [1..NoOfRules] of List(TruthVal),
             condVals:array [1..NoOfRules] of TruthVal,
             s:AbstSched):Status;
var  i        : Nat;
     ev, cv   : TruthVal;
     a        : Action;
     eventVals: array [1..NoOfRules] of TruthVal;
while s != [] do {
    <ev,cv,a>:= head s;
    s        := tail s;
    deltaVals:= INFER_DELTAS(deltaVals,deltaQueries,<ev,cv,a>);
    eventVals:= INFER_EVENTS(eventQueries,a,deltaVal_a);
    condVals := INFER_CONDS(condVals,condQueries,a,deltaVal_a);
    for i := 1 to NoOfRules do
        if eventVals[i] != False and condVals[i] != False then
            s := [<eventVals[i],condVals[i],a> | a <- actions[i]]
                 ++ s;
}
return(DefiniteTermination);
```

---

date statements occur, i.e. when event relations are non-empty, regardless of whether the database has changed.

[4] Since rules are considered in increasing order of priority in the for loop, actions of higher priority rules will be placed in front of actions of lower priority ones.

We observe the syntactic similarity between `execRules` and INC. In fact, INC can be considered to be performing an *abstract interpretation* of `execRules` (see [5] for theoretical foundations). The abstract schedule is a list of triples:

```
type AbstSched = List(TruthVal,TruthVal,Action)
```

As well as each action, it records the truth values of the event and condition queries when the rule fired. This is because INC places rules on the schedule if their event and condition queries are inferred to be True or Unknown, and the imprecision caused by the latter case needs to be carried forward into the subsequent inferencing process. Thus, the variables `ev` and `cv` above are the truth values of the rule's event and condition queries when the rule action was placed on the schedule, and `a` is the actual action. The variable `deltaVal_a` denotes the current value of the delta query corresponding to the action `a`.

The database state is abstracted by two arrays which contain the truth values of all the rule conditions and rule delta queries w.r.t. the current database state:

```
var condVals  : array [1..NoOfRules] of TruthVal;
var deltaVals : array [1..NoOfRules] of List(TruthVal);
```

where the type `truthVal` consists of three constants `True`, `False` and `Unknown`.

By *rule delta query* we mean the query that defines the value of the positive or negative delta relation that results when a rule action is executed. In particular, for an insertion $+R \leftarrow query$ the rule delta query is $query - R$ while for a deletion $-R \leftarrow query$ it is $query \cap R$. A rule in general has a list of actions, and hence a list of corresponding delta queries and delta query truth values. We assume the following global variable contains the rules' delta queries:

```
var deltaQueries :array[1..NoOfRules] of List(Query);
```

The `condVals` record whether a rule condition is currently True, False or Unknown. The `deltaVals` record whether a rule action would have a semantic effect (i.e. produce a change in the database) were it to be executed. So, instead of using an actual database with relations containing tuples as does `execRules`, INC uses a coarser view of the database to perform inferencing about how the actual rule execution might proceed.

`condVals` and `deltaVals` need to be maintained in synch with the current database state during actual rule execution. This is done by modifying `execRules` as follows:

(a) When a rule is triggered within the `for` loop and its condition query is then evaluated, the resulting truth value (True or False) will be recorded in the corresponding entry of the `condVals` array.

(b) Condition queries that are not evaluated within the `for` loop (because the rule has not been triggered) will have truth values inferred for them using incremental evaluation techniques (see Section 3.1 for details of these);

(c) New truth values for all the delta queries are similarly inferred on each iteration of the `while` loop.

Notice that under (a) condition queries will be assigned a value of either True or False while under (b) and (c) condition and delta queries may be assigned an Unknown truth value.

INC calls three functions to repeatedly infer the next round of truth values for the rules' delta queries, event queries and condition queries. INFER_DELTAS takes the current values of the delta queries, the delta queries themselves, and the triple `<ev,cv,a>` currently at the head of the schedule and infers new truth values for the delta queries. INFER_EVENTS takes the event queries, the current action a, and the current value of the delta query corresponding to a, `deltaVal_a`, and infers the truth values of the event queries. Finally, INFER_CONDS takes the current truth values of the condition queries, the condition queries themselves, the current action a, and its corresponding delta query value, `deltaVal_a`, and infers the new truth values of the condition queries. The inferencing techniques employed by all three functions are described in Section 3.1 below.

If INC terminates from a given initial action and database state, we can infer that `execRules` would also terminate from that initial action and database state. This is reflected by INC's return status of `DefiniteTermination`.

As it stands, INC may of course fail to terminate. There are several possible ways to force it to do so: place an upper limit on the number of iterations of its `while` loop, or implement a check for the occurrence of repeating states, or both of these. We discuss these methods further in Section 4. With any of these approaches, the status returned by INC would be `PossibleNonTermination`.

3.1 The INFER Functions

The three INFER functions invoked by INC use incremental techniques to deduce a new truth value for a query from its old truth value. Suppose we have an event, condition or delta query q and an update occurs in the database. What new truth value will be inferred for q ? If an inclusion occurs into a relation r referenced by q, then the new truth value of q is inferred using the following rules:

Rule Inc1: If the previous truth value of q was T and r doesn't occur in q or occurs only positively, then the new truth value of q is T.

Rule Inc2: If the previous truth value of q was F and r doesn't occur in q or occurs only negatively, then the new truth value of q is F.

Rule Inc3: Otherwise, the new truth value of q is U.

Similarly, if an exclusion occurs from a relation r referenced by q, then the new truth value of q is inferred using the following rules:

Rule Excl1: If the previous truth value of q was T and r doesn't occur in q or occurs only negatively, then the new truth value of q is T.

Rule Exc2: If the previous truth value of q was F and r doesn't occur in q or occurs only positively, then the new truth value of q is F.

Rule Exc3: Otherwise, the new truth value of q is U.

In the above rules, r can be either a user-defined relation or a delta relation since both of these may appear in condition queries and delta queries. For a user-defined relation, inclusions and exclusions will occur via the explicit insertions and deletions specified in the rule actions or in the top-level transaction. For a delta relation, inclusions and exclusions will occur implicitly. In particular, a delta relation $\triangle R$ $(\triangledown R)$ will undergo an implicit inclusion whenever an insertion (deletion) occurs on R, and will then undergo an implicit exclusion in the next action executed that is not an insertion (deletion) on R.

An action a has a special effect on its own delta query dq_a as given by the following rules, where an action $\pm R \leftarrow query$ is *idempotent* if R does not appear within *query*, otherwise it is *non-idempotent*:

Rule Own1: If the old truth value of dq_a was F, then the action a will not execute and so the new truth value of dq_a is also F.

Rule Own2: If a is idempotent and the old truth value of dq_a was U or T then the new truth value of dq_a is F.

Rule Own3: If a is non-idempotent and the old truth value of dq_a was U or T then the new truth value of dq_a is U.

The INFER_DELTAS function calculates the new truth value for the delta query, dq_a, associated with the action a as follows, where infer_own performs inferences according to Rules Own1-3 [5]:

```
newDeltaVal_a = ev & cv & infer_own(dq_a,oldDeltaVal_a,a)
```

For all other delta queries dq_i, their new truth value is the same as their old truth value if newDeltaVal_a is False or if dq_i is independent of the action a (i.e. the relation in the head of a does not appear in dq_i). Otherwise, the new truth value of dq_i is determined as follows, where infer_normal performs inferences according to Rules Inc1-3 and Excl-3:

```
newDeltaVal_i = ev & cv & infer_normal(dq_i,oldDeltaVal_i,a)
```

The INFER_EVENTS function calculates the new truth value for each event query eq_i as follows, where infer_event returns T if the action a matches the event query eq_i and F otherwise:

```
newEventVal_i = newDeltaVal_a & infer_event(eq_i,a)
```

Finally, the INFER_CONDS function calculates the new truth value for each condition query cq_i. The new truth value of cq_i is the same as its old truth value if deltaVal_a is False or if cq_i is independent of a. Otherwise the new truth value of cq_i is given by:

```
newCondVal_i = newDeltaVal_a & infer_normal(cq_i,oldCondVal_i,a)
```

---

[5] Here, & is a 3-valued logic conjunction operator:

&	T	F	U
T	T	F	U
F	F	F	F
U	U	F	U

Example 1. Consider the 6 rules below[6]:

Rule	Event	Condition	Action(s)	Delta Query(s)
r_1	$ins(R_4)$	$R_4 \bowtie R_5$	$-R_3 \leftarrow R_8; +R_6 \leftarrow R_4 \bowtie R_5$	$R_3 \cap R_8; (R_4 \bowtie R_5) - R_6$
r_2	$ins(R_6)$	$R_4 - R_3$	$+R_3 \leftarrow R_4 - R_3$	$(R_4 - R_3) - R_3$
r_3	$ins(R_3)$	$R_4 \bowtie R_1$	$-R_1 \leftarrow R_9 \bowtie (R_5 - R_4)$	$(R_9 \bowtie (R_5 - R_4)) \cap R_1$
r_4	$del(R_1)$	$true$	$-R_0 \leftarrow R_5$	$R_0 \cap R_5$
r_5	$del(R_0)$	$true$	$+R_0 \leftarrow R_2 \cap \bigtriangledown R_0$	$(R_2 \cap \bigtriangledown R_0) - R_0$
r_6	$ins(R_0)$	$R_7 \bowtie R_8$	$-R_0 \leftarrow R_3$	$R_0 \cap R_3$

These rules are non-terminating, since r_5 and r_6 could trigger each other infinitely. We will see, however, that knowledge about the initial truth values of the condition and delta queries means that we can predict that the rules will terminate for the current database instance.

Consider the trace given below of successive iterations of the **while** loop in INC, starting from the abstract database state shown in the first line. Recall that a triple $<$T,T,a$>$ on the abstract schedule indicates an action, a, whose corresponding event and condition queries were both True at the time the action was placed on the schedule. **a_i** denotes the action of rule r_i (for a single-action rule) while **a_i_j** denotes the jth action of rule r_i (for a multi-action rule).

Note that all actions except r_2's are idempotent, so that the delta queries of all other rules are made False by the execution of their actions. Step 1 shows an initial abstract database state where r_1 was triggered. In step 3 r_2 has fired; the deltaVals of r_1 have become False due to the idempotence property of r_1's actions. In step 4 r_3 has fired; the first deltaVal of r_1, the deltaVal of r_5 and the condVal of r_2 have all become Unknown due to the execution of a_2. In step 5 r_4 has fired. In step 6 r_5 has fired. In step 7 r_6 has become triggered; however, since the condVal of r_6 is False, it will not fire. Thus INC terminates after the execution of five rules.

Step	deltaVals	condVals	abstract schedule
1	[[T,T],T,T,T,T,F]	[T,T,T,T,T,F]	[$<$T,T,a_1_1$>$,$<$T,T,a_1_2$>$]
2	[[F,T],T,T,T,T,F]	[T,T,T,T,T,F]	[$<$T,T,a_1_2$>$]
3	[[F,F],T,T,T,T,F]	[T,T,T,T,T,F]	[$<$T,T,a_2$>$]
4	[[U,F],U,T,T,T,U]	[T,U,T,T,T,F]	[$<$T,T,a_3$>$]
5	[[U,F],U,F,T,T,U]	[T,U,U,T,T,F]	[$<$T,T,a_4$>$]
6	[[U,F],U,F,F,T,U]	[T,U,U,T,T,F]	[$<$T,T,a_5$>$]
7	[[U,F],U,F,U,F,U]	[T,U,U,T,F,F]	[]

We thus infer that the actual rule execution will also terminate after executing these rules, at most (in fact we can infer that it will execute *precisely* this sequence of rules because no triggered rule has an Unknown event, condition, or

---

[6] For reasons of brevity, we use the relational algebra notation for this and subsequent examples, rather than SQL. In this and subsequent examples, all the rules are statement-level rules, unless otherwise stated.

delta query). Thus, checking for the k limit during the subsequent actual rule execution can be turned off since we know that this rule execution will terminate.

4   Detecting Possible Non-termination

Both the actual rule execution and the abstract semantics of INC suffer from the drawback that the **while** loop may fail to terminate. One way of preventing this for the actual rule execution would be to maintain a history of states and to check for the reoccurrence of a past state, where a "state" consists of the current database and current action to be executed.

Due to the size of real databases, this may not be a feasible extension to execRules, although work in [7] shows how to improve its efficiency. However, checking for repeating states is also possible in INC and moreover is much less costly in this case. The "state" now consists of the triple <ev,cv,a> which is currently at the head of the abstract schedule, and the current truth values of the rule conditions and rule delta queries. The history is a list of such states and is maintained by prefixing the current state to the history on each iteration of the **while** loop. An extra test is added to the **while** loop to test if the current state is equal to a state in the history — note that this is just a simple syntactic equality:

```
history := [];
while s != [] do {
    <ev,cv,a>:= head s;
    s         := tail s;
    if member(<deltaVals,condVals,<ev,cv,a>>,history) then
        return(PossibleNonTermination);
    history  := [<deltaVals,condVals,<ev,cv,a>>] ++ history;
    deltaVals:= INFER_DELTAS(deltaVals,deltaQueries,<ev,cv,a>);
    eventVals:= ... as before ... }
return(DefiniteTermination);
```

There is a bounded number of possible distinct states that INC can reach, of the order of NoOfRules$*3^{\text{NoOfQueries}}$ (since there are NoOfRules rules and NoOfQueries condition and delta queries each of which can take one of three truth values). The extended INC function is thus guaranteed to terminate since a repeating state will eventually occur if execution proceeds for long enough. Notice that this is even true for rules that are non-function-free. In contrast, in the actual rule execution, a repeating state may never occur if the rule language is able to create new constants.

Example 2. Consider the following two rules:

Rule	Event	Condition	Action	Delta Query
r_1	$del(R_3)$	$R_8 \bowtie R_4$	$+R_3 \leftarrow R_5$	$R_5 - R_3$
r_2	$ins(R_3)$	$R_5 - R_4$	$-R_3 \leftarrow R_4$	$R_4 \cap R_3$

We trace through an execution of INC in the same way as before:

Step	deltaVals	condVals	abstract schedule
1	[T,T]	[T,T]	[<T,T,a_1>]
2	[F,T]	[T,T]	[<T,T,a_2>]
3	[U,F]	[T,T]	[<T,T,a_1>]
4	[F,U]	[T,T]	[<U,T,a_2>]
5	[U,F]	[T,T]	[<U,T,a_1>]
6	[F,U]	[T,T]	[<U,T,a_2>]

Notice that both rule actions are idempotent. Step 1 shows an initial abstract database state where r_1 has fired. In step 2 r_2 has fired. The two rules continue to fire in turn during steps 3 to 6. In step 3 r_2's action makes r_1's delta query Unknown and in step 4 r_1's action makes r_2's delta query Unknown. The state in step 6 is a repetition of that in step 4 and so INC terminates with a status of PossibleNonTermination. It is therefore not safe to ignore the default value of the k limit during the subsequent actual rule execution.

In summary, if INC returns PossibleNonTermination, then we perform actual rule execution with the default k limit (k_{def}). Otherwise, if INC returns DefiniteTermination after l iterations, then we perform rule execution with the k limit set to l. If $l > k_{def}$, then we will have prevented an unnecessary abort of rule execution. If $l \leq k$ or PossibleNonTermination was returned by INC, then running INC will have brought no benefits, but since the cost of INC is low (see Section 5) there will have been negligible impact on system performance. A final point to note is that adding new rules to the rule set is easily accomplished: extra entries just need to be created for these rules in the condVals and deltaVals arrays and their starting values set to Unknown.

5   Evaluation

Cost and Effectiveness of the Method. We have extended the PFL active database system [17] with the dynamic rule analysis method described here. The history of abstract database states is stored in main memory as a list of arrays of truth values. The time cost incurred is primarily dependent on the cost of (a) performing the INFER functions and (b) scanning the history for a repeating state. The cost of (a) is negligible. With our present simple encoding of the history, the cost of (b) grows quadratically with the length of the history and on a mid-range Pentium machine reaches 0.5 seconds at a history length of approximately 500 and 1 second at a history length of approximately 1500 Clearly, more sophisticated encodings of the history would improve these times.

The main space cost incurred is by the history. This is bounded by the number of different states that can occur, of the order of $\text{NoOfRules} * 3^{\text{NoOfQueries}}$. This could be very large if NoOfRules is greater than 10 (say). In practice an upper limit, L, will be imposed on history length, determined by the time cost of searching for repeating states[7]. We conjecture setting L to a relatively high number (2 to 3 orders of magnitude larger than the default k limit) will be sufficient to detect most cases of definite termination, and our experiments with synthetic sets of rules indicate that this is indeed the case. [8]

Relationship to Transaction Execution. We now consider how our dynamic analysis approach integrates with the overall system behaviour. This behaviour can be divided into two modes, transaction mode and rule execution mode. In transaction mode, transactions are submitted to the database and are executed. The truth values of the condition queries and delta queries are maintained in synch with the updates made by the transaction, using the same incremental evaluation techniques as used during INC. If a rule is triggered within a transaction, the system enters rule execution mode. This consists of executing INC followed the actual rule execution. After termination of rule execution, the system reverts to transaction mode again.

Integration with Other Methods. Extra knowledge about properties of the rule set may be available and it is possible to incorporate this into the INC algorithm. Firstly, we may know from prior static analysis that execution is guaranteed to terminate when certain rules are reached, in which case INC need not continue if it reaches one of these rules. Secondly, we can utilise human-aided analysis in the inference procedure. For instance, rules may be *self disactivating* (i.e. their condition is always made False by their action) and this knowledge can be used for more accurate inferencing. Inferencing can also be made more precise by applying containment and satisfiability tests to determine whether actions will ever have an effect on condition and delta queries. Finally, there is also scope for improving inferencing using knowledge about global properties of rules (e.g. event based stratifications of rule sets as in [6]).

Relationship to SQL3. The rule execution semantics of `execRules` undertake a **semantic, set-oriented** triggering of rules. It is semantic triggering in the sense that rule event queries are delta relations, and rules are triggered if these delta relations are non-empty. In contrast, SQL3's statement-level triggers undertake a **syntactic** triggering of rules i.e. rules are triggered when update statements occur irrespective of whether they cause any change to the database.

Our semantics are easily modified to model execution of SQL3 statement-level AFTER triggers. The condition parts of rules need to be encoded within the bodies of the rule actions and not evaluated within the `for` loop of `execRules`. This causes rule conditions to be evaluated with respect to the database state that the action will be executed on, rather than the database state when the rule was triggered. We use a schedule to store triggered rule actions, rather than SQL3's *trigger execution contexts* (TECs), but the effect is the same. The event parts of rules now need to be event relations (*insEventR* or *delEventR*) rather than delta relations ($\triangle R$ or $\triangledown R$). Incremental inferencing proceeds as

---

[7] Note that L should not be confused with the default k limit for actual rule execution.
[8] Of course it may be tempting to just use a default k limit set to some high number e.g. 1000, but this would result in wasted execution when the rules are non-terminating.

with semantic triggering, except now all delta query values are assumed to be always True and event query values will be either True or False (never Unknown).

SQL3's BEFORE triggers are not significant for the purposes of termination analysis since they cannot trigger any other trigger. We have also ignored the checking of integrity constraints and have assumed that these will not be violated (for the purposes of termination analysis the worst-case scenario is that no integrity constraints are violated and no aborts occur).

Our rule execution semantics are set-oriented rather than instance-oriented and thus do not directly model the behaviour of SQL3's row-level triggers. However, `execRules` is easily extended to also support row-level triggers, as follows. If a rule `i` has fired and it is a row-level rule then for each tuple `t` ∈ `eval(eventQueries[i])` a list of actions is placed on the schedule, obtained from `actions[i]` by substituting each occurrence of `eventQueries[i]` in the body of the actions by the singleton set `{t}`.

The question is how should INC be modified, and in particular how many copies of each rule action should be placed on the abstract schedule ? The solution is to dynamically place as many copies as are required until either a repeating state is reached or definite termination can be concluded.

So we recursively invoke INC from the current abstract database state, db_0, with a schedule consisting of 1 copy of the rule action. Either a repeating state will be encountered or definite termination will be inferred. In the former case, we are done and the overall result of INC is possible non-termination. In the latter case we examine if the abstract database state now reached, db_1 say, is the same as db_0. If so, we are done and we can infer definite termination of the execution of this row-level rule and continue processing the rest of the schedule. Otherwise, we recursively invoke INC again from db_1 with a schedule again consisting of 1 copy of the rule action. We continue recursively invoking INC in this way, obtaining a sequence of database states db_0, db_1, db_2, ... db_i, until either possible non-termination results from the ith invocation or db_i is equal to some prior db_j. In the former case the overall result of INC will be possible non-termination. In the latter case we can infer definite termination of the execution of this row-level rule and continue processing the rest of the schedule.

Example 3. Consider the rule set and initial abstract database state of Example 1, but now make rule 5 a row-level rule. Execution is the same as in Example 1 for steps 1-4. At step 5, an action is placed on the schedule, corresponding to a single instance of r_5's action, and INC is recursively invoked with this singleton schedule; at step 6, r_6's condition is false, so the schedule becomes empty and the recursive invocation of INC terminates. INC is then re-invoked recursively, with another instance of r_5's action. Again this recursive invocation terminates, this time with the same state as in Step 6. We thus conclude that execution of the row-level rule r_5 terminates. The overall execution of INC thus terminates. So, checking for the k limit during the subsequent actual rule execution can be turned off since we know that this rule execution will terminate.

Step	deltaVals	condVals	abstract schedule
1	$[[T,T],T,T,T,T,F]$	$[T,T,T,T,T,F]$	$[<T,T,a\_1\_1>,<T,T,a\_1\_2>]$
2	$[[F,T],T,T,T,T,F]$	$[T,T,T,T,T,F]$	$[<T,T,a\_1\_2>]$
3	$[[F,F],T,T,T,T,F]$	$[T,T,T,T,T,F]$	$[<T,T,a\_2>]$
4	$[[U,F],U,T,T,T,U]$	$[T,U,T,T,T,F]$	$[<T,T,a\_3>]$
5	$[[U,F],U,F,T,T,U]$	$[T,U,U,T,T,F]$	$[<T,T,a\_4>]$
6	$[[U,F],U,F,F,T,U]$	$[T,U,U,T,T,F]$	$[<T,T,a\_5>]$
7	$[[U,F],U,F,U,F,U]$	$[T,U,U,T,T,F]$	$[]$
8	$[[U,F],U,F,U,T,U]$	$[T,U,U,T,T,F]$	$[<T,T,a\_5>]$
9	$[[U,F],U,F,U,F,U]$	$[T,U,U,T,T,F]$	$[]$

Example 4. Consider the next rule set. Suppose that r_1 is a row-level rule, r_2, r_3 and r_4 are statement-level rules and that r_3 has higher priority than r_2.

Rule	Event	Condition	Action	Deltaval
r_1	$del(R_3)$	$R_8 \bowtie R_4$	$+R_3 \leftarrow R_5 \cap \triangledown R_3$	$(R_5 \cap \triangledown R_3) - R_3$
r_2	$ins(R_3)$	$R_5 - R_3$	$-R_6 \leftarrow R_4$	$R_6 \cap R_4$
r_3	$ins(R_3)$	$R_1 - R_6$	$-R_7 \leftarrow R_4$	$R_7 \cap R_4$
r_4	$del(R_7)$	$true$	$-R_7 \leftarrow R_3 \bowtie R1 \bowtie R_7$	$R_7 \cap (R_3 \bowtie R_1 \bowtie R_7)$

Consider the following execution trace of INC from the stated initial state. Note that the actions of rules r_1, r_2 and r_3 are idempotent. Rule r_1 is assumed to be initially triggered and INC is recursively invoked with a single instance of its action on the schedule. This invocation terminates at step 3. Another recursive invocation of INC is performed at step 4. This time both r_2 and r_3 are triggered and their actions placed on the schedule in order of priority. Execution continues and a repeating state is found at steps 7 and 8. We therefore conclude the set of rules is possibly non-terminating from this initial state:

Step	DeltaVals	condVals	abstract schedule
1	$[T,T,T,T]$	$[T,T,F,T]$	$[<T,T,a\_1>]$
2	$[F,T,T,T]$	$[T,U,F,T]$	$[<T,U,a\_2>]$
3	$[F,F,T,T]$	$[T,U,U,T]$	$[]$
4	$[T,F,T,T]$	$[T,U,U,T]$	$[<T,T,a\_1>]$
5	$[F,F,T,T]$	$[T,U,U,T]$	$[<T,U,a\_3>,<T,U,a\_2>]$
6	$[F,F,F,U]$	$[T,U,U,T]$	$[<U,T,a\_4>,<T,U,a\_2>]$
7	$[F,F,U,U]$	$[T,U,U,T]$	$[<U,T,a\_4>,<T,U,a\_2>]$
8	$[F,F,U,U]$	$[T,U,U,T]$	$[<U,T,a\_4>,<T,U,a\_2>]$

Remark. If rule r_1 had been statement-level, then execution would have halted at step 3 and definite termination from the initial state concluded.

6   Related Work

Most previous work on termination analysis for active rules has dealt with static analysis. In [1], triggering graphs were first presented and later refined in in [11] and [13], where techniques for removing paths are shown. Generalisations using a method called rule reduction are described in [7]. If one were to extend this method to allow incorporation of knowledge about constraints known to hold in the database (e.g. truth values of conditions), then the result would be quite similar to the approach we have described in this paper. The idea of using abstract interpretation to assist with rule analysis was first presented in [2] and extended to a more complex language in [4]. In [4] complex, and potentially expensive, abstractions are used without any knowledge about the initial database state, whereas here we use a simple, and cheap, abstraction together with some knowledge about the initial database state.

The principal previous work in dynamic analysis is [7], where checking is performed at run-time to see whether a repeating database state has occurred in a history of previous states. In principle, the method is totally precise. However, it is restricted to function-free rules. Also, even with the optimisations presented, it is potentially quite expensive to store the history of database states. Moreover, for real-time applications it is less applicable if one needs to detect loops in a timely manner i.e. before having needlessly executed rules.

Our inferencing depends on deducing new query values from old ones in the presence of updates, and we can make use of previous techniques such as [15, 8, 16, 9, 10]. These techniques were developed for use in query optimisation. Here we have applied them instead to analysis, our focus being on when the values of queries should to be incrementally inferred and with what input, rather than how the inference should be done. Finally, optimisation of triggers based on execution flow is treated in [14], but there it is the execution context of a transaction program, not the rules themselves, which is of interest.

7   Summary and Further Work

We have examined the problem of dynamically enforcing termination of active rules. Rather than aborting rule execution after a fixed number of rule firings, we have described an approach which dynamically infers this limit. The advantage of this is that more terminating rule execution sequences can be allowed to proceed without being aborted prematurely. The algorithms required are cheap since they only operate on synthetic databases, and are thus immediately usable in practical systems. There are a number of directions of further work:

Improving the Precision of INC. INC loses precision when condition or delta queries have an Unknown value, which may result in INC returning `PossibleNonTermination` where `execRules` would terminate. This can be alleviated in two ways. (a) condition/delta queries that have a current value of Unknown can be evaluated during periods of DBMS inactivity (and thus be updated to True or False), so that the input to the next invocation of INC is made more precise. (b) INC can be interleaved with phases of actual rule execution e.g. if actual rule execution reaches k, rather than giving up and aborting INC can be reinvoked to see more accurate inferences can be made. In particular, if definite termination can now be concluded from the new abstract database state, then the actual rule execution can be allowed to proceed to termination.

Improving the Precision of the INFER Functions. Rather than just recording the truth value of condition and delta queries, we could record truth values for their sub-queries also. For even more precision, we could use even more detailed information, such as the number of tuples that made a condition true. **Other Analysis Questions.** The thrust of this paper has been towards termination enforcement. However, our techniques are also applicable to other analysis questions that involve reachability e.g. would a given rule eventually be triggered during rule processing on the current database ?
Using Definite Analysis Information for Rule Optimisation. Suppose we infer from INC that certain rules are guaranteed to have a definitely True or False condition at particular points in the rule execution sequence (e.g. as in Example 1). Then can then use this knowledge to optimise the subsequent actual rule execution sequence by turning off condition evaluation at those points.

References

1. A. Aiken, J. Widom, and J. M. Hellerstein. Static analysis techniques for predicting the behavior of active database rules. *ACM TODS*, 20(1):3–41, 1995.
2. J. Bailey, L. Crnogorac, K. Ramamohanarao, and H. Søndergaard. Abstract interpretation of active rules and its use in termination analysis. In *Proc. 6th ICDT, LNCS 1186*, pages 188–202, 1997.
3. J. Bailey, G. Dong, and K. Ramamohanarao. Decidability and undecidability results for the termination problem of active database rules. In *Proc. of PODS'98*.
4. J. Bailey and A. Poulovassilis. Abstract interpretation for termination analysis in functional active databases. *J. of Intell. Info. Systems*, 12(2/3):243–273, 1999.
5. J. Bailey and A. Poulovassilis. An abstract interpretation framework for termination analysis of active rules. In *Proc. 7th DBPL*, September 1999.
6. E. Baralis, S. Ceri, and S. Paraboschi. Modularization techniques for active rules design. *ACM TODS*, 21(1), 1996.
7. E. Baralis, Ceri. S., and S. Paraboschi. Compile-time and runtime analysis of active behaviors. *IEEE TKDE*, 10(3):353–370, 1998.
8. E. Baralis and J. Widom. Using delta relations to optimize condition evaluation in active databases. In *Proc. 2nd RIDS, LNCS 985*, pages 292–308, Athens, 1995.
9. T. Griffin and B. Kumar. Algebraic change propagation for semijoin and outerjoin queries. *ACM SIGMOD Record*, 27(3):22–27, 1998.
10. T. Griffin, L. Libkin, and H. Trickey. A correction to "Incremental recomputation of active relational expressions". *IEEE TKDE*, 9(3):508–511, 1997.
11. A. Karadimce and S. Urban. Refined triggering graphs: A logic based approach to termination analysis in an active oo database. In *Proc. of ICDE96*, pages 384–391.
12. K. Kulkarni, N. Mattos, and R. Cochrane. Active database features in SQL3. In N. Paton, editor, *Active Rules in Database Systems*, pages 197–219. 1999.
13. S. Y. Lee and T. W. Ling. A path removing technique for detecting trigger termination. In *Proc. 6th EDBT*, pages 341–355, Valencia, 1998.
14. F. Llirbat, F. Fabret, and E. Simon. Eliminating costly redundant computations from SQL trigger executions. In *Proc. ACM SIGMOD*, pages 428–439, 1997.
15. X. Qian and G. Wiederhold. Incremental recomputation of active relational expressions. *IEEE TKDE*, 3(3):337–341, 1991.
16. D. Quass. Maintenance expressions for views with aggregation. In *Proc. Workshop on Materialised Views: Techniques and Applications*, pages 110–118, 1996.
17. S. Reddi, A. Poulovassilis, and C. Small. PFL: An active functional DBPL. In N. Paton, editor, *Active Rules in Database Systems*, pages 297–308. 1999.

Constraint-Based Termination Analysis for Cyclic Active Database Rules[*]

Saumya Debray[1] and Timothy Hickey[2]

[1] Department of Computer Science
The University of Arizona, Tucson, AZ 85721, USA
debray@cs.arizona.edu
[2] Michtom School of Computer Science
Brandeis University, Waltham, MA 02454, USA
tim@cs.brandeis.edu

Abstract. There are many situations where cyclic rule activations—where some set of active database rules may be activated repeatedly until the database satisfies some condition—arise naturally. However, most existing approaches to termination analysis of active rules, which typically rely on checking that the triggering graph for the rules is acyclic, cannot infer termination for such rules. We present a constraint-based approach to termination analysis that is able to handle such cyclic rule activations for a wide class of rules.

1   Introduction

Active databases, which are conventional databases extended with a mechanism to create and execute production rules that manipulate the state of the database, have attracted considerable interest in recent years. Such rules provide a general mechanism for a number of database features such as integrity constraint checking and view maintenance, and simplify building and reasoning about database applications.

In general, rule activations in active databases can "cascade," i.e., the execution of an active rule can cause a change in the database state that causes another rule to be executed; the resulting change can then cause the activation of a third rule; and so on. Ensuring that such cascaded rule activations do not go on forever therefore becomes of fundamental importance. Analyses that examine a set of active rules to determine whether rule activations will terminate are called *termination analyses.*

Almost all of the work to date on termination analysis for active databases (see Section 6) relies on checking that a directed graph called the "triggering graph" for a set of rules is acyclic. The essential intuition this expresses is that a rule should not be able to cause itself to be (re-)activated, either directly or indirectly. The differences between various proposals for such analyses lie in the sets of edges they are able to eliminate from the triggering graph before this

---

[*] This work was supported in part by the National Science Foundation under grants CCR-9711166, CDA-9500991, and ASC-9720738.

J. Lloyd et al. (Eds.): CL 2000, LNAI 1861, pp. 1121–1136, 2000.

acyclicity check. In most of these proposals, the underlying sets of rules being considered satisfy the property of not being self-activating in this manner, and the analyses themselves focus on identifying and eliminating edges that could introduce spurious cycles into the triggering graph.

There are, however, many situations where it is natural to have a rule that can activate itself, but where such self-activations are guaranteed to eventually terminate. As an example, suppose we have a rule stating that, whenever an employee in a firm gets a raise that causes his salary to exceed his manager's salary, the manager should also get a commensurate raise. This rule can be self-activating, since the raise given to an employee can cause his manager to be given a raise, which in turn can cause the manager's manager to get a raise, and so on. However, it is not difficult to see that, under realistic assumptions, such a cycle of rule activations cannot go on for ever.

Throughout this paper, we use the following example, taken from Chapter 2 of a text by Zaniolo *et. al.* [24].

Example 1. The following rule, defined by a budget-conscious manager, imposes a salary reduction of 10% on every employee in an organization whenever the average salary exceeds a threshold (in this case 100):

```
rule SalaryControl on Emp
when inserted, deleted, updated(Sal)
if (Select Avg(Sal) from Emp) > 100
then update Emp
     set Sal = 0.9*Sal
```

Notice that this rule can be activated if an employee is hired with a high initial salary; if the initial salary is high enough, one round of salary reductions may not suffice to satisfy the termination condition, so the rule may be activated again. Eventually, however, the average salary must fall below 100, causing the rule activations to terminate.

While this rule seems "obviously terminating," reasoning about such rules can be quite subtle. For example, consider a rule that is identical to that shown above, the only difference being that the activation condition is

```
if (Select Avg(Sal) from Emp) > 0 then ...
```

This rule is structurally very similar to that of Example 1, with a decreasing value for the average salary and a lower bound on how far it can decrease. It is, nevertheless, non-terminating. As another example, consider a rule that is identical to that of Example 1, with the only difference being that the action is to set each employee's salary to 0.9*Sal + Bonus, where Bonus is some constant. In this case, it turns out that the rule is terminating if Bonus < 10, and nonterminating if Bonus ≥ 10. What these examples illustrate is that any termination analysis that aims to handle such cyclic rule activations must be able to analyze the effects of cyclic rule execution with a fairly high degree of precision.

2   Preliminaries

2.1   Active Rules

We consider *Event-Condition-Action* (ECA) rules: a rule is triggered when certain *events* specified in the rule occur, and provided that their (optional) *conditions* hold; when a rule so triggered is executed, the *actions* specified in the rule are carried out. For concreteness we use the syntax and semantics of the Starburst rule system [23]: a rule is assumed to have the structure

> rule *RuleName* on *Relation*
> when *EventList*
> if *C* then *Action*

where *EventList* specifies a set of events that cause the rule to be triggered. The execution of a triggered rule involves the evaluation of the condition C, and if this evaluates to *true*, carrying out the actions specified in the list *Action*. The condition C, which determines when the rule is activated, is referred to as the *activation condition* of the rule; we sometimes also use the term *termination condition* for the rule to refer to the condition $\neg C$.

Since the handling of aggregation operations is more or less orthogonal to the main focus of this paper, we make the simplifying assumption that any aggregation operations in active rules are applied to the entire relation, i.e., there is no aggregation over partitions of the relation computed using constructs such as the 'group by' clause of SQL. The basic idea is that if a rule computes an aggregate operation f on an attribute A of a relation R, we handle this using a dummy relation R_A_f containing a single tuple that has a single attribute whose value is that of the operation f applied to attribute A of R. Changes to the relation R through *insert*, *delete*, or *update* operations—including those in active rules—are considered to also modify such dummy relations appropriately, albeit in a conservative manner: that is, unless the new value of the aggregate value can be predicted, its value is considered to be unknown and represented in the dummy relation using a null value.

2.2   Constraint Systems

For the purposes of this paper, *constraints* are first-order formulae over a signature Σ, such that: the binary predicate symbol '=' is in Σ; there are constraints that are identically true and identically false; and the class of constraints is closed under variable renaming, conjunction, and existential quantification. A *constraint system* is a system for maintaining and manipulating constraints over a *constraint domain* $\mathcal{D}$, which is essentially a (first-order) structure, i.e., a universe D together with an appropriate assignment of functions and relations over D to the symbols in Σ. Operations on constraints supported by the constraint system are assumed to include [17]:

- A test for *consistency* or *satisfiability*: $\mathcal{D} \models (\exists) c$.
- A test for *implication* (i.e., *entailment*) of one constraint by another: $\mathcal{D} \models c_0 \Rightarrow c_1$.

- The *projection* of a constraint c_0 onto variables $\bar{x}$ to obtain a constraint c_1 such that $\mathcal{D} \models c_1 \Leftrightarrow (\exists \bar{y}) c_0$, where $\bar{y} = vars(c_0) - \bar{x}$ is the set of variables in c_0 except for those mentioned in $\bar{x}$.

It should be noted that typical constraint logic programming systems, such as CLP($\mathcal{R}$) [16] and SICStus Prolog [20] (see also the survey by Jaffar and Maher [17]), support this level of functionality.

In particular, we focus on the CLP(F) constraint system [13], which is powerful enough for our needs and whose implementation is freely available. This is a constraint system over the reals that supports, in addition to the usual arithmetic and comparison operators, the functions $abs(x)$, $exp(x)$, $log(x)$, x^n, x^y, as well as the trigonometric functions $sin(x)$, $cos(x)$, $tan(x)$ and their inverses. Our implementation of this system uses interval constraints, and handles these functions using a reimplementation of the standard math library based on interval arithmetic. A detailed discussion of this system is omitted due to space constraints: for our purposes it suffices to note that the constraint solver is queried with a quantifier-free first-order conjunction $Q(x_1, \ldots, x_n)$, interpreted as the question "*do there exist any $x_1, \ldots, x_n$ such that $Q(x_1, \ldots, x_n)$?*" The solver responds either with a set of real intervals $I_1, \ldots, I_n$, interpreted as "*if there exist any $x_1, \ldots, x_n$ such that $Q(x_1, \ldots, x_n)$, then for all such values it must be the case that $x_1 \in I_1$ and $\ldots$ and $x_n \in I_n$*," or indicates that there are no values for the variables x_i that satisfy $Q(\cdots)$. A fundamentally important aspect of the system is that the constraint system is provably sound [13, 14], i.e., if the solver returns such a set of intervals $I_1, \ldots, I_n$ for a query $Q(x_1, \ldots, x_n)$, then it is guaranteed that for every solution $\hat{x}_1, \ldots, \hat{x}_n$ to the query it is the case that $\hat{x}_i \in I_i$. However, completeness is not guaranteed in general, i.e., just because the solver returns a set of intervals does not imply that these are the minimal intervals containing all solutions to the query.

3   Annotated Triggering Graphs

Many termination analyses proposed in the literature use the notion of triggering graphs. A triggering graph is a directed graph where each vertex represents a rule and where there is an edge from vertex r_i to vertex r_j if the action of rule r_i can cause rule r_j to become triggered [8]. We generalize this notion to that of "annotated triggering graphs," which additionally incorporate information, at each vertex, about the change(s) resulting from the activation of the corresponding rule. To this end, we first define how such changes might be represented.

Definition 1. [Bounds Function] *A bounds function over a schema S maps each attribute of S to a pair $\langle lo, hi \rangle$ where each of lo and hi is either $\bot$ or a linear expressions over (numerical) attributes in S.*

If a bounds function maps an attribute to $\langle lo, hi \rangle$, this indicates that lo is a lower bound on the values of that attribute while hi is an upper bound, with a value of $\bot$ indicating a complete lack of knowledge (i.e., indicating that we cannot say anything about the values for the corresponding attribute), and non-$\bot$ values indicating definite knowledge. Note that these bounds are not restricted to be numbers, but may in general be expressions that depend on the values for other attributes.

Definition 2. [Annotated Triggering Graph] *Given a set of rules R with schema S, an annotated triggering graph is a pair $(G, \mathcal{F})$ where $G = (V, E)$ is a conventional triggering graph, and $\mathcal{F}$ maps each vertex in V to a bounds function over S.*

Thus, at each vertex of an annotated triggering graph, each attribute is mapped to a pair of expressions that specify upper and lower bounds on the values of that attribute. As an example, the rule in Example 1 would associate, with the vertex corresponding to the rule, the bounds function $[Sal \mapsto \langle 0.9 * Sal, 0.9 * Sal \rangle]$ (attributes that are not explicitly mentioned are assumed to not have changed, and are therefore mapped to themselves). This indicates that the result of the activation of the rule is to update each tuple so that the value of its Sal attribute is 90% of its old Sal value, while the other attribute values are left unchanged.

3.1   Constructing Annotated Triggering Graphs

This section describes a simple algorithm for constructing annotated triggering graphs. It is quite conservative in its treatment of bounds, and can almost certainly be improved to increase its precision. Consider a rule

```
rule RuleName on R
when ...
if ...
then update R'
    set x = φ(y₁,...,yₙ) where Cond
```

The first question we consider is whether all of the tuples in R' will be modified. If the final **where** clause is absent, or $Cond$ is identically true, then we know that all tuples in R' will have the value of attribute x set to $\varphi(y_1, \ldots, y_n)$. So in this case the bounds function maps x to $\langle \varphi(y_1, \ldots, y_n), \varphi(y_1, \ldots, y_n) \rangle$.

Otherwise, if it is possible that only some of the tuples will be updated, we attempt to determine the relationship of the value of the expression $\varphi(y_1, \ldots, y_n)$ with that of x. Let $\mathcal{C}_0$ be a conjunction of constraints on the possible values for various attributes, obtained from domain information for the database schema as well integrity constraints on the database ($\mathcal{C}_0$ is a global constraint and need be computed only once, at the beginning of the analysis). We then construct a constraint $\mathcal{C} \equiv \mathcal{C}_0 \wedge [z = \varphi(y_1, \ldots, y_n) - x]$, where z is a new variable not appearing in $\mathcal{C}_0$, and examine whether or not certain constraints on z are entailed by $\mathcal{C}$ (see Section 2.2 for our assumptions regarding entailment operations in constraint systems). We consider the following possibilities:

- $\mathcal{C}$ entails $z \geq 0$. This means that the value of x is non-decreasing as a result of the update. Since it is possible that only some of the tuples will be updated, an upper bound on the x attribute value is given by $\varphi(y_1, \ldots, y_n)$, while a lower bound is given by x. Thus, in this case we have the bounds function $[x \mapsto \langle x, \varphi(y_1, \ldots, y_n) \rangle]$.

- $\mathcal{C}$ entails $z \leq 0$. This means that the value of x is non-increasing. Reasoning as in the previous case, we get the bounds function $[x \mapsto \langle \varphi(y_1, \ldots, y_n), x \rangle]$.
- If neither of these previous two cases holds, we conclude that nothing can be said about the value of x after the update. The resulting bounds function is $[x \mapsto \langle \perp, \perp \rangle]$.

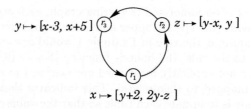

Fig. 1. An example of a cycle in an annotated triggering graph

3.2   Reasoning about Annotated Triggering Graphs

Once we have constructed an annotated triggering graph for a set of rules, we examine any cycles in this graph to determine the net effect of going around the cycle once. Intuitively, what we need to do is to somehow compose the bounds functions at each of the vertices in the cycle. Before discussing the details of how this should be done, we consider an example. Consider the cycle consisting of three vertices, shown in Figure 1. Suppose we wish to determine an upper bound on the change in the value of x at vertex r_1 when we go around the cycle once. Let the upper bound on x be denoted by x_{max}: after the execution of r_1, we use the upper bound on x, from the bounds function at this vertex, to obtain the constraint $x_{max} = 2y - z$. After the execution of rule r_2, the new value of z has bounds $y - x \leq z \leq y$. Since z appears with a negative coefficient in the expression $2y - z$, we use the lower bound to obtain the constraint $z = y - x$. Composition (i.e., conjunction) of constraints then yields $x_{max} = 2y - z \wedge z = y - x$; projecting on x_{max} yields $x_{max} = y + x$. Finally, at vertex r_3, the bounds on y are $x - 3 \leq y \leq x + 5$; this time, since the coefficient of y is positive in the expression $y + x$, we use the upper bound $x + 5$. As before, we compose constraints to obtain $x_{max} = y + x \wedge y = x + 5$; this is then projected on x_{max} to yield $x_{max} = 2x + 5$. Thus, the change in the value of x when we go around this cycle once is (at most) $2x + 5$.

This example illustrates how we summarize the effects of a cycle. To estimate an upper bound on the value of x at a vertex r after going around the cycle (the case for lower bounds is analogous), we start with the constraint $x_{max} = E$, where E gives the upper bound on x after r's execution. We then work our way around the cycle: at each vertex we take the conjunction of the current constraint on x_{max} and constraints on the variables occuring in it, obtained from the bounds on these variables at that vertex given by the annotated triggering graph; the resulting constraint is then projected on x_{max}. During this process, we use the lower bound for a variable if it occurs negatively in the constraint associated with x_{max}, and the upper bound if it occurs positively.

Given a constraint C and a set of variables[1] $X = \{x_1, \ldots, x_n\}$, we use the notation $\exists_X C$ to denote the constraint obtained by projecting away the variables in X, i.e., $\exists x_1 x_2 \cdots x_n C$. Let $vars(E)$ denote the variables appearing in an expression E. Given an annotated triggering graph $(G, \mathcal{F})$ with schema S and a vertex r in G, let $\mathcal{F}(r)(v) = \langle lo_v^{(r)}, hi_v^{(r)} \rangle$ for any $v \in S$. We can then formalize the procedure sketched above as follows.

- *Processing a single vertex r.* Given a constraint $C \equiv x_{max} = E$, let C' be the constraint

$$C' = \bigwedge_{v \in vars(E)} \{v = e \mid e = \begin{cases} lo_v^{(r)} & \text{if } v \text{ appears negatively in } E \\ hi_v^{(r)} & \text{if } v \text{ appears positively in } E \end{cases} \}.$$

Since bounds functions map variables to linear expressions (Definition 1), each variable occurs at most once in E. Thus, C' imposes a single (equality) constraint on any such variable, and therefore is satisfiable.

The result of propagating C through the vertex r is then given by

$$\mathsf{ProcVertex}(r, C) = \exists_{vars(E)}(C \wedge C').$$

- *Processing a sequence of vertices.* The result of propagating a constraint C through a sequence of vertices s is given by $\mathsf{ProcVertexSeq}(s, C)$, where:

$$\mathsf{ProcVertexSeq}(\varepsilon, C) = C$$
$$\mathsf{ProcVertexSeq}(rs', C) = \mathsf{ProcVertexSeq}(s', \mathsf{ProcVertex}(r, C)).$$

Here, ε denotes the empty sequence while rs' denotes the sequence whose first element is r and the remaining sequence is s'.

- *Processing a cycle.* Given a cycle $r_1 r_2 \cdots r_n r_1$, an upper bound on the change in the value of a variable x on going around the cycle once is given by

$$\mathsf{ProcCycle}(x, s) = \mathsf{ProcVertexSeq}(s, `x_{max} = x\text{'}).$$

where $s = r_1 r_2 \cdots r_n$.

The determination of a lower bound on the change in the value of a variable is analogous.

Since bounds functions map variables to linear expressions (Definition 1), the procedure described above for computing $\mathsf{ProcCycle}(x, s)$ for a cycle s is essentially involves composing a sequence of linear functions, and therefore yields a linear expression of the form $ax + E$. The effect on the value of x of going around the cycle n times can then be expressed as a difference equation $x_n = a x_{n-1} + E$ where x_i represents the value of x after i iterations around the cycle.[2] In general,

---

[1] Since our approach uses constraints on attribute values, we treat attributes as the variables in such constraints. In the remainder of the paper, therefore, we will use the terms *attribute* and *variable* interchangeably.

[2] Again, note that this represents an upper bound on x, so strictly speaking we should write $x_n \leq a x_{n-1} + E$. However, since we are concerned with proving termination in the worst case, when this maximum is actually realized, we simply use the equality.

the procedure described can yield a system of simultaneous linear difference equations. However, it is always possible to reduce a system of linear difference equations to a single linear difference equation in one variable [18], so it suffices to consider the solution of a single linear difference equation in one variable.

3.3   Approximate Solution of Difference Equations

Having obtained a difference equation as discussed above, we consider how it may be solved. The automatic solution of general difference equations is a difficult problem, but there is a wide class of equations that can be solved automatically, using either characteristic equations or generating functions [9, 15, 19]. For the purpose of analysis of active database rules, however, we additionally require that the solution method used be efficient, even if this means sacrificing precision in some cases. For this reason, we use a table-driven method for computing an upper bound to the actual solution. Our approach is to use a "library" of difference equation templates together with a symbolic solution for each such template [12, 10, 11]. The idea is to use pattern matching to identify a template that matches the equation obtained from the analysis described in Section 3.2. Once a match is obtained against a template, the solution to the equation can then be obtained by substituting into the symbolic solution for that template. In general, the library of difference equation templates will contain many different entries, and the pattern matching process will try to match a given equation against these templates in increasing order of the "size" of their solutions. If the equation cannot be matched against any template in the library, we attempt to use simplifying approximations, as described below. If no match can be obtained even after any applicable simplifying approximations, we give up and return the value $\perp$, indicating that we cannot say anything about the solution.

The idea can be illustrated by an example. Suppose that the difference equation library has the template:

$$x_n = Ax_{n-k} + B$$

together with the symbolic solution

$$x_n = (x_0 + \tfrac{B}{A-1})A^{n/k} - \tfrac{B}{A-1}, \qquad \text{where } x_0 \text{ is the initial value of } x.$$

Given an equation $x_n = 0.9x_{n-1}$, pattern matching against this template succeeds with $A = 0.9$, $B = 0$, $k = 1$; substituting these values into the symbolic solution yields the solution $x_n = 0.9^n x_0$.

If the difference equation at hand cannot be matched against any template in the library, we attempt to approximate it in a way that is conservative, i.e., termination inferred from the approximating equation (as discussed in the next section) must imply termination of the original equation. Space constraints preclude a detailed discussion of such approximations: we outline the general ideas and illustrate them with an example. Suppose we have the difference equation $x_n = 0.8x_{n-1} - 0.15x_{n-2}$, and are trying to simplify it so as to match against the template shown above. To do this, we use the activation condition on x (see Section 2.1), obtained from the rule(s) involved in the cycle, to determine (i) whether the values of x are bounded above or below; and (ii) whether the values of the x_i are positive or negative. This is done using the entailment operation of the constraint system, in a manner very similar to that discussed in Section 3.1. For example, suppose that for this particular case we have the activation condition $x > 100$. Then, we have the following:

(*i*) The termination condition for the rule is $x \leq 100$, i.e., we have a lower bound on the value of x below which the rule will not be activated. This implies that we can use an upper bound on the actual difference equation for termination analysis. In other words, if we can construct a difference equation $y_n = f(\cdots)$ such that $y_n \geq x_n$ for all $n \geq 0$, and can use this equation to determine that eventually the values of y_n will satisfy the termination condition for the rule, then we can conclude that the original variable x_n would eventually satisfy the termination condition of the rule as well. If the termination condition implied an upper bound for x, then we would, analogously, construct an approximation that is a lower bound on x_n.

(*ii*) The activation condition $x > 100$ implies that x is positive. This, in turn, implies that the expression $0.8x_{n-1}$ is an upper bound on the expression $0.8x_{n-1} - 0.15x_{n-2}$.

We therefore use the equation $x_n = 0.8x_{n-1}$ to approximate (from above) the original equation. The approximating equation can now be successfully matched against the template shown above.

3.4   Extensions

The discussion thus far has focused on numerical attributes and update operations. This section discusses how it can be extended to handle rules that manipulate certain kinds of non-numerical attributes, as well as to the use of operations other than updates, i.e., insertion and deletion of tuples.

Our approach can be readily extended to any non-numeric domain S that has a partial order $\preceq$ such that the poset $(S, \preceq)$ has no infinite descending chains. For any element s in such a domain S, let *height(s)* denote the length of the longest chain from any minimal element of S to s. For termination analysis, we use the *height* function to map domain values to numbers, then formulate and reason about difference equations as discussed. Thus, suppose we have the rule

Whenever a professor A gets a raise, any professor in the same department who is more senior than A must also get a [commensurate] raise.

Assuming that the "*more senior than*" relation is a partial order with no infinite chains, we can show that this rule—which can be self-activating—will nevertheless eventually terminate. Notice that, unlike the approach of Weik and Heuer [22], the poset $(S, \preceq)$ need not be a lattice: for example, in the rule above, we do not require the existence of a unique seniormost professor.

The discussion in Section 3.1 on the construction of annotated triggering graphs focuses on update operations. This can be extended to handle insertion and deletion operations by reasoning about difference equations involving aggregate values such as the number of tuples in a relation. In the absence of any additional information, we can, at the very least, use the dummy relation

R_Count, for handling the aggregation operation Count on a relation R (see Section 2), to monitor the number of tuples in R: the insertion of a tuple into R causes this value to increase by 1, the deletion of a tuple causes it to decrease by 1, and updates leave it unchanged. As an example, this can be used to infer termination of a cycle along which two tuples are deleted from a relation and one tuple inserted: we would obtain a difference equation stating that there is a net reduction of 1 tuple in the size of the relation each time around the cycle, and use this to determine that the deletions must eventually stop. This approach can be improved further using additional semantic information about the database, e.g., from integrity constraints.

4 Static Termination Analysis

The approach described in the previous section allows us to obtain an (upper bound) solution to a difference equation describing the effects of a cycle in the triggering graph. Ultimately, however, we are interested not so much in the solutions to these equations, but rather in determining whether or not the rule activations eventually terminate. Suppose that the activation condition for the rule under consideration is $C(x)$. We use the constraint solver determine an interval within which all of the values of n for which $C(x_n)$ is true, i.e., for which the rule will be activated, must lie; termination can then be inferred by examining this interval. This is done as follows:

1. We add constraints expressing upper and lower bounds on the value of x_0, denoted by MAXVAL and MINVAL, obtained from domain information for the database schema as well as any applicable integrity constraints; if there are no applicable constraints, these can simply be the largest and smallest numerical values representable on the system. Moreover, if $C(x_0)$ is false the cycle of active rules will not be initially triggered (see Section 2.1), so we may assume that $C(x_0)$ holds: this provides additional constraints on the values of x_0. Let the conjunction of these constraints on the possible values of x_0 be denoted by $Bounds(x_0)$.
2. Suppose the difference equation library associates, with the equation template we have matched, the solution $x_n = \mathcal{E}(n, x_0)$, where $\mathcal{E}(\cdots)$ is some expression involving n and x_0. We then solve the following constraint for n:

$$(\exists x_0, x_n, n)[Bounds(x_0) \wedge x_n = \mathcal{E}(n, x_0) \wedge n \geq 0 \wedge C(x_n)]. \qquad (1)$$

If the activation cycle is non-terminating then the constraint (1) will be true for all $n \geq 0$. The constraint solver will return an interval $I \subset [0, \infty]$ (or, if metalevel solvers are used [14], a union I of intervals) and soundness of the solver implies that all n which satisfy this constraint must lie in I. If I is a *proper* subset of $[0, \infty]$ which omits some positive integer m, then termination (in at most m steps) has been proved. If, on the other hand, $I = [0, \infty]$, then nothing has been proved, and rule activation may indeed be nonterminating.

Returning to the rule in Example 1, the difference equation we obtain is $x_n = 0.9x_{n-1}$. For the rule under consideration, we have $C(x) \equiv x > 100$. Suppose that in the system under consideration, MAXVAL $= 10^{100}$, which means $Bounds(x_0) \equiv \text{`}x_0 > 100 \wedge x_0 \leq 10^{100}\text{'}$. We therefore solve the constraint

$$x_0 > 100 \wedge x_0 \leq 10^{100} \wedge x_n = 0.9^n * x_0 \wedge n \geq 0 \wedge x_n > 100.$$

In this case, the constraint solver yields the solution $n < 2142$.[3]

Notice that the constraint solver gives much more information than simply whether or not the cycle will terminate: it tells us that termination will occur after at most 2142 iterations of the cycle. This may seem high, but it is a result of the very large bound on the initial value x_0: it corresponds to starting out with an average salary of 10^{100}. If tighter bounds are available on the value of x_0, then the bound on the maximum number of iterations of the cycle can be correspondingly tightened. For example, suppose we know, from the integrity constraints on the database, that the maximum (and hence the average) salary cannot exceed 100,000: the bound we get in this case is $n < 66$. Information about the maximum number of iterations of a cycle can be a useful design and/or debugging tool for the database designer, e.g., for detecting inadvertently omitted integrity constraints. It can also be useful, as discussed at the end of the next section, in application areas such as soft real-time systems, where we may be interested not just in whether a rule activation terminates, but also the maximum number of iterations it may execute.

Recall that a cycle in a directed graph is *simple* if no vertex in the cycle is also part of a different cycle. The following theorem gives the soundness of our termination analysis:

Theorem 1. *The procedure described for termination analysis is sound provided that all cycles in the triggering graph are simple. In other words, if the analysis infers that a cycle terminates, then it in fact terminates (equivalently, any cycle that may not terminate is inferred to be non-terminating).*

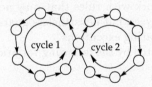

Fig. 2. An example of a non-simple cycle

The reason for the qualification that cycles should be simple is shown in Figure 2. The vertex in the center is part of two different cycles, so it is possible to have an execution where we go around cycle 1 some number of times, then around cycle 2 some number of times, then back around cycle 1, and so on. It may happen that each of the two cycles shown, considered on its own, can be shown to be terminating, but the two taken together do not terminate: this can happen, for example, if cycle 1 inserts some tuples into a relation until a maximum count is

---

[3] Actually, the solution it returns is the interval [0,2141.725842024721714551560581]. In our current implementation the execution time for this is about 10 ms.

reached, while cycle 2 deletes tuples from that relation until a minimum count is reached. We believe that our results can be extended to non-simple cycles provided that the cycles don't "interfere" with each other, in the sense that one of them increases a value that is decreased by the other. We are currently looking into how our ideas may be extended to deal with arbitrary cycles.

Finally, the discussion of the way in which the solution to a difference equation is used for termination analysis can be used to guide the construction of the difference equation library. In particular, it makes no sense to have a very precise solution to a particular equation template if the constraint system is not powerful enough to handle that solution. Thus, knowing the capabilities of the constraint system, we may choose to associate "approximate solutions"—i.e., upper and lower bounds, intended to be used as discussed at the end of Section 3.3—that we know can be handled by by the constraint system, if the exact solution cannot be handled by it.

5 Dynamic Termination Analysis

There may be situations where the approach described in the previous section does not work, i.e., we are unable to prove, statically, that a cyclic rule activation will necessarily terminate. This may happen either because the cycle is, in fact, potentially non-terminating, or because the constraint system is not powerful enough to solve the constraint (1) sufficiently precisely. Conventional static termination analyses would then reject the rule set for not being provably terminating. An alternative, however, would be to use dynamic termination analysis [6], where we insert code into the appropriate active rules to determine, when the rule is activated, whether that particular activation of the rules can be guaranteed to terminate. The latter approach gives us greater flexibility in handling rules, by allowing us to work with rules that may not be provably terminating via static termination analyses, but nevertheless guarantee that at runtime there will not be any nonterminating executions.

The idea can be illustrated by the following variation to Example 1 mentioned at the end of Section 1:

```
if (Select Avg(Sal) from Emp) > 100
then update Emp
     set Sal = 0.9*Sal + Bonus
```

This rule will terminate if **Bonus** < 10; for values of **Bonus** ≥ 10 the rule is nonterminating. Thus, if the value of **Bonus** is not known statically (e.g., if it is computed dynamically based on other values in the database), it will not be possible to prove the termination of this rule statically. Instead of rejecting the rule, however, we can introduce code into it to carry out dynamic termination analysis: the result would be to allow rule activation for situations where the value B of **Bonus** guarantees termination and rejecting it for values that do not. Suppose that at runtime, this rule is activated with $x_0 = 10,000$ and **Bonus** $= 9$. Then, given the static solution (see Section 3.3) $x_n = (x_0 - \frac{B}{0.1}) * 0.9^n + \frac{B}{0.1}$ for the difference equation for the corresponding cycle, and the value $B = 9$, this runtime check would use the constraint solve to solve for n in the constraint

$$x_n = (x_0 - \tfrac{B}{0.1}) * 0.9^n + \tfrac{B}{0.1} \wedge x_0 = 10000 \wedge B = 9 \wedge n \geq 0 \wedge x_n > 100.$$

In this case, the $\mathsf{CLP(F)}$ constraint solver infers the bound $n < 66$, which means that termination (in at most 66 steps) can be guaranteed. On the other hand, if at runtime we have $\mathsf{Bonus} = 10$, the constraint solver infers the bound $n \in [0, +\infty]$, correctly indicating that the rule activation may not terminate.

An interesting aspect of this kind of dynamic termination analysis is that it allows runtime decisions based not just on whether or not a cycle terminates, but, if we wish, the maximum number of iterations that may be executed. This can be used for controlling rule activation in active databases within soft real-time systems. For example, suppose that based on runtime monitoring of rule activations, we decide that a particular cycle can be allowed to iterate at most 50 times if the timing constraints are to be satisfied. Using our approach, we can test for this before the rule is activated: this allows more flexible systems (cyclic activations are permitted) but at the same time improves resource utilization ("bad" rule activations are rejected ahead of time, instead of having to be aborted if they are found to be running too long).

The overhead of dynamic termination analysis for cycles can be reduced significantly by observing that, once we have verified that a sequence of cyclic rule activations will eventually terminate, it is not necessary to test it again and again as we go around the cycle during that sequence of rule activations. The dynamic termination check can therefore be moved out of the cycle, in a manner similar to the optimization of invariant code motion out of loops commonly carried out in compilers [1].

6   Related Work

There is a significant body of literature on termination analysis for active database rules. Among the earliest of these is the work of Aiken *et al.* [2], who proposed using triggering graphs to reason about termination; this approach has subsequently been refined and improved by various authors [4, 5, 7, 21, 22]. The general idea here is to use acyclicity of the triggering graph to infer termination; the relative precision of different analyses depend on their use of different techniques to remove edges from the triggering graph prior to the acyclicity test.

Weik and Heuer describe an approach to identify terminating cycles in triggering graphs [22]. They consider lattice-structured domains: a cycle is then inferred to be terminating if it represents an increasing operation in the lattice (i.e., values get mapped to "higher" values according to the lattice ordering) with a non-decreasing step size, and there is an upper bound on the resulting values (and dually with decreasing operations). While their goals are similar to ours, the details are very different. Their approach is unable to infer termination for rules such as that in Example 1, since the step size of the operation in this example does not satisfy their criterion for being non-increasing. Moreover, as discussed in Section 3.4, our approach does not require lattice-structured domains.

Bailey *et al.* use abstract interpretation for termination analysis of active rules [3]. The idea is to reason about sequences of database states using an "approximate semantics," and use fixpoint computation (over a lattice) to handle cycles. The algorithm described by these authors does not have any knowledge of arithmetic operations, and so cannot infer termination of rules such as that in Example 1. A more fundamental problem is the issue of termination of the termination analysis itself. The usual approach taken in the abstract interpretation literature for proving termination of analyses is to assume that the abstract domain is Noetherian, i.e., does not contain any infinite ascending chains; such an assumption, while not explicitly stated, seems necessary for the work of Bailey *et al.* as well. This requirement restricts the structure of the abstract domains they are able to use. The restriction seems especially problematic for situations such as those considered here, where we have numeric domains such as the integers and reals, and where it may not be *a priori* obvious which subsets of these domains may be relevant for a particular rule set. This problem does not arise with our approach because we do not attempt to construct fixpoints iteratively. For this reason, we believe that the approach described in this paper is more precise than that of Bailey *et al.*.

Baralis *et al.* discuss the problem of dynamic termination analysis [6]. Their approach is based on the idea of monitoring rule activations at runtime to detect situations where a database state is repeated during execution, thereby indicating nontermination. This is a sufficient condition for nontermination in general, and is necessary and sufficient for "function-free" rules, which do not introduce any new values into the database. The runtime monitoring of database states can be quite expensive, and Baralis *et al.* propose a number of optimizations to their basic scheme to reduce this cost. Their approach differs from ours in two important ways. First, our approach does not involve keeping track of (representations or encodings of) previously encountered database states, and so can be made more efficient. Second, cyclic activations involving real numbers, as illustrated by the examples considered in this paper, may introduce new values into the database (e.g., the series of values 0.9, 0.9^2, 0.9^3, ...), and so are not function-free; for such rules, the technique of Baralis *et al.* give a sufficient condition for nontermination but not a necessary one. This means that, at least in principle, there may be nonterminating executions that will not be detected as nonterminating by their analysis; however, such executions will be detected as nonterminating by the approach described in this paper.

The table-driven approach described here for approximate solution of difference equations was developed by us in the context of optimized execution of parallel logic programs [10]. We have subsequently used it for query size analysis for recursive rules in deductive databases [11] and for estimating the computational cost of recursive logic programs [12]. Caslog, a system for cost analysis of logic programs that is based on this work, is available via anonymous FTP from ftp://ftp.cs.arizona.edu/caslog, and is part of the CIAO-Prolog distribution available at http://www.clip.dia.fi.upm.es. Our implementation of the CLP(F) constraint system is freely available at http://www.cs.brandeis.edu/~tim/clip.

7 Conclusions

Most existing approaches to termination analysis of active database rules rely on verifying that the triggering graph for those rules is acyclic. Because of this, they are unable to handle rules whose triggering graphs are inherently cyclic. Such rules can, nevertheless, be useful because they allow us to express, in a straightforward and natural way, situations that involve the repeated application of a set of active rules until some desired state is reached. This paper describes a constraint-based approach that can be used for termination analysis in such cases. The basic idea is to use a notion of *annotated triggering graphs* to capture the effect of going around a cycle in the triggering graph once, use this to estimate what happens after n executions of the cycle, and verify from this that the cyclic rule activation will eventually terminate. The idea can be readily generalized to allow dynamic termination testing, thereby allowing the analysis to cope with both proof systems that are not sufficiently powerful, and with rules that terminate sometimes but not necessarily always.

Acknowledgements

We are grateful to Elena Baralis for pointers to related work.

References

1. A. V. Aho, R. Sethi and J. D. Ullman, *Compilers – Principles, Techniques and Tools*, Addison-Wesley, 1986.
2. A. Aiken, J. M. Hellerstein, and J. Widom, "Static Analysis Techniques for Predicting the Behavior of Active Database Rules", *ACM Transactions on Database Systems*, vol. 20 no. 1, pp. 63–84, March 1995.
3. J. Bailey, L. Crnogorac, K. Ramamohanarao, and H. Søndergaard, "Abstract Interpretation of Active Rules and Its Use in Termination Analysis", *Proc. 6th. International Conference on Database Theory*, 1997.
4. E. Baralis, S. Ceri, and J. Widom, "Better Termination Analysis for Active Databases", *Proc. First International Workshop on Rules in Database Systems*, Aug. 1993, pp. 163–179.
5. E. Baralis, S. Ceri, and S. Paraboschi, "Improved Rule Analysis by means of Triggering and Activation Graphs", *Proc. 2nd. International Workshop on Rules in Database Systems* (RIDS), Sept. 1995.
6. E. Baralis, S. Ceri and S. Paraboschi, "Compile-Time and Runtime Analysis of Active Behaviors", *IEEE Transactions on Knowledge and Data Engineering* vol. 10 no. 3, May/June 1998, pp. 353–370.
7. E. Baralis and J. Widom, "Better Static Rule Analysis for Active Database Systems", *ACM Transactions on Database Systems*, 2000 (to appear).
8. S. Ceri and J. Widom, "Deriving Production Rules for Constraint Maintenance", *Proc. 16th. VLDB Conference*, Aug. 1990, pp. 566–577.
9. J. Cohen and J. Katcoff, "Symbolic Solution of Finite-Difference Equations," *ACM Transactions on Mathematical Software* 3, 3 (Sept. 1977), pp. 261–271.
10. S. K. Debray, N. Lin and M. Hermenegildo, "Task Granularity Analysis in Logic Programs," *Proc. ACM SIGPLAN'90 Conference on Programming Language Design and Implementation*, June 1990, pp. 174–188.

11. S. K. Debray and N. Lin, "Static Estimation of Query Sizes in Horn Programs," *Proc. Third International Conference on Database Theory*, Paris, France, December 1990, pp. 514–528.

12. S. K. Debray and N.-W. Lin, "Cost Analysis of Logic Programs", *ACM Transactions on Programming Languages and Systems* (**15**) 5, Nov. 1993, pp. 826–875.

13. T. J. Hickey, "Analytic Constraint Solving and Interval Arithmetic", *Proc. 27th. ACM Symp. on Principles of Programming Languages*, Jan. 2000, pp. 338–351.

14. T. J. Hickey, "CLIP: A CLP(Intervals) Dialect for Metaleve Constraint Solving", *Proc. PADL'00*, LNCS vol 173, Jan. 2000, pp. 200-214.

15. J. Ivie, "Some MACSYMA Programs for Solving Recurrence Relations," *ACM Transactions on Mathematical Software* 4, 1 (March 1978), pp. 24–33.

16. J. Jaffar, S. Michaylov, P. Stuckey, and R. Yap, "The CLP($\mathcal{R}$) Language and System", *ACM Transactions on Programming Languages and Systems* vol. 14 no. 3, July 1992, pp. 339–395.

17. J. Jaffar and M. J. Maher, "Constraint Logic Programming: A Survey", *J. Logic Programming* vol. 19.20, May/July 1994, pp. 503–581.

18. H. Levy and F. Lessman, *Finite Difference Equations*, Sir Isaac Pitman & Sons, London, 1959.

19. M. Petkovsek, *Finding Closed-Form Solutions of Difference Equations by Symbolic Methods*, PhD Thesis, Carnegie Mellon University, 1991.

20. Swedish Institute of Computer Science, *SICStus Prolog User Manual*, Release 3.8, Oct. 1999.

21. A. Vaduva, S. Gatziu, and K. R. Dittrich, "Investigating Termination in Active Database Systems with Expressive Rule Languages", *Proc. 3rd International Workshop on Rules in Database Systems*, June 1997.

22. T. Weik and A. Heuer, "An Algorithm for the Analysis of Termination of Large Trigger Sets in an OODBMS", *Proc. International Workshop on Active and Real-Time Database Systems*, June 1995.

23. J. Widom, "The Starburst Active Database Rule System", *IEEE Transactions on Knowledge and Data Engineering*, 8(4):583-595, August 1996.

24. C. Zaniolo, S. Ceri, C. Faloutsos, R. T. Snodgrass, V. S. Subramanian, and R. Zicari, *Advanced Database Systems*, Morgan Kaufman, 1997.

A Formal Model for an
Expressive Fragment of XSLT

Geert Jan Bex[1], Sebastian Maneth[2*], and Frank Neven[1**]

[1] Limburgs Universitair Centrum, Universitaire Campus
Dept. WNI, Infolab, B-3590 Diepenbeek, Belgium
{gjb,frank.neven}@luc.ac.be
[2] Leiden University, LIACS, PO Box 9512
2300 RA Leiden, The Netherlands
maneth@liacs.nl

Abstract. The aim of this paper is two-fold. First, we want to show that the recent extension of XSL with variables and passing of data values between template rules has increased its expressiveness beyond that of most other current XML query languages. Second, in an attempt to increase the understanding of this already wide-spread but not so transparent language, we provide an essential and powerful fragment with a formal syntax and a precise semantics.

1 Introduction

XSL [6] is a current W3C [8] proposal for an XML extensible stylesheet language. Its original primary role was to allow users to write transformations of XML to HTML, thus describing the presentation of XML documents. Nowadays, many people use XSL as their basic tool for XML to XML transformations which renders XSL into an XML query language. It has been noted by the database community [9, 1], though, that the transformations XSL can express are rather limited. For instance, XSL does not have joins or skolem-functions (and, hence cannot do sophisticated grouping of output data). In other words, XSL lacks the most basic property any query language should have: it is not relationally complete. However, as the language is still under development, some features have changed over time. Recently various extensions were added to the language [7]. The most apparent ones being the addition of *variables* and *parameter passing* between template rules. We show that these additions, together with the use of modes (which are actually states as used in finite state machines and which were already defined in earlier versions of XSL) render XSL into a powerful query language. Indeed, XSL not only becomes relationally complete, but it can do explicit grouping (with or without skolem functions), it can simulate regular path expressions, and it can simulate most other current XML query languages.

---

* The work of this author was supported by the EC TMR Network GETGRATS.

** Research Assistant of the Fund for Scientific Research, Flanders. Work partly performed while visiting the University of California, San Diego.

J. Lloyd et al. (Eds.): CL 2000, LNAI 1861, pp. 1137–1151, 2000.

Actually together with the addition of the new features, XSL was split into two parts: XSL Transformations (XSLT) [7] and XPath [5]. The latter contains the description of XSL's associated pattern language, while the former defines the real transformation language. To emphasize that we are focusing on the *transformation* part, with the new features, we refer to XSL by XSLT in the rest of this paper.

The main source for the definition of XSLT is its specification [7] which is a bit difficult to read, especially when one only wants an impression of how the language works or what it is capable of. To remedy this, we define an abstract formal model of XSLT incorporating most of its features, but all of those which are necessary to simulate, say, XML-QL. The purpose of this model is two-fold: (*i*) the clean and formal semantics provides the necessary mathematical model for studying properties of XSLT; (*ii*) our formal model abstracts away from the actual syntax of XSLT and emphasizes on its features in such a way that the interested reader can get a feeling of the language and what it is capable of.

We use this model to gain some insight in XSLT. First, we obtain that XSLT can compute all unary monadic second-order (MSO) structural properties. In brief, MSO is first-order logic (FO) extended with set quantification and is an expressive and versatile logic: on trees, for instance, it captures many robust formalisms, like regular tree languages [20], query automata [16], finite-valued attribute grammars [18, 15], ... By structural patterns we mean MSO without joins, that is, we cannot check whether the values of two attributes are the same (see Section 4 for details). In fact, Neven and Schwentick [17] showed that, already w.r.t. structural patterns, MSO is more expressive than FO extended with various kinds of regular path expressions. Thus, as most current XML query languages are based on FO extended with regular path expressions, this already indicates that XSLT cannot be simulated by, say, XML-QL.

Next, we study the expressivenesss of XSLT. To study decidability of type checking, Milo, Suciu, and Vianu [13] defined the k-pebble tree-transducer as a formalism capturing the expressiveness of all existing XML query languages, including XML-QL [9], XQL [19], Lorel [2], StruQL [11], UnQL [4] and the previous version of XSL. Their model does not take value equation into account (needed for joins, for instance) but can easily be modified to do so. We obtain that XSLT can simulate this model. For more concrete simulations, we refer the interested reader to [3], were we show how the XML-QL queries in [9] can be expressed in actual XSLT.

We want to emphasize that we do *not* provide a model for all of XSLT. For instance, we excluded for-loops and variables can only be instantiated by data values (not by result tree fragments or node-sets). The idea is that we want to use variables as a look-ahead or to fetch data values occurring 'far' from the current node. The resulting language is, hence, not Turing complete. The study of the properties of our formal model, however, is beyond the scope of the present

```
<!DOCTYPE organization [
    <!ELEMENT organization   group+ topmgrs>
    <!ELEMENT topmgrs        employee+>
    <!ELEMENT group          (mgr group+) | employee+>
    <!ELEMENT mgr            employee>
    <!ATTLIST employee       id  ID  #REQUIRED>
    <!ATTLIST group          id  ID  #REQUIRED>
]>
```

Fig. 1. A DTD describing an organization.

paper. The most important fact is that the defined language is more expressive than the previous version of XSL [9, 1] as it is capable to do joins.[1]

The rest of the paper is structured as follows. In Section 2, we introduce the important features of XSLT by means of two examples. In Section 3, we define our formal model. Finally, in Section 4 we obtain our expressibility results.

2   XSLT by Example

A basic XSLT program is a collection of *template rules* where each such rule consists of a *matching pattern*, a *mode* (which indicates the (finite) state the computation is in), and a *template* (see, for example, the program in Figure 2). The computation on a document t starts at its root in the starting mode[2] and proceeds roughly as follows. When the computation arrives at a node, say u, in a certain mode, say q, the program tries to find a template rule with mode q and whose matching pattern matches u.[3] If it finds such a template rule, the program executes the corresponding template. The latter usually instructs XSLT to produce some XML output and at various positions in this XML output to selects lists of nodes for further processing (we refer to patterns that select nodes for further processing as *selecting patterns*). Each of these selected nodes are then processed independently as before. Finally, the documents that are constructed by these subprocesses are inserted in at the positions where the subprocesses were generated.

To illustrate the new features of XSLT we use the DTD in Figure 1. It describes an organization as a sequence of groups together with a list of top managers. Each group has an ID, consists of a manager and a list of other groups, or just consists of a list of employees. For simplicity we identify employees by their ID. The XSLT program in Figure 2 computes pairs (e_1, e_2) of employees,

---

[1] In previous work we defined a formal model for the version of XSL not incorporating data values [12].

[2] Actually, modes are optional, but for convenience we assume every template has one and there is a start mode.

[3] Usually, and in all our examples, such a matching pattern only refers to the label of the current node. In fact, we show in Section 4 that such patterns suffice.

```xml
<xsl:template match="organization" mode="start">
    <result>
        <xsl:apply-templates select="/organization/topmgr/employee"
                    mode="selecttopmgr"/>
    </result>
</xsl:template>

<xsl:template match="employee" mode="selecttopmgr">
    <xsl:variable name="varID">
        <xsl:value-of select="@id"/>
    </xsl:variable>
    <xsl:if test="$varID != 'Bill'">
        <xsl:apply-templates mode="display"
            select="//group[mgr/employee[@id=$varID]]/group//employee">
            <xsl:with-param name="varID" select="$varID"/>
        </xsl:apply-templates>
    </xsl:if>
</xsl:template>

<xsl:template match="employee" mode="display">
    <xsl:param name="varID"/>
    <pair>
        <xsl:attribute name="topmgrID">
            <xsl:value-of select="$varID"/>
        </xsl:attribute>
        <xsl:attribute name="employeeID">
            <xsl:value-of select="@id"/>
        </xsl:attribute>
    </pair>
</xsl:template>
```

Fig. 2. An XSLT program computing the query of Section 2.

where e_1 is a top manager different from `Bill` and is a direct or indirect manager of e_2. Pairs are encoded simply by a `pair` element with attributes `topmgrID` and `employeeID` (cf. Figure 4).

On the face of it, the program just makes a join between the list of top managers and the group managers, that is, the ones occurring in the top manager list and the ones occurring as a manager of a group. However, it does so in a rather direct and procedural way. In brief, the XSLT program starts by applying the first template rule at the root in mode start. This rule selects each top manager (in mode `selecttopmgr`). In particular, the pattern `/organization/topmgr/employee` is matched against the current node which is labeled by `organization` and then selects all `employee` children of all `topmgr` children (the symbol / means 'child of'). For each selected employee (in mode `selecttopmgr`), the second template rule is applied which stores the employee's ID, say e_1, in the variable `varID` and verifies, by using the latter, whether e_1

```
<organization>
    <group id="HR">
        <mgr><employee id="Bill"/></mgr>
        <group id="HR-prod">
            <mgr><employee id="Edna"/></mgr>
            <group id="HR-prod-empl">
                <employee id="Kate"/>
                <employee id="Ronald"/>
            </group>
        </group>
        <group id="HR-QA">
            <mgr><employee id="John"/></mgr>
            <group id="HR-QA-empl">
                <employee id="Jane"/>
                <employee id="Jake"/>
            </group>
        </group>
    </group>
    <topmgr>
        <employee id="Bill"/>
        <employee id="John"/>
    </topmgr>
</organization>
```

Fig. 3. An XML document conforming to the DTD of Figure 1.

is different from Bill. If so, it selects all the descendants of the group manager who have an ID e_1 (in mode `display`). In particular, the selection pattern in the second template rule says 'select all employees that are descendants of a group that itself is a child of a group whose manager has the same ID as the one stored in the variable `varID` (the symbol // means 'descendant of'; the expression between the brackets '[...]' is a filter on group elements). In this latter selection the XSLT program passes the ID e_1 along as a parameter. Next, for each employee e_2 selected by the latter selection, the program outputs an element `pair` with attribute values e_1 and e_2 for the attributes `topmgrID` and `employeeID`, respectively.

```
<result>
    <pair topmgrID="John" employeeID="Jane"/>
    <pair topmgrID="John" employeeID="Jake"/>
</result>
```

Fig. 4. The output of the XSLT program of Figure 2 on the document of Figure 3.

The above program is not the 'best' way in XSLT to compute the desired query, but it nicely illustrates the three most important features of XSLT: modes, variables, and passing of data values. Let us discuss these briefly:

(i) Modes enable XSLT to act differently upon arrival at the same element types. For instance, as described above, when our program arrives at an employee element, its action depends on the actual mode, `select` or `display`, this element was selected in.

(ii) Variables can be used for two purposes. The most apparent one, which is illustrated by the above query, is that they allow to perform joins between data values. A less apparent application is to use them as a 'look-ahead'. In Figure 5, we give a fragment of an XSLT program evaluating a binary tree, representing a Boolean circuit, to its truth value. Essentially, the use of variables allows for a bottom-up computation. The restriction to binary trees is just for expository purposes. In fact, it can be shown that XSLT can evaluate any bottom-up tree automaton over unranked trees [14]. In brief, when arriving at an or-labeled node, the program returns the correct truth value based upon the truth values of the first and second subtree.

(iii) Passing of data values to other template rules can be crucial for performing joins if the items that have to be joined are 'far' apart. Moreover, when node IDs are present in the XML document,[4] we can use this mechanism to place 'pebbles' on the input document which enables us to do complicated grouping operations.

It are exactly these three features which render XSLT into a quite powerful transformation language.

In the next section, we give an abstract formal syntax for XSLT. First of all, we restrict matching patterns to test only the label of the current node (as is already the case in Figure 2). This is no restriction, as Theorem 8 shows that we can test many properties of the current node in the body of the template rule. Further, we divide a template rule into two parts: the *variable definition part* and the *construction part*. Variables can only be assigned data values. In particular, a variable can be defined as the value of some attribute of the current node or by an XSLT apply-templates statement that will return exactly one data value. We will refer to such special templates as *selection template rules*. In the construction part of the template rule, the actual output is defined relative to some conditions on the values of the variables, the parameters, the attribute values of the current node, and possibly whether the current node is the root, a leaf, or the first or last child of its parent.

3   A Formal Model for XSLT

3.1   Trees and Forests

We start with the necessary definitions regarding trees and forests over a finite alphabet Σ (the symbols in Σ correspond to the element names of the XML

---

[4] If not, XSL is capable of generating them itself (see Section 4).

```
<xsl:template match="or">
  <xsl:variable name="arg1">
    <xsl:apply-templates select="./*[1]"/>
  </xsl:variable>
  <xsl:variable name="arg2">
    <xsl:apply-templates select="./*[2]"/>
  </xsl:variable>
  <xsl:choose>
    <xsl:when test="($arg1 = 'false') and ($arg2 = 'false')">
      <xsl:value-of select="'false'"/>
    </xsl:when>
    <xsl:otherwise>
      <xsl:value-of select="'true'"/>
    </xsl:otherwise>
  </xsl:choose>
</xsl:template>
```

Fig. 5. The fragment of an XSLT program evaluating tree-structured Boolean circuits that takes care of *or*-nodes.

document the tree represents). To use these trees as adequate abstractions of actual XML documents, we extend them with attributes that take values from an infinite domain $\mathbf{D} = \{d_1, d_2, \dots\}$.

The set of Σ-forests, denoted by $\mathcal{F}_\Sigma$, is inductively defined as follows: every $\sigma \in \Sigma$ is a Σ-forest; if $\sigma \in \Sigma$ and $f \in \mathcal{F}_\Sigma$ then $\sigma(f)$ is a Σ-forest; if $f_1, \dots, f_n \in \mathcal{F}_\Sigma$ then $f_1 \cdots f_n$ is a Σ-forest. A Σ-*tree* is a Σ-forest of the form $\sigma(f)$. We denote the set of all Σ-trees by $\mathcal{T}_\Sigma$. Note that there is no a priori bound on the number of children of a node in a forest. In the following, whenever we say tree or forest, we always mean Σ-tree and Σ-forest.

The reason we consider forests is that even when we use XSL for tree to tree transformations only, we sometimes need to specify template rules that construct forests.

For every forest $f \in \mathcal{F}_\Sigma$, the *set of nodes of f*, denoted by Nodes(f), is the subset of $\mathbb{N}^*$ inductively defined as follows: if $f = \sigma(t_1 \cdots t_n)$ with $\sigma \in \Sigma$, $n \geq 0$, and $t_1, \dots, t_n \in \mathcal{T}_\Sigma$, then Nodes$(f) = \{\varepsilon\} \cup \{iu \mid i \in \{1, \dots, n\}, u \in \text{Nodes}(t_i)\}$. If $f = t_1 \cdots t_n$, then Nodes$(f) = \{iu \mid i \in \{1, \dots, n\}, u \in \text{Nodes}(t_i)\}$. Thus, for a tree the node ε represents its root and ui represents the i-th child of u. Further, for a forest the node iu represents the node u of the i-th tree in the forest.

Next, we add XML attributes to the above defined attributes. To this end, for the rest of the paper, we fix a finite set of attributes A. An *attributed forest with domain S* is a pair $(f, (\lambda_a^f)_{a \in A})$ with $f \in \mathcal{F}_\Sigma$ and where for each $a \in A$, $\lambda_a^f : \text{Nodes}(f) \mapsto S$ is a (partial) function assigning a value in S to each node of f. The set of all attributed forests with domain S, is denoted by $\mathcal{F}_\Sigma^S$. For S we will usually take $\mathbf{D}$. However, to create output in template rules we will use attributed forests over $\mathbf{D} \cup \{x_1, \dots, x_n\}$ where the variables refer to those defined by the variable defining part of the template. Of course, in real XML documents, usually, not all element types have the same set of attributes. Obviously, this is just a convenient, not a necessary restriction. In an analogous way one can define the set of attributed trees, denoted by $\mathcal{T}_\Sigma^\mathbf{D}$. For a set B, $\mathcal{F}_\Sigma^\mathbf{D}(B)$ denotes the set of attributed forests f over $\Sigma \cup B$ such that symbols of B may only appear at the leaves of f. Below, B will be the set of apply template expressions.

In our formal model we abstract away from a particular selection pattern language. Recall that XSLT uses the pattern language described in XPath [5] (see [21], for a formal semantics). Patterns can be rather involved as illustrated by the second template rule in Figure 2 where the pattern depends on the value of the variable varID. In addition, patterns can also be moving instructions like select parent, left sibling, right sibling, or first child. Actually, the proof of Theorem 9 indicates that such local selections only are enough to simulate all existing XML query languages. In the following, we assume an infinite set of variables $\mathcal{X}$. We define a pattern over the variables $X \subseteq \mathcal{X}$ as a function $(\mathcal{T}_\Sigma^\mathbf{D} \times (X \mapsto \mathbf{D})) \mapsto (\mathbb{N}^* \mapsto 2^{\mathbb{N}^*})$ and denote the set of all patterns over X by $\mathcal{P}_\Sigma^X$. The idea is as follows. Let p be a pattern, t be a tree, and γ be a variable assignment (for the variables in p). Then $p(t, \gamma)(u)$ is the set of selected nodes when the pattern is applied at node u.

3.2   Syntax

Definition 1. An *XSLT program* is a tuple $P = (\Sigma, \Delta, M^c, M^s, \text{start}, R)$, where

- Σ is an alphabet of *input symbols*;
- Δ is an alphabet of *output symbols*;
- M^c and M^s are finite sets of *construction* and *selection modes*;
- start $\in M^c$ is the *start* mode; and
- R is a finite set of *construction* and *selection template rules* (to be defined below).

As mentioned at the end of section 2, we distinguish between two types of template rules: *constructing* and *selecting* ones. The former are used to create output. So, the result of applying these is a forest. The latter are used to fetch data values. So, each one returns exactly one domain element. The mode will determine the nature of the template: constructing or selecting.

Definition 2. A *construction apply-templates-expression* r (at-expression for short) is of the form $q(p, \bar{z})$, where $q \in M^c$, p is a pattern and $\bar{z}$ is a possibly empty sequence of variables in $\mathcal{X}$ and domain elements in $\mathbf{D}$. A *selection at-expression* is defined as a constructing one with the restriction that $q \in M^s$ and p only selects single nodes, that is, for every tree t, each assignment of variables γ, and each node u of t, $p(t, \gamma)(u)$ is a singleton set. We denote the set of construction (selection) at-expression by $\mathcal{AT}^c$ ($\mathcal{AT}^s$).

For instance, the apply-templates expression in the second template of Figure 2 is a constructing one and corresponds in our model to the expression

$$\text{display}(p, \text{varID}),$$

with p the pattern

$$//\texttt{group[mgr/employee[@id=varID]]/group//employee}.$$

Note that application of this pattern eventually leads to the generation of a pair element. So the expression is constructing in the sense that it eventually will produce output.

Definition 3. An *attribute expression* is an expression of the form $a(.)$ where a is an attribute. An *atomic test* is one of the following: (i) an expression of the form $x = y$ where x and y are attribute expressions, variables, or domain elements; or, (ii) an expression of the form root, leaf, first-child, or last-child. Finally, a *test* is a Boolean combination of atomic tests.

During a computation the expressions $a(.)$ will evaluate to the value of the attribute a of the current node. Further, root, leaf, first-child, last-child evaluate to true whenever the current node is the root, a leaf, the first or the last child of its parent. Selection template rules are defined next. Recall that they output one domain element.

Definition 4. Let $q \in M^s$ and $\sigma \in \Sigma$. A (q, σ)-*selection template rule* is of the form

template $q(\sigma, x_1, \ldots, x_n)$
    vardef
        $y_1 := r_1; \ldots; y_m := r_m$
    return
        if c_1 then $z_1; \ldots;$ if c_k then z_k
end

where $n, m \geq 0$, $k \geq 1$; and,

- all x's and y's are variables (the former are parameters while the latter are local variables);
- each $r_i \in \mathcal{AT}^s$ or is an attribute expression; further, if $r_i \in \mathcal{AT}^s$ then every variable occurring in it is among $y_1, \ldots, y_{i-1}, x_1, \ldots, x_n$;
- all c_i are tests containing only variables in $X := \{x_1, \ldots, x_n, y_1, \ldots, y_m\}$; and
- every z_i is a domain element, a variable in X, or a selecting at-expression with the restriction that all variables occurring in it should belong to X.

Definition 5. Let $q \in M^c$ and $\sigma \in \Sigma$. A (q, σ)-*construction template rule* is of the same form as a selection rule only now each z_i is a forest in $\mathcal{F}_\Sigma^{\mathbf{D} \cup \mathcal{X}}(\mathcal{AT}^c)$ (recall that these are forests where attributes take values in $\mathbf{D} \cup \mathcal{X}$ and where leaves may be labeled with constructing at-expression) with the restriction that each variable occurring in an at-expression occurring at a leaf of z_i should be in X.

To keep the model total and deterministic we require the existence of exactly one (q, σ)-template rule for each mode and each σ. Further, to ensure that an XSLT program generates tree to tree translations, we require that each z_i in a (start, σ)-construction template rule is a tree (rather than a forest).

Example 6. We illustrate the above by translating the program in Figure 2 into our syntax. The patterns p_1 and p_2 refer to the patterns in the first and second template rule, respectively. In the second template rule display(p_2,varID) is the tree consisting of one node labeled with display(p_2,varID); further, ε denotes the empty tree. In the last rule, **pair[topmgr→varID; employeeID→myID]** denotes the tree t consisting of one node where $\lambda^t_{\texttt{topmgrID}}(\varepsilon) :=$ varID and $\lambda^t_{\texttt{employeeID}}(\varepsilon) :=$ myID. For readability, we omitted the test 'if true then'. All modes are constructing.

template start(organization)
    return
        result(selecttopmgr(p_1))
end;

template selecttopmgr(employee)
    vardef
        varID := id(.);
    return
        if varID $\neq$ Bill then display(p_2,varID);
        if varID = Bill then ε
end;

template display(employee,varID)
    vardef
        myID := id(.);
    return
        pair[topmgrID→varID; employeeID→myID]
end;

3.3 Semantics

To define the semantics we need the following. Let $\bar{w}$ consist of a sequence of variables of $\mathcal{X}$ and domain elements. For a function $\gamma : \mathcal{X} \mapsto \mathbf{D}$, we denote by $\bar{w}[\gamma]$ the sequence of domain elements obtained from $\bar{w}$ by replacing each occurrence of the variable x in $\bar{w}$ by $\gamma(x)$. By $x_1 \backslash d_1, \dots, x_n \backslash d_n$ or $\bar{x} \backslash \bar{d}$ we denote the function that maps each x_i to d_i.

We next define the semantics of an XSLT program P on a tree t. Thereto, we need the following concept. A *local configuration* is an element of Nodes(t) $\times$ $(M^c \cup M^s) \times \mathbf{D}^*$. Intuitively, $\theta := (u, q, d_1, \dots, d_n)$ means that the program has selected node u in mode q with values $\bar{d}$ as parameters. For ease of presentation, we define the result of P on θ, denoted by $P^t(\theta)$, in a direct and procedural way. The latter has the advantage over the usual definition, in terms of rather complicated but formally more correct rewrite relations, that it is more transparent. The drawback is that it does not deal with the border case when XSLT programs get into infinite cycles. However, it should be clear that $P^t(\theta)$ is undefined whenever one of the generated subprocesses computes forever. We defer the formal semantics in terms of rewrite relations to the full version of the paper. We distinguish between two cases. In both of these, let the label of u be σ.

– Suppose q is a selection mode. Then $P^t(\theta) \in \mathbf{D}$. Let the (q, σ)-template rule be of the form as specified in Definition 4, where each r_i is $q_i(p_i, \bar{x}'_i)$ or the attribute expression $a_i(.)$.

Intuitively, this template is evaluated as follows. First, the values of the variables $y_1, \ldots, y_n$, are defined. Such a value can be an attribute value of the current node or can be defined by invoking an at-rule that will compute the desired data value. The output then is determined by z_i where c_i is the first test that evaluates to true.

Suppose the variables $y_1, \ldots, y_m$ get assigned the domain values $e_1, \ldots, e_m$, respectively. That is,

- if r_i is an at-expression, then $e_i := P^t(v_i, q_i, \bar{x}'_i[\gamma_i])$, where γ_i maps each x_j to d_j, for $j = 1, \ldots, n$, and y_j to e_j for $j = 1, \ldots, i-1$, and v_i is the node selected by p_i, that is, $p_i(t, \gamma_i)(u) = \{v_i\}$; or
- if r_i is an attribute expression, then $e_i := \lambda^t_{a_i}(u)$.

Next, suppose c_i is the first condition that evaluates to true by interpreting each y_j by e_j, x_j by d_j, $a(.)$ by $\lambda^t_a(u)$, and root, leaf, first-child, last-child by true iff u is the root, a leaf, the first or the last child of its parent, respectively. To ensure that the translation is total, we require that at least one such c_i exists.[5] Then, z_i determines the output value in the following way. If z_i is a constant, a variable, or an attribute expression then $P^t(\theta)$ equals the corresponding value. If z_i is a selecting at-expression $q'(p, \bar{w})$, then $P^t(\theta) := P^t(v, q', \bar{w}[\bar{x}\backslash\bar{d}, \bar{y}\backslash\bar{e}])$ where v is the node selected by p, that is, $p(t, [\bar{x}\backslash\bar{d}, \bar{y}\backslash\bar{e}])(u) := \{v\}$.

– Suppose q is a construction mode. Then $P^t(\theta) \in \mathcal{F}^{\mathbf{D}}_\Sigma$. Let the (q, σ)-template rule be of the form as specified in Definition 5. Suppose the variables $y_1, \ldots, y_m$ get assigned the values $e_1, \ldots, e_m$, as described above, and c_i is the first condition that evaluates to true. Then z_i determines the output value in the following way. Recall that z_i is forest in $\mathcal{F}^{\mathbf{D}\cup\mathcal{X}}_\Sigma(\mathcal{AT}^c)$, that is, a forest where attributes take values in $\mathbf{D} \cup \mathcal{X}$ and where leaves may be labeled with constructing at-expression. $P^t(\theta)$ is the forest obtained from z_i by replacing

- every occurrence of a y_j and a x_j as the value of some attribute by the data values e_j and d_j, respectively;
- every occurrence $q'(p', \bar{w})$ of an at-expression at a leaf of z_i by the forest

$$P^t(u_1, q', \bar{w}[\bar{x}\backslash\bar{d}, \bar{y}\backslash\bar{e}]) \cdots P^t(u_\ell, q', \bar{w}[\bar{x}\backslash\bar{d}, \bar{y}\backslash\bar{e}]),$$

---

[5] Obviously, one could also add an 'otherwise' construct rather than having this condition.

where $p'(t, [\bar{x}\backslash\bar{d}, \bar{y}\backslash\bar{e}])(u) = \{u_1, \ldots, u_\ell\}$ and $u_1 \prec \ldots \prec u_\ell$ (here $\prec$ denotes document order). Recall that each $P^t(u_i, q', \bar{w}[\bar{x}\backslash\bar{d}, \bar{y}\backslash\bar{e}])$ returns an attributed forest.

The *initial* local configuration is defined as $\theta_{\text{start}} := (\varepsilon, \text{start})$.

Definition 7. *The* result *of an XSLT program P on a tree t, denoted by $P(t)$, is defined as $P^t(\theta_{start})$.*

3.4   Some Remarks

We conclude this section with some remarks. First, we note that XSLT does not make the explicit distinction between constructing and selecting template rules, or even, between the variable definition part and the constructing part of a template rule. However, we feel that by making this explicit, programming becomes more structured. On the other hand, we did not incorporate everything XSLT has to offer. For instance, we refrained from including for-loops. Nevertheless, we show in the next section that we have captured a powerful fragment capable of simulating most existing XML query languages and even more.

4   Expressiveness

We next show that XSLT is capable of computing very expressive structural patterns. Thereto, we first say how we view attributed trees as logical structures (in the sense of mathematical logic [10]) over the binary relation symbols E and $<$, and the unary relation symbols $(O_\sigma)_{\sigma\in\Sigma}$. The domain of t, viewed as a structure, equals the set of nodes of t, i.e., $\text{Nodes}(t)$. E is the edge relation and equals the set of pairs $(v, v \cdot i)$ for every $v, v \cdot i \in \text{Nodes}(t)$. The relation $<$ specifies the ordering of the children of a node, and equals the set of pairs $(v \cdot i, v \cdot j)$, where $i < j$ and $v \cdot j \in \text{Nodes}(t)$. For each σ, O_σ is the set of nodes that are labeled with a σ. The logic MSO* is MSO over the above vocabulary (with MSO defined in the usual way, see, e.g., [10]) extended with atomic formulas of the form $a(x) = d$, where a is an attribute and $d \in \mathbf{D}$. Denote the latter atomic formula by φ. Its semantics is then defined as follows $t \models \varphi[u]$ iff $\lambda_a^t(u) = d$, that is, the attribute a of u has value d. Note that we do not allow atomic formulas of the form $a(x) = b(y)$, so we do not allow joins. Note further that no quantification over $\mathbf{D}$ is allowed.

Clearly, MSO* can define all XPath matching patterns. The next theorem says that XSLT is capable of expressing all unary MSO* patterns. In particular, this means that one does not need matching patterns in templates. That is, XSLT actually allows to specify rules like

```
<xsl:template match="p" mode="q">
```

where p is a matching pattern rather than just a label. It means that a rule can only be applied on nodes that satisfy p. The next theorem implies that one can test for p in the body of the template rule and, hence, does not need matching patterns. Due to space limitations we omit the proof. We refer the interested reader to [14].

Theorem 8. *Let $\varphi(x)$ be an MSO* formula. There exists an XSLT program P and a mode q_φ such that $P^t(u, q_\varphi) = \text{true}$ iff $t \models \varphi[u]$.*

To study decidability of type checking, Milo, Suciu, and Vianu [13] defined the k-pebble tree-transducer as a formalism capturing the expressiveness of most existing XML query languages. Such transducers transform binary trees into other binary trees.[6] We next describe such deterministic transducers with *equality tests on data values*. The k-pebble deterministic tree-transducer uses up to k pebbles to mark certain nodes in the tree. Transitions are determined in a unique way by the current node symbol, the current state (or mode), the presence/absence of the various pebbles on the current node, and equality tests on the attribute values of the nodes the pebbles are located on. Pebbles are ordered and numbered from 1 to k. The machine can place pebbles on the root, move them around, and remove them (actually, the use of the pebbles is restricted by a stack discipline which ensures that the model does not become too powerful, that is, accepts non-tree-regular languages). There are move transitions and output transitions. Move transitions are of the following kind: move-to-parent, move-to-first-child, move-to-last-child, move-to-left-sibling, move-to-right-sibling, remain-and-change-state, place-new-pebble, and pick-current-pebble. There are two kinds of output transitions. A binary output outputs a Σ-symbol σ, possibly with attributes defined as an attribute value of a pebbled node, and spawns two computation branches that compute, independently of each other, the left and the right subtree of σ. Both branches inherit the positions of all pebbles on the input and do not communicate with each other, that is, each branch moves the pebbles independently of the other. In a nullary output, the node being output is a leaf of the output tree, again possibly with attributes, and the computation halts.

It should be clear that, apart from the pebbles, the above described model is extremely close to XSLT: XSLT is equiped with modes (states), can do local movements and the simple output transitions. Under the assumption that each node has a unique id, XSLT can also simulate pebbles.[7] Indeed, we just use k variables x_1 up to x_k, where at each time instance x_i contains the id of the node on which the i-th pebble is located. The above discussion immediately leads to the next theorem which implies that XSLT can simulate most other current

---

[6] When proving properties of XML transformations, restricting to binary trees is usually sufficient as unranked ones can be encoded into ranked ones; of course, this is not the case when one tries to define a formal model for XSLT which works directly on unranked trees.

[7] Actually, this assumption is not necessary as XSLT is equiped with the function generate-id(.) which generates a unique id for the current node. Furthermore, this id only depends on the current node, that is, when invoked for the same node several times it will return the same value. So there is no need to store the node id's; they can be computed on demand.

XML query languages, like for instance, XML-QL [13] . We refer the interested reader to [3] were we show how the XML-QL queries in [9] can be expressed in actual XSLT.

Theorem 9. *XSLT can simulate k-pebble deterministic tree-transducers with equality tests on data values.*

We point out that non-deterministic tree-transducers can be simulated by giving a non-deterministic semantics to XSLT in the obvious way.

5   Discussion

The present paper shows that the recent additions to XSLT render it into a powerful transformation language. We are rather hesitant, however, to accept or promote XSLT as the standard XML *query* language. Our main objection is that XSLT is much too procedural for a query language and therefore too difficult for the average user. On the other hand, as indicated by its widespread use, XSLT is highly adequate for the simple transformations it was intended for (recall that XSL was originally intended just for XML to HTML transformations). These simple XSLT programs are typical one pass transformations from the root to the leaves of the document. Performing joins and doing complicated grouping operations seem to require XSLT programs to traverse the input document many times in several directions and are therefore more difficult to write, especially for people with little programming experience.

Acknowledgements

The last author thanks Bertram Ludäscher, Dan Suciu, and Victor Vianu for encouraging and helpful discussions.

References

1. S. Abiteboul, P. Buneman, and D. Suciu. *Data on the Web : From Relations to Semistructured Data and XML*. Morgan Kaufmann, 1999.
2. S. Abiteboul, D. Quass, J. McHugh, J. Widom, and J. L. Wiener. The lorel query language for semistructured data. *International Journal on Digital Libraries*, 1(1):68–88, 1997.
3. G. J. Bex, S. Maneth, F. Neven. Examples of translations from XML-QL to XSLT. http://www.luc.ac.be/~gjb/xml-ql2xslt.html.
4. P. Buneman, S. Davidson, G. G. Hillebrand, and D.Suciu. A query language and optimization techniques for unstructured data. In *Proceedings of the 1996 ACM SIGMOD International Conference on Management of Data*, volume 25:2 of *SIGMOD Record*, pages 505–516. ACM Press, 1996.
5. J. Clark. XML Path Language (XPath). http://www.w3.org/TR/xpath.
6. J. Clark and S. Deach. Extensible stylesheet language (XSL). http://www.w3.org/TR/WD-xsl.

7. James Clark. XSL transformations version 1.0. `http://www.w3.org/TR/xslt`, November 1999.
8. World Wide Web Consortium. Extensible Markup Language (XML). `http://www.w3.org/XML/`.
9. A. Deutsch, M. fernandez, D. Florescu, A. Levy, D. Maier, and D. Suciu. Querying XML data. *Data Engineering Bulletin*, 22(3):10–18, 1999.
10. H.-D. Ebbinghaus and J. Flum. *Finite Model Theory*. Springer, 1995. `http://www-db.research.bell-labs.com/user/simeon/xquery.html`, 1999.
11. M. F. Fernandez, D. Florescu, J. Kang, A. Y. Levy, and D. Suciu. Catching the boat with strudel: Experiences with a web-site management system. In L. M. Haas and A. Tiwary, editors, *SIGMOD 1998, Proceedings ACM SIGMOD International Conference on Management of Data*, pages 414–425. ACM Press, 1998.
12. S. Maneth and F. Neven. Structured document transformations based on XSL. To appear in the proceedings of the Seventh International Workshop on Database Programming Languages, *Lecture Notes in Computer Science*, 1999.
13. T. Milo, D. Suciu, and V. Vianu. Type checking for XML transformers. To appear in the *Proceedings of the Nineteenth ACM Symposium on Principles of Database Systems*. ACM Press, 2000.
14. F. Neven. *Design and Analysis of Query Languages for Structured Documents — A Formal and Logical Approach*. Doctor's thesis, Limburgs Universitair Centrum (LUC), 1999.
15. F. Neven. Extensions of attribute grammars for structured document queries. To appear in the proceedings of the Seventh International Workshop on Database Programming Languages, *Lecture Notes in Computer Science*, 1999.
16. F. Neven and T. Schwentick. Query automata. In *Proceedings of the Eighteenth ACM Symposium on Principles of Database Systems*, pages 205–214. ACM Press, 1999.
17. F. Neven and T. Schwentick. Expressive and efficient pattern languages for tree-structured data. To appear in the *Proceedings of the Nineteenth ACM Symposium on Principles of Database Systems*. ACM Press, 2000.
18. F. Neven and J. Van den Bussche. Expressiveness of structured document query languages based on attribute grammars. In *Proceedings of the Seventeenth ACM Symposium on Principles of Database Systems*, pages 11–17. ACM Press, 1998.
19. J. Robie. The design of XQL. `http://www.texcel.no/whitepapers/xql-design.html`, 1999.
20. W. Thomas. Languages, automata, and logic. In G. Rozenberg and A. Salomaa, editors, *Handbook of Formal Languages*, volume 3, chapter 7. Springer, 1997.
21. P. Wadler. A formal semantics of patterns in XSLT. Markup Technologies, 1999.

On the Equivalence of XML Patterns

Peter T. Wood

Department of Computer Science, King's College London
Strand, London WC2R 2LS, UK
ptw@dcs.kcl.ac.uk

Abstract. Patterns for matching parts of XML documents are used in
a number of areas of XML document management: in links between documents, in templates for document transformation, and in queries for
document retrieval. The W3C has defined XSLT patterns as a common
sub-language for all these applications. We study the equivalence problem for XSLT patterns by defining a logic-based data model for XML and
a semantics for XSLT patterns in terms of Datalog programs. Although
uniform equivalence of Datalog programs is not sufficient to capture the
equivalence of programs derived from XSLT patterns, we nevertheless
show that equivalence can be decided by a variant of the chase process using embedded tuple-generating dependencies. One advantage of
this approach is that the method can easily be extended to determine
equivalence when documents are known to satisfy constraints imposed
by document type definitions.

1 Introduction

In structured document representation and processing, the need to refer to or
select parts of documents arises frequently. This might be in order to specify a
link from one document to a part of another, to match document elements in
order to transform them using a stylesheet, or to query documents to find those
elements matching a given pattern. For XML documents, these requirements can
be addressed by XPointer [16], XSL [17] and, for example, XQL [11], respectively.

XPointer, XSLT (the transformation sub-language of XSL) and XQL share a
common core pattern language, which we will refer to as *XSLT patterns*. When
applying an XSL stylesheet to a document, for example, one of these patterns p
can either be used to find elements x in the document which *match* the pattern,
or be applied in the context of some element in order to *select* other elements.

Example 1. Consider an XML document d representing a UML statechart diagram. Some of the possible element names in d are CompositeState, State,
Transition, ActionSequence and Event. The simplest form of XSLT pattern
is an element name. For example, the pattern State *matches* all elements in
d whose name is State. If the same pattern were applied in the context of an
element e, it would *select* the child elements of e whose name is State.

More complicated patterns are built from simpler ones using operators such
as /, [] and //. Patterns which appear inside the operator [] are known as

J. Lloyd et al. (Eds.): CL 2000, LNAI 1861, pp. 1152–1166, 2000.

qualifiers. For example, in the context of element e, (i) `State/Transition` selects `Transition` elements which are children of `State` elements which are children of e, (ii) `State[Transition]` selects `State` elements which are children of e and have *some* `Transition` element as a child, (iii) `State[Transition]` `[ActionSequence]` selects `State` elements which are children of e and have as children *both* a `Transition` element and an `ActionSequence` element, and (iv) `CompositeState//State` selects `State` elements which are *descendents* of `CompositeState` elements which are children of e. □

In this paper, we study the equivalence problem for XSLT patterns by considering containment between patterns. We say that pattern p_2 *contains* pattern p_1, written $p_1 \subseteq p_2$, if, for all documents d, the set of elements in d matched by p_2 contains the set matched by p_2. Patterns p_1 and p_2 are *equivalent*, written $p_1 \equiv p_2$, if $p_1 \subseteq p_2$ and $p_2 \subseteq p_1$. The motivation for studying equivalence is the possibility of replacing patterns by simpler, equivalent ones when linking, transforming or querying XML documents.

Example 2. Consider the XSLT patterns
$p_1 = $ `State[ActionSequence/Event][ActionSequence]`,
$p_2 = $ `State[ActionSequence/Event]`, $p_3 = $ `State[ActionSequence]`, and
$p_4 = $ `State`. Examples of containments are $p_1 \subseteq p_2 \subseteq p_3 \subseteq p_4$. It is also easy to see that $p_2 \subseteq p_1$; hence, $p_1 \equiv p_2$ and the expression `[ActionSequence]` is redundant in p_1. □

The definition of equivalence of XSLT patterns relies on knowing their semantics when applied to XML documents. Wadler has recently proposed a formal XML data model and given a denotational semantics for XSLT patterns [14]. We rephrase his model and semantics in terms of Datalog. In particular, we represent an XML document as a set of facts and so-called model rules, and for each XSLT pattern p, derive a Datalog program which defines the semantics of p. The containment and equivalence of XSLT patterns is then defined by the containment and equivalence of their associated Datalog programs.

Each XSLT pattern in Example 2 corresponds to a non-recursive Datalog program, so testing containment is no harder than testing containment of conjunctive queries [1]. However, patterns which use the // operator give rise to recursive Datalog programs, where, in general, containment is undecidable [13]. In [12], Sagiv defined the stronger notion of *uniform containment* of Datalog programs, showed that it is decidable, and gave an algorithm for minimizing a Datalog program under uniform equivalence. Given programs P_1 and P_2 corresponding to patterns p_1 and p_2, respectively, if we can show that P_2 uniformly contains P_1, written $P_1 \subseteq^u P_2$, then we can conclude that $p_1 \subseteq p_2$.

Example 3. Let Datalog programs P_5 and P_6 correspond to the XSLT patterns $p_5 = $ `CompositeState//State//Event` and $p_6 = $ `CompositeState//Event`, respectively. In Section 5, we show that $P_5 \subseteq^u P_6$; hence $p_5 \subseteq p_6$. □

Unfortunately although showing uniform containment is sufficient to show containment, it is not always necessary, even for the restricted class of Datalog programs which correspond to XSLT patterns. In other words, there are pairs of patterns p_1 and p_2 for whose programs P_1 and P_2 it is the case that $P_1 \subseteq P_2$, but $P_1 \not\subseteq^u P_2$.

Example 4. The symbol * in an XSLT pattern matches any element name. Consider the XSLT patterns $p_7 = $ CompositeState//*/Transition and $p_8 = $ CompositeState/*//Transition, along with their corresponding programs P_7 and P_8. It turns out that $P_7 \equiv P_8$ and hence $p_7 \equiv p_8$, but that $P_7 \not\equiv^u P_8$ and $P_8 \not\subseteq^u P_7$. Note that the equivalence only holds because of the use of * in p_7 and p_8. For patterns $p_9 = $ CompositeState//State/Transition and $p_{10} = $ CompositeState/State//Transition, it is the case that $p_9 \not\equiv p_{10}$. □

In [12], Sagiv introduced a procedure which can sometimes be used to show containment of recursive Datalog programs when uniform containment does not hold. The procedure requires finding an appropriate set of *tuple-generating dependencies* (tgds), and may not terminate. We show that, for Datalog programs P_1 and P_2 corresponding to XSLT patterns, Sagiv's procedure need only use a fixed set of two tgds and is guaranteed to decide whether $P_1 \subseteq P_2$.

It may be argued that the scope for the kinds of simplifications suggested in the above examples may be limited in practice, and that defining the equivalence of XSLT patterns in terms of equivalence of Datalog programs is unnecessarily complicated. We believe, however, that when documents satisfy a given *document type definition* (DTD), the potential for pattern simplification will be far greater, not least because people authoring or querying documents may not take the trouble to find out or understand the constraints imposed on documents by the DTD. Mapping XSLT patterns to Datalog programs gives us a well-defined framework within which to study equivalence under various DTD constraints. Some of these constraints have been identified by Böhm *et al.* [3], while their connection to tgds and query optimization has been described in [15].

In the next section, we discuss research which is related to the present paper. In Section 3, we cover the necessary background on containment of Datalog programs. This is followed in Section 4 by the definition of our logic-based data model for XML as well as the syntax and Datalog semantics of XSLT patterns. The main results concerning containment and equivalence of XSLT patterns are presented in Section 5. The final section gives conclusions and directions for further research.

2   Related Work

In common with the present paper, Neven and Van den Bussche study the translation of structured document queries into deductive rules [9]. Their queries, however, are based on Boolean-valued attribute grammars, and their main concern is with defining the correct semantics for the deductive rules. They do not consider equivalence of queries.

Maneth and Neven define a document transformation language $\mathcal{DTL}^{reg}$ which is based on XSL and uses regular expressions as the pattern language [8].

Although they do address the issue of equivalence of selection patterns, regular expressions are not sufficient to capture the expressiveness of patterns in XSLT.

Containment of conjunctions of regular path queries is proved decidable in [4, 5]. Conjunctions of regular path queries are sufficiently similar to XSLT patterns that it is probable that the decidability of equivalence for the latter follows from the decidability of equivalence for the former. However, our main contribution is not that containment for XSLT patterns is decidable, but that the chase procedure using embedded tuple-generating dependencies can be used as a decision procedure for containment of Datalog programs derived from XSLT patterns.

Although not the main focus of the present paper, results on query rewriting using constraints derived from document type definitions (DTDs) are also relevant [3, 6, 10, 15]. Böhm *et al.* [3] optimise expressions in the PAT algebra using DTD constraints. These constraints are similar to those which we proposed independently in [15], where we show that they correspond to tuple-generating dependencies when documents are viewed as relational structures.

Papakonstantinou and Vassalos study rewriting a query expressed in a language called TSL in terms of a set of views [10]. They include some rewritings based on DTD constraints similar to some of those in [15]. Liefke, on the other hand, is concerned with using DTD constraints to rewrite queries concerning the *order* of elements in XML documents [6], a property we do not represent in our model.

We are not aware of any work on the equivalence of XSLT patterns in general. Wadler has recently given a denotational semantics for XSLT patterns [14], which he uses to prove the equivalence of three particular pairs of patterns. We will reformulate his semantics in terms of Datalog programs in Section 4.3. Finally, we draw heavily on Sagiv's results on equivalence of Datalog programs [12]. We review these in the next section.

3   Containment of Datalog Programs

Containment of Datalog programs has been studied extensively by Sagiv [12]. We summarise his definitions and results in this section, following his notation, except that we use either upper-case letters or mixed-case strings as predicate names, lower-case letters as variables, and upper-case strings as constants.

Datalog programs comprise both *extensional* and *intensional* predicates. A *relation* q for a predicate Q is a set of *ground* atoms of Q. If $q_1, \ldots, q_n$ are relations for the predicates $Q_1, \ldots, Q_n$, respectively, then $\langle q_1, \ldots, q_n \rangle$ denotes their union.

Let P be a program with extensional predicates $E_1, \ldots, E_n$ and intensional predicates $I_1, \ldots, I_m$. The *input* to program P is the *extensional database* (EDB) $\langle e_1, \ldots, e_n \rangle$, where each e_i is a relation for E_i, $1 \leq i \leq n$. The *output* computed by P, denoted $P(\langle e_1, \ldots, e_n \rangle)$, is a relation for each intensional predicate, which is called the *intensional database* (IDB), although, to simplify notation, we will define the output to be both the EDB and IDB, called the *database* (DB). Also in order to define uniform containment, we need to view the input to P as comprising both an EDB $\langle e_1, \ldots, e_n \rangle$ and an IDB $\langle i_1, \ldots, i_m \rangle$. In this case, the output computed by P is denoted $P(\langle e_1, \ldots, e_n, i_1, \ldots, i_m \rangle)$.

Let P_1 and P_2 be programs with extensional predicates $E_1, \ldots, E_n$ and intensional predicates $I_1, \ldots, I_m$. Program P_1 *contains* program P_2, written $P_2 \subseteq P_1$, if for all EDBs $\langle e_1, \ldots, e_n \rangle$, it is the case that $P_2(\langle e_1, \ldots, e_n \rangle) \subseteq P_1(\langle e_1, \ldots, e_n \rangle)$. Programs P_1 and P_2 are *equivalent*, written $P_1 \equiv P_2$, if $P_1 \subseteq P_2$ and $P_2 \subseteq P_1$.

Program P_1 *uniformly contains* program P_2, written $P_2 \subseteq^u P_1$, if for all pairs of an EDB $\langle e_1, \ldots, e_n \rangle$ and an IDB $\langle i_1, \ldots, i_m \rangle$, it is the case that

$$P_2(\langle e_1, \ldots, e_n, i_1, \ldots, i_m \rangle) \subseteq P_1(\langle e_1, \ldots, e_n, i_1, \ldots, i_m \rangle).$$

Programs P_1 and P_2 are *uniformly equivalent*, written $P_1 \equiv^u P_2$, if $P_1 \subseteq^u P_2$ and $P_2 \subseteq^u P_1$.

Uniform containment implies containment, but the converse does not necessarily hold. Also it is known that containment of Datalog programs in general is undecidable [13], while uniform containment is decidable [12].

Example 5. Let P_1 be the program

$$anc(x, y) : - par(x, y).$$
$$anc(x, y) : - anc(x, z), anc(z, y).$$

and P_2 be the program

$$anc(x, y) : - par(x, y).$$
$$anc(x, y) : - par(x, z), anc(z, y).$$

Then $P_1 \equiv P_2$, but $P_1 \not\equiv^u P_2$. Although $P_2 \subseteq^u P_1$, it can be seen that $P_1 \not\subseteq^u P_2$ by taking the input to be the empty relation for *par* and some nonempty relation for *anc* which is not transitively closed [12]. □

A DB $P(\langle e_1, \ldots, e_n, i_1, \ldots, i_m \rangle)$ is a *model* of P if

$$\langle e_1, \ldots, e_n, i_1, \ldots, i_m \rangle = P(\langle e_1, \ldots, e_n, i_1, \ldots, i_m \rangle).$$

Let $M(P)$ denote the set of all models of P. Two programs are equivalent if for all EDBs the programs have the same minimal model which contains the EDB. Two programs are uniformly equivalent if they have the same set of models. Uniform containment can be characterized in terms of containment of models as follows:

$$P_2 \subseteq^u P_1 \iff M(P_1) \subseteq M(P_2).$$

Testing $M(P_1) \subseteq M(P_2)$ and hence $P_2 \subseteq^u P_1$ can be done by a variant of the *chase* process [7]. The following algorithm decides whether $P_2 \subseteq^u P_1$ by checking whether, for all rules r of P_2, $r \subseteq^u P_1$.

Algorithm 1. Given programs P_1 and P_2, test whether $P_2 \subseteq^u P_1$.

1. For each rule r of P_2, test whether $r \subseteq^u P_1$ as follows:
   (a) Replace each variable x in r by a unique constant $\theta(x)$ not already in r or P_1.
   (b) Form a database d from the atoms in the body of r; that is, if $p(x_1, \ldots, x_k)$ is an atom, then $p(A_1, \ldots, A_k)$ is in the EDB, where $A_i = \theta(x_i)$, $1 \le i \le k$.
   (c) Apply the rules of P_1 to the database d. If the head predicate of r, with variables replaced by their corresponding constants, is inferred, then $r \subseteq^u P_1$; else not.
2. If $r \subseteq^u P_1$ for each rule r in P_2, then $P_2 \subseteq^u P_1$; otherwise $P_2 \not\subseteq^u P_1$. □

Examples using the above algorithm are given in Section 5.

When uniform containment between programs does not hold, Sagiv has shown that Algorithm 1 can sometimes still be used to show containment when constraints in the form of tuple-generating dependencies are present [12].

A *tuple-generating dependency* (tgd) [2] is a formula of the form

$$\forall \bar{x} \exists \bar{y} [\psi_1(\bar{x}) \to \psi_2(\bar{x}, \bar{y})]$$

where $\bar{x}$ and $\bar{y}$ are vectors of variables and both ψ_1 and ψ_2 are conjunctions of atoms. As is common, we will write tgds without the quantifiers.

A DB d *satisfies* a tgd τ if for every instantiation θ of the universally quantified variables which makes the left-hand side of τ comprise ground atoms of d, the right-hand side of τ can also be be instantiated to ground atoms of d by extending θ to an instantiation of all the variables of τ. A DB d satisfies a set T of tgds if d satisfies each tgd in T. The set of all DBs satisfying a set T of tgds is denoted by $SAT(T)$.

Program P_1 *uniformly contains* P_2 *over* $SAT(T)$, written $P_2 \subseteq^u_{SAT(T)} P_1$, if $P_2(d) \subseteq P_1(d)$ for all DBs $d \in SAT(T)$. Program P preserves T if $P(d) \in SAT(T)$ for all DBs $d \in SAT(T)$.

The procedure for showing containment of programs in the presence of tgds outlined below includes generating the so-called *preliminary* DB for a program P and DB d. This is the DB which includes d and all atoms obtained by applying those rules of P whose bodies comprise only EDB predicates to d.

In order to show that $P_2 \subseteq P_1$ in the presence of a set T of tgds, it suffices to show that the following four conditions, the first two of which show that $P_2 \subseteq^u_{SAT(T)} P_1$, are satisfied:

1. $SAT(T) \cap M(P_1) \subseteq M(P_2)$.
2. P_1 preserves T.
3. For all EDBs d, programs P_1 and P_2 have the same preliminary DB.
4. All the preliminary DBs satisfy T.

The first step can be performed by a modified version of Algorithm 1 which applies both P_1 and T to the body of each rule of P_2. Applying a set of tgds to the body of a rule is similar to applying a rule, except that existentially quantified variables on the right-hand side of a tgd give rise to *null values*, denoted by δ_i for some i, in the atoms added to the DB.

Example 6. The DB $\{anc(A,B), par(A,C)\}$, where A, B and C are constants, satisfies the tgd

$$anc(x,y) \rightarrow par(x,z).$$

Applying the tgd to the DB results in the atom $par(A,\delta_0)$, where δ_0 is a null value, being added to the DB.   □

As stated by Sagiv [12], the above procedure has a number of drawbacks. Firstly, it is not clear how to find a suitable set of tgds for a pair of programs. Secondly, the procedure for testing steps (1) and (2) may not terminate if the answer is negative. However, in Section 5, we show that, for Datalog programs derived from XSLT patterns, step (3) is always true, as well as that a fixed set of two tgds ensures both that steps (2) and (4) always hold and that the procedure for step (1) always terminates.

4   XML and XSLT Patterns

Wadler has described a data model for XML and a denotational semantics for XSLT patterns [14]. In this section, we adapt these to a logic-based setting. In the first subsection, we present the XML data model in such a way that an XML document corresponds to a Datalog program. In the second, we present the syntax of XSLT patterns as defined by Wadler. In the third subsection, we define the semantics of XSLT patterns so that each pattern can be modelled as a Datalog program.

4.1   XML Data Model

An XML document comprises a number of nodes, represented by the unary predicate *isNode*. Because we study the equivalence problem for only a subset of XSLT patterns in this paper, we will simplify the XML data model accordingly. Essentially the only nodes appearing in an XML document we are interested in are those which are element nodes; we do not consider XSLT patterns which refer to nodes which are attributes, text, comments or processing instructions. There is, however, a distinguished node called the root node which is different from the document element node which contains all the other nodes [14][1]. Hence, each node is either the root node or an element node, as indicated by the unary predicates: *isRoot* and *isElement*.

$$isNode(x) :- isRoot(x).$$
$$isNode(x) :- isElement(x).$$

---

[1] One reason for this definition, is in order to be able to define the '.' pattern in XSLT.

The following predicates relate nodes to other nodes in the document: $par(x, y)$ is true if node x is the parent of node y in the document, and $root(x, y)$ is true if x is the root of the document and y is a node.

$$root(x, y) : - \ isRoot(x), isNode(y).$$

In general, the predicate *name* is used for the names of nodes. Because we have only elements in our model, $name(x, y)$ is true if element x has name y.

Example 7. Consider an XML document representing a statechart diagram which has a `StatechartDiagram` element d which in turn contains two `State` elements s_1 and s_2, with s_2 containing a `Transition` element. From now on, we will abbreviate element names by using only the upper-case letters in the names, so `StatechartDiagram` will be abbreviated as SD and `Transition` as T, for example. The parent of element node d is the distinguished root node r. The EDB representing this document is $\{isRoot(r), \ isElement(d), \ isElement(s_1), \ isElement(s_2), \ isElement(t), \ name(d, SD), \ name(s_1, S), \ name(s_2, S), \ name(t, T), \ par(r, d), \ par(d, s_1), \ par(d, s_2), \ par(s_2, t)\}.$ □

The XML data model imposes a number of constraints on documents. Each node has at most one name and at most one parent. If we define the predicate *anc* as the reflexive, transitive closure of *par*:

$$anc(x, x) : - \ isNode(x).$$
$$anc(x, y) : - \ par(x, y).$$
$$anc(x, y) : - \ anc(x, z), anc(z, y).$$

then it must be the case that the root is an ancestor node of every node, that is,

$$isRoot(x) \wedge isNode(y) \rightarrow anc(x, y).$$

4.2 Syntax of XSLT Patterns

We now turn to the definition of the abstract syntax of XSLT patterns [14], although we consider only a subset of possible patterns in this paper. The syntax of a pattern p is given by the following grammar:

$$p ::= /p \mid //p \mid p/p \mid p//p \mid p[p] \mid n \mid *$$

where n denotes an element name which is represented as a string. We do not consider selection patterns $p|p$, `@n`, `@*`, `text()`, `comment()`, `pi(n)`, `pi()`, `id(p)`, `id(s)`, `ancestor(p)`, `ancestor-or-self(p)`, '`.`' or '`..`'. The only qualifier (in square brackets) we consider is one which is itself a selection pattern. In general, a qualifier may contain Boolean connectives, equality tests for the values of nodes, and tests regarding order of nodes.

In fact, the above syntax is more permissive than that actually allowed. For example, the patterns $/p$ and $//p$ can appear only at the beginning of a complete pattern or the beginning of a qualifier.

4.3   Semantics of XSLT Patterns

Below we give a Datalog semantics for the subset of XSLT patterns defined above. As stated in the introduction, a pattern p can be used either for matching elements x, denoted by $match_p(x)$ below, or for selecting elements y in the context of elements x, denoted $select_p(x, y)$ below.

Given a pattern p, we can produce a Datalog program representing the semantics of $match_p(x)$ or $select_p(x, y)$ by recursively decomposing p, generating a Datalog rule for each sub-pattern in p. In what follows, predicate names $select_p$ and $select_q$, for $p \neq q$, are considered to be different.

$$match_p(x) : - \, root(y, x), anc(y, z), select_p(z, x).$$
$$select_{/p}(x, y) : - \, root(z, x), select_p(z, y).$$
$$select_{//p}(x, y) : - \, root(z, x), anc(z, w), select_p(w, y).$$
$$select_{p_1/p_2}(x, y) : - \, select_{p_1}(x, z), select_{p_2}(z, y).$$
$$select_{p_1//p_2}(x, y) : - \, select_{p_1}(x, z), anc(z, w), select_{p_2}(w, y).$$
$$select_{p_1[p_2]}(x, y) : - \, select_{p_1}(x, y), select_{p_2}(y, z).$$
$$select_n(x, y) : - \, par(x, y), name(y, n).$$
$$select_*(x, y) : - \, par(x, y).$$

The final program for a pattern is given by the rules generated by the decomposition, along with the rules for $isNode$, $root$ and anc, which we call the *model* rules, defined in Section 4.1.

Example 8. Consider the pattern SD/CS[S]//CS used for selection. The corresponding Datalog program (assuming left-to-right decomposition) is

$$select_{SD/CS[S]//CS}(x, y) : - \, select_{SD}(x, z), select_{CS[S]//CS}(z, y).$$
$$select_{CS[S]//CS}(x, y) : - \, select_{CS[S]}(x, z), anc(z, w), select_{CS}(w, y).$$
$$select_{CS[S]}(x, y) : - \, select_{CS}(x, y), select_S(y, z).$$
$$select_{SD}(x, y) : - \, par(x, y), name(y, SD).$$
$$select_{CS}(x, y) : - \, par(x, y), name(y, CS).$$
$$select_S(x, y) : - \, par(x, y), name(y, S).$$

□

Since we do not allow alternation in patterns, we can always replace all *select* atoms by their definitions to get a single select rule, along with the model rules. For example, the six rules of Example 8 can be replaced by the single rule

$$select_{SD/CS[S]//CS}(x, y) : - \, par(x, z), name(z, SD), par(z, v), name(v, CS),$$
$$par(v, u), name(u, S), anc(v, w),$$
$$par(w, y), name(y, CS).$$

From now on, we will assume that programs derived from select patterns comprise only a single *select* rule.

5   Containment of XSLT Patterns

In this section, we study the containment problem for XSLT patterns. Let p_1 and p_2 be XSLT patterns. From the definition of $match_p$ in terms of $select_p$ given in Section 4.3, it is clear that the program for $match_{p_1}$ is equivalent to that for $match_{p_2}$ if and only if the program for $select_{p_1}$ is equivalent to that for $select_{p_2}$. So from now on, the meaning given to a pattern p will be taken to be the program P derived for $select_p$. We will say that P is the program *corresponding* to p.

For patterns p_1 and p_2, we say that p_1 *contains* p_2, written $p_2 \subseteq p_1$, if and only if $P_{p_2} \subseteq P_{p_1}$, where P_{p_i} is the program corresponding to pattern p_i. As a shorthand, we will usually write P_i instead of P_{p_i}. Patterns p_1 and p_2 are *equivalent*, written $p_1 \equiv p_2$, if $p_1 \subseteq p_2$ and $p_2 \subseteq p_1$.

Containment and uniform containment coincide for non-recursive Datalog programs, so we can use Algorithm 1 from Section 3 to determine containment of XSLT patterns which do not use the // operator.

Example 9. Referring back to Example 2, let $p_1 = $ S[AS/E][AS] and $p_2 = $ S[AS/E]. We will show that $p_1 \equiv p_2$ by showing that $P_1 \equiv P_2$. Program P_1 is

$$select_{S[AS/E][AS]}(x, y) : - \ par(x, y), name(y, S), par(y, v), name(v, AS),$$
$$par(v, u), name(u, E), par(y, w), name(w, AS).$$

while P_2 is

$$select_{S[AS/E]}(x, y) : - \ par(x, y), name(y, S), par(y, v), name(v, AS),$$
$$: - \ par(v, u), name(u, E).$$

For the purpose of showing containment and equivalence, we now assume that predicates $select_p$ and $select_q$, for arbitrary XSLT patterns p and q, are the same, and refer to them both simply as $select$.

We first show that $P_1 \subseteq P_2$. P_1 comprises only a single rule[2], so we form a DB from the atoms in the body of the rule by mapping each variable to a unique constant. This gives DB as $\{par(X, Y), name(Y, S), par(Y, V), \ name(V, AS),$ $par(V, U), name(U, E), par(Y, W), name(W, AS)\}$. Applying the rule of P_2 to this database allows us to infer $select(X, Y)$, the head of the rule comprising P_1. We conclude that $P_1 \subseteq P_2$.

We now show that $P_2 \subseteq P_1$. The DB from the atoms in the body of the only rule in P_2 is $\{par(X, Y), name(Y, S), par(Y, V), name(V, AS), par(V, U),$ $name(U, E)\}$. We can apply the rule of P_1 to DB by mapping x to X, y to Y, u to U, v to V and w to V, thus inferring the instantiated head of the rule in P_2. We conclude that $P_2 \subseteq P_1$; hence $P_1 \equiv P_2$ and $p_1 \equiv p_2$.   □

XSLT patterns which use the // operator give rise to recursive Datalog queries, where, in general, there is a distinction between containment and uniform containment. If we can show uniform containment using Algorithm 1, then we know that containment also holds.

---

[2] The model rules are unreachable.

Example 10. Let us consider the XSLT patterns $p_5 = \texttt{CS//S//E}$ and $p_6 = \texttt{CS//E}$ from Example 3. We will show that $P_5 \subseteq^u P_6$. Program P_5 comprises the rule r_5

$$select_{CS//S//E}(x, y) : -\, par(x, z), name(z, CS), anc(z, u), par(u, v), name(v, S),$$
$$anc(v, w), par(w, y), name(y, E).$$

along with the model rules, while P_6 comprises the rule r_6

$$select_{CS//E}(x, y) : -\, par(x, z), name(z, CS), anc(z, w), par(w, y), name(y, E).$$

along with the model rules. Recall that the model rules for *anc* are

$$anc(x, x) : -\, isNode(x).$$
$$anc(x, y) : -\, par(x, y).$$
$$anc(x, y) : -\, anc(x, z), anc(z, y).$$

Consider rule r_5 of P_5. The DB d from the body of r_5 is $\{par(X, Z), name(Z, CS),$ $anc(Z, U), par(U, V),\ name(V, S), anc(V, W), par(W, Y), name(Y, E)\}$. We now apply the rules of P_6 to d. The second *anc* rule of P_6 allows us to add $anc(U, V)$ to $P_6(d)$. Using the third *anc* rule, we get $anc(Z, V)$, and then $anc(Z, W)$ in $P_6(d)$. Now, using r_6, we get $select(X, Y)$ in $P_6(d)$. We conclude that $r_1 \subseteq^u P_6$. Since the other rules of P_5 are identical to rules in P_6, we have that $P_5 \subseteq^u P_6$.

□

As we claimed in the introduction, showing uniform containment is not always necessary in order to show containment, even for the restricted programs which correspond to patterns. This is illustrated in the following example.

Example 11. Consider the XSLT patterns $p_7 = \texttt{CS//*/T}$ and $p_8 = \texttt{CS/*//T}$ from Example 4. To simplify the subsequent explanation, we will instead use the patterns $p_7 = \texttt{*//*/*}$ and $p_8 = \texttt{*/*//*}$, although the same results hold. Program P_7 comprises the rule r_7

$$select_{*//*/*}(x, y) : -\, par(x, z), anc(z, u), par(u, v), par(v, y).$$

while P_8 comprises the rule r_8

$$select_{*/*//*}(x, y) : -\, par(x, z), par(z, u), anc(u, v), par(v, y).$$

each augmented with the model rules. It is not hard to see that $P_7 \equiv P_8$ if we view them as regular path queries over a tree structure, all of whose edges are labelled with the symbol p, representing the relation *par*. Program P_7 corresponds to the regular expression $p \cdot p^* \cdot p \cdot p$, while P_8 corresponds to the regular expression $p \cdot p \cdot p^* \cdot p$. However, $P_7 \not\subseteq^u P_8$. The DB d from P_7 is $\{par(X, Z), anc(Z, U), par(U, V), par(V, Y)\}$. By applying the second *anc* rule from P_8, we can derive $anc(U, V)$. However, there is no way to derive $par(Z, U)$ which is needed in order to derive the instantiated head of rule r_7. DB d is a counterexample to the claim that $P_7 \subseteq^u P_8$, since $P_7(d)$ includes $select(X, Y)$ while $P_8(d)$ does not. A similar argument shows that $P_8 \not\subseteq^u P_7$.

□

Recall the procedure from Section 3 for showing the containment of Datalog programs using a set T of tuple-generating dependencies (tgds). We will prove below that, for programs derived from patterns, the procedure always terminates and is a sound and complete method for deciding containment. We first show that three of the steps in the procedure are always satisfied, starting with step (3). We assume we are dealing only with recursive programs.

Lemma 1. *Let P_1 and P_2 be recursive programs derived from XSLT patterns. For all EDBs d, P_1 and P_2 have the same preliminary DB.*

Proof. Recall that the preliminary DB is the DB which includes d and all atoms obtained by applying those rules of the program whose bodies comprise only EDB predicates to d. In the case of a recursive program P derived from a pattern, the only such rules are model rules which are the same for every program.   □

We will show that using the set T comprising the two tgds τ_1 and τ_2 defined below in the containment procedure of Section 5 is sufficient to prove the containment of any two programs generated from XSLT patterns. The tgd τ_1 is

$$par(x, z) \land anc(z, y) \to anc(x, w) \land par(w, y)$$

while τ_2 is

$$anc(x, w) \land par(w, y) \to par(x, z) \land anc(z, y).$$

We now prove that step (4) of the procedure is always satisfied by T.

Lemma 2. *Let P be a recursive program derived from an XSLT pattern, $T = \{\tau_1, \tau_2\}$ be the set of tgds defined above, and d an EDB. The preliminary DB of P and d satisfies T.*

Proof. Let the preliminary DB d' of P include $par(X, Z)$ and $anc(Z, Y)$, the left-hand side of tgd τ_1. Then d' must also include $anc(X, Z)$ by the second rule for anc. For d' to include $anc(Z, Y)$, d must include $par(Z, Y)$. Since $d \subseteq d'$, d' includes the instantiated right-hand side of τ_1, namely, $anc(X, Z)$ and $par(Z, Y)$; hence d' satisfies τ_1.

A similar argument holds for τ_2, so we conclude that d' satisfies T.   □

Step (2) of the procedure requires that we show that program P preserves the set T of tgds. In general, it is not known whether there is a proof procedure for showing that P preserves a set of tgds. However, if we can show that P preserves T *non-recursively*, then we can conclude that P preserves T. Applying a program P *non-recursively* to a DB d, denoted $P^n(d)$, means applying it only to the ground atoms of d. The P *preserves T non-recursively* if $\langle d, P^n(d) \rangle \in SAT(T)$ for all $d \in SAT(T)$. Once again, this can be shown using a variant of the chase process.

Lemma 3. *Let P be a recursive program derived from an XSLT pattern, and $T = \{\tau_1, \tau_2\}$ be the set of tgds defined above. Then P preserves T.*

Proof. Consider the tgd τ_1. We first instantiate the left-hand side of τ_1 by replacing each variable with a distinct constant not already in P. This gives $par(X, Z)$, which becomes part of the EDB d, and $anc(Z, Y)$, which becomes part of $P^n(d)$. Next we look for a way in which τ_1 could be violated by P. This happens if it is possible for the left-hand side of τ_1 to be generated by P without the right-hand side being generated. So we need to consider all ways in which $anc(Z, Y)$ can be produced when P is applied non-recursively to d. This can be in one of two ways: by applying the second or third rule for anc.

Consider the second rule. In order for $anc(Z, Y)$ to be produced, $par(Z, Y)$ must be in d. Now, since d satisfies T, we apply the tgds of T to d. This produces nothing new since there is no anc atom in d. Next we apply P non-recursively to d to get $P^n(d)$. Since $d = \{par(X, Z), par(Z, Y)\}$, we get $P^n(d) = \{anc(X, Z), anc(Z, Y)\}$. Finally, we need to check whether $\langle d, P^n(d)\rangle$ satisfies τ_1. This is indeed the case since the instantiation of the left-hand side of τ_1 can be extended such that the right-hand side of τ_1 becomes a subset of $\langle d, P^n(d)\rangle$, namely, $\{anc(X, Z), par(Z, Y)\}$.

Consider the third rule for anc in P. In order for $anc(Z, Y)$ to be produced, $anc(Z, W)$ and $anc(W, Y)$ must be in d, for some constant W. So $d = \{par(X, Z), anc(Z, W), anc(W, Y)\}$. Applying the tgds of T to d adds $anc(X, \delta_0)$ and $par(\delta_0, W)$ followed by $anc(\delta_0, \delta_1)$ and $par(\delta_1, Y)$ to d, for some null values δ_0 and δ_1. Applying P non-recursively to d yields, among others, $anc(X, \delta_1)$, which, along with $par(\delta_1, Y)$ gives an instantiated right-hand side of τ_1.

A similar argument shows that P preserves τ_2, so P preserves T.   □

Before proving that step (1) of the procedure is necessary for containment to hold, we consider again the programs of Example 11.

Example 12. Consider the programs P_7 and P_8 from Example 11. Recall that the database d from P_7 is $\{par(X, Z), anc(Z, U), par(U, V), par(V, Y)\}$. Using tgd τ_2, allows us to add $par(Z, \delta_1)$ and $anc(\delta_1, V)$ to d. Now P_8 can derive $select(X, Y)$; hence $SAT(T) \cap M(P_8) \subseteq M(P_7)$. The preceding lemmas then allow us to conclude that $P_7 \subseteq^u_{SAT(T)} P_8$ and $P_7 \subseteq P_8$.   □

Lemma 4. *Let P_1 and P_2 be recursive programs derived from XSLT patterns, and $T = \{\tau_1, \tau_2\}$ be the set of tgds defined above. If $P_2 \subseteq P_1$, then $SAT(T) \cap M(P_1) \subseteq M(P_2)$.*

Proof. (Informal sketch) Let r_1 and r_2 be the non-model rules in P_1 and P_2, respectively. The crucial part of the proof is showing that if a maximal chain s of *par* and *anc* atoms in r_1 "contains" a chain t of *par* and *anc* atoms in r_2, applying the tgds in T and the model rules to the DB formed from t will produce a chain of *par* and *anc* atoms to which there is a containment mapping from s.

For chain s to contain chain t, there must be at least as many *par* atoms in t as in s. In addition, there must be as many *name* atoms associated with variables in *par* atoms in t as there are in s, and the names used in these atoms in t must be equal to the associated names in s. If there are more *par* atoms in t than in s, then we can apply the second *anc* rule to produce a chain t' in DB with the same number of *par* atoms as in *s*. We apply the rule only to those *par* atoms which are either not associated with *name* atoms or are associated with *name* atoms which are not needed for the containment mapping from *s*. If there are the same number of *par* atoms in *s* and *t*, then $t' = t$.

Now if there are more *anc* atoms in t' than *s*, we can use the tgds in *T* along with the third *anc* rule to produce a chain t'' in DB which has both the same number of *anc* atoms as in *s* and in the same positions in the chain. On the other hand, if there are fewer *anc* atoms in t' than *s*, we can use the tgds and the first *anc* rule to produce t''.   □

We can also show that it is sufficient to apply the tgds in *T* only a number of times which is quadratic in the number of atoms in *P*. This, along with the preceding lemmas and results of Sagiv [12], give us the following theorem.

Theorem 1. *Sagiv's procedure provides a sound and complete method for deciding containment of Datalog programs derived from XSLT patterns.*

6   Conclusion

We have defined a logic-based model for XML and a semantics for XSLT patterns based on a translation to Datalog. This provided us with a framework within which to study the problem of equivalence of XSLT patterns by studying the equivalence of the corresponding Datalog programs. Although equivalence is undecidable for Datalog programs in general, the simple form of programs derived from XSLT patterns suggested that the decidable property of uniform equivalence might suffice. However, we showed that not every containment between such programs is also a uniform containment. Nevertheless, we proved that the procedure defined by Sagiv [12] which, in general, can only sometimes be used to show containment of programs using tuple-generating dependencies (tgds) and the chase process is in fact a sound and complete decision procedure for programs derived from XSLT patterns.

This framework will allow us to study the equivalence of broader classes of XSLT patterns, as well as equivalence of patterns in the presence of constraints imposed on documents by document type definitions (DTDs). For example, it may be the case in a DTD *D* for UML statechart diagrams that an `Action` (*A*) element can only appear as part of an `ActionSequence` (*AS*) element. This constraint can be expressed by the tgd τ

$$name(x, A) \rightarrow name(y, AS) \land par(x, y)$$

which in turn allows us to show using the chase that the (abbreviated) XSLT patterns `AS/A` and `*/A` are equivalent on databases (documents) satisfying τ and hence on those satisfying *D*. Similar constraints include those in which an element must have another element as a child or as a descendent.

An example of a more complicated constraint in a DTD for statecharts might be that the only path from a `Transition` element to an `Action` is via a `TransitionLabel` element and an `ActionSequence` element. On documents which are valid with respect to this DTD, the (abbreviated) patterns `T//A` and `T/TL/AS/A` are equivalent; in other words, the Datalog program corresponding to the former pattern is bounded.

Future work involves devising algorithms for deciding equivalence for wider classes of XSLT patterns and under various classes of DTD constraints, as well as determining the computational complexity of the associated decision problems.

References

1. A. V. Aho, Y. Sagiv, and J. D. Ullman. Equivalences among relational expressions. *SIAM J. Computing*, 8(2):218–246, 1979.
2. C. Beeri and M. Y. Vardi. A proof procedure for data dependencies. *J. ACM*, 31(4):718–741, 1984.
3. K. Böhm, K. Aberer, M. T. Özsu, and K. Gayer. Query optimization for structured documents based on knowledge on the document type definition. In *Proc. Advances in Digital Libraries*, pages 196–205. IEEE Press, 1998.
4. D. Calvanese, G. de Giacomo, and M. Lenzerini. On the decidability of query containment under constraints. In *Proc. Seventeenth ACM Symp. on Principles of Databases Systems*, pages 149–158. ACM Press, 1998.
5. D. Florescu, A. Y. Levy, and D. Suciu. Query containment for conjunctive queries with regular expressions. In *Proc. Seventeenth ACM Symp. on Principles of Databases Systems*, pages 139–148. ACM Press, 1998.
6. H. Liefke. Horizontal query optimization on ordered semistructured data. In *Proc. WebDB'99: Int. Workshop on the Web and Databases*, pages 61–66, 1999.
7. D. Maier, A. O. Mendelzon, and Y. Sagiv. Testing implications of data dependencies. *ACM Trans. on Database Syst.*, 4(4):455–469, 1979.
8. S. Maneth and F. Neven. Structured document transformations based on XSL. In *Proc. Database Programming Languages*, 1999.
9. F. Neven and J. Van den Bussche. On implementing structured document query facilities on top of a DOOD. In *Proc. 5th Int. Conf. on Deductive and Object-Oriented Databases*, pages 351–367, 1997.
10. Y. Papakonstantinou and V. Vassalos. Query rewriting for semistructured data. In *Proc. ACM SIGMOD Int. Conf. on Management of Data*, pages 455–466, 1999.
11. J. Robie, J. Lapp, and D. Schach. XML query language (XQL). In *Proc. QL'98— The Query Languages Workshop*, 1998.
12. Y. Sagiv. Optimizing Datalog programs. In J. Minker, editor, *Foundations of Deductive Databases and Logic Programming*, pages 659–698. Morgan Kaufmann, 1988.
13. O. Shmueli. Decidability and expressiveness aspects of logic queries. In *Proc. Fifth ACM Symp. on Principles of Databases Systems*, pages 237–249, 1986.
14. P. Wadler. A formal semantics of patterns in XSLT. In *Markup Technologies 99*, 1999.
15. P. T. Wood. Optimizing web queries using document type definitions. In *ACM CIKM'99 2nd International Workshop on Web Information and Data Management (WIDM'99)*, pages 28–32. ACM Press, 1999.
16. World Wide Web Consortium. XML pointer language (XPointer). http://www.w3.org/TR/WD-xptr, March 1998.
17. World Wide Web Consortium. Extensible stylesheet language (XSL). http://www.w3.org/TR/WD-xsl, 1999.

Querying XML Specified WWW Sites:
Links and Recursion in XML-GL*
(Extended Abstract)

Barbara Oliboni and Letizia Tanca

Politecnico di Milano - Dipartimento di Elettronica e Informazione
Piazza Leonardo da Vinci, 32 - 20133 Milano
{oliboni,tanca}@elet.polimi.it

Abstract. In this paper we present XML-GL^{rec}, an extended version of the graphical query language for XML documents XML-GL. XML-GL allows to extract and restructure information from XML specified WWW *documents*. XML-GL^{rec} also allows to represent XML simple links and generic recursive queries, thus permitting to query *whole XML specified WWW sites* in a simple and intuitive way.

1 Introduction

XML [W3C98a] was born as a simplification of SGML [ISO8879], a general document markup language initially conceived for document bases; following a recommendation of the World Wide Web Consortium, XML is now spreading out as a standard for the representation of semistructured documents on the Web. Indeed, unlike HTML tags, which are mainly designed to represent hypertext presentation features, XML tags can be appropriately defined by the document writer to represent information semantics, by giving a formal description of data content. Accordingly, a host of researchers is now working with the objective of defining appropriate syntaxes and semantics for querying XML documents ([DFF+98], [GMW99], [AM98], [W3C98b]).

XML was initially conceived as a document representation standard, thus little attention was given to the definition of links between documents, which are, in contrast, the main distinctive feature of the WWW and of hypermedia in general. Some proposals have been made for XML extensions [W3C98c], but none of the XML query languages defined to this moment addresses the problem of querying several documents related to one another by XML links.

In this paper we present XML-GL^{rec}, an extended version of XML-GL, a graph-based query language for extracting information from XML *documents* and for restructuring such information into novel XML documents [CCD+99]. The current version of XML-GL allows to query XML specified WWW *documents*: we extend XML-GL by allowing to *represent XML simple links, and recursive queries through IDREFS and XML simple links*.

* This research has been funded by the Italian MURST 1999 project Data-X

J. Lloyd et al. (Eds.): CL 2000, LNAI 1861, pp. 1167–1181, 2000.

In order to achieve this, we first introduce a syntactic extension of XML-GL which supports XML link specification; then, we provide a semantics for this new version, in particular allowing for the specification of generic recursive queries, by translating XML-GL^{rec} into the graph-based, logical language G-Log [PPT95], whose expressive power allows recursion on any type of binary relationship between objects. We believe that our work has an interest in two respects: first of all, we are here persisting with our purpose of adopting graph based query language for making query formulation easier for the end user; this is ever more interesting in the semistructured and XML context, where information is very naturally represented as graphs or trees. Second, our translation into G-Log makes immediately available for XML-GL^{rec} some results on G-Log [CDQT98] which allow the definition of parametric semantics. This semantics is based on the notion of *graph bisimulation*, and defines different levels of matching of the query graph to the instance graph, which correspond to stricter or looser requirements on topological similarity.

2   XML-GL

In this section we present a simplified version of the language XML-GL, which excludes specific constructs for computation. Our objective in extending this version of XML-GL is to query whole XML WWW sites, thus in the next section we add constructs to represent XML links and support recursion through such links.

2.1   The XML-GL Data Model

The Data Model of XML-GL is quite intuitive, and dictated by the formal structure of XML itself. With XML-GL, graphical notations and constructs are introduced to the end of representing exactly those concepts which are present in the XML formalism. Since a (set of) XML document(s) is often associated with a DTD, which dictates its syntactic structure, we also represent DTD's graphically: we depict XML DTD's (Fig. 1.a), documents, and queries (Fig. 1.b) by means of *XML graphs*.

An *XML graph* is a directed labeled graph $\langle N, A \rangle$, where:

- N is a (finite) set of labeled nodes, representing XML elements. Nodes in N are partitioned into two disjoint sets: E is the set of *element nodes* and P is the set of *property nodes*. Nodes in P are further partitioned into two disjoint sets: *attribute nodes* and *content nodes*. Nodes in E are labeled by the name of the element they represent, and sometimes by the URL of the document they refer to. The special label ANY can be used as a node label. Nodes in P are labeled by a string denoting a type-name and optionally by a string denoting a constant value. Property nodes do not have outgoing arcs. In Fig. 1.a an example of XML element is "Company". The element "Company" has an attribute node: "ID" and three content nodes: "Found_year", "Name" and "Type".

- A is a set of labeled arcs (n, λ, n'), where λ is the arc label and $n, n' \in N$. Arcs in A are partitioned into two disjoint sets: the set C of *containment* arcs and the set R of *reference* arcs. Arcs in R are labeled by the name of the IDREF attribute, while all arcs in C share the same label $CONT$, which may be omitted. The graph $\langle N, C \rangle$, i.e. the projection of the XML graph on its containment arcs, is acyclic. Arcs are represented as arrows connecting nodes, labeled in case of reference arcs. Reference arcs may be connected to element nodes of any type, including the element nodes labeled ANY. Cardinality and optionality are represented as annotations to the corresponding reference or containment arc, in a similar way as in the Entity-Relationship model. Cardinality (1:1) is taken as default, when not explicitly represented.
- For every node n in E, a total order is defined on the set of *element* and *content* nodes directly reachable from n (children nodes). For each given node, the order of its children is represented by marking the first outgoing arc with a small trait and ordering the other outgoing arcs counterclockwise.
- A set $XOR \subseteq 2^C$ is defined, which identifies sets of containment arcs which are in mutual exclusion. A set of containment arcs outgoing from an element in mutual exclusion is denoted by a segment labeled XOR crossing them.

The following topological constraints apply to each XML graph representing an *XML DTD*: property nodes cannot have a label denoting their value; reference arcs can only be directed to nodes labeled ANY; and no element node is replicated.

The following topological constraints apply to XML graphs that represent *XML documents*: no node labeled ANY is allowed; mutual exclusion and cardinality constraints do not appear in instance graphs; and each element node in the graph may have *at most one ingoing containment arc*. Moreover, if a document is associated to a DTD $\mathcal{D}$, then it must *conform* to $\mathcal{D}$. For example, the DTD of Fig.1.a represents the ownership relationship between companies. Each company is represented by ID, foundation year, name and type and is linked to its owned companies.

2.2   Query Language

The typical structure of an XML-GL query on a set of XML documents is a pair of sets of graphs. The graph(s) on the left side indicates information to be extracted from the document collection and properties such information must verify. The graph(s) on the right side indicates which elements retrieved in the left-hand part should appear in the result, and dictates how to construct or restructure the information to be produced as output. Accordingly, an XML-GL query consists of four parts:

1. The *extract* part identifies the scope of the query, by indicating both the target documents and the target elements inside these documents.
2. The *match* part (optional) specifies logical conditions that the target elements must satisfy in order to be part of the query result.

3. The *clip* part specifies the sub-elements of the extracted elements that satisfy the match part to be retained in the result.
4. The *construct* part (optional) specifies the *new* elements to be included in the result document and their relationships to the extracted elements; the same query can be formulate with different construction parts, to obtain results formatted differently. The construct part allows both the creation of new elements, the definition of new links, and the restructuring of local information to a given element.

Formally, an XML-GL query is a triple (LHS, RHS, M), where LHS, RHS are two disjoint sets of XML-GL graphs, called the *left hand side* and *right hand side* of the query, respectively and M is a correspondence between nodes in LHS and nodes in RHS, called *binding*.

Visually, the left-hand-side and right-hand-side of an XML-GL query are displayed side by side and separated by a vertical line. The correspondence of nodes in M is denoted either by labeling corresponding nodes in the LHS and in the RHS with the same name or by drawing unlabeled non-directed edges (called *binding edges*) between corresponding nodes. The left-hand-side graph(s) conveys the extract and match parts, while the right-hand-side graph(s) expresses the clip and construct parts.

Additional notations and specific topological constraints are needed to specify queries by means of XML graphs: new types of nodes, arcs and labels are defined.

- *Constructor nodes* are special nodes for building new elements. They are further distinguished into *list nodes* (denoted by triangles) and *index (or grouping) nodes* (denoted by rectangles containing horizontal lines). Both types of nodes may have an optional label. List and grouping nodes appear only in the RHS.
- *Anonymous nodes*, unlabeled, may appear both in the LHS and RHS, and are equivalent to nodes with the ANY label; they stand for elements of any type.
- *Kleene star arcs* are containment arcs in the LHS or RHS labeled by an asterisk. They represent the transitive closure of the *containment* relation, i.e., paths of any length between two elements.
- *GROUP_BY arcs* (grouping binding) are labeled by the string *GROUP_BY*.
- *Predicate labels* are labels that can be applied to a property node in the LHS of the query; they are further distinguished into *compare-to-value* predicate labels (e.g. $>$ 5 or $=$ "Sar$"), and *compare-to-property* predicate labels (e.g., ">", "<"). Compare-to-property labels apply to property nodes shared by two or more elements in the LHS.
- Nodes and arcs in the LHS can be *dashed* to represent *negative conditions*. Solid arcs of the LHS may only connect solid nodes, whereas dashed arcs may connect solid and/or dashed nodes. For example, a dashed arc between two solid nodes requires the absence of a containment or reference relationship between two elements.
- Mutual exclusion and cardinality constraints cannot appear in the LHS graphs.

- Property nodes in the LHS may be pointed to by arcs coming from two different element nodes: this notation is used for a compare-to-property predicates label to represent a *join* between elements, and the related comparison predicate.
- An unlabeled *binding edge* may connect RHS and LHS nodes according to the binding correspondence M.

An XML-GL query is *simple* if its LHS and its RHS graph consist of a single connected component. Otherwise an XML-GL query is *complex*.

An example of simple XML-GL query is depicted in Fig. 1.b, finding all the *company* elements that don't produce *flowers* and have the foundation year greater than 1999. In the result the company *name* and *type* are retained.

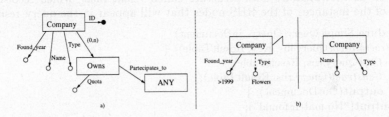

Fig. 1. XML-GL representation of an XML DTD (a) and simple XML-GL query (b)

2.3   Operational Semantics of XML-GL

In this section we describe the operational semantics of XML-GL and the algorithm for evaluating XML-GL queries. The operational semantics of a simple XML-GL query is based on the extract-match-clip-construct paradigm, and described by the following general algorithm [C99]. The most significant part of the algorithm is the *extract-match* procedure, strongly based on the formal notion of *matching* defined as follows:

Definition 1. (Node Match) Let $D = \langle N_D, A_D \rangle$ be an XML document graph, $L = \langle N_L, A_L \rangle$ be the LHS graph of an XML-GL query and $n_d, n'_d \in N_D$, $n_l \in N_L$, then n_d **type-matches** n_l (denoted $n_d \approx n_l$), iff they are both elements, or content nodes or attribute nodes, and either node-label$(n_d) =$ node-label(n_l) or node-label$(n_l) =$ "ANY" and n_d **matches** n_l (denoted $n_d \equiv n_l$), iff any of the following conditions holds:

1. $n_d \approx n_l$ and content-label$(n_d) =$ content-label(n_l) or
2. predicate-label(n_l) is a compare-to-value predicate label, and predicate-label(n_l)(content-label(n_d)) $= true$ or
3. predicate-label(n_l) is a compare-to-property predicate label, and there are two element nodes $e_d, e'_d \in N_D$ and other two ones $e_l, e'_l \in N_L$ such that $e_d \approx e_l$, $e'_d \approx e'_l$, and $(e_d, CONT, n_d) \in A_D$, $(e'_d, CONT, n'_d) \in A_D$, $(e_l, CONT, n_l) \in A_L$, $(e'_l, CONT, n_l) \in A_L$ and predicate-label(n_l)(content-label(n_d), content-label(n'_d)) $= true$.

Definition 2. (Graph Match) Let $L = \langle N_L, A_L \rangle$ be a LHS graph of an XML-GL query Q; let $D = \langle N_D, A_D \rangle$ be the input document graph.
Let $\phi : N_L \to N_D$ and $\psi : A_L \to A_D$ be two mappings between the two graphs. Then the subgraph $\langle \phi(N_L), \psi(A_L) \rangle$ of D is called a *match* of L in D iff the following conditions hold:
1. for each $n \in N_L$ $\phi(n) \equiv n$.
2. for each arc $(n_1, \lambda, n_2) \in A_L$, $\lambda \neq$ "$*$", with $n_1, n_2 \in N_L$,
$\psi(n_1, \lambda, n_2) = (\phi(n_1), \lambda, \phi(n_2))$.
3. for each arc $(n_1, *, n_k) \in A_L$ there is a sequence of arcs
$(\phi(n_1), CONT, n'_2), (n'_2, CONT, n'_3), ... (n'_{k-1}, CONT, \phi(n_k))$ in A_D.

The query evaluation algorithm takes as input the simple query and the document graph and gives as output another document graph. The algorithm relies on an intermediate data structure called *result table*, which records the OIDs of the instances of the RHS nodes that will appear in the query result.

Procedure *SimpleQuery*(Query, InDocument)
if (*ExtractMatch*(Query.lhs, Key, ResultTable)) {
      Clip(Query.rhs, ResultTable);
      Construct(Query.rhs, ResultTable);
      output(OutDocument); }
else output("No match found");
EndProcedure;

The procedure *SimpleQuery* takes as input the query and the input document graph and returns the query result as an XML graph. It starts from an empty result table and populates it with the data of the result, by performing three steps:

1. Extract-Match step. Procedure *ExtractMatch* takes as input the LHS of a query, its key nodes[1] and the (initially empty) result table. It finds all the possible matches and updates the result table by recording the OIDs of the key nodes of the matches; it returns a boolean value that states if at least one match has been found ([C99], [OT00a]).
2. Clip step. Procedure *Clip* takes as input the RHS of a query and the result table, which has been populated by procedure *ExtractMatch*. It returns the result table updated with the values of the OIDs of the non-invented nodes.
3. Construct step. Procedure *Construct* takes as input the RHS of a query and the result table, which has been populated by procedures *ExtractMatch* and *Clip*. It returns the result table updated with the values of the OIDs of the invented nodes. For each invented node of the RHS the result table is updated according to the type of node. Next, the output document graph is constructed starting from the query-result table.

Since a complex query is equivalent to multiple simple queries, complex query evaluation is obtained by computing a set of simple queries, each composed of one LHS graph and one RHS graph, and then by combining their result. We call such queries *components* of the complex query.

---

[1] The set of LHS nodes connected to the RHS by a binding edge, which will be the ones "transferred" to the RHS.

3 XML-GL^{rec}: Querying Web Sites

In this section we introduce some notations which allow the expression of generic queries to whole XML-specified WWW sites. In order to represent simple links, we add to set A of XML-GL arcs the *Href arcs*, which are arcs labeled by the string "Href". They may connect an XML element to any node and represent a simple link.

3.1 XML Links in XML-GL^{rec}

XML Linking Language (XLink) [W3C98c] allows to insert elements into XML documents in order to create and describe links between resources. XLink provides a framework for creating both basic unidirectional links and more complex linking structures, but in this paper we consider only *simple links*. A simple link is a link that associates exactly two resources, one local and one remote, and implicitly provides a single traversal arc from the local resource to the remote one. This could represent, for example, the name of a product appearing in text that is linked to information about the product. A simple link may be declared as an XML element or as a set of attributes in another XML element. A sample declaration for an element named *xlink:index* is the following, showing beside an XML document using it:

```
<!ELEMENT xlink:index ANY>          | <xlink:index>
<!ATTLIST xlink:index               |   href="/products/Ulysses.xml"
  href CDATA               #REQUIRED |   role="product"
  role NMTOKEN             #IMPLIED  |   title="Info about Ulysses"
  title CDATA              #IMPLIED  |   show="replace"
  show (embed|new|replace) #IMPLIED  |   actuate="onRequest"> Ulysses
  actuate (onLoad|onRequest) #IMPLIED > | </xlink:index> by J. Joyce.
```

In this document we have, in an index of books, the title "Ulysses", which is a simple link to another XML document containing information about that book. A sample declaration for an element that uses the link attributes is:

```
<!ELEMENT productlink ANY>
<!ATTLIST productlink
    xlink:type (simple)              #FIXED "simple"
    xlink:href CDATA                 #REQUIRED
    xlink:role NMTOKEN               #FIXED "product"
    xlink:title CDATA                #IMPLIED
    xlink:show (embed|new|replace)   #FIXED "replace"
    xlink:actuate (onLoad|onRequest) #FIXED "onRequest" >
```

In this case we do not have an XML element representing a simple link, but the information about the link is annexed to a normal XML element, so that the XML element "productlink" contains its attributes and the link attributes. Note that in this case the link attribute contains the information about the link type and this attribute is fixed to "simple". The following example shows an XML document using this declaration:

```
<productlink
    href="/product/Ulysses.xml"
    title="Info about Ulysses"> Ulysses </productlink> by J. Joyce.
```

We represent the simple links by an arc labeled with "Href". The Href arc starts from the link element and points to an anonymous node. In Figure 2 each DTD represents a document type, and the corresponding documents may be linked by simple links. In the DTD1 the link is represented by the *Product_list* element, which contains its attribute *Type_name* and the link attributes *xlink:type*, *xlink:role*, *xlink:title*, *xlink:show*, *xlink:actuate* and the *Href* arc, which points to an element *ANY*. In DTD2 the links are represented by *Made_by* and *Component* elements. Each link element contains the link attribute *role*, *title*, *show* and *actuate* and has an *Href* arc which points to an element *ANY*. This representation is consistent with a link from documents of type DTD1 to documents of type DTD2 through *Product_list*: in this case the link attributes are annexed to the element *Product_list*. We represent the XML link as an arc labeled *Href* that points to an *ANY* element. Note that, as is also the case with IDREF arcs, the DTD cannot provide information about which element type is referred to by the *Href* attribute.

The representation is also consistent with a link from documents of type DTD2 to documents of type DTD3 through *Made_by* towards *Company*. The element *Made_by* is a simple link and has the link attribute and the arc labeled *Href* which points to an *ANY* element. In DTD2 there is also another link, and it is represented by the element *Component*: through this link each product can be linked to the products that compose it. Again, this cannot appear at the DTD level, where link destination element types cannot be specified. An interesting remark is that queries which involve *Href* and *IDREF* arcs must necessarily be *blind*, that is, they cannot take advantage of a complete information about the documents' structures, even when the DTDs are known.

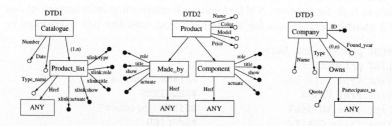

Fig. 2. An example of site DTDs

3.2   Some Examples of Recursive Queries

From the definition of XML-GL of Section 2 we can notice that the initial version of the language [CCD+99] allows some form of recursion by means of the Kleene star arcs which, in practice, express the transitive closure of the *contains* relation.

However, while this is enough when querying single documents or even sets of documents which are related by join conditions, it becomes too restrictive when we want to traverse XML-specified WWW sites. Moreover, note that in XML, whenever we want to define a symmetrical relationship between two elements, we are obliged to use IDREF attributes because the containment relationship is directed; the recursive extension will also be useful in order to traverse sequences of IDREF related elements. Accordingly, we extend the XML-GL semantics with recursion on any kind of relationship, including IDREF and LINK arcs. The first query of Fig. 3 on the DTD of Fig. 1.a finds all the companies owned by a certain company and the second query defines as *allies* the pairs of companies where the first refers to the second via the relationship "involved_in" and vice-versa.

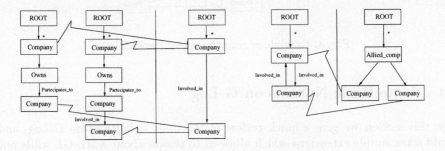

Fig. 3. Example of recursive query through idrefs

The semantics of queries like the first in Figure 3 is intuitively understandable: the leftmost graph of the LHS represents the *base recursion step*, and defines a relationship "involved_in" between two companies, if one is owned by the other. The second graph of the LHS defines the recursive rule: whenever one company is related to another one by "involved_in", and is at the same time owned by a third company, then the latter is also related by the relation "involved_in" with the first. This is a typical complex query, and is based on the general XML-GL principle that a RHS element with multiple bindings coming from the LHS expresses union. Accordingly, a definition as that of Figure 3 appears as most natural, but is not captured by the algorithm of the Section 2.3, which does not perform recursive calls to its procedures. In order to give a formal semantics to such kinds of queries, we rely on the translation of XML-GL^{rec} to G-Log [PPT98], which has all the expressive power needed for recursive computations.

While the query in Figure 3 is a recursive query through an IDREF arc, the query in Figure 4, on the DTD of Fig. 2, is a recursive query through a simple link. We define a new node with label "composed" and a new arc with label "Href". The leftmost graph of the LHS represents the base recursion step and defines a new link between two products, if one is composed by the other. The second graph of the LHS is the recursive rule. Thus the final result is the new element "composed" which is directly linked to all its components. Note that in both the queries of Figures 3 and 4, the ROOT nodes and their outgoing arcs with label "*" are reported in the CLIP part, because the existing links must be kept in the result of each recursive step, so that each step can be applied to the result of the previous step.

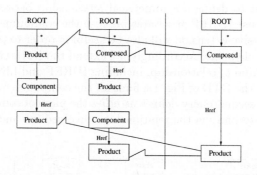

Fig. 4. Example of recursive query through links

4   Some Basic Notions on G-Log

In this section we give a quick review of the basic definitions on G-Log, and add some simple extensions which allow us to reason about XML-GL while not affecting the G-Log semantics as defined in [PPT95]. We refer to Generative G-Log, a reduced version of G-Log with the same expressive power [PPT98].

In G-Log, *directed labeled graphs* are used as the formalism to specify and represent schemata, instances and programs. The *nodes* of the instance graphs stand for objects and the *edges* indicate relationships between objects. We distinguish two kinds of nodes: *printable nodes*, also called *slots*, depicted as ellipses, indicate objects with a representable value; *non-printable nodes*, depicted as rectangles, indicate abstract objects. A *G-Log schema* contains information about the structure of the database and includes the (types of) objects that are allowed, how they can be related and what values they can take. We add to the set of *object labels* of Generative G-Log the special label "DUMMY". A G-Log schema, representing the same information as the running example, is shown in Fig.5. A *G-Log instance* is a directed labeled graph where printable nodes' values are specified; note that missing information is modeled by allowing the instance to lack some of the nodes defined at the schema level. *G-Log queries* (rules) are also represented as (set of) graphs. Like Horn clauses, rules in G-Log represent implications. To distinguish the body of the rule from the head in the graph P representing the rule, the part of P that corresponds to the body is colored red, and the part that corresponds to the head is green. Rules in Generative G-Log can also contain negation in the body: solid lines represent positive information and dashed red lines represent negative information. A query is a set of rules defined over a *source schema* S_1 and whose result instance has *target schema* S_2. Intuitively, a G-Log rule is "applied" by "embedding" its red part as a subgraph into the input instance; wherever we find an embedding, we extend that part of the instance with a piece of graph matching the green part. The concept of embedding defined in the sequel extends [PPT98] in order to deal with DUMMY nodes and DUMMY arcs in the red part and with predicates defined on slots. The algorithm itself is the same, and can be found in [PPT98]. Examples of G-Log rules are the ones of Figure 7, obtained as translations of the first XML-GL rule of Figure 3. Since this paper is black and white, we use thin lines for red nodes and edges and thick lines for green ones.

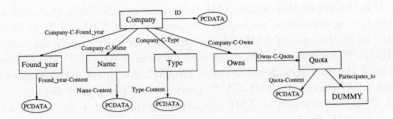

Fig. 5. The G-Log schema correspondent to the DTD of Fig.1.a

An *embedding* i of a subgraph $P = (N_P, E_P)$ in an instance $I = (N_I, E_I)$ is a total mapping $i : N_P \to N_I$ such that:

- $\forall n \in N_P$: if $label(n) \neq$ "DUMMY", then $label(i(n)) = label(n)$;
- $\forall n \in N_P$: if $label(n) =$ "DUMMY", then $label(i(n)) \in N_I$;
- $\forall n \in N_P$: if n has a print label, then $print(i(n)) = print(n)$;
- $\forall(n, arc\_label, n') \in E_P$: if $arc\_label \neq$ "DUMMY",
  then $(i(n), arc\_label, i(n')) \in E_I$;
- $\forall(n, DUMMY, n') \in E_P$: then $\exists\ arc\_label : (i(n), arc\_label, i(n')) \in E_I$;
- $\forall(n, arc\_label, n') \in E_P$ such that $label(n), label(n')$ are slot labels:
  if $label(arc\_label)$ is a comparison predicate then $(print(i(n))\ label(arc\_label)$
  $print(i(n')))$ is TRUE.

Thus, in a G-Log rule a DUMMY entity can be mapped to any node and a DUMMY arc can be mapped to any arc. It is easy to observe that this definition is extraordinarially similar to the definition of *XML-GL match* given in Section 2.3. The semantics of a G-Log program P can be described as a relation $Sem_{G-Log}(P)$ between G-Log instances:

$$Sem_{G-Log}(P) = \{(I, I') :\ I' \text{ is the result of the application of } P \text{ to } I\}$$

where the application of P to I consists in recursively applying the rules of P, i.e. by embedding all the red parts of the rules of P into I, and extending I with the green parts of these rules, until no more extensions can be made. The semantics of G-Log is described as a relation because it is non-deterministic: given an initial instance I, the application of a program may yield different resulting instances.

5   XML-GL^{rec} to G-Log

In an analogous way to the definition of G-Log semantics, we define the execution of an XML-GL^{rec} query Q on a set of XML valid documents as an application $Sem_{XML-GL^{rec}}(Q)$, from a (set of) XML documents, represented as XML graphs, to a unique *resulting* XML document, i.e.

$$Sem_{XML-GL^{rec}}(Q) : 2^{\mathcal{D}} \longrightarrow \mathcal{D}$$

where $\mathcal{D}$ is the set of all possible XML document graphs. Note that, differently from the G-Log semantics, we require the semantics of XML-GL^{rec} to be deterministic, as in the case of XML-GL. In order to formally specify the semantics of XML-GL^{rec} we define a correspondence between XML-GL^{rec} and G-Log. We define both the correspondence between an XML document graph and a G-Log instance, and between an XML-GL^{rec} query and a G-Log program.

Let $\mathcal{D}$ be the domain of XML document graphs and $\mathcal{I}$ be the domain of G-Log instances. Then,

$$\tau : 2^{\mathcal{D}} \longrightarrow \mathcal{I}$$

is a function that associates to a set of XML document graphs a G-Log instance.

Let $\mathcal{Q}$ be the domain of XML-GL^{rec} queries and $\mathcal{P}$ be the domain of G-Log programs. Then,

$$\mu : \mathcal{Q} \longrightarrow \mathcal{P}$$

is a function that associates to an XML-GL^{rec} query a G-Log program. The μ function maps each XML-GL element into a G-Log element and each XML-GL arc into a G-Log arc. Moreover, since XML-GL arcs are not labeled, it creates a label for each G-Log arc. The μ function takes into account the order of XML-GL elements, thus by translating from XML-GL into G-Log we allow to compute queries with an ordered semantics. In fact the algorithm for evaluating of XML-GL queries does not take into account ordered semantics. For a formal description of functions τ and μ see [OT00b].

We are also interested to the inverse transformation of this function that associates to a G-Log instance a single XML-GL^{rec} document graph, defined as:

$$\tau^{-1} : \mathcal{I} \longrightarrow \mathcal{D}$$

Note that τ^{-1} is well defined because τ is a one-to-one function [OT00b].

Now we explain the diagram of Fig. 6. The right part of the diagram represents the XML-GL^{rec} semantics: starting from a set of XML-GL^{rec} documents $(D_1, D_2, \ldots, D_n)$ the application of an XML-GL^{rec} query Q yields a resulting XML document graph D.

The upper left part of the diagram represents the G-Log semantics: given an initial G-Log instance I the application of a G-Log program P returns a set of resulting final G-Log instances $(I'_1, I'_2, \ldots, I'_n)$. Since XML-GL is a deterministic language, we want to keep this feature also in XML-GL^{rec}. Function *choose* takes care of getting rid of the non-determinism introduced in G-Log by new node invention. Function *choose* selects the instance which corresponds to the

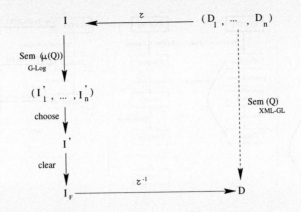

Fig. 6. Translation of XML-GL^{rec} into G-Log and vice-versa

result of the XML-GL^{rec} query: it takes as input the set of resulting G-Log instances $(I'_1, I'_2, \ldots, I'_n)$ and appropriately chooses one instance I' on the basis of the constructor nodes:

$$choose : 2^{\mathcal{I}} \longrightarrow \mathcal{I}$$

If the constructor node is an *element node*, then the function chooses the instance $I' = (N, E)$ where N has the highest cardinality; if it is a *list node*, then the function chooses the instance where N has the lowest cardinality; finally, if it is a *group by* node, then the function chooses the instance where $|N|$ equals the number of different values that the "group by" attribute assumes in the resulting document, and groups values accordingly. Now the instance I' corresponds to the result of the corresponding XML-GL^{rec} query, but still contains a set of *service nodes* ("EX-PTR" and "CLIP" nodes) that we add in the translation from XML-GL^{rec} to G-Log. We eliminate such nodes by using the *clear* function:

$$clear : \mathcal{I} \longrightarrow \mathcal{I}$$

The semantics of XML-GL^{rec} $Sem_{XML-GL^{rec}}(Q)$ applied to a set of documents $(D_1, D_2, \ldots, D_n)$ is thus defined as the result obtained by transforming $(D_1, D_2, \ldots, D_n)$ and Q via functions τ and μ respectively, into a G-Log instance and program, and by applying first $Sem_{G-Log}(\mu(Q))$ and subsequently functions *choose* and *clear* to the G-Log instances obtained, and finally by transforming the instance I_F into an XML-GL^{rec} document graph D via τ^{-1}.

Note that so far, by using the *choose* function, we have taken care of the non-determinism introduced by new object invention. To take care of the non-determinism caused by recursive XML-GL^{rec} queries containing negation, we consider the correspondent G-Log programs, construct the *dependency graphs* in order to check if they are *stratified*, and accept only XML-GL^{rec} programs that give stratified G-Log programs [CGT90].

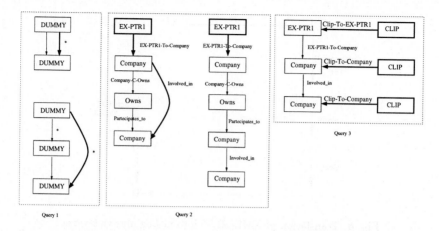

Fig. 7. From XML-GL^{rec} to G-Log: translation of the first query of Fig. 3

Now, we state a theorem establishing that the semantics of XML-GL^{rec} defined through the commutative diagram reduces to the semantics of XML-GL as defined in [CCD+99]:

Theorem 1. The commutative diagram in Fig. 6 is correct on XML-GL, i.e.

$$\tau^{-1}(clear(choose(Sem_{G-Log}(\mu(Q))))) = Sem_{XML-GL}(Q)$$

if Q is an XML-GL query and $I = \tau(D_1, \ldots, D_n)$.

The proof of this theorem [OT00b] is made by induction on the number of nodes and on the number of graphs, and based on the similarity between the concept of *matching* in XML-GL and *embedding* in G-Log.

6   Conclusions

We have presented XML-GL^{rec}, an extended version of the graphical query language for XML documents XML-GL, which allows to extract and restructure information from XML specified WWW *documents* connected by simple links. XML-GL^{rec} also allows to represent generic recursive queries, which should allow for querying *whole XML specified WWW sites* in a simple and intuitive way. The translation of XML-GL^{rec} into G-Log is in itself interesting for us, because we want to extend to XML-GL some results obtained on the positive fragment of G-Log, where a new semantics has been imposed based on the notion of *bisimulation* [CDQT98]. In a future work we will investigate the applications of such results, which are related to the possibility of graduating graph matchings in order to obtain more or less flexible semantics. A precise definition of a general XML-GL^{rec} evaluation algorithm, which is here still quite abstract, will also constitute our future work.

Acknowledgements

We would like to thank Ernesto Damiani, Sara Comai and Nico Lavarini for the useful discussions on this work.

References

[AM98]   G. O. Arocena, A. O. Mendelzon. WebOQL: Restructuring Documents, Databases and Webs. *Proc. ICDE'98*, 1998.

[C99]   S. Comai. Graphical Query Languages for Semi-structured Infomation. *Ph.D. Thesis*, 1999.

[CCD+99]   S. Ceri, S. Comai, E. Damiani, P. Fraternali, S. Paraboschi, L. Tanca. XML-GL: a graphical language for querying and restructuring XML documents. *Proceedings of the eight International World Wide Web Conference WWW8*, Toronto, Canada, May 1999.

[CDQT98]   A. Cortesi, A. Dovier, E. Quintarelli, L. Tanca. Operational and Abstract Semantics of a Query Language for Semi-Structured Information. *Proceedings of 6th International Workshop on Deductive Databases and Logic Programming DDLP'98*. GMD Report 22, 1998.

[CGT90]   S. Ceri, G. Gottlob, L. Tanca. Logic Programming and Databases. *Springer Verlag*, 1990.

[DFF+98]   A. Deutsch, M. Fernandez, D. Florescu, A. Levy, D. Suciu. XML-QL: A Query Language for XML. *Proc. QL'98 - The Query Languages Workshop*, 1998.

[GMW99]   R. Goldman, J. McHugh, J. Widom. From Semi-structured Data to XML: Migrating the Lore Data Model and the Query Language. *Proc. Webdb'99*, 1999.

[ISO8879] ISO (International Organization for Standardization). ISO 8879:1986(E). Information processing – Text and Office Systems – Standard Generalized Markup Language (SGML). First edition – 1986-10-15. [Geneva]: International Organization for Standardization, 1986.

[OT00a]   B. Oliboni, L. Tanca. Querying XML specified WWW sites: links and recursion in XML-GL. *Proc. SEBD 2000*, giugno 2000.

[OT00b]   B. Oliboni, L. Tanca. Querying XML specified WWW sites: links and recursion in XML-GL. *Technical Report, Politecnico di Milano, 2000*.

[PPT95]   J. Paredaens, P. Peelman, L. Tanca. G-Log a declarative graph-based language. *IEEE Tans. on Knowlwdge and Data Eng.*, 1995.

[PPT98]   J. Paredaens, P. Peelman, L. Tanca. Merging graph-based and rule-based computation: The language G-Log. *Data & Knowledge Engineering* 25, p. 267–300, 1998.

[W3C98a]   The World Wide Web Consortium. Extensible Markup Language 1.0. Feb. 1998. http://www.w3.org/TR/REC-xml

[W3C98b]   The World Wide Web Consortium. Query Language 98. Dec. 1998. http://www.w3.org/TandS/QL/QL98/

[W3C98c]   W3C Working Draft. XML Linking Language (XLink). Dec. 1999. http://www.w3c.org/TR/1999/WD-xlink-19991220

A Heuristic Approach for Converting HTML Documents to XML Documents

Seung-Jin Lim and Yiu-Kai Ng

Computer Science Department, Brigham Young University
Provo, Utah 84602, U.S.A.
{ng,sjlim}@cs.byu.edu

Abstract. XML is rapidly emerging, and yet there still exist numerous HTML documents on the Web. In this paper, we present a heuristic approach for converting HTML documents to XML documents. During the conversion process, we eliminate all the HTML elements in an HTML document from the resulting XML document since these elements are designed for the display of data exclusively, but retain the character data of each element along with the implicit hierarchy among the data. The proposed conversion approach extracts the data hierarchy of HTML documents as closely as possible with no human intervention. The approach can be adopted to construct the data hierarchy of an HTML document and to collect data in HTML documents into an XML repository.

1 Introduction

Since Extensible Markup Language (XML) was introduced in 1996 and became the official W3C Recommendation in 1997, it has been emerging as a de facto standard in electronic data exchange quickly. At present, there are still a large number of new and existing HTML documents, either dynamically created via CGI-like technologies or statically created, on the Web. It is worth to migrate existing HTML documents to XML documents to avoid inefficiency and additional complexity for managing documents in two different formats. Migration of dynamic HTML documents to XML can be done easily by modifying the respective CGI-like modules. It is, however, more time consuming to migrate static HTML documents to XML unless conversion tools are provided.

In this paper, we present a heuristic approach, called *Html2Xml*, to convert HTML documents to XML documents. We consider the following two issues:

- First, in the resultant XML document, it is desirable to just retain data and exclude HTML tags that are contained in the source HTML document since the primary role of HTML tags is to merely define the display, i.e., the "look-and-feel," of data.
- Second, the explicit or implicit data hierarchy of the source HTML document should be determined and preserved in the resultant XML document.

Consider the body block of the HTML document, *Utah County Demographic Analysis 1996* (UCDA), as shown in Figure 1. According to the container-content constraint specified in HTML grammar, Figure 2(a) shows a typical hierarchy of the body block of UCDA. In Figure 2(a), the hierarchy of the data, such as the

J. Lloyd et al. (Eds.): CL 2000, LNAI 1861, pp. 1182–1196, 2000.

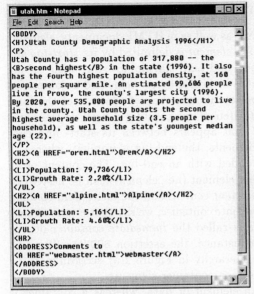

Fig. 1. Body block of utah.htm

population and growth rate of a city in Utah County, is interleaved with HTML tags such as Bs, ULs, and LIs. As a result, the data content of the first paragraph (P) yields three leaf nodes in the hierarchy since it is divided into three parts by B. Because of the separation, the association between a city name and its population and growth rate is not clearly shown in the figure. We believe the hierarchy in Figure 2(b) depicts the relationship among the data "better" than that of Figure 2(a) since in Figure 2(b) population 79,736 is tied with its city "Orem" and population 5,161 is tied with its city "Alpine" according to the container-content relationship.

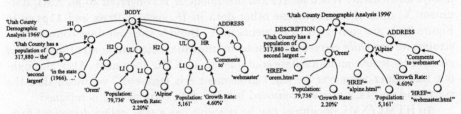

(a) The document hierarchy (DOH) generated by the HTML grammar

(b) The desired data hierarchy (DAH)

Fig. 2. Two different hierarchies of the HTML document in Figure 1

Our Html2Xml approach is based on the notion of *data hierarchy* (DAH). The DAH of an HTML document H is a tree representation of the data in H, with the exclusion of most of the HTML elements in H. Also, data in a DAH are identified by their hierarchical relationships with other data without using HTML elements. In this regard, the notion of DAH distinguishes itself from other approaches [1, 2, 6, 7] where manipulation of HTML elements is indispensable in the process of locating a particular data item. Furthermore, our Html2Xml approach does not require any knowledge of the structure of a source HTML document beforehand, and we generate the XML representation of all the data, rather than a selected portion, in an HTML document with no human intervention, which is required in [10].

We proceed to present our results as follows. In Section 2, we include preliminary definitions that are used for further discussions in this paper. In Section 3, we introduce our approach for converting HTML documents to XML documents. In Section 4, we give the concluding remarks.

2   HTML/XML Documents

There are two major constructs in XML as well as in HTML documents: elements and character data (data in short). An *element* is delimited by its *start-tag* and *end-tag*, unless it is an empty element, and text that do not start with '<' are *character data*. Moreover, an element is identified by its *name* and accompanied with an *attribute list* of zero or more attributes, each of which is of the form *attribute name = value*. (For a data item *d*, we consider *d* itself as the name of *d*.) An element contains *content* that appears between its start- and end-tags. For some non-empty HTML elements, the end-tag is implicit, whereas a non-empty XML element is always ended with an end-tag. The content of an HTML/XML element is either another element (i.e., elements can be nested) or character data. We call the former *element content* and the latter *data content*. Also, given an element *e* and its immediate content *c*, we say that *e immediately contains c*, denoted by $e \leftarrow c$, and *e* is called the *immediate container* of *c* or *c* is the *immediate content* of *e*. For instance, the assertion BODY ← UL ← LI ← *'Population: 5,161'* holds for the hierarchy in Figure 2(a) according to the HTML grammar. Empty elements are non-container elements.

Recall that a content is either an element or data, whereas a container is always an element. When an HTML document *H* is converted to an XML document *X*, data that encompass other data in *H*, such as Orem and Alpine in Figure 2(a), are converted to elements in *X*. Besides the container-content constraint, we use *child element* to denote an immediate element content and *parent element* to denote an immediate container in an XML document. Also, throughout this paper whenever we say "an element *e* is removed," we mean that the start- and end-tags of *e* are removed but the data content of *e* is retained.

An HTML/XML document can be perceived as a tree, called *document hierarchy (DOH)*, where a node denotes an element or data component, and edges are determined by the container-content relationships among nodes. If each node in a DOH *D* exclusively represents an HTML/XML data or an XML element, we call *D* a *data hierarchy* (DAH), denoted DAH_D.

Definition 1. Given an HTML/XML document *D*, the *document hierarchy* (DOH) of *D* is a tree, denoted $DOH_D = (V, E, g)$, where (i) a node in *V* denotes an element *e* or a character data *d* in *D* and is labeled by the name of *e* or *d*, respectively[1]. For any node *n* and its child nodes n_1, n_2, ..., n_m, n_j appears before n_k in the left-to-right, top-to-bottom manner in *D* if $1 \leq j < k \leq m$. The root node V_R in *V* is the BODY element if *D* is an HTML document, or the first element appeared after the prolog block if *D* is an XML document; (ii) *E* is a finite set of directed edges; and (iii) $g : E \rightarrow V \times V$ is the *edge definition function* such that $g(e) = (v_1, v_2)$ if $v_2 \leftarrow v_1$. □

According to Definition 1, the hierarchy shown in Figure 2(a) is the DOH of utah.htm, where the name of each leaf node is surrounded by ' '. To reference an element or data *v* in a hierarchy where *v* belongs, we define the *context* of *v*.

---

[1] Since we guarantee one-to-one relationships between *D* and DOH_D, we interchangeably use the nodes in DOH_D and the elements/data in *D*, as well as *D* and DOH_D.

Definition 2. Given a set S of elements or data that are hierarchically structured, the *context* of an element or data v in S is defined as $X_v = N_v$, if v is the root node of the hierarchy; otherwise, $X_v = X_{v'}.N_v$, where N_v is the *name* of v and $X_{v'}$ is the *context* of the predecessor of v in the hierarchy. (The dot '.' in $X_{v'}.N_v$ is the *dot* operator which is the separator of $X_{v'}$ and N_v.) □

The context of a node v in a DOH is the concatenation of the names of v and its ancestors along the path from the root node, and each distinct name is delimited by '.' from its adjacent names. Furthermore, using an ordered list of context of the leaf nodes in a DOH, we can represent the DOH as a string. We adopt the convention $A.(B, C)$ for $(A.B, A.C)$, where $(A.B, A.C)$ is an ordered list of context. In addition, if sibling nodes share the same name, we append an index number to their names, such that *node*[1] denotes the first node with the name *node*, according to their order of appearance in the source document.

Consider the hierarchy in Figure 2(b). Using the context of each leaf node, the data in the subtree rooted at **Alpine** can be expressed as follows:

('Utah County Demographic Analysis 1996'.'Alpine'.'HREF="alpine.html"',
'Utah County Demographic Analysis 1996'.'Alpine'.'Population: 5,161',
'Utah County Demographic Analysis 1996'.'Alpine'.'Growth Rate: 4.60%') =
'Utah County Demographic Analysis 1996'.'Alpine'.(
  'HREF="alpine.html"', 'Population: 5,161', 'Growth Rate: 4.60%')

3 Construction of the Data Hierarchy of an HTML Document

We now present our approach for constructing the data hierarchy (DAH), which captures the hierarchical relationships among the data contents, of a given HTML document D. The construction process of DAH_D includes (i) the exclusion of HTML elements from D and (ii) the refinement of the container-content relationships among the data in D.

3.1 Exclusion of HTML Elements

Among the defined HTML elements, the role of some elements is to define the block structure of data (called *type 1*), whereas others are to define the cosmetic style of the rendered data in a Web browser exclusively (called *type 2*).

We group HTML elements into type 1 and type 2 based on whether they form blocks of data such that one block is distinguishable from another hierarchically. Table 1 shows the grouping which follows the widely-supported HTML 3.2 [8]. Note that the primary role of text-level elements is to define the style of data, and they do not contribute to the formation of a hierarchical block with the exception of **A**. (**A** is considered as type 1 since any data d appeared in a linked document from another HTML document D are subordinate to D and **A** is a lead to d.) Also, we include into type 2 head-related elements, as well as all the non-container elements among the rest of the HTML elements. *Head-related* elements are type 2 elements since no data is presented in the head block, and all *empty* elements are excluded from type 1 as well since they contain no data. *Form-related* and *Java applet-related* elements are also excluded from type 1 since they

Table 1. Two groups of HTML elements, type 1 and type 2

HTML elements			type 1	type 2
head content				TITLE, META, ISINDEX, BASE, LINK, SCRIPT, STYLE, META
body content	headings		H1, H2, H3, H4, H5, H6	
	block-level		UL, OL, DIR, MENU, LI, DL, DT, DD, P, DIV, TR, TABLE, TH, TD, CAPTION, CENTER, BLOCKQUOTE	ISINDEX, HR, XMP, LISTING, PLAINTEXT
	text-level	font		TT, I, B, U, STRIKE, BIG, SMALL, SUB, SUP
		phrase		EM, STRONG, DFN, CODE, SAMP, KBD, VAR, CITE
		special	A	IMG, APPLET, FONT, BR, BASEFONT, SCRIPT, MAP
		form		FORM, INPUT, SELECT, OPTION, TEXTAREA
	client-side image maps			MAP, AREA
	Java applet			APPLET, PARAM
	address		ADDRESS	

† META with *name* attribute="keywords" and $< BODY >$ are considered as type 1, while other METAs, $< HTML >$, $< HEAD >$, and $<! >$ are treated as type 2 elements.

are used to query data rather than to present data. Among the elements that do not appear in Table 1, we exclude HTML and HEAD from type 1 but retain BODY as type 1 to ensure that the resulting DAH of an HTML document is a tree.

Note that table-related elements were not included in the earlier version of HTML specification and were added later to present data in a tabular form. They are the most versatile among the HTML elements in organizing data hierarchically and are treated as type 1. We emphasize HTML tables since they are very capable in presenting data hierarchically, and most of the data generated dynamically through CGI-like programs are presented in HTML tables.

Given an HTML document D, we first remove the HTML elements of type 2 from D and the resulting document is called an *approximated* document. For example, after B is removed from utah.htm, the content of P is restored as a paragraph in the approximated utah.htm, and HR is also removed hereafter.

3.2 Edge Definition Function of DAH

During the process of defining edges, we apply four *hierarchy resolution rules* to D which provide the mechanism for refining the hierarchy of D. The first rule describes how to handle an anchor A and its data in our Html2Xml approach.

Rule 1. Given an ordered list of container-content relationships ($p \leftarrow C_1, p \leftarrow$ A $\leftarrow C_2, p \leftarrow C_3$), where p is the parent of C_1, A, and C_3, A is an anchor element, and C_i ($1 \leq i \leq 3$) is a data item, the *edge definition function g* of DAH yields $p \leftarrow C \leftarrow HREF$, where $HREF$ is the *name* and *value* pair of the HREF attribute in A, and $C = concat(concat(C_1, C_2), C_3)^2$. Hereafter, A is removed. □

---

² $Concat(s_1, s_2) = trim(s_1 +$ s $+ s_2)$, where s_1 and s_2 are strings, s is a space, $+$ is a string concatenation operator, and *trim* removes any leading and trailing spaces.

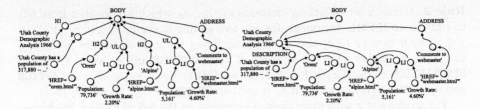

(a) Modified DOH after Rule 1 is applied

(b) Modified DOH after Rule 2 is applied to the DOH in Figure 3(a)

Fig. 3. Evolving DOHs

By Rule 1, we restore the data that might have been fragmented by A, and retain the HREF attribute of A as a placeholder for the data in the linked document.

Consider the ADDRESS element in utah.htm as shown in Figure 2(a) whose content is separated into three parts. By Rule 1, we obtain two edges such that ADDRESS ← 'Comments to webmaster' ← 'HREF="webmaster.html"'. Also, H2[1] ← A[1] ← 'Orem' yields H2[1] ← 'Orem' ← 'HREF="orem.html"', and H2[2] ← A[2] ← 'Alpine' yields H2[2] ← 'Alpine' ← 'HREF="alpine.html"'. Figure 3(a) shows the modified DOH after Rule 1 has been applied to the approximated utah.htm.

Next, we refine the hierarchy of the nodes at the same level in the current DOH. In this process, we adopt the precedence spectrum as shown in Figure 4, where items on the left of '≫' have higher precedence than that on the right.

We place headings higher than other body content elements since they are headings of the text blocks that appear next to the headings, and H1 has higher precedence than H6. Since the roles of OL, DL, DIR, and MENU are similar to that of UL, they have the same precedence. (In fact, DIR, MENU, and UL are treated the same in many Web browsers.) The roles of DIV, CENTER, and BLOCKQUOTE are similar, and hence we place them at the same precedence level. (In fact, CENTER is identical to DIV whose ALIGN attribute value is CENTER.) All these elements, along with ADDRESS, have the same precedence as P and TABLE since none of these elements is subordinate to one another. Since LI is used as a content of UL, OL, DIR and MENU, DT is used as a content of DL, and CAPTION is a content of TABLE according to the HTML specification, we place these elements at the next level in the precedence spectrum. DD is placed at the next level for a similar reason. TR, on the other hand, should have the same precedence as CAPTION according to the HTML specification; however, we place it at a level lower than CAPTION since we consider the content of CAPTION as the title of the entire table. The respective precedence of TR, TH and TD are obvious according to the container-content specification of these elements.

High   *Low*

$$H1 \gg H2 \gg H3 \gg H4 \gg H5 \gg H6 \gg \begin{pmatrix} \text{P, UL, OL, DL, DIR, MENU,} \\ \text{ADDRESS, DIV, CENTER,} \\ \text{BLOCKQUOTE, TABLE} \end{pmatrix} \gg \begin{pmatrix} \text{LI, DT,} \\ \text{CAPTION} \end{pmatrix} \gg \begin{pmatrix} \text{DD,} \\ \text{TR} \end{pmatrix} \gg \begin{pmatrix} \text{TH,} \\ \text{TD} \end{pmatrix}$$

Fig. 4. Precedence among HTML elements

Rule 2. Given a set of sibling elements e_1, ..., e_n which are located from left to right in an HTML document, for any two sibling elements e_i and e_j ($1 \leq i < j \leq n$) such that $e_i \leftarrow c_1$ and $e_j \leftarrow c_2$, applying the *edge definition function* g to e_1, ..., e_n yields (i) $c_1 \leftarrow e_j \leftarrow c_2$, if e_j is ADDRESS and $e_i \gg e_j$, (ii) $c_1 \leftarrow$ DESCRIPTION $\leftarrow c_2$, if e_j is P and $e_i \gg e_j$, (iii) $e_i \leftarrow e_j \leftarrow c_2$, if e_i is CAPTION and e_j is TR, or (iv) $c_1 \leftarrow c_2$, if e_j is neither ADDRESS, P nor TR and $e_i \gg e_j$.

For an element e with more than one element on the left of e which has higher precedence than e, we retain only the edge between the element of the highest precedence and e if e is ADDRESS; otherwise, we retain the edge between e and the nearest element to e. Hereafter, any empty HTML elements are removed. □

By Rule 2, the contents of a set of sibling elements are refined, if necessary. Note that we treat ADDRESS separately since it has a unique role, such as authorship and contact details for the source HTML document. We rename P elements as DESCRIPTIONs until the construction of an XML document X is completed since they play special roles during the construction of X. We will discuss CAPTION and TR in details in the next section.

Consider the DOH in Figure 3(a) and apply Rule 2 to the child elements of BODY. Since H1 $\gg$ P, 'Utah County Demographic Analysis 1966' $\leftarrow$ DESCRIPTION $\leftarrow$ 'Utah County has a population of ...' by Rule 2(ii). Consider P and H2[1]. Since H2 $\gg$ P but P appears before H2[1], the contents of these elements are not rearranged. However, since H1 $\gg$ H2, 'Utah County Demographic Analysis 1966' $\leftarrow$ 'Orem' $\leftarrow$ 'HREF="orem.html"' by Rule 2(iv). Now, compare H2[1] and UL[1]. Since H2 $\gg$ UL, ('Orem' $\leftarrow$ LI[1], 'Orem' $\leftarrow$ LI[2]) by Rule 2(iv), and eventually ('Orem' $\leftarrow$ LI[1] $\leftarrow$ 'Population: 79,736', 'Orem' $\leftarrow$ LI[2] $\leftarrow$ 'Growth Rate: 2.20%'). H2[2] and UL[2] are processed similarly. Figure 3(b) shows the modified DOH after Rule 2 has been applied. Note that ADDRESS is retained and LI[1] (LI[3], respectively) cannot be resolved against LI[2] (LI[4], respectively) since LI[1] and LI[2] (LI[3] and LI[4], respectively) have the same precedence.

Rule 3. Given a container-content relationship $e_1 \leftarrow e_2 \leftarrow e_3$, where e_2 is neither ADDRESS, a table-specific element, nor DESCRIPTION attached by P, the *edge definition function* g of DAH produces $e_1 \leftarrow e_3$. □

By now, the hierarchies of all the sibling elements in the DOH should have been refined. Any remaining HTML elements in the DOH, with the exception of ADDRESS and table-specific elements (to be discussed in Section 3.3), can be safely removed since they do not contribute to the determination of the data hierarchy of the given HTML document.

Consider the DOH in Figure 3(b). After applying Rule 3, LI[1], LI[2], LI[3], LI[4], and BODY are removed, and the resulting hierarchy is as shown in Figure 2(b) which is the resulting DAH for utah.htm since no HTML table is contained in utah.htm.

Rule 4. If a DOH which is modified by Rule 3 is a forest, then $t \leftarrow n_1$, $t \leftarrow n_2$, ..., $t \leftarrow n_k$, where t is the content of the TITLE element of the source HTML document and n_1, ..., n_k are the root nodes in DOH. □

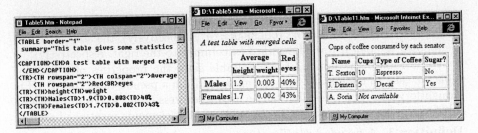

(a) The source code of HTML Table 1 as shown in Figure 5(b)

(b) HTML Table 1 with heading rows & columns

(c) HTML Table 2 with a heading row

Fig. 5. Two typical types of HTML tables

Rule 4 ensures that the resulting DAH is a tree. The content of the TITLE element is chosen to be the root in the DAH since it is the only required element in an HTML document H and provides an indication regarding what H is about.

3.3 Edge Definition Function for Table-Specific Elements

Among the table-specific elements, TR determines the number of rows, and TH and TD determine the number of columns in an HTML table (tables in short). THs are used for declaring table headings and TDs for asserting data of table cells. The data contents of TD elements are called *table data*. In contrast, the data contents of TH elements are column or row headings that are not considered as table data. However, data of either element is rendered in a Web browser.

There are a few popular types of HTML tables with respect to headings: (i) tables that have at least one heading row at the top and at least one heading column on the left, such as HTML Table 1 as shown in Figure 5(b) in [9]. We call this type of tables *column-row-wise*. (ii) Tables that contain at least one heading row at the top without heading columns, such as HTML Table 2 as shown in Figure 5(c) [9]. We call this type of tables *column-wise*. In a column-wise table, the heading rows yield the schema of the table. (iii) Other than these two types of tables, we notice that a large number of tables do not make use of table-related elements other than TABLE and TD. We, however, draw from our analysis a conclusion that the creator of this type of tables often implicitly designates the first row as a heading. Hence, we treat this type of tables as column-wise.

Two attributes of TH and TD, ROWSPAN and COLSPAN, play significant roles in determinating the data hierarchy of a table. Consider the source code of a table shown in Figure 5(a). It has four rows (i.e., four TRs) as rendered in Figure 5(b). (The source code shown in the figure is the original code which includes EM and BR before the approximation of the table is performed.) Note that the first TR contains three TH elements, implying that the row is a heading which includes three cells (i.e., three columns). The second row, on the other hand, contains two TH elements, implying that there are two heading cells, whereas each of the last two TRs contains one TH and three TDs, implying that there is one heading cell on the left followed by three data cells in each row. Apparently, the numbers of columns of the first two rows are not equal, nor with that of the last two rows. It is not clear which cell in one row belongs to the same column with a cell in another row until we take ROWSPANs and COLSPANs into consideration. When a TH or TD includes ROWSPAN="n" (COLSPAN="n", respectively), the associated cell is supposed to span n rows downward (n columns to the right, respectively).

We introduce the notion of pseudo-table since the properties of a pseudo-table are easy to understand and the mapping from a pseudo-table to a DAH is straightforward. A pseudo-table can be used to express either a column-row-wise table or a column-wise table with the table-specific elements mentioned above.

Definition 3. A *pseudo-table* $T = \{(a_{1,1}, \ldots, a_{1,n}), (a_{2,1}, \ldots, a_{2,n}), \ldots, (a_{m,1}, \ldots, a_{m,n})\}$ with column headings $C_1, \ldots, C_n$ and caption C, is a two-dimensional table, where each column heading C_i ($1 \leq i \leq n$) or table data $a_{i,j}$ ($1 \leq i \leq m$, $1 \leq j \leq n$) may be null. If a column heading or table data o is null, then the name of the object representing o is the empty string. Data values of rows i and j of the first column in T are different if $i \neq j$. □

Recall that the hierarchy of HTML elements and data in a DOH is determined by their container-content relationships. The hierarchy of a pseudo-table, however, is defined over its caption, column headings and table data. Since column headings and table data may be null in a pseudo-table, we consider a special case: given the container-content relationships $o_1 \leftarrow o_2 \leftarrow o_3$, where o_i ($1 \leq i \leq 3$) is either a column heading or table data, $o_1 \leftarrow o_2 \leftarrow o_3$ is reduced to $o_1 \leftarrow o_3$ if the name of o_2 is the empty string.

Rule 5. Given an n-ary pseudo-table $T = \{(a_{1,1}, \ldots, a_{1,n}), (a_{2,1}, \ldots, a_{2,n}), \ldots, (a_{m,1}, \ldots, a_{m,n})\}$ with column headings $C_1, \ldots, C_n$ and caption C, the *edge definition function* g yields $V_R \leftarrow C_1 \leftarrow a_{i,1} \leftarrow C_j \leftarrow a_{i,j}$ ($1 \leq i \leq m, 2 \leq j \leq n$), where V_R is labeled C if C is not empty, or is labeled "Table", otherwise. □

Since the caption of a pseudo-table T provides a short description on what the table is about, we choose the caption as the name for the root node of T (and hence the corresponding DAH). If CAPTION is missing, the root node of the corresponding pseudo-table is named "Table" simply to indicate the corresponding DAH is an HTML table. Furthermore, according to Rule 5, a DAH contains subtrees rooted at $a_{1,1}, \ldots, a_{m,1}$ with the constraints $V_R \leftarrow C_1 \leftarrow a_{i,1}$ ($1 \leq i \leq m$). This is because each row in T can be uniquely identified from the other rows by the first column (i.e., $a_{i,1}$) in T (see Definition 3). Figure 6 shows the transformation between a pseudo-table and its corresponding DAH according to Rule 5. (Rule 5 indeed states how to construct the hierarchy of the components in a pseudo-table in order to obtain the corresponding DAH.) Figure 7 (Figure 8, respectively) shows how to map a column-wise HTML (column-row-wise, respectively) table to a pseudo-table.

Colspan and Rowspan. An HTML table may not have the same number of THs or TDs in each row, and COLSPANs and ROWSPANs play an important role in mapping such an HTML table to a pseudo-table. If a TH or TD contains COLSPAN = "n", the particular cell of the TH or TD is to be expanded to $n-1$ more columns, starting from the current cell in the current row. Hence, at the current row, we insert $n-1$ cells to the right of the current cell and replicate the data content of the current cell $n-1$ times to the new cells. If a TH element contains ROWSPAN = "n", the particular cell of the TH element is to be expanded to the next $n-1$

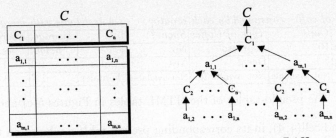

Fig. 6. A pseudo-table T and its corresponding DAH

$h_{1,1}$	$\cdots$	$h_{1,n}$
$\vdots$		$\vdots$
$h_{k,1}$	$\cdots$	$h_{k,n}$
$d_{k+1,1}$	$\cdots$	$d_{k+1,n}$
$\vdots$		$\vdots$
$d_{k+m,1}$	$\cdots$	$d_{k+m,n}$

$\Longleftrightarrow$

$C_1 =$	$\cdots$	$C_n =$
$h_{1,1}.....h_{k,1}$	$\cdots$	$h_{1,n}.....h_{k,n}$
$a_{1,1} = d_{k+1,1}$	$\cdots$	$a_{1,n} = d_{k+1,n}$
$\vdots$		$\vdots$
$a_{m,1} = d_{k+m,1}$	$\cdots$	$a_{m,n} = d_{k+m,n}$

A single dot (.) is the dot operator as presented in Definition 2.

Fig. 7. Mapping from a column-wise HTML table to a pseudo-table

$hh_{1,1}$		$\cdots$		$hh_{1,n}$
$\vdots$				$\vdots$
$hh_{k,1}$		$\cdots$		$hh_{k,n}$
$hv_{k+1,1}$	$\cdots$ $hv_{k+1,l}$	$d_{k+1,l+1}$	$\cdots$	$d_{k+1,l+n-1}$
$\vdots$	$\vdots$	$\vdots$		$\vdots$
$hv_{k+m,1}$	$\cdots$ $hv_{k+m,l}$	$d_{k+m,l+1}$	$\cdots$	$d_{k+m,l+n-1}$

$\Longleftrightarrow$

$C_1 =$	$\cdots$	$C_n =$
$hh_{1,1}.....$		$hh_{1,n}.....$
$hh_{k,1}$		$hh_{k,n}$
$a_{1,1} = hv_{k+1,1}.$	$\cdots$	$a_{1,n} =$
$....hv_{k+1,l}$		$d_{k+1,l+n-1}$
$\vdots$		$\vdots$
$a_{m,1} = hv_{k+m,1}.$	$\cdots$	$a_{m,n} =$
$....hv_{k+m,l}$		$d_{k+m,l+n-1}$

A single dot (.) is the dot operator as presented in Definition 2.

Fig. 8. Mapping from a column-row-wise HTML table to a pseudo-table

rows. For that we insert $n-1$ cells beneath the current TH cell in the current column, and push the data content h of the current cell all the way down to the $(n-1)$th new cell, rather than replicating h to the underneath rows $n-1$ times. As a result, h appears at the $(n-1)$th new cell, and each of the cells above the $(n-1)$th new cell in the same column is left as the empty string. This is necessary for retaining the correct association among the table data across all the rows in a column. On the other hand, if ROWSPAN is contained in a TD, we insert $n-1$ new cells underneath the current TD cell, and replicate the data content of the TD to the inserted cells since each table data in different rows of the same column is meant to represent a data entry with the same content. After COLSPANs and ROWSPANs are processed, the corresponding table conforms to the specification of a pseudo-table as stated in Rule 5.

Consider the table in Figure 5(c) and suppose the cell at the ith row and the jth column is denoted by $cell(i, j)$. Note that "Not available" appears across the last three column spaces of the forth row of the table due to COLSPAN="3" in cell$(4, 2)$ (the source code is not included in this paper due to page limit), and hence we replicate "Not available" of cell$(4, 2)$ to the next two inserted cells

Cups of coffee consumed by each senator				A test table with merged cells			
Name	Cups	Type of Coffee	Sugar?		Average. height	Average. weight	Red eyes
T. Sexton	10	Espresso	No				
J. Dinnen	5	Decaf	Yes	Males	1.9	0.003	40%
A. Soria	Not available	Not available	Not available	Females	1.7	0.002	43%

Fig. 9. The pseudo-tables of the HTML tables in Figures 5(c) and 5(b)

cell$(4,3)$ and cell$(4,4)$, in its corresponding pseudo-table as shown on the left in Figure 9.

In the following example, we demonstrate the process of constructing the DAH (via the pseudo-table) of the HTML table shown in Figure 5(b).

Consider the source code in Figure 5(a). The first and third TH both contain ROWSPAN="2". Thus, the null data of the first TH is pushed down to the next row in the corresponding pseudo-table T. At a glance, it may look like that this action has no effect to the table since the pushed-down value is a null data. Indeed, with this action, the pushed-down null data is inserted into cell$(2,1)$ in T and subsequently the TH with *height* (*weight*, respectively) is moved to the new location which is cell$(2,2)$ (cell$(2,3)$, respectively) in T. This is desirable since the correct association among "height," "weight," and other table data are now in place in T. In addition, the second TH contains COLSPAN = "2" and subsequently its data content "Average" is replicated once to the right in the same row in T, and "Red eyes", which is originally in the third TH, is moved to the forth column and then pushed onto the forth column of the next row in T since ROWSPAN = "2".

Recall that EM and BR, as shown in the source code in Figure 5(a), should have already been removed after the approximation of the table by Rule 5. Also, there are two heading rows in T and each C_i $(1 \leq i \leq 4)$ is determined by the concatenation of the data contents of the two rows in the ith column. As a result, C_1 is the empty string, $C_2 = $ Average.height, $C_3 = $ Average.weight, and $C_4 = $ 'Red eyes'. Furthermore, the caption of T is the caption of the HTML table in Figure 5(a). The resulting pseudo-table T is as shown on the right in Figure 9.

We map the resulting pseudo-table T to the DAH. Since T contains the caption C, 'A test table with merged cells', C forms the root node of the DAH according to Rule 5. Next, consider C_1. Since C_1 is empty, we skip C_1 in the hierarchy $V_R \leftarrow C_1 \leftarrow a_{i,1} \leftarrow \ldots$ and create two child nodes of C by using $a_{1,1}$ (Males) and $a_{2,1}$ (Females). The rest of the cells $a_{i,j}$ $(1 \leq i \leq 2, 2 \leq j \leq 4)$ in the last two rows of T yield nodes and edges in DAH_T as follows: $a_{1,1} \leftarrow C_2 \leftarrow a_{1,2}; a_{1,1} \leftarrow C_3 \leftarrow a_{1,3}; a_{1,1} \leftarrow C_4 \leftarrow a_{1,4}; a_{2,1} \leftarrow C_2 \leftarrow a_{2,2}; a_{2,1} \leftarrow C_3 \leftarrow a_{2,3}; a_{2,1} \leftarrow C_4 \leftarrow a_{2,4}$. We render the resulting DAH in WebView [4], as shown under "[ROOT=E:\Table5.xml]" in the left pane of Figure 10. Note that the association of a table data D with another can be conceived by examining the context of D. For instance, 'A test table with merged cells'.Males.Average.height.'1.9' captures the data hierarchy of "1.9".

3.4   DAH to XML

According to the XML recommendation [3], an XML document consists of three consecutive blocks: (i) a prolog, (ii) a data block of one or more XML elements,

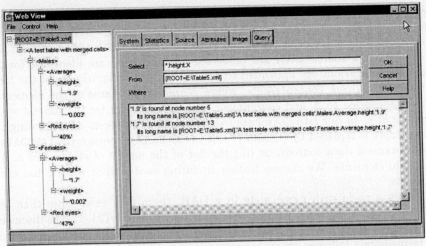

Fig. 10. DAH of the HTML table in Figure 5(a), rendered in WebView

and (iii) an optional miscellaneous block. The major components of a prolog include an XML declaration, followed by a document type declaration (DTD). A DTD provides the grammar of a class of XML documents, and the second block (i.e., *data block*), where the actual data are contained, must conform to the grammar. The optional third block contains miscellaneous data such as comments which is not the primary focus of this paper.

An XML document X is *well-formed* if X contains an XML declaration and all the markups are properly nested with no overlap. Furthermore, a well-formed XML document X is *valid* if X includes the DTD with which X complies. Violations of these constraints are treated differently. If an XML document X violates the well-formedness constraint, *fatal* error is invoked and a normal process on X must terminate, whereas a violation of the validity constraint is only considered as an error, and the document can still be processed normally. Thus, our emphasis in generating XML documents is on well-formed XML documents.

The well-formedness property of the resulting XML document X converted from an HTML document is guaranteed by our Html2Xml approach using a stack machine Σ [4]. In our Html2Xml approach, the processing thread enters a new element whenever it processes a new node n in a DAH. For n, there are two cases to be considered: (i) n is a child node of the previously processed node n_0, or (ii) n is a sibling node of n_0. In case (i), the stack symbol of n is pushed on Σ, on top of the stack symbol of n_0, and in case (ii) the stack symbol of n_0 is first popped and then the stack symbol of n is pushed onto Σ. Moreover, if n is a leaf node in the DAH, no stack operation is performed but the name of n is appended to X as the data content of the element whose stack symbol is still at the top of Σ. With that we guarantee that X is well-formed.

Document Type Declaration. DTD can be internal, external, or both. In our Html2Xml approach, we generate external DTDs. Using a stack machine Σ (as discussed earlier), an external DTD D for an XML document X is created while X is generated. At the beginning of the process, D is initialized by the text declaration `<?xml encoding="UTF-8"?>`, where `"UTF-8"` can be replaced by other encoding names such as `"UTF-16"` or `"ISO-10646-UCS-4"`. As the nodes in a source DAH are processed and elements are identified for X, element declarations are appended to D. An element declaration is of the form `<!ELEMENT` $Name$ $contentspec$`>`, where $Name$ is the name of the element e that is appended to X and $contentspec$ is the placeholder for the content specification of e. In our Html2Xml approach, during the process of generating X, $contentspec$ is replaced by (i) `(EMPTY)`, if e is an empty element; (ii) `(#PCDATA)`, if e contains a data content; or (iii) the list of the names of children of e, if e has child elements. We discuss further updating $contentspec$ when e has child elements.

Given a node with name `node` in a DAH, there may exist more than one child node with the same name, such as `cnode[1]`, `cnode[2]`, ..., as discussed in Section 2. If so, `cnode` in $contentspec$ of `<!ELEMENT node` $contentspec$`>` can be immediately followed by an occurrence symbol '?', '*' or '+', which denotes that the preceding content particle, i.e., `node`, of the respective symbol may occur once or more times (+), zero or more times (*), or at most once (?). Note that the implications of these three symbols are not distinct. For instance, if `cnode` occurs just once, either `<!ELEMENT node (cnode)?>`, `<!ELEMENT node (cnode)*>`, `<!ELEMENT node (cnode)+>`, or even `<!ELEMENT node (cnode)>` is a valid declaration. In our Html2Xml approach, `(cnode)` will be appended to the resulting XML document if `cnode` occurs just once in the source DAH, or `(cnode)*` will be appended if `cnode` occurs more than once.

Along with the update of $contentspec$ in an element declaration, we need to consider attribute list declarations of an element e as well if e accompanies any attribute. When an element e is found to accompany attributes of the form $attr_i = attrVal_i$ $(i \geq 1)$, this information is added after the element declaration of e in the DTD as `<!ATTLIST` e $attr_i$ $AttType$ $DefaultDecl$`>` for each $attr_i$, where $AttType$ is `CDATA` which denotes that the corresponding attribute is of string type, and $DefaultDecl$ is `#IMPLIED` which denotes that no default value is provided for the attribute. Note that $attr_i$ may appear more than once with different values val_1, val_2, ..., val_n $(1 \leq n)$. In such a case, $(attrVal_i)$ is first bound to (val_1), then to $(val_1 \mid val_2)$ when val_2 is identified, and so forth while the DAH is processed. Eventually, $(attrVal_i)$ is bound to $(val_1 \mid val_2 \mid \ldots \mid val_n)$.

Applying algorithm Dah2Xml[3] to the DAH in Figure 2(b) yields the resulting XML document X as shown below.

```
<?xml version="1.0" ?>
<!DOCTYPE UtahCountyDemographicAnalysis1996 SYSTEM
 "UtahCountyDemographicAnalysis1996.dtd">
<UtahCountyDemographicAnalysis1996 AddressDescription="Comments to
webmaster" AddressLink="webmaster.htm">
 <DESCRIPTION>Utah County has a population of 317,880--...</DESCRIPTION>
 <Orem Link="orem.htm"><Population:79,736/><GrowthRate:2.20%/></Orem>
 <Alpine Link="alpine.htm"><Population:5,161/><GrowthRate:4.60%/></Orem>
</UtahCountyDemographicAnalysis1996>
```

---

[3] Algorithm Dah2Xml is not included in this paper but can be found in [5].

Also, the resulting DTD D of the DAH is shown below.

```
<?xml encoding="UTF-8"?>
<!ELEMENT UtahCountyDemographicAnalysis1996 (DESCRIPTION, Orem, Alpine)>
<!ATTLIST UtahCountyDemographicAnalysis1996 AddressDescription CDATA #IMPLIED>
<!ATTLIST UtahCountyDemographicAnalysis1996 AddressLink CDATA #IMPLIED>
<!ELEMENT DESCRIPTION (#PCDATA)>
<!ELEMENT Orem (Population:79,736, GrowthRate:2.20%)>
<!ATTLIST Orem Link CDATA #IMPLIED>
<!ELEMENT Population:79,736 (EMPTY)>
<!ELEMENT GrowthRate:2.20% (EMPTY)>
<!ELEMENT Alpine (Population:5,161, GrowthRate:4.60%)>
<!ATTLIST Alpine Link CDATA #IMPLIED>
<!ELEMENT Population:5,161 (EMPTY)>
<!ELEMENT GrowthRate:4.60% (EMPTY)>
```

Recall that 'Utah County Demographic Analysis 1996' is the root node of the DAH. It forms the root element of X and D is named after it by default. Since ADDRESS is treated as an attribute list of its parent element in X, the subtree rooted at ADDRESS is converted to the AddressDescription and AddressLink attributes of the root in X. In addition, DESCRIPTION, Orem, and Alpine are attached to X as the immediate contents of the root since they are child nodes of the root in the DAH. Note that the child node of DESCRIPTION in the DAH is a leaf node, and hence the *contentspec* of the DESCRIPTION element is declared as (#PCDATA) in D, and the *contentspec* of any leaf node is (EMPTY). Also, each HREF node is converted as an attribute to its parent element.

As another example, the XML document and its DTD of the DAH as shown in the left pane of Figure 10, where table-specific elements are involved, are

```
<?xml version="1.0" ?>
<!DOCTYPE ATestTableWithMergedCells SYSTEM "ATestTableWithMergedCells.dtd">
<ATestTableWithMergedCells>
    <Males>
        <Average><height>1.9</height><weight>0.003</weight></Average>
        <RedEyes>40%</RedEyes>
    </Males>
    <Females>
        <Average><height>1.7</height><weight>0.002</weight></Average>
        <RedEyes>43%</RedEyes>
    </Females>
</ATestTableWithMergedCells>

<?xml encoding="UTF-8"?>
<!ELEMENT ATestTableWithMergedCells (Males, Females)>
<!ELEMENT Males (Average, RedEyes)>
<!ELEMENT Average (height, weight)>
<!ELEMENT RedEyes (#PCDATA)>
<!ELEMENT height (#PCDATA)>
<!ELEMENT weight (#PCDATA)>
<!ELEMENT Females (Average, RedEyes)>
```

3.5   Implementation of the Html2Xml Approach

Portions of the proposed conversion approach, which includes the approximation (discussed in Section 3.1) and table-specific elements (discussed in Section 3.3), have been implemented as a Java class using JDK 1.1.7. The Java class generates the data hierarchy of any given HTML table T in the lexical form whose representation is similar to the ordered list of the data context in T. For rendering and querying DOHs and DAHs graphically, WebView [4] can be used.

4   Concluding Remarks

We have presented a heuristic approach to convert HTML documents to XML documents. XML is rapidly emerging but there are still numerous existing HTML documents. It is desirable to convert these HTML documents to XML documents rather than to obsolete them or maintain documents of two different specifications. During the process of conversion, we eliminate all the HTML elements in a source HTML document from the resultant XML document. The approach for constructing the data hierarchy, as a part of our conversion approach, can be used for extracting the data hierarchy of an HTML document. Our approach can be used by existing wrappers and integrators (in data warehousing systems), which frequently access large number of HTML tables for extracting hierarchically structured data to automate the data acquisition process for XML repositories.

References

1. G. Arocena and A. Medelzon. WebOQL: Restructuring Documents, Databases and Webs. In *Proceedings of the 14th ICDE*, 1998.
2. P. Atzeni and G. Mecca. Cut and Paste. In *Proceedings of the 16th Intl. Symposium on Principles of Database Systems*, pages 144–153, 1997.
3. T. Bray, J. Paoli, and C. Sperberg-McQueen. Extensible Markup Language (XML) 1.0 W3C Recommendation 10-February-1998, February 1998.
4. S.-J. Lim and Y.-K. Ng. WebView: A Tool for Retrieving Internal Structures and Extracting Information from HTML Documents. In *Proceedings of the 6th International Conference on Database Systems for Advanced Applications (DASFAA '99)*, pages 71–80, April 1999.
5. S.-J. Lim and Y.-K. Ng. A Heuristic Approach for Converting HTML Documents to XML Documents. http://lunar.cs.byu.edu/paper.html, July 2000.
6. A. Mendelzon, G. Mihaila, and T. Milo. Querying the World Wide Web. In *Proceedings of the Conf. on Parallel & Distributed Info. Systems*, 1996.
7. A. Mendelzon and T. Milo. Formal Models of Web Queries. In *Proceedings of the 16th Intl. Symposium on PODS*, pages 134–143, 1997.
8. D. Raggett. HTML 3.2 Reference Specification. http://www.w3.org/TR/REC-html32, January 1997.
9. D. Raggett, A. Hors, and I. Jacobs. HTML 4.0 Specification – W3C Recommendation. http://www.w3.org/TR/REC-html40, April 1998.
10. A. Sahuguet and F. Azavant. Looking at the Web through XML-glasses. In *Proceedings of the 4th Intl. Conf. on Cooperative Info. Systems*, 1999.

Specification of an Active Database System Application Using Dynamic Relation Nets

Laurent Allain[1] and Pascal Yim[2]

[1]Institut Supérieur d'Electronique du Nord, Département Informatique
41 Boulevard Vauban, F-59046 Lille Cedex, France
laurent.allain@isen.fr
[2]Ecole Centrale de Lille, LAIL UPRESA 8021, BP 48
F-59650 Villeneuve d'Ascq Cedex, France
pascal.yim@ec-lille.fr

Abstract. This paper describes a new kind of specification of an active database system application based on the Dynamic Relation Nets, which are themselves derived from high-level Petri nets. We introduce the capability of a Dynamic Relation Net to describe both static and dynamic aspects of a system, and show how such a formalism may be used to specify ECA-rules. This model uses the graphical advantages of Petri nets as a visual interface with the user and inherits the precision of formal languages based on the set theory by describing unambiguously management rules of information systems. The derived tool, namely NetSpec, provides the designer with the ability to focus on the design rather than the implementation, since there is no imperative code to produce while in the design phase of an application.

1   Introduction

An active database system extends a pre-existing database model (generally relational or object-oriented) with some variant of a common paradigm of computation: *event-condition-action* (ECA) *rules*. An *event* represents some occurrence in the database; this may be either an access or modification to a specific data item managed by the database or an external occurrence such as the state of a clock. The occurrence of such an event triggers the checking of a *condition*: this is a boolean-valued query over the database having no side effects. If this query returns *true*, an *action* will be performed: this can be any operation expressible in the database [1].

A number of designs and implementations of active databases now exists [2]. A designer or programmer might wish to see the aspects of active rules formally defined, essentially to see how far the available formal definition methodologies are able to characterize them [3]. These aspects include the following criteria: underlying data model, partial correctness, total correctness, transactional properties, structure of events, and implementation environment. Concurrently, a large number of formal methodologies currently in use can be evaluated, according to at least six criteria: modularization, abstraction of data model, tool support, executable model, temporal description capability, and relevant experience. Such methodologies are algebraic specification [4], denotational semantics [5], set-theoretic modeling [6][7],

J. Lloyd et al. (Eds.): CL 2000, LNAI 1861, pp. 1197-1209, 2000.

higher-order logic [8], constructive logics [9], temporal logics [10], Petri nets [11], process algebra [12], and statecharts [13].

Three objectives are achieved in this paper: present general considerations about ECA-rules, discuss analysis of Dynamic Relation Nets and their potential forward the modeling of ECA-rules, and introduce our own system prototype.

2   ECA-Rules

In an active database system, ECA-rules usually take the form:

```
on event
if condition
then action
```

An *event* happens instantaneously at specific points in time. For example, in a relational model, database events are relative to actions such as *insert*, *delete*, and *update*. Temporal events are related to a clock, and may be absolute or relative. Finally, explicit events are those events that are detected along with their parameters by application programs. All of these types of events are *primitive* events and can be combined together with event operators to form *composite* events [14].

A *condition* is a simple query over the database. In other words, a condition returns a boolean value, that is true if the query has produced a set containing at least one row of data.

An *action* is executed if the condition is satisfied. The action part of the rule usually inserts, deletes, or updates data.

If the event part of the rule does not exist, we call such a rule *pattern-based*, and if the condition part does not exist, we call such a rule *event-based*.

ECA-rules are usually processed using the following algorithm, derived from the *recognize-act* cycle of expert systems [15]:

```
initial match //execute rule conditions
repeat until no rule conditions produce tuples
   perform conflict resolution //pick a triggered rule
   act //execute the rule's action for all tuples
        //produced by the condition
   match //test rule conditions
end
```

In the *match* phase, rule patterns are matched against data to determine which rules are triggered and for which instantiations. The entire set of triggered rule instantiations is named the *conflict set*, and one instantiation is chosen from this set using a conflict resolution strategy. In the *act* phase, the selected rule's action is executed for all tuples of the selected instantiation, then the cycle repeats.

The choice of which rule to execute when multiple rules are triggered is named conflict resolution. In many active database systems this choice is made more or less arbitrarily: random [16], numeric priorities [17], partial order [18], based on coupling modes [19], concurrent execution [20].

Each time a rule is fired, there is an *instantiation* associated with that execution: a data item, or combination of items, that matches the rule's pattern. At execution time, the values of the instantiated items can be referenced in the rule's action through the use of variables specified in the rule's pattern. That is, at run-time, variables are *bound* in the pattern and passed to the action.

Coupling modes [21] determine how rule events, conditions, and actions relate to database transactions. Generally, rule conditions are evaluated and actions are executed in the same transaction, but it is not always the case. Associated with each rule is an *E-C* coupling mode and a *C-A* coupling mode, where *E*, *C*, *A* denote the events, conditions and actions respectively. Each coupling mode is either *immediate*, indicating immediate execution, *deferred*, indicating execution at the end of the current transaction, or *decoupled* (detached), indicating execution in a separate transaction. For each of the combinations of coupling modes, it is relatively easy to construct an active database application for which the behavior seems most appropriate [22].

3   Dynamic Relation Nets

By using an homogeneous formalism, the power of the Dynamic Relation Net (*DRN*) approach resides in the integration of both static and dynamic aspects of an information system. So, describing bag constraints, markings and transitions, precisely and fully describes both structure and behavior of the system. Abstraction of this new formalism is guaranteed by a purely formal description of the system behavior by using a semantics based on Z [6]. However, notice that the Z syntax never appears on the net itself and that the annotations are limited to sets of elementary constraints. We will no more discuss the use of Z in *DRN* in this paper, but the reader may find some additional informations in [23].

In practice, a *DRN* is a graphical tool where places (also named bags) depicted as circles, are used to represent availability of resources, transitions depicted as bars or rectangles, model the events, and edges indicate the relationship between places and transitions. Tokens in places and their flow regulated by firing transitions add dynamics to the *DRN*.

Initially, a *DRN* is defined by a tuple ($P, T, E, N, W, D, C_T, C_M, M_0$) where:

- P, T, and E are finite and disjoined sets of *places* (bags), *transitions*, and *edges*,
- $N : E \rightarrow (P \times T) \cup (T \times P)$ is a function mapping each edge to an *input node* and to an *output node*,
- $W : E \rightarrow \leq \cup \{*\}$ is a function associating a *weight* to each edge,
- $D : E \rightarrow \{$ production$\lfloor$, consumption $\lceil$, information $\}$, negative information $\lfloor \}$ is a function associating a type to each edge,
- $C_T : T \rightarrow F$ associating a formula to each transition, also named a *transition constraint*,
- C_M is a formula, named a *marking constraint*,
- $M_0 : P \rightarrow X$ is a function mapping each place to a set expression, satisfying the marking constraint.

Some special considerations must be understood from this definition of a *DRN*, which imply tokens, constraints, and edge types and weight. As in high-level Petri nets, tokens are distinguishable, structured, and updatable. That is, tokens are defined by attributes of various types (Fig. 1 shows an example).

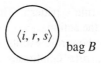

Fig. 1. An example of a token definition. Tokens residing inside bag B have three attributes, the types of which are *integer*, *real*, and *string of characters*. Each attribute is named as a field in a structure of a classical programming language. We will further reference individual attributes by expressions $B.i$, $B.r$, and $B.s$

Constraints in a *DRN* are expressions (C_M and C_T) based on token attributes. They can be instantiated and evaluated (see Fig. 2). Marking constraints apply to bags. Transition constraints apply to transitions. Possible constraints are:

- a key constraint, for which two or more tokens cannot reside inside the same bag if one or more of their attributes values are equal (the keys themselves which are underlined to be recognizable, i.e. $\langle \underline{i}, r, s \rangle$),
- a bag constraint, for which a token can take place into a bag only if one or more of its attribute values are adequate,
- a marking constraint, which is a global constraint over the entire net, and can express interactions between different bags at any time,
- a transition constraint, for which a token is removed from a bag only if its attributes have correct values,
- a transition constraint, for which a new token is produced into a bag with new attribute values.

New edge types are *information* depicted as $\}$ and *negative information* depicted as $\lfloor$. An information edge allows to check the presence of a token inside a bag without any consumption, while negative information allows to detect the absence of a token inside a bag. These detections are based on constraints against token attribute values, so the negative information edge cannot be compared to the inhibitor edge of classical Petri nets. Examples of these edges are shown in Fig. 3.

The last interesting feature of a *DRN* is the capability to annotate an edge with a weight denoted *, meaning that a finite set of tokens can circulate over such an edge at the time the transition is fired (set-oriented firing). It is important to notice that we cannot know anything about the cardinality of such a set at design time. However, it will be the greatest possible at execution time, as shown in Fig. 4.

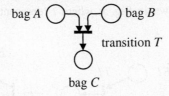

Fig. 2. Assuming bag A retains tokens $\langle x \rangle$, bag B retains tokens $\langle y \rangle$, bag C retains tokens $\langle z,t \rangle$ with a constraint key on z, and a bag constraint such as $(C.z > C.t)$. Initial marking is (all attribute types are integers): bag A contains tokens $\langle 1 \rangle$, $\langle 2 \rangle$, and $\langle 3 \rangle$, bag B contains token $\langle 3 \rangle$, and bag C contains nothing. Let transition T constraint be defined by $(A-.x<4) \wedge (B-.y>0) \wedge (C+.z=B-.y) \wedge (C+.t=A-.x)$. According to the meaning of the different constraints, $\langle 1 \rangle$ will be removed from A and <3> will be removed from B and $\langle 3,1 \rangle$ will be produced into C, or $\langle 2 \rangle$ will be removed from A and <3> will be removed from B and $\langle 3,2 \rangle$ will be produced into C, depending on the first choice done in the selection of a token from A. Notice that both tokens $\langle 3,1 \rangle$ and $\langle 3,2 \rangle$ cannot be produced into bag C because of the constraint key on z, and that $\langle 3,3 \rangle$ cannot be produced because of the bag constraint on C

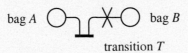

Fig. 3. Assuming the same definitions of bags A and B, a transition constraint such as $(A?.x=B\sim.y)$, and an initial marking of $\langle 1 \rangle$ into A, then $\langle 1 \rangle$ will be not be removed from A but will only be checked and the transition will be crossed if and only if no token equal to $\langle 1 \rangle$ exists inside bag B

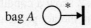

Fig. 4. Assuming the same definition of bag A, an initial marking of $\langle -1 \rangle$, $\langle 0 \rangle$, $\langle 1 \rangle$, $\langle 2 \rangle$, and a transition constraint such as $(A^*-.x>0)$, the set of two tokens $\{\langle 1 \rangle,\langle 2 \rangle\}$ will be removed from A at the time the transition is fired

4   Specifying ECA-Rules with Dynamic Relation Nets

Although *DRNs* have not primarily been created to model ECA-rules, we can easily use them to do that. If conditions and actions are obviously recognizable in constraints, events are worth receiving some particular explanations.

4.1   Events

Constraints in a *DRN* extend the definition of an event, which becomes relative to a specific marking of the net: the existence (or absence) of a token inside a bag may be considered as an event, and attribute values too. In a *DRN*, we can also easily detect composite events [24], as shown in Fig. 5, where *t* represents the time of an event occurrence.

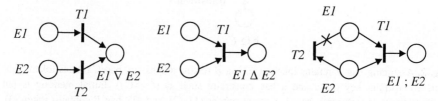

Fig. 5. Detection of composite events in a *DRN*. *Disjunction* of two events *E1* and *E2*, denoted *E1∇E2* occurs when *E1* occurs or *E2* occurs: *T1*: $(E1∇E2)+.t = E1-.t$ and *T2*: $(E1∇E2)+.t = E2-.t$. *Conjunction* of two events *E1* and *E2*, denoted *E1∆E2* occurs when both *E1* and *E2* occur, irrespective of their order of occurrence: *T1*: $(E1∆E2)+.t = MAX(E1-.t, E2-.t)$. *Sequence* of two events *E1* and *E2*, denoted *E1;E2* occurs when *E2* occurs provided *E1* has already occurred ; this implies that the time of occurrence of *E1* is guaranteed to be less than the time of occurrence of *E2*: *T1*: $(E1;E2)+.t = MAX(E1-.t, E2-.t)$ and *T2*: $E1~.t \leq E2-.t$

4.2   Conditions

A condition in a *DRN* can be modeled with a transition constraint. Such a constraint checks for the existence of tokens (consumption and information edges) or the absence of tokens (negative information edge). For example, the two first anded terms of the constraint of the transition *T* in Fig. 2 show a condition. Furthermore, bag and key constraints can also model a condition: the act phase of the ECA-rule cannot be executed if these constraints are not satisfied. We will see in the next paragraph that a part of a condition might also appear inside the action itself. Note that variables, i.e. token attributes, are bound while in the evaluation phase of a condition, to be passed to the act phase as parameters.

4.3   Actions

An action, specified by a transition constraint, is executed if all conditions return a true value. It consists of two phases: the consumption of all tokens referenced in the conditions (only those circulating over consumption edges), and the production of new tokens. In the latter case, a production constraint allows us to determine new token attribute values. These new values may be specified as constants of various types, or by using the binding capability between conditions and actions.

A new feature of *DRNs* is that the new attribute values can be reevaluated themselves to satisfy some constraint. If this second "condition" returns a false boolean value, the transition cannot be crossed and the act phase will not be executed, as shown in Fig. 6.

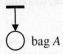
bag A

Fig. 6. Condition inside a production constraint. Assuming bag A retains tokens $\langle x,y \rangle$, and a new token receives attribute values $\langle 3,2 \rangle$ by any way. If the production constraint contains $A+.x=A+.y$ (which is obviously false), the transition cannot be crossed.

5   Implementation Issues

We have decided to implement our complete system *NetSpec* on the basis of a layered architecture, that means, to use an existing non-active DBMS (in our case DB2) and to add a monitor layer that is responsible for providing active capability [25].

As shown in Fig. 7, the application layer allows to design a *DRN* with a graphical tool, to store its definition, then to analyze and translate its definition to a set of executable programs (formally the job of the *DRN* compiler). A run-time library (the situation monitor layer), independent of the application itself, is responsible for providing rule processing (rule ordering based on conflict resolution).

5.1   Special Considerations

However, special considerations must be understood if we want to model ECA-rules by the way of *NetSpec*:

- Events are not managed as in the definition of ECA-rules because the existence (the absence) of a token, as well as its attribute values, can be specified directly in the condition. So, ECA-rules supported by *NetSpec* are pattern-based only,
- The act phase of the recognize-act cycle operates only for one tuple rather than for all of those, to avoid a set-oriented firing of transitions [26] as in Petri nets,
- *DRNs* do not allow to specify a conflict resolution strategy: a transition may be fired as soon as it has been triggered. So, the design of a transition constraints is very important if we want to obtain a deterministic behavior of the net. With *NetSpec*, conflict resolution is implemented by using numeric priorities, of three different types: fixed priorities (the match phase checks the rule conditions in a specific order), rotating priorities (a triggered rule will receive the lowest priority for the next match phase), and iterative priorities (a triggered rule will receive the highest priority for the next match phase, allowing an equivalent of set-oriented firing. We can also specify no conflict resolution, since *NetSpec* now supports multitasking (all transitions are modeled by concurrent processes),
- Finally, the only coupling mode supported when using conflict resolution is the deferred one. In fact, immediate C-A coupling mode may cause problems (causally dependent constraints), and detached C-A coupling mode is reserved for multitasking mode. Practically, on the match and act phases, queries of types delete (for consumption) and insert (for production) are generated, but will be executed at

the end of the transaction, in that order, to avoid token duplication in the case of an update of attribute values.

These restrictions are not developed in this paper, because our purpose is first to show that *DRNs* have enough potential toward the design side of an ADBMS-based application.

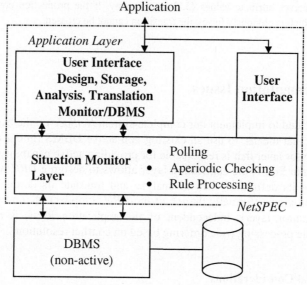

Fig. 7. The layered active database architecture of NetSpec

5.2   Dynamic Relation Net Compiler

The main job of the situation monitor layer is to provide rule processing. In fact, the main difficulty is for the *DRN* compiler, to order the evaluation of all constraints over the net [27].

For a transition, the input part (from bags to a transition) will be evaluated first, beginning with variables circulating over edges of weight $\in$ $\leq$, i.e. variables well known. For one tuple of the result, variables circulating over edges of weight * are evaluated (the result is a multiset). Last, this multiset is checked for its cardinality. The output part (from a transition to bags) is then computed to generate new token attribute values. These values are optionally checked for compatibility (condition into an action) and finally, bag constraints and key constraints are evaluated. If all of these constraints are satisfied, the transition can be crossed and the update of the net is done by the way of insert and/or delete queries. Last resort, if a marking constraint over the entire net is specified, it will be checked and the transaction will be committed if this constraint is satisfied, or canceled (rollbacked) if not.

As an example, consider the *DRN* shown in Fig. 8. For this *DRN*, bags *A*, *B*, *C*, *D* contain tokens $\langle x \rangle$, $\langle y \rangle$, $\langle z \rangle$, $\langle t \rangle$ respectively. The instantiations of tokens are $\langle 1 \rangle \langle 2 \rangle$ for *A*, $\langle 2 \rangle$ for *B*, $\langle 1 \rangle \langle 1 \rangle \langle 2 \rangle$ for *C*, and $\langle 1 \rangle$ for *D*. The constraints of this net are:

- $A{-}.x = B{\sim}.y$
- $A{-}.x = C^{*}{-}.z$
- $card(C^{*}{-}) > 1$
- $D{+}.t = sum(C^{*}{-}.z) + A{-}.x$
- a key constraint on *D*, relative to the *z* attribute
- a bag constraint on *D*: *t* mod 2 = 1
- a marking constraint: $card(D) \leq 1$

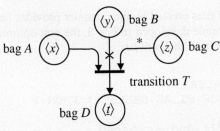

bag *A* — transition *T* — bag *B* — bag *C* — bag *D*

Fig. 8. An hypothetical *DRN* with several consumption edges, a production edge, a *-weighted information edge and a negative information edge

The processing phases of this ECA-rule will be:

- $A{-}.x = B{\sim}.y$ is evaluated and gives $A{-}.x = \langle 1 \rangle$ since *B* does not contain $\langle 1 \rangle$
- $A{-}.x = C^{*}{-}.z$ is evaluated and gives the greatest set $C^{*}{-} = \{\langle 1 \rangle, \langle 1 \rangle\}$
- $card(C^{*}{-}) > 1$ is evaluated and gives *TRUE*, since it is equal to 2
- $D{+}.t = sum(C^{*}{-}.z) + A{-}.x$ is computed and gives $D{+}.t = \langle 3 \rangle$ $(1 + 1 + 1 = 3)$
- bag constraint on *D* is evaluated and gives *TRUE*, since 3 mod 2 = 1
- key constraint on *D* is evaluated and gives *TRUE*, since bag *D* does not contain $\langle 3 \rangle$
- so, $\langle 1 \rangle$ is removed from *A* and removed 2 times from *C*, and $\langle 3 \rangle$ is produced into *D*. *B* remains unchanged
- marking constraint over the net gives *FALSE*, since $card(D)$ is now equal to 2, so the whole transaction is canceled

5.3   Code Generation Example

From a *DRN* specification, either created by the way of the graphical tool or directly written in the native language of NetSpec, the compiler creates two executable files. The former of these two files is a script that contains commands used to create the database itself. With a relational data model, bags are implemented by tables, each record of which (row) keeps one token, which attributes are columns of the row. For example, the bag *A* of Fig. 3 will be created by:

```
CREATE TABLE A ( INT PK_A, INT X, PRIMARY KEY(PK_A) )
```

Notice that the primary key *PK_A* is automatically inserted by the compiler to avoid duplication of tokens having no key constraint and receiving same attribute values at run-time. So, such tokens can be distinguished without ambiguity inside database queries. This primary key is invisible for the designer and is reserved for internal use only.

Transition constraint queries can also be created as views at this time. These views are relative to the input part of such a constraint (only those generating well known variables):

```
CREATE VIEW V ( PK_A,X )
        AS SELECT PK_A, X FROM A
            WHERE ( X NOT EXISTS IN SELECT Y FROM B )
```

The latter of the two files created by the compiler provides functions used for rule processing. For the example developed in Fig. 8, the non-optimized code (and so not very powerful!) of the transition *T* will be:

```
begin
  crossed ← FALSE
  DECLARE CURSOR C1 AS SELECT * FROM V
  OPEN C1
  while ¬EOF(C1) and ¬crossed
    FETCH C1 INTO :pk_a,:x
    SELECT COUNT(*) INTO :count FROM C WHERE Z=:x
    if count > 1 then
      SELECT SUM(Z) INTO :sum FROM C WHERE Z=:x
      t ← sum + x
      if t mod 2 = 1 then
        SELECT COUNT(*) INTO :count FROM D WHERE T=:t
        if count = 0 then
          DELETE FROM A WHERE PK_A=:pk_a
          DELETE FROM C WHERE Z=:x
          INSERT INTO D VALUES(:t)
          SELECT COUNT(*) INTO :count FROM D
          if count = 0 then
            COMMIT WORK
            crossed ← TRUE
          else ROLLBACK WORK fi
        fi
      fi
    fi
  endwhile
  CLOSE C1
end
```

6   Conclusion

In this paper, we have described the implementation of our approach in active database systems, based on the Dynamic Relation Nets. Our system, *NetSpec*, automatically generates the imperative code of the computational part of an ADBMS based application, by the way of a new modeling language that makes abstraction of classical programming.

However, *NetSpec* has enlightened some problems that do not exist in the *DRN* theory. First of all and the most important one, a *DRN* may have concurrent transitions whose constraints are not exclusive. Such a configuration introduces a non-deterministic behavior of the net. *NetSpec* uses priorities to resolve conflicts between triggered transitions, as many of the existing ADBMS. However, the "programming style" has a possible influence on the model, because the designer can choose its priority type.

Another problem is the necessity to build a coherent development tool, especially with a debugger (see Fig. 9). In fact, the fired transitions of a *DRN* introduce the same consequences of the fired ECA-rules in ADBMS: transitions (as ECA-rules) behavior may be complex and not easily understood. The designer of an application must be able to directly influence the transition firing, to solve terminations and deadlocks. This is an objective of our future directions.

We have highlighted three main qualities for a processing model: processing abstraction, dynamic behavior and graphical representation. We have defined a model closely related to high-level Petri Nets. Dynamic Relations Nets allow within a unique graphical representation the specification of data, processing, events and constraints. Annotations of the net use a set based abstract language. Constraints arise from three levels: from places (related to the notion of abstract type), from markings (we can then express global constraints between places), and from transitions (in order to specify processing as state transformations).

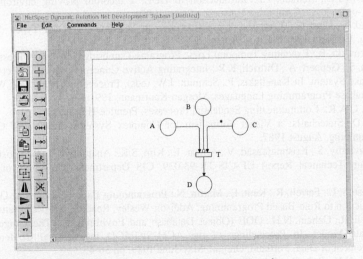

Fig. 9. A sample screen of the NetSpec prototype development tool

The definition of *DRNs* is now complete. We have not developed here a true method built around *DRNs*. A reverse design study gave birth to new ideas especially related to valid schema transformations, allowing a gradual materialization from an abstract model to an operational one, as with the B method. In fact, the non-deterministic behavior remains a critical aspect: a *DRN* must satisfy some properties so the implementation (for example with NetSpec) fits the initial specifications. Therefore, we will concentrate on applying proof tools related to Z and B to our model. Our future works will be based on a set of tools designed to build and to validate a general method usable on non obvious applications. We hope to create a set of consistent design tools, dedicated to processing specifications.

References

1 Dittrich, K.R., Gatziu, S., Geppert, A.: The Active Database Management System Manifesto. Proceedings of the 2nd Workshop on Rules in Databases, Athens, Greece, September 1995. pp 3-20.

2 Paton, N.W., Diaz, O., Williams, M.H., Campin, J., Dinn, A., Jaime, A.: Dimensions of Active Behaviour. In Paton, N.W., Williams, M.H. (eds): Proceedings of the 1st International Workshop on Rules in Database Systems. Springer-Verlag, 1995. pp. 40-57.

3 Campin, J., Paton, N.W., Williams, M.H.: A Structured Specification of an Active Database System. Computing & Electrical Engineering Department, Heriot-Watt University, Riccarton, Edinburgh. October 1994.

4 Goguen, J.A., Winkler, T.: Introducing OBJ. Technical Report SRI-CSL-88-9, SRI International, Stanford, August 1988.

5 Schmidt, D.A.: Denotational Semantics: a Methodology for Language Development. Allyn and Bacon, 1986.

6 Spivey, J.M.: The Z Notation: a reference manual. Prentice-Hall, second edition, 1992.

7 Jones, C.B.: Systematic Software Development Using VDM. Prentice-Hall, 1990.

8 Gordon, M.J.C., Melham, T.F.: Introduction to HOL: a theorem proving environment for higher-order logic. Cambridge University Press, 1993.

9 Coquand, T., Huet, G.: A theory of constructions. In Semantics of Data Types. Springer-Verlag, 1985. pp 95-120.

10 Moszkowski, B.: Executing Temporal Logic Programs. Cambridge University Press, 1986.

11 Gatziu, S., Geppert, A., Dittrich, K.R.: Integrating Active Concepts into an Object-Oriented Database System. In Kanellakis, P., Schmidt, J.W. (eds), Proceedings of the 3rd Workshop on Database Programming Languages. Morgan-Kaufmann, 1991.

12 Hoare, C.A.R.: Communicating Sequential Processes. Prentice-Hall, 1984.

13 Harel, D.: Statecharts: a Visual Formalism for Complex Systems. Science of Computer Programming, August 1987.

14 Chakravarthy, S., Krishnaprasad, V., Anwar, E., Kim, S.K.: Anatomy of a Composite Event Detector. Technical Report UF-CIS-TR-93-039, CIS Department, University of Florida, 1993.

15 Brownston, L., Farrell, R., Kant, E., Martin, N.: Programming Expert Systems in OPS5: An Introduction to Rule-Based Programming. Addison-Wesley, Reading, Massachusetts, 1985.

16 Agrawal, R., Gehani, N.H.: ODE (Object Database and Environment): The Language and the Data Model. In Proceedings of the ACM-SIGMOD International Conference on Management of Data, Portland, Oregon, May-June 1989. pp 36-45.

17 Hanson, E.N.: Rule Condition Testing and Action Execution in Ariel. In Proceedings of the ACM-SIGMOD International Conference, June 1992. pp 49-58.

18 Widom, J., Cochrane, R.J., Lindsay, B.G.: Implementing Set-Oriented Production Rules As An Extension To Starburst. In Proceedings of the 17th International Conference on Very Large Data Bases (VLDB), Barcelona, Spain, 1991. pp 275-285.

19 Gatziu, S., Geppert, A., Dittrich, K.R.: The SAMOS Active DBMS Prototype. Technical Report 94.16, Institut für Informatik, Universität Zürich Switzerland, 1994.

20 Chakravarthy, S.: HiPAC: A Research Project in Active, Time-Constrained Database Management, Final Report. Technical Report XAIT-89-02, Xerox Advanced Information Technology, Cambridge, Massachussets, August 1989.

21 McCarthy, D.R., Dayal, U.: The Architecture of an Active, Object-oriented Database Management System. In Proceedings of the ACM-SIGMOD International Conference on Management of Data Vol. 18 No. 2, Portland, Oregon, May/June 1989. pp 215-224.

22 Hanson, E.N., Widom, J.: An Overview of Production Rules in Database Systems. Technical Report UF-CIS 92-031, CIS Department, University of Florida, October 1992.

23 Cadivel, C., Lefort, A., Yim, P.: Process Modeling in Information System by Formal Net. In IEEE International Conference on Systems, Man and Cybernetics, Vancouver Canada, October 22-25 1995.

24 Gatziu, S., Dittrich, K.R.: Detecting Composite Events in an Active Database System using Petri Nets. In Proceedings of the 4th International Workshop on Research Issues in Data Engineering: Active Database Systems, Houston, Texas, February 1994. pp. 2-9.

25 Chakravarthy, S.: Architectures and Monitoring Techniques for Active Databases: an Evaluation. Technical Report UF-CIS-TR-92-041, CIS Department, University of Florida, 1992.

26 Kiernan, G., de Maindreville, C., Simon, E.: Making Deductive Database a Practical Technology: A Step Forward. In Proceedings of the ACM SIGMOD International Conference on Management of Data, May 1990.

27 Allain, L.: Contribution à la Modélisation et à la Spécification: Réseaux Formels et Bases de Données Actives. Thèse de Doctorat en Productique, Automatique et Informatique Industrielle, LAIL UPRESA 8021, EC-Lille, Université des Sciences et Technologies de Lille, France, 1999.

Invariance, Maintenance, and Other Declarative Objectives of Triggers – A Formal Characterization of Active Databases

Mutsumi Nakamura[1] and Chitta Baral[2]

[1] Department of CSE, University of Texas at Arlington
Arlington, TX 76019, USA
nakamura@cse.uta.edu
[2] Department of CSE, Arizona State University
Tempe, AZ 85287, USA
chitta@asu.edu

Abstract. In this paper we take steps towards a systematic design of active features in an active database. We propose having declarative specifications that specify the objective of an active database and formulate the correctness of triggers with respect to such specifications. In the process we distinguish between the notions of 'invariance' and 'maintenance' and propose four different classes of specification constraints. We also propose three different types of triggers with distinct purposes and show through the analysis of an example from the literature, the correspondence between these trigger types and the specification classes. Finally, we briefly introduce the notion of k-maintenance that is important from the perspective of a reactive (active database) system.

1   Introduction and Motivation

Many commercial database systems (such as Oracle, Sybase, IBM's DB2-V2, etc.) and the database standard SQL3 incorporate *active features* – namely *constraints* (also referred to as *integrity constraints*) and *triggers*. Due to these active features explicit update requests to the database may have several consequences from the request being refused (as it may violate 'integrity constraints'), to the request being fulfilled with slight changes (as modified through 'before triggers'), to additional changes triggered by cascade deletes and inserts used in the processing of some constraints and/or firing of 'after triggers'.

Although originally, integrity constraints were thought of as *declarative* constraints about database states and defined which database states were valid and which were not, with the presence of cascade operations in the SQL3 constraints and the use of after triggers to maintain the integrity of the data, there is currently little tradition (except in [CF97] and few other cases) of using or following standard software engineering practices of separating specification from implementation when designing and developing active databases. This means that

J. Lloyd et al. (Eds.): CL 2000, LNAI 1861, pp. 1210–1224, 2000.
© Springer-Verlag Berlin Heidelberg 2000

often active database developers do not even *specify* what the purpose of the active features of their database are. Thus there is no way to *verify* the correctness of the active features. We believe this is one of the reasons why many companies balk at using the active features of a database.

Our goal in this paper is to take steps towards developing a systematic approach to the design of active databases. In the process we will develop several language constructs that can be used in specifying the purpose of an active database; formulate the correctness of the procedural triggers with respect to declarative specifications; and develop guidelines that match the procedural aspects with the declarative aspects.

One major hindrance in this pursuit has been the multitude of syntax and semantics (and their complexity) associated with the various different implementation of active rules [WC96,Pat98] and the complexity of their semantics. In this paper we will follow the SQL3 standard (and the DB2-V2 implementation) to some extent and make certain simplifications.

1.1   The Declarative Notions

The basic goal of the active features of a database is to constrain the evolution of the database. Based on analyzing a large class of active database examples, we have identified four kind of constraints: *state invariance constraints; state maintenance constraints (or quiescent state constraints); trajectory invariance constraints; and trajectory maintenance constraints.*

In the above constraints there are two dimensions: (i) state vs trajectory (ii) invariance vs maintenance. Intuitively, in state constraints we are concerned about the integrity about particular states, while the trajectory constraints focus on the trajectory of evolution of the database. On the other hand, invariance constraints worry about all states of the database, while the maintenance constraints focus only on the quiescent states.

Definition 1 (State Constraints). *[ADA93]* A *state constraint* γ_s on a database scheme R, is a function that associates with each database r of R a boolean value $\gamma_s(r)$. A database r of R is said to *satisfy* γ_s if $\gamma_s(r)$ is true and is said to *violate* γ_s if $\gamma_s(r)$ is false. In the former case, it is also said that γ_s holds in r. A database r is said to satisfy a set of state constraints if it satisfies each element of the set.   □

Definition 2 (Trajectory Constraints). A *trajectory constraint* γ_t on a database scheme R, is a function that associates with each database sequence Υ of R a boolean value $\gamma_t(\Upsilon)$. A database sequence Υ of R is said to *satisfy* γ_t if $\gamma_t(\Upsilon)$ is true and is said to *violate* γ_t if $\gamma_t(\Upsilon)$ is false. In the former case, it is also said that γ_t holds in Υ. A database sequence Υ is said to satisfy a set of trajectory constraints if it satisfies each element of the set.   □

Often static integrity constraints are expressed through sentences in propositional logic or first-order predicate calculus while we need temporal operators to express trajectory constraints. We further discuss this in Section 3.

1.2   The Procedural Features of an Active Database

In SQL3 (and DB2-V2) the active features are: *Constraints; Before triggers; and After triggers.*

The constraints in DB2-V2 are of the kinds: NOT NULL constraints, column defaults, unique indexes, check constraints, primary key constraints, and foreign key constraints. Among these, the NOT NULL constraints, unique indexes, check constraints, primary key constraints and some of the foreign key constraints (with NO ACTION or RESTRICT in the action part) *refuse updates* that violate the constraints. These correspond to the state invariance constraints mentioned in the previous section.

On the other hand column default constraints and the foreign key constraints with CASCADE or SET NULL in the action part accept the updates but make additional changes. The former correspond to the state invariance constraints, while the later correspond to the state maintenance constraints.

The before triggers act on the update request directly (instead of the updated database) and modify it if necessary while the after triggers are triggered by the update request and can either refuse the update (through a rollback) or force additional changes. Here, the former can implement state and trajectory invariance constraints, while the later can implement any of the four types of constraints.

From the above analysis, it seems that certain specifications such as a state maintenance constraint can be implemented in multiple ways, through a DB2-V2 constraint or through after triggers. But the trigger processing architecture treats DB2-V2 constraints very differently from after triggers. Thus it becomes very difficult to formulate and verify the correctness of the DB2-V2 (or SQL3) active features with respect to specifications mentioned in Section 1.1.

We propose a different class of active features that are close to the SQL3 features, but that are *distinct* in terms of their goals. Our class consists of three kind of procedural features (triggers): *refusal triggers, wrapper triggers*, and *maintenance triggers*.

Intuitively, *the refusal triggers* when triggered refuse the update that caused the triggering. Thus refusal triggers can express not only after triggers with refuse actions, but also NOT NULL constraints, unique indexes, check constraints, primary key constraints, and foreign key constraints with NO ACTION or RE-STRICT in the action part. The *wrapper triggers*, wrap the update request by additional changes and thus can express both before triggers and column default constraints. The *maintenance triggers*[1] trigger additional updates and thus can express both after triggers with similar purpose, and foreign key constraints with CASCADE or SET NULL in the action part.

---

[1] In Section 4 we will further divide maintenance triggers to two classes: short-term and long-term. This becomes necessary when we need to worry about reactive response to update requests.

Our division of the triggers into the above three classes makes them distinct in terms of what they set out to achieve. This is different from the active features in DB2-V2 and SQL3 where there is overlapping of goals making it difficult in designing active databases and formulating their correctness.

2   Actions, Events, and Triggers

In this section we describe the necessary mechanism for reasoning about actions and events which we will then use to formulate correctness of triggers with respect to declarative specifications.

2.1   Actions and Effects

Intuitively, an action when executed in a world changes the state of the world. In databases, an action can take several meanings; from the basic *insert*, *delete* and *update* actions to SQL update statements. In this paper by an action we will usually refer to an uninterruptable transaction.

To specify the effects of an action on a database we borrow constructs from the specification language $\mathcal{A}$ [GL93] and our earlier work in [BL96,BLT97]. In the following by a fluent we will mean a database fact, and by a fluent literal we will mean either a database fact or its negation. Effects of actions are specified through effect axioms of the following form:

$$a(\overline{X}) \textbf{ causes } f(\overline{Y}) \textbf{ if } p_1(\overline{X_1}), \ldots, p_n(\overline{X_n}) \tag{2.1}$$

where $a(\overline{X})$ is an action and $f(\overline{Y}), p_1(\overline{X_1}), \ldots, p_n(\overline{X_n})$ are fluent literals ($n \geq 0$). $p_1(\overline{X_1}), \ldots, p_n(\overline{X_n})$ are called *preconditions*. The intuitive meaning of (2.1) is that in any state of the active database execution in which $p_1(\overline{X_1}), \ldots, p_n(\overline{X_n})$ are true, the execution of the action $a(\overline{X})$ causes $f(\overline{Y})$ to be true in the resulting state. A word of caution is needed regarding the *safeness* [Ull88] of variables in the   *causal law* . The preconditions $p_1(\overline{X_1}), \ldots, p_n(\overline{X_n})$ will be evaluated as regular queries in the database and $a(\overline{X})$ is an action that could be invoked by a user or an active rule. Thus, variables appearing in $\overline{Y}$ or in any negated fluent in the preconditions must also appear in one of the positive fluents in the precondition. If there are variables in $\overline{X}$ that do not appear in any of the positive fluents in the preconditions these arguments must be ground at the time of the invocation of the action, otherwise there will be an error in the execution. Moreover, the variables are *schema variables*, and intuitively an effect axiom with variables represents the set of ground effect axioms where the variables are replaced by ground terms in the domain.

Two effect axioms with preconditions $p_1, \ldots, p_n$ and $q_1, \ldots, q_m$ respectively are said to be *contradictory* if they describe the effect of the same action a on complementary fs, and $\{p_1, \ldots, p_n\} \cap \{\overline{q_1}, \ldots, \overline{q_m}\} = \emptyset$

A *state* is a set of fluent names. Given a fluent name f and a state σ, we say that f *holds* in σ if $f \in \sigma$; $\neg f$ *holds* in σ if $f \notin \sigma$. A *transition function* is a mapping

Φ of the set of pairs (a, σ), where a is an action name and σ is a state, into the set of states.

A collection of effect axioms (EA) for various actions in our world – with no contradictory effect axioms in them, define a transition function from the set of actions and the set of database states to the set of database states.

For every action a and every state σ,

$$\Phi(a, \sigma) = (\sigma \cup \sigma') \setminus \sigma'',$$

where σ' (σ'') is the set of fluent names f such that EA includes an effect proposition describing the effect of action a on f (respectively, $\neg f$) whose preconditions hold in σ.

We now show how the effect of simple actions such as *insert*, *delete* and *update* can be specified using effect axioms.

$$insert(R(t)) \textbf{ causes } R(t) \tag{2.2}$$

$$delete(R(t)) \textbf{ causes } \neg R(t) \tag{2.3}$$

$$update(R(t), R(t')) \textbf{ causes } R(t') \textbf{ if } R(t) \tag{2.4}$$

$$update(R(t), R(t')) \textbf{ causes } \neg R(t) \textbf{ if } R(t) \tag{2.5}$$

We now show how we can specify the effect of actions corresponding to more complex transactions:

Example 1. Consider another transaction a_2 from [Cha96]:

UPDATE parts
SET qonorder = qonhand,
    qonhand = qonorder
WHERE partno = 'P207';

Its effects can be described in our language through the following effect propositions:

a_2 **causes** $parts(P207, Descr, qonhand, qonorder)$ **if**
$$parts(P207, Descr, qonorder, qonhand)$$

a_2 **causes** $\neg parts(P207, Descr, qonhand, qonorder)$ **if**
$$parts(P207, Descr, qonhand, qonorder) \qquad \square$$

To reason about the effect of a sequence of actions on a database σ, we need to extend the function Φ, to allow sequence of actions as its first parameter. This extension is defined as follows:

- $\Phi([], \sigma) = \sigma$, and
- $\Phi([\alpha|a], \sigma) = \Phi(a, \Phi(\alpha, \sigma))$.

2.2   Events and ECA Rules

Triggers (or active rules) in active databases are normally [WC96] represented as a triple consisting of *events, conditions and actions*. In most active database architectures, the sequence of actions that have been executed since the last evaluation point are evaluated to decide on what events have taken place. These events together with the valuation of the condition with respect to the current database state determine whether a particular ECA active rule should be triggered or not.

Different active databases allow different event sets and have different ways of evaluating the events. In the simplest case, the events can be the set of *inserts* and *deletes* explicitly performed by the last action. On the other hand, in Starburst [Wid96] events are defined in terms of the net effects of a sequence of transitions. To allow the flexibility of defining a set of events and computing them from a sequence of actions we use the notion of event definitions from [BLT97].

An *event definition* proposition is an expression of the form:

$$e(\overline{X}) \textbf{ after } a(\overline{W}) \textbf{ if } e_1(\overline{Y_1}), \ldots, e_m(\overline{Y_m}), q_1(\overline{Z_1}), \ldots, q_n(\overline{Z_n}) \qquad (2.6)$$

where $e(\overline{X}), e_1(\overline{Y_1}), \ldots, e_m(\overline{Y_m})$ are event literals[2] and $q_1(\overline{Z_1}), \ldots, q_n(\overline{Z_n})$ are fluent literals. This proposition says that the execution of the action $a(\overline{W})$ ordered in a state in which each of the fluent literals $q_i(\overline{Z_i})$ is true *and* each of the event literals $e_j(\overline{Y_j})$ is true generates the event literal $e(\overline{X})$ if the event literal is positive, or removes the event from the set of current events if the event literal $e(\overline{X})$ is negative. If the execution is ordered in a state in which some of the $q_i(\overline{Z_i})$ or $e_j(\overline{Y_j})$ does not hold then (2.6) has no effect. Each of the (schema) variables appearing in $\overline{X}$ or in a negated event or fluent literals, has to appear either in $\overline{W}$ or in a positive event/fluent literal.

The default assumption is that the event *persists* from one state to another, with two possible exceptions: either the event is *consumed* by an active rule (see below), or the event is removed by an action based on the specification of an event definition. For example, if we have an expression $\neg e_1 \textbf{ after } a_1$, the execution of the action a_1 will cause the event e_1 not to be present in the resulting state. Hence, the meaning of "an event is true in a given state" is: the event was induced (i.e. generated) in some state prior to the given one and the event persisted, or the event was induced by an execution of an action in the previous state.

Example 2 (Events in Starburst). In Starburst net effects (or events) are expressed in words through the following conditions:

- If a tuple is inserted and then updated, it is considered an insertion of the updated tuple.

---

[2] Like fluent literals, an event literal is an event or its negation.

- If a tuple is updated and then deleted, it is considered as a deletion of the original tuple.
- If a tuple is updated more than once, it is considered as an update from the original value to the newest value.
- If a tuple is inserted and then deleted, it is not considered in the net effect at all.

These four premises can be encoded through event definitions as follows:

$$
\begin{aligned}
e\_add(H) &\quad \textbf{after} \quad upd(G, H) \; \textbf{if} \; e\_add(G) \\
\neg e\_add(G) &\quad \textbf{after} \quad upd(G, H) \; \textbf{if} \; e\_add(G) \\
e\_del(G) &\quad \textbf{after} \quad del(F) \; \textbf{if} \; e\_upd(G, F) \\
\neg e\_upd(G, F) &\quad \textbf{after} \quad del(F) \; \textbf{if} \; e\_upd(G, F) \\
e\_upd(G, I) &\quad \textbf{after} \quad upd(H, I) \; \textbf{if} \; e\_upd(G, H) \\
\neg e\_upd(G, H) &\quad \textbf{after} \quad upd(H, I) \; \textbf{if} \; e\_upd(G, H) \\
\neg e\_add(G) &\quad \textbf{after} \quad del(G) \; \textbf{if} \; e\_add(G)
\end{aligned}
\tag{2.7}
$$

In the above example, at the first glance it appears that our notation is more verbose than the original rules. For each of the first three rules we needed two event definition propositions. This is because *we assume that events have inertia*. This assumption actually cuts down in writing individual event definition propositions encoding the persistence of each event due to actions that do not affect it. For example we do not need to explicitly write:

$$
e\_add(H) \; \textbf{after} \; del(G) \; \textbf{if} \; e\_add(H), H \neq G
$$

We characterize events using the function Ξ whose input is a set of events, a state, and an action and the output is a set of events. More formally, let $E^+(E, \sigma, a) = \{\, e : \text{there is an event definition proposition of the form } e \; \textbf{after} \; a$ $\textbf{if} \; e_1, \ldots e_m, q_1, \ldots, q_n \text{ where } e_1, \ldots, e_m \text{ hold in } E \text{ and } q_1, \ldots, q_n \text{ hold in } \sigma \,\}$; and let $E^-(E, \sigma, a) = \{\, e : \text{there is an event definition proposition of the form } \neg e \; \textbf{after} \; a \; \textbf{if} \; e_1, \ldots e_m, q_1, \ldots, q_n \text{ where } e_1, \ldots, e_m \text{ hold in } E \text{ and } q_1, \ldots, q_n$ hold in $\sigma \,\}$. $\Xi(E, \sigma, a)$ is then defined as follows:

$$
\Xi(E, \sigma, a) = (E \cup E^+(E, \sigma, a)) \setminus E^-(E, \sigma, a)
$$

To be able to compute events with respect to a sequence of actions we extend Ξ as follows:

- $\Xi(E, \sigma, [\,]) = E$, and
- $\Xi(E, \sigma, [\alpha | a]) = \Xi(\Xi(E, \sigma, \alpha), \Phi(\alpha, \sigma), a)$.

2.3   Characterizing Database Evolution Due to ECA Rules

As mentioned in Section 1.2, we have three kinds of triggers: wrapper triggers, refusal triggers and maintenance triggers. We represent each of them through ECA rules but distinguish them by the action part. In wrapper triggers the action part is a *wrapping function* ω which maps an action sequence and a database state to an action sequence. Intuitively, for a single action a, by $\omega(a, \sigma) = a'$ we mean that a' is the action obtained by wrapping a with ω in state σ. In refusal triggers the action part is the special action $REFUSE$ and in maintenance triggers the action part could be an arbitrary sequence of actions. Thus an ECA rule is a triple $\langle e, c, \alpha \rangle$, where e is an event in our language, c is a temporal formula about the database history, and α is either a wrapping function, the special action REFUSE, or a sequence of actions. Often we will represent a single action as the ECA rule $\langle \emptyset, True, a \rangle$.

In this subsection our goal is to give a formal characterization of the evolution of a database due to a sequence of actions in presence of a set of ECA rules. In our characterization we strive to keep a balance between not making the semantics too complicated and at not losing expressibility. We now give an intuitive description of our characterization.

Intuitively, after the action sequence (with necessary modifications due to wrapper triggers) is executed the set of events corresponding to that sequence of actions are evaluated. Then the ECA rules that match with the events are identified. We assume (as in many implemented systems [Cha96]) that there is a total ordering among the ECA rules with the condition that refusal triggers have higher priority than maintenance triggers. Using this total ordering a priority list of the identified ECA rules is created. Then the condition parts of the ECA rules in the priority list are evaluated in the order of their priority and if the condition evaluates to be true, the action part is executed. Since the action part may trigger additional ECA rules, an important concern is how these ECA rules are assimilated into the already existing prioritized list of ECA rules. Two straightforward approaches are to view the list as a stack where newly triggered ECA rules are pushed onto the top of the stack, or to view the list as a queue where newly triggered ECA rules are put at the end of the queue. In both cases, among the newly added rules, the wrapper triggers have the highest priority, the refusal triggers have the second highest priority and the maintenance triggers have the lowest priority.

So after the execution of the action part of the currently considered ECA rule, the newly triggered ECA rules are put into the priority list and the evaluation of the ECA rules in the modified list are again done based on their priority. This loop of executing the action part of the currently chosen ECA rule, updating the list of ECA rules, and evaluating the list to find the next ECA rule, continues until the list is empty. During the execution when faced with a trigger whose action part is REFUSE, the database is rolled back.

We now formally define the function $\Psi(\sigma, \alpha, List)$, where σ is a database state, α is a sequence of actions and $List$ is a prioritized list of ECA rules that are yet to be processed, and the output of the function is a sequence of database states. Once we define this function, the evolution of a database state σ due to an action sequence α, can then be expressed by $\Psi(\sigma, \alpha, [\,])$. (For lack of space we only consider the simple case where there are no triggers with REFUSE in their action part.)

Definition 3. [Evolution due to Actions and Triggers]

1. $\Psi(\sigma, \alpha, List) = \sigma$ if σ is a state, α is an empty sequence, and $List = [\,]$.
2. $\Psi(\sigma, \alpha, List)$ is an empty list if σ is undefined.
3. $\Psi(\sigma, \alpha, List) = \sigma \circ \Upsilon$ if
   (a) $\sigma' = \Phi(\omega(\alpha), \sigma)$, where ω is the composition of the wrapping functions of the before triggers triggered by the events in $\Xi(\emptyset, \sigma, \alpha)$. (If there are no before triggers triggered by the events in $\Xi(\emptyset, \sigma, \alpha)$ then ω is the identity function; i.e., $\forall \alpha. \omega(\alpha) = \alpha$).
   (b) $List_1$ is the list obtained by adding the new ECA rules triggered by the events in $\Xi(\emptyset, \sigma, \omega(\alpha))$ to $List$ and *adjusting the priorities*,
   (c) eca is the ECA rule with the highest priority in the priority list $List_1$,
   (d) α' is the action part in eca,
   (e) $List_2 = List_1 \setminus \{eca\}$, and
   (f) $\Psi(\sigma', \alpha', List_2) = \Upsilon$. $\square$

Because of the second condition above, when $\Phi(\omega(\alpha), \sigma)$ is undefined we obtain Υ as an empty list, and then $\Psi(\sigma, \alpha, List)$ is a sequence of length one with σ as the only element. Rollbacks can be accounted for by having an additional parameter in Ψ which stores the initial state, where the database should be rolled back to when a trigger with REFUSE in its action part is triggered.

2.4   Correctness of ECA Rules

Our next step is to formally define when a set of ECA rules are correct with respect to invariant and maintenance constraints. For state maintenance constraints, intuitively, the correctness means that the ECA rules force the database to evolve in such a way that the final state that is reached is a state where all the state maintenance constraints are satisfied. For state invariant constraints, intuitively, the correctness means that the ECA rules force the database to evolve in such a way that the state invariance constraints are satisfied in all states of the trajectory.

Since our ultimate goal is to be able to use this definition to verify the correctness, we add another dimension to the definition: *the class of exogenous actions that we consider;* where exogenous actions are the actions that outside users are allowed to execute on the database. It should be noted that the action part of the ECA rules may have actions other than the exogenous actions.

We now formally define correctness with respect to state invariant and maintenance constraints.

Definition 4. Let Γ_{si} be a set of state invariant constraints, Γ_{sm} be a set of state maintenance constraints, A be a set of exogenous actions, and T be a set of ECA rules. We say T is correct with respect to $\Gamma_{si} \cup \Gamma_{sm}$ and A, if for all database states σ where the constraints in Γ_{si} and Γ_{sm} hold, and for all action sequences α consisting of exogenous actions from A,

- all the states in the sequence $\Psi(\sigma, \alpha, [\,])$ satisfy the constraints in Γ_{si}; and
- the last state of the evolution given by $\Psi(\sigma, \alpha, [\,])$ satisfies the constraints in Γ_{sm}. □

To expand the Definition 4 to define correctness with respect to trajectory constraints we need to consider a larger evolution window where the database evolves through several exogenous requests each consisting of a sequence of (exogenous) actions. For this we use the notation σ_α to denote the last state of the evolution given by $\Psi(\sigma, \alpha, [\,])$. We use the notation $\sigma_{(\alpha_1, \alpha_2)}$ to denote the last state of the evolution given by $\Psi(\sigma_{\alpha_1}, \alpha_2, [\,])$, and similarly define $\sigma_{(\alpha_1, \ldots, \alpha_i)}$.

Definition 5. Let Γ_{si} be a set of state invariant constraints, Γ_{sm} be a set of state maintenance constraints, Γ_{ti} be a set of trajectory invariant constraints, Γ_{tm} be a set of trajectory maintenance constraints, A be a set of exogenous actions, and T be a set of ECA rules. We say T is correct with respect to $\Gamma_{si} \cup \Gamma_{sm} \cup \Gamma_{ti} \cup \Gamma tm$ and A, if for all database states σ where the constraints in Γ_{si} and Γ_{sm} hold, and for all action sequences $\alpha_1, \ldots, \alpha_n$ consisting of exogenous actions from A,

- all the states in the sequences
  $\Psi(\sigma, \alpha_1, [\,]), \Psi(\sigma_{\alpha_1}, \alpha_2, [\,]), \ldots, \Psi(\sigma_{(\alpha_1, \ldots, \alpha_{n-1})}, \alpha_n, [\,])$ satisfy the constraints in Γ_{si};
- all the states $\sigma_{\alpha_1}, \ldots, \sigma_{(\alpha_1, \ldots, \alpha_n)}$ satisfy the constraints in Γ_{sm};
- the trajectory obtained by concatenating $\Psi(\sigma, \alpha_1, [\,])$ with $\Psi(\sigma_{\alpha_1}, \alpha_2, [\,])$, $\ldots, \Psi(\sigma_{(\alpha_1, \ldots, \alpha_{n-1})}, \alpha_n, [\,])$ satisfy the constraints in Γ_{ti}; and
- the trajectory $\sigma, \sigma_{\alpha_1}, \ldots, \sigma_{(\alpha_1, \ldots, \alpha_n)}$ satisfies the constraints in Γ_{tm}. □

Example 3. Consider the relational Schema:

$Employee(Emp\#, Name, Salary, Dept\#)$
$Dept(Dept\#, Mgr\#)$

We have two state maintenance constraints:
(i) If (e, n, s, d) is a tuple in $Employee$ then there must be a tuple (d', m') in $Dept$ such that $d = d'$.
(ii) If (d, m) is a tuple in $Dept$, then there must be a tuple (e', n', s', d') in $Employee$ such that $d = d'$ and $m = e'$

The only allowable exogenous action is $del(Employee(E, N, S, D))$.

The set of maintenance triggers that can be shown to be correct with respect to the above maintenance constraints and exogenous actions consists of the following trigger.

• For any Delete (e, n, s, d) from $Employee$, if (d, e) is a tuple in $Dept$, delete that tuple from $Dept$ and delete all tuples of the form (e', n', s', d') from $Employee$, where $d = d'$. □

We can now make the formal claim that the above maintenance triggers are correct with respect to the above mentioned state maintenance constraints and exogenous actions.

3   Elaborating on Our Abstractions

In Section 1.1 we defined state constraints and trajectory constraints as boolean functions on database states and sequences of database states respectively. Our next concern is how to represent such functions parsimoniously. One approach is to use logical constructs. In this section we introduce several language constructs that we proposed to use in specifying state and trajectory constraints and show their use through examples.

We start with a description of the mail order business active database from [Cha96]. To save space and to make it readable without knowing the syntax of triggers in DB2-V2, we describe the triggers of this active database in words, and not in the syntax of DB2-V2.

3.1   The Tables

The five tables that are mentioned in the database in [Cha96] and their attributes are:

Cust(C#, Cname, Caddr, Baldue, Creditlmt)
Suppl(S#, Sname, Saddr, Amtowed)
Inv(It#, Iname, S#, Qonhand, Unitsalpr, Qonorder, Unitorderpr, Orderthreshold, Minorder)
Purch(Orddate, Ordtime, S#, It#, Qordered, Dtrecvd, Qrcvd, Unitpr)
Sales(Sldate, Sltime, C#, It#, Qsold, Unitpr, Totalsale)

3.2   A Subset of the Triggers

Due to lack of space we only consider two of the eight triggers given in [Cha96], and identify the state and trajectory constraints corresponding to these triggers.

– (PT1: a wrapper trigger)
  When *inserting* into the *Purch table* modify the tuples (to be inserted) so that for any It#, the values for S# and Unitpr are the values for S# and Unitorderpr for that It# in the Inv table. (Note that because of the constraints associated with the Purch table that allow Orddate and Ordtime to get the current date and time by default, It# and Qordered are the only pieces of information required to do insertions into the Purch table.)
– (PT2 – a maintenance trigger)
  After *inserting* an order for an It# to *Purch*, update the Inv table by increasing the Qonorder (in the tuple with that It#) by Qordered.

The Corresponding Constraints. We first list the constraints in a high level language that we developed and then explain the meaning of the constructs in this language.

- (C1) **ForAll** $It\#. Inv.S\# = Purch.S\#$ **is invariant**
- (C2) **ForAll** $It\#. Inv.Unitorderpr = Purch.Unitpr$ **is invariant**
- (C3) **newtuple** $Purch$ **requires** $Orddate = Currentdate$ and $Ordtime = Currenttime$
- (C4) **ForAll** $It\#. Purch.Sum(Qordered) - Purch.Sum(Qrcvd) = Inv.Qonorder$ **is maintained**

Among the above constraints, the first two are state invariant constraints, the second is a trajectory invariant constraint, and the third is a state maintenance constraint. These constraints can be specified in first-order logic with temporal and aggregate constructs. We specify them using such constructs below with the assumption that all free variables are universally quantified and all the existentially quantified variables are denoted by underscores "_".

- (C1') $(Inv(It\#, \_, S_1, \_, \_, \_, \_, \_, \_) \wedge Purch(\_, \_, S_2, It\#, \_, \_, \_, \_))$ $\Rightarrow (S_1 = S_2)$
- (C2') $(Inv(It\#, \_, \_, \_, \_, \_, UOP_1, \_, \_) \wedge Purch(\_, \_, \_, It\#, \_, \_, \_, UP_2))$ $\Rightarrow (UOP_1 = UP_2)$
- (C3') $(\neg Purch(OD, OT, S\#, It\#, \_, \_, \_, \_) \wedge$ **nexttime** $(Purch(OD, OT, S\#, It\#, \_, \_, \_, \_))) \Rightarrow$ **nexttime** $(OD = date \wedge OT = time)$
- (C4.1') $R_1(It\#, Sum\_Qord) = {}_{It\#}\mathcal{G}_{Sum\ Qordered}(Purch)$

  (C4.2') $R_2(It\#, Sum\_Qrcvd) = {}_{It\#}\mathcal{G}_{Sum\ Qrcvd}(Purch)$

  (C4') $(quiescent \wedge R_1(It\#, Sum\_Qord) \wedge R_2(It\#, Sum\_Qrcvd) \wedge$ $Inv(It\#, \_, \_, \_, \_, \_, Qonorder, \_, \_, \_)) \Rightarrow (Sum\_Qord - Sum\_Qrcvd = Qonorder)$

The first order formulas (C1') and (C2') are low level representations of the state invariant constraints (C1) and (C2) respectively. The temporal formula (C3') is a low level representation of the trajectory invariant constraints (C3) and the temporal operator **nexttime** in (C3') has the usual FTL (future temporal logic) [CT95] meaning. Next we have the formulas (C4.1'), (C4.2') containing grouping aggregation expressions using the notation[3] from the text book [SKS96], and

---

[3] In this notation the general form is: ${}_{G_1, G_2, \dots, G_n}\mathcal{G}_{F_1\ A_1, F_2\ A_2, \dots, F_m\ A_m}(E)$, where E is any relational-algebra expression, $G_1, \dots, G_n$ constitute a list of attributes on which to group, each F_i is an aggregate function, and each A_i is an attribute name. The meaning of the operation is defined as follows. The tuples in the result of expression E are partitioned into groups such that:

(i) All tuples in a group have the same values for $G_1, \dots, G_n$.

(ii) Tuples in different groups have different values for $G_1, \dots, G_n$.

The groups now can be identified by the values of the attributes $G_1, \dots, G_n$ of the relation, and for each group $(g_1, \dots, g_n)$, the result has a tuple $(g_1, \dots, g_n, a_1, \dots, a_m)$ where, for each i, a_i is the result of applying the aggregate function F_i on the multi-set of values for the attribute A_i in the group.

(C4') which are a low level representation of the state maintenance constraint (C4). Note the difference between (C4') and (C1'-C2'). Since the former is a maintenance constraint, we use the proposition *quiescent* in the left hand side of the implication, meaning that the implication only holds in quiescent states. On the other hand the implications in (C1'-C2') must hold in all states.

Proposition 1. Let DB be the schema declaration in Section 3.1, and the only allowable exogenous action is 'Insert into Purch with Dtrecvd and Qrcvd as null, and Qordered as a positive value'. Then in the context of DB the set of triggers {PT1,PT2}, is correct w.r.t. the set of constraints {C1, C2, C3, C4}, and the above mentioned exogenous action.   □

4   Interrupting Exogenous Updates

So far we have (implicitly) assumed that if new exogenous update requests come in when the active database system is in the midst of processing ECA rules due to a previous exogenous update, the new requests are kept in hold until the processing (due to the previous update) comes to an end. Such an assumption is perhaps acceptable when the exogenous updates are not that frequent and/or trigger processing is not that time consuming, and *there is no guaranteed quality of service requirement*.

With the popularity of e-commerce where updates to the database would often be due to e-transactions over the web, companies may require a guaranteed quality of service requirement. In particular, they may require *immediate response to requests*. In such a case, it may be a good idea to partition *maintenance triggers* to two kinds *short term* and *long term*, with the idea that in order *to give reactive response to new update requests, processing of long term maintenance triggers may be postponed in favor of processing the new update request*.

The formulation of correctness in such a case becomes tricky, and we have made a small start in that direction. In this we only consider condition-action triggers, and consider all triggers to be *long term*. Before we get to our definition of correctness in such cases, we have the following notation. Let T be a set of condition-action triggers, and σ be a database state. By $\Xi_T(\sigma)$ we denote the action of the trigger which has the highest priority among the triggers whose conditions are satisfied in σ. We also have the following additional notations:

- $\Xi_T^0(\sigma) = \Xi_T(\sigma)$ and $\sigma_T^0 = \sigma$.
- $\Xi_T^{k+1}(\sigma) = \Xi_T(\sigma_T^{k+1})$ and $\sigma_T^{k+1} = \Phi(\Xi_T^K(\sigma), \sigma_T^k)$.

Definition 6 (k-Maintenance). Let T be a set of condition-action triggers, Γ be a set of long term maintenance constraints, S be a set of states, and A be a set of allowable exogenous actions.

By $Closure(S, T, A)$ we denote the smallest set of states that is a superset of S and that satisfies the properties that if $\sigma \in S$, then for an exogenous action a from A, $\Phi(a, \sigma) \in S$, and $\Phi(\Xi_T(\sigma), \sigma)) \in S$.

We say T k-maintains the maintenance constraints Γ from S and A, if for each state σ in S, the sequence $\sigma_T^0, \ldots, \sigma_T^k$ satisfies Γ.   □

Intuitively, the notion of k-maintenance means that the active database system will get back to consistency (with respect to Γ) if it is given a window of opportunity of processing k triggers without any outside interference in terms of new update requests.

An important aspect of such a notion of k-maintainability is that in reactive (active database) systems, if we know that our system is k-maintainable, and each transition takes say t time units, then we can implement a transaction mechanism that will regulate the number of exogenous actions allowed per unit time to be $\frac{1}{k \times t}$. On the other hand, given a requirement that we must allow m requests (exogenous actions) per unit time, we can work backwards to determine the value of k, and then find a set of triggers to make the system k-maintainable.

5   Conclusion and Future Work

In this paper we have taken several steps towards the systematic design of active features in an active database. The main steps that we have taken are identifying a few constructs for specification, classifying triggers into distinct classes based on their purpose, linking the trigger classes with the specification classes, formulating correctness of triggers with respect to a given specification, elaborating our formulation through examples and briefly introducing the notion of k-maintainability.

Due to space limitations we were not able to detail our formulation (especially, the prioritization used in defining Ψ and the differentiation between row and statement triggers) and show the design methodology with respect to a large example. In the full version we will show how our formulation in this paper can be used in systematically developing the triggers for the complete example in [Cha96], starting from a specification which is not given in [Cha96]. Our main future work will be to develop composition methods and theorems so that given sets of triggers T_1 and T_2 that are correct with respect to specifications S_1 and S_2 respectively, we can construct triggers that are correct with respect to $S_1 \cup S_2$. We also plan to identify additional specification constructs with matching trigger sub-classes, and further elaborate on our notion of k-maintainability.

References

[ADA93] P. Atzeni and V. De Antonellis. *Relational database theory.* The Benjamin/Cummings publishing company, 1993.

[BL96] C. Baral and J. Lobo. Formal characterization of active databases. In *Proc. of International Workshop on Logic in Databases – LID'96 (LNCS 1154)*, pages 175–195, 1996.

[BLT97] C. Baral, J. Lobo, and G. Trajcevski. Formal characterization of active databases: Part II. In *DOOD 97*, 1997.

[CF97]   S. Ceri and P. Fraternali. *Designing database applications with objects and rules – the IDEA methodology.* Addison-Wesley, 1997.

[Cha96]   D. Chamberlin. *Using the new DB2: IBM's Object-relational database system.* Morgan Kaufmann, 1996.

[CT95]   J. Chomicki and D. Toman. Implementing temporal integrity constraints using an active dbms. *IEEE transactions on knowledge and data engineering,* 1995.

[GL93]   M. Gelfond and V. Lifschitz. Representing actions and change by logic programs. *Journal of Logic Programming,* 17(2,3,4):301–323, 1993.

[Pat98]   N. Paton. *Active rules in database systems.* Springer-Verlag, 1998.

[SKS96]   A. Silberschatz, H. Korth, and S. Sudershan. *Database System Concepts.* McGraw Hill, 3rd edition, 1996.

[Ull88]   J. Ullman. *Principles of Database and Knowledge-base Systems, volume I.* Computer Science Press, 1988.

[WC96]   J. Widom and S Ceri, editors. *Active Database Systems - Triggers and Rules for advanced database processing.* Morgan Kaufmann, 1996.

[Wid96]   J. Widom. The Starbust rule system. In J. Widom and S Ceri, editors, *Active Database Systems,* pages 87–110. Morgan Kaufmann, 1996.

Fluents: A Refactoring of Prolog for Uniform Reflection and Interoperation with External Objects

Paul Tarau

Department of Computer Science, University of North Texas
P.O. Box 311366, Denton, Texas 76203
tarau@cs.unt.edu

Abstract. On top of a simple kernel (Horn Clause Interpreters with LD-resolution) we introduce **Fluents**, high level stateful objects which empower and simplify the architecture of logic programming languages through reflection of the underlying interpreter, while providing uniform interoperation patterns with object oriented and procedural languages. We design a Fluent class hierarchy which includes first-class stateful objects representing the meta-level Horn Clause Interpreters, file, URL, socket Readers and Writers, as well as data structures like terms and lists, with high-level operations directly mapped to iterative constructs in the underlying implementation language. Fluents melt naturally in the fabric of Logic Programming languages and provide elegant composition operations, reusability, resource recovery on backtracking and persistence. The Web site of our Kernel Prolog prototype, http://www.binnetcorp.com/kprolog/Main.html allows the reader to try out online the examples discussed in this paper.
Keywords: Logic Programming Language Design and Implementation, Interoperation of Declarative and Stateful Languages, Meta-Programming and Reflection

1 Introduction

Despite significant syntactic, semantic and implementational variations, Logic Programming languages share a common kernel: *Horn Clause Resolution*[1], a semantically and operationally well understood calculus. As it is the case with pure functional programming languages, this calculus allows reasoning with referentially transparent, stateless entities.

However, the resolution process as such, is obviously not stateless, as it proceeds in time, step by step. If we want to preserve the ability to *reflect* in the object language the resolution process provided by the underlying interpreter, even simple abstractions like the sequence of alternative answers computed by the interpreter, will require non-trivial additional programming language constructs. While implementing reflection mechanisms, a careful language designer

---

[1] The most commonly used variation is Prolog's LD-resolution which combines a depth-first search rule with a left-to-right selection rule.

J. Lloyd et al. (Eds.): CL 2000, LNAI 1861, pp. 1225–1239, 2000.

will be quickly faced with the need to pass Occam's razor to keep in check the explosion of redundant ontology.

Evolving algebras [6] have shown that programming languages can be seen as a combination of a basic, *terminating step* and some form of *iterative closure* operation. Linear logic [5, 1] has provided a more accurate description of the state of the proof process, with emphasis on seeing formulas as *resources*, with special notation indicating if they are unique or reusable.

Independently, the same need for *state representation with minimal new ontology* arises from the need for simplified *interoperation* of declarative languages with conventional software and operating system services which often relay on stateful entities.

Through constructs ranging from plain file or socket streams in C, to lazy list streams in languages like Scheme, iterators in Java or C++, monadic constructs [18, 2] in Haskell or in λ-Prolog, declarative I/O in Mercury [12], share the need for *abstracting away the nature of the stepping process* in a (finite or infinite, actual or generated as needed) sequence. Moreover, in the case of a declarative language implemented in a procedural or object oriented language, a uniform reflection mechanism is needed, for consistent modeling of stateful external objects providing native services.

This paper will introduce a concept of first class *fluents* on top of Horn Clauses with LD-Resolution to provide reflection of the underlying interpreter and interoperation with external stateful components, in a uniform way.

When seen from inside an Interpreter, other Interpreters will appear as instances of Fluents (Sources) producing a stream of answers. Through a set of suitable abstractions, they will be put to work as reusable components cooperating through independent resolution processes.

We will also describe a set of Fluent constructors which create Fluents from conventional data structures like lists, strings, files, terms and clauses and then provide Fluent Composers - allowing to elegantly combine them as building blocks for software components.

We will provide two compact meta-interpreters showing how backtracking and forward derivation can both be reflected (and controlled) at source level.

As a practical outcome, we provide a redesign of some key Prolog built-ins, of possible use in the next iteration of the ISO Prolog standardization process.

2   First Class Horn Clause Interpreters

2.1   Fluents: From Reflection to Interoperation with External Objects

We will build *Kernel Prolog* as a collection of Horn Clause Interpreters running LD-resolution on a default clause database and calling built-in operations. Each of them has a constructor which initializes them with a *goal* and an *answer pattern*. In fact, they will be seen as possibly infinite *sources of answers* which can be explored one by one. The object encapsulating the state of the interpreter is very similar to a file descriptor encapsulating the advancement of a file reader. We will call such stateful entities evolving in time *Fluents*.

Kernel Prolog Interpreters will possess, through built-in calls, the ability to create and query other Interpreters, as part of a general mechanism to a manipulate **Fluents**. *Fluents* encapsulating interpreters, like any other stateful objects, will have their independent life-cycles.

This general mechanism will allow Kernel Prolog interpreters to interoperate with the underlying object oriented implementation language, which will provide to and request from the interpreters, various services through a hierarchy of **Fluents**.

2.2   Interpreters as Answer Sources

Answer Sources can be seen as generalized iterators, allowing a given program to control answer production in another. Each Answer Source works as a separate Horn Clause LD-resolution interpreter (a very compact Java implementation of such an interpreter is given in the APPENDIX).

The **Answer Source** constructor initializes a new interpreter.

`answer_source(AnswerPattern,Goal,AnswerSource)`

creates a new Horn Clause solver, uniquely identified by **AnswerSource**, which shares code with the currently running program and is initialized with resolvent **Goal**. **AnswerPattern** is a term, usually a list of variables occurring in **Goal**.

The **get/2** operation (to be provided by all **Sources**, see section 3) is used to retrieve successive answers generated by an Answer Source, on demand.

`get(AnswerSource,AnswerInstance)`

tries to harvest the answer computed starting from **Goal**, as a instance of **AnswerPattern**. If an answer is found, it is returned as **the(AnswerInstance)**, otherwise **no** is returned. Note that once **no** has been returned, all subsequent **get/2** on the same **AnswerSource** will return **no**. Returning distinct functors in the case of success and failure allows further case analysis in a pure Horn Clause style, without needing Prolog's CUT operation. Bindings are not propagated to the original **Goal** or **AnswerPattern** when **get/2** retrieves an answer, i.e. **AnswerInstance** is obtained by first standardizing apart (renaming) the variables in **Goal** and **AnswerPattern**, and then backtracking over its alternative answers in a separate Prolog interpreter. Therefore, backtracking in the caller interpreter does not interfere with the new Answer Source's iteration over answers. Note however that backtracking over the Answer Source's creation point as such, makes it unreachable and therefore subject to garbage collection.

Finally, an Answer Source is stopped with the **stop** operation (implemented by all **Sources**, see section 3).

`stop(AnswerSource)`

The **stop/1** operation is called automatically when no more answers can be produced as well as through the Fluent's **undo** operation on backtracking.

3   Fluent Classes and their Operations

After seeing how AnswerSources encapsulate interaction with an interpreter, we will proceed with building a class hierarchy which generalizes this interaction pattern to external objects. The crux of this design is to make stateful external objects and interpreters communicate with a given interpreter in a uniform way. This turns out to be a very natural process, as modern "pattern aware" [4] object oriented design usually results in "interpreter-like" classes providing their services through high level abstractions. For instance, the Java classes in the Collections framework (JDK 1.2 and later), closely model set and finite function mathematics and are usable without any reference to "data-structure level" implementation detail.

We will first describe the root of our hierarchy, the **Fluent** class, then give some examples of simple Fluents and operations on Fluents.

Fluents are created with specific *constructors*, usually by converting from other Fluents or conventional Prolog data structures like Terms, Lists or Databases. All **Fluents** are enabled with a **stop/1** operation which releases their resources (most **Fluents** also call **stop** on backtracking, through their internal **undo** operation).

In our Java based reference implementation, the Fluent class looks as follows:

```
// Constructor, which adds this Fluent to the parent's trail.
class Fluent extends SystemObject {
  Fluent(Prog p) {trailMe(p);}

  // add the fluent to the parent Interpreter's Trail
  protected void trailMe(Prog p) {
    if(null!=p) p.getTrail().push(this);
  }

  // usable (through overriding) to release resources
  // and/or stop ongoing computations
  public void stop() {}

  // release resources on backtracking, if needed
  protected void undo() {stop();}
}
```

Sources are **Fluents** enabled with an extra **get/2** operation. Typical **Sources** are Horn Clause Interpreters, File, URL or String Readers, Fluents built from Prolog lists, Fluents iterating over data structures like Vectors or Hashtables or Queues in the underlying implementation language. Note that the constructor **Fluent(Prog p)** is trailed on the caller program **p**'s trail, and provides an **undo** operation to be called by **p** on backtracking, to release resources through the Fluent's **stop** method.

The Source abstract class looks as follows:

```
abstract class Source extends Fluent {

  Source(Prog p) {super(p);}

  abstract public Term get();
}
```

Sinks are fluents enabled with an extra **put/2** and **collect/2** operation. Typical Sinks are **ClauseWriters** or **CharWriters** targeted to TermCollectors (implemented as a Java **Vectors** collecting Prolog terms), **StringSinks** (implemented as a Java **StringBuffers** collecting String representations of Prolog terms).
The Sink abstract class looks as follows:

```
abstract class Sink extends Fluent {

  Sink(Prog p) {super(p);}

  // sends T to the Sink for tasks as accumulation or printing
  abstract public int put(Term T);

  // returns data previously sent to the Sink
  // (if collection ability is present)
  public Term collect() {return null;}
}
```

Not surprisingly, *even Prolog databases* are first class citizens implemented as extensions of **Sources** which provide **add/2, remove/2, collect/2** operations.
Fluents can be seen as *resources* which go through state transitions as a result of **put/2, get/2** and **stop/1** operations. They end their life cycle in a stopped state when all the data structures and/or threads they hold are freed.

3.1   Fluent Composers

Fluent composers provide abstract operations on **Fluents**. They are usually implemented with lazy semantics.
For instance, **append_sources/3** creates a new **Source** with a **get/2** operation such that when the first **Source** is stopped, iteration continues over the elements of the second **Source**.
Compose_sources/3 provides a cartesian product style composition, the new **get/2** operation returning pairs of elements of the first and second **Source**.
Reverse_source/2 builds a new Source **R** from a (finite) Source **F**, such that **R**'s **get/2** method returns elements of **F** in reverse order.
Split_source/3 is a cloning operation creating two **Source** objects identical to the **Source** given as first argument. It allows writing programs which iterate over a given **Source** multiple times.

Sources and Sinks are related through a **discharge(Source,Sink)** operation which sends all the elements of the **Source** to the given **Sink**. This allows for instance copying in a generic way a stream of answers of an Interpreter as well as data coming from a URL, through a socket, to a file, without having to iterate explicitly or know details on how data is actually produced and what its concrete representation is.

3.2   Fluent Modifiers

Fluent modifiers allow dynamically changing some attributes of a give Fluent. For instance **set_persistent(Fluent,YesNo)** is used to make a Fluent survive failure, by disabling its **undo** method, which, by default, applies the Fluent's **stop** method on backtracking.

4   Source Level Extensions through New Definitions

To give a glimpse to the expressiveness of the resulting language, we will now introduce, through definitions in Kernel Prolog, a number of built-in predicates known as "impossible to emulate" in Horn Clause Prolog (except by significantly lowering the level of abstraction and implementing something close to a Turing machine).

4.1   Negation and once/1

These constructs are implemented simply by discarding all but the first solution produced by a Solver.

```
% returns the(X) or no as first solution of G
first_solution(X,G,Answer):-
  answer_source(X,G,Solver),
  get(Solver,Answer),
  stop(Solver).

% succeeds by binding G to its first solution or fails
once(G):-first_solution(G,G,the(G)).

% succeeds without binding G, if G fails
not(G):-first_solution(_,G,no).
```

4.2   Reflective Meta-interpreters

The simplest meta-interpreter **metacall/1** just reflects backtracking through **element_of/2** over deterministic Answer Source operations.

```
metacall(Goal):-
  answer_source(Goal,Goal,E),
  element_of(E,Goal).
```

```
element_of(I,X):-get(I,the(A)),select_from(I,A,X).
```

```
select_from(_,A,A).
select_from(I,_,X):-element_of(I,X).
```

We can see **metacall/1** as an operation which fuses two orthogonal language features provided by Answer Sources: *computing an answer of a Goal*, and *advancing to the next answer*, through the source level operations **element_of/2** and **select_from/3** which 'borrow' the ability to backtrack from the underlying interpreter. The existence of this simple meta-interpreter indicates that **answer_sources** lift expressiveness of first-order Horn Clause logic significantly.

Note that **element_of/2** *works generically on* **Sources** *and is therefore re usable, for instance, to backtrack over the character codes of a file or a URL.*

After showing that we can emulate metacalls, we will use, for convenience, variables directly in predicate call position.

Note also that an Answer Source enumerates elements of the transitive closure of the *clause unfolding* relation [15, 16].

If our interpreter can access a single unfolding step through a similar Fluent, a *finer grained meta-interpreter* can be built as follows. Let's introduce a new Fluent,

```
unfolder_source(Clause,Source)
```

which, given a Clause produces a stream of clauses obtained by unfolding the first atom on the right side against a matching clause in the database. Each step is described through an (associative) clause composition operation $\oplus$ as follows:
    Let $A_0\text{:-}A_1,A_2,\ldots,A_n$ and $B_0\text{:-}B_1,\ldots,B_m$ be two clauses (suppose $n > 0, m \geq 0$). We define

$$(A_0\text{:-}A_1,A_2,\ldots,A_n) \oplus (B_0\text{:-}B_1,\ldots,B_m) = (A_0\text{:-}B_1,\ldots,B_m,A_2,\ldots,A_n)\theta$$

with $\theta = \text{mgu}(A_1,B_0)$. If the atoms A_1 and B_0 do not unify, the result of the composition is denoted as $\perp$ (failure). Furthermore, we consider $A_0\text{:-}\texttt{true},A_2,\ldots,A_n$ to be equivalent to $A_0\text{:-}A_2,\ldots,A_n$, and for any clause C, $\perp \oplus C = C \oplus \perp = \perp$. As usual, we assume that at least one operand has been renamed to a variant with variables standardized apart.

We can now build a meta-interpreter which implements the transitive closure of the unfolding operation $\oplus$ (provided as the get/2 operation of an Unfolder Source in the underlying implementation language), combined with backtracking trough **element_of/2**.

```
unfold_solve(Goal):-unfold(':-'(Goal,Goal),':-'(Goal,true)).
```

```
unfold(Clause,Clause).
```

```
unfold(Clause,Answer):-
  unfolder_source(Clause,Unfolder),
  element_of(Unfolder,NewClause),
  unfold(NewClause,Answer).
```

Note that this meta-interpreter will provide both backtracking and recursion for implementing Prolog's LD-resolution search. Clearly, alternative search mechanisms can be programmed quite easily.

4.3   If-then-else

Once we have *first_solution* and *metacall* operations, emulating if-then-else is easy.

```
% if Cond succeeds executes Then otherwise Else
if(Cond,Then,Else):-
  first_solution(successful(Cond,Then),Cond,R),
  select_then_else(R,Cond,Then,Else).

select_then_else(the(successful(Cond,Then)),Cond,Then,_):-Then.
select_then_else(no,_,_,Else):-Else.
```

4.4   All-Solution Predicates

All-solution predicates like findall/3 can be obtained by collecting answers through recursion.

```
% if G has a finite number of solutions
% returns a list Xs of copies of X each
% instantiated correspondingly
findall(X,G,Xs):-
  answer_source(X,G,E),
  get(E,Answer),
  collect_all_answers(Answer,E,Xs).

% collects all answers of a Solver
collect_all_answers(no,_,[]).
collect_all_answers(the(X),E,[X|Xs]):-
  get(E,Answer),
  collect_all_answers(Answer,E,Xs).
```

Note that, again, the **collect_all_answers** operation is generic, and works on any **Source**. This suggest providing a built-in Source-to-List converter **source_list/2** which can be made more efficient in the underlying implementation language where iteration replaces **collect_all_answers/3**'s recursion while also the eliminating interpretation overhead.

The alternative definition of findall/3 becomes simply:

```
findall(X,G,Xs):-
  answer_source(X,G,Solver),
  source_list(Solver,Xs).
```

4.5   Term Copying and Instantiation State Detection

As standardizing variables apart upon return of answers is part of the semantics of `get/2`, term copying is just computing a first solution to `true/0`. Implementing `var/1` uses the fact that only free variables can have copies unifiable with two distinct constants.

```
copy_term(X,CX):-first_solution(X,true,the(CX)).
var(X):-copy_term(X,a),copy_term(X,b).
```

The previous definitions have shown that the resulting language subsumes (through user provided definitions) constructs like negation as failure, if-then-else, once, **copy_term**, **findall** - this justifies its name *Kernel Prolog*. As Kernel Prolog contains negation as failure, following [3] we can, in principle, use it for an executable specification of full Prolog.

4.6   Implementing Exceptions

While it is possible to implement exceptions at source level as shown in [17], through a continuation passing program transformation (binarization), an efficient, constant time implementation can simply allow the interpreter to return a new answer pattern as indication of an exception. We have chosen this implementation scenario in our Kernel Prolog compiler which provides a **return/1** operation to exit an engine's emulator loop with an arbitrary answer pattern, possibly before the end of a successful derivation.

```
throw(E):-return(exception(E)).

catch(Goal,Exception,OnException):-
  answer_source(answer(Goal),Goal,Source),
  element_of(Source,Answer),
  do_catch(Answer,Goal,Exception,OnException,Source).

do_catch(exception(E),_,Exception,OnException,Source):-
  if(eq(E,Exception),
    OnException % call action if matching
    throw(E)    % throw again otherwise
  ),
  stop(Source).
do_catch(the(Goal),Goal,_,_,_).
```

The **throw/1** operation returns a special exception pattern, while the **catch/3** operation stops the engine, calls a handler on matching exceptions or re-throws non-matching ones to the next layer.

5   Built-Ins as a Library of Fluents

Modular extension of Kernel Prolog through new built-ins is based on an Object Oriented hierarchy of Fluents.

5.1   Lists and Terms as Source Fluents

Sequential Prolog data structures are mapped to Fluents naturally. For instance, **list_source/2** creates a new Fluent based on a List, such that its **get/2** operation will return one element of the list at a time. Similarly **term_source/2** creates a Fluent from an N-argument compound term, such that its **get/2** method will return first its function symbol then each argument. They are directly usable for composition/decomposition operations like **univ/2** (also known as =../2):

```
univ(T,FXs):-if(var(T),list_to_fun(FXs,T),fun_to_list(T,FXs)).

list_to_fun(FXs,T):-list_source(FXs,I),source_term(I,T).
fun_to_list(T,FXs):-term_source(T,I),source_list(I,FXs).
```

As they can be converted easily to/from Prolog data-structures, Fluents are usable as *canonical representation for data objects* as well as for *computational processes* (like in the case of **answer_sources**). *Fast iteration on Fluents, using loops over efficient native data structures in the implementation language, replace recursion in the object language.* This makes it possible to build high performance Fluent based logic programming implementations in relatively slow languages like Java (preliminary benchmarks indicate that our ongoing Jinni 2000 implementation is within an order of magnitude of the fastest C-based Prolog implementations, and it is likely to match quite closely slower ones like SWI Prolog). Interoperation with external objects is also simpler as implementation language operations can be applied to Fluents directly.

5.2   File, URL, and Database I/O in Kernel Prolog

File and URL I/O operations are provided by encapsulating Java's Reader and Writer classes as Fluents. Clause and character Readers are seen as instances of Sources and therefore benefit from Source composition operations. Moreover, Prolog operations traditionally captive to predefined list based implementations (like DCGs) can be made generic and mapped to work directly on Sources like file, URL and socket Readers.

Dynamic clause databases are also made visible as **Fluents**, and reflection of the interpreter's own handling of the Prolog database becomes possible. As an additional benefit, multiple databases are provided, to simplify adding module, object or agent layers at source level. By combining database and communication (socket or RMI) Fluents abstractions like mobile code are built easily and naturally.

5.3   Memoing Fluents

Most Fluents are designed, by default, to be usable only once, and to release all resources held (automatically on backtracking or under programmer's control when their **stop** operation is invoked). While Fluent operations like split fluent/3 can be used[2] to duplicate most Source Fluents, the following alternative provides a more efficient alternative.

A **Memoing Fluent** is built on top of a Source Fluent by progressively *accumulating* computed values in a List or dynamic array. A Memoing Fluent can be shared between multiple consumers which want to avoid recomputation of a given value.

5.4   Fluent Based Lazy Lists

Lazy Lists can be seen as an instance of Memoing Fluents: they accumulate successive values of a Source Fluent in a (reusable) list. The simple Lazy List abstraction in our reference implementation works as follows:

```
source_lazy_list(Source, LazyList)
```

creates a new LazyList object from a Source object:

```
lazy_head(LazyList, LazyHead)
```

extracts the current head element of the list. Iteration over the list is provided by

```
lazy_tail(LazyList, LazyTail)
```

which returns LazyTail, a new lazy list encapsulating the next stage of the Source fluent.

While complete automation of lazy lists through a form of attributed variable construct is possible, we have chosen a simpler implementation scenario based on the previously described operations, mainly because overriding unification with execution of an arbitrary procedure would introduce potential *non-termination* - something which would break the very idea of keeping the execution mechanism as close as possible to basic Horn Clause resolution, as available in classic Prolog.

Based on these operations, a lazy **findall/3** is simply:

```
% creates lazy list from an answer source
lazy_findall(X,G,LazyList):-
  answer_source(X,G,S),
  source_lazy_list(S,LazyList).
```

In fact, the behavior of the lazy list encapsulating **lazy findall**'s advancement on alternative solutions produced by an Answer Source, is indistinguishable from a lazy list constructed from an ordinary **list source**:

---

[2] The astute reader might notice that Linear Logic provers provide similar operations. This is by no means accidental, a resource conscious proof procedure will usually provide explicit means to implement multiple use of a resource.

```
% creates a lazy list from a List
lazy_list(List,LazyList):-
  list_source(List,S),
  source_lazy_list(S,LazyList).
```

The following operations are centered around the **lazy_tail/3** advancement operation, which produces a lazily growing reusable list. This list is explored with **lazy_element_of/2** in a way similar to the way ordinary lists are explored with **member/2** and ordinary Sources are explored with **element_of/2**.

```
% explores a lazy list in a way compatible with backtracking
% allows multiple 'consumers' to access the list, end ensures that
% the lazy list advances progressively and consistently
lazy_element_of(XXs,X):-
  lazy_decons(XXs,A,Xs),
  lazy_select_from(Xs,A,X).
```

```
% backtracks over the lazy list
lazy_select_from(_,A,A).
lazy_select_from(XXs,_,X):-lazy_element_of(XXs,X).
```

```
% returns a head/tail pair of a non-empty lazy list
lazy_decons(XXs,X,Xs):-
  lazy_head(XXs,X),
  lazy_tail(XXs,Xs).
```

A minor change in Prolog's chronological backtracking is needed however: only the creation point of the lazy list is subject to trailing, and the complete lazy list is discarded at once. This is achieved in our reference implementation by giving to each lazy list its own (dynamically growing) trail, and by providing an **undo** operation which rewinds the trail completely when backtracking passes the lazy list object's creation point.

6   Related Work

Similar to the Answer Sources described in this paper, *engine* constructs have been part of systems like Oz [11, 10] BinProlog [13] and Jinni [14].

The main differences with Oz engines are:

- while Oz designers have chosen not to handle backtracking in exchange for the ability of sharing variables between different threads, Kernel Prolog provides *encapsulated backtracking*, local to a given **Answer Source**
- Oz engines are not separated from the underlying multi-threading model, they are not simple Horn Clause processors, they are part of Oz's computation spaces - which include threads and constraint stores
- in Oz, answers are returned only when a computation space is stable - the engine mechanism in Oz is overloaded as a synchronization device - which in our case is an orthogonal concept

– Oz engines have been designed for a different purpose, i.e. to program alternative search algorithms or for local constraint propagation, while our objective is a uniform reflection mechanism for multiple first order Horn Clause interpreters and interoperation with (other) external stateful objects

Fluents share some design objectives with Haskell's IO Monad approach [9] - which essentially encapsulates the state of the external world in a single stateful entity on which IO operates as a sequence of transitions. Our fluents can be seen as an abstraction for multiple stateful worlds organized as a typed inheritance hierarchy and specialized toward *source* and *sink* roles - corresponding to abstract *read* and *write* operations. Note however that some sink fluents provide a **collect** operation allowing to build new sources. Arguably, fluents offer a more flexible management of input and output flows than the monolithical IO Monad. In fact, John Hughes recent proposal to replace monads with the more powerful concept of arrow [7] with emphasis on directionality hints towards possible evolution towards a fluent-like concept.

Java's own design of Reader and Writer class trees and the ability to transform streams into new streams with stronger properties or elements of a different granularity (which in fact serves as the implementation bases for some of our fluents, behind the scenes) and its recently introduced Collection framework [8] also show convergence towards similar design patterns.

Our previous work on the Jinni agent programming language [14] and Bin-Prolog [13] has described similar engine constructs. However, the key idea of seeing engines as instances of Fluents, the separation of engines from the multi-threading mechanism, the reconstruction of Prolog's built-ins as a hierarchy of Fluent classes and the interoperation of external objects encapsulated as Fluent instances are definitely new.

New languages based on relatively pure subsets of Prolog like Mercury [12] have been designed as targets of more efficient implementation technologies and for their reliability in building large software systems. While Horn Clauses with negation have been extensively studied and some of the techniques described in this paper might be well known to experienced Prolog programmers, the very idea of systematically exploring the gains in expressive power as a result of having multiple pure Prolog interpreters as first order objects, has not been explored yet, to our best knowledge.

7   Future Work

We have recently finished the first cut of a fast WAM based implementation of Kernel Prolog in Java and integrated it with the interpreter described in this paper. Preliminary benchmarks indicate being constantly within one order of magnitude from the fastest C-based Prolog implementations.

This opens the door for a number of real-life software applications.

The advent of component based software development and intelligent appliances requiring small, special purpose, self contained, still powerful processing elements, makes Kernel Prolog an appealing implementation technique for building logic programming components. In particular, in the case of small, wireless interconnected devices, subject to severe memory and bandwidth limitations, compact and orthogonally designed small language processors are instrumental.

Our ongoing commercial Palm Prolog and Prolog-in-Java implementations use respectively C and Java variants of a fast Horn Clause LD-resolution WAM emulator based on the Kernel Prolog design described in this paper. This high-performance Kernel Prolog compiler (subject of an upcoming paper) will also provide support for Agent Classes - a new form of code structuring which promises to bring logic programming to functionality beyond the usual object oriented Prolog extensions, within a declarative framework.

Here are a few open issues and some other ongoing or projected Kernel Prolog related developments:

- executable specification of ISO Prolog in terms of Kernel Prolog
- a study of Kernel Prolog's invariance under program transformations (unfolding)
- type checking / type inference mechanisms for Kernel Prolog
- lightweight engine creation and engine reuse techniques for Kernel Prolog
- Kernel Prolog as a basis of embedded Prolog component technology and Prolog based Palm computing

8   Conclusion

We have provided a design for the uniform interoperation of Horn Clause Solvers with stateful entities (Fluents) ranging from external procedural and object oriented language services like I/O operations, to other, 'first class citizen' Horn Clause Solvers. As a result, a simplified Prolog built-in predicate system has emerged.

By collapsing the semantic gap between Horn Clause logic and (most of) the full Prolog language into three surprisingly simple, yet very powerful operations, we hope to open the doors not only for an implementation technology for a new generation of lightweight Prolog processors but also towards a better understanding of the intrinsic elegance hiding behind the core concepts of the logic programming paradigm.

Our Horn Clause Solvers encapsulated as Fluents provide the ability to communicate between distinct OR-branches as an practical alternative to the use assert/retract based side effects, in implementing all-solution predicates. Moreover, lazy variants of all solution predicates are provided as a natural extension to Fluent based lazy lists.

Finally, high level Fluent Composers allow combining component functionality in generic, data representation independent ways.

References

1. J.-M. Andreoli and R. Pareschi. Linear objects: Logical processes with built-in inheritance. In D.H.D. Warren and P. Szeredi, editors, *7th Int. Conf. Logic Programming*, Jerusalem, Israel, 1990. MIT Press.
2. Yves Bekkers and Paul Tarau. Monadic Constructs for Logic Programming. In John Lloyd, editor, *Proceedings of ILPS'95*, pages 51–65, Portland, Oregon, December 1995. MIT Press.
3. P. Deransart, A. Ed-Dbali, and L. Cervoni. *Prolog: The Standard.* Springer-Verlag, Berlin, 1996. ISBN: 3-540-59304-7.
4. E. Gamma, R. Helm, R. Johnson, J. Vlissides, and G. Booch. *Design Patterns : Elements of Reusable Object-Oriented Software.* Professional Computing. Addison-Wesley, 1995. ISBN: 0201633612.
5. J.-Y. Girard. Linear logic. *Theoretical Computer Science*, (50):1–102, 1987.
6. Yuri Gurevich. Evolving algebras: An attempt to discover semantics. *Bulletin of the EATCS*, 43:264–284, 1991.
7. John Hughes. Generalizing Monads to Arrows. Technical report. available from: http://www.cs.chalmers.se/~rjmh/Arrows/.
8. Sun Microsystems. The Java Collections Framework. Technical report. available from: http://java.sun.com/products/jdk/1.2/docs/guide/collections/.
9. Simon Peyton Jones and John Hughes. Haskell 98: A Non-strict, Purely Functional Language. Technical report, February 1999. available from: http://www.haskell.org/onlinereport/.
10. Christian Schulte. Programming constraint inference engines. In Gert Smolka, editor, *Proceedings of the Third International Conference on Principles and Practice of Constraint Programming*, volume 1330 of *Lecture Notes in Computer Science*, pages 519–533, Schloß Hagenberg, Austria, October 1997. Springer-Verlag.
11. Christian Schulte and Gert Smolka. Encapsulated search in higher-order concurrent constraint programming. In Maurice Bruynooghe, editor, *Logic Programming: Proceedings of the 1994 International Symposium*, pages 505–520, Ithaca, NY, USA, November 1994. The MIT Press.
12. Zoltan Somogyi, Fergus Henderson, and Thomas Conway. The Mercury Language Web Site. 1998. http://www.cs.mu.oz.au/research/mercuryl.
13. Paul Tarau. BinProlog 7.0 Professional Edition: Advanced BinProlog Programming and Extensions Guide. Technical report, BinNet Corp., 1998. Available from http://www.binnetcorp.com/BinProlog.
14. Paul Tarau. Inference and Computation Mobility with Jinni. In K.R. Apt, V.W. Marek, and M. Truszczynski, editors, *The Logic Programming Paradigm: a 25 Year Perspective*, pages 33–48. Springer, 1999. ISBN 3-540-65463-1.
15. Paul Tarau and M. Boyer. Nonstandard Answers of Elementary Logic Programs. In J.M. Jacquet, editor, *Constructing Logic Programs*, pages 279–300. J.Wiley, 1993.
16. Paul Tarau and Michel Boyer. Elementary Logic Programs. In P. Deransart and J. Maluszyński, editors, *Proceedings of Programming Language Implementation and Logic Programming*, number 456 in Lecture Notes in Computer Science, pages 159–173. Springer, August 1990.
17. Paul Tarau and Veronica Dahl. Logic Programming and Logic Grammars with First-order Continuations. In *Proceedings of LOPSTR'94, LNCS, Springer*, Pisa, June 1994.
18. Philip Wadler. Monads and composable continuations. *Lisp and Symbolic Computation*, pages 1–17, 1993.

So Many WAM Variations, So Little Time

Bart Demoen[1] and Phuong-Lan Nguyen[2]

[1] Department of Computer Science, K.U. Leuven
Celestijnenlaan 200A, B-3001 Leuven, Belgium
bmd@cs.kuleuven.ac.be
[2] Institut de Mathematiques Appliquées, Université Catholique de l'Ouest
Place André Leroy 3, 49008 Angers, France
nguyen@ima.uco.fr

Abstract. The WAM allows within its framework many variations e.g. regarding the term representation, the instruction set and the memory organization. Consequently several Prolog systems have implemented successful variants of the WAM. While these variants are effective within their own context, it is difficult to assess the merit of their particular variation. In this work, four term representations that were used by at least one successful system are compared empirically within dProlog, one basic implementation which keeps all other things equal. We also report on different implementation choices in the dProlog emulator itself. dProlog is reasonably efficient, so it makes sense to use it for these experiments.

1 Introduction

The WAM (see [1,16]) has been the basis for many Prolog systems, also the most successful ones. It leaves open certain issues like the implementation of cut, dynamic code etc. but even when it specifies other issues, there are variations that can still pass for the WAM in the broad sense. Examples are optimizations like instruction compression, new ways to propagate the read-write mode, the organization of the stacks or a different tagging schema. Another variation - the one of interest here - concerns the term representation itself: the WAM initializes permanent variables on the local stack when possible, while other implementations have chosen to globalize permanent variables on their first occurrence (BIM_Prolog always, AQUARIUS [15] under certain conditions) and consequently do not have to deal with *unsafe* variables; PARMA [14] represents the binding between two free variables differently from the WAM and has constant time dereferencing; BinProlog [13] employs a *tag on data* schema instead of the WAM *tag on pointer* schema. Each of these WAM variations was effective within its own context: BIM_Prolog used native code generation (not common in 1985 !); BinProlog binarizes clauses before compiling them [12]; PARMA and AQUARIUS rely on abstract interpretation for their top speed. Because the implementation context of these term representations was different from each other and from the original WAM, it is not at all clear how they really compare, i.e. there has been no empirical study of the impact of changing within a single efficient system one term representation into another one while *all others things*

J. Lloyd et al. (Eds.): CL 2000, LNAI 1861, pp. 1240–1254, 2000.

are kept equal. We intend to do exactly that: evaluate empirically and compare directly within the same basic implementation the four above mentioned term representations.

Such an experiment only makes sense if the basic Prolog implementation is reasonably complete and fast. Yap [4] or SICStus Prolog [3] could have served as a good starting point for the experiment. However, adapting such systems is very time consuming and that was one reason for starting almost from scratch: because of our prior involvement with XSB (see e.g. [7]), we borrowed the XSB compiler (see [17]), for the generation of abstract machine code (XSB is largely WAM based) and we built a new emulator. This permitted us to redo partly the experiment reported on in [4] and at the same time benefit from its advice, investigate the potential for speeding up the Prolog part of XSB and build the basis for a dedicated Prolog system for inductive learning applications [6]. It also gave us the chance to satisfy a private curiosity regarding an unusual term representation for integers and floating point numbers, and a different layout of environments: these are reported on later.

We named the resulting Prolog system **dProlog**[1]. dProlog is complete enough to bootstrap itself but hardly more complete than needed for the experiment.

We decided to stay in the emulator business as [4], but since it clearly doesn't make sense to study the impact of changes in a slow system we wanted dProlog to be in the same ball park as SICStus Prolog emulated with all bells and whistles (i.e. using gcc extensions). The SICStus Prolog emulator is not the fastest around: Yap [4] beats SICStus Prolog consistently. So we decided to borrow from Yap techniques applicable at the C-level as well as the abstract machine code level. As a consequence dProlog performs as good as Yap for certain benchmarks - especially smaller ones - but given our choice of XSB for generating the abstract machine code, dProlog has not a chance to get always on par with SICStus Prolog. Still, we felt that the initial goal was met close enough. We report on the aspect of performance compared to other systems in section 4, mainly because it shows that our emulator is of sufficient quality to make the results of the experiments relevant.

We also experimented with implementation choices within the emulator itself. Therefore we have set up dProlog so that it can be installed in 6 different basic emulator modes depending on two parameters: the first parameter sets the number of opcode fields in each instruction; it is either *1* - as is customary - and then the read-write mode in the unify-instructions is explicitly tested by means of the WAM S register; or it is *2*, in which case the read-write mode is propagated by using the first opcode field in read mode and the second in write mode (see [4] for more detail). The second parameter can orthogonally be set to *switch*, *jump_table* and *threaded* which is a similar choice as in SICStus *THREADED = 0,1 or 2*. The latter two require GNU cc. We report on the effects (time and space) of these six modes in section 5.

Section 6 reports on choices in the implementation of the emulator: the assignment of a hardware register to the WAM program counter, binding calls,

---

[1] http://www.cs.kuleuven.ac.be/~md/dProlog for source code and benchmarks

conditional trailing, trail overflow checking and 28 versus 32 bit integers. In the same section, we also report on the effect of several instruction compressions.

The initial version of dProlog (with all the above variations) always globalizes permanent variables on their first occurrence: we will refer to it as the **heap_vars** version. We then created three more versions: we will refer to them as **wam_vars**, **parma_vars** and **tag_on_data**. They differ from the heap_vars dProlog in only one aspect: wam_vars initializes permanent variables on the local stack whenever possible, exactly as in the WAM, and thus knows *unsafe* variables (see [1]); parma_vars uses the variable representation as in [14]; tag_on_data uses the representation as in BinProlog [13], but without term compression. Parma_vars and tag_on_data also always globalize permanent variables: BinProlog, the only other Prolog system using the tag-on-data representation, doesn't even have a local stack and the intricacies of having PARMA variables also in the local stack reported in [11] scared us off. All these different representations are shortly explained in section 3. We report on the impact of these changes in section 7.

We start with an overview of the XSB compiler and dProlog in section 2.

All the experiments were performed on a Pentium II, 260MHz, 128Mb.

2   The XSB Compiler and dProlog

XSB supports HiLog and tabling, both of which we were not interested in for this experiment: consequently, we have removed most of the code in the XSB compiler that deals with these extensions. They do not interfere with the compilation of ordinary Prolog programs. Also *call specialization*[2] was switched off. The XSB compiler can generate indexing for any argument (depending on declarations); we have disabled the index declaration and specialized all indexing instructions to the first argument. Overall, the XSB compiler generates reasonable to good code, but some basic choices in the compiler are bad for performance, especially within an emulator: (1) the activation of a predicate can cause the creation of two choice points [2]; this slows down some benchmarks; in particular *sdda*, *meta_qsort*, and also to a lesser extent *boyer*; (2) the convention for in-lined built-ins is that their arguments are put in the argument registers 1 up to the arity of the built-in; sometimes up to three *movreg* instructions are generated before and after the call to a built-in; the twin calls to functor/3 in *boyer* are a good example of this inefficiency; (3) register allocation is far from optimal; this results in badly compiled arithmetic (among other things); e.g. the inner loop of *tak* contains at least five instructions that would have been avoided with a better register allocation; (4) XSB does not treat void variables in a special way; this slows down a.o. *zebra*.

The basic structure of the XSB compiler was not changed: variable classification, built-in calling convention, the indexing schema, register allocation etc. were not touched. We made five changes: (1) the generation of the *test_heap* instruction - the entry point of each predicate in the current implementation of

---

[2] a predicate specialization according to (partially instantiated) call patterns that appear in the same module

XSB which tests for heap overflow - was suppressed, and its functionality moved to the *call* and *execute* instructions; (2) in order to provide for native size floating point numbers and integers small changes were necessary: see later; (3) XSB uses specialized instructions for the atom []; this specialization was switched off; (4) we have added some peephole optimizations for instruction compression and added a few instruction specializations (section 6.2); (5) we have specialized the XSB *switch_on_term* instruction to lists; this was important for testing an optimization referred to later as *switch* (section 6.2); this does not affect other issues: in our tagging schema, the list and compound test have the same cost.

XSB has only *truncated* integers (28 bits on a 32-bit machine). We implemented both truncated integers and *full* integers, i.e. 32 bits. The latter need changes in the generated code, since a 32-bit integer must always reside on the heap. We give the two instruction streams for the head of the clause

truncated ints	full ints
getstr f/2, A1	getstr f/2, A1
uninumcon 9	unitvar A2
unicon a	unicon a
	getint A2, 9

head(f(9, a)). The overhead of full integers comes from its higher heap consumption and from extra emulator cycles. This will be clear in the benchmarks. Floating point numbers in dProlog are never truncated and always require the above transformation.

All versions of dProlog have the following characteristics: (1) separate stacks for environments and choice points; (2) no environment trimming: the XSB compiler does not generate the information to do it; the local stack grows towards the heap and environments are put upside-down (see [9]); this can result in less testing during trailing, but in an extra comparison when binding two free variables; (3) no tidying of the trail during cut; (4) no trail overflow testing: see section 6 for explanation and the effect on speed of trail overflow testing; all other overflow testing is done in software; (5) dProlog deals with hash collisions in the indexing code when using hashing by a try-retry-trust chain, just like XSB does; (6) floating point operations are not IEEE compliant.

3 The Three Term Representations on the Heap in dProlog

The heap_vars and wam_vars term representation on the heap is the same: the difference is in *where* permanent variables are initialized. Heap_vars does that always on the heap; wam_vars in the environment when possible. Tag_on_data and parma_vars are really different. So, we can speak of *three* heap term representations. The next figure shows the representation of the list [a, b] in the tag_on_data schema to the right and in the other schemas to the left. Each heap cell consists of a tag (P,S,L,A,I or F) and a pointer or value. An empty tag or value field means it is never inspected.

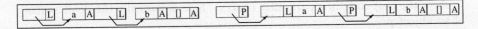

Tag_on_data uses one heap cell more per cons than the other representations. In the tag_on_data schema as implemented in BinProlog, the list constructor is treated as any other constructor. We have instead chosen to specialize the representation of lists within the tag_on_data philosophy, because that results in exactly the same abstract machine instructions being executed in all variants of dProlog. The next figure shows compound terms, variables and numbers in $f(X, g(X), 666, 3.14)$. Note how the PARMA representation of two bound free variables creates a cycle instead of a chain of references.

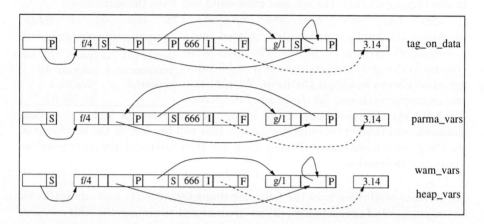

Pointers (to the heap and local stack) are always aligned on a 4 byte boundary, so the tags on pointers (P, S and L) can be 2 bits without restricting the range of pointers. The dProlog tags are as follows (only the significant lower bits are given):

P (ref) = 00	S (struct) = 01	L (list) = 11
A (atom) = 0110	I (integer) = 1010	F (float) = 1110

The representation of floating point numbers is a bit unusual: the number is put on the heap, and its (F-tagged) offset from the start of the heap is used as its entry; the dashed pointer symbolizes the offset. This representation is also used for full integers. We have since long wanted to use such a representation (offsets instead of pointers) and now understand better the consequences. The main issues are: (1) some routines (like general unify) need to know the start of the heap; if the implementation needs to be re-entrant, it means that this start of heap must be passed as an argument; (2) copying terms (with numbers) becomes a bit more involved if the region one copies to (or from) is not contiguous (like for instance in findall buffers); (3) a sliding garbage collection algorithm needs an extra mark bit since numbers on the heap are not preceded by a header; (4) retaining sharing during copying is nearly impossible. We recommend this representation to nobody.

Dereferencing in the three representations is different. Without an attempt to show the best code in a particular context, here is basically the dereferencing of an object p:

parma_vars	if (ref(p)) p = *p;
wam_vars and heap_vars	while (ref(p)) { if (p == *p) break; p = *p; }
tag_on_data	while (ref(p)) { if (p == *p) break; q = p; p = *p; }

In tag_on_data, the value of q might be needed after deref: if after deref, p contains an S-tagged value, $q + 1$ points to the first argument of the structure.

In parma_vars dereferencing is a constant time operation. When two free variables are bound to each other, they must be tested for equality. [11] reports this as a drawback of parma_vars, but the truth is that – as was noted during the HAL project in which also the PARMA representation is used (see [5]) – testing for equality of two free variables in parma_vars might require less steps than in the other representations. Also, there exist programs for which the WAM is quadratic and PARMA linear in the input.

4   Comparing dProlog with Other Prolog Systems

We compare dProlog with other well-known and/or relevant systems on a set of benchmarks taken from [15]. The compiler of dProlog compiling itself (with output suppressed - input performed with *get0/1* and a reader in Prolog) is added as a medium sized more realistic benchmark: it consists of about 5000 lines of code. Times are always in 1/100s of a second. Sizes in tables are always in units of 4 bytes and represent the maximal stack usage during the running of all the benchmarks above the size figure in the same table; the code size includes also the compiler and toplevel. We repeated each benchmark in a failure driven way; the repetition factor is mentioned in the table: sdda(1200) means that a timing is shown for repeating *sdda* 1200 times. Each such repetition was performed four times; the first timing is always ignored (it is often an out-lier either way) and the smallest timing of the remaining three is reported. For dProlog, we show here only the mode *threaded with two opcodes + all other defaults* (see section 6) for heap_vars. We use an older SICStus version because it was our initial target and the most recent release (3.8.1) is significantly slower.

SICStus Prolog, Yap and XSB all implement wam_vars, while BinProlog obviously implements tag_on_data. SICStus and Yap (as dProlog) use gcc specific features, while XSB and BinProlog use only ANSI-C. Yap uses a single stack for choice points and environments, like the WAM.

5   Comparing the Six Basic Modes of dProlog

Table 2 shows the results of running dProlog in its six basic modes on the standard set of benchmarks. The modes are indicated as *switch* (for a C switch), *jump* (for a jump table) and *threaded* (for the threaded implementation) and the suffix *1* or *2* indicates whether read-write propagation is done as in the WAM (1) or with two operation codes (2) as described in [4].

The stack sizes are the same for all modes and not included in the table. The code sizes for switch1 and jump1 must be equal, and also the code sizes for switch2 and jump2. The fact that the code sizes for switch1 and switch2 are exactly the same is a coincidence: the instruction layout is such that each instruction has a spare byte.

Table 1. Comparing dProlog with other systems

	dProlog 1	SICStus 3#5	Yap4.2.1	XSB 2.1	BinProlog 6.84
boyer(1)	40	34	32	95	106
browse(1)	48	47	30	95	147
cal(10)	77	69	68	140	105
chat(5)	45	55	43	77	98
crypt(200)	53	57	41	108	79
ham(2)	59	74	54	137	146
meta_qsort(125)	51	42	34	118	150
nrev(5000)	43	66	45	227	88
poly_10(10)	32	27	23	64	58
queens_16(2)	88	88	44	180	148
queens(10)	106	141	91	260	241
reducer(20)	19	13	10	37	35
sdda(1200)	40	33	29	70	75
send(10)	49	48	28	85	124
tak(10)	73	77	53	159	208
zebra(30)	82	82	63	139	173
compile(1)	776	914	739	1774	2074

The positive effect of using two opcodes (or two addresses in the case of threading) for read-write propagation is not as good as one might hope. We think the main reason is that the WAM non-read-write propagation with the S register, performs quite well on modern architectures with pre-fetching and branch prediction. The increased code size probably does not matter: this was confirmed by other experiments that are not reported on here.

It might seem strange that switch2 performs worse than switch1: we have tried three variants of switch2 and the results were always similar. Compared to switch1, switch2 requires extra jumps and/or increases register pressure even on instructions that have no read-write variant. This is not true when comparing jump1 with jump2 or threaded1 with threaded2.

6 The Effect of Features and Optimizations in dProlog

The next tables only contain figures that relate to the heap_vars version of dProlog. The general setup is that the default settings are compared with a version in which one (or sometimes more) features are introduced or disabled. We first show variations in the implementation of the emulator itself (section 6.1) and variations in the generated abstract machine code (section 6.2).

6.1 Variations in the Implementation of the Emulator

Table 3 shows the variation of features in the emulator itself. An absent size figure means it is the same as for the default version. The explanation of the columns is:

- **default**: the default for dProlog is threaded, two opcodes, bind call, truncated integers, local pc = bx, with conditional trailing, no trail overflow check and with all instruction specializations and compressions

Table 2. The six basic modes of dProlog - heap_vars

	switch1	switch2	jump1	jump2	threaded1	threaded2
boyer	54	67	44	44	40	40
browse	81	95	51	50	48	48
cal	87	105	87	87	78	77
chat	54	64	48	47	46	45
crypt	70	84	57	56	52	53
ham	99	115	66	65	60	59
meta_qsort	76	89	56	55	52	51
nrev	130	157	45	43	46	43
poly_10	46	56	36	34	33	32
queens_16	118	141	100	98	89	88
queens	176	211	113	110	107	106
reducer	26	30	20	20	19	19
sdda	51	62	41	42	41	40
send	70	85	59	60	49	49
tak	101	125	78	78	73	73
zebra	103	113	85	83	83	82
code	48251	48251	48251	48251	73104	77038
compile	1094	1324	827	808	786	776
code	50202	50202	50202	50202	77826	81692

- **no bind call**: usually the call instruction refers to a predicate table to find the entry point of the predicate to be called; this makes the implementation of debugging and reconsult easier; in its default mode however, dProlog puts the address of the entry point directly in the call (and execute) instruction; we name this *bind call*; supporting debugging and reconsult under this schema adds a little implementation complexity and is not fully done in dProlog; this column shows the effect of not binding calls: although binding calls looks a priori like an optimization, its effect varies and is not large; this is in part caused by the fact that in dProlog the lookup of the entry of a predicate, is very simple: only one indirection is needed
- **always trail**: this column represents unconditional trailing; its effect depends on the kind of benchmark (a benchmark where each potential trailing is actual, obviously benefits from deleting the test) but is never large except for *nrev*; we also give the maximal trail usage for comparison
- **trail overflow test**: by default, dProlog allocates enough space for the trail (as much as the heap in heap_vars and tag_on_data, six times as much in parma_vars, as much as heap and local stack together in wam_vars), so that trail overflow testing is not necessary [3]; however, the space penalty can be too high; so it is worth looking at the potential performance gain; the effect is quite high on some benchmarks, but overall small
- **full integers**: many implementations sacrifice the range of integers for the benefit of their compact representation: XSB represents integers with just 28 bits, as in the default mode of dProlog; dProlog can also run in a mode with 32 bit integers: this column shows the performance penalty both space and time wise; the relatively bad performance can be partly explained by the particular representation used for full integers, relying on a heap offset; another reason is the suboptimal abstract machine code for full integers (see section 2)
- **glob bx, glob bp, register, no reg decl**: as advised in [4] we assigned the WAM program counter (pc) to a hardware register; [4] does not report that there

---

[3] this "optimization" came up during working with Paul Tarau but might be folklore

are several choices: one can reserve the hardware register locally to the emulator loop or globally in the whole of the implementation; and different choices as to which hardware register is used are possible; our default choice is to assign the program counter locally to the hardware register bx: *loc bx*; the meaning of *glob bx* and *glob bp* follows; we also tried just declaring the program counter locally as a register or giving no directions to the C compiler at all.

Table 3. The effect of emulator properties in dProlog

	default	no bind call	always trail	check tr overflow	full integers	glob bx	glob bp	register	no reg decl
boyer	40	40	40	41	45	40	40	41	41
browse	48	47	47	50	49	47	47	50	49
cal	77	78	79	79	91	78	78	77	78
chat	45	45	45	45	47	45	45	44	44
crypt	53	52	54	51	62	52	52	52	51
ham	59	61	62	62	60	59	59	64	65
meta_qsort	51	51	52	52	51	51	51	51	51
nrev	43	46	53	44	44	43	43	52	51
poly_10	32	32	33	32	33	31	31	31	31
queens_16	88	90	90	88	108	88	88	90	90
queens	106	105	107	103	108	103	103	107	107
reducer	19	19	19	19	19	18	18	19	19
sdda	40	41	41	40	41	40	40	41	40
send	49	49	50	55	60	49	49	54	54
tak	73	74	72	74	93	75	75	74	74
zebra	82	83	83	86	86	81	81	85	85
heap	448296	-	-	-	674911	-	-	-	-
trail	57677	-	403043	-	-	-	-	-	-
code	77038	-	-	-	77761	-	-	-	-
compile	776	779	787	787	844	769	796	785	785
heap	1369456	-	-	-	5972416	-	-	-	-
trail	227623	-	854611	-	-	-	-	-	-
code	81692	-	-	-	82198	-	-	-	-

The table indicates that assigning the WAM program counter to a global bx register (the Yap choice is global bp) performs best, followed closely by the local bx register. One should not take this as a general truth: it will depend on factors beyond control like the C compiler and the particular way of writing C code in the emulator. Rather one should take this as an indication that exploring the alternatives might be worthwhile. We made local bx our default because it performs well while being local. Note that also just declaring the program counter as a register without assigning it to any particular hardware one, performs quite well, with the additional advantage that it is fully ANSI.

6.2   Variations on the Abstract Machine Code

We report here on variations in the generated abstract machine code: the columns in table 4 show the timings when one or more instruction compression or specialization is turned *off*. Note that even though some instructions are not generated when some optimizations were turned off, all instructions are present in the emulator at all times.

The XSB compiler performs one particular instruction compression during its peephole optimization: the sequence *getlist,unitvar,unitvar* is compressed to *getlist_tvar_tvar*; append/3 in particular benefits. Table 4 mentions it as *getlist*. We implemented two more instruction compressions and two specializations:

- **dealloc**: compresses the instruction sequence *deallocate, proceed* into one (new) instruction *dealloc_proceed*, the sequence *deallocate, execute* into *deallex* and *deallocate, builtin, proceed* into *builtin, dealloc_proceed*;
- **uni**: two subsequent *unitva** instructions are compressed to one instruction; this leads to four instructions *uni_tvaX_tvaY* where X and Y can be *r* or *l*; Yap also performs this compression;
- **try**: specialized versions for the *try, retry* and *trust* instructions are generated for predicates with arities 2 and 3; Yap does this for 0 up to 4;
- **switch**: this specialization exists in Yap and in some other forms in other implementations; if the list exit of a *switch_on_list* instruction points to the corresponding *getlist* instruction, a specialized *switch* instruction is generated which in the list exit jumps directly to the read-mode of the instruction *following* the *getlist*

Table 4. Variations of abstract machine code in dProlog

	default	try	dealloc	switch	getlist	uni	switch getlist	switch uni	getlist uni	switch getlist uni
boyer	40	42	40	40	40	40	40	40	40	40
browse	48	49	49	47	49	50	49	48	50	51
cal	77	80	77	77	77	77	77	77	77	77
chat	45	45	45	44	45	45	45	46	46	46
crypt	53	53	53	54	55	52	54	54	55	55
ham	59	66	59	59	66	61	66	61	70	70
meta_qsort	51	54	51	50	51	54	51	54	54	54
nrev	43	43	43	50	43	54	50	62	54	62
poly_10	32	32	32	32	32	33	32	33	33	33
queens_16	88	89	88	92	89	90	92	92	92	94
queens	106	115	105	106	106	107	108	108	113	116
reducer	19	19	19	19	19	19	18	19	20	19
sdda	40	41	41	40	41	40	41	40	41	41
send	49	49	49	46	49	49	49	49	49	49
tak	73	73	73	73	73	73	73	73	73	73
zebra	82	82	82	82	84	83	84	82	87	87
code	77038	77474	77477	77005	77317	78355	77317	78289	78913	78913
compile	776	785	782	776	782	789	784	787	796	796
code	81692	82236	82209	81641	82184	83177	82184	83075	84161	84161

The specialization *try* and compression *dealloc* are each independent of all the other transformations; they are performed in the order: *switch, getlist, uni*. A *switch* specialization prevents a *getlist* compression of the corresponding getlist instruction, but still allows the *uni* compression of the instructions after the getlist. Likewise, a *getlist* compression clearly prevents the application of *uni* compression on the unify instructions after the getlist. Since the interaction of these three transformations is tricky, we give all seven possibilities (together with the default, that makes 8).

7   Comparing Four Term Representation Schemas

Table 5 shows the execution times and some stack sizes for the four term representations mentioned in section 3. Every version here has the same default settings as in 6.1. Only heap and trail sizes are mentioned, as the choice point stack, local stack and the code size are the same for all four versions.

A priori, one can reason that heap_vars and parma_vars must consume the same amount of heap, while tag_on_data potentially consumes more (due to the absence of an optimized list representation) and wam_vars consumes less because some objects only ever live on the local stack. For the trail, one expects heap_vars and tag_on_data to trail exactly the same cells, while both wam_vars and parma_vars trail potentially more. Indeed, when a variable is bound to a non-variable in parma_vars all the cells in the chain representing the variable are bound and subject to trailing. Note also that in parma_vars trailing one cell needs two entries on the trail stack. It is clear that wam_vars must (conditionally) trail on globalizing a permanent variable. But even for permanent variables that are never globalized, wam_vars potentially trails more than heap_vars.

The figures in table 5 are in accordance with the above reasoning. However, for the smaller benchmarks, the difference in trail usage between parma_vars and the others is very small, which confirms the common knowledge that var-var bindings are uncommon ... for small benchmarks. The *compile* benchmark shows a different picture.

The huge difference between the heap usage of wam_vars and the others is striking. Even though 99% of the difference is caused by the double calls to functor/3 and arg/3 in *boyer*, and a better built-in calling convention would reduce the difference to almost zero, in general this extra heap consumption is a drawback for any schema that always globalizes variables.

In order to reduce the potential bias in common operations towards one particular term representation, we have tried for each version several ways to write (in C) the dereference operation: each version is run with the best (sometimes more than one) we found for it. For the wam_vars version, we have specialized the trailing test whenever possible.

Tag_on_data is clearly the loser. On the small benchmarks, wam_vars comes out as the winner with heap_vars a close second; parma_vars suffers badly from its disadvantages on some of the small benchmarks. On *compile* parma_vars wins, albeit with a small margin: the high number of trail entries (almost triple of heap_vars) indicates that more var-var bindings occur here and that is where parma_vars is at its strongest.

8   Related Work

[4] is worth mentioning because it gives good advice on implementing an emulator for Prolog. We have followed it to a large extent and we did benefit a lot from it. In fact, most of the advice we put to scrutiny turned out to be excellent, even though we were working in the context of a different abstract machine code generator and a different stack layout. So, our work is in line with [4], redoing partly its experiment in a different setting. [4] does not stress the importance

Table 5. Four schemas for term representation

	heap_vars	wam_vars	parma_vars	tag_on_data
boyer	40	38	40	42
browse	48	46	46	53
cal	77	75	77	77
chat	45	44	46	47
crypt	53	52	52	54
ham	59	58	60	64
meta_qsort	51	48	54	53
nrev	43	44	47	56
poly_10	32	31	34	34
queens_16	88	85	90	90
queens	106	103	113	113
reducer	19	18	21	21
sdda	40	42	43	44
send	49	45	52	49
tak	73	71	75	73
zebra	82	82	97	90
heap	448296	144069	448296	448366
trail	57677	58635	115366	57677
compile	776	776	773	840
heap	1369456	862479	1369505	1647279
trail	227623	237689	642356	227633

of the quality of the generated machine code, probably because its compiler - although not sophisticated - is of sufficient quality. We think that a decent compiler is very essential for speed. Also, [4] does not provide any insight in the importance of the double opcode schema for read-write mode propagation, which we do in section 5. Finally, [4] was not aimed at providing empirical data on alternative term representations. In fact, no such work exists as far as we know. Alternative term representations were always implemented in combination with other features which can obscure in unknown ways the effect of the choice of the term representation.

As far as "paper" comparisons is concerned: [11] describes nicely the issues involved in implementing PARMA variables and relates them to the WAM, but as the authors note themselves, it is impossible to conclude with any confidence how within the same implementation these two alternatives would compare. [13] compares only minimally tag-on-data with the usual WAM representation and focuses on the issue of term compression and stack usage.

9 Conclusion and Future Work

We have gathered experimental data on how four term representations that are easily compatible with the WAM compare and about choices in the implementation of the abstract machine compiler and emulator. One conclusion is that the tag_on_data representation seems the least attractive from the performance point of view. Its main attraction is in the fact that since pointers are tag-less, the address space is not restricted and that one can have up to 32 tag bits in the data, a luxury that can make any implementor's mouth water. Admittedly, we have not implemented term compression, but since [13] does not report a significant speedup related to term compression and sometimes even a slowdown, we feel that our conclusion holds. The situation with parma_vars is more complicated: first of all, one must realize that for admittedly artificial examples, parma_vars can perform arbitrarily better than the other version. Moreover, while parma_vars performs worse on the smaller benchmarks, it performs better on the one benchmark that makes more use of the full potential of the Prolog variable. The figures give a slight preference to wam_vars time wise over heap_vars, and space wise wam_vars clearly wins, modulo the remarks made in section 7. However, other considerations could make one prefer heap_vars. E.g. in the context of SLG-WAM, the trail *must* be tidied on cut as far as the local stack trailed entries goes. But tidying the trail has bad worst case complexity. Then choosing for a heap_vars schema seems suddenly quite attractive given the small time penalty. In any case, such tradeoffs should be made by the implementor and might be based on the figures here or after having seen the actual implementation of dProlog.

We have put a lot of effort into avoiding bias towards any one version of dProlog. In particular, we have made sure that in all versions the same abstract machine code is executed instruction by instruction, that the stack layout is the same, that the number of times the general unification is called is the same, that the indexing (in particular the occurrence and treatment of hash collisions) is the same etc. [4] When comparing the four term representation each within a different context, it will be next to impossible to keep all the above factors the same. However, one might also see this uniformity as a drawback: each of the term representations might benefit in a different way from a particular action, e.g. dereferencing during a particular instruction might be good in wam_vars but not in parma_vars. We are aware of the fact that given much more time, we can improve each of the four versions; but we are not aware of having favored any particular one. We have even put effort in providing each version with its best dereferencing macro and tag testing sequence.

The figures in section 6 give a good indication on which specializations, compressions and emulator optimizations are interesting and also uncover weaknesses in the XSB compiler. Our experience has been used in a partial redesign of XSB.

The experiments might show different results on other processors. Since dProlog is portable the experiments can be redone for other platforms. Still, some extra work is required, mainly because one must assign hardware registers to WAM registers carefully.

Like [4] we found that a fast emulator is a combination of the following factors: (1) a good discipline for writing C code, (2) selective use of gcc features, (3) a decent basic abstract machine code generator, (4) some instruction compression, (5) some instruction specialization. In dProlog, we were missing mostly item 3: while [4] claims for instance that a sophisticated register allocation (see e.g. [8]) is not needed, we found that bad register allocation as in XSB, is a real

---

[4] the number of times dereferencing is performed is *not* the same: wam_vars and parma_vars have by necessity more than heap_vars (about 6% for the benchmark suite); tag_on_data has marginally less because of a different optimal sequence of instructions in the switchonlist instruction

drawback. Also the following two points are very important in our opinion: single level indexing is to be preferred over double level indexing (see also [2]); and secondly the basic mechanism for (in-lined) built-ins must suit the emulator: the XSB mechanism leads to more register shuffling and executed emulator cycles.

One can wonder whether redoing the effort described in [4] in a different context is relevant: we think that redoing it in exactly the same context would have been meaningless. Our work shows that the advice of [4] is useful elsewhere.

Directly related to dProlog, there is ample work for speeding up the implementation. Apart from issues mentioned before, we think two more points are worth exploring further: specialization of built-ins (e.g. functor/3 is almost always called in one of two basic modes and the compiler usually knows which because of the var-val distinction) and instruction compression over predicate boundaries: the *call* or *execute* instructions transfer very often to the same instructions. We experimented shortly with both, but gathered until now insufficient systematic data to report on them.

More generally, there are still many things worth investigating within a fixed implementation context: there is for instance no hard comparative data on entirely different tagging schemas, e.g. like the one SICStus Prolog is using. Other issues are the implementation of general unify (with support for cyclic terms or occurs check), optimal abstract machine code for arithmetic, calling of built-ins, the use of type or mode information in an emulator (as in [10]) and many more. Also different allocation schemas within a WAM-like implementation can and should be experimented with, together with different garbage collection strategies and principles. Inspiration here might come from the implementation of other programming languages. The problem with memory management experiments is however that an entirely new type of benchmarks is needed.

We will definitely continue using dProlog for experimenting and gathering information on the implementation of WAM variants and beyond.

Acknowledgements

We thank the XSB team – in particular David S. Warren and Kostis Sagonas – for making their compiler and system available, and for explanations. We are also grateful to Vitor S. Costa and Paul Tarau for making their systems freely available and for help in using them.

References

1. H. Aït-Kaci. *Warren's Abstract Machine: A Tutorial Reconstruction.* The MIT Press, Cambridge, Massachusetts, 1991.
2. M. Carlsson. *Freeze, Indexing and Other Implementation Issues in the WAM.* Proceedings of the 4th International Conference on Logic Programming, Melbourne, 1987, pp 40-58
3. M. Carlsson. *Design and Implementation of an Or-Parallel Prolog Engine.* PhD thesis, The Royal Institute of Technology (KTH), Stokholm, Sweden, Mar. 1990.
4. V. S. Costa, *Optimising Bytecode Emulation for Prolog.* Proceedings of PPDP'99, LNCS 1702, Springer-Verlag, 261-277, September, 1999.

5. B. Demoen, M. García de la Banda, W. Harvey, K. Marriott, and P. Stuckey. *Herbrand Constraint Solving in HAL*. Proceedings of the International Conference on Logic Programming 1999, Las Cruces, New Mexico, ed. D. De Schreye, MIT Press, pp. 260–274

6. B. Demoen, G. Janssens, H. Vandecasteele. *Executing Query Flocks for ILP*. Proceedings of BENELOG'99, Maastricht, 5 November 1999

7. B. Demoen, K. Sagonas. *Heap Garbage Collection in XSB: Practice and Experience* Proceedings of the Second Int. Workshop on Practical Aspects of Declarative Languages, Boston, Jan. 2000, pp. 93–108

8. G. Janssens, B. Demoen, A. Mariën. *Improving the register allocation in WAM by reordering unification*. Int. Conference & Symposium on Logic Programming, Seattle, Washington aug 1988, pp. 1388-1402

9. A. Mariën, B. Demoen. *On the management of E and B in WAM*. Proceedings of the North American Conference on Logic Programming, Cleveland, Ohio, oct 1989, pp. 1030-1047

10. Phuong-Lan Nguyen. *Optimisation du Code produit par un Compilateur Prolog*. Rapport de DEA, ENSIMAG, Laboratoire de Génie Informatique, Grenoble, 1988

11. T. Lindgren, P. Mildner, and J. Bevemyr. *On Taylor's scheme for unbound variables*. Technical report, UPMAIL, October 1995.

12. P. Tarau. *Program Transformations and WAM-support for the Compilation of Definite Metaprograms*. In A. Voronkov, editor, Logic Programming, RCLP Proceedings, number 592 in Lecture Notes in Artificial Intelligence, pages 462-473, Berlin, Heidelberg, 1992. Springer-Verlag.

13. P. Tarau and U. Neumerkel. *A Novel Term Compression Scheme and Data Representation in the BinWAM*. Proceedings of Programming Language Implementation and Logic Programming, sept. 1994, Springer, LNCS 844, pp. 73–87

14. A. Taylor. *PARMA–bridging the performance gap between imperative and logic programming*. Journal of Logic Programming, 29(1–3), 1996.

15. P. Van Roy. *Can Logic Programming Execute as Fast as Imperative Programming ?* Report 90/600, UCB/CSD, Berkeley, California 94720, Dec 1990.

16. D. H. D. Warren. *An Abstract Prolog Instruction Set*. Technical Report 309, SRI International, Menlo Park, U.S.A., Oct. 1983.

17. See http://www.cs.sunysb.edu/~sbprolog/.

A Module Based Analysis for Memory Reuse in Mercury[*]

Nancy Mazur, Gerda Janssens, and Maurice Bruynooghe

Department of Computer Science, K.U.Leuven
Celestijnenlaan, 200A, B–3001 Leuven, Belgium
{nancy,gerda,maurice}@cs.kuleuven.ac.be

Abstract. In previous work Bruynooghe, Janssens and Kågedal developed a live-structure analysis for Mercury which detects memory cells available for reuse. Separate compilation of modules is an essential ingredient of a language such as Mercury which supports programming in the large. Hence, to be practical, a live-structure analysis also has to be module based. This paper develops a modular live-structure analysis and extends it with a modular reuse analysis. It also describes preliminary results obtained with a first prototype of the module based analysis.

1 Introduction

In declarative languages, the programmer is liberated from the low level details of memory management such as allocation of memory and destructive updates of data structures. The price to pay for this convenience is a loss of performance due to the run-time overhead of garbage collection, due to an increased number of cache misses (caused by the loss of locality of data structures) and due to the overhead of creating new data structures (creating a new version of a data structure is typically more expensive than updating an existing one).

There has been a lot of research on methods to overcome this handicap and improve the memory management, both for logic programming languages [5, 12, 14], as for functional programming languages [10, 19]. Some approaches depend on a combination of special language constructs and analysis [17, 1, 21], others are solely based on compiler analyses [7, 11, 20]. At least in logic programming, none of the analysis based methods has reached the maturity of becoming part of a widely distributed implementation, so this largely remains an unsolved problem.

A language as Mercury, a logic language with declarations [17], offers a partial solution through the availability of destructive input *di* and unique output *uo* modes; however the use of these modes is cumbersome for the programmer. Moreover it does not fit into the declarative programming paradigm. Hence we believe it is a useful research goal to develop a reuse analysis for Mercury. In addition, mastering it for Mercury should be a useful stepping stone for developing such an analysis for systems such as Ciao Prolog [9] where declarations are

---

[*] This work has been supported by the GOA project LP$^+$, the ESPRIT project ARGo, and the FWO-Vlaanderen.

J. Lloyd et al. (Eds.): CL 2000, LNAI 1861, pp. 1255–1269, 2000.

optional and where one has to cope with the impurities of Prolog and HAL [6] which is a constraint language having many similarities with Mercury.

Mulkers et al. [14] have developed an analysis for Prolog which detects when memory cells become available for reuse; however the lack of declarations and the impurity of Prolog make it rather infeasible to obtain acceptable analysis times and to integrate it in a Prolog compiler. In [3] Bruynooghe et al. have adapted the analysis for a Mercury-like language with type, mode and determinism declarations; the analysis takes also backtracking into account (the original work relied on the trail to restore overwritten data structures on backtracking). The paper only briefly sketches some preliminary ideas about how to make the analysis modular. Modularity is essential for the analysis to be practical as it is infeasible to analyse large programs (e.g. the Mercury compiler) as a single unit. The concept of modules is an integral part of the Mercury support for *programming in the large* and even simple applications import predicates from libraries. Moreover, Mercury compiles each module of a program separately, hence an analysis which has to become part of the compiler better does the same. This paper presents a module based analysis for memory reuse as a two step analysis where a so called default liveness analysis of the procedures exported by the module is followed by a reuse analysis. Results obtained by a prototype are presented. Finally the paper suggests also some solutions w.r.t. the creation of multiple versions for procedures.

The paper is a reworking and elaboration of [13] where the non modular default analysis was first described. Modularisation of analysis is also a current research issue in the Ciao Prolog project. A discussion of possible approaches which have quite some parallels with our work is in [15].

Section 2 recalls the basics of the work described in [3]. Section 3 develops module based liveness analysis. Section 4 reports on the results obtained with our prototype analysis system. We conclude with a brief discussion in Section 5.

2   Background

2.1   Abstract Interpretation

The analysis system in [3] uses the top-down abstract interpretation framework of [2]. Abstract interpretation mimics concrete execution by replacing the program's operations on concrete data with abstract operations over data descriptions. The analysis of a predicate, given abstract information about the predicate's arguments (*call pattern*), computes abstract information for each program point, and a final abstract description of the state of the variables at the exit point (*exit pattern*). For each predicate call, abstract information from the caller's context is mapped onto information relevant for the called predicate (*procedure entry*), thus obtaining the call pattern of that predicate. The called predicate is analysed w.r.t. this call pattern. The obtained exit pattern will be used to compute the abstract state of the program point following the predicate call (*procedure exit*). The analysis uses fixpoint iteration to cope with recursion.

2.2   Mercury

Mercury [8] is a logic programming language with types, modes and determinism declarations. Its type system is based on a polymorphic many-sorted logic and its mode-system does not allow the use of partially instantiated structures.

Our analysis is performed at the level of the *High Level Data Structure* (HLDS) constructed by the Mercury compiler. Within this structure, predicates are *normalized*, i.e. all atoms appearing in the program have distinct variables as arguments, and all unifications $X = Y$ are explicited as one of (1) a test $X == Y$, (2) an assignment $X := Y$, (3) a construction $X \Leftarrow f(Y_1, \ldots, Y_n)$, or (4) a deconstruction $X \Rightarrow f(Y_1, \ldots, Y_n)$. Within the HLDS, the atoms of a clause body are –if needed– reordered such that the body is well moded.

Just like in the HLDS we will use the notion of a *procedure*, i.e. a combination of one predicate with *one* mode, and thus talk about the analysis of a procedure.

2.3   Types and Selectors

Using a simple example, we recall some basics about types.

The polymorphic type $list(T)$ is defined as: `list(T)--->[] ; [T|list(T)]`. This type is obtained by applying a *type constructor* (`list`) on zero or more types or type variables (here type variable `T`). Its definition is given by the right hand side of the above expression and consists of one or more alternatives. Each alternative is a distinct *type functor* applied to zero or more types or type variables (`[]` has zero arguments, the list constructor has two, namely `T` and `list(T)`). A *type tree* is a possibly infinite graphical representation of a type definition. A finite *type graph* is obtained by imposing that two type nodes on the same branch from the root are the same when they are labelled with the same type. The graph of `list(T)` is shown in Fig. 1: it has two type nodes (`list(T)` and `T`) and two functor nodes (`[]` and `[.]`).

Type selectors are used to select type nodes in type graphs. The empty selector is denoted by ϵ; with t a type, t^ϵ selects the root node of its type graph. If t_0^s selects a node of type t_1 in the type graph of t_0 and one of the alternatives defining t_1 has a type functor f/n then $t_0^{s.(f,j)}$ with $j \leq n$ selects the type node which is the jth child of the functor node labeled f/n that is a child of t_1.

With recursive types, several selectors can select the same node in a type graph. This equivalence is denoted with $s_1 \equiv s_2$, with s_1 and s_2 selectors. Using "." as list constructor, $list(T)^{(.,2)}$ and $list(T)^\epsilon$ both select the root node. Our analysis always simplifies selectors, hence will replace the former by the latter.

Terms also have a tree representation and nodes of the term tree can be mapped to type nodes of the corresponding type tree. With X a variable which has a term of type t as value and with s a selector for t, X^s denotes the nodes in the term tree of X which are mapped to t^s. We refer to the memory cells implementing these nodes as the *data structure* of X^s. X^ϵ selects (at least) the root node of the term tree. This root node is the *top-level data structure* of X.

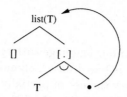

Fig. 1. Type graph of list(T)

2.4   Liveness Analysis

Our liveness analysis exploits the mode, type and determinism information available in the HLDS of Mercury programs. It can be applied on any sequential logic programming language where this information is available through declarations or analysis. Due to the absence of partially instantiated data structures every unification can be reduced to one of the cases in Section 2.2. Although the analysis can handle full unification, the ultimate reuse will depend on the presence of deconstruction/construction pairs. With less precise modes, less of these pairs occur in the code.

The liveness analysis of [3] computes in each program point which data structures are live. Calling the program point under consideration the *current* program point and the atom following it the *current* atom, a data structure is **live** in the *current* program point if –given the bindings of the program variables before executing the current atom– the data structure is reachable

- either from a program variable occurring in an atom following the *next* program point (hence it will possibly be accessed while continuing the execution after successful completion of the current atom).
- or from a program variable which will possibly be accessed after the backtracking which would occur if the execution of the current atom fails.

Liveness is expressed as a set of elements X^s. That X^s is live in program point p means that the data structure(s) selected by X^s in the current value of the variable X will probably be accessed after executing the current atom.

The liveness set in a program point p is computed from two components:

- A binary relation $ALIAS$. Tuples in this relation are of the form (X^s, Y^t). The intuitive meaning is: if data structure X^s is live then Y^t is *possibly* live and, if Y^t is live, then X^s is *possibly* live[1]. The relation is not transitive as we maintain only one $ALIAS$ relation in each program point, hence it is possible that (X^s, Y^t) holds due to one computation path and (Y^t, Z^r) due to another incompatible computation path, while (X^s, Z^r) does not

---

[1] Possibly because the analysis makes approximations and may overestimate the $ALIAS$ relation. Also reflexive tuples exist, e.g. $(X^{(\cdot,1)}, X^{(\cdot1)})$ with X of type list expresses: if one element of the list is live then others are possibly live, in other words the value of X is a list with possibly several occurrences of the same element.

hold. When, due to a unification or a procedure call, new $ALIAS$ tuples are derived then an *alternating closure* which alternates over new and old tuples is used to update the $ALIAS$ relation. The $ALIAS$ relation consists of a global component GA containing the aliases between input arguments of the procedure that existed prior to calling the analysed procedure and a local componant LA_p giving the aliases created by executing the procedure up to the program point p. The whole $ALIAS$ relation is then given by the alternating closure of both components, i.e. $ALIAS_p = Altclos(GA, LA_p)$.

- A set IN_USE. It is the union of two sets. The first, $LIVE_0$, is a global component which contains elements X^s expressing that X^s is live due to the context of the caller. In other words, X^s will probably be accessed after completion (with success or failure) of the current procedure. It is called $LIVE_0$ because it is derived from the liveness which exists in the program point where the analysed procedure is called. The second set, LU_p, is a local component containing elements X^ϵ for every variable which can be accessed after completing the execution of the current atom (with success or failure).

The set $LIVE_p$ describing the liveness in a program point is obtained by using the implications in $ALIAS_p$ to extend the initial liveness set given by IN_USE_p. More formally, defining

$$\mathcal{L}(L, A) = \begin{array}{l} \{X^s | X^s \in L\} \\ \cup \, \{X^s | Y^t \in L \text{ and } (Y^{t.t_1}, X^s) \in A\} \\ \cup \, \{X^{t.s_1} | Y^{s.s_1} \in L \text{ and } (Y^s, X^t) \in A\} \end{array} \tag{1}$$

we have

$$LIVE_p = \mathcal{L}(IN\_USE_p, ALIAS_p) \tag{2}$$

where $IN\_USE_p = LIVE_0 \cup LU_p$ and $ALIAS_p = Altclos(GA, LA_p)$. For more technical details we refer to [3].

2.5 Reuse Analysis

The liveness analysis computes a safe approximation of the liveness, hence a data structure which is not live is –if reachable at all– only reachable from the program variables in the current atom. The interesting case is when the current atom is a deconstruction $X \Rightarrow f(X_1, \ldots, X_n)$ and X^ϵ is not live in the current program point. Then, [3] the data structure X^ϵ is *available for reuse* in the program point following the deconstruction as it is no more reachable from any accessible program variable. If, within the procedure, the deconstruction is followed by a construction $Y \Leftarrow f(Y_1, \ldots, Y_n)$ then the top level of X can be used to construct Y and we say that there is *direct* reuse (of X^ϵ) in the analysed procedure. We say that a procedure has *indirect* reuse if it calls a procedure q/m and q/m allows for (in the context of that call) direct or indirect reuse. To distinguish this phase from the liveness analysis, we call it the *reuse analysis*. When analysing the program as a single unit, this pass requires no fixpoint iteration as it only has to verify whether deconstruction/construction pairs are fitted for reuse.

2.6   Using the Analysis Results

Which deconstruction/construction pairs are suited for reuse can be returned to the compiler as an extra piece of information in the HLDS code. The work of Taylor [18] could be adapted to perform the actual reuse. Actually this should be easier than the current approach which still requires a non-trivial local analysis of the programmer-provided di/uo annotations.

An important point to recall is that procedures can be called with different call patterns and that one obtains a form of multiple specialisation as described in [16]. Eventually, although having different call patterns, two versions may end up with identical direct and indirect reuse, hence should be merged in a single version. Such version control is discussed in [16]. As also explained there, the analysis has two phases. In our case, the first phase performs the liveness analysis and constructs a table with call/exit patterns (a pattern consists of the $ALIAS$ relation and the IN_USE set). This phase requires fixpoint iteration to handle recursive procedures. The second phase performs a single pass over the program, generates the required versions for each procedure and checks whether deconstruction/construction pairs satisfy the reuse condition. It also takes care that each procedure call calls the proper version.

3   Module Based Analysis

For separate compilation of modules Mercury uses interfaces which are created during compilation and which contain the needed information of the exported predicates. Mutual dependencies are not a problem as all relevant information about exported procedures is in the obligatory declarations. However, mutual dependencies pose a problem during abstract interpretation of mutually recursive predicates defined in different modules. This problem is discussed in Sect.3.3. For the time being, we assume a tree structure for the calling hierarchy between modules.

3.1   Modular Liveness Analysis

The domain of the liveness analysis is suited for a so called goal independent analysis [4]. Starting the analysis of a procedure p/n with an empty $LIVE_0$ and an empty GA component, one obtains as exit pattern the $ALIAS$ relation describing the possible aliases created between the arguments of p/n due to the execution of p/n. Similarly, one obtains the IN_USE component describing the arguments of p/n in use due to the execution of p/n (which are nothing else than the data structures in the arguments which could be needed when backtracking returns control to p/n). This goal independent information about p/n suffices to perform the liveness analysis of a procedure q/m calling p/n. Combining the goal independent exit pattern of p/n with the liveness information of the point before the call to p/n, one can compute the liveness in the program point following p/n^2. Storing the call/exit patterns of exported predicates in the module interface, modules importing predicates can be analysed by accessing their call/exit pattern in the corresponding interfaces. Hence a goal independent liveness analysis can be performed in a modular way.

3.2   Modular Reuse Analysis

For a truly modular analysis, the reuse analysis must also be modular. Problem is that reuse is not goal independent. One useful property is that the amount of reuse decreases monotonically with increases of $LIVE_0$, the liveness in the caller's context and GA, the aliases in the caller's context. Hence performing a reuse analysis based on a goal independent liveness analysis of a procedure exported from a module gives a maximal amount of reuse. However, it is unlikely that an actual call will ever have $LIVE_0 = \emptyset$. At least the output arguments of the procedure will be in $LIVE_0$[3]. This suggests the following approach for analysing procedures exported from a module: besides the standard Mercury code without reuse, a version with reuse is generated. It is created starting from a liveness analysis of these procedures which are initialised with $GA = \emptyset$ and $LIVE_0 = \{X^\epsilon | X \ is \ an \ output \ argument\}$ (called the *default liveness analysis*). The standard reuse analysis is applied on the outcome of this analysis and results in code with reuse annotations for the exported procedure and for the internal procedures called by them. When calling an imported procedure, one can check whether the caller's context meets the assumption for reuse, i.e. whether there are no aliases between the (input) arguments of the procedure and none of the input arguments is live. If so, the version with reuse can be called; if not, the version without reuse is called. In what follows, we call the default liveness analysis of the procedures exported by a module followed by the reuse analysis the *default analysis* of the module.

The above approach is overly pessimistic. Consider predicate *append* with mode (in,in,out). The default analysis reveals that the backbone of the first input list can be reused for constructing the output list. Calls with the elements of the first input list live, or with the second input list live do not meet the requirement for using the reuse version. However, performing the analysis for such call patterns reveals that reuse is still possible. Intuitively, the reuse version of *append* can be called when the backbone of the first input list is not live. More generally, the problem to be addressed is: which results about the default analysis should be stored and how to check that a particular call meets the requirements to call the reuse version resulting from the default analysis.

---

[2] Although the $ALIAS$ component is not idempotent, $Altclos(ALIAS, ALIAS) \neq ALIAS$, there is no loss of precision with respect to a goal dependent analysis. This is because the aliases created during the analysis of p/n depend only on the mode declared for p/n, not on the call pattern of p/n.

[3] Making a call and not using some of the outputs is not impossible; however, we consider it part of a preceding source level specialisation step to create a special version of the procedure with the unneeded outputs eliminated.

3.2.1   Conditions for Reuse. In what follows, a component is given a subscript i when its value depends on the program point i. It is given a superscript da or gd when its value differs between the default and the goal dependent analysis.

Consider the following program fragment:

```
q(Q1,...,Qn) :- ... ; X => f(...), ...
```

Performing a default liveness analysis for q/n, formula (2) applied at program point i yields the live set

$$LIVE_i^{da} = \mathcal{L}(LU_i \cup LIVE_0^{da}, LA_i) \tag{3}$$

where $LIVE_0^{da} = \{Q_i^\epsilon | Q_i$ is an output argument of $q\}$ and LU_i, LA_i are respectively the local use and the local aliases at i. The top level of X becomes available for reuse when $X^\epsilon \notin LIVE_i^{da}$. A goal-dependent analysis of q/n computes

$$LIVE_i^{gd} = \mathcal{L}(LU_i \cup LIVE_0^{gd}, Altclos(LA_i, GA^{gd})) \tag{4}$$

with $LIVE_0^{gd}$ the initial liveness of q/n and GA^{gd} the initial aliases of q/n. We want to check whether reuse is still possible without performing a goal dependent analysis for q/n. To do so, we first present a theorem which addresses a slightly more general situation. First we introduce some new notation.

- With R a relation over (a set from) a domain of data structures and V a set of variables, $R|_V$ denotes the restriction of the relation to the variables in V.
- With D a set of data structures, V a set of variables and LA_i the local aliases at a program point i, D_i^V is the abbreviation for $\mathcal{L}(D, LA_i)|_V$, i.e. the restriction to V of the data structures reachable from the set D due to the aliases in LA_i.

Theorem 1. *Given a procedure with head variables $\mathcal{H}$ and local aliases LA_i and local use LU_i at program point i. Let D be a set of data structures from the procedure. If*

$$X^s \in D \text{ implies } X^s \notin \mathcal{L}(LU_i \cup LIVE_0^{da}, LA_i) \tag{5}$$

$$Y^t \in D_i^{\mathcal{H}} \text{ implies } Y^t \notin \mathcal{L}(LIVE_0^{gd} \cup LU_i^{\mathcal{H}}, Altclos(GA^{gd}, LA_i|_{\mathcal{H}})) \tag{6}$$

then

$$X^s \in D \text{ implies } X^s \notin \mathcal{L}(LU_i \cup LIVE_0^{gd}, Altclos(GA^{gd}, LA_i)) \tag{7}$$

Proof. Note that GA^{gd} and $LIVE_0^{gd}$ contain only data structures from $\mathcal{H}$. Assume $X^s \in \mathcal{L}(LU_i \cup LIVE_0^{gd}, Altclos(GA^{gd}, LA_i))$. $X^s \in LU_i \cup LIVE_0^{gd}$ is in contradiction with conditions (5) ($X^s \notin LU_i$) and (6) (if $X^s \in LIVE_0^{gd}$ then $X \in \mathcal{H}$ but then $X^s \in D_i^{\mathcal{H}}$) of the theorem. Hence there must be a path starting in $Z^t \in LU_i \cup LIVE_0^{gd}$, alternating over GA^{gd} and LA_i and ending in X^s (according to (1)). We perform a case analysis and show that each case is inconsistent with the conditions of the theorem.

– $Z \notin \mathcal{H}$ (hence $Z^t \in LU_i$)
  - path of length 1: $(Z^t, X^s) \in LA_i$ and thus (5) is violated for X^s.
  - path of length > 1: The first edge in the path is of the form $(Z^t, Y_1^{s_1})$ and belongs to LA_i; moreover (the path alternates with GA^{gd}) $Y_1 \in \mathcal{H}$ hence $Y_1^{s_1} \in LU_i^{\mathcal{H}}$. From the assumption it follows that $(Y_1^{s_1}, X^s) \in Altclos(GA^{gd}, LA_i)$, hence an alternating path $(Y_1^{s_1}, Y_2^{s_2}), \ldots, (Y_n^{s_n}, X^s)$ with $Y_1, \ldots, Y_n \in \mathcal{H}$ exists. If $X^s \in \mathcal{H}$ then we have $(Y_1^{s_1}, X^s) \in Altclos(GA^{gd}, LA_i|_{\mathcal{H}})$ and (6) is violated for X^s. Otherwise $X^s \notin \mathcal{H}$, hence $Y_n^{s_n} \in D_i^{\mathcal{H}}$ and $(Y_1^{s_1}, Y_n^{s_n}) \in Altclos(GA^{gd}, LA_i|_{\mathcal{H}})$ hence (6) is violated for Y^{s_n}.

– $Z \in \mathcal{H}$ (hence $Z^t \in LU_i|_{\mathcal{H}} \cup LIVE_0^{gd}$)
  - path of length 1: Either $(Z^t, X^s) \in GA^{gd}$ or $(Z^t, X^s) \in LA_i$. In the former case, $(Z^t, X^s) \in Altclos(GA^{gd}, LA_i|_{\mathcal{H}})$ and (6) is violated for X^s. In the latter case, either $Z^t \in LU_i$ and (5) is violated for X^s or $Z^t \in LIVE_0^{gd}$, hence also $Z^t \in D_i^{\mathcal{H}}$ and condition (6) is violated for Z^t.
  - path of length > 1: $(Z^t, X^s) \in Altclos(GA^{gd}, LA_i)$ hence there is an alternating path $(Y_1^t, Y_2^{s_2}), \ldots, (Y_n^{s_n}, X^s)$ with $Z = Y_1$ and $Y_1, \ldots, Y_n \in \mathcal{H}$. If $X^s \in \mathcal{H}$ then $(Y_1^t, X^s) \in Altclos(GA^{gd}, LA_i|_{\mathcal{H}})$ and condition (6) is violated for X^s. Otherwise $X^s \notin \mathcal{H}$, hence $Y_n^{s_n} \in D_i^{\mathcal{H}}$ and $(Y_1^t, Y_n^{s_n}) \in Altclos(GA^{gd}, LA_i|_{\mathcal{H}})$ hence condition (6) is violated for $Y_n^{s_n}$.

□

With $D = \{X^\epsilon\}$, the set of data structures potentially available for reuse, condition (5) verifies whether X^ϵ is available for reuse in the default analysis, while condition (7) verifies whether X^ϵ is available for reuse in the goal dependent analysis. Hence, given that reuse is possible in the default case, the theorem says that the latter condition can be replaced by condition (6) which is a condition involving only head variables. It suffices to store the relations/sets $LA_i|_{\mathcal{H}}$, $D_i^{\mathcal{H}}$ and $LU_i^{\mathcal{H}}$ (the *reuse information*) in the module interface to allow a caller to check whether it can call the reuse version of the imported procedure q/n.

Consider $append(A, B, C)$ with mode (in,in,out), $\mathcal{H} = \{A, B, C\}$ and $LIVE_0^{da} = \{C^\epsilon\}$. The default analysis computes in the point preceding $A \Rightarrow \ldots$ that $D = \{A^\epsilon\} = D_i^{\mathcal{H}}$, $LA_i|_{\mathcal{H}} = \emptyset$ and $LU_i^{\mathcal{H}} = \{B^\epsilon, C^\epsilon\}$. Consider a call with $LIVE_0^{gd} = \{A^{(.,1)}, C^\epsilon\}$ and $GA^{gd} = \emptyset$. Condition (6) becomes: $Y^t \in D_i^{\mathcal{H}}$ implies $Y^t \notin \mathcal{L}(\{A^{(.,1)}, B^\epsilon, C^\epsilon\}, \emptyset)$ which is satisfied.

We also have to address the problem of verifying whether a version with indirect reuse can be called. Consider the following fragment:

```
r(R1,...,Rm) :- ... ; q(X1,...,Xn), ...
q(Q1,...,Qn) :- ... ; X => f(...), ...
```

To verify that the default version of r/m can call the version of q/n with reuse at program point i, one should check that the data structures in $D' = \rho(D_i^{\mathcal{H}_q})$ (ρ renames the variables in the head of q/n into the variables in the call to q/n) are not live, taking into account $LA'_j = LA_j \cup \rho(LA_i|_{\mathcal{H}})$ as local aliases and

$LU'_j = LU_j \cup \rho(LU_i^{\mathcal{H}})$ as local use (this is the rephrasing of (6) to the context of program point j). If this indirect reuse is possible in the default case, then the reuse information over the variables of r/m ($LA'_j|_{\mathcal{H}_r}$, $D'_j{}^{\mathcal{H}_r}$, and $LU'_j{}^{\mathcal{H}_r}$) can be computed. A caller to r/m can use the version of r/m with indirect reuse in q/m if (6) is satisfied for the reuse information of r/m. Repeating this, the reuse information can be propagated up to the level of the exported predicates. Note that here fixpoint iteration is needed to handle recursive procedures (the reuse information of a recursive procedure is needed while computing it).

3.2.2   Version Control. The default analysis of an exported procedure may reveal more than one point for reuse: there can be several deconstruction/construction pairs allowing reuse as well as indirect reuse through calls to procedures with reuse. For each case of reuse, a relation $LA_i|_{\mathcal{H}}$ and sets $D_i^{\mathcal{H}}$ and $LU_i^{\mathcal{H}}$ are obtained so that the condition for the particular reuse can be tested by a caller. (The reuse is unconditional when $D_i^{\mathcal{H}}$ is empty.) If all conditions are satisfied then the version of the exported procedure which performs all the reuses can be called. If one of the conditions is violated, should one give up all reuse and call the version without any reuse? Ideally one should call a version which performs all the other reuses. This would require to create 2^n versions of the procedure when there are n places with (different) conditional reuse. This becomes infeasible for large n. Experience will have to show whether many cases of conditional reuse show up in a single procedure. If so, some pragmatic solutions will have to be worked out. Several scenarios are feasible:

- Only make 2 versions, one without any conditional reuse and one with all conditional reuses.
- Provide the programmer with a pragma to express interest in the reuse of a data structure. Then only the versions with conditional reuse involving these data structures are created. Such a pragma should still be much less tedious to use than *di/uo* declarations.
- Make versions on demand: reuse code is only generated if a call occurs for which a particular set of reuse conditions is satisfied. This scenario breaks with the strict modularity of the compilation process. Also, versions created on demand for the compilation of another module may finally never be called from the main program.
- Create all possible versions and add a final *global* analysis pass: once all modules of a program are analysed, a final global compilation can be performed, which, starting from the top-level module, makes a single pass over the whole program (and thus compiled code), and links those versions of the procedures which are actually needed into the final compiled code. While this solution also departs from the strict modularity principle, once modules are compiled with all their multitude of procedure versions, these modules will not have to be recompiled if used for other programs.

3.3   Circular Dependencies between Modules

A problematic circular dependency exists when predicates that depend on each other are distributed over different modules. Several solutions with different computational costs are feasible (see also the discussion in [15]).

- When importing a procedure from a module which cannot be analysed due to a circular dependency, a worst case assumption can be made for the liveness (all arguments are live) and for the aliasing (all pairs of data structures with compatible types are aliases) of the imported procedure. This allows to continue the analysis of the current module but gives a suboptimal result.
- Another solution is to make a best case assumption (only the output arguments are live and there are no aliases) and to reanalyse the current module when this assumption turns out to be false. So a fixpoint iteration across modules will be necessary.
- A third solution is to load all dependent modules and analyse them together as one module. If the module is too large, the call graph of its procedures could be used to split it into parts that can be compiled separately.

4   Experimental Results

A prototype of the modular analysis has been implemented. The first phase performs a default liveness analysis of the exported procedures and the second phase uses its results to perform a reuse analysis. It creates for each exported procedure two versions (unless both versions are identical): one version with unconditional reuse only (or none at all) and a version with all possible reuse. For the latter version, the reuse information is also computed. It allows callers to verify whether they meet the conditions for reuse.

4.1   Benchmarks and Results

The following modules are analysed: basic library modules for tree and list manipulation (assoc_list, bintree, bool, bt_array, list, set_ordlist, tree234), library modules which import procedures from the basic ones (bag, bintree_set, eqvclass, graph, group, map, multi_map, queue, set, set_unordlist), a module of the industrial users of Mercury in the ESPRIT project ARGo (argo_cnters) and modules from the Mercury compiler (labelopt, llds, opt_util). In table 1 the library modules are in the upper part and the other modules in the lower part.

Time The time in seconds of the default liveness analysis[4].
Pr The number of procedures in the module.
Xp The number of exported procedures.
CR The number of exported procedures for which conditional reuse is detected.

---

[4] The analysis is done with a generic abstract interpretation tool written in Prolog, using Master Prolog, release 4.1 ERP on a UltraSPARC-IIi (333MHz) with 256MB RAM, using SunOS Release 5.7, under a usual workload.

Table 1. Results; "-" means not applicable.

module	Time	Pr	Xp	CR	UR	NR	Cnd	pol	DC	%DR	Lc	%LR	Ec	EcR	%ER
assoc_list	0.27	7	6	5	0	1	2.40	1.00	7	100	7	86	10	0	-
bag	2.46	26	24	17	10	5	4.95	1.19	4	100	29	90	70	25	100
bintree	1.37	30	19	6	2	11	3.00	1.03	17	100	56	43	33	0	-
bintree_set	0.16	23	21	11	6	9	1.08	1.04	1	100	16	75	26	6	100
bool	0.01	5	5	2	0	3	2.00	1.00	2	100	2	100	0	0	-
bt_array	5.97	37	17	6	4	9	1.75	2.30	38	97	137	55	181	0	-
eqvclass	1.55	21	12	4	4	4	1.00	1.19	5	100	27	78	37	12	100
graph	6.96	26	14	6	6	6	0.75	1.38	9	100	42	33	51	12	100
group	1.95	20	11	2	4	7	0.50	1.25	4	100	27	41	27	8	100
list	1.84	66	56	34	3	22	1.76	1.21	46	91	111	64	38	2	100
map	6.69	42	38	16	4	18	3.65	1.24	2	100	39	54	56	16	100
multi_map	1.95	36	33	11	6	16	2.82	1.03	1	0	13	46	48	21	100
queue	0.18	12	11	5	1	6	2.80	1.00	4	100	2	100	12	8	100
set	0.08	27	27	6	0	21	1.00	1.00	0	-	0	-	27	6	100
set_ordlist	0.52	31	29	6	0	23	1.00	1.16	7	0	41	2	19	6	100
set_unordlist	0.34	30	27	13	3	14	1.15	1.10	1	100	25	64	12	6	100
tree234	1140	74	20	10	1	9	5.55	1.14	283	88	443	71	136	0	-
argo_cnters	4.79	18	1	0	1	0	0.00	1.00	32	100	41	29	56	0	-
labelopt	12.00	6	2	2	1	0	2.00	2.00	2	100	17	88	13	9	78
llds	0.08	7	7	0	0	7	-	1.00	0	-	6	0	2	0	-
opt_util	2028	73	46	20	8	23	2.04	1.47	48	83	284	28	70	24	100

UR The number of exported procedures for which unconditional reuse is detected. (The two types of reuse can occur in the same procedure.)

NR The number of exported procedures without reuse.

Cnd The average number of reuse conditions for exported procedures with conditional reuse. Some conditions might be equal (i.e. different sources of reuse might produce exactly the same reuse information). The number of reduced conditions is not available here.

pol The average polyvariance resulting from the liveness analysis, i.e. the average number of call patterns per procedure.

DC The number of deconstruction/construction pairs in the analysed module.

%DR The percentage of deconstruction/construction pairs resulting in direct reuse.

Lc The number of calls to procedures internal at the module.

%LR The percentage of Lc that calls a version with reuse.

Ec The number of calls to imported procedures.

EcR The number of calls to imported procedures for which a reuse version exists.

%ER The percentage of EcR that calls a version with reuse. ("-" if EcR=0).

4.2   Discussion

– In most cases the analysis time is of the same order as the compilation time of the module. In a few cases it is rather large (tree234 and opt_util). We do not consider these times as unbearable, especially for library modules which have to be compiled only once. Modules importing them need only to consult the module interface. Our prototype leaves room for much improvement and it is a topic of further research to consider alternative representations of the *ALIAS* information and to develop appropriate widenings. Our reuse analysis is not yet fine-tuned enough to report reuse analysis times. In most cases the time needed for it is comparable to the time for the default liveness. We believe it should only be a small fraction of the total analysis time, especially in cases where the default analysis time is large.

– Reuse versions are created for a large fraction of exported predicates. Even unconditional reuse is quite frequent. This is an indication that our analysis is able to find an interesting amount of reuse.

– The average number of reuse conditions is in general small. However for bag and tree234 the average is about 5 conditions. In tree234 there is a procedure with 12 conditions. Yet some of these conditions appear to be equivalent, and upon simplification, the total set of different conditions is reduced to only 3. It seems not feasible to create a version for each of the combinations of reuse. It requires further experimentation to find out how many of the conditions are satisfied by typical calls to procedures with many conditions and what are good strategies for version creation (see discussion in 3.2.2).

– The polyvariance is in general low. The multiple specialisation inherent at the analysis does not result in an explosion of versions of the same procedure.

– Quite a large fraction of deconstruction/construction pairs result in direct reuse. If no direct reuse is detected, it is either because no reuse is possible or because the analysis is too imprecise. It requires hand analysis to find out what is the real cause; it is not feasible to analyse this on a large scale.

– Versions of local procedures with reuse are quite frequently called.

– Although the total number of calls to imported procedures (Ec) looks high with regard to the number of calls to such procedures for which a reuse version exists (EcR), most of the calls happen to be I/O related, or integer-operations, hence are to procedures which cannot have reuse versions.

4.3   Effect on the Performance of Mercury Programs

There is yet no version of the Mercury compiler which makes use of the reuse analysis. However, Taylor [18] has implemented structure reuse for a separate distribution of the Mercury compiler. It is based on the *di/uo* annotations provided by the programmer. Hand translating the reuse annotations in *di/uo* annotations, we did a few experiments.

For *argo_cnters*, a benchmark counting various properties in a file, this comparison revealed a speedup of up to 30% depending on the size of the input. Comparing memory usage yields an improvement of 50% (7 mega-words compared to 14 mega-words in the non-optimized version). Other programs (too small to be included in table 1), like *nrev* (naive reverse of a large list of integers), and *insert* (inserting elements in a binary tree) reveal speedups up to 75%, and memory savings up to 85%. The latter programs were also used as benchmarks in [18]. The *di/uo* annotations considered there correspond to the reuse annotations we derived.

5   Conclusion

This paper describes how the liveness analysis of [11] can be extended into a modular reuse analysis for Mercury. The reuse analysis discovers when data structures become garbage and allows the compiler to reuse them. The concepts can be adapted for other sequential logic programming languages such as Ciao Prolog and HAL; however, one can expect that less precise type, mode and determinism information will result in less reuse.

The contribution of this paper is to develop a modular reuse analysis which can become part of module compilation. While this was fairly straightforward for the liveness analysis —liveness analysis is fitted for goal independent analysis—, it was a nontrivial task for reuse analysis. A major contribution is a theorem which allows to transform a condition verifying whether data structures become available for reuse at some program point into a condition over the head variables of the procedure which can be verified by the caller of the procedure. This is the basis to derive conditional reuse for procedures exported by a module. Storing the necessary information in the module interface, other modules importing the procedure can easily verify whether they can call a version with reuse or not.

The paper also reports on experiments done with a prototype. Our results are promising; a substantial number of opportunities for reuse are detected and a few experiments show that they can have a substantial impact on performance and memory consumption. The results are encouraging enough to start the development of an analyser in Mercury itself which can become a component of the Mercury compiler. Much more extensive experiments will localise the remaining problems. We expect that we will be confronted with too bulky aliasing information and will have to consider more compact representation for it and/or appropriate widening operators. The issue of multiple specialisation will also need further investigation. We also have to incorporate language features ignored so far such as higher order predicates and type classes.

References

1. Yves Bekkers and Paul Tarau. Monadic constructs for logic programming. In John Lloyd, editor, *Proceedings of the International Symposium on Logic Programming*, pages 51–65, Cambridge, December 4–7 1995. MIT Press.
2. Maurice Bruynooghe. A practical framework for the abstract interpretation of logic programs. *Journal of Logic Programming*, 10(2):91–124, February 1991.
3. Maurice Bruynooghe, Gerda Janssens, and Andreas Kågedal. Live-structure analysis for logic programming languages with declarations. In L. Naish, editor, *Proceedings of the Fourteenth International Conference on Logic Programming (ICLP'97)*, pages 33–47, Leuven, Belgium, 1997. MIT Press.
4. M. Codish, M. Bruynooghe, M. García de la Banda, and M. Hermenegildo. Exploiting goal independence in the analysis of logic programs. *Journal of Logic Programming*, 32(3):247–261, September 1997.
5. Saumya K. Debray. On copy avoidance in single assignment languages. In David S. Warren, editor, *Proceedings of the Tenth International Conference on Logic Programming*, pages 393–407, Budapest, Hungary, 1993. The MIT Press.

6. B. Demoen, M. García de la Banda, W. Harvey, K. Marriott, and P. Stuckey. An overview of HAL. In *Proceedings of the International Conference on Principles and Practice of Constraint Programming*, pages 174–188, Virginia, USA, October 1999. Springer Verlag.

7. G. Gudjonsson and W. Winsborough. Update in place: Overview of the Siva project. In D. Miller, editor, *Proceedings of the International Logic Programming Symposium*, pages 94–113, Vancouver, Canada, 1993. The MIT Press.

8. Fergus Henderson, Thomas Conway, Somogyi Zoltan, and Jeffery David. The mercury language reference manual. Technical Report 96/10, Dept. of Computer Science, University of Melbourne, February 1996.

9. M. V. Hermenegildo, F. Bueno, G. Puebla, and P. López. Program analysis, debugging, and optimisation using the Ciao preprocessor. In D. De Schreye, editor, *Logic programming, Proc. of the 1999 Int. Conf. on Logic Programming*, pages 52–66, Las Cruces, NM, December 1999. MIT-Press.

10. S. B. Jones and D. Le Métayer. Compile-time garbage collection by sharing analysis. In *Proceedings of the Conference on Functional Programming Languages and Computer Architecture '89, Imperial College, London*, pages 54–74, New York, NY, 1989. ACM.

11. Andreas Kågedal and Saumya Debray. A practical approach to structure reuse of arrays in single assignment languages. In Lee Naish, editor, *Proceedings of the 14th International Conference on Logic Programming*, pages 18–32, Cambridge, July 8–11 1997. MIT Press.

12. Feliks Kluźniak. Compile-time garbage collection for ground Prolog. In Robert A. Kowalski and Kenneth A. Bowen, editors, *Proceedings of the Fifth International Conference and Symposium on Logic Programming*, pages 1490–1505, Seattle, 1988. MIT Press, Cambridge.

13. N. Mazur, G. Janssens, and M. Bruynooghe. Towards memory reuse for Mercury. In *Proc. Int. Workshop on Implementation of Declarative Languages (IDL'99)*, Paris, September 1999.

14. Anne Mulkers, Will Winsborough, and Maurice Bruynooghe. Live-structure dataflow analysis for Prolog. *ACM Transactions on Programming Languages and Systems*, 16(2):205–258, March 1994.

15. G. Puebla and H. Hermenegildo. Some issues in analysis and specialisation of modular programs. In M. Leuschel, editor, *Optimisation and Implementation of Declarative Programs, (WOID'99), a ICLP'99 workshop*, 1999. 17 pages.

16. G. Puebla and M. Hermenegildo. Abstract multiple specialisation and its application to program specialisation. *The Journal of Logic Programming*, 41:279–316, November-December 1999.

17. Zoltan Somogyi, Fergus Henderson, and Thomas Conway. The execution algorithm of Mercury, an efficient purely declarative logic programming language. *The Journal of Logic Programming*, 29(1–3):17–64, October-December 1996.

18. Simon Taylor. Optimization of Mercury programs. Honours report, Department of Computer Science, University of Melbourne, November 1998.

19. Mads Tofte and Talpin Jean-Pierre. Region-based memory management. *Information and Computation*, 132(2):109–176, 1997.

20. K. Ueda. Linearity analysis of concurrent logic programs. In M. Leuschel, editor, *Optimisation and Implementation of Declarative Programs, (WOID'99), a ICLP'99 workshop*, 1999. 14 pages.

21. Philip Wadler. The essence of functional programming. In *Conference Record of the Nineteenth Annual ACM SIGPLAN-SIGACT Symposium on Principles of Programming Languages*, pages 1–14, Albequerque, New Mexico, January 1992.

Mode Checking in HAL

María García de la Banda[1], Peter J. Stuckey[2],
Warwick Harvey[1], and Kim Marriott[1]

[1] Monash University, Clayton 3168, Australia
{mbanda,wharvey,marriott}@csse.monash.edu.au
[2] University of Melbourne, Parkville 3152, Australia
pjs@cs.mu.oz.au

Abstract. Recent constraint logic programming (CLP) languages, such as HAL and Mercury, require type, mode and determinism declarations for predicates. This information allows the generation of efficient target code and the detection of many errors at compile-time. However, mode checking in such languages is difficult since the compiler is required to appropriately re-order literals in the predicate's definition for each predicate mode declaration. The task is further complicated by the need to handle complex instantiations which interact with type declarations, higher order functions and predicates, and automatic initialization of solver variables. Here we give the first formal treatment of mode checking in strongly typed CLP languages which require reordering of clause body literals during mode checking. We also sketch the mode checking algorithms used in the HAL compiler.

1 Introduction

While traditional logic and constraint logic programming (CLP) languages are untyped and unmoded, recent languages such as Mercury [13] and HAL [4] require type, mode and determinism declarations for (exported) predicates and functions. This information allows the generation of efficient target code (e.g. mode information provides a substantial speed improvement [3]), improves robustness and facilitates efficient integration with foreign language procedures. Here we describe our experience with mode checking in the HAL compiler.

HAL is a CLP language designed to facilitate "plug-and-play" experimentation with different solvers. To achieve this it provides support for user-defined constraint solvers, global variables and dynamic scheduling. Mode checking in HAL is one of the most complex stages in compilation. It requires the compiler to appropriately re-order literals in the body of each rule. Since predicates can be given multiple mode declarations, the compiler mode checks each of these modes and creates a specialized *procedure* (i.e. performs multi-variant specialization). Three issues make mode checking even more difficult. First, instantiations (which describe the possible states of program variables) may be very complex and interact with the type declarations. Second, accurate mode checking of higher order functions and predicates is difficult. Third, the compiler needs to handle automatic initialization of solver variables.

J. Lloyd et al. (Eds.): CL 2000, LNAI 1861, pp. 1270–1284, 2000.

Here we formalize mode checking in the context of strongly typed CLP languages which may need reordering of clause body literals during mode checking. In order to do this we introduce "ti-trees", which are a kind of labelled deterministic regular tree. We also describe the mode checking algorithms currently used in the HAL compiler. Since HAL and the logic programming language Mercury share similar type and mode systems,[1] much of our description and formalization also applies to mode checking in Mercury (which has not been previously described). However, there are significant differences: HAL requires the automatic initialization of solver variables and handles a limited form of polymorphic mode checking. Furthermore, determining the best reordering in HAL is more complex than in Mercury because the order in which constraints are solved can have a greater impact on efficiency [9]. On the other hand, Mercury's mode system allows the specification of information about data structure liveness and usage.

Mode inference and checking of logic programs has been a fertile research field for many years. However, starting with [11,2], almost all research has focused on mode checking/inference in traditional logic programming languages where the analysis assumes the given literal ordering is correct, only simple instantiations are used and higher-order predicates are largely ignored. Regular trees have been used before in logic programming to define types, e.g. [6], and instantiations, e.g. [8], usually in the context of inference of information. Here, although we use regular trees to formalize types, our type analysis [5] is based on a Hindley-Milner approach. A key difference with previous work (in particular [8]) is that we describe instantiations for polymorphic types, including higher-order objects. The only other work on mode checking in strongly typed logic languages with reorderable clause bodies is that of [12].

2   The HAL Language

In this section we provide an overview of the HAL language. The basic syntax follows the standard CLP syntax, with variables, rules and predicates defined as usual (see, for example, [10] for an introduction to CLP). HAL supports integer, float, string and char data types and terms over these types. However, the base language support is limited to assignment, testing for equality, and construction and deconstruction of ground data. More sophisticated constraint solving requires the programmer to import a constraint solver for the type. In the case of terms, the declaration :- herbrand f/n. indicates that the system should use a Herbrand solver for terms of type $f(T_1, \ldots, T_n)$. Types with an associated constraint solver are called *solver types*.

Programmers may annotate predicate definitions with type, mode and determinism declarations. Types specify the representation format of program variables. For example, the type system in HAL distinguishes between constrained integers (cint) and standard numerical integers (int) since these have a different representation. Type definitions are (polymorphic) regular tree type statements.

---

[1] In part, because HAL is compiled to Mercury.

Instantiations specify the possible values, within a type, that a program variable may have. The *base* instantiations are new, old and ground. A variable is new if it has not been seen by any constraint solver, old if it has, and ground if it is known to take a fixed value. For data structures such as lists of solver variables, more complex instantiations may be used. A mode is of the form $Inst_1 \rightarrow Inst_2$ where $Inst_1, Inst_2$ describe the *call* and *success* instantiations, respectively. The standard modes are mappings from one base instantiation to another: we use two letter codes (oo, no, og, gg=in, ng=out) based on the first letter of the instantiation, e.g. ng is new→ground. Every constraint solver is required to provide an initialization predicate, init/1, with mode no. Determinism declarations describe how many answers a procedure may have: nondet means any number of solutions; multi at least one solution; semidet at most one solution; det exactly one solution; failure no solutions; and erroneous a runtime error.

```
:- typedef list(T) -> ([];[T|list(T)]).
:- instdef elist -> [].
:- instdef nelist -> [ground|list(ground)].
:- instdef list(I) -> ([];[I|list(I)]).
:- modedef out(I) -> (new -> I).
:- modedef in(I) -> (I -> I).

:- pred push(list(T),T,list(T)).
:- mode push(in,in,out(nelist)) is det.
push(S0,E,S1) :- S1 = [E|S0].
:- pred pop(list(T),T,list(T)).
:- mode pop(in,out,out) is semidet.
:- mode pop(in(nelist),out,out) is det.
pop(S0,E,S1) :- S0 = [E|S1].
:- pred empty(list(T)).
:- mode empty(in) is semidet.
:- mode empty(out(elist)) is det.
empty(S) :- S = [].
```

Consider the following HAL program implementing a polymorphic stack using lists. The first line defines a (parametric) list type. The next three lines define instantiations: elist describes empty lists, nelist describes non-empty ground lists, and list(I) describes lists of elements with instantiation I. Note the deliberate reuse of the type name. The next two lines are mode definitions, defining macros for modes. The out(I) mode requires a new object on call and returns an object with instantiation I. The in(I) mode requires instantiation I on call and has the same instantiation on success. The next three lines define predicate push/3. The first line is a type declaration (polymorphic in element type T). The second is a mode declaration specifying that the first two arguments must be ground on call, the third returns a non-empty ground list, and the determinism is det. The remaining lines similarly define pop/3 and empty/1. Note that each has two modes of usage.

3   Type, Instantiation, and Type-Instantiation Trees

This section formalizes type and instantiation definitions in terms of deterministic regular trees. It then introduces type-instantiation (ti-) trees which combine type and instantiation information and are the basis for mode checking in HAL.

Regular Trees: Regular trees are a well understood formalism (see, for example, [7]) but algorithms for them are surprisingly hard to find in the literature: [8]

gives algorithms for ordering ($\preceq$) and lower bound ($\sqcap$), while [1] give algorithms for (polymorphic) non-deterministic regular trees.

A signature Σ is a set of pairs f/n where f is a symbol and $n \geq 0$ is the integer arity of f. Let $\tau(\Sigma)$ denote the set of all ground terms (the Herbrand Universe) over Σ. We assume (for simplicity) that Σ contains at least one constant (i.e. arity 0) symbol.

A *(deterministic) regular tree* r over some signature Σ is a rooted directed graph with the following properties:

1. Each node a has a label denoted $label(a)$ and has $deg(a)$ outgoing edges labelled $1, \ldots, deg(a)$.
2. There are two classes of nodes: *functor nodes* and *set nodes*. Consider a node a with $label(a) = f$ and $deg(a) = n$. If a is a functor node then $f/n \in \Sigma$ and each outgoing edge ends at a set node. If a is a set node then $f \in Set$, all outgoing edges end at functor nodes, and these functor nodes refer to distinct function symbols, i.e. for each two children a_i and a_j, either $label(a_i) \neq label(a_j)$ or $deg(a_i) \neq deg(a_j)$. For standard regular trees $Set = \{OR\}$.
3. The root node is a set node.
4. Each node is reachable from the root node.

Note that regular trees are bipartite: set nodes alternate with functor nodes.

We use paths (sequences of integers) to refer to nodes in a regular tree: If r is a regular tree, $r.\epsilon$ refers to the root of r, while if $r.p$ refers to node a, then $r.p.i$ refers to the node reached from a by following the edge labelled i. Each path p in a regular tree r defines a subset $[\![r.p]\!]$ of $\tau(\Sigma)$. This is the least set satisfying:

$$[\![r.p]\!] = \begin{cases} \bigcup\{[\![r.p.i]\!] \mid 1 \leq i \leq deg(r.p)\}, & \text{if } label(r.p) = OR \\ \{f(t_1, \ldots, t_n) \mid f = label(r.p), \; n = deg(r.p), \\ \quad \text{and } t_i \in [\![r.p.i]\!] \text{ for } 1 \leq i \leq n\}, & \text{otherwise.} \end{cases}$$

We extend this notation by defining the *meaning* of regular tree r as $[\![r]\!] = [\![r.\epsilon]\!]$.

Example 1. Consider the signature $\{[]/0, \text{`.'}/2, a/0, b/0, c/0, d/0\}$ and the associated regular trees r_{1a} and r_{1b} shown in Figure 1(a) and (b), respectively. The tree r_{1a} defines lists of as, bs and cs. The notation $r_{1a}.2.2.2.1.2$ refers to the node labelled b. The tree whose root is $r_{1a}.2.1$ defines the set of terms $\{a, b, c\}$, while r_{1b} defines even length lists of bs, cs and ds.

The $[\![\cdot]\!]$ function induces a partial order on regular trees: $r_1 \preceq r_2$ iff $[\![r_1]\!] \subseteq [\![r_2]\!]$. With the addition of $\bot$, the least regular tree, and $\top$, the greatest regular tree, the partial order gives rise to a lattice over the regular trees. We use $\sqcap$ to denote the meet (i.e. greatest lower bound) operator in this lattice, and $\sqcup$ to denote the join (i.e. least upper bound) operator. We have that $[\![r_1 \sqcap r_2]\!] = [\![r_1]\!] \cap [\![r_2]\!]$. Because we restrict ourselves to deterministic regular trees the join is inexact: $[\![r_1 \sqcup r_2]\!] \supseteq [\![r_1]\!] \cup [\![r_2]\!]$.

Example 2. Consider the regular trees r_{1a} and r_{1b} illustrated in Figure 1. Their meet $r_{1a} \sqcap r_{1b}$ is shown in Figure 1(c). Their join $r_{1a} \sqcup r_{1b}$ is shown in Figure 1(d).

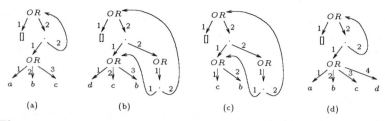

Fig. 1. Regular trees for lists of as, bs, cs and ds and their meet and join.

Type Trees: Types in HAL are formalized using (possibly polymorphic) deterministic regular trees. We assume a fixed signature Σ_{term} of term constructors.

A *type constructor* f is a functor of some arity. A *type expression* (or simply *type*) is either a type variable v or a term of the form $f(t_1, \ldots, t_n)$ where f is an n-ary type constructor, and $t_1, \ldots, t_n$ are type expressions. A *type definition* for f is of the form

:- typedef $f(v_1, \ldots, v_n)$ -> $(f_1(t_1^1, \ldots, t_{m_1}^1); \cdots; f_k(t_1^k, \ldots, t_{m_k}^k))$.

where $v_1, \ldots, v_n$ are distinct type variables, $\{f_1/m_1, \ldots, f_k/m_k\} \subseteq \Sigma_{term}$ are distinct term constructor/arity pairs, and $t_1^1, \ldots, t_{m_k}^k$ are type expressions involving at most variables $v_1, \ldots, v_n$.

Every type t has a corresponding regular tree r defined as follows: If t is a type variable v then r is a singleton set node with label v and no children. We thus need to add to *Set* (the set of possible labels for set nodes) an infinite number of type variables. Conceptually, a type variable is simply a place holder which can be substituted with a type expression. Otherwise, t is of the form $f(e_1, \ldots, e_n)$, where f is defined by a type definition of the form above. Let θ be the substitution $\{v_1 \mapsto e_1, \ldots, v_n \mapsto e_n\}$. Then r has as root an OR labelled node a with k functor nodes as children. The jth child of a is labelled f_j and has m_j children. The lth child of $r.j$ is the tree corresponding to the type $\theta(t_l^j)$.

A type can be understood in a "naive" set-theoretic manner as the meaning of its associated regular tree. From now on we will not distinguish between types and their corresponding regular trees. For example, we will use the notation $[\![t]\!]$ on a variable-free type t to refer to the set of terms defined by its corresponding regular tree. For simplicity, we will ignore the built-in types **float**, **int**, **char** and **string** whose treatment does not significantly complicate mode checking.

Example 3. Given the type definition: :- typedef abc -> a ; b ; c. the corresponding regular tree to type list(abc) is shown in Figure 1(a). The meaning, $[\![\text{list(abc)}]\!]$, is the set of lists of as, bs and cs. The regular tree corresponding to the type expression list(T) is shown in Figure 2(a).

Instantiation Trees: Instantiation definitions look like type definitions, the only difference being that the arguments are instantiations rather than types. However, they should not be confused: a type describes the representation format for a variable and is thus invariant over the life of the variable, while an instantiation describes at a particular point in execution how constrained a variable is and what values it may have been bound to.

An *instantiation constructor* g is a functor of some arity. An *instantiation expression* (or simply *instantiation*) is either a base instantiation (one of **ground**, **old** or **new**), an instantiation variable w, or a term of the form $g(i_1, \ldots, i_n)$ where g is an n-ary instantiation constructor, and $i_1, \ldots, i_n$ are instantiation expressions. A *instantiation definition* for g is of the form:

:- **instdef** $g(w_1, \ldots, w_n)$ -> $(g_1(i_1^1, \ldots, i_{m_1}^1); \cdots; g_k(i_1^k, \ldots, i_{m_k}^k))$.

where $w_1, \ldots, w_n$ are distinct instantiation variables, $\{g_1/m_1, \ldots, g_k/m_k\} \subseteq \Sigma_{term}$ are distinct term constructors, and $i_1^1, \ldots, i_{m_k}^k$ are instantiation expressions other than **new**,[2] involving at most the variables $w_1, \ldots, w_n$.

HAL requires instantiations appearing in a predicate mode declaration to be variable-free. As a result, mode checking only deals with variable-free instantiations. Thus, from now on we will assume all instantiations are variable free. We can associate a slightly extended form of regular tree with a variable-free instantiation, analogously to how we associate a regular tree to a type. The only differences are that there are no nodes labelled by instantiation variables and that we require new set node labels $\{\text{new}, \text{old}, \text{ground}\} \in Set$ to express the base instantiations. Each of these set nodes has no outgoing arcs and any **new** node must be the only node in its regular tree.

Type-Instantiation Trees: The type information of a variable x can be combined with an instantiation for x to give even more detailed information about the possible values x can take at a particular program point. To do this, we define a function $rt(t, i)$ from a type expression t and a variable-free instantiation expression i to a *type-instantiation regular tree* (or *ti-tree*).

The base instantiation **ground** represents all elements of the type but indicates that the program variable is bound to a unique value. Hence, if t is a variable-free type, $rt(t, \text{ground})$ is simply t. Otherwise, $rt(t, \text{ground})$ is obtained from t by replacing each node labelled by a type variable v by a node labelled $\text{ground}(v)$ with no children. Conceptually, this new node represents the tree $rt(t', \text{ground})$ obtained if v were replaced by the variable-free type t'.

The base instantiation **old** represents all elements of the type, including the possibility that the program variable may still not have a unique value for those parts of the type which are solver types (i.e. have an associated solver). The regular tree $rt(t, \text{old})$ is obtained from t by (a) adding a new child labelled $old_{t'}$ to any OR node corresponding to a solver type t', and (b) replacing the nodes labelled with a type variable v by a node labelled $\text{old}(v)$ with no children.

Example 4. Suppose that list types are solver types but that the type **abc** is not. Then $rt(\text{list(abc)}, \text{old})$ $(= olabc1)$ is the regular tree shown in Figure 1(a), but with an extra (third) child of the root labelled $old_{\text{list(abc)}}$. The set $[\![olabc1]\!]$ includes terms $\{[], [a|old_{\text{list(abc)}}], [b], [b, a, c, a|old_{\text{list(abc)}}]\}$. The symbol $old_{\text{list(abc)}}$ represents possible positions of **list(abc)** variables.

Suppose **abc** is a solver type but list types are not, then $rt(\text{list(abc)}, \text{old})$ $(= olabc2)$ is again the tree shown in Figure 1(a), but with a new (fourth) child of the non-root OR node labelled old_{abc}. It is shown in Figure 2(c). The set $[\![olabc2]\!]$

---

[2] In HAL (and Mercury) uninitialized (**new**) data cannot appear in data structures.

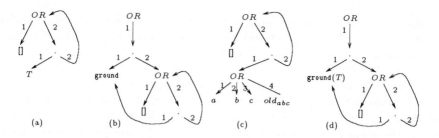

Fig. 2. Trees list(T), nelist, rt(list(abc), old) and rt(list(T), nelist).

includes terms $\{[], [a], [old_{abc}, b, old_{abc}]\}$. Note that the two occurrences of the symbol old_{abc} do not necessarily represent the same variable.

The base instantiation **new** cannot exist as part of another instantiation. Thus, the regular tree $rt(t, \mathbf{new})$ is a singleton node with no incoming or outgoing edges, labelled new_t. This is true regardless of whether t is a variable or not.

We have now defined the result of $rt(t, i)$ whenever i is a base instantiation. In the case of non-base instantiations, rt is defined analogously to the $\sqcap$ operation.

A ti-tree is thus a regular tree where $\Sigma = \Sigma_{term} \cup \{old_t | t \text{ is a type expression}\}$ and $Set = \{OR\} \cup \{\mathbf{ground}(v), \mathbf{old}(v) \mid v \text{ is a type variable}\} \cup \{new_t \mid t \text{ is a type expression}\}$. We extend the partial ordering and hence meet and join on regular trees to ti-trees by taking into account the "is more constrained" partial order on the base instantiations. The extension is as follows. For the case of the singleton new_t: $new_t \preceq r$ iff $r = new_t$; $new_t \sqcup new_t = new_t$; $new_t \sqcup r = \top$ when $r \neq new_t$ (no representable upper bound); $new_t \sqcap r = r$ for any r^3 (usually representing when a variable is first instantiated to r). Let us now consider $\mathbf{ground}(v)$ and $\mathbf{old}(v)$. We assume mode checking occurs after type analysis and, thus, we know the code is type-correct and we can assume we have the most specific type description for each program variable. As a result, we will only compare nodes containing the same type variable v. Therefore, we only need note that $\mathbf{ground}(v) \preceq \mathbf{old}(v)$, and the meet and join operations follow in the natural way.

Example 5. Assume abc is a solver type and list types are not. The regular trees in Figures 2(a), (b), (c) and (d) correspond to type list(T), instantiation nelist, and ti-trees rt(list(abc), old) and rt(list(T), nelist), respectively.

Finally, we introduce the concept of a *type-instantiation state* (or *ti-state*) $\{x_1 \mapsto r_1, \ldots, x_n \mapsto r_n\}$, which maps program variables to ti-trees. We can extend operations on ti-trees to ti-states over the same set of variables in the obvious manner. Given ti-states $TI = \{x_1 \mapsto r_1, \ldots, x_n \mapsto r_n\}$ and $TI' = \{x_1 \mapsto r'_1, \ldots, x_n \mapsto r'_n\}$ then $TI \preceq TI'$ iff $r_l \preceq r'_l$ for all $1 \leq l \leq n$, $TI \sqcap TI' = \{x_l \mapsto r_l \sqcap r'_l \mid 1 \leq l \leq n\}$ and $TI \sqcup TI' = \{x_l \mapsto r_l \sqcup r'_l \mid 1 \leq l \leq n\}$.

---

3 This interpretation of $\sqcap$ does not agree with the ordering, instead it gives the correct answer when we use $\sqcap$ to create new instantiations during mode checking.

4 Basic Mode Checking

Mode checking is a complex process which aims to reorder body literals in order to satisfy the mode constraints provided by each mode declaration, thus generating different code for each mode declaration.

Before performing mode checking, the HAL compiler normalizes the program (i.e. rewrites it to a form where each atom has distinct variables as arguments and each equality is either of the form $x = y$ or $x = f(x_1, \ldots, x_n)$, where $x, y, x_1, \ldots, x_n$ are distinct variables) and performs type checking (and inference) so the type of each program variable is known.

We shall now explain mode checking by showing how to check whether each program construct is schedulable for a given ti-state and, if so, what the resulting ti-state is. If the program construct is not schedulable for the given ti-state it may be reconsidered after other constructs are scheduled. We assume that before checking each construct for initial ti-state TI, we extend TI so that any variable of type t local to the construct is assigned the ti-tree new_t.

Equality: Consider the equality $x_1 = x_2$ where x_1 and x_2 are variables of type t and current ti-state $TI = \{x_1 \mapsto r_1, x_2 \mapsto r_2\} \cup RTI$ (where RTI is the ti-state for the remaining variables). The two standard modes of usage for such an equality are **copy** (:=) and **unify** (==). If exactly one of r_1 and r_2 is new_t (say r_1), **copy** $x_1 := x_2$ can be performed and the resulting ti-state is $TI' = \{x_1 \mapsto r_2, x_2 \mapsto r_2\} \cup RTI$. If both are not new_t then **unify** $x_1 == x_2$ is performed and the resulting instantiation is $TI' = \{x_1 \mapsto r_1 \sqcap r_2, x_2 \mapsto r_1 \sqcap r_2\} \cup RTI$. If neither of the two modes of usage apply, the literal is not schedulable (yet).

Consider the equality $x = f(x_1, \ldots, x_n)$ where $x, x_1, \ldots, x_n$ are variables with types $\{x \mapsto t, x_1 \mapsto t_1, \ldots, t_n \mapsto t_n\}$ and current ti-state $TI = \{x \mapsto r, x_1 \mapsto r_1, \ldots, x_n \mapsto r_n\} \cup RTI$. Its two standard modes of usage are: **construct** (:=) and **deconstruct** (=:). The **construct** mode applies if r is new_t and none of the r_j are new_{t_j}. The resulting ti-state is $TI' = \{x \mapsto r', x_1 \mapsto r_1, \ldots, x_n \mapsto r_n\} \cup RTI$ where r' is the ti-tree defined by $OR \to_1 f(r_1, \ldots, r_n)$. The **deconstruct** mode applies if each r_j is new_{t_j} and r is not new_t and has no child old_t (i.e. it is definitely bound to some functor). If r has a child tree of the form $f(r'_1, \ldots, r'_n)$ the resulting ti-state is $TI' = \{x \mapsto r, x_1 \mapsto r'_1, \ldots, x_n \mapsto r'_n\} \cup RTI$. If r has no child tree of this form, the resulting ti-state is the same but with $r'_j = \bot, 1 \leq j \leq n$, indicating that the **deconstruct** must fail. If some of the variables x_j are **new** (i.e. $r_j = new_{t_j}$) and some are not (say $x_{k_1}, \ldots, x_{k_m}$), the compiler decomposes the equality constraint into a **deconstruct** followed by new equalities by introducing fresh variables, e.g. $x = f(x_1, \ldots, fresh_{k_j}, \ldots), \ldots, x_{k_j} = fresh_{k_j}, \ldots$. These new equalities are handled as above.

Example 6. Assume X and Y are ground lists and A is **new**. Scheduling the goal `Y = [A|X]` results in the code `Y =: [A|F]`, `X == F`.

The above uses of **deconstruct** are guaranteed to be safe at runtime. One difference between HAL and Mercury is that HAL allows the use of the **deconstruct** mode when x is **old** (i.e. $r = rt(t, \text{old})$). In this case r has a child node of the form $f(r'_1, \ldots, r'_n)$ and we proceed as in the previous paragraph. Note that this is where the HAL mode system is weak (i.e. run-time mode errors can occur), since if at run-time x is a variable the **deconstruct** will abort if it cannot initialize all of $x_1, \ldots, x_n$.

Example 7. Assuming `abc` is not a solver type but lists are, the following program may detect a mode error only at run-time:
```
:- pred p(list(abc), abc).
:- mode p(oo, out) is semidet.
p(X,Y) :- X = [Y|_].
```
The equation is schedulable as a deconstruct since X is old. However, if at run-time X is not bound when p is called, the deconstruct will generate a run-time error since it cannot initialize Y.

Predicates: Consider the predicate call $p(x_1, \ldots, x_n)$ where $x_1, \ldots, x_n$ are variables with type $\{x_1 \mapsto t_1, \ldots, x_n \mapsto t_n\}$ and current ti-state $TI = \{x_1 \mapsto r_1, \ldots, x_n \mapsto r_n\} \cup RTI$, and p has mode declaration $p(c_1 \to s_1, \ldots, c_n \to s_n)$ where c_j, s_j are the call and success instantiations, respectively, for argument j.

The predicate call can be scheduled if for each $j \in \{1..n\}$ the current ti-state is stronger than (defines a subset of) the calling ti-state required for p, i.e. $r_j \preceq rt(t_j, c_j)$. If the predicate is schedulable for this mode the new ti-state is $TI' = \{x_1 \mapsto r_1 \sqcap rt(t_j, s_1), \ldots, x_n \mapsto r_n \sqcap rt(t_n, s_n)\} \cup RTI$. The predicate call can also be scheduled if for each j such that $r_j \not\preceq rt(t_j, c_j)$ then $rt(t_j, c_j) = new_{t_j}$. For each such j, the argument x_j in predicate call $p(x_1, \ldots, x_{j-1}, x_j, x_{j+1}, \ldots, x_n)$ is replaced by $fresh_j$, where $fresh_j$ is a fresh new program variable, and the equation $fresh_j = x_j$ is added after the predicate call.

If multiple modes of the same predicate are schedulable, we choose a mode with calling ti-state CTI (defined as $\{x_1 \mapsto rt(t_1, c_1), \ldots, x_n \mapsto rt(t_n, c_n)\}$) such that, for each other schedulable calling ti-state CTI', $CTI' \not\preceq CTI$.

Conjunctions, Disjunctions and If-Then-Elses: To determine if a conjunction $G_1, \ldots, G_n$ is schedulable for initial ti-state TI we choose the left-most goal G_j which is schedulable for TI and compute the new ti-state TI_j. This default behavior schedules goals as close to the user-defined left-to-right order as possible. If the state TI_j assigns $\perp$ to any variable, then the subgoal G_j must fail and hence the whole conjunction is schedulable. The resulting ti-state TI' maps all variables to $\perp$, and the final conjunction contains all previously scheduled goals followed by `fail`. If TI_j does not assign any variable to $\perp$ we continue by scheduling the remaining conjunction $G_1, \ldots, G_{j-1}, G_{j+1}, \ldots, G_n$ with initial ti-state TI_j. If all subgoals are eventually schedulable we have determined both an order of evaluation for the conjunction and a final ti-state.

To determine if a disjunction $G_1; \cdots; G_n$ is schedulable for initial ti-state TI we check whether each subgoal G_j is schedulable for TI and, if so, compute each resulting ti-state TI_j, obtaining the final ti-state $TI' = \bigsqcup_{j \in \{1..n\}} TI_j$. If this ti-state assigns $\top$ to any variable or one of the disjuncts G_j is not schedulable then the whole disjunction is not schedulable.

To determine whether an if-then-else $G_i \to G_t; G_e$ is schedulable for initial ti-state TI, we determine first whether G_i is schedulable for TI with resulting ti-state TI_i. If not, the whole if-then-else is not schedulable. Otherwise, we try to schedule G_t in state TI_i (resulting in state TI_t say) and G_e in state TI (resulting in state TI_e say). The resulting ti-state is $TI' = TI_e \bigsqcup TI_t$. If one of G_t or G_e is not schedulable or TI' includes $\top$ the whole if-then-else is not schedulable.

Mode Declarations: To check if a predicate with head $p(x_1, \ldots, x_n)$ and declared (or inferred) type $\{x_1 \mapsto t_1, \ldots, x_n \mapsto t_n\}$ satisfies the mode declaration $p(c_1 \to s_1, \ldots, c_n \to s_n)$, we build an initial ti-state $TI = \{x_1 \mapsto rt(t_1, c_1), \ldots, x_n \mapsto rt(t_n, c_n)\}$ to analyse the body of the predicate (multiple rules are treated as a disjunction). The mode declaration is correct if everything is schedulable with final ti-state $TI' = \{x_1 \mapsto s'_1, \ldots, x_n \mapsto s'_n\}$ and for each argument variable $1 \le i \le n$, $s'_i \preceq rt(t_i, s_i)$. A mode error results if some s'_i is not strong enough or if the body is not schedulable (in which case the compiler reports an error about the least subpart of the goal which is not schedulable.)

Example 8. Consider mode checking of the following code:
```
:- pred dupl(list(T), list(T)). %% duplicate top of stack
:- mode dupl(in(nelist), out(nelist)) is det.
dupl(S0, S) :- S0 = [], S = [].
dupl(S0, S) :- pop(S0, A, S1), push(S0, A, S).
```
We start by constructing the initial ti-state $TI = \{S0 \mapsto r_{2d}, S \mapsto new_{list(T)}\}$ where $r_{2d} = rt(\texttt{list}(T), \texttt{nelist})$ is the tree shown in Figure 2(d). Checking the first disjunct (rule) we have $S0 = []$ schedulable as a deconstruct. The resulting ti-state assigns $\bot$ to $S0$, thus the whole conjunction is schedulable with $TI_1 = \{S0 \mapsto \bot, S \mapsto \bot\}$. Checking the second disjunct, we first extend TI to map A to new_T and $S1$ to $new_{list(T)}$. Examining the first literal $\texttt{pop(S0,}$ $\texttt{A, S1)}$ we find that both modes declared for $\texttt{pop/3}$ are schedulable. Since the second mode has more specific calling instantiations, it is chosen and the ti-trees for A and $S1$ become $\texttt{ground}(T)$ and $rt(\texttt{list}(T), \texttt{ground})$, respectively. Now the second literal is schedulable obtaining for S the ti-tree r_{2d}. Restricting to the original variables the final ti-state is $TI_2 = \{S0 \mapsto r_{2d}, S \mapsto r_{2d}\}$. Taking the join $TI' = TI_1 \sqcup TI_2 = TI_2$. Checking this against the declared success instantiation we find the declared mode correct. The code generated for the procedure is:
```
dupl_mode1(S0, S) :- fail.
dupl_mode1(S0, S) :- pop_mode2(S0, A, S1), push_mode1(S0, A, S).
```
where $\texttt{pop\_mode2/3}$ and $\texttt{push\_mode1/3}$ are the procedures associated to the second and first modes of the predicates, respectively.

Our algorithm does not track variable dependencies and thus it might obtain a final ti-state weaker than expected. This can be overcome by adding a definite sharing and/or a dependency based groundness analysis to the mode checking phase. In practice, however, it seems these kinds of modes are rarely used.

5   Automatic Initialization

Many constraint solvers require solver variables to be initialized before they can be used in constraints. Thus, explicit initializations for local variables may need to be introduced. This is not only a tedious exercise for the user, it may even be impossible for multi-moded predicate definitions since each mode may require different initialization instructions. Therefore, the HAL mode checker automatically inserts variable initializations when required. Hence, whenever a literal cannot be scheduled because there is a requirement for an argument of type t to be $rt(t, \text{old})$ when it is new_t and t is a solver type, then the init/1 predicate for type t can be inserted to make the literal schedulable.

Unfortunately, unnecessary initialization may slow execution and introduce unnecessary variables (when it interacts with implied modes). Hence, we would only like to add those initializations required so that mode checking will succeed. The HAL mode checker implements this by first trying to mode the procedure without allowing initialization. If this fails it tries to find the leftmost unscheduled literal, starting from the previous partial schedule, which can be scheduled with initialization. If such a literal is found the appropriate initialization calls are added, the literal is scheduled, and then scheduling continues once more trying to schedule without initialization. If there are no literals schedulable with initialization the whole conjunct is not schedulable. This two-phase approach is applied at every conjunct level individually.

Example 9. Consider the following program where cint is a solver type:

```
:- pred length(list(cint),int).
:- mode length(out(list(old)),in) is semidet.
length(L,N) :- N = 0, L = [].
length(L,N) :- N > 0, N = N1 + 1, L = [V|L1], length(L1,N1).
```

In the first phase the second rule is not schedulable since L = [V|L1] cannot be a **construct** (V is new) or a **deconstruct** (L is new). In the second phase we try to schedule the remaining unscheduled literal, which can be managed by initializing V, obtaining:

```
length(L,N) :- NN := 0, NN == N, L := [].
length(L,N) :- N > 0, N1 := N - 1, length(L1,N1), init(V), L := [V|L1].
```

The initialization policy above is not always optimal. We are investigating more informed policies which give a better tradeoff between adding constraints as soon as possible and delaying constraints until they can be tests or assignments.

6   Higher-Order Terms

Higher-order programming is particularly important in HAL because it is the mechanism used to implement dynamic scheduling, which is vital in CLP languages for extending and combining constraint solvers. Higher-order programming introduces two new kinds of literals: construction of higher-order objects and higher-order calls. A higher-order object is constructed using an equation of the form $h = p(x_1, \ldots, x_k)$ where $h, x_1, \ldots, x_k$ are variables and p is an n-ary predicate with $n \geq k$. The variable h is referred to as a higher-order object. Higher-order calls are literals of the form $\text{call}(h, x_{k+1}, \ldots, x_n)$ where

$h, x_{k+1}, \ldots, x_n$ are variables. Essentially, the `call/n` literal supplies the $n - k$ arguments missing from the higher-order object h.

The *higher-order type* of a higher-order object h is of the form $pred(t_{k+1}, \ldots, t_n)$ where $pred/m$ is a special type construct and $t_{k+1}, \ldots, t_n$ are types. It provides the types of the $n - k$ arguments missing from h. The higher-order instantiation of h is of the form $pred(c_{k+1} \to s_{k+1}, \ldots, c_n \to s_n)^4$ where $pred/m$ is a special instantiation construct and $c_j \to s_j$ are call and success instantiations. It provides the modes of the $n - k$ arguments missing from h.

We extend our earlier definitions involving regular trees by introducing a new node labelled *pred* which has $n - k$ children for a higher-order object of type $pred(t_{k+1}, \ldots, t_n)$. The jth child node of *pred* is labelled $type_j$ and has exactly one child which is the type of the jth missing argument of the predicate. The $type_j$ functor nodes are not usually written when referring to the type and are there simply to keep the regular tree graphs bipartite. In the regular tree associated with a higher-order instantiation (or type-instantiation) the jth child node of *pred* is labelled $\to_j$ and has exactly two children: the call c_j and success s_j instantiations (resp. ti-trees).

Example 10. Consider the goal ?- H = code('a'), map(H,[7,0,11],S). and program:
```
:- pred map(pred(A,B), list(A), list(B)).
:- mode map(in(pred(in,out) is det), in, out) is det.
map(H, [], []).
map(H, [A|As], [B|Bs]) :- call(H,A,B), map(H,As,Bs).
:- pred code(char,int,char).
:- mode code(in,in,out) is det.
code(C1,I,C2) :- C2 = chr(ord(C1) + I).
```
The `map/3` predicate takes a higher-order predicate with two missing arguments with types A and B and modes `in` and `out`, respectively. This predicate is applied to a list of As, returning a list of Bs. The literal H = code('a') builds a higher-order object which calls the `code` predicate with first argument 'a'. The type-instantiation of H, `pred(int::in,char::out)`, is represented by the regular tree shown in Figure 3(b).

As discussed in the next section, HAL treats the mode and determinism of higher order terms as if they were part of the "type". This means that, for example, in a list of higher-order objects, all elements must have the same mode and determinism. This makes sense since otherwise after removing an element from the list it cannot be called as we have lost its mode and determinism.[5] This simplifies mode checking since, as a result, the only comparable ti-trees with root labelled *pred* must be identical.

We extend rt so that $rt(pred(t_1, \ldots, t_n), \mathbf{ground})$ and $rt(pred(t_1, \ldots, t_n), \mathbf{old})$ are new singleton nodes labelled $\mathbf{ground}(pred(t_1, \ldots, t_n))$ and $\mathbf{old}(pred(t_1, \ldots, t_n))$

---

[4] In practice, the determinism also appears in the higher-order instantiation.

[5] Mercury treats this differently: two higher-order objects with different mode and/or determinism information can be placed in the same list, but an error will occur when calling an element removed from this list.

t_n)), respectively. These nodes act like $\mathbf{ground}(v)$ and $\mathbf{old}(v)$ but they can also be compared with more complicated ti-trees (with root nodes labelled $pred$) of the same type. We define $r \preceq \mathbf{ground}(pred(t_1, \ldots, t_n)) \preceq \mathbf{old}(pred(t_1, \ldots, t_n))$ for any ti-tree r of the form $pred(c_1 \rightarrow_1 s_1, \ldots, c_n \rightarrow_n s_n)$ where $s_j \preceq t_j$, $1 \leq j \leq n$.

Intuitively, a higher-order equation $h = p(x_1, \ldots, x_k)$ is schedulable if h is **new** and $x_1, \ldots, x_k$ are at least as instantiated as the call instantiations of one of the modes declared for p/n. If this is true for more than one mode, an ambiguity is reported. If it is not true for any mode, the equation is delayed until the arguments become more instantiated. Note that the instantiation of each x_j is unchanged and, in fact, will not be updated when the call to h is made. Hence, higher-order objects lose precision of mode information. This would lead to erroneous mode information if some x_j is **new**. Hence, the call is not schedulable if this is the case. The HAL compiler warns if the declared mode of p used in the higher-order call may have lost instantiation information.

A higher-order call $\mathbf{call}(h, x_{k+1}, \ldots, x_n)$ is schedulable if $x_{k+1}, \ldots, x_n$ are at least as instantiated as the call instantiations of the arguments of the higher-order type-instantiation previously assigned to h. If this is not true, the call is delayed until the arguments become more instantiated. Just as for normal predicate calls, *implied modes* are also possible where if h requires one of the x_l to be **new** and it is not, we can replace it in the $\mathbf{call}$ literal by a fresh variable $fresh_l$ and a following equation $fresh_l = x_l$.

7   Polymorphism and Modes

Interfaces for storing polymorphic objects lose substantial information about the instantiations of retrieved items (they are only known to be **ground** or **old**). The problem is more severe for higher-order objects because then we do not have enough information for the higher-order object to be used (called).

Example 11. Consider the following goal:
```
?- empty(S0), I0 = code('a'), push(S0,I0,S1), pop(S1,I,S2), map(I,[7],S).
```
When item I is extracted from the list we know it is a **ground** object of type $\mathbf{pred(int,char)}$. Since the mode and determinism information of I has been lost, it cannot be used in $\mathbf{map}$ and a mode error results.

We could overcome this problem by having a special version of each predicate for the case of higher-order predicates. But this defeats the purpose of the abstract data type. Our approach is to use polymorphic type information to recover the lost mode information. This is an example of "Theorems for Free" [14]: since polymorphic code can only copy[6] terms with polymorphic type it cannot create instantiations and, hence, the output instantiations of polymorphic arguments must result from the calling instantiations of non-output arguments. Thus, they must be at least as instantiated as the join of the input instantiations.

---

[6] In HAL and Mercury it can also unify such terms, but this only creates more instantiated modes.

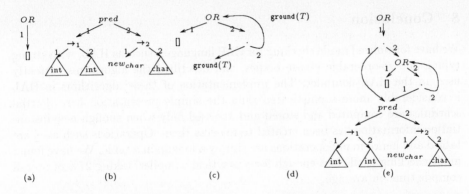

Fig. 3. Gaining information from polymorphic types.

To recover instantiation information we extend mode checking for procedures with polymorphic types to take into account the extra mode information that is implied by the polymorphic type. Due to space considerations we simply illustrate this by an example.

Example 12. Assume we are scheduling the push/3 literal in the goal:
?- empty(S0), I0 = code('a'), push(S0,I0,S1), pop(S1,I,S2), map(I,[7],S).
for current ti-state $\{$S0 $\mapsto$ elist, I0 $\mapsto$ $pred(\text{int} \to_1 \text{int}, new_{char} \to_2 \text{char})\}$, the remaining variables being new. The ti-trees r_{3a} and r_{3b} corresponding, respectively, to S0 and I0 are illustrated in Figure 3(a) and (b). The ti-trees defined by the type and mode declarations for the first two arguments of push/3, $rt(\text{list}(T), \text{ground})$ and $rt(T, \text{ground})$, are shown in Figure 3(c) and (d). The literal is schedulable. Computation of the output instantiation proceeds by finding corresponding sub-graphs in the formal and actual input instantiations where the former is labelled with $\text{ground}(T)$. This comparison of sub-graphs in Figures 3(c) and (d) with the ti-trees of Figure 3(a) and (b), respectively, gives that $\text{ground}(T)$ is matched by r_{3b}. Hence in the output instantiation, the only $\text{ground}(T)$ nodes must come from this input instantiation. Thus the success instantiation for the third argument is $rt(\text{list}(T), \text{nelist})$ (see Figure 2(d)) with the $\text{ground}(T)$ node replaced by r_{3b}. The result (the output instantiation of S1) is shown in Figure 3(e). Note that the mode information of the higher-order term is preserved.

There is a caveat which currently prevents this method from being more widely used in HAL. HAL currently assumes that a program variable with variable type may indeed be a solver type and hence can be initialized. This means polymorphic code can introduce the instantiation old for polymorphically typed code thus destroying the correctness of the "theorem for free". Thus, this enhanced polymorphic mode checking cannot be used when a matching type is a solver type. However, it is, of course, correct for higher-order types. When type classes are fully integrated in the compiler they will eliminate the assumption above thus removing the caveat.

8   Conclusion

We have formalized mode checking for CLP languages, such as HAL, with strong typing and re-orderable clause bodies, and described the algorithms currently used in the HAL compiler. The implementation of these algorithms in HAL is considerably more sophisticated than the simple presentation here. Partial schedules are computed and stored and accessed only when enough new instantiation information has been created to reassess them. Operations such as $\preceq$ are tabled and hence many operations are simply a lookup in a table. We have found mode checking is efficient enough for a practical compiler, taking 27% of overall compile time on average.

Acknowledgements

We would like to thank Bart Demoen for his contributions to the HAL mode system, and Fergus Henderson and Zoltan Somogyi for discussions of the Mercury mode system and the present paper.

References

1. A. Aiken and B.R. Murphy. Implementing regular tree expressions. In *Proc. of the 5th FPCA*, LNCS, 427–447. Springer-Verlag, 1991.
2. S. K. Debray. Static Inference of Modes and Data Dependencies in Logic Programs. *ACM Transactions on Programming Languages and Systems*, 11(3):418–450, 1989.
3. B. Demoen, M. García de la Banda, W. Harvey, K. Marriott, and P.J. Stuckey. Herbrand constraint solving in HAL. In *Proc. of ICLP*, 260–274. MIT Press, 1999.
4. B. Demoen, M. García de la Banda, W. Harvey, K. Marriott, and P.J. Stuckey. An overview of HAL. In *Proc. of CP99*, LNCS. Springer-Verlag, October 1999.
5. B. Demoen, M. García de la Banda, and P.J. Stuckey. Type constraint solving for parametric and ad-hoc polymorphism. In *Proc. of 22nd ACSC*, 217–228. Springer-Verlag, 1999.
6. T. Fruüwirth, E. Shapiro, M. Vardi, and E. Yardeni. Logic programs as types for logic programs. In *Procs. IEEE Symp. on Logic in Computer Science*, 1991.
7. F. Gecseg and M. Steinby. *Tree Automata*. Academei Kaido, Budapest, 1984.
8. G. Janssens and M. Bruynooghe. Deriving descriptions of possible value of program variables by means of abstract interpretation. *JLP*, 13:205–258, 1993.
9. K. Marriott and P. Stuckey. The 3 R's of Optimizing Constraint Logic Programs: Refinement, Removal, and Reordering. In *Proc. of 19th POPL*, 334–344. 1992.
10. K. Marriott and P.J. Stuckey. *Programming with Constraints: an Introduction*. MIT Press, 1998.
11. C.S. Mellish. Abstract Interpretation of Prolog Programs. *Abstract Interpretation of Declarative Languages*, 181–198, 1987.
12. Z. Somogyi. A system of precise modes for logic programs. In *Proc. of 4th ICLP*, 769–787, MIT Press, 1987.
13. Z. Somogyi, F. Henderson, and T. Conway. The execution algorithm of Mercury: an efficient purely declarative logic programming language. *JLP*, 29:17–64, 1996.
14. P. Wadler. Theorems for free. In *FPCA '89 Conference on Functional Programming Languages and Computer Architecture*, 347–359. ACM, 1989.

The Impact of Cache Coherence Protocols on Parallel Logic Programming Systems*

Inês de Castro Dutra[1], Vítor Santos Costa[1], and Ricardo Bianchini[1,2]

[1] COPPE Systems Engineering, Federal University of Rio de Janeiro
Rio de Janeiro, Brazil 21945-970
{ines,vitor,ricardo}@cos.ufrj.br
[2] Department of Computer Science, Rutgers University
Piscataway, NJ 08854-8019

Abstract. In this paper we use execution-driven simulation of a scalable multiprocessor to evaluate the performance of the Andorra-I parallel logic programming system under invalidate and update-based protocols. We use two versions of Andorra-I. One of them was originally designed for bus-based multiprocessors, while the other is optimised for scalable architectures. We study a well-known invalidate protocol and two different update-based protocols. Our results show that for our sample logic programs the update-based protocols outperform their invalidate-based counterpart for the original version of Andorra-I. In contrast, the optimised version of Andorra-I benefits the most from the invalidate-based protocol, but a hybrid update-based protocol performs as well as the invalidate protocol in most cases. We conclude that parallel logic programming systems can consistently benefit from hybrid update-based protocols.

Keywords: Logic programming, parallelism, cache coherence protocols, DSM architectures, performance evaluation

1 Introduction

One of the most important advantages of logic programming is the availability of several forms of implicit parallelism that can be naturally exploited on shared-memory multiprocessors. These forms include: or-parallelism, as exploited in the systems Aurora [17] and Muse [1]; independent and-parallelism, as in &-Prolog [12] and &-ACE [11]; dependent and-parallelism, as in Parlog's JAM [6], KLIC [26], and DDAS [25]; data-parallelism, as in Reform Prolog [4]; and combined and–or parallelism, as in Andorra-I [24], Penny [19], and ACE [10]. All these systems have been able to obtain good performance on early bus-based systems, such as the Sequent Symmetry multiprocessors.

As modern architectures are developed and the gap between CPU and memory speeds widens, the issue arises of whether the current parallel logic programming systems can also perform well on the new, scalable, architectures. In

---

* This work was sponsored by CNPq, Brazilian Research Council.

J. Lloyd et al. (Eds.): CL 2000, LNAI 1861, pp. 1285–1299, 2000.

modern multiprocessors, performance depends heavily on the miss rates and may be limited by the communication overhead that is involved in sharing writable data.

Sharing in parallel logic programming systems occurs under several circumstances. The use of logical variables for communication in dependent and-parallel applications, for instance, is an example of producer–consumer sharing of data. A second major form of sharing, migratory sharing, arises from synchronisation between processors. Synchronisation occurs in tasks such as fetching work from other processors, and on being the leftmost goal or branch to execute cuts or side-effects.

The sharing of writable data structures introduces the problem of coherence between the processors' caches. Most parallel machines have used a write invalidate (WI) protocol [9] in order to keep caches coherent. In this protocol, whenever a processor writes a data item, copies of the cache block containing the item in other processors' caches are invalidated. If one of the invalidated processors later requires the same item, it will have to (re)fetch it from the writer's cache.

Write update (WU) protocols [18] are the main alternative to invalidate-based protocols. In WU protocols, whenever an item is written, copies of the new value are sent to the other processors that share the item, so that it does not have to be (re)fetched on a later access.

The tradeoff between WI and WU protocols is then clear: WI protocols usually involve more cache misses but less communication than WU protocols. Thus, the performance of parallel logic programming systems on modern multiprocessors will depend heavily on the sharing behavior of these systems and how well it matches the underlying cache coherence protocol. We are interested in exactly this interplay between sharing behavior and coherence protocol.

To address this issue, we use execution-driven simulation of a scalable multiprocessor running the Andorra-I parallel logic programming system [24]. We simulate three different coherence protocols: a well-known invalidate protocol and two update-based protocols. Andorra-I is an ideal subject for our experiments because it supports two rather different forms of parallelism in logic programs: and-parallelism and or-parallelism. We experiment with two versions of Andorra-I. One of them was originally designed for bus-based multiprocessors, while the other has been optimised for scalable architectures [21].

Our results show that for our sample logic programs the update-based protocols outperform their invalidate-based counterpart for the original version of Andorra-I. The detailed analysis of these results shows a hybrid form of WU performing better than WI both for or-parallel and and-parallel benchmarks. In contrast, we find that the optimised version of Andorra-I benefits the most from the invalidate-based protocol, but the hybrid protocol performs as well as the invalidate protocol in most cases. We conclude that parallel logic programming systems can consistently benefit from the hybrid update-based protocol and that multiprocessors designed for running these systems efficiently should adopt some form of this protocol.

Our approach contrasts with previous studies of the performance of coherence protocols for parallel logic programming systems. Tick and Hermenegildo [28] studied caching behaviour of independent and-parallelism in bus-based multiprocessors. Other researchers have studied the performance of parallel logic programming systems on scalable architectures, such as the DDM [20], but did not evaluate the impact of different coherence protocols. Our initial work studied the impact of different cache coherence protocols for the original, non-optimised, Andorra-I version, using a limited benchmark set and a relatively small data cache [22]. We next performed a detailed analysis of the WI protocol based on the Andorra-I data areas [23], which led us to proposing optimisations that improved the speedup of the WI protocol by more than 100% for some applications [21]. In this study we address the question of how the original and the optimised versions of Andorra-I perform under the various coherence protocols. We use a set of benchmarks that covers both and-parallelism and or-parallelism, with examples of scalable and non-scalable applications.

The remainder of the paper is organised as follows. Section 2 describes the Andorra-I parallel logic programming system and the techniques we used to optimise its performance for scalable architectures. Section 3 presents the methodology used to obtain our results. Section 4 describes our benchmark set. Section 5 presents speedup results for the or-parallel, and-parallel, and combined parallel benchmarks ran on both versions of Andorra-I under all protocols, and evaluates the performance of the protocols. Finally, section 6 draws our conclusions and suggests future work.

2   Andorra-I

2.1   Overview

The Andorra-I parallel logic programming system is based on the Basic Andorra Model [30]. The system was developed at the University of Bristol by Beaumont, Dutra, Santos Costa, Yang, and Warren [24,32]. To the best of the authors' knowledge, Andorra-I was the first parallel logic programming system that exploited both and- and or-parallelism, and yet could run real-world applications with significant parallel performance. This is the main motivation for using this system in our experiments.

Andorra-I employs a very interesting method for exploiting and-parallelism in logic programs, namely to execute *determinate* goals first and concurrently, where determinate goals are the ones that match at most one clause in a program. Thus, Andorra-I exploits determinate dependent and-parallelism. Eager execution of determinate goals can result in a reduced search space, because unnecessary choicepoints are eliminated. The Andorra-I system also exploits or-parallelism that arises from the non-determinate goals. Its implementation is influenced by JAM [7] when exploiting and-parallelism, and by Aurora [17] when exploiting or-parallelism.

A processing element that performs computation in Andorra-I is called a *worker*. In practice, each worker corresponds to a separate processor. Andorra-I is designed in such a way that workers are classified into *masters* and *slaves*. One master and zero or more slaves form a *team*. Each master in a team is responsible for creating a new choicepoint, while slaves are managed and synchronised by their master. Workers in a team cooperate with each other in order to share available and-work. Different teams of workers cooperate to share or-work. Note that workers arranged in teams share the same set of variables used in a given branch of the search tree.

Most of the execution time of workers should be spent executing *engine* code [33], i.e., performing reductions. Andorra-I is designed in such a way that data corresponding to each worker is as local as possible, so that each worker tries to find its own work without interfering with others. Scheduling in Andorra-I is demand-driven, that is, whenever a worker runs out of work, it enters a *scheduler* to find another piece of available work.

The or-scheduler is responsible for finding or-work, i.e., an unexplored alternative in the or-tree. Our experiments used the Bristol or-scheduler [3], originally developed for Aurora. The strategy used by the Bristol scheduler concentrates on mandatory work, choosing work from the richest worker. If there is no mandatory work available, speculative work is chosen in a leftmost order.

The and-scheduler is responsible for finding eligible and-work, which corresponds to a goal in the run queue (list of goals not yet executed) of a worker in the same team. Each worker in a team keeps a run queue of goals. This run queue of goals has two pointers. The pointer to the head of the queue is only used by the owner. The pointer to the tail of the queue is used by other workers to "steal" goals when their own run queues are empty. If all the run queues are empty, the slaves wait either until some other worker (in our implementation, the master) creates more work in its run queue or until the master detects that there are no more determinate goals to be reduced and it is time to create a choicepoint.

Workers can migrate between teams and change from master to slave and vice-versa through the reconfigurer [8].

2.2   Two Versions of Andorra-I

We used in our experiments two versions of Andorra-I. The first was originally written for early bus-based machines, while the second has been optimised for modern scalable architectures.

The second version of Andorra-I optimises the original version of the system using the following 5 techniques: (1) trimming of shared variables (removal of all variables from the source code that are not relevant to the main execution of the programs and that generate a surprising amount of read misses, e.g., statistical shared counters and debugging variables), (2) data layout modification (this optimisation includes mainly padding and field reordering in order to reduce the amount of false sharing on some data areas in Andorra-I), (3) privatisation of shared data structures, (4) lock distribution, and (5) elimination of locking in scheduling. Shared variable trimming and the modification of the data layout produced the greatest improvements under a WI protocol. These optimisations were performed after a careful analysis of the data areas in the Andorra-I execution [21].

3   Methodology

We use a detailed on-line, execution-driven simulator that simulates a 24-node, DASH-like [16], directly-connected multiprocessor. Each node of the simulated machine contains a single processor, a write buffer, cache memory, local memory, a full-map directory, and a network interface. The simulator was developed at the University of Rochester and uses the MINT front-end [29] to simulate the MIPS architecture, and a back-end [5] to simulate the memory and interconnection systems.

We simulate a WI protocol and two different WU-based protocols. Our WI protocol keeps caches coherent using the DASH protocol with release consistency [16]. In our WU implementation, a processor writes through its cache to the home node. The home node sends updates to the other processors sharing the cache block, and a message to the writing processor containing the number of acknowledgments to expect. Sharing processors update their caches and send an acknowledgment to the writing processor. The writing processor only stalls waiting for acknowledgments at a lock release point.

Our WU implementation includes two optimisations. First, when the home node receives an update for a block that is only cached by the updating processor, the acknowledgment of the update instructs the processor to retain future updates since the data is effectively private. Second, when a parallel process is created by *fork*, we flush the cache of the parent's processor, which eliminates useless updates of data initialised by the parent but not subsequently needed by it.

In order to reduce the number of update messages of the WU protocol, we experiment with a dynamic hybrid protocol (WUh2) [14] based on the coherence protocols of the bus-based multiprocessors using the DEC Alpha AXP21064 [27]. In these multiprocessors, each node makes a local decision to invalidate or update a cache block when it sees an update transaction on the bus. We associate a counter with each cache block and invalidate the block when the counter reaches the threshold. References to a cache block reset the counter to zero. We used counters with a threshold of 2 updates.

4   Applications

4.1   And-Parallel Applications

We used two examples of and-parallel applications, the clustering algorithm for network management from British Telecom, bt-cluster, and a program to calculate approximate solutions to the traveling salesperson problem, tsp. The clustering program receives a set of points in a three dimensional space and groups these points into *clusters*. Basically, three points belong to the same cluster if the distance between them is smaller than a certain limit. And-parallelism in this case naturally stems from running the calculations for each point in parallel. The test program uses a cluster of 400 points as input data. This program has very good and-parallelism, and, being completely determinate, no or-parallelism. The traveling salesperson program is based on a Reform Prolog [4] benchmark that finds an approximate solution for the TSP problem in a graph with 24 nodes. To obtain best performance, the Andorra-I team rewrote the original applications to make them determinate-only computations.

4.2   Or-Parallel Applications

We use two or-parallel applications. Our first application, chat80, is an example from the well-known natural language question-answering system chat-80, written at the University of Edinburgh by Pereira and Warren [31]. This version of chat-80 operates on the domain of world geography. The program chat80 makes queries to the chat-80 database. This is a small scale benchmark with good or-parallelism, and it has been traditionally used as one of the or-parallel benchmarks for both the Aurora and Muse systems. The second application, floorplan, is an example query for a knowledge-based system for the automatic generation of floor plans [15]. The input to this program is a set of desired rooms and their sizes with restrictions on windows facing north, south, etc. We ran this application for 9 different rooms with different restrictions. This application should at least in principle have significant or-parallelism.

4.3   And/Or-Parallel Applications

We used a program (called flypan) to generate naval flight allocations, based on a system developed by Software Sciences and the University of Leeds for the Royal Navy. It is an example of a real-life resource allocation problem. The program allocates airborne resources (such as aircraft) whilst taking into account a number of constraints. The problem is solved by using the technique of active constraints as first implemented for Pandora [2]. In this technique, the co-routining inherent in the Andorra model is used to activate constraints as soon as possible. The program has both or-parallelism, arising from the different possible choices, and and-parallelism, arising from the parallel evaluation of different constraints. The input data we used for testing the program consists of 11 aircrafts, 36 crew members and 10 flights needed to be scheduled. The degree of and- and or-parallelism in this program varies according to the queries, but all queries give rise to more and-parallelism than or-parallelism.

5   Results: The Impact of Different Coherence Protocols

In this section we present speedup results for Andorra-I under the three protocols, WI, WU and WUh2. We present results for the two versions of Andorra-I:

orig, the original version, and optim, the version optimised for a scalable architecture.

All results, except for the or-parallel applications, were obtained using the reconfigurer to automatically adapt to the available parallelism. The or-parallel applications used a fixed all-masters configuration. Also, we obtained times for the *first* run of an application (results would be somewhat better for other runs).

5.1   The orig Version

Figures 1, 2, 3, 4, and 5 show the speedups for all protocols with the Andorra-I orig version. We can observe that the hybrid protocol becomes the best for all applications as we increase the size of the multiprocessor up to 24 processors.

Among the and-parallel applications, bt-cluster exhibits excellent and-parallelism, resulting in fairly good speedups under WUh2. WI achieves its best speedup of 11.3 with 24 processors, while WU achieves its best speedup of 8.5 with 16 processors. WUh2 achieves its best speedup of 15.9 for 24 processors yielding an improvement of 40% over the WI protocol and 97% over the WU protocol.

Figure 2 shows that tsp achieves worse speedups than bt-cluster. The main reason for this result is the sharing behaviour of these applications. Under the WI protocol and 16 processors, for instance, tsp issues 26 million references to shared memory with a cache miss rate of 3%, while bt-cluster issues 27 million references to shared memory with a cache miss rate of only 1.6%.

It is interesting to observe that the performance of the WU protocol is better than that of the WI protocol for the tsp application, but not for the bt-cluster application. Recall that pure WU can reduce the miss rate with respect to WI but can also generate heavy coherence traffic in doing so. For tsp, WU reduces the miss rate substantially without a significant increase in network traffic. More specifically, the miss rate of tsp is reduced from 3% under WI to 0.7% under WU on 16 processors, while the corresponding amount of network traffic increases from 148 MBytes to only 180 MBytes (a 22% increase), respectively. The WU protocol does not behave as nicely for bt-cluster. For this application, the miss rate is reduced from 1.6% under WI to 0.9% under WU again on 16 processors, while the network traffic increases from 71 MBytes to 313 MBytes (a 4-fold increase), respectively.

The performance of the or-parallel applications is similar, with floorplan (figure 5) achieving better performance than chat-80 (figure 4). WU again performs better than WI for the or-parallel applications, chat-80 and floorplan. The reason for the better performance of the WU protocol for these applications is that most sharing misses are due to false sharing and WU usually performs better for this kind of sharing pattern.

The application flypan is not much affected by any protocol. As can be observed from figure 3, this application achieves maximum speedup of 5 for 16 and 24 processors. Its execution is dominated by parallel overheads. In particular, flypan spends a significant amount of time in the and-scheduler trying to find

Fig. 1. Speedup of `bt-cluster` on the original system

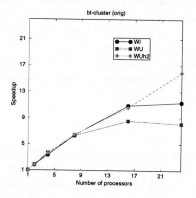

Fig. 2. Speedup of `tsp` on the original system

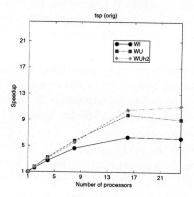

Fig. 3. Speedup of `pan2` on the original system

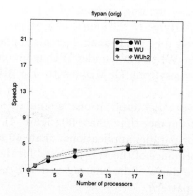

Fig. 4. Speedup of `chat-80` on the original system

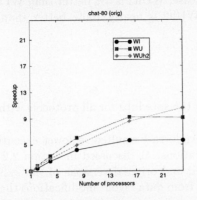

Fig. 5. Speedup of `floorplan` on the original system

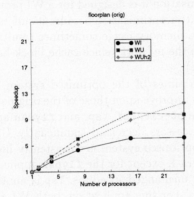

available and-work. This causes a degradation in performance as we increase the number of processors, which does not allow the application to scale well.

Table 1. Improvements of WUh2 over WI and WU

Applications	WUh2/WI	WUh2/WU
bt-cluster	1.40	1.97
tsp	1.79	1.23
flypan	1.05	1.21
chat-80	1.88	1.16
floorplan	1.86	1.18

WUh2 is the best protocol for the original version of Andorra-I. The overall improvements of WUh2 over the WI and WU protocols on 24 processors are shown in table 1. In the worst case, WUh2 is 5% better than WI and 16% better than WU. In the best case, WUh2 is nearly 100% better than WU and 88% better than WI.

5.2   The optim Version

Figures 6, 7, 8, 9, and 10 show the speedups for all protocols with the Andorra-I optim version.

The optimised version of Andorra-I resulted in lower execution times than the original code for all applications. As discussed in section 2.2 the major differences between the optimised and original versions of the system stem from trimming shared variables and from data layout modifications that reduced false sharing at the cost of increasing memory usage (e.g., by using padding). The first optimisation was particularly effective for or-parallel benchmarks and benefits all protocols. The second optimisation was designed for a WI protocol. WU does not benefit as much from this latter optimisation because it suffers less with false sharing than WI and the extra memory usage sometimes results in more data and coherence messages sent to the network (since cache block-based coalescing of messages becomes ineffective).

Even though the execution times of the optimised system are lower, the speedups it achieves not always improve upon those of the original system. More specifically, the speedups of the bt-cluster, tsp, and flypan applications under the WU protocol on 24 processors decreased significantly. Under the other protocols, the speedup of the optimised system is consistently higher than that of the original version of Andorra-I, except for the flypan application for which WI and WUh2 exhibit roughly unchanged speedups. Tsp is another interesting application in terms of speedup. For this application, both WI and WUh2 saturate at a speedup of 12 on 16 processors, while the speedup of these protocols increases up to 24 processors for all the other applications.

Overall, the best performance is now obtained with the WI protocol, since the optimised version of Andorra-I almost completely eliminates false sharing. Nevertheless, the performance of WUh2 is virtually indistinguishable from that of WI for all but one application, bt-cluster. For this application, WI reaches a speedup of 20 on 24 processors, while WUh2 performs about 25% worse. Out of all applications, the best performance is obtained by the or-parallel benchmark floorplan, where speedups are almost linear for all protocols (20-fold speedup for 24 processors). Performance is also quite good for chat-80 under the WI and WUh2 protocols, as both protocols obtain a speedup of 18 on 24 processors.

6   Conclusions and Future Work

We studied the performance of the Andorra-I parallel logic programming system under different cache coherence protocols for distributed shared-memory machines. We experimented with two versions of Andorra-I: the original system

Fig. 6. Speedup of `bt-cluster` on the optimised system

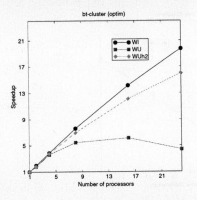

Fig. 7. Speedup of `tsp` on the optimised system

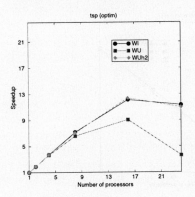

Fig. 8. Speedup of `pan2` on the optimised system

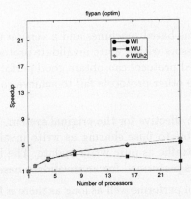

which was destined for early initialisation purposes and a subset that was mostly shared for inter/intra processes data. The data involved are not shared, but rather lead a significant amount of private values and obtained good performance; the high response of $WUh2$, while the other protocols had to maintain a security good performance.

$WUh2$ and protocol is quite effective for the optimal system but this is because this protocol is not as vulnerable as the other ones as within candidate and data flow operations its much preserves $WUh2$ and is a more effective. It is the protocol also benefits from optimisations.

The same invalidate protocol performs in one case as seen in both false sharing. The difficult and that reason it is therefore important to study the memory access pattern of the application and how the pass sequence is so sharing. The implies a way detailed understanding of the interaction between workload application, hypervisor and parallel architecture. We performed such a study in [2].

Fig. 9. Speedup of `chat-80` on the optimised system

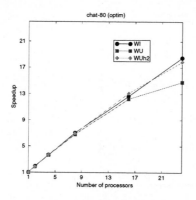

Fig. 10. Speedup of `floorplan` on the optimised system

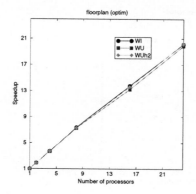

which was designed for early bus-based machines and a version that was an optimised for scalable multiprocessors with a write invalidate protocol. Our results show that a hybrid update-based protocol can obtain good performance for both versions of Andorra-I, while the other protocols fail to achieve consistently good performance.

The hybrid protocol is quite effective for the original system. This is because this protocol is not as vulnerable to false sharing as write invalidate and does not generate as much network traffic as pure write update. The hybrid protocol also benefits from optimisations performed for an invalidate-based machine.

The write invalidate protocol performs well as long as there is little false sharing. To obtain good performance it is therefore important to study the memory access patterns of the application and how they can generate false sharing. This requires a very detailed understanding of the interplay between parallel application, C compiler, and parallel architecture. We performed such a study in [21].

The write update protocol's main advantage is that it is not as vulnerable to false sharing as the write invalidate protocol. Unfortunately, Andorra-I is a memory intensive system and can saturate the network under this protocol. This problem is most remarkable in the optimised version, because padding was used to reduce false sharing.

We will be performing a similar analysis for other parallel logic programming systems. Besides confirming the generality of our claims, such an analysis will give us further insight into the current performance and scalability of parallel logic programming systems.

Acknowledgments

The authors would like to thank Leonidas Kontothanassis and Jack Veenstra for their help with the simulation infrastructure used in this paper. The authors would also like to thank Rong Yang, Tony Beaumont, D. H. D. Warren for their work in Andorra-I that made this work possible. We would like to thank Dr. László Kovács who kindly sent us his source code of the `floorplan` program used in this work. Vítor Santos Costa and Inês Dutra would like to thank the CNPq CLoP^n project.

References

1. Khayri A. M. Ali and Roland Karlsson. The Muse Or-parallel Prolog Model and its Performance. In *Proceedings of the 1990 North American Conference on Logic Programming*, pages 757–776. MIT Press, October 1990.

2. Reem Bahgat. Solving Resource Allocation Problems in Pandora. Technical report, Imperial College, Department of Computing, 1990.

3. Anthony Beaumont, S. Muthu Raman, and Péter Szeredi. Flexible Scheduling of Or-Parallelism in Aurora: The Bristol Scheduler. In Aarts, E. H. L. and van Leeuwen, J. and Rem, M., editor, *PARLE91: Conference on Parallel Architectures and Languages Europe*, volume 2, pages 403–420. Springer Verlag, June 1991. Lecture Notes in Computer Science 506.

4. Johan Bevemyr, Thomas Lindgren, and Håkan Millroth. Reform Prolog: The Language and its Implementation. In *Proceedings of the Tenth International Conference on Logic Programming*, pages 283–298. MIT Press, June 1993.

5. R. Bianchini and L. I. Kontothanassis. Algorithms for Categorizing Multiprocessor Communication Under Invalidate and Update-Based Coherence Protocols. In *Proceedings of the 28th Annual Simulation Symposium*, April 1995.

6. J. A. Crammond. *Implementation of Committed Choice Logic Languages on Shared Memory Multiprocessors*. PhD thesis, Heriot-Watt University, Edinburgh, May 1988. Research Report PAR 88/4, Dept. of Computing, Imperial College, London.

7. J. A. Crammond. The Abstract Machine and Implementation of Parallel Parlog. Technical report, Dept. of Computing, Imperial College, London, June 1990.

8. I. C. Dutra. *Distributing And- and Or-Work in the Andorra-I Parallel Logic Programming System*. PhD thesis, University of Bristol, Department of Computer Science, February 1995. available at http://www.cos.ufrj.br/~ines.

9. James R. Goodman. Using Cache Memory to Reduce Processor-Memory Traffic. In *Proceedings of the 10th International Symposium on Computer Architecture*, pages 124–131, 1983.

10. Gopal Gupta, M. V. Hermenegildo, E. Pontelli, and V. Santos Costa. ACE: And/Or-parallel Copying-based Execution of Logic Programs. In *Proceedings of the Eleventh International Conference on Logic Programming*, Italy, June 1994.

11. Gopal Gupta, Enrico Pontelli, and Manuel Hermenegildo. &ACE: A High Performance Parallel Prolog System. In *Proceedings of the First International Symposium on Parallel Symbolic Computation, PASCO'94*, 1994.

12. M. V. Hermenegildo and K. Greene. &-Prolog and its Performance: Exploiting Independent And-Parallelism. In *Proceedings of the Seventh International Conference on Logic Programming*, pages 253–268. MIT Press, June 1990.

13. Markus Hitz and Erich Kaltofen, editors. *Proceedings of the Second International Symposium on Parallel Symbolic Computation, PASCO'97*, July 1997.

14. A. R. Karlin, M. S. Manasse, L. Rudolph, and D. D. Sleator. Competitive snoopy caching. *Algorithmica*, 3:79–119, 1988.

15. L. Kovács. An Incremental Prolog System development for the Floor Plan Design by Dissecting. In *Proceedings of the International Conference on Practical Application of Prolog*, volume 2, 1992.

16. D. Lenoski, J. Laudon, K. Gharachorloo, A. Gupta, and J. Hennessy. The Directory-Based Cache Coherence Protocol for the DASH Multiprocessor. *Proceedings of the 17th ISCA*, pages 148–159, May 1990.

17. Ewing Lusk, David H. D. Warren, Seif Haridi, et al. The Aurora Or-parallel Prolog System. *New Generation Computing*, 7(2,3):243–271, 1990.

18. E. M. McCreight. The Dragon Computer System, an Early Overview. In *NATO Advanced Study Institute on Microarchitecture of VLSI Computers*, July 1984.

19. Johan Montelius. Penny, A Parallel Implementation of AKL. In *ILPS'94 Post-Conference Workshop in Design and Implementation of Parallel Logic Programming Systems, Ithaca, NY, USA*, November 1994.

20. S. Raina, D. H. D. Warren, and J. Cownie. Parallel Prolog on a Scalable Multiprocessor. In Peter Kacsuk and Michael J. Wise, editors, *Implementations of Distributed Prolog*, pages 27–44. Wiley, 1992.

21. V. Santos Costa and R. Bianchini. Optimising Parallel Logic Programming Systems for Scalable Machines. In *Proceedings of the EUROPAR'98*, pages 831–841, Sep 1998.

22. V. Santos Costa, R. Bianchini, and I. C. Dutra. Evaluating the Impact of Coherence Protocols on Parallel Logic Programming Systems. In *Proceedings of the 5th EUROMICRO Workshop on Parallel and Distributed Processing*, pages 376–381, 1997. Also available as technical report ES-389/96, COPPE/Systems Engineering, May, 1996.

23. V. Santos Costa, R. Bianchini, and I. C. Dutra. Parallel Logic Programming Systems on Scalable Multiprocessors. In *Proceedings of the 2nd International Symposium on Parallel Symbolic Computation, PASCO'97 [13]*, pages 58–67, July 1997.

24. V. Santos Costa, D. H. D. Warren, and R. Yang. Andorra-I: A Parallel Prolog System that Transparently Exploits both And- and Or-Parallelism. In *Third ACM SIGPLAN Symposium on Principles & Practice of Parallel Programming*, pages 83–93. ACM press, April 1991. SIGPLAN Notices vol 26(7), July 1991.

25. Kish Shen. *Studies of And/Or Parallelism in Prolog*. PhD thesis, Computer Laboratory, University of Cambridge, 1992.

26. T. Chikayama, T. and Fujise, and H. Yashiro. A Portable and Reasonably Efficient Implementation of KL1. In *Proceedings of the Eleventh International Conference on Logic Programming*, June 1993.

27. Charles P. Thacker, David G. Conroy, and Lawrence C. Stewart. The alpha demonstration unit: A high-performance multiprocessor for software and chip development. *Digital Technical Journal*, 4(4):51–65, 1992.

28. Evan Tick. *Memory Performance of Prolog Architectures*. Kluwer Academic Publishers, Norwell, MA 02061, 1987.

29. J. E. Veenstra and R. J. Fowler. MINT: A Front End for Efficient Simulation of Shared-Memory Multiprocessors. In *Proceedings of the 2nd International Workshop on Modeling, Analysis and Simulation of Computer and Telecommunication Systems (MASCOTS '94)*, 1994.

30. David H. D. Warren. The Andorra model. Presented at Gigalips Project workshop, University of Manchester, March 1988.

31. David H. D. Warren and Fernando C. N. Pereira. An Efficient Easily Adaptable System for Interpreting Natural Language Queries. Technical Note, Dept of AI, University of Edinburgh, 1981.

32. Rong Yang, Tony Beaumont, Inês Dutra, Vítor Santos Costa, and David H. D. Warren. Performance of the Compiler-Based Andorra-I System. In *Proceedings of the Tenth International Conference on Logic Programming*, pages 150–166. MIT Press, June 1993.

33. Rong Yang, Vítor Santos Costa, and David H. D. Warren. The Andorra-I Engine: A parallel implementation of the Basic Andorra model. In *Proceedings of the Eighth International Conference on Logic Programming*, pages 825–839. MIT Press, 1991.

Data Protection by Logic Programming

Steve Barker

University of Westminster, London W1M 8JS, U.K.
barkers@westminster.ac.uk

Abstract. This paper discusses the representation of a variety of *role-based access control (RBAC)* security models in which users and permissions may be assigned to roles for restricted periods of time. These security models are formulated as logic programs which specify the security information which protects data, and from which a user's permission to perform operations on data items may be determined by theorem-proving. The representation and verification of integrity constraints on these logic programs is described, and practical issues are considered together with the technical results which apply to the approach.

1 Introduction

Role-based access control (RBAC) is an approach to representing security requirements in which individuals are assigned to roles in an organization and are thereby authorized to perform the actions associated with these roles. For example, membership of a *doctor* role in a medical environment enables a member of *doctor* to read a patient's medical history if this permission has been assigned to the *doctor* role. Members of different roles (e.g. the *nurse* role) will have different sets of permissions on objects.

RBAC is increasingly being recognized as a practical security policy to adopt [20]. Supporting temporal authorizations has also been identified as important in practice [5]. It follows then that temporal authorization in *RBAC* is important to study if one is interested in practical security issues.

There are many situations in which users and permissions may need to be assigned to roles for limited periods of time. For example, a contract programmer may need to be assigned to the *programmer* role for the length of their contract, whilst the *programmer* role itself may need to be constrained to exercising permissions on data objects for the duration of time allocated to a project which uses these objects. Temporal authorizations are also important for applications like workflow systems, and can limit the damage intruders may cause if they are able to gain unauthorized access to information [19].

Thus far, temporal authorization has been studied under the assumption that a *discretionary access control (DAC)* policy is to be used [5]. In this context, certain subjects may grant permissions to others for a certain duration; these permissions are automatically removed on the expiration of the interval of time for which they were initially permitted.

J. Lloyd et al. (Eds.): CL 2000, LNAI 1861, pp. 1300–1314, 2000.
© Springer-Verlag Berlin Heidelberg 2000

It is increasingly being recognized, however, that supporting *DAC* alone is insufficient in practice. Many organizations now require facilities for formulating security requirements using *RBAC* [14], and want the flexibility to be able to specify *RBAC, DAC* or *mandatory access control (MAC)* policies as needs demand. Since *RBAC* subsumes *DAC* and *MAC* [3], it is especially important to consider temporal *RBAC* models since temporal *DAC* and *MAC* are special cases. However, despite its practical importance, no temporal *RBAC* model has thus far been described in the literature.

In this paper, we show how logic programs which incorporate the *Simplified Event Calculus (SEC)* [17] may be used to specify any number of *RBAC* security theories which support time-constrained permissions and membership of roles. We believe that there are a number of important reasons why such logic programs are of particular value for representing *RBAC* security models with temporal authorizations: they enable a wide range of security requirements to be represented in a high-level language and as an executable specification which may be formally verified as satisfying organizational, administrative, user and technical requirements prior to implementation; they have well-defined semantics; and sound, complete, terminating and efficient proof methods are known to exist for classes of logic program in which realistic temporal *RBAC* security theories may be specified. More generally, we believe that clausal form logic has an important part to play in formally treating a number of fundamental notions in *RBAC* that are currently not well-defined.

The rest of this paper is organized in the following way. In Section 2, we show how an *RBAC* model can be represented as a logic program, an *RBAC security theory*. In Section 3, a brief introduction to the *SEC* is given. Section 4 describes the representation of an example *RBAC* security theory with time-constrained access rights, a *temporal RBAC (TRBAC)* theory. In Section 5, a theorem-proving approach for determining access permissions from a *TRBAC* theory is discussed. In Section 6, the representation and checking of integrity constraints on *TRBAC* theories are considered. Finally, in Section 7, some conclusions are drawn, and suggestions are made for further work.

2   Representing RBAC as a Logic Program

In our approach, a *security administrator (SA)* represents an *RBAC* security model as a set of normal clauses, a *normal clause theory* or a *normal logic program* [16]. A *normal clause* has the form: $H \leftarrow L1, L2, ..., Ln$. Here, the *head* of the clause, H, is an atom and $L1, L2, ..., Ln$ is a conjunction of *literals* which comprise the *body* of the clause. A literal is an atomic formula or its negation. Negation in this paper is *negation as failure (NAF)* [8], and the negation of the atom A is denoted by *not A*. A clause which has an empty set of literals in its body is an *assertion* or a *fact*; a *query* or *goal clause* is expressed in the following (denial) form: $\leftarrow L1, L2, ..., Ln$.

Variables which appear in a literal are assumed to be universally quantified. Henceforth, we will denote variables by using terms in the upper case. In this paper, constants are the only type of function which are admitted and are denoted by letters which appear in the lower case. We also require that clauses be *ranged restricted*. A finite logic program LP is *range-restricted* iff for all clauses in LP, every variable in the head of the clause also appears in the body, and every variable that appears in a negative literal in the body of the clause also appears in a positive literal in the body.

The example $RBAC$ security theories we consider are based on the family of $RBAC$ models from [20]. That is, we assume that an $RBAC$ theory includes role and permission assignments ($RBAC_0$), and may additionally include specifications of role hierarchies ($RBAC_1$) or constraints ($RBAC_2$). $RBAC_3$ subsumes $RBAC_1$ and $RBAC_2$ and hence supports both role hierarchies and constraints. As we will show, temporal versions of any of these $RBAC$ models may be represented as logic programs.

In our approach, a SA may create and destroy roles, and they may assign users (i.e. those who request access to data items) and access permissions (e.g. to read or write a data item) to a role or remove them from a role. A SA is also responsible for specifying role hierarchies and the constraints on an $RBAC$ theory. A SA will also maintain three unary relations $role(X)$, $user(X)$, and $permission(X)$ to, respectively, record the (disjoint) sets of roles, users and permissions which constitute the universe of discourse for an $RBAC$ security theory. These relations are important for validating security specifications. To simplify the discussion that follows, we do not consider the specific permissions a SA must have in order to perform these administrative tasks.

In $RBAC$, when an authenticated user, U, is assigned to a role, R, U automatically acquires the permissions associated with R. In our representation of an $RBAC$ theory as a logic program, to record the assignment of users to a role, a SA will include definitions of the binary relation $ura(U,R)$ in an $RBAC$ security theory. Here, ura is shorthand for *user-role assignment*. Similarly, definitions of the ternary relation $rpa(R,P,O)$ may be used by a SA to specify that the permission to perform a P operation on an object O is assigned to a role R. In this case, rpa stands for *role-permission assignment*.

To see what is involved in specifying ura and rpa definitions, consider the following (simple) scenario:

> Sue is assigned to role *r2*, and *r2* is authorized to read object *o1*. Write access on an object implies read access.

To represent this information, a SA will include the following security specifications in an $RBAC$ theory (where ';' is used to separate clauses):

$ura(sue,r2)\leftarrow; \; rpa(r2,read,o1)\leftarrow; \; rpa(R,read,O)\leftarrow rpa(R,write,O)$

Role hierarchies are used to represent the fact that senior roles may inherit the (positive) permissions assigned to roles which are junior to them in the hierarchy (but not conversely). For example, suppose that the *top manager* role is described in a role hierarchy as being senior to a *middle manager* role which, in turn, is senior to a *office worker* role. If a member of *middle manager* has been assigned the permission to read the personal files of members of *office worker* then members of *top manager* also have this permission. Although the unconstrained upward inheritance of positive permissions may not always be appropriate, we do not address this issue in this paper.

To represent an $RBAC_1$ role hierarchy in our approach, a SA uses a set of ground instances of a binary relation to describe the pairs of roles which are involved in a "seniority" relationship in the partial order which represents a role hierarchy. In this case, the partial order is represented by the pair $(R,>)$ where R is a set of roles and $>$ is a "senior to" relation.

In more formal terms, a role $R1$ is *senior to* role $R2$ in a role hierarchy, RH, iff there is a path from $R1$ to $R2$ in RH such that $R1 > R2$ holds in the partial order describing RH. The reflexive, antisymmetric and transitive *senior to* relation (i.e. $>$) may be defined in terms of an irreflexive and intransitive relation "directly senior to". The *directly senior to* relation, denoted by $\rightarrow$, may be defined (since $>$ is not dense) in the following way (where $\land$ is logical 'and', $\neg$ is classical negation, and Ri ($i \in \{1,2,3\}$) is an arbitrary role from $Role(X)$):

$$\forall R1,R2\ [R1 \rightarrow R2 \text{ iff } R1 > R2 \land R1 \neq R2 \land$$
$$\neg\exists R3[R1 > R3 \land R3 > R2 \land R1 \neq R3 \land R2 \neq R3]]$$

To see how a role hierarchy may be represented as part of an $RBAC_1$ theory, consider the following instance (in which ri, $i=(1..5)$, is a role identifier and $ri \rightarrow rj$ denotes that ri is directly senior to rj ($j \in \{2,..,5\}$)):

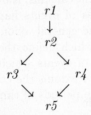

This instance of a role hierarchy may be represented in an $RBAC_1$ security theory by the following set of *d-s* facts (where *d-s* is short for *directly senior to*):

$\{d\text{-}s(r1,r2)\leftarrow;\ d\text{-}s(r2,r3)\leftarrow;\ d\text{-}s(r2,r4)\leftarrow;\ d\text{-}s(r3,r5)\leftarrow;\ d\text{-}s(r4,r5)\leftarrow\}$
We also require the following set of clauses which define the *senior-to* relation as the reflexive transitive closure of the *d-s* relation (where '_' is a "don't care"/anonymous variable):
senior-to(R1,R1)←*d-s(R1,_)*
senior-to(R1,R1)←*d-s(_,R1)*
senior-to(R1,R2)←*d-s(R1,R2)*
senior-to(R1,R2)←*d-s(R1,R3),senior-to(R3,R2)*

The definition of *senior-to* is used in the *permitted* rule that follows:

$$permitted(U,P,O) \leftarrow ura(U,R1), senior\text{-}to(R1,R2), rpa(R2,P,O)$$

The *permitted* rule specifies that a user U has the permission to perform a P operation on O if U is assigned to a role $R1$ which is senior to a role $R2$ to which the P permission on O has been assigned and is therefore inherited by $R1$.

A special role *public* may be used to specify public access on objects. For that, we may add a *d-s(r_i,public)* assertion for each $r_i \in Role(X)$ such that $\neg\exists r_j[r_i \rightarrow r_j]$ holds in a role hierarchy (where $r_j \in Role(X)$). Appropriate *rpa(public,P,O)* definitions may then be added to the security specification to record that the P permission on O is assigned to *public*.

In our approach, object, permission, and group hierarchies can be defined in the same way as role hierarchies, and restrictions on permission inheritance, like allowing *private roles* [20], can easily be accommodated.

Constraints on $RBAC_2$ and $RBAC_3$ theories are discussed in Section 6, after we have considered the use of the *SEC* for temporal $RBAC_1$ security theories.

3   The Simplified Event Calculus (SEC)

The *SEC* is a restricted form of the original *Event Calculus* [17] which has proved to be useful for treating a number of practical problems involving reasoning about time and events (e.g. [10], [13]).

The *SEC*, like the original event calculus, is based on the use of normal clause logic to specify the consequences of events happening in a world of interest. The basic idea is to combine the general axioms of the event calculus with a set of domain-specific axioms, which define the initiation and termination of relationships, and a description of events which have occurred in the world a theory describes. From this set of axioms the consequences of events occurring may be derived together with the periods of time for which these consequences hold.

The *SEC* only permits forward persistence and is based on the simplifying assumption that complete information exists about events, including the times at which they happen. Under this assumption (an entirely reasonable one in the context of security theories), a single persistence axiom is all that is required to specify that an initiated relationship, Q, continues to persist until an event occurs to terminate it. The core axiom of the *SEC* capturing this notion may be expressed thus (where $<$ is 'earlier than'):

$(C0)\ holdsat(Q,T) \leftarrow happens(E1,T1), initiates(E1,Q), T1 < T,$
$\qquad\qquad \neg\exists E2, T2[happens(E2,T2), terminates(E2,Q), T1 < T2, T2 \leq T]$

More fully, $C0$ expresses that a relationship Q holds at a time point T if an event $E1$ happened which initiated Q (i.e. made Q true) at an earlier point in time *T1*, and no intervening event *E2* has terminated *Q* (i.e. made *Q* false) subsequent to its initiation.

4   Formulating $TRBAC_1$ as a Logic Program

When checking a request by a user *U* to perform a *P* action on an object *O*, the key issue to decide is whether this action is authorized, according to a $TRBAC_1$ theory, at the time *T* at which *U*'s access request is made. For this, we include the following core *permitted* axiom in our example $TRBAC_1$ theory, a variant of the *C0* axiom of the *SEC*:

(C1) permitted(access(U,P,O),T)←happens(E1,T1),initiates(E1,ura(U,R1)),
$\qquad\qquad\qquad\qquad\quad$ *T1 < T,happens(E2,T2),*
$\qquad\qquad\qquad\qquad\quad$ *initiates(E2,rpa(R2,P,O)),*
$\qquad\qquad\qquad\qquad\quad$ *T2 < T,senior-to(R1,R2),*
$\qquad\qquad\qquad\qquad\quad$ *not ended(ura(U,R1),T,T1),*
$\qquad\qquad\qquad\qquad\quad$ *not stopped(E1,ura(U,R1),T),*
$\qquad\qquad\qquad\qquad\quad$ *not ended(rpa(R2,P,O),T,T2),*
$\qquad\qquad\qquad\qquad\quad$ *not stopped(E2,rpa(R2,P,O),T)*

The reading of the *C1* rule is as follows: at the time *T* (taken from the "system clock") at which *U* requests *P* access on *O*, a *permitted(access(U,P,O),T)* query is performed by the security system. *U* will be authorized to execute the requested *P* action if a security event (defined below) has occurred which initiated a period of time during which *U* is assigned to role *R1*, *R1* has inherited, from some role, *R2*, the permission to perform the *P* operation on *O* which has been assigned to *R2*, the assignment of *U* to *R1* has been terminated by neither a security event nor the expiration of *U*'s assignment to *R1*, and the *P* permission on *O* for *R2* has neither been terminated by a security event nor the expiration of a period of time for which the role *R2* was authorized to perform the *P* action on *O*.

As we will see, the security events which may occur in our $TRBAC_1$ model result in a user or a permission being assigned or removed from a role. A *SA* creates a role by simply adding a reference to it in the *d-s* assertions which form part of a $TRBAC_1$ security theory. Conversely, a role is destroyed by a *SA* removing all references to the role in a $TRBAC_1$ security theory (and removing the role from *Role(X)*). The create and destroy actions are not treated as events since they do not have times associated with them; when a role is created (destroyed) it is assumed to exist (not to exist) indefinitely into the future.

The definitions of *ended* and *stopped* in *C1* are as follows:

(C2) ended(ura(U,R1),T,T1)←happens(E2,T2),
$\qquad\qquad\qquad\qquad\qquad$ *terminates(E2,ura(U,R1)),T1 < T2,T2 ≤ T*

(C3) ended(rpa(R2,P,O),T,T2)←happens(E3,T3),
$\qquad\qquad\qquad\qquad\qquad$ *terminates(E3,rpa(R2,P,O)),T2 < T3,T3 ≤ T*

(C4) stopped(E1,ura(U,R1),T)←stop(E1,T1),T1 ≤ T

(C5) stopped(E2,rpa(R2,P,O),T)←stop(E2,T1),T1 ≤ T

The axioms $C2$ and $C3$ are used to deal with the ending of an access permission as a consequence of an event occurring that terminates it; $C4$ and $C5$ respectively deal with the cases where a user's time-constrained membership of a role expires, and where a permission which has been assigned to a role is stopped as a result of the expiration of the period of time for which it was initially allowed.

The set of axioms $C=\{C1,C2,C3,C4,C5\}$ is an essential part of our example $TRBAC_1$ security theory. For a particular instance of this theory, a set of *initiates* and *terminates* rules is added to C. These *initiates* and *terminates* rules are specified by a SA, and define the consequences of performing a security action which is supported in a $TRBAC_1$ model. The events which affect a $TRBAC_1$ security theory are those which result in a user or a permission being assigned to a role or removed from that role. For the former we need the following *initiates* rules ($A1$ and $A2$), and for the latter we need the *terminates* rules ($A3$ and $A4$) which follow:

(A1) initiates(E,ura(U,R))←user(E,U),role(E,R),act(E,ura)

(A2) initiates(E,rpa(R,P,O))←role(E,R),permission(E,P),object(E,O),act(E,rpa)

(A3) terminates(E,ura(U,R))←user(E,U),role(E,R),act(E,revokeura)

(A4) terminates(E,rpa(R,P,O))←role(E,R),
   permission(E,P),object(E,O),act(E,revokerpa)

When considered in relation to the core axioms, the rule $A1$ expresses that an event which involves specifying that U is assigned to role R initiates (i.e. makes true) *ura(U,R)*. Similarly, $A2$ expresses that an event in which R is assigned the P permission on object O initiates *rpa(R,P,O)*. Conversely, $A3$ specifies that *ura(U,R)* is terminated (i.e. is made false) by an event in which U is removed (i.e. revoked) from R, and $A4$ represents that *rpa(R,P,O)* is terminated by the occurrence of an event which removes the permission to perform a P operation on O from R. Henceforth, we will use A to denote the set of axioms, $A=\{A1,A2,A3,A4\}$.

In addition to the core *initiates* and *terminates* axioms in A, it is possible to define any number of implicit assignments of users and permissions to roles by defining *initiates* in terms of *initiates* or *terminates* or *terminates* in terms of *terminates* or *initiates*. For instance, to express that "write permission implies read permission" the following rule may be included in a $TRBAC_1$ theory:

initiates(E,rpa(R,read,O))←initiates(E,rpa(R,write,O))

The *initiates* and *terminates* rules which are included in a $TRBAC_1$ theory are used with a set of ground, binary assertions which describe a history of user-role or permission-role assignment events. The permissions we allow a SA to assign to roles are read and write permissions on objects. In $RBAC$, the permissions allocated to a role are application-specific, and often quite different to read and write. However, these two operations will be sufficient to demonstrate what our approach entails, and how it can be extended to accommodate any number of operations.

To see what is involved in recording user and permission assignments to a role, suppose an event, *e1* (say), happens on 01/09/99 and involves indefinitely assigning a user, Bob, to the role, *r1*. To represent this, the following *security event description* is included as part of our example $TRBAC_1$ security theory (where *max* is the maximum permitted chronon in the domain on which the system time line is defined):

$\{happens(e1,01/09/99)\leftarrow; act(e1,ura)\leftarrow;$
$\qquad\qquad\qquad\qquad user(e1,bob)\leftarrow; role(e1,r1)\leftarrow; stop(e1,max)\leftarrow\}$

We call a set of security event descriptions an *authorization history*. To see what is involved in their representation, consider the following scenario:

The role *r1* is assigned a write permission on the object *o1* on 10/09/99, the user Jim is assigned to the role *r3* on 20/09/99, *r3* is assigned a read permission on *o1* on 03/10/99, but only until 20/12/99, the user Sue is assigned to the role *r2* on 10/11/99, but only until 31/01/00, and Jim is removed from role *r3* on 03/12/99.

To represent this information the required authorization history, *H*, is:

$\{happens(e2,10/09/99)\leftarrow; act(e2,rpa)\leftarrow; role(e2,r1)\leftarrow;$
$\qquad\qquad\qquad object(e2,o1)\leftarrow; permission(e2,write)\leftarrow; stop(e2,max)\leftarrow\}$

$\{happens(e3,20/09/99)\leftarrow; act(e3,ura)\leftarrow;$
$\qquad\qquad\qquad\qquad user(e3,jim)\leftarrow; role(e3,r3)\leftarrow; stop(e3,max)\leftarrow\}$

$\{happens(e4,03/10/99)\leftarrow; act(e4,rpa)\leftarrow; role(e4,r3)\leftarrow; object(e4,o1)\leftarrow;$
$\qquad\qquad\qquad\qquad permission(e4,read)\leftarrow; stop(e4,20/12/99)\leftarrow\}$

$\{happens(e5,10/11/99)\leftarrow; act(e5,ura)\leftarrow; user(e5,sue)\leftarrow;$
$\qquad\qquad\qquad\qquad role(e5,r2)\leftarrow; stop(e5,31/01/00)\leftarrow\}$

$\{happens(e6,03/12/99)\leftarrow; act(e6,revokeura)\leftarrow; user(e6,jim)\leftarrow; role(e6,r3)\leftarrow\}$

Notice that there is no *stop* time associated with acts of revocation (a revocation corresponds to a *stop* at the time the revocation *happens*), and that *max* is used to denote that the relationships in the security event description are assumed to persist until the maximum future time point is reached.

In implementations of our approach, a history of user-role and permission-role assignments and revocations is maintained. Maintaining this history is useful for a number of reasons: it makes it possible to express authorization derivation rules based on a user's past history of role and permission assignment, it enables the initiation of assignments of users and permissions to roles to be defined in terms of terminating events, it enables a variety of temporal constraints to be expressed on a $TRBAC$ theory, and it is useful for auditing purposes. An alternative approach is for the SA to perform a physical deletion to remove, from an authorization history, an event description which initiated a user or permission assignment to a role as soon as a decision to revoke these assignments is made. Similarly, it is possible for an event description to be physically deleted as soon as the current time exceeds the *stop* time in the event description. If physical deletion of event descriptions is to be used then the axioms defining our $TRBAC_1$ theory may be modified to take any such policy into account. Whilst physical deletion is always used to remove event descriptions which refer to roles or users which have ceased to be relevant to the security of the system, other choices of delete policy will depend on application-specific requirements.

It should be noted that the type of object, $o1$, to be protected from unauthorized access requests will depend on the type of objects our approach is used to protect. For instance, $o1$ could be a UNIX file, a base table or view in a relational database or an EDB or IDB predicate in a deductive database. Note also that: a *security event validation procedure* is used to ensure that an authorization history is syntactically and semantically meaningful; proactive authorizations may be included in an authorization history; and a much finer time granularity than the DAY type we have assumed thus far would be expected to be available in practice.

5   Access Control by Theorem-Proving

Our example $TRBAC_1$ security theory includes the core set of axioms, C, the definition of *senior-to*, the *initiates* rules ($A1$ and $A2$), and the *terminates* rules ($A3$ and $A4$). To this set of axioms, the application-specific authorization history and d-s clauses may be added to form a particular instance of a $TRBAC_1$ security theory. Henceforth, we will denote an arbitrary instance, T_i, of our $TRBAC_1$ security theory by $TRBAC_1(T_i)$; specific instances of a $TRBAC_1$ theory will be denoted by substituting a natural number for the subscript i in T_i. The instance of the $TRBAC_1$ security theory outlined in the previous section will be denoted by T_1. We will assume that $TRBAC_1(T_1)$ includes H, the authorization history from Section 4, and the d-s facts from Section 2.

As we will see, any application-specific instance of our example $TRBAC_1$ security theory can be represented in a subset of normal clause logic for which (safe) *SLDNF-resolution* is sound and complete with respect to Clark's 2-valued *completion* semantics [8]. It follows then that SLDNF-resolution may be used for deciding questions about a user's access permissions on data items from a $TRBAC_1$ theory. In our approach therefore, at the time T at which user U

requests P access on an object O, an SLDNF-derivation for the goal clause $\leftarrow permitted(access(U,P,O),T)$ is performed on the $TRBAC_1$ theory.

If $TRBAC_1(T_i) \cup \{\leftarrow permitted(access(U,P,O),T)\}$ has an *SLDNF-refutation* then, from the soundness of SLDNF-resolution [16], we have: $comp(TRBAC_1(T_i))$ $\models permitted(access(U,P,O),T)$. In this case, U's request at time T to perform the P operation on O is authorized. Conversely, if $TRBAC_1(T_i) \cup \{\leftarrow permitted(access(U,P,O),T)\}$ has a *finitely-failed SLDNF-tree* then $comp(TRBAC_1(T_i))$ $\models \neg permitted(access(U,P,O),T)$, and U is not authorized to perform the P action on O at time T. Soundness ensures that no unauthorized access is permitted.

The set of axioms in $C \cup A$ together with the *senior-to* relation, forms an *allowed* [16] and *call-consistent* [15] theory, the application-specific d-s and authorization history comprise a set of positive assertions, $\leftarrow permitted$ $(access(U,P,O),T)$ is allowed and always ground when it is selected for evaluation with respect to $TRBAC_1(T_i)$, and $TRBAC_1(T_i)$ is *strict* [2] with respect to $\leftarrow permitted(access(U,P,O),T)$. From the results in [22], it therefore follows that SLDNF-resolution is complete, with respect to Clark's semantics, for evaluating access requests on $TRBAC_1(T_i)$. That is, if $comp(TRBAC_1(T_i))$ $\models permitted(access(U,P,O),T)$ (resp., $comp(TRBAC_1(T_i))$ $\models \neg permitted$ $(access(U,P,O),T))$ then $TRBAC_1(T_i)) \cup \{\leftarrow permitted(access(U,P,O),T)\}$ has an SLDNF-refutation (resp., a finitely-failed SLDNF-tree). Completeness ensures that authorized access requests are never denied.

Before giving an example of the use of SLDNF-resolution for access control, certain practical issues need to be mentioned. In implementations of our approach we store *senior-to* as a *materialized relation* [1]. Although the costs involved in updating *senior-to* will be increased in this case, in practice the additional update costs are small relative to the savings in access costs. Similarly, ground instances of *initiates* and *terminates* may be dynamically asserted to avoid their recomputation in processing subsequent access requests. This type of lemma generation increases the size of the security theory, but it does have the advantage of permitting proofs on a $TRBAC_1$ theory to be efficiently performed since ground assertions are used, almost entirely, in the process. Various other optimizations are also possible.

In implementations of $RBAC$ it is usually the case that in addition to U being recorded as being assigned to role R and R having been assigned the permission to perform a P operation on O, for U to be able to execute a P act on O, U is also required to have activated R at the time of U's request to perform the P action on O. In our approach, role activation/deactivation is managed in the following way. Definitions of a binary relation $active(U,R)$ are included, by a SA, in a $TRBAC$ theory to specify the set of roles the user U is permitted to activate. Thereafter, a ground instance of an $initiates(E,active(U,R),T)$ fact is dynamically asserted into a $TRBAC$ theory at the time T (taken from the system clock) at which a request by U to activate role R has been verified as being authorized. In this case, E is instantiated with a system generated event identifier. Conversely, the appropriate instance of an $initiates(E,active(U,R),T)$ assertion is physically deleted as soon as U deactivates R.

Example (Determining Access Rights on $TRBAC_1(T_1)$)
Suppose that, on 01/12/99, Sue requests read access on the object *o1*. Assuming that Sue has activated the necessary roles, then for $\{\leftarrow permitted(access(sue, read, o1), 01/12/99)\}$ we have the following (abbreviated) SLDNF-refutation (in which each predicate name is the first character of the corresponding predicate name in *C1*):

$$\leftarrow p(access(sue, read, o1), 01/12/99)$$
$$\downarrow$$
$$\leftarrow i(E1, ura(sue, R1)), i(E2, rpa(R2, read, o1)), h(E1, T1),$$
$$T1 < 01/12/99, h(E2, T2), T2 < 01/12/99, s\text{-}t(R1, R2),$$
$$not\ e(ura(sue, R1), 01/12/99, T1), not\ s(E1, ura(sue, R1), 01/12/99),$$
$$not\ e(rpa(R2, read, o1), 01/12/99, T2), not\ s(E2, rpa(R2, read, o1), 01/12/99)$$
$$\downarrow$$
$$\cdot$$
$$\downarrow$$
$$\leftarrow not\ e(ura(sue, r2), 01/12/99, 10/11/99), not\ s(e5, ura(sue, r2), 01/12/99),$$
$$not\ e(rpa(r3, read, o1), 01/12/99, 03/10/99), not\ s(e4, rpa(r3, read, o1), 01/12/99)$$
$$\downarrow$$
$$success$$

It should be clear that, at 01/12/99, all of the negated subgoals in the SLDNF-derivation succeed since: Sue's membership of the role *r2* has not been ended by a revocation; the read permission on *o1* has not been revoked for role *r3*; Sue's assignment to *r2* has not been stopped as a result of the expiration of a period of time for which she was assigned to *r2*; and the assignment of the read permission on *o1* for role *r3* has not expired by 01/12/99.

In contrast, on 20/12/99 the read permission on *o1* expires for role *r3*, and, thereafter, Sue does not inherit this permission from another role in the role hierarchy for T_1. As such, she is unable to read *o1* on 21/12/99 (say). In terms of SLDNF-resolution, the subtree for $\leftarrow s(e4, rpa(r3, read, o1), 21/12/99)$ on $TRBAC_1(T_1)$ has an SLDNF-refutation, and hence $\leftarrow p(access(sue, read, o1), 21/12/99)$ is finitely failed.   ◇

We have used SLDNF-resolution in our example of access request checking since (being the standard procedural semantics for PROLOG) it is the best-known proof method for query evaluation on $TRBAC_1$ theories. Moreover, the constraint checking methods we refer to in the next section are SLDNF-based. We have also used Clark's completion in our discussion since this is the standard declarative semantics for SLDNF-resolution, and is used to define integrity constraint satisfaction. It should be clear, however, that other declarative or procedural semantics may be used instead of completion and SLDNF-resolution. In fact, *XSB* [21] is used in implementations of our approach. Hence, instead of using SLDNF-resolution and Clark's completion, SLG-resolution may be used to evaluate *permitted* queries and to compute the well-founded partial model of a $TRBAC_1$ theory.

Since $TRBAC_1$ theories satisfy the *bounded-term-size property*, SLG-resolution is guaranteed to terminate for such theories [7]. Moreover, from the results in [7], SLG-resolution is sound and search space complete, with respect to the well-founded model of a $TRBAC_1$ theory, for all non-floundering queries. The problem of incompleteness due to floundering does not arise in any instance of our example $TRBAC_1$ theory since every clause is range-restricted and *permitted* queries on a $TRBAC_1$ theory are only ever positive.

Every instance of our example $TRBAC_1$ theory is also *locally stratified*. The well-founded model of a $TRBAC_1$ theory is total in this case, and equivalent to both the perfect model and the unique 2-valued stable model of the theory. Having a total semantics is important (especially, if a *closed access policy* [6] is to be adopted) since every ground instance of *permitted(access(U,P,O),T)* should be either true or false (but not both) in a $TRBAC_1$ theory.

In addition to its attractive soundness, completeness and termination properties, SLG-resolution is a particularly efficient method of computation to use with $TRBAC_1$ theories. Since $TRBAC_1$ theories are function-free, SLG-resolution has polynomial time data complexity for evaluating $\leftarrow permitted(access(U,P,O),T)$ queries [7]. Moreover, since our $TRBAC_1$ theories are locally stratified, SLG is more efficient than it is for computation on arbitrary function-free logic programs, since the number of transformation rules required to generate answer clauses is reduced from that required in the general case.

6   Integrity Constraints and TRBAC Theories

Integrity constraints have been suggested to be a principal motivation for $RBAC$ [20]. Constraints are necessary for expressing high-level organizational policy and general security principles. In this section we consider how constraints on $RBAC$ security models may be represented in clausal form logic, and how they may be checked by using SLDNF-based methods whenever changes are made to the application-specific information contained in an $RBAC$ (or $TRBAC$) theory. We believe that clausal form logic satisfies the fundamental criteria, identified in [20], which candidate languages for constraint representation in $RBAC$ must satisfy: that they have a well-defined formal semantics, and are sufficiently powerful to represent the wide range of constraints which are likely to need to be specified on realistic $RBAC$ theories.

Whilst $RBAC_2$ models permit integrity constraints to be expressed, we will consider the more general case of $RBAC_3$. The latter permits $RBAC$ security theories to include both integrity constraints and role hierarchies. Moreover, since $TRBAC_3$ subsumes $RBAC_3$ we will only refer to the former. Henceforth, we will denote an arbitrary $TRBAC_3$ security theory, T_i, by $TRBAC_3(T_i)$.

Integrity constraints may be expressed in denial form viz: $\leftarrow L1,L2,...,Ln$ (where Li, $i=(1..n)$, is a literal). The denial $\leftarrow L1,L2,...,Ln$ may be read as stating that it is impossible for the conjunction of literals $L1,L2,...,Ln$ to be simultaneously "true" in a $TRBAC$ security theory. For instance, the denial $\leftarrow d\text{-}s(R1,R2), d\text{-}s(R2,R1), R1{\neq}R2$ represents the constraint that it is impossible for a $TRBAC_3$ theory to include a set of $d\text{-}s$ facts which record that role $R1$ is senior to $R2$ and $R2$ is senior to $R1$ (where $R1$ and $R2$ are distinct roles). A set of integrity constraints, IC, on $TRBAC_3(T_i)$ is satisfied iff $comp(TRBAC_3(T_i))$ $\cup\ IC$ is consistent [18].

Notice that, since denials may be expressed using constants or variables, it is possible for a SA to make the constraints on a $TRBAC_3$ theory as specific or as general as is required. However, we believe that the constraints should be written in their most general form, and should be specialized as needs be by including instances of application-specific assertions in a $TRBAC_3$ theory.

To illustrate what is involved in the representation of constraints on a $TRBAC_3$ theory, we consider the specification of two fundamental types of $RBAC$ constraint: *static separation of duties (ssd)* and *dynamic separation of duties (dsd)*. A *ssd* constraint prevents a user being recorded in a security theory as being assigned to any pair of roles which are specified as being mutually exclusive (i.e. statically separated). A *dsd* constraint prevents a user being *active* in a pair of roles, specified as being dynamically separated, at the same point in time.

To specify a *ssd* constraint, a SA will include ground instances of a binary relation $ssd(R1,R2)$ in a $TRBAC_3$ theory (where $R1$ and $R2$ are distinct roles from the domain defined by $Role(X)$). More specifically, if r_i and r_j $(i{\neq}j)$ are instances of roles (where $r_i, r_j \in Role(X)$) and are to be specified as being statically separated then a SA will include the assertions $ssd(r_i, r_j)$ and, because of the symmetry of the *ssd* relation, $ssd(r_j, r_i)$ in a $TRBAC_3$ theory. The *ssd* constraint can then be specified thus (where $currenttime(T)$ is used to extract the "current time" from the system clock):

$$\leftarrow currenttime(T), happens(E1,T1), T1 < T, act(E1,ura), user(E1,U), role(E1,R1),$$
$$happens(E2,T2), T2 \leq T, act(E2,ura), user(E2,U), role(E2,R2),$$
$$E1{\neq}E2, ssd(R1,R2), stop(E1,T3), stop(E2,T4), T < T3, T < T4$$

The *ssd* constraint will be checked each time an attempt is made to insert an event description involving $ura(E,R)$ into an authorization history.

Similarly, to specify a *dsd* constraint a SA will include $dsd(r_i, r_j)$ and, due to the symmetry of *dsd*, $dsd(r_j, r_i)$ $(i{\neq}j)$ assertions for any pair of roles r_i and r_j $(r_i, r_j \in Role(X))$ which are to be recorded as being dynamically separated in a $TRBAC_3$ theory. The *dsd* constraint can then be specified thus:

$$\leftarrow initiates(E1, active(U,R1), T1),$$
$$initiates(E2, active(U,R2), T2), dsd(R1,R2), T1 < T2$$

The *dsd* constraint will be checked whenever an $initiates(E, active(U,R), T)$ fact is dynamically inserted into a $TRBAC_3$ theory after a user U's request to activate a role R has been determined to be authorized.

A variety of SLDNF-based methods may be used for constraint checking on $TRBAC_3$ theories (e.g. [18], [9]), and have attractive technical properties for such theories. For instance, the *SLIC (Selection-driven Linear resolution procedure for Integrity Checking)* method from [9] is sound, and shares the same completeness results as SLDNF-resolution. On the latter point, the argument we gave in the previous section can be extended to give a completeness result for *SLIC* used for constraint checking on a $TRBAC_3$ theory. Note also that, from the results in [9], since all (realistic) $TRBAC_3$ theories are *confined*, termination of (fair) *SLIC* is guaranteed. Moreover, since constraint checks will predominantly involve using ground assertions and since none of the axioms in $C \cup A$ are involved in testing for constraint violations, it follows that constraint checking can be efficiently performed on a proper subset of a $TRBAC_3$ theory.

7   Conclusions and Further Work

We have shown how a range of $TRBAC$ (and hence $RBAC$) security models can be represented as logic programs and how proof methods used in logic programming can be used to decide whether a user's requests to access data items are authorized or not. We have also demonstrated that it is possible to represent and to enforce high-level security requirements expressed via integrity constraints written in clausal form logic. Since DAC and MAC security policies are special cases of $RBAC$, it follows that logic programming may be used to represent security theories with temporal authorizations which are based on any of the three main classes of access policy. Our approach also provides a SA with a general methodology which may be used to develop a range of $TRBAC$ security models. This methodology involves extracting user requirements and formulating them as a security specification written in clausal form logic, then translating this specification into an implementation which enables access requests to be determined to be authorized (or not) by theorem-proving on the resulting theory.

Whilst the expressive power of normal clause logic is important for enabling a wide range of security requirements to be specified, in further work we want to investigate sublanguages and special purpose implementations which might enable realistic security theories to be expressed, but which may be more efficient to compute with. In future work, we also intend to investigate the specification and implementation of large-scale $TRBAC$ models with a commercial organization, and how the work presented in this paper can be combined with our recent work on deductive database security [4].

References

1. Abiteboul, S., Hull, R., and Vianu, V., *Foundations of Databases*, Addison-Wesley, 1995.
2. Apt, K., Blair, H., and Walker, A., Towards a theory of declarative knowledge, in J. Minker (Ed.), *Foundations of Deductive Databases and Logic Programming*, Morgan-Kaufmann, 1988.
3. Barker, S., Security policy specification in logic, *International Conference on Artificial Intelligence*, 2000.
4. Barker, S., Protecting deductive databases from unauthorized retrievals, *To Appear*.
5. Bertino, E., Bettini, C., Ferrari, E., and Samarati, P., A temporal access control mechanism for database systems, *IEEE Trans. on KDE*, 8(1), 1996.
6. Castano, S., Fugini, M., Martella, G., and Samarati, P., *Database Security*, Addison-Wesley, 1994.
7. Chen, W., Swift., T., and Warren, D., Efficient top-down computation of queries under the well-founded semantics, *JLP*, 24, 1995.
8. Clark, K., Negation as failure, in H. Gallaire and J. Minker(Eds), *Logic and Databases*, Plenum, 1978.
9. Decker, H., and Celma, M., A slick procedure for integrity checking in deductive databases, *ICLP*, 1994.
10. Eshghi, K., Abductive planning with the event calculus, *ICLP*, 1988.
11. Griffiths, P. P., and Wade, B.W., An authorization mechanism for relational database systems, *ACM TODS*, 1(3), 1976.
12. Jajodia, S., Samarati, P., Subrahmanian, V., and Bertino, E., A unified framework for enforcing multiple access control policies in *Proc. ACM SIGMOD International Conference on Management of Data*, 1997.
13. Kowalski, R., Database updates in the Event Calculus, *JLP*, 12, 1992.
14. Kuhn, D. R., Mutual exclusion of roles as a means of implementing separation of duty in role-based access control systems, *Proc. 2nd ACM Workshop on Role-Based Access*, 1997.
15. Kunen, K., Signed data dependencies in logic programs, *JLP*, 7, 1989.
16. LLoyd, J., *Foundations of Logic Programming*, Springer, 1987.
17. Sadri, F. and Kowalski, R., Variants of the event calculus, *ICLP*, 1995.
18. Sadri, F. and Kowalski, R., A theorem-proving approach to database integrity in *Foundations of Deductive Databases and Logic Programming*, J. Minker (Ed.), Morgan-Kaufmann, 1988.
19. Sandhu, R., Coyne, E., Feinstein, H., and Youman, C., Role-Based access control: a multi-dimensional view, *Proc. 10th Annual Computer Security Applications Conf.*, 1994.
20. Sandhu, R., Coyne, E., Feinstein, H., and Youman, C., Role-Based access control models, *IEEE Computer*, 1996.
21. Sagonas, K., Swift, T., Warren, D., Freire, J., Rao. P., The XSB System, Version 2.0, Programmer's Manual, 1999.
22. Shepherdson, J., Negation as failure, completion and stratification in D. Gabbay et al. (Eds), *Handbook of Logic in AI and Logic Programming, Volume 5, Logic Programming*, Oxford, 1997.

A Deterministic Shift-Reduce Parser Generator for a Logic Programming Language

Chuck Liang

Department of Computer Science, Trinity College
300 Summit St., Hartford, CT 06106-3100, USA
chuck.liang@mail.trincoll.edu

Abstract. This paper addresses efficient parsing in the context of logical inference for the purpose of using logic programming languages in compiler writing. A bottom-up, deterministic parsing mechanism is formulated for "bounded right context" grammars, a subclass of LR(k) grammars with characteristics amenable to declarative parser specification. A working parser generator for λProlog is described, although the basic parsing mechanism is applicable to logic programming in general.

1 Introduction

The overall aim of this paper is to use logic programming as a practical instrument for compiler writing and other activities concerning programming languages and systems. Many declarative methods in logic programming (e.g., higher order abstract syntax) have been developed for the representation and analysis of programming language constructs. However, logic programming is still not as widely used as conventional languages in compiler writing. One reason for this has been the lack of general and efficient parsing schemes. Parsing in Prolog has traditionally focused on a range of issues broader than programming languages (e.g., natural language processing). In such a context, generality often takes precedence over determinism. The well-known definite clause grammars (DCG, [13]) have a wide range of application. In a system using depth-first proof search however, DCGs represent a top-down, recursive-descent parsing mechanism that suffers from non-determinism and non-termination. Some of these problems are alleviated by alternative implementations and optimization techniques of logic programming. They alone, however, can not replace all efficient parsing strategies, such as the use of lookahead symbols and precedence functions. Although DCGs have been used in compiler writing, extensive grammar specialization and other techniques are generally required (e.g. to deal with left-recursion and associativity) before syntax can be parsed deterministically.

Bottom-up parsing in Prolog has also been studied. In fact, shift-reduce parsing of *any* context free grammar can be formulated by the following pair of rules (which are meant to be read bottom-up):

$$\frac{\alpha t \triangleleft w}{\alpha \triangleleft tw} \; Shift \qquad \text{and} \qquad \frac{\alpha A \triangleleft w}{\alpha \gamma \triangleleft w} \; Reduce, \; A \to \gamma \text{ is a production}$$

J. Lloyd et al. (Eds.): CL 2000, LNAI 1861, pp. 1315–1329, 2000.

The ◁ symbol separates the parse stack from the remaining input. α and w are schematic variables representing sequences of symbols[1]. These rules can be directly encoded as Horn Clauses with the bottom sides at the head of each clause. However, this "universal parser" will behave non-deterministically for all but the simplest grammars. Similar formulations of Earley's Algorithm also exist (see [14, 15]). Even LR-style parsing in Prolog has some precedents (e.g., [5, 12]). The aims of most such efforts, however, are again not specific to compiler construction (with the noted exception of [3] - see Section 7 for further discussion). As a consequence, these works are usually not concerned with the exact non-deterministic *choice points* of a grammar, namely reduce-reduce and shift-reduce conflicts. For example, in [12] non-determinism was *intentionally* preserved in order to process a larger class of logic programs. Unambiguous parser generation as required in compiler writing requires that non-deterministic choice points be identified and resolved.

One obvious solution to providing a deterministic parser for logic programming would be to directly implement the LR parsing algorithms described in compiler texts using brute-force methods. Such an approach, however, would derive few advantages from the use of logic programming and the resulting parser will little resemble its declarative grammar. Furthermore, this type of approach may not necessarily preserve all the advantages of LR parsing (e.g., "fast table lookup" may have no meaning). Declarative programming is better suited for implementing *deductive systems*, and would benefit from studies of parsing in this context.

In this paper we reconsider a class of context free grammars that are closely related to LR grammars and are likewise capable of describing all deterministic context-free languages. These grammars exhibit characteristics that can be used to formulate a parsing strategy in the framework of logical inference. The inference rules for these parsers are specialized versions of the two basic "shift and reduce" rules above. However, they will be *deterministic* in the sense that at most one rule is applicable at any time, and *linear* in the sense that every rule has at most one recursive premise. They are also terminating. Efficient shift-reduce parsing is thus manifested as logic programming.

2   Bounded Right Context and LR Grammars

The type of grammar we consider suitable for formulating deterministic parsing *as deduction* are known as *bounded right context* (BRC) grammars, introduced by Floyd [4]. The principal characteristic of a BRC grammar is that the unique "handle" of a bottom-up, rightmost derivation step can be determined by looking *ahead* some k symbols to the right (the remaining input), and looking *back* some l symbols to the left (the stack). The better known $LR(k)$ grammars also require lookaheads of k symbols to the right, but look back at the *entire* stack. Implementations of LR parsers rely on deterministic finite state machines to

---

[1] The representation of parsers in the style of logical inference rules was introduced in [14].

keep track of stack contents. *All BRC grammars are also LR grammars and all LR grammars have BRC equivalents that recognize the same language* (see [10, 7]). The essential difference between BRC grammars and LR grammars that are not already BRC can be illustrated by the following $LR(0)$ grammar:

$$S \rightarrow aA \mid bB$$
$$A \rightarrow (A) \mid x$$
$$B \rightarrow (B) \mid x$$

A "reduced-reduce" conflict would exist between $A \rightarrow x$ and $B \rightarrow x$ unless one keeps track of whether an 'a' or a 'b' was the first symbol read. This is the critical information maintained by the $LR(0)$ state machine of this grammar. An equivalent BRC grammar, preserving the distinction between A and B, can be given as follows:

$$S \rightarrow aA \mid bB$$
$$A \rightarrow (A) \mid x$$
$$B \rightarrow PB) \mid x$$
$$P \rightarrow ($$

That is, by *looking back* one symbol to the left, one can now determine the same "state" information, which is now carried by the non-terminal symbol P. State machine generation for this grammar can be avoided.

Because BRC grammars are subsumed by the larger LR class, their development as a tool for parser specification was appearantly halted. It is not our intention here to compete with other parsing algorithms, except we note that most implementations of LR parsing are also restricted to subclasses (SLR and LALR). Our reason for resurrecting the BRC subclass is that the trade-off they offer compared to general LR grammars is a positive one *in the context of logic programming*. Due to the lack of arrays, pointers and mutable variables, the computation of state information necessary for efficient LR parsing is precisely the kind of programming that many current declarative languages are not best suited for. Logic programming is better suited for the specification of *deductive* systems. The simplification afforded by BRC grammars can be used to formulate deterministic parsing as such a system, one that can take advantage of the declarative syntax and unification capabilities of logic programming.

An indication of the practical suitability of BRC grammars for use in compiling is that every LR grammar that appears in the most popular compiler texts (including [1] and [2]) are in fact also BRC grammars. When required, the modifications needed to form BRC grammars from LR grammars are usually few and similar to that of the above example (a more practical example is given in Section 3.2). General algorithms for translating LR grammars into BRC equivalents also exist (see [6]). We shall also introduce a simplification of BRC grammars that also suffices for most parsing needs in Section 5.1.

3   Formal Definitions

The following technical presentation assumes a basic familiarity with bottom-up parsing concepts such as provided in compiler texts (e.g. [1,2]). A more detailed introduction to the theory of deterministic languages and parsing can be found in [8]. We briefly state some basic definitions.

A context-free grammar is a tuple (V, Σ, P, S), where V represents a finite set of grammar symbols and $\Sigma \subset V$ a set of "terminal" symbols. P is a finite set of "productions" of the form $A \to \gamma$ where $A \in N = V - \Sigma$ (the non-terminals) and $\gamma \in V^*$. $S \in N$ is the designated "start symbol." A *rightmost derivation* step is of the form $\alpha A w \Longrightarrow_r \alpha \beta w$ where $\alpha \in V^*$, $w \in \Sigma^*$ and $A \to \beta \in P$. Derivation in arbitrary numbers of steps are represented by $\overset{*}{\Longrightarrow}_r$ and $\overset{+}{\Longrightarrow}_r$. If $\gamma \overset{*}{\Longrightarrow}_r \epsilon$, the empty sequence, then γ is said to be *nullable*. We also confine our discussion to *reduced* context-free grammars where for all $A \in V$, $S \overset{*}{\Longrightarrow}_r \alpha A \beta \overset{*}{\Longrightarrow}_r w$ such that $w \in \Sigma^*$. In other words, all grammar symbols are reachable from the start symbol and every symbol derives a sequence of terminal symbols. We also exclude grammars where $A \overset{+}{\Longrightarrow}_r A$ is possible for any non-terminal A. Reduced grammars allowing such derivations are necessarily ambiguous.

If $S \overset{*}{\Longrightarrow}_r \gamma$ then γ is a *right sentential form* of the grammar. If $S \overset{*}{\Longrightarrow}_r \alpha A w$ and $\alpha A w \Longrightarrow_r \alpha \beta w$ then any prefix of $\alpha \beta$ is a *viable prefix*, and $A \to \beta$ is called the *handle* of $\alpha \beta w$ at position $\alpha \beta$. The handle identifies which production to apply in reverse (and where) in a bottom-up, rightmost derivation.

Let $last_l(\gamma)$ be the length-l suffix of γ (or γ if γ contains less than l symbols), and let $first_k(\gamma)$ be defined in the usual way: the set of length-k prefixes of terminal sequences derivable from γ (or length $k' < k$ sequences if γ derives a string of length k'). Formally, a context free grammar (V, Σ, P, S) is of type $BRC(l, k)$ if the following condition holds (from [7]):

1. $S \overset{*}{\Longrightarrow}_r \alpha A w \Longrightarrow_r \alpha \beta w$,
2. $S \overset{*}{\Longrightarrow}_r \alpha_2 A_2 w_2 \Longrightarrow_r \alpha_2 \beta_2 w_2 = \sigma \beta u$ such that $\sigma \beta$ is a prefix of $\alpha_2 \beta_2$, and
3. $first_k(w) = first_k(u)$ and $last_l(\alpha) = last_l(\sigma)$

implies

$$A \to \beta = A_2 \to \beta_2 \quad \text{and} \quad \alpha_2 \beta_2 = \sigma \beta.$$

If we restrict the preconditions of the definition so that $\alpha = \sigma$ (which would also make redundant the "lookback" condition $last_l(\alpha) = last_l(\sigma)$), then this definition would be equivalent to that of $LR(k)$ grammars ([10]). Thus it is easy to see why every $BRC(l, k)$ grammar is immediately an $LR(k)$ grammar. Furthermore, BRC grammars are capable of generating the same set of languages as LR grammars, namely all deterministic context-free languages ([10,7]). In particular, every $LR(k)$ grammar has an equivalent $BRC(1, k)$ grammar and every deterministic language has a $BRC(1, 1)$ grammar. Our formulation below, however, is generalized to $BRC(l, k)$ grammars.

3.1   Valid Handles and Inference Rules

The intended meaning of a shift-reduce *parsing judgement* of the form $\alpha \lhd w$, seen in Section 1, is that α is a viable prefix of right sentential form αw of the grammar under consideration. α will be used to represent a sequence of grammar symbols and w a sequence of terminal grammar symbols.

The symmetrical nature of BRC grammars suggests that we augment each grammar with an implicit production $S' \rightarrow \$_0 S \$_1$, where $\$_0$ and $\$_1$ are unique symbols representing "begin of file" and "end of file" respectively. The $\$_0$ symbol ensures that lookback sequences are never empty.

We define a *contexted handle* of a grammar to be a triple $(\beta_l, A \rightarrow \gamma, a_k)$ such that $A \rightarrow \gamma$ is a production, β_l are either l grammar symbols or $l' < l$ symbols beginning with $\$_0$, and a_k are either k terminal symbols or $k' < k$ terminal symbols ending in $\$_1$. Contexted handles (with fixed l and k) are "valid" if they satisfy the following:

Definition 1. *(Valid (l, k) Handles)*
Given a grammar (V, Σ, P, S) augmented with $S' \rightarrow \$_0 S \$_1$,

1. $(\$_0, S \rightarrow \gamma, \$_1)$ *is a valid handle for each production $S \rightarrow \gamma$.*
2. *if $(\beta_l, A \rightarrow \sigma B \gamma, a_k)$ is a valid handle, $\beta_l' = last_l(\beta_l \sigma)$, and $a_k' \in first_k(\gamma a_k)$, then $(\beta_l', B \rightarrow \rho, a_k')$ is a valid handle for each production $B \rightarrow \rho$.*

We emphasize that unlike $first_k$, $last_l$ need not be a set since the lookback may contain non-terminal as well as terminal symbols.

Valid handles characterize the right sentential forms of a grammar up to a "bounded context," as formalized by the following lemma (it's implied here that $\alpha = \epsilon$ if β_l begins with $\$_0$, and analogously for w):

Lemma 2. $(\beta_l, A \rightarrow \gamma, a_k)$ *is a valid (l, k) handle of a grammar if and only if $S' \overset{*}{\Longrightarrow}_r \alpha \beta_l A a_k w$ for some $\alpha \in V^*$ and $w \in \Sigma^*$.*

Proof: by induction on the length of rightmost derivations and the definition of valid handles. □

The computation of valid handles is similar to the computation of the "follow" set described in compiler texts, except that the left and right contexts of non-terminal symbols are kept tract of simultaneously. That is, we can compute the handles by starting with $(\$_0, S \rightarrow \gamma, \$_1)$ and follow the above inductive definition until a closure is formed (the computation is also bounded by l, k and the number of productions and symbols in the grammar). We shall describe the formation of valid handles further in Section 5.

A grammar with a set of valid handles gives rise to a set of *canonical* inference rules as defined below.

Definition 3. *(Canonical Inference Rules)*
Given the valid (l, k) handles of a grammar:

- *The implicit production $S' \to \$_0 S \$_1$ yields two special rules:*

$$\frac{\$_0 a \; \lhd \; a'_{k-1} w}{\$_0 \; \lhd \; a a'_{k-1} w} \; Shift \;, \; a a'_{k-1} \in first_k(S), \quad and \quad \frac{}{\$_0 S \; \lhd \; \$_1} \; Accept$$

- *For each valid handle $(\beta_l, A \to \gamma, a_k)$ there exists a rule*

$$\frac{\alpha \beta_l A \; \lhd \; a_k w}{\alpha \beta_l \gamma \; \lhd \; a_k w} \; Reduce$$

Here, α and w are schematic variables ranging over arbitrary sequences of grammar symbols and terminal grammar symbols respectively.
- *For each valid handle $(\beta_l, A \to \gamma, b_k)$ where $\gamma = G_1 \ldots G_n$ for $G_1, \ldots, G_n \in V$ and $n > 1$, and for each i such that $1 \leq i < n$ where G_{i+1} is not nullable, there exists a rule[2]*

$$\frac{\alpha \beta_l G_1 \ldots G_i a \; \lhd \; a'_{k-1} w}{\alpha \beta_l G_1 \ldots G_i \; \lhd \; a a'_{k-1} w} \; Shift \;, \; a a'_{k-1} \in first_k(G_{i+1} \ldots G_n b_k)$$

Here, if $k = 0$ (no lookahead) then the $first_k$ side condition is omitted as long as $a \neq \$_1$. If $k = 1$ (one lookahead) then, since G_{i+1} is non-nullable, the side condition simplifies to $a \in first(G_{i+1})$.

The *first* relation can be pre-computed so it is not necessarily a costly condition to verify.(and if all shift rules are collapsed into one default rule in actual parser code, the *first* condition becomes unnecessary).

Determinicity of the canonical inference rules can be checked by pairwise unification of their bottom sides, which should share no common instance. Formally, A *reduce-reduce* conflict between two distinct inference rules exists if they are of the forms

$$\frac{\alpha \beta_l A \; \lhd \; a_k w}{\alpha \beta_l \gamma \; \lhd \; a_k w} \; Reduce \quad and \quad \frac{\alpha' \beta'_l A' \; \lhd \; a_k w'}{\alpha' \beta'_l \gamma' \; \lhd \; a_k w'} \; Reduce$$

such that $\alpha \beta_l \gamma = \alpha' \beta'_l \gamma'$ for some α and α'. This condition can be checked by unification where α and α' are free variables. For example, a reduce-reduce conflict exists between one rule having bottom side $\alpha a a A$ and another one have $\alpha' a A$, since $\alpha' = \alpha a$ is possible.

Similarly, a *shift-reduce* conflict exists between any two rules of the forms

$$\frac{\alpha \beta_l A \; \lhd \; a a'_{k-1} w}{\alpha \beta_l \gamma \; \lhd \; a a'_{k-1} w} \; Reduce \quad and \quad \frac{\alpha' \beta'_l \gamma' a \; \lhd \; a'_{k-1} w'}{\alpha' \beta'_l \gamma' \; \lhd \; a a'_{k-1} w'} \; Shift$$

---

[2] It can be shown that G_{i+1} is nullable only if $G_{i+1} \Rightarrow_r B\sigma$ such that $B \to \epsilon$ is a production and σ is nullable. But then the valid handles for $B \to \epsilon$ will inherit the same lookback and lookahead symbols from G_{i+1}. Adding a shift rule at this point will thus result in a shift-reduce conflict with $B \to \epsilon$.

if $\alpha\beta_l\gamma = \alpha'\beta_l'\gamma'$ for some α and α'.

We say that a set of canonical inference rules are *deterministic* if there exist no shift-reduce or reduce-reduce conflicts.

3.2   Examples

The correctness of this parsing scheme is addressed in section 4, but first we give some examples of grammars and their encoding as bottom-up inference rules.

The following simple grammar requires a single lookback symbol for determinism:

$$S' \to \$_0 A \$_1$$
$$A \to Aa \mid a$$

This $BRC(1,0)$ (and thus $LR(0)$) grammar has the valid handles (the lookahead components are omitted):

- $(\$_0, A \to Aa)$
- $(\$_0, A \to a)$

These in turn give rise to the following deterministic inference rules

$$\frac{\$_0 A \vartriangleleft w}{\$_0 Aa \vartriangleleft w} R \qquad \frac{\$_0 A \vartriangleleft w}{\$_0 a \vartriangleleft w} R \qquad \frac{\$_0 At \vartriangleleft w}{\$_0 A \vartriangleleft tw} S \qquad \frac{\$_0 t \vartriangleleft w}{\$_0 \vartriangleleft tw} S \qquad \frac{}{\$_0 A \vartriangleleft \$_1} A$$

Without the lookback symbol $\$_0$, there would exist a reduce-reduce conflict between the productions $A \to Aa$ and $A \to a$. Note also that, since no lookaheads are needed, the shift rules need not consider which symbol is being shifted (as long as it's not $\$_1$).

The following grammar (with implicit production for S' omitted) requires both a lookback and a lookahead and is of type $BRC(1,1)$. The lack of either would lead to reduce-reduce conflicts between $A \to c$ and $B \to c$ and a nondeterministic parser:

$$S \to aAd \mid aBe \mid bAe \mid bBd$$
$$A \to c$$
$$B \to c$$

With both lookback and lookahead, non-conflicting reduce rules for the A and B productions are derived:

$$\frac{\alpha a A \vartriangleleft dw}{\alpha ac \vartriangleleft dw} R \qquad \frac{\alpha a B \vartriangleleft ew}{\alpha ac \vartriangleleft ew} R \qquad \frac{\alpha b A \vartriangleleft ew}{\alpha bc \vartriangleleft ew} R \qquad \frac{\alpha b B \vartriangleleft dw}{\alpha bc \vartriangleleft dw} R$$

The final example shows where in the syntax of a programming language do BRC grammars differ from general LR grammars. Consider a language with function *definitions* of the form `function f(x) = ...` and function *calls* of the form `f(a)`. A possible source of conflict is that in the definition header `x` can only be an individual identifier, whereas in a function call `a` can be an arbitrary expression. A possible LR grammar for this syntax would be

$$F \rightarrow function\ id(id)\ =\ E$$
$$E \rightarrow id\ |\ E+T\ |\ (E)\ |\ \ldots$$

Without the *function* keyword, a shift-reduce conflict would result when reading an identifier (id) inside parentheses. A BRC grammar would require the following modification:

$$F\ \rightarrow\ Gid)\ =\ E$$
$$G\ \rightarrow\ function\ id($$
$$E\ \rightarrow\ id\ |\ E+T\ |\ (E)\ |\ \ldots$$

The unique non-terminal symbol G allows inference rules to distinguish the appropriate context using a single lookback:

$$\frac{\alpha Gid)\ \triangleleft\ w}{\alpha Gid\ \triangleleft\ )w}\ Shift \qquad \frac{\alpha(E\ \triangleleft\ )w}{\alpha(id\ \triangleleft\ )w}\ Reduce$$

This modification is essentially the same as for the example in Section 2, and all required modifications we have encountered are of this nature. Only two modifications of this type were required in defining a BRC grammar for an experimental imperative language. Occassional grammar modifications, including such seemingly redundant productions, are sometimes also needed for the SLR and LALR simplifcations of LR parsing. Users of any parser generator must be aware of the requirements of the underlining grammar formalism.

4   Correctness

The formal correctness of our deductive parsing mechanism consists of lemma 2 plus the following results. We use "deduction" to mean the application of a sequence of inference rules and "derivation" to mean rightmost derivations of grammar symbols.

Lemma 4. *If there is a deduction of $\alpha\ \triangleleft\ w$ from $\$_0 S\ \triangleleft\ \$_1$ then α is a viable prefix and αw is a right sentential form of the grammar.*

Proof: by induction on the height of deductions, appealing to lemma 2. □

Lemma 5. *If $S' \overset{*}{\Longrightarrow}_r \alpha A w$, then there is a deduction from $\$_0 S\ \triangleleft\ \$_1$ of $\alpha A\ \triangleleft\ w$*

Proof: by induction on the length of rightmost derivations, appealing to lemma 2. □

These "soundness and completeness" lemmas are better understood *top-down*, although they are meant to establish the correctness of a bottom-up parsing strategy, which is formalized by the following theorem:

Theorem 6. *A grammar is $BRC(l,k)$ if and only if its canonical inference rules are deterministic.*

Proof: The forward direction is proved by contradiction. Using the previous lemmas, it is seen that a reduce-reduce conflict entails the existence of two right sentential forms that satisfy the preconditions of the definition of BRC grammars but contradict the requirement that $A \to \beta = A_2 \to \beta_2$. Similarly, a shift-reduce conflict contradicts the requirement that $\alpha_2\beta_2 = \sigma\beta$: $\sigma\beta$ will remain a *proper* prefix of $\alpha_2\beta_2$. For the reverse direction, it can be shown that if $\sigma\beta$ is a proper prefix of $\alpha_2\beta_2$ then at some earlier point in the bottom-up inference of a terminal sequence the same reduce rule was applicable, and by determinism will entail a different sentential form from $\alpha_2\beta_2w_2{}^3$. Once we know that $\alpha_2\beta_2 = \sigma\beta$, $A \to \beta = A_2 \to \beta_2$ follows directly from the absence of reduce-reduce conflicts. □

Termination of bottom-up deductions is complicated by the presence of ϵ-productions (since they can expand the size of the stack). It can be shown that termination for grammars without ϵ-productions does not require determinism (because we assume that $A \xLongrightarrow{+}_r A$ is not possible). However, without any lookbacks or lookaheads, any grammar with an ϵ-production has infinite deductions in reverse. The general termination result is state thus:

Theorem 7. *There are no infinite deductions in reverse for the canonical inference rules of a $BRC(l, k)$ grammar.*

Proof: It suffices to show that there can not be an infinite sequence of reduce steps between shifts. Since reduce rules derive from valid handles, if there is such an infinite sequence then, using lemma 2, it can be shown that there is also an infinite sequence of reductions in reverse for some right sentential form. This contradicts determinism and lemma 5. □

5   Handle Merging

Two valid handles of the form $(b, A \to \gamma, a)$ and $(b, A \to \gamma, a')$ can be merged to form one set of inference rules without introducing new conflicts, since either lookahead will cause the same action. The merged handle would have the form $(b, A \to \gamma, \{a, a'\})$. Handles of the form $(b', A \to \gamma, a)$ and $(b, A \to \gamma, a)$ can similarly be merged safely. Handles of the form $(b, A \to \gamma, a)$ and $(b', A \to \gamma, a')$, however, can not in general be merged without causing new conflicts (consider the second example of Section 3.2). In the representation of valid handles we can therefore use sets for both the lookbacks and lookaheads. Handle merging is an important implementation-wise feature because it significantly reduces the number of inference rules needed.

For example, consider the following $BRC(1, 1)$ grammar:

$$S' \to \$_0 S \$_1$$
$$S \to L = R \mid R$$

---

³ This argument uses the fact that in reduced grammars all sentential forms derive terminal sequences, and that grammars where $A \xLongrightarrow{+}_r A$ is possible are excluded.

$$L \to *R \mid id$$
$$R \to L$$

There are sixteen valid handles of this grammar, but they can be safely merged into the following eight handles:

- $(\{\$_0\}, S \to L = R, \{\$_1\})$, $(\{\$_0\}, S \to R, \{\$_1\})$
- $(\{*, \$_0\}, L \to *R, \{=, \$_1\})$, $(\{*, \$_0\}, L \to id, \{=, \$_1\})$
- $(\{=\}, L \to *R, \{\$_1\})$, $(\{=\}, L \to id, \{\$_1\})$
- $(\{*\}, R \to L, \{\$_1, =\})$, $(\{\$_0, =\}, R \to L, \{\$_1\})$

These merged handles give rise to inference rules with extra side conditions, such as

$$\frac{abL \ \triangleleft \ aw}{ab * R \ \triangleleft \ aw} R, b \in \{*, \$_0\}, a \in \{=, \$_1\})$$

Note that the *union* of all lookaheads of the valid handles of $L \to id$ and $L \to *R$ is exactly the "follow" set of L, and similarly for S and R. We exploit this characteristic in the next section.

5.1   Simple BRC

For $BRC(1, 1)$ grammars, the number of inference rules resulting from the (merged) valid handles is comparable to the number of states in the finite automaton of a $LR(1)$ parser[4]. The previous section suggests a technique that is analogous to "SLR" parsing in relation to $LR(1)$ parsing: we allow valid handles of the form $(b, A \to \gamma, a)$ and $(b', A \to \gamma, a')$ to be merged into $(\{b, b'\}, A \to \gamma, \{a, a'\})$. This will ensure that the number of merged handles is always the same as the number of productions of the grammar (minus the initial production for S'). Conflicts introduced by this type of merging can still be detected and resolved by other means (e.g., the user can be prompted to choose which action should be given preference). We say that a grammar is a *Simple BRC* (SBRC) grammar if the resulting set of inference rules derived from the "simply-merged" handles remain deterministic. The following grammar is often used as a standard example of bottom-up parsing:

$$S' \to \$_0 E \$_1$$
$$E \to E + T \mid T$$
$$T \to T * F \mid F$$
$$F \to (E) \mid id$$

The fully merged valid handles of this grammar are:

- $(\{\$_0, (\}, E \to E + T, \{\$_1, +, \}))$, $(\{\$_0, (\}, E \to T, \{\$_1, +, \})$
- $(\{\$_0, (, +\}, T \to T * F, \{\$_1, +, *, \}))$, $(\{\$_0, (, +\}, T \to F, \{\$_1, +, *, \})$
- $(\{\$_0, (, +, *\}, F \to (E), \{\$_1, +, *, \}))$, $(\{\$_0, (, +, *\}, F \to id, \{\$_1, +, *, \})$

---

[4] Each rule roughly corresponds to an occurrence of a "kernel item" in a DFA state.

The inference rules derived from these handles remain deterministic. Note in particular the absence of $+$ among the lookbacks of the handles for $E \to T$, and the absence of $*$ from the lookbacks for $T \to F$. This ensures that $E + T$ (or $T * F$) on top of the stack would not be reduced erroneously to $E + E$ (or $T * T$). The lookaheads of each handle is exactly the *follow* set of the left-hand side non-terminal symbol of the associated production. The lookbacks of each handle would correspond to a left-side analogy of *follow* (which we call the *before set*). Thus a SBRC parser generator need only compute the first, follow, and before relations in order to generate the merged handles from which inference rules can be derived. Experiments have shown that this technique, combined with operator precedence and associativity declarations and user-resolved shift-reduce conflicts, suffices to yield a useful parser generator for many purposes.

6   A Parser Generator

We now describe aspects of a working parser generator in a logic programming language[5]. Both the full $BRC(1,1)$ and the simple BRC methods have been implemented. The SBRC method has sufficed for most examples we've tried so far, and is currently being further developed. The programming language is $\lambda Prolog$ (*Teyjus* implementation [11]). The choice of this language has to do with the semantic actions of a parser (they can generate *higher-order abstract syntax*), and not with any aspect of our parsing mechanism in particular. λProlog properly embeds Horn Clause Prolog. Notationally, application in λProlog is written in curried form: (f a b) instead of f(a,b).

The input to the parser generator is itself a λProlog file (module) where a grammar is declared by a clause such as the following:

```
cfg   % attributed context free grammar for online calculator
[
rule ((ae R) ==> [iconst R2]) (R is R2),
rule ((ae R3) ==> [lparen,(ae R1),rparen]) (R3 is R1),
rule ((ae R4) ==> [(ae A4),plust,(ae B4)]) (R4 is (A4 + B4)),
rule ((ae R5) ==> [(ae A5),minust,(ae B5)]) (R5 is (A5 - B5)),
rule ((ae R6) ==> [(ae A6),timest,(ae B6)]) (R6 is (A6 * B6)),
rule ((ae R7) ==> [(ae A7),dividet,(ae B7)]) (R7 is (A7 div B7)),
rule ((ae R8) ==> [(ae A8),expt,(ae B8)]) (power A8 A8 B8 R8)
].
```

The implicit production for S' is internal. The symbols ae, iconst, minust, plust, lparen, etc., are grammar symbols. A grammar symbol can be a function symbol with distinct variables, representing semantic attributes, as its arguments. Each production is represented by a **rule** term with the infix symbol

---

[5] The full implementation, which also includes a semi-universal lexical analyzer, plus several larger examples and additional notes are available from the homepage at http://www2.trincoll.edu/~cliang/parsergen, or by contacting the author.

==> seperating the non-terminal from a list of right hand side symbols. The last component of a `rule` term is a semantic action in the form of a λProlog goal (which takes the place of C code in Yacc). Unlike Yacc-style generators, a separate parser is not needed for the grammar specification.

It is required that no attribute variable in a list of productions appear more than once, except in the semantic action goals. Also, only variables can appear as attribute arguments in a production. Without such restrictions, the grammar may become context *sensitive* (DCGs have the same problem).

Valid handles are generated by forming a closure of triples following the inductive definition as described in the foregoing. The *first* relation needed for lookaheads is pre-computed and written to the parser file as atomic clauses (for efficient lookup). The detection of reduce-reduce and shift-reduce conflicts proceeds directly from the valid handles (except we consider each "`member`" of the lookbacks and lookaheads of a merged handle by virtue of Prolog's backtracking using negation-as-failure).

The generated representation of parsing judgements are four-place predicates of the form `parse Stack Input Result Rule_Type` where `Stack` and `Input` are lists, and `Rule_Type` is a string that's either `"shift"`, `"reduce"`, `"accept"`, `"special"`, or `"error"`. `Result` is instantiated by the `"accept"` rule to the start symbol of the grammar along with its attribute (usually the abstract syntax tree). For example, a merged handle such as $(\{b\}, p \to qr, \{a1, a2\})$ can be represented by the clauses

```
parse [q,b|Stack] [r|Input] Result "shift" :-
  parse [r,q,b|Stack] Input Result Nextrule.
parse [r,q,b|Stack] [A|Input] Result "reduce" :-
  member A [a1,a2], (semantic_action),
  parse [p,b|Stack] [A|Input] Result Nextrule.
```

Semantic action goals are added to reduce rules in the obvious way.

6.1 Operator Precedence and Associativity

The grammar shown in the `cfg` clause, used in an implementation of an "online calculator" however, is ambiguous as defined and the parser generator outputs the messages[6]:

```
Computing Valid Handles...
No reduce-reduce conflicts.
**Shift-Reduce conflict with  ae _63 ==> ae _85 :: plust :: ae _87
:: nil  exists
 when top of stack is of form  ae _683 :: plust :: ae _694 ::
bofs :: _68306
 and lookahead symbol is  plust
Do you want to (s)hift or (r)educe (default is shift):
```

---

[6] Symbols such as _85 are internally generated logic variables. "::" is alternative notation for the list constructor |. bofs is $\$_0$.

As with Yacc-style generators, shift-reduce conflicts caused by ambiguity concerning operator precedence and associativity can be resolved by supplementary declarations. This feature is easily incorporated into our parser generator by clauses illustrated by the following examples:

```
binaryop plust (ae X) (ae Y) "left" 3.
binaryop timest (ae X) (ae Y) "left" 2.
```

These clauses declare which grammar symbols are to be regarded as operators (on certain kinds of expressions) as well as their associativity and precedence level. Ambiguity caused by these operators are then resolved by "special" clauses at the beginning of the file. This feature requires the use of ! in the parser (otherwise non-determinism due to backtracking will become possible). For example, Binary operator associativity is resolved by the following clause, which redirects a goal to a shift or reduce rule:

```
parse [Ea,OP,Eb|Alpha] [OP|Beta] Result "special" :-
  binaryop OP Ea Eb Assoc Prec, !,
  ( (Assoc = "left",
     parse [Ea,OP,Eb|Alpha] [OP|Beta] Result "reduce");
    (Assoc = "right",
     parse [Ea,OP,Eb|Alpha] [OP|Beta] Result "shift")).
```

Unary and implicit operators are handled similarly. A default "error" clause is also placed at the end of the file to report failure.

The parser displays messages for remaining conflicts as illustrated above. Reduce-reduce conflicts result in failure. Remaining shift-reduce conflicts are resolved by user input, producing "special" clauses that redirect goals matching the form of the conflicts to "shift" or "reduce" rules.

Another simplification (currently unimplemented) is to collapse all shift rules into a simple default rule, which is used only if no reduce rule is applicable. This simplification however, means that a shift is always possible and errors will not be reported until the end of the file has been reached. This problem can be largely solved if the default shift rule is aware of the maximum number of terminal symbols on the right-hand side of any grammar production (which limits the number of symbols that can be shifted before a reduce rule must be applied).

7 Related Work

In Section 1 we have already discussed the relationship between our approach and some other works on parsing in logic programming. A close precedent to the type of work presented here, however, is that of Cohen and Hickey [3], who described strategies for parsing in Prolog with similar goals. They showed how to compute grammar properties such as "first" and "follow" succinctly, and gave enough details for building LL(1) parsers in Prolog. A formulation of deterministic bottom-up parsing was proposed based on "weak-precedence grammars." However, this formulation is incomplete: an extra condition that excludes productions with right-hand sides ending in the same symbol must be enforced, otherwise non-determinism of the reduce-reduce type may persist[7]. This extra condition however, further restricts the type of grammars that can be used with their technique. Nevertheless, the ultimate aims of this paper is very much in the same spirit as [3].

8   Conclusion

When faced with the need for a generic parsing tool appropriate for use in compiler writing, the logic programmer can consider several alternatives. DCGs are general, but non-deterministic. Using an existing parser generator in an alien language is another alternative. It is technically possible to extract the parse table from code generated by Yacc and use it in a Prolog parser. However, it is difficult to see how such a process can be automated, especially when declarative semantic attributes must be attached to grammar symbols. A forced implementation of established LR parsing algorithms is also possible, and would at least allow semantic actions to be defined in the native language. If such a tool already exists for the declarative language in question, then it may seem needless to examine another grammar formalism. However, when faced with the task of developing a parser generator from scratch, it is valid to address the fact that certain aspects of general LR parsing renders its formulation as declarative, logical clauses highly awkward. Aspects of LR parsing that give it its efficiency also may not translate into anything meaningful in a logic programming context. Perhaps future logic programming languages, such as those based on linear logic, can give declarative formulations of the kind of computation required by general LR parsing. But the past also deserves some consideration. The almost-forgotten class of BRC grammars were never considered in the light of logic programming. BRC grammars, and our SBRC grammars, offer simplifications of LR parsing that are conducive to logic programming, just as LALR and SLR grammars are appropriate simplifications for conventional languages.

Our parser generator has been used in the implementation of an experimental imperative language (with static scoping, functions and types). A parser for most of λProlog itself was also generated. An experimental interpreter for core SML in λProlog is currently being developed. Additionally, it has been used for purposes other than compiling as part of an interactive theorem prover for translating the syntax of various "object-logics" into λProlog host syntax[8].

This paper has intentionally not addressed the detailed representation of semantic attributes and actions. We have completely separated the basic parsing mechanism so that it can be incorporated into a variety of declarative settings. However, it was the desire to reason with a new class of abstract syntax, namely

---

[7] Consider the grammar $(S \rightarrow aB \mid cA, \quad A \rightarrow ab, \quad B \rightarrow b)$ in relation to the formulation of weak-precedence parsing in [3].

[8] Please see accompanying homepage for more details on these applications (http://www2.trincoll.edu/~cliang/parsergen/).

higher order abstract syntax, that truely motivated this work. It is hoped that the availability of this parsing tool will facilitate the exploration of a host of possible applications of declarative programming in general, and of higher order logic programming in particular.

For future work on the parser generator we plan to improve its performance and usability, especially in the form of additional **"error"** clauses for error correction.

Acknowledgments

Support for this work was provided by Dale Miller at the Pennsylvania State University. The author also wishes to thank Jeremie Wajs for testing the parsers.

References

1. A. V. Aho, R. Sethi, and J. Ullman. *Compilers: Principles, Techniques, and Tools.* Addison-Wesley, 1986.
2. A. W. Appel. *Modern Compiler Implementation in ML.* Cambridge University Press, 1998.
3. J. Cohen and T. Hickey. Parsing and compiling using prolog. *ACM Transactions on Programming Languages and Systems,* 9(2):125–163, 1987.
4. R. Floyd. Bounded context syntactic analysis. *Communications of the ACM,* 7(2):62–67, 1964.
5. S. Fong. *Computational Properties of Principle-Based Grammatical Theories.* PhD thesis, MIT, June 1991.
6. S. L. Graham. On bounded right context languages and grammars. *SIAM Journal on Computing,* 3(3):224–254, 1974.
7. M. Harrison and I. Havel. On the parsing of deterministic languages. *Journal of the ACM,* 21(4):525–548, 1974.
8. M. A. Harrison. *Introduction to Formal Language Theory.* Addison-Wesley, 1978.
9. R. Ochitani K. Uehara and O. Kakusho. A bottom-up parser based on predicate logic. *IEEE Proceedings, International Symposium on Logic Programming,* pages 220–227, 1984.
10. D. E. Knuth. On the translation of languages from left to right. *Information and Control,* 8(6):607–639, 1965.
11. G. Nadathur and D. Mitchell. System description: Teyjus—a compiler and abstract machine based implementation of λProlog. In *Automated Deduction–CADE-13,* Springer-Verlag LNAI no. 1632, pages 287–291, July 1999.
12. U. Nilsson. AID: an alternative implementation of DCGs. *New Generation Computing,* 4:383–399, 1986.
13. F. Pereira and D. Warren. Definite clause grammars for language analysis. *Artificial Intelligence,* 13:231–278, 1980.
14. F. Pereira and D. Warren. Parsing as deduction. In *21st Annual Meeting of the Association for Computational Linguistics,* pages 137–144, 1983.
15. Shieber S., Schabes Y., and Pereira F. Principles and implementation of deductive parsing. Technical Report TR-11-94, Center for Research in Computing Technology, Harvard University, December 1998.

A Logic Programming Application for the Analysis of Spanish Verse

Pablo Gervás

Departmento de Inteligencia Artificial
Universidad Europea de Madrid
Villaviciosa de Odón, Madrid 28670
pg2@dinar.esi.uem.es

Abstract. Logic programming rules are provided to capture the rules governing formal poetry in Spanish. The resulting logic program scans verses in Spanish to provide their metric analysis. The program uses DCG grammars to model the division of each word into syllables, and additional predicates are employed to define metric phenomena such as synaloepha, syllable count of a verse, rhyme of a word... The system is tested over a set of Spanish Golden Age sonnets and shown to give reasonable results, providing a very useful pegdagogical application for teaching Spanish poetry.

1 Introduction

Logic programming has provided many tools for natural language processing (see [1, 11]). It has been applied with success in various fields like generation, understanding, parsing, and semantic representation. The present paper extends the application of logic programming to natural language processing beyond everyday language. Logic programming rules are provided to capture the rules governing formal poetry in Spanish. The resulting logic program scans verses in Spanish to provide their metric analysis. As such it constitutes a useful tool for literary study of Spanish poetry, or as a pedagogical tool for teaching students how Spanish poetry is analysed. The system is tested over a set of Spanish Golden Age sonnets and shown to produce good results.

The system has immediate aplication as a pedagogical tool to help in the process of teaching Spanish poetry and metric at school and university level. As well as scanning metrically a set of verses, the system allows easy location of places where the poet has used poetic licenses such as hiatus, dieresis and syneresis, thereby providing a good tool for stylistic analysis of texts.

2 Description of the Problem

Formal poetry in Spanish is governed by a set of rules that determine a valid verse form and a valid strophic form. A given poem can be analysed by means of these rules in order to establish what strophic form is being used. Another

J. Lloyd et al. (Eds.): CL 2000, LNAI 1861, pp. 1330–1344, 2000.

set of rules is applied to analyse (or *scan*) a given verse to count its metrical syllables. This paper presents a logic programming application that carries out this analysis. The program uses DCG grammars to model the division of each word into syllables, and additional predicates are employed to define metric phenomena such as synaloepha, syllable count of a verse, rhyme of a word...

2.1   Parsing the Syllables in a Word

As a starting point the process of scanning a verse requires a preliminary decomposition of the verse into syllables. These syllables, as understood by the layman with no notions of formal analysis of poetry, do not match metric syllables, but they constitute the starting point of the analysis. The Spanish language presents advantages over other languages in this respect in the sense that one can work out the division of a word into syllables algorithmically from the way it is written. The process of parsing the list of letters corresponding to a word in order to generate a list of syllables applies a set of ortographical rules governing the way letters are grouped together into syllables (see [8, 7]). These rules have to be taken into account when parsing automatically. The next step in the process of scanning a verse is to take into account metric considerations that transform this initial list of syllables into metric syllables, and to generate a count of metric syllables in the verse. These processes depend on the position of the stressed syllables of each word.

2.2   Locating Stressed Syllables

The accents that need to be counted are not those that are usually represented by a slanted dash over a word. Every word has its own prosodic accent, and this is placed over the *sílaba tónica*, the one that carries the stress when it is pronounced. Spanish does have a set of rules that allow automatic location of the stressed syllable of a word from its written form (see [8]). This is important because it allows analysis with no need for a lexical entry for each word in the verse.

According to the distance from the stressed syllable to the end of the word, words are classified into three different types:

- *palabras agudas*, or oxytone words, those in which the stressed syllable is the last syllable of the word
- *palabras llanas* , or paroxytone words, those in which the stressed syllable is the one before the last syllable of the word
- *palabras esdrújulas* , or proparoxytone words, those in which the stressed syllable lies two syllables from the end of the word

2.3   Metric Syllable Count

In working out the count of metric syllables of a verse the concept of syllable involved differs slightly from its everyday equivalents. A metric syllable does not always match the corresponding morphological syllable. When a word ends in a vowel and the following word starts with a vowel, the last syllable of the first word and the first syllable of the following word constitute a single syllable. This is known as *synaloepha* (see [7], or [13] for an overview in English), and it is one of the problems that we are facing.

For instance, the following list of syllables for a verse

bás - te - te a - mor lo que ha por mi pa - sa - do
13 syllables

turns into the list of metric syllables:

bás - te - te_ a - mor lo que _ ha por mi pa - sa - do
11 syllables

because it shows two instances of synaloepha (marked in bold).

Another phenomenon that affects the syllable count is given by the position of the accent of the last word a verse (see [7], or [13] for an overview in English). If the last word is a *palabra llana* (stress one syllable from the end) the verse is considered to have as many metric syllables as it has morphological syllables.

to - dos sen - ti - dos hu - ma - nos
8 metric syllables

If the last word is a *palabra aguda* (stress right at the end) the verse is considered to have one more metric syllable than it has morphological syllables.

A - sí, con tal en - ten - der
7 + 1 = 8 metric syllables

If the last word is a *palabra esdrújula* (stress two syllables from the end) the verse is considered to have one metric syllable less than it has morphological syllables.

A - mor, tus fuer - zas rí - gi - das
8 - 1 = 7 metric syllables

2.4   Distribution of Stressed Syllables

The considerations presented so far describe how a division of a verse into metric syllables and the corresponding metric syllable count is obtained. Formal analysis of poetry also studies the position of stressed syllables over a verse. For the verse to sound pleasing, the prosodic accents must be distributed according to precise patterns. This distribution of prosodic patterns provides the quality of being pleasant to the ear.

For instance, for an eleven syllable long verse to sound pleasing, it needs some of the stressed syllables of its words to fall on certain specific positions. It is not necessary for the stressed syllables of every word in the verse to be in specific positions. It is enough for certain strategic syllabic positions within the verse to have a stressed syllable. There are four accepted combinations that produce the required prosodic effect (see [7, 13]).

1) Stressed syllables fall on positions 1, 6 and 10. The verse is then referred as an *endecasílabo enfático*. In the following examples, one such verse is first given in its original form, followed by a divided version in which words have been split up into syllables and syllables from adjoining words are linked together whenever *synaloepha* has occurred. Syllabic positions are numbered in the line below, and stressed syllables falling in key positions are marked out in bold

$$\begin{array}{ccccccccccc} \textbf{bás-} & \text{te-} & \text{te\_} & \text{a-} & \textbf{mor} & \text{lo} & \textbf{que} & \_ & \textbf{ha} & \text{por mi pa-} & \textbf{sa-} & \text{do} \\ 1 & 2 & 3 & 4 & 5 & & 6 & & 7 & 8 \; 9 & 10 & 11 \end{array}$$

2) Stressed syllables fall on positions 2, 6 and 10. The verse is then referred as an *endecasílabo heroico*. For instance "en verdes hojas vi que se tornaban":

$$\begin{array}{ccccccccccc} \text{en-} & \textbf{ver-} & \text{des} & \text{ho-} & \text{jas} & \textbf{vi} & \text{que} & \text{se} & \text{tor-} & \textbf{na-} & \text{ban} \\ 1 & 2 & 3 & 4 & 5 & 6 & 7 & 8 & 9 & 10 & 11 \end{array}$$

3) Stressed syllables fall on positions 3, 6 and 10. The verse is then referred as an *endecasílabo melódico*. For instance"a la entrada de un valle, en un desierto":

$$\begin{array}{ccccccccccc} \text{a} & \text{la\_} & \text{en-} & \textbf{tra-} & \text{da} & \text{de\_} & \text{un} & \textbf{va-} & \text{lle\_} & \text{en un de-} & \textbf{sier-} & \text{to} \\ 1 & & 2 & 3 & 4 & 5 & & 6 & 7 & 8 \; 9 & 10 & 11 \end{array}$$

4) Stressed syllables fall on positions 4, 6 or 8, and 10. The verse is then referred as an *endecasílabo sáfico*. For instance, the verse "que con lloralla cresca cada día":

$$\begin{array}{ccccccccccc} \text{que} & \text{con} & \text{llo-} & \textbf{ra-} & \text{lla} & \textbf{cres-} & \text{ca} & \text{ca-} & \text{da} & \textbf{dí-} & \text{a} \\ 1 & 2 & 3 & 4 & 5 & 6 & 7 & 8 & 9 & 10 & 11 \end{array}$$

Once a verse has been scanned, and the stressed syllables have been located for every word in the verse, analysis of the positions of stressed syllables is a simple matter.

2.5 Extracting Word Rhyme

In order to identify the strophic form of a given poem it is important to identify the rhyme of each verse. In Spanish (see [7, 13]) the last vowel of the verse and all the following letters (both vowels and consonants) are the same in verses that rhyme. The rules described in the previous sections also allow determination of the set of letters at the end of the word that constitute its rhyme.

2.6   Related Work

Work along similar lines has been carried out for Italian Renaissance poetry [9], French [3], Middle Indo-Aryan [4], and Old English [2]. In particular, [9] discusses the need for metrically scanned electronic versions of classical texts, and discusses the severe limitations of automatic procedures for marking accents and counting syllables in the case of Italian. As a conclusion of this discussion, an interactive program is suggested as the best means of scanning the text metrically. Similar difficulties are met in [3] while dealing with French text. French requires prior specific transcription of the written text into phonemes before the metrical analysis can be carried out. The study of Middle Indo-Aryan Prakrit in [4] presents an additional problem due to the fact that a special character set is required for the language, so the text must be first be transcribed onto Roman script. The work carried out on Old English in [2] concentrates on analysis of phonological patterning, with particular emphasis on alliteration.

Spanish does not present as many difficulties as Italian or French, because the phonetics of a word can be unambiguously obtained from its written form. This includes word accents, since the language provides special means of representing accents graphically. However, Spanish presents the additional difficulty of allowing a number of poetic licenses concerning metrical scansion. This implies that scansion of Spanish verse cannot be decided unambiguously without resorting to the context. A verse scanned as 12 syllables may be re-interpreted as 11 syllables long if it appears in the context of a poem built solely of 11 syllable long verses, provided that the right conditions for poetic licence to occur are met.

Existing work on analysis of Spanish poetical texts, such as [10], applies computational techniques to six main streams of research: sentential analysis, word length analysis, running words analysis, word frequency analysis, use of words analysis, and cluster analysis. At present we are not aware of any work that concentrates specifically on the metrical analysis of Spanish verse.

3   The Logic Programming Implementation

The analyser presented in this paper is implemented in SWI Prolog (see [12]). In order to carry out the whole set of analyses required to decide whether a given text is a correct poem, verses must be treated as lists of words, words must be treated as lists of characters (later as lists of syllables) and syllables as lists of characters. Prolog provides very useful mechanisms to process such a representation. In this program, Definite Clause Grammars (DCG) (see [5]) have been used to encode the different stages of analysis. A detailed description of the implementation of each step is given below.

The predicate that carries out the analysis of a single verse is implemented as a predicate **analysis**. The predicate **analysis** obtains the following information from a verse represented as a list of words: number of syllables after applying all the rules, list of syllables in the verse, list of positions of stressed syllables, and rhyme of the verse.

For instance, for the following call:

```
?- analysis([Cerrar,podra_,mis,ojos,la,postrera],N,Ls,La,Ri).
```

the system would return the following results:

```
N = 11
Ls = [Ce,rrar,po,dra_,mis,o,jos,la,pos,tre,ra]
La = [2,4,5,6,8,10]
Ri = era
```

These items are obtained in two stages. To carry out the task in hand, the system needs to know the following information about each word in the verse: number of syllables, list of syllables in the word, position of stressed syllable of the word, and rhyme of the word.

The first step during analysis is to check whether such information is available in the system vocabulary (a database of facts) for all the words in the verse. If data are missing for a given word of the verse, they are worked out from the word using the rules as described below. The system adds this information to the database of vocabulary facts available for metric analysis.

The second step starts when all data are available. The verse is analysed recursively, using the data worked out for each word, and applying the metric rules to scan the verse properly. Two types of analysis are possible: finding the list of syllables of a word (and therefore the metric syllable count for the verse), or finding the list of positions of stressed syllables (which determines the correctness of the verse).

The division of the general process into two different stages gives the system exceptional flexibility when confronted with new texts. On the one hand, any unfamiliar word appearing in the text can be analysed to obtain the required data. On the other hand, the system may resort to previously stored analysis to avoid recomputation of the data for a specific word. This may have a dual effect on the efficiency of the system, transferring the load from computation time to memory requirements. And additional advantage lies in the fact that there are many exceptions to the general rules implemented in the system. The rules capture the general pattern of word formation of the Spanish language, but many words borrowed from other languages but now fully accepted do not conform to these rules. The particular structure proposed allows the relevant data for problematic to be loaded into the system prior to its use, therefore avoiding errors during the analysis due to exceptions to the rules appearing in a text.

The rest of this section provides brief descriptions of the different processes involved in the analysis.

3.1   Syllabic Analysis of a Word: Word Syllable Parser

The Word Syllable Parser module takes as an input the list of characters of the word to be analysed. The complete operation is carried out in three stages of parsing.

Parsing Character Type. The first parse classifies each character (or group of two characters) into one of 14 different categories according to its ability to combine with other characters to form basic sound groups (double consonants, consonants that can group with other consonants, high, low or middle vowels). Information about vowel classification plays an important role in sorting out syllable boundaries in diphthongs (see [7,13] for details). For instance, an r following an r is grouped into a single rr 'double consonant' group. This grouping is carried out by a DCG of 4 basic rules and 63 rules describing terminals. This proliferation of rules for terminals is due to the fact that both upper and lower case characters must be taken into account, and combinations of these in cases of double consonants. Only the simplest examples of the grammar are presented here. There are many variations and many exceptions to each rule (u after q acts as a single consonant, ns at the end of a syllable cannot be separated, double consonants ch, rr, ll and pr need separate rules...).

Terminal elements of the grammar are defined as facts of the form:

```
vowel(va([a]))-->[a].              /* a */
vowel(vm([e]))-->[e].              /* e */
vowel(vc([i]))-->[i].              /* i */
vowel(vu([u]))-->[u].              /* u */

consonant(n([n]))-->[n].
consonant(cp([p]))-->[p].          /* p */
consonant(cl([l]))-->[l].          /* l */
consonant(c([v]))-->[v].

double_consonant(cd([c,h]))-->[c,h].   /* ch */
double_consonant(cd([r,r]))-->[r,r].   /* rr */
```

Vowels are classified into high (i,u), middle (e,o) or low (a). This information is required to work out the behaviour of diphthongs (see [8]). Groups of different vowels are grouped together into a single syllable (a dyphthong) when certain circumstances are met. These circumstances are specified in terms of whether the group of vowels is made up of different combinations of vowels from one group or another, and whether the corresponding vowels are stressed or not. The rules for the grouping of vowels into dyphthongs requrie this information at a later stage, so the distinction is noted during this stage of the analysis.

The vowel u requires special treatment because it also acts as auxiliary to consonants g and q.

Consonants are classified according to their ability to form different letter groups either with other consonants (groups ns, *r, *l...) or with specific vowels (groups qu, gu...). Letters with different combination properties are identified as members of the specific group and marked as such at this stage. In each case, a functor is generated that identifies the type of letter considered, and contains the letter itself (in list format if it is a complex letter such as a double consonant) as an argument.

The rules of the grammar simply parse the input assigning categories to each group of letters:

```
parse_letters([])-->[].
parse_letters([X|Rest])-->double_consonant(X),
                          parse_letters(Rest).
parse_letters([X|Rest])-->consonant(X),
                          parse_letters(Rest).
parse_letters([X|Rest])-->vowel(X),
                          parse_letters(Rest).
```

Parsing Character Groups. The second parse operates over the output of the first and joins together basic sound groups that make up either a consonantal group or a vowel group. For instance, *pr*, *gl*, *ns*, group together as consonants; and vowels are grouped into diphthongs or triphthongs according to the rules. This DCG has 60 rules. The basic rule for this level of analysis (identifying groups of consonants and groups of vowels) is defined as:

```
group_letters([])-->[].
group_letters([X|Rest])-->group(X),group_letters(Rest).
```

The rest of the rules take the form:

```
group(cons(X))-->[cd(X)].
group(cons(X))-->[c(X)].

group(gv(X))-->[va(X)].
group(gv([A,B]))-->[vc([A]),vm([B])].
```

Certain cases require a step of look-ahead in order to make the right decision. For instance, the rules for *g*, *u* combinations before *i* and *e* (in which cases the *u* is silent); or cases where a certain combination of vowels forming a diphthong is broken by the graphic accent of *tilde*[1]. For instance, the combination of a low vowel and a stressed high vowel, such as ...*aí*... does not form a dyphthong and should be parsed into two syllables, whereas the combination of a stressed low vowel and a high vowel, such as ...*ái*... does, and should be parsed into the same syllable.

```
group(cons([G,U]), [gr([G]),vu([U]),vm([e])|X],[vm([e])|X]).
group(cons([G,U]), [gr([G]),vu([U]),vc([i])|X],[vc([i])|X]).
```

```
% dyphthong
group(gv([A,T,B]))-->[va([A]),ac([T]),vu([B])].
```

```
% no dyphthong (requires lookahead)
group(gv(A),[va(A),vc(B),ac(T)|X],[vc(B),ac(T)|X]).
```

---

[1] The *tilde* is represented in the system as an ac(T) functor.

The examples presented here are only a selection of particular instances of the type of rule discussed in each case.

Parsing Syllables. The third parse takes as input the list of consonant and vowel groups and tacks together those that form valid syllables. This DCG has 14 rules. The basic structure of this grammar is:

```
find_syllables --> syllable,find_syllables.
find_syllables --> [],!.

syllable -->initial_consonant,vowel_group,final_consonant.
syllable -->initial_consonant,vowel_group.
syllable -->vowel_group,final_consonant.
syllable -->vowel_group.
```

These rules include an additional argument which returns the list of the syllables found for the word, each one converted into a Prolog atom.

Locating the Stressed Syllable of a Word. Simple Prolog predicates carry out the task of locating the stressed syllable of a given word, taking as input the list of syllables. The representation in use includes a notation symbol for the tilde, used in Spanish orthography to help locate stressed syllables using a few simple rules. This rules are taught to every primary school student (and forgotten regrettably fast!). For a detailed reference, see [8].

Extracting the Rhyme of a Word. The rhyme of a word is given by the fragment of the word that lies beyond the last stressed vowel of the word. The rhyme of each word is obtained by a predicate `obtain_rhyme` that operates over the list of syllables for that word. Taking into account the location of the stress in the word, it truncates the stressed syllable to obtain its tail (from the stressed vowel to the end) and it appends to it all the remaining syllables to the end of the word. The procedure is made up of three rules. Each rule deals with one possible stress pattern for the word. Every rule works by locating the last stressed syllable, applying the predicate `end_of_syllable` (which returns the portion of the syllable which lies beyond the last stressed vowel), and joins it together with any remaining syllables between the stressed syllable and the end of the word.

The information about the rhyme of a word is also included in the fact stored for it in memory. Therefore, during the metric analysis of a verse, identifying the rhyme of a word involves just querying the vocabulary database.

Managing the Vocabulary Database. The system operates with a vocabulary database that is declared in the form of Prolog facts. When the system reads a word, whether during selection of rhymes or during the writing of a draft, it consults the vocabulary database. If the word is not found, the required procedures are invoked to obtain the necessary information.

This information is stored as facts of the form:

```
known_word(1,ar,[ce,rrar],no,no,cerrar).
```

where: the first argument 1 shows the position of the stressed syllable from the end of the word, ar   is the rhyme of the word, [ce,rrar]is the list of syllables of the word, the first no indicates whether the word starts with a vowel, the second no indicates whether the word ends with a vowel, and the final argument cerrar is the word itself, to be used as key when retrieving the rest of the information.

If a given word in the text was not present could not be found in the database, the results of the analysis are declared in memory in the same format as existing items in the database. At the end of a session, the system allows the updated database to be saved. This makes the result of all new words that have been already parsed available in database form for later analyses.

This method allows the option of starting the system with an empty vocabulary database each time (thereby optimising memory use), or to build the vocabulary database incrementally by loading a previous version before the analysis of each new text. This second option implies growing memory requirements for subsequent executions, but improves the computational efficiency of the analysis. It has the additional advantage of progressively building a vocabulary database of metrically analysed Spanish words.

3.2   Metric Analysis of a Verse: The Metric Syllable Counter

The metric syllable counter is defined as a set of Prolog predicates that operate recursively over the list of words in a verse. All the information about the division into syllables and the location of the stressed syllable obtained for a given word during previous two stages is declared in memory as Prolog facts. In this way, while processing each word in the verse the syllable counter has access to the list of syllables of the word and the position of the stressed syllable. From this information it can also determine easily whether a word starts or ends with a vowel.

Counting the Metric Syllables in a Verse. The predicate word_analysis works out the scansion of the verse and it returns a list of metric syllables corresponding to that verse, as well as the number of syllables found in the verse.

A simple predicate synaloepha implements the decision rule for synaloepha, and appends two contiguous syllables whenever necessary. This is done by means of two auxiliary predicates (start_vowel y end_vowel) that identify whether a word starts or ends with a vowel. When processing a word, the final syllable of the previous word is carried over, together with a variable indicating whether it ended in a vowel or not. The last syllable of the previous word is treated as if it were part of the word. According to the variable one or the other rule of the procedure is used. If synaloepha takes place, the rule that requires the previous word to end in a vowel simply acts as an interface, calling the other version with the corresponding alterations of the list of parameters: the number of syllables found so far is reduced by one, and the last syllable of the previous word and the first syllable of the present one are fused into a single syllable. Since this operation is carried out recursively, two syllables appended in this way may yet be appended to a third one if the conditions are right. This is quite common when one vowel articles such as *a* occur between words that finish and start with vowels. This method requires special attention to be paid to border situations. For the first call (at the beginning of a verse) an additional ghost syllable must be added. This ghost syllable must be eliminated from the final list of syllables at the end. In the same way, for the last call (which would given the empty list as a result) the last syllable of the previous word must be returned as sole member of the list of syllables found, to ensure that it is not lost.

The predicate `reevaluate` takes into account the effect on the count of metric syllables of the verse (as opposed to prosodic ones) of the position of the stressed syllable of the last word. It has three different versions, one for each possible pattern of stress placement. They all carry out basic arithmetic operations over the resulting number of syllables: subtract one if the last word is proparoxytone, leave as it is for a paroxytone word, add one for an oxytone word.

A similar predicate, `accent_analysis`, operating over the same list of words for the verse and using the information facts in memory for each word, translates the list of words into a list of stressed syllable positions. This process is parallel to the one carried out when creating the list of syllables, with a numerical counter taking the part of the syllables.

Using Results to Validate a Verse. Over the results of the analysis, a diagnostic of the correctness of the verse can be obtained by pattern matching with a set of valid patterns declared in memory. The predicate `conclusions` takes the obtained results and works out whether the verse under analysis is valid as *endecasílabo*. If it is, the type of *endecasílabo* is identified by checking the positions of the stressed syllables.

In the example above, the verse:

Cerrar podrá mis ojos la postrera

is an *endecasílabo heróico*, because it is eleven syllables long ($N = 11$)and its list of positions of stressed syllables ($La = [2,4,5,6,8,10]$) contains the key positions 2, 6, 10.

4   Evaluation of the System

The system has been evaluated over a set of classical poems. The number of incorrect analyses is worked out as a percentage. Specific sources of error are identified and their contribution to the general error is discussed. In each case, possible solutions are discussed.

4.1   The Choice of Test Data

The system has been tested over a set of 64 classic Spanish Golden Age sonnets (taken from [6]). These sonnets were fed to the system in separate files containing the sonnets by different authors. The system output a file with the syllable count, list of syllables, list of stressed positions, and rhyme for each of the given verses. Sonnets were chosen as benchmark poems because they have a very rigid formal structure. Every verse in a Spanish sonnet must be 11 syllables long according to the rules. Over the resulting files, verses that had been assigned by the system a syllable length other than 11 were hand checked for errors.

4.2   The Results

The results obtained are presented in table 1.

Table 1. Raw Results

Author	Sonnets	Verses	Errors	% Error
Quevedo	21	294	31	89.5
Lope	16	224	17	92.4
Góngora	11	154	19	87.7
Garcilaso	8	112	21	81.3
Boscán	3	42	2	95.2
Aldana	5	70	11	84.3
Totals	64	896	101	88.7

4.3   The Problem of Poetic License

A poet is allowed a number of poetic licences to make the verses fit into the metric structure. These poetic licences are known as *syneresis*, *dieresis*, and *hiatus* (see [13] for details). Of these, *dieresis* allows a diphthong to be broken (adding one syllable to a given word), *syneresis* allows an illegal diphthong to be created (subtracting a syllable to a word), and *hiatus* allows synaloepha to be broken (adding a syllable to a given verse). Resolving issues of poetic license presents special problems because the main idea behind the concept is too allow the same verse to be parsed as having a certain length in one specific context and as having a different one in another. This is achieved by overlooking or enforcing two different metric rules: the rules for synaloepha and the rules for dyphthong formation. Two syllables that might constitute synaloepha (or two vowels making a dyphthong) and be parsed as one under normal conditions can exceptionally be broken up if the poet needs an extra syllable to his verse at that stage, resulting in hiatus (or dieresis). Alternatively, syllables (or vowels) that would be parsed as separate may be parsed as a unit if the poet wants one syllable less, resulting in hiatus (or syneresis). The fact that correct solutions are context dependent means that they cannot be implemented for isolated verses, but only when verses are scanned as part of a whole poem, in which case, the metric rules for the poem impose specific lengths on verse. In a wider setting, these poetic licenses can easily be solved by rephrasing synalopeha and dypththong rules as defeasible inferences (or simply allowing the implicit backtracking in Prolog to find the alternative solution).

The system as it stands allows easy location of poetic licenses, which gives added-value when analysing poetry. The results for poetic licenses obtained for the test data are presented in table 2. The number of poetic licenses taken in each set of poems is listed for each kind. The percentage of error when problems of poetic license are discounted is also shown. A great improvement in system efficiency is appreciated.

Table 2. Poetic Licenses

Author	Verses	Hiatus	Dieresis	Syneresis	Total	Real % error
Quevedo	294	5	1	1	7	97.6
Lope	224	6	2	1	9	96.0
Góngora	154	3	4	4	11	92.9
Garcilaso	112	10	2	2	14	87.5
Boscán	42	0	0	0	0	100
Aldana	70	2	3	1	6	91.4
Totals	896	26	12	9	47	94.8

4.4   Detected Errors and Planned Improvements

The most important source of real errors is the conjunction y, which can act both as a vowel and as a consonant. This creates problems when determining whether synaloepha is possible or not between words. The rules for synaloepha must be redesigned to acoutn for these variations.

The remaining errors can be attributed to exceptions in diphthong formation rules. Although there are generally accepted rules governing diphthong formation, certain cases constitutes exceptions (for historical or etymological reasons). Foreign words that have been accepted into Spanish also constitute exceptions to the syllabic rules. The fact that the system keeps a database of facts for the words in its vocabulary allows exceptions to the rules to be declared directly into the database. In this way, known exceptions can be included from the start, thereby improving the accuracy of the system.

Table 3 shows final results for the system once problems of poetic licence and probles related with conjunction are excluded.

Table 3. Final Results

Author	Sonnets	Verses	Y Errors	% Error
Quevedo	21	294	20	98.6
Lope	16	224	7	99.6
Góngora	11	154	8	100
Garcilaso	8	112	6	99.1
Boscán	3	42	2	100
Aldana	5	70	5	100
Totals	64	896	48	99.3

5   Conclusions and Further Work

Several conclusions can be drawn from the above observations. On one hand, the logic programming tools used to implement the system have demonstrated their power and flexibility in coping with a complex problem of symbolic processing. On the other hand, the system shows potential both in the fields of literary analysis of large texts, and in the field of teaching.

5.1   Advantages of Logic Programming for the Task

The problem tackled in this paper presented a complex structure of several layers of analysis (at character level, at character group level, at syllable level, at the level of words in a verse), each implemetned as a DCG. Solutions with fewer layers are possible, and some have been tested during the development of the system, but were rejected because of the excessive amount of backtracking required whenever information from bottom layers affects the decision process in top layers.

The declarative nature of logic programming, and the modular design of the program (with general rules set distinctly apart from specific data for a given word in the vocabulary database) allows very easy encoding of exceptions. It also allows the system to act both as a parsing tool and as a vocabulary database generator. None of these advantages would have been available in an imperative implementation of the system, even though such an implementation would possibly carry out the parsing problem more efficiently if all the different cases were coded. The modularity of the program allows easy modification and might allow reuse of some parts of the code for languages with similar phonetic structure.

5.2   The System as a Practical Tool

The system is shown to give very good results over a basic sample. Although a considerably bigger sample would be required for a proper validation of the system, the fact that different authors (and therefore different vocabulary and different use of poetic licence) are involved improves the significance of the result.

It is also important to note that although the system is based on linguistic rules for contemporary Spanish, the results are good even when applied to the work of Sixteenth Century poets – which speakers of modern Spanish sometimes find obscure. This shows that the system is not dependent on the specific database of vocabulary facts that it starts with, and it can reasonably be expected to cope with new words however alien to contemporary speakers (as long as they conform to the rules).

The system may be put to practical use as an autonomous analysis tool (as a first approximation to block analysis of texts), or as a pedagogical tool in teaching environments. As extensions of this line of work, a complete system for the analysis of poems, including a diagnostic of strophic form is under development at present. Additional issues such as modelling the described forms of poetic license during the analysis are being considered.

References

1. Allen, J. : Natural Language Understanding, London, Benjamin/Cummings (1995).
2. Barquist, C.R., Shie, D.L.: Computer Analysis of Alliteration in Beowulf Using distinctive Feature Theory. Oxford Journal of Literary and Linguistic Computing, vol. 6, no. 4 (1991).
3. Beaudoin, V., Yvon,F.: The Metrometer: a Tool for Analysing French Verse. Oxford Journal of Literary and Linguistic Computing, vol. 11 no. 1 (1996).
4. Ousaka, Y., Yamazaki, M.: Automatic Analsyis of the canon of Middle Indo-Aryan by personal computer. Oxford Journal of Literary and Linguistic Computing, vol. 9, no. 2 (1994).
5. Pereira, F.C.N. and Warren, D.H.D.: Definite Clause Grammars for Language Analysis: a Survey of the Formalism and Comparison with Augmented Transition Networks. Artificial Intelligence, vol. 13, no. 3 (1980).
6. Pérez de la Cruz Molina, J.L., personal web page,
   http://www.lcc.uma.es/personal/cruz/sonetos/pral.html
7. Quilis, A.: Métrica española, Ariel, Barcelona (1985).
8. Real Academia Española (Comisión de Gramática): Esbozo de una nueva gramática de la lengua española, Espasa-Calpe, Madrid (1986).
9. Robey, D.: Scanning Dante's the Divine comedy: a computer Based approach. Oxford Journal of Literary and Linguistic Computing, vol. 8, no. 2 (1993).
10. Stratil, M., Oakley, R.J.: A Disputed Authorship Study of Two Plays Attributed to Tirso de Molina. Oxford Journal of Literary and Linguistic Computing, vol. 2, no. 3 (1987).
11. Saint-Dizier, P. Advanced Logic Programming for Language Processing, London, Academic Press (1994).
12. Wielemaker, Jan, http://swi.psy.uva.nl/usr/jan/SWI-Prolog.html
13. Wiliamsen, V.G. and Abraham, J.T., Association for Hispanic Classical Theater web page, ftp://listserv.ccit.arizona.edu/pub/listserv/comedia/poetic1.html

A Documentation Generator
for (C)LP Systems

Manuel Hermenegildo

Department of Computer Science, Technical U. of Madrid (UPM)
herme@fi.upm.es

Abstract. We describe lpdoc, a tool which generates documentation manuals automatically from one or more logic program source files, written in Ciao, ISO-Prolog, and other (C)LP languages. It is particularly useful for documenting library modules, for which it automatically generates a rich description of the module interface. However, it can also be used quite successfully to document full applications. A fundamental advantage of using lpdoc is that it helps maintaining a true correspondence between the program and its documentation, and also identifying precisely to what version of the program a given printed manual corresponds. The quality of the documentation generated can be greatly enhanced by including within the program text *assertions* (declarations with types, modes, etc. ...) for the predicates in the program, and *machine-readable comments*. One of the main novelties of lpdoc is that these assertions and comments are written using the Ciao system *assertion language*, which is also the language of communication between the compiler and the user and between the components of the compiler. This allows a significant synergy among specification, debugging, documentation, optimization, etc. A simple compatibility library allows conventional (C)LP systems to ignore these assertions and comments and treat normally programs documented in this way. The documentation can be generated interactively from emacs or from the command line, in many formats including texinfo, dvi, ps, pdf, info, ascii, html/css, Unix nroff/man, Windows help, etc., and can include bibliographic citations and images. lpdoc can also generate "man" pages (Unix man page format), nicely formatted plain ASCII "readme" files, installation scripts useful when the manuals are included in software distributions, brief descriptions in html/css or info formats suitable for inclusion in on-line indices of manuals, and even complete WWW and info sites containing on-line catalogs of documents and software distributions. The lpdoc manual, all other Ciao system manuals, and parts of this paper are generated by lpdoc.

1 Introduction

lpdoc is an *automatic program documentation generator* for (C)LP systems. Its main functionality is to generate a reference manual automatically from one or more source files of (constraint) logic programming systems. It has been developed as part of the Ciao Prolog [1] program development environment, but it can also be used to document source files of almost any other (ISO-)Prolog-like [6] (C)LP system. lpdoc is particularly useful for documenting library modules,

J. Lloyd et al. (Eds.): CL 2000, LNAI 1861, pp. 1345–1361, 2000.
© Springer-Verlag Berlin Heidelberg 2000

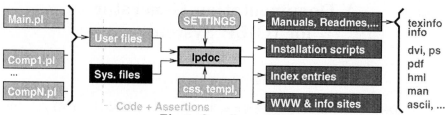

Fig. 1. Overall operation

for which it automatically generates a rich description of the module interface. However, it can also be used quite successfully to document full applications.

The operation of lpdoc is illustrated in Figure 1. lpdoc combines the information from a number of user and system files (as specified in a user-provided configuration file –SETTINGS in Figure 1)[1] and produces manuals in a number of formats (texinfo, dvi, ps, pdf, info, html/css, ascii, Windows help, etc.) which can include bibliographic citations and images (if the target supports them). In addition to full manuals, lpdoc can also generate nicely formatted plain ASCII "readme" files, man pages (Unix manual page format), as well as brief descriptions in html or emacs info formats suitable for inclusion in an on-line *master index* of applications. Using these index entries, lpdoc can create and maintain fully automatically WWW and info sites containing pointers to the on-line versions of the documents it produces. Similarly, it can be used to generate software distribution sites. lpdoc also generates installation scripts for the manuals it produces, which simplify the process of creating a distribution of the corresponding software package. Finally, it is also possible to start a number of *viewers* directly from lpdoc in order to quickly browse the manuals produced. The documentation can be generated interactively from emacs or from the command line in a documentation directory containing configuration files.

The quality of the documentation generated can be greatly enhanced by including within the program text *assertions* (declarations with types, modes, and other properties) for the predicates in the program, and *machine-readable comments* (in the "literate programming" style [11,4]). The assertions and comments included in the source file need to be written using the Ciao *assertion language* [12,10,13]. This is *one of the main novelties of* lpdoc. The fact that this assertion language also serves as the communication vehicle between the compiler and the user and between the components of the compiler allows a significant synergy among specification, debugging, analysis, optimization, and, thanks to lpdoc, program documentation. As we will see, lpdoc understands natively this language and can thus provide accurate information and relate both the the formal and the textual aspects of properties with the assertions in which they occur.

In order to make the discussion self-contained, an example of source code and the output produced by lpdoc is included at the end of the paper. However, since it is difficult to show significant output from the system in the space available, the

---

[1] It also possible to use files written in GNU texinfo format as part of the lpdoc input (useful when gradually converting a manual from this popular format to lpdoc).

reader is invited to look at actual manuals generated by lpdoc for reference while reading the paper. In particular, the lpdoc manual [9] and all other Ciao system manuals are generated by lpdoc. The Ciao manuals and other lpdoc-generated manuals can be found on-line at http://www.clip.dia.fi.upm.es/Software, http://www.clip.dia.fi.upm.es/Software/Ciao, and http://www.clip.dia.fi.upm.es/Software/Beta (registration as a Beta tester is needed for access to the latter). In fact, all these WWW sites are automatically generated and maintained by lpdoc as well.

2   Generating a Manual

We now describe, from the user's point of view, the process of generating a manual (semi-)automatically from a set of source files, installing them in a public area, and accessing them on line.

Documentation can be generated fully automatically from within emacs (e.g., from the Ciao emacs-based program development environment) or calling lpdoc from the command line. The process starts (automatically in the former case or by hand in the latter) by creating a directory (e.g., doc) in which the documentation will be built. This directory is usually placed in the top directory of the distribution of the application or library to be documented and will contain the (automatically generated) manuals as well as scripts for installation of such manuals during the installation of the software package. Typically, almost all files in this directory will be automatically generated by lpdoc, which also takes care of cleaning up this directory of intermediate files before distribution of the software, leaving only the manuals in the selected formats. The configuration file of Figure 1, normally named *SETTINGS*, also resides in this directory. This file is written in Prolog syntax, possibly using Ciao syntactic enhancements (in particular, the functional notation is often useful in this context).

A manual can be generated either from a single source file or from a set of source files. In the latter case, one of these files should be chosen to be the *main file*, and the others will be the *component files*. The main file is the one that will provide the title, author, date, summary, etc. to the entire document. In principle, any set of source files can be documented, even if they contain no assertions or comments. However, the presence of these will greatly improve the documentation (see Section 3).

The name of main file is specified in the SETTINGS file by defining a fact of a predicate main. Facts of a (possibly empty) predicate components define the component files which will generate the different chapters of the manual. Facts of a predicate filepaths are used to define all the directories where the previously mentioned files can be found. Similarly, facts of the predicate systempaths are used to list all the *system* directories where system files used by the files being documented can be found. This is needed because on startup lpdoc has *no default search paths for files* defined, not even those defined by default in the Prolog system under which it was compiled (typically Ciao). This has the important consequence that it allows documenting Prolog systems other than that under which `lpdoc` was compiled. The effect of putting a path in `systempaths` instead of in `filepaths` is that the modules and files in those paths are documented as *system modules* (this is useful when documenting an application to distinguish its parts from those which are in the system libraries).

These are the only settings which are strictly needed in order to generate a manual. However, many aspects of the generated manuals can be controlled through additional configuration parameters. For example, it is possible to control what is included in the different files and how: whether to include bug information or not, comments associated to version changes and/or to patches, author info, detailed explanation of predicate argument modes, starting page number, etc. It is also possible to define the set of formats (`dvi`, `ps`, `pdf`, `ascii`, `html`, `info`, `manl`, ...) in which the documentation should be generated by default (however, a manual in any of the supported formats can be generated on demand by typing "lpdoc *format*"). In particular, selecting `htmlindex` and/or `infoindex` requests the generation of (parts of) a master index to be placed in an installation directory and which provide pointers to the documents generated.

A predicate `indices` determines a list of indices to be included at the end of the document. These can include indices for defined predicates, modules, properties, types, concepts, files, etc. The contents of these indices are afterwards used for several purposes in on-line documents. In particular, `lpdoc` includes an `emacs` library for automatically locating any part of the manual related to the symbol (predicate, flag, property, type, etc.) under the cursor ("help for symbol under cursor") and also performing automatic completion of partially typed names of predicates, types, etc. This is very useful when typing the name of a library predicate: it is possible to complete the name and also locate in one step the corresponding page in the on-line manual generated by `lpdoc`.

It is possible to define a predicate `bibfile` containing paths of *.bib files*, i.e., files containing *bibliographic entries* in BiBTeX format. If citations are used in the text (using the `@cite` command) these will be the files in which the citations will be searched for. All the references in all component files will appear together in a *References* appendix at the end of the manual (the `-norefs` option prevents generation of the 'References' appendix). It is also possible to select different levels of verbosity during processing, from pretty silent –more or less only a couple of messages per file–, to quite verbose, reporting the files visited and the predicates being documented on the fly. The latter is obviously quite useful for debugging.

Once the manual has been generated in the desired formats, `lpdoc` can also install them in a different area, specified by a predicate `docdir` in the `SETTINGS` file. As mentioned before, `lpdoc` can generate directly brief descriptions in html or `emacs` info formats suitable for inclusion in an on-line index of applications. In particular, if the `htmlindex` and/or `infoindex` options are selected, then `lpdoc` will create the installation directory, place the documentation in the desired formats in this directory, and produce and place in the same directory suitable `index.html` and/or `dir` files. These files will contain some basic info on the manual (extracted from the summary and title, respectively) and include pointers to the relevant documents which have been installed. The appearance of the actual indices created (e.g., `index.html`) can be controlled via templates and style sheets, specified in the configuration file. Several manuals, coming from different `doc` directories, can be installed in the same `docdir` directory. In this case, the descriptions of and pointers to the different manuals will be automatically combined (appearing in alphabetic order) in the `index.html` and/or `dir` indices, and a *contents area* will appear at the beginning of the *html index page*. In the same way, facilities are provided for de-installation of manuals from the `docdir` area.

3   Enhancing the Documentation Being Generated

`lpdoc` will generate quite useful information from standard program files: e.g., exported predicates with their arity, characteristics of these predicates –dynamic, multifile, ...–, other modules used, required libraries, and, if available, types and other properties, etc. However, the quality of the documentation generated can be greatly enhanced by including within the program text *assertions*, and *machine-readable comments*.

Assertions are declarations which are included in the source and provide information regarding certain characteristics of the program. Typical assertions include type declarations, modes, general properties (such as *does not fail*), etc. For our purposes, we can consider standard compiler directives (such as `dynamic/1`, `op/3`, `meta_predicate/1`...), also as assertions. When documenting a module, `lpdoc` will use the assertions associated with the module interface to construct a textual description of this interface. In principle, only the exported predicates are documented, although any predicate can be included in the documentation by explicitly requesting it (by using a particular `comment/2` declaration –see below). Judicious use of these assertions allows at the same time documenting the program code, documenting the external use of the module, and greatly improving the debugging process. The latter is possible because the assertions provide the compiler with information on the intended meaning or behavior of the program (i.e., the specification) which can be checked at compile-time (by a preprocessor/static analyzer) and/or at run-time (via checks inserted by the same preprocessor) –see [8] for details.

Machine-readable comments are also declarations included in the source program but which contain additional information intended to be read by humans (this is where the connection with the *literate programming* style of Knuth [11, 4] is closest). These declarations are ignored by the compiler in the same way as classical comments. Thus, they can be used to document the program source in place of (or in combination with) the normal comments typically inserted in the code by programmers. However, because they are more structured and they are machine-readable, they can also be used to improve the automatic generation of printed or on-line documentation. Typical such comments include module title, author(s), bugs, changelog, etc. Judicious use of these comments allows enhancing at the same time the documentation of the program text and the manuals generated.

As mentioned before, lpdoc requires these assertions and comments to be written using the Ciao system *assertion language* [12, 10, 13].[2] Comments have the general form:

```
:- comment(CommentType, CommentData).3
```

where generally the first argument states the type of comment and the second one the comment itself, written in a particular markup language which is very similar to texinfo and LaTeX (see Section 7). Examples of comments are:

```
:- comment(title,"Complex numbers library").
:- comment(summary,"Provides an ADT for complex numbers.").
:- comment(ctimes(X,Y,Z),"@var{Z} is @var{Y} times @var{X}.").
```

An example of an assertion is:

```
:- pred qsort(X,Y) : list(X) => sorted(Y)
                # "@var{Y} is a sorted permutation of @var{X}.".
```

which states that in the calls to predicate qsort/2 the first argument should be a list and, upon exit, the second argument should be sorted. There is also a textual *assertion comment*, written using the same markup language as in comment/2. The properties list/1 and sorted/1 used in the assertion might be declared as such with the following assertions (we are also including the actual definitions for illustration purposes):

```
:- prop sorted(X) # "@var{X} is sorted.".
sorted([]).
sorted([_]).
sorted([X,Y|R]) :- X < Y, sorted([Y|R]).

:- regtype list(X) # "@var{X} is a list.".
list([]).
list([_|T]) :- list(T).
```

(list is actually a particular case of property: a *regular type*). Space limitations unfortunately do not allow a description of the assertion language. See the appendices for more examples and [12, 10, 13] for details.

4   Overall Structure of the Generated Documents

If the manual is generated from a single main file (i.e., components is empty), then the document generated will be a flat document containing no chapters. If the manual is generated from a main file and one or more components, then the main file will be used to generate the cover and introduction, while each of the component files will generate a separate chapter. The contents of each chapter will reflect the contents of the corresponding component source file.

---

[2] A simple compatibility library can be used so that programs documented using assertions and comments can be loaded by traditional (constraint) logic programming systems which lack native support for them. Using this library, such assertions and comments are simply ignored by the compiler.

[3] For brevity, also :- doc(...,...). can be used.

If a `.pl` file does not define the predicates `main/0` or `main/1`, it is assumed to be a *library* and information on the interface (e.g., the predicates exported by the file, the name of the module and usage if it is a module, etc. –the API), is produced by default. If, on the contrary, the file defines the predicates `main/0` or `main/1`, it is assumed to be an *application* and no description of the interface is generated. Instead, usage information is produced. Any combination of libraries and/or main files of applications can be used arbitrarily as components or main files of an `lpdoc` manual (see the `lpdoc` manual [9] for interesting combinations). A `:-comment(filetype,`*filetype*`).` declaration can be used to defeat these rules.

In any case, a cover is generated with the title, authors, summary, version, etc. of the whole manual, which are those of the main file. Then comes the table of contents, whose level of detail can also be controlled via options. This is followed by the sections or chapters corresponding to the file or files being documented. Finally, the manual ends with the selected indices, list of references, etc.

5   Structure of Chapters

The structure of the individual chapters depends also on whether they are applications or libraries. In the case of libraries, the structure is as below. Note that inclusion of many of the following items can be turned on or off and can be configured in several ways through options. Examples of a source file and the chapter generated for it (under a particular set of options) are listed in appendices A and B, for illustration while reading the following items.

- Chapter title, from a `title` comment, such as the line:
  `:- comment(title,"The classical quick-sort").`
  in the example. If the file is the main file, the title text (a documentation string) will also be used in the cover page and also as the description of the manual in on-line indices. If no such comment exists, then a suitable one is generated from the module or file name. Also, a `subtitle` comment is allowed.
- Authors, which are obtained from `author` comments, such as:
  `:- comment(author,"Alan Robinson").`
  There can be more than one of these declarations per module (normally, one per author). These are followed by copyright info (from `copyright` comments) and version info (from changelog comments). If the file is part of a bigger package, then both the file version (i.e., when last changed) and the overall system versions are documented.
- Chapter introduction, taken from a `summary` comment or from a `module` comment, if no summary is available (see also the example).
- A usage and interface section, which is typically generated without any need for comment declarations, and includes:
  - Module usage info, stating whether it is a module, a user file, a package [2], etc., and how it is to be loaded. These automatically generated loading instructions can be replaced by more specific ones by means of a `usage` comment.

- List of exported predicates. These are classified by kind: normal predicates, multifile predicates, regular types, properties, declarations, etc.
- The list of other modules used. These are separated into *User*, *System* and, optionally, *Engine* libraries[4] (this division is controlled by the paths in SETTINGS). It is possible to optionally prevent the information on *System* and/or *Engine* libraries used from being included in the manual. Note that this information is useful because it allows the user of a library to see which other libraries it will load, and thus the impact that it will have on the size of the executable.

- A section with overall information on the library, taken from the module comment, if available (and if this comment was not already used before).
- A section documenting new declarations [2] defined (Ciao-specific).
- A section documenting the predicates (including regular types and properties) exported by the library (e.g., qsort/2, list/1, and sorted/1 in the example). In principle, all exported predicates are documented. However, it is possible to prevent documentation on a predicate from appearing in the manual by using a hide comment (useful, e.g., for low-level predicates which are exported but are not meant to be used directly).
- A section documenting the multifile predicates defined by the library.
- Possibly a section documenting some internal predicates (or regular types or properties) defined by the library. In principle internal (local) predicates are not documented, but documentation of an internal predicate can be forced by using a doinclude comment. This is the case for partition/4 in the example. This is useful for example when generating "internals" manuals or implementation chapters for inclusion in larger documents.
- Optionally, a section with known bugs, i.e., those present in bug comments (see the example).
- Optionally, a section with a list of changes, those present in version comments (see the example). It is possible to list only comments associated with major version changes an leave out minor changes ("patches"). This allows writing version comments which are internal, i.e., not meant to appear in the manual. Code is provided for maintaining version numbers automatically with emacs, or they can also be maintained with other tools such as standard version control systems.
- Reexported predicates, i.e., predicates which are exported by a module m1 but defined in another module m2 which is used by m1, are normally not documented in the original module, but instead a simple reference is included to the module in which they are defined. This is useful if the documentation for the referred module is included in the same document. Otherwise, using a comment/2 declaration with doinclude in the first argument and the predicate descriptor in the second forces the documentation to be included in the referring module. This is often useful when documenting a library made of several components: typically there is a principal module, which is the one

---

[4] In Ciao, engine libraries contain builtins that are always present in any executable, independently of whether they are imported or not from the program.

which users will do a `use_module/1` of, and which exports or reexports all the predicates which define the library's user interface. It is then often best to include in the manual this main file only, with the appropriate `doincludes`.

If the chapter is documenting an application, then no module interface information is included in the documentation, but it still contains title, authors, version, summary, usage information, body, bugs, changelog, etc.

6   Documentation on Predicates, Properties, etc.

We now describe how individual predicates, declarations, properties, etc. are documented. This is done in essentially the same way, independently of whether they appear in the export list or they are internal predicates. The documentation is obviously more detailed if more information is available on the predicate in the form of assertions and comments.

If the program does not contain any declarations for the predicate, a line is output documenting that this is a predicate of the given name and arity and a simple comment is included saying that there is no further documentation available. Note that this means for example that the predicate will appear in the index, and also that its name will be available for command completion within `emacs`.

If the predicate is declared to be a property or regular type, then this fact is included in the documentation. If there is no textual comment available for it, then its actual definition is included in the documentation (see `list/1` in the example). Otherwise, the comment is used (as with `sorted/1` in the example).

If an overall comment (a `comment/2` declaration) is available for a predicate, it is used as a general explanation (see the general comment for `qsort/2` in the example). If any assertions are present, they are documented in mostly textual form. In particular, if `pred` declarations are present, each of them is considered a possible conceptual *usage* (i.e., a particular way in which the predicate is intended to be used) and is documented as such (e.g., the two `pred` declarations for `qsort/2` in the example). Also, if a comment appears in the `pred` declaration, it is associated with the usage (as opposed to the general comment above).

The syntactic sugar which can be used with the assertions (e.g., property macros [12, 13]) can be either kept as is or expanded when documentation is generated. In the example, having chosen the corresponding option, the *modes* (which are "property macros" in the Ciao assertion language) used in `partition/4` have been spelled out in the documentation. Note that the parametric type `list/2` used (e.g., in `list(X,num)`) is assumed to be imported by default.

A point of particular interest is that if a textual comment is available in the definition of a property or regular type (such as for `sorted` in the example) then *this text is used when the property itself is used elsewhere in an assertion.* An example is the use of `sorted` in the two usages for `qsort/2`. This also occurs if the property is imported from another module: the comment is read from that module (actually, from the module's .asr interface file) [14].[5]

7   Documentation Strings

As shown in previous examples, the character strings which can be used in machine readable comments (comment/2 declarations) and assertions can include certain *formatting commands* ("markup"). The syntax of all the formatting commands is: @*command* (followed by either a space or {}), or @*command*{*body*} where *command* is the command name and *body* is the (possibly empty) command body. Also, a command may have several bodies, as in: @*command*{*body1*}{*body2*}.

In order to make it possible to produce documentation in a wide variety of formats, the command set is kept small. The names of the commands are intended to be reminiscent of the commands used in the LaTeX text formatting system, except that "@" is used instead of "\". Note that "\" would need to be escaped in ISO-Prolog strings, which would make the source less readable.[6] Given that space restrictions do not allow a full description of the command set, we provide a general description by categories.

There are a number of *indexing commands* which are used to mark certain words or sentences in the text as concepts, names of predicates, libraries, files, etc. and which then get indexed and cross-referenced in hypertext formats. There are also *referencing commands* which are used to introduce *bibliographic citations* and *references* to sections, urls, email addresses, etc. A set of *formatting commands* are provided which allow typesetting certain words or sentences in a special fonts/faces, build itemized lists, introduce sections, include verbatim examples, cartouches, etc. There are also special commands for generating *accented* and *special* characters. A number of *inclusion commands* (@include, @includedef,...) allow inserting code or strings of text as part of the documentation. The latter may reside in external files or in the file being documented. The former must be part of the module being documented. There are also commands for inserting and scaling images.

8   Other Issues

Separating the documentation from the source file: Sometimes one would not like to include long introductory comments in the module itself but would rather have them in a different file. This can be done quite simply by using the @include command mentioned above. For example, the following declaration:

```
:- comment(module,"@include{Intro.lpdoc}").
```

---

[5] This occurs in the example with list/2, which is in the lists library.

[6] @ is familiar to texinfo users and, in any case, many ideas in LaTeX were taken from scribe, where the escape character was indeed "@"!

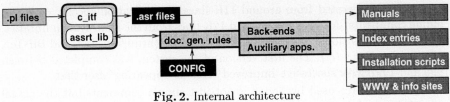

Fig. 2. Internal architecture

will include the contents of the file `Intro.lpdoc` as the module description.

Alternatively, sometimes one may want to generate the documentation from a completely different file. Assuming that the original module is `m1.pl`, this can be done by calling the module containing the documentation `m1_doc.pl`. This `m1_doc.pl` file is the one that will be included the `lpdoc` `SETTINGS` file, instead of `m1.pl`. `lpdoc` recognizes and treats such `_doc` files specially so that the name without the `_doc` part is used in the different parts of the documentation, in the same way as if the documentation were placed in file `m1`.

Generating auxiliary files (e.g., READMEs): Using `lpdoc` it is often possible to use a common source for documentation text which should appear in several places. For example, assume a file `INSTALL.lpdoc` contains text (with `lpdoc` formatting commands) describing an application. This text can be included in a section of the main file documentation as follows:

```
:- comment(module,"... @section{Installation instructions}
                       @include{INSTALL.lpdoc} ...").
```

At the same time, this text can be used to generate a nicely formatted `INSTALL` file in ASCII, which can perhaps be included in the top level of the application's source directory. To this end, an `INSTALL.pl` file is constructed as follows:

```
:- include(library([assertions])).
:- comment(title,"Installation instructions").
:- comment(module,"@include{INSTALL.lpdoc}").
main. %% forces file to be documented as an aplication
```

Then, the ASCII `INSTALL` file will be generated by simply running `lpdoc ascii` in a directory with a `SETTINGS` file where `MAIN` is set to `INSTALL.pl` (these steps can be performed automatically in the interactive environment).

9   System Architecture and Implementation

Space limitations only allow us to sketch the architecture and implementation of the system.[7] `lpdoc` is implemented in (Ciao-)Prolog and compiled into a standalone Ciao executable. Executable size is around 300K for the dynamic version and 2.7Mbytes for the fully static version (including WAM engine). The

---

[7] Details can be found in the comments within the source files of the system, which, when printed out using `lpdoc` constitute the system's internals manual.

executable is generated from around 11K lines of application-specific code (including comments/documentation) and 12K lines from the Ciao system libraries, plus some 1K additional lines of miscellaneous code (html/css, TeX and BiBTeX styles, emacs lisp, etc.). The first version of the system was completed between 1996 and 1997 with successive improved versions appearing after that.

Since the source used by lpdoc is not just simple comments but the actual code of the modules (e.g., the assertions, the module declarations, exports, imports, dynamic declarations, syntax extensions, mode definitions, etc., and even the source code) lpdoc requires a *full reader*. This is specially true for the full Ciao system source language, which is designed to be very extensible [2]. Also, the reader (and the overall system) must be *adaptable* to different operator definitions and sets of built-ins so that different flavors of Prolog and other (C)LP languages can be supported. Finally, because the design objective was to be able to document very large systems in an efficient way, processing of the source files, including module interface information, declarations, comments, assertions, etc. needs to be *highly incremental*.

At the level of source file processing, the objectives are achieved in a relatively straightforward way thanks to the Ciao assertion processing library (see Figure 2), itself an instance of the c_itf low-level generic modular processing library [3]. For each documented file, and transitively for other files used by the one being documented, the library reads all the information, normalizes the assertions, and saves them in .asr and .itf cache files. This process is only repeated on a needed basis when a source file is modified. The syntax extensions and builtins "seen" during the processing of a file can be controlled by setting the lpdoc load paths (systempaths and filepaths –see Section 2) so that files containing the appropriate syntax extension definitions and the documentation for the builtins are "seen" by lpdoc (see [2] for details).

Once it has read the information for a file and its auxiliary files, lpdoc uses a number of documentation generation rules (also written in Prolog and part of which are defined in a configuration file) to implement the documentation actions outlined in previous sections. Documentation is in general first generated in an internal format (basically, the language of Section 7), and then converted by a number of backends in Prolog and/or auxiliary (publicly available) applications (TeX, dvi2ps, etc.) into manuals in the different formats, index entries, installation scripts, etc. It is quite easy to add new backends. The generation of the documentation files is also partly incremental, in that a documentation cache file (currently in GNU texinfo format)[8] is kept for each Prolog file being documented and which only changes as needed by any changes in the source files. Thus, a form of "separate documentation" (in the same sense as "separate compilation") is achieved. Early versions used makefiles for dependency tracking in this process, while more recent versions do the job in Prolog using the ciao make library, which has greatly increased portability. Unfortunately some of the auxiliary tools currently used by lpdoc are difficult to make incremental,

---

[8] See "The GNU Texinfo Documentation System" manual for more info on this format, widely used in the GNU project and on Linux and other Unix systems.

although this is not a real problem in practice. For example, the Ciao reference manual is generated from approx. 180 source Prolog files and a corresponding number of cache `texinfo` files, producing 50K lines of `texinfo` code and 550 busy A4 pages. Regenerating the `dvi` file after changing a single file (e.g., the `lists` library) takes only 10% of the time needed to generate the whole manual from scratch.

One of the most complicated issues has been to generate consistent documentation and support as many common features as possible across many different formats. For example, supporting citations using BiBTeX files was tricky because few of the underlying formats were capable of this (the solution was to bridge the missing capabilities in Prolog).

10   Related Work

We are not aware of other automatic documentation systems that have all the capabilities of `lpdoc`. There are some systems which allow interspersing TeX and Prolog in a source file in the style of Knuth's original formulation of literate programming.[9] While these systems are quite useful, we believe that `lpdoc` goes beyond them in that a significant part of the documentation is generated essentially automatically by modules of the compiler, and that the assertion language used is shared with other program development tools, which makes them quite useful beyond just documentation. ICON and Perl have some (limited) facilities for merging documentation and programs. Perhaps the closest tool to `lpdoc` is the `javadoc` documentation system for Java [7] (the development of `lpdoc` and `javadoc` started about the same time and independently). As `lpdoc`, `javadoc` uses information which is typically read and/or derived by the compiler (types, class structure, etc.), allows including textual comments with (HTML) markup, and can be extended via *doclets*. `javadoc` seems to have concentrated on producing good HTML output, while `lpdoc` aims to produce consistent documentation across a large number of different formats. Because of the tight integration with the language, `javadoc` cannot be used well for Prolog programs (in the same way as `lpdoc` would certainly not be as effective as `javadoc` for Java programs). Also, we feel that the markup language and, specially, the assertion language and the way properties can be used in documentation, are richer in `lpdoc`. Also, `lpdoc` is not limited to documenting APIs, i.e., it can also include source code in the generated documents, create indices, maintain web and info sites, etc.

11   Conclusions

Since the first "production" versions of the `lpdoc` system became available [9], we have applied it in a number of scenarios. We have used it to document all the components of the Ciao Prolog development environment, libraries for SICStus

---

[9] See `ftp://ftp.dante.de/tex-archive/macros/latex/contrib/other/gene/pl.tar.gz` for a good example.

and CHIP, standalone Prolog applications, and even applications not written in Prolog. It has certainly proven very useful for documenting library modules. However, we have also found it quite useful for generating "internals" and also user manuals of applications and project reports. Because the system can not only generate manuals in many formats, but also maintain documentation and software distribution sites, we have found ourselves using it for documenting and building such sites for a number of applications which, as mentioned above, were not even written in Prolog.

We have found that, with a bit of practice, one can write assertions and comments that at the same time document the program code, document the external use of the library, and greatly improve the debugging and maintenance cycles. One of the fundamental practical advantages observed when using lpdoc to document programs is that it is much easier to maintain a true correspondence between the program and its documentation, and to identify precisely to what version of the program a given printed manual corresponds. Furthermore, another fundamental advantage comes from the fact that the assertions are designed to be checkable in part, either statically or dynamically [10, 8], so that the documentation also achieves a certain degree of certification. While in the Ciao system writing assertions is optional (in contrast to, e.g., Mercury [15]), the fact that they will generate a good part of the manual encourages programmers to write them, and this in turn helps developing programs faster, because more errors are detected early on.

lpdoc is publicly available.[10] The system is currently undergoing further development in several directions, such as, for example, reducing the need for auxiliary applications (so that it is portable to more platforms) or improving the emacs-based interactive environment. As mentioned previously, with a simple compatibility library it is relatively easy to make traditional (constraint) logic programming systems (in which new declarations can be defined) accept programs adorned with Ciao-style assertions and comments, so that they are ignored during compilation but lpdoc (and the Ciao preprocessor!) can be used on them. As mentioned above, we have done this for SICStus and CHIP. It should not be too difficult to modify the front end for other type/assertion languages, such as those used in Mercury [15] and HAL [5] (this is under study at least in the case of HAL), or even non LP-based languages (which would, however, need a specific front-end).

Acknowledgements: The design of the lpdoc system has benefitted from suggestions made by CLIP group members and users of Ciao Prolog which are too many to mention here (acknowledgements are given in the reference manual and source files). This document has benefitted from detailed comments from Daniel Cabeza, Per Cederberg, and the anonymous referees. The author would also like to thank the PC for deciding to accept this paper, despite its perhaps somewhat atypical nature. The development of lpdoc has been funded in part by CICYT project EDIPIA (TIC99-1151).

---

[10] See http://www.clip.dia.fi.upm.es/Software .

References

1. F. Bueno, D. Cabeza, M. Carro, M. Hermenegildo, P. López-García, and G. Puebla. The Ciao Prolog System. Reference Manual. TR CLIP3/97.1, School of Computer Science, Technical University of Madrid (UPM), August 1997.
2. D. Cabeza and M. Hermenegildo. A New Module System for Prolog. In *International Conference on Computational Logic, CL2000*, LNCS. Springer-Verlag, July 2000. To appear.
3. D. Cabeza and M. Hermenegildo. The Ciao Modular, Standalone Compiler and Its Generic Program Processing Library. In *Special Issue on Parallelism and Implementation of (C)LP Systems. To appear*, Electronic Notes in Theoretical Computer Science. Elsevier - North Holland, 2000.
4. D. Cordes and M. Brown. The Literate Programming Paradigm. *IEEE Computer Magazine*, June 1991.
5. B. Demoen, M. Garcia de la Banda, W. Harvey, K. Marriott, and P. Stuckey. Herbrand Constraint Solving in HAL. In *Int. Conf. on Logic Programming*. MIT Press, Cambridge, MA, U.S.A., November 1999.
6. P. Deransart, A. Ed-Dbali, and L. Cervoni. *Prolog: The Standard*. Springer-Verlag, 1996.
7. Lisa Friendly. The Design of Distributed Hyperlink Program Documentation. In *Int'l. WS on Hypermedia Design*, Workshops in Computing. Springer, June 1996. Available from http://java.sun.com/docs/javadoc-paper.html.
8. M. Hermenegildo, F. Bueno, G. Puebla, and P. López-García. Program Analysis, Debugging and Optimization Using the Ciao System Preprocessor. In *1999 International Conference on Logic Programming*, pages 52–66, Cambridge, MA, November 1999. MIT Press.
9. M. Hermenegildo and The CLIP Group. An Automatic Documentation Generator for (C)LP – Reference Manual. The Ciao System Documentation Series–TR CLIP5/97.3, Facultad de Informática, UPM, August 1997.
10. M. Hermenegildo, G. Puebla, and F. Bueno. Using Global Analysis, Partial Specifications, and an Extensible Assertion Language for Program Validation and Debugging. In K. R. Apt, V. Marek, M. Truszczynski, and D. S. Warren, editors, *The Logic Programming Paradigm: a 25–Year Perspective*, pages 161–192. Springer-Verlag, July 1999.
11. D. Knuth. Literate programming. *Computer Journal*, 27:97–111, 1984.
12. G. Puebla, F. Bueno, and M. Hermenegildo. An Assertion Language for Debugging of Constraint Logic Programs. In *ILPS'97 WS on Tools and Environments for (C)LP*, October 1997. ftp://clip.dia.fi.upm.es/pub/papers/assert/lang_tr_discipldeliv.ps.gz
13. G. Puebla, F. Bueno, and M. Hermenegildo. An Assertion Language for Debugging of Constraint Logic Programs. In P. Deransart, M. Hermenegildo, and J. Maluszynski, editors, *Analysis and Visualization Tools for Constraint Programming*, LNCS. Springer-Verlag, 2000. To appear.
14. G. Puebla and M. Hermenegildo. Some Issues in Analysis and Specialization of Modular Ciao-Prolog Programs. In *Special Issue on Optimization and Implementation of Declarative Programming Languages*, volume 30 of *Electronic Notes in Theoretical Computer Science*. Elsevier - North Holland, March 2000.
15. Z. Somogyi, F. Henderson, and T. Conway. The execution algorithm of Mercury: an efficient purely declarative logic programming language. *JLP*, 29(1–3), October 1996.

Note: Most CLIP group publications are available from
http://www.clip.dia.fi.upm.es

A   An Example: Source

```
:- module(sort,[qsort/2,list/1,sorted/1],[assertions,regtypes,isomodes]).
:- use_module(library(lists),[append/3]).
:- comment(title, "The classical quick-sort").
:- comment(module,"This library provides a naive implementation of
   quick-sort and some associated types and properties.").

:- comment(qsort(X,Y),"@var{Y} is a sorted permutation of @var{X}.").
:- pred qsort(X,Y) : list(X) => sorted(Y)
        # "This is the normal use.".
:- pred qsort(X,Y) : (list(X), sorted(Y))
        # "Checking that @var{Y} is a sorted permutation of @var{X}.".
qsort([],[]).
qsort([X|L],R) :-
   partition(L,X,L1,L2), qsort(L2,R2), qsort(L1,R1), append(R1,[X|R2],R).

:- pred partition(+list(num),+num,-list(num),-list(num)).
:- comment(doinclude,partition/4).
partition([],_B,[],[]).
partition([E|R],C,[E|Left1],Right):-
        E < C, !, partition(R,C,Left1,Right).
partition([E|R],C,Left,[E|Right1]):-
        E >= C, !, partition(R,C,Left,Right1).

:- prop sorted(X) # "@var{X} is sorted.".
sorted([]).
sorted([_]).
sorted([X,Y|R]) :- X < Y, sorted([Y|R]).

:- regtype list/1.
list([]).
list([_|T]) :- list(T).

:- comment(bug, "Code uses @pred{append/3}, which is inefficient.").
:- comment(version_maintenance,on).
:- comment(version(0*1+1,1999/10/11,03:19*00+'CEST'),
   "Already made the first change...   (Manuel Hermenegildo)").
:- comment(version(0*1+0,1999/10/11,03:18*29+'CEST'),
   "File created. (Manuel Hermenegildo)").
```

B   The Classical Quick-Sort

Version: 0.1#1 (1999/10/11, 3:19:0 CEST)

This library provides a naive implementation of quick-sort and some associated types and properties.

B.1   Usage and Interface (sort)

> - **Library Usage:**
>   ```
>   :- use_module(library(sort)).
>   ```

- **Exports:**
  - *Predicates:*
    qsort/2.
  - *Properties:*
    sorted/1.
  - *Regular Types:*
    list/1.
- **Other Modules Used:**
  - *System Library Modules:*
    lists.

B.2 Documentation on Exports (sort)

qsort/2:   PREDICATE

qsort(X,Y): Y is a sorted permutation of X.
Usage 1: qsort(X,Y)

- *Description:* This is the normal use.
- *Should hold at call time:* list(X).
- *Should hold upon exit:* Y is sorted (sorted/1).

Usage 2: qsort(X,Y)

- *Description:* Checking that Y is a sorted permutation of X.
- *Should hold at call time:* list(X) (list/1), Y is sorted (sorted/1).

list/1:   REGTYPE

A regular type, defined as follows:
list([]).
list([_1|T]) :-
       list(T).

sorted/1:   PROPERTY

Usage: sorted(X)
- *Description:* X is sorted.

B.3 Documentation on Internals (sort)

partition/4:   PREDICATE

Usage:
- *Should hold at call time:* Arg1 is a list of nums (list/2), Arg2 is a number (list/2), Arg3 is a free variable (var/1), Arg4 is a free variable (var/1).
- *Should hold upon exit:* Arg3 is is a list of nums (list/2), Arg4 is is a list of nums (list/2).

B.4 Known Bugs and Planned Improvements (sort)
- Code uses append/3, which is inefficient.

B.5 Version/Change Log (sort)
- **Version 0.1#1 (1999/10/11, 3:19:0 CEST)**
  Already made the first change... (Manuel Hermenegildo)
- **Version 0.1 (1999/10/11, 3:18:29 CEST)**
  File created. (Manuel Hermenegildo)

Psychiatric Diagnosis from the Viewpoint of Computational Logic

Joseph Gartner[1], Terrance Swift[2], Allen Tien[3],
Carlos Viegas Damásio[4], and Luís Moniz Pereira[4]

[1] Medicine Rules Inc, 25 East Loop Rd, Stony Broon, NY 11794
agartner@earthlink.net
[2] Department of Computer Science, SUNY at Stony Brook, Stony Brook, NY
tswift@cs.sunysb.edu
[3] Medical Decision Logic Inc 7921 Ruxway Rd, Baltimore MD 21204-3515
atien@jhmi.edu
[4] A.I. Centre, Faculdade de Ciências e Tecnologia
Universidade Nova de Lisboa, 2825-114 Caparica, Portugal
{cd,lmp}@di.fct.unl.pt

Abstract. While medical information systems have become common in
the United States, commercial systems that automate or assist in the
process of medical diagnosis remain uncommon. This is not surprising,
since automating diagnosis requires considerable sophistication both in
the understanding of medical epidemeology and in knowledge representation techniques. This paper is an interdisciplinary study of how recent
results in logic programming and non-monotonic reasoning can aid in
psychiatric diagnosis. We argue that to logically represent psychiatric
diagnosis as codified in the *Diagnostic and Statistical Manual of Mental Disorders, 4th edition* requires abduction over programs that include
both explicit and non-stratified default negation, as well as dynamic
rules that express preferences between conclusions. We show how such
programs can be translated into abductive frameworks over normal logic
programs and implemented using recently introduced logic programming
techniques. Finally, we note how such programs are used in a commercial
product *Diagnostica*.

1 Introduction

Medical information systems have become an active area of software development
in the United States, with a market of over 10 billion dollars per year. Typically,
these systems have as their goals either to cut the costs of medical treatment or
to ensure that treatments are performed in a standard, well-documented manner. Traditional medical information systems may have considerable complexity
and most often address problems such billing or shift-scheduling; problems related to workflow management such as monitoring of treatment plans; or image
processing. However, commercial systems that partially automate the process of
medical diagnosis are uncommon, partly because the process of medical reasoning is difficult to automate. The purpose of the *Diagnostica* system developed

J. Lloyd et al. (Eds.): CL 2000, LNAI 1861, pp. 1362–1376, 2000.

by Medicine Rules, Inc is twofold. As a research system, it explores how psychiatric assessment can be represented by extensions of classical logic and serves as a focus of an interdisciplinary collaboration between computer scientists and research psychiatrists. Just as importantly, as a commercially available product Diagnostica seeks to aid psychiatrists, psychologists and psychiatric social workers in diagnosing patients in an efficient and systematic manner.

Accurate diagnoses can be difficult to make, even for a trained psychiatrist. For instance a confused, elderly patient could suffer either from Alzheimer's Dementia or a Major Depressive Disorder (sometimes colloquially called *pseudodementia*). In the latter case, the patient may be treatable with medication; in the former case the patient may not be. Similarly, it may be difficult to determine whether a child has Attention Deficit Disorder (treated by medication) or an Adjustment Disorder (treated by therapy or by changing the child's environment). Diagnostic procedures concerning such disorders have been codified by the American Psychiatric Association in the fourth edition of its reference book *Diagnostic and Statistical Manual of Mental Disorders*, or *DSM-IV* [7], which is widely used in the United States. These procedures specify various *criteria* that a patient must satisfy in order to meet a diagnosis for a mental disorder. As an example, criteria for Asperger's Disorder, a Childhood Pervasive Development Disorder, is shown in Figure 1. As terminology we use the term *criterion* to specify both the conditions comprising a rule (e.g. criteria 1–5 in Figure 1) and the "symptoms" that the patient exhibits, e.g. criteria 1.a–1.d in Figure 1 which are sometimes called *base criteria*.

Criterion 1 reflects the *polythetic* nature of psychiatric diagnoses, in which there need be no essential characteristic or criterion of a diagnosis. Instead, multiple prototypes with varying features are used to group together a wide range of disparate phenomena into a diagnosis. At the same time there may be a significant amount of symptom overlap between different diagnoses. For instance, the failure to develop peer relationships can, under different circumstances, indicate schizophrenia, autism, and many other disorders. The issues of multiple prototypes and symptom overlaps leads to occasional difficulty and even ambiguity in distinguishing between the 618 DSM-IV diagnoses, as in the cases mentioned above. Because of these complications, while most American psychiatrists use DSM-IV, few use it to its full advantage. Studies have shown that clinical psychiatrists err in using DSM-IV by not considering all possible diagnoses, while research psychiatrists err by not excluding diagnoses quickly enough.

As indicated by Figure 1, DSM-IV diagnostic rules have a clear formulation that lends itself to coding as a logic program: thus a patient meets criteria for a diagnosis if the body of the diagnosis, expressed as a logical rule, is satisfied. However, the logical formulation and implementation of DSM-IV is not always straightforward, and includes the need to exclude certain diagnoses in order to prove other diagnoses, the need to represent incomplete knowledge, and the need for hypothetical reasoning during diagnosis. This paper explores how recently introduced techniques in logic programming and non-monotonic reasoning can be used to represent aspects of diagnosis as codified in DSM-IV. Specifically:

1. Qualitative impairment in social interaction, as manifested by at least two of the following
   (a) marked impairment in the use of multiple nonverbal behaviors such as eye-to-eye gaze, facial expression, body postures, and gestures to regulate social interaction;
   (b) failure to develop peer relationships appropriate to developmental level
   (c) a lack of spontaneous seeking to share enjoyment, interest,m or achievements with other people (e.g. by a lack of showing, bringing, or pointing out objects of interest to other people).
   (d) lack of social or emotional reciprocity
2. Restricted repetitive and stereotyped patterns of behavior, interests, and activities, as manifested by at least one of the following:
   (a) encompassing preoccupations with one or more stereotyped and restricted patterns of interest that is abnormal either in intensity or focus
   (b) apparently inflexible adherence to specific nonfunctional routines or rituals.
   (c) stereotyped and repetitive motor mannerisms (e.g., hand or finger flapping or twisting, or complex whole-body movements)
   (d) persistent preoccupation with parts of objects
3. The disturbance causes clinically significant impairment in social, occupational, or other important areas of functioning
4. There is no significant clinical delay in cognitive development or in the development of age-appropriate self-help skills, adaptive behavior (other than in social interaction) and curiosity about the environment in childhood.
5. Criteria are not met for another Pervasive Development Disorder or Schizophrenia

Fig. 1. A Diagnostic Criterion for Asperger's Disorder

– We show that modeling DSM-IV requires non-stratified negation in order to handle ambiguities in its formulation; we argue that both default and explicit negation are required to codify DSM-IV as is a provision for hypothetical reasoning.

– We show how practical diagnosis using DSM-IV can be based on interpreting non-stratified negation in DSM-IV through the well-founded semantics [16] augmented by a novel form of preference logic whose semantics we define.

– We describe how the Diagnostica system is based on a partial implementation of these techniques, and discuss an important use for abduction to construct differentials for diagnoses.

Section 2 discusses the knowledge representation problems of DSM-IV in detail. Section 3 shows how these problems can be addressed in an abductive framework that includes logical preferences; while Section 4 provides a 3-valued semantics for these logical preferences and compares it to other semantics in the literature. For readability by non-specialists, nearly all discussion of the semantics of our Preference Logic Programs is confined to Section 4. However, we employ standard logic programming terminology throughout.

2   The Nature of Knowledge in DSM-IV

From the perspective of knowledge representation, several factors distinguish the process of psychiatric assessment.

Exclusion Criteria. In making a diagnosis, a psychiatrist may need to ensure that certain criteria are fulfilled, while others are excluded. One example of an *exclusion criterion* is criterion 5 for Asperger's disorder (Figure 1) which specifies that criteria must not be met for Schizophrenia or for any other Pervasive Development Disorder (a class that includes Autism, Retts, Childhood Disintegrative Disorder, Asperger's, and Pervasive Development Disorder Not Otherwise Specified). Exclusion criteria occur frequently in DSM-IV diagnosis, with some variability in the phrasing of the negative conditions. Other exclusion criteria may state that "criteria are not better accounted for" by another diagnosis or class of diagnoses, (e.g. in Major Depressive Disorder a criterion requires that symptoms be not better accounted for by Schizophrenia) or that a patient has "not ever" experienced a syndrome (e.g. in Major Depressive Disorder a criterion requires verification that a patient has not ever had a manic episode).

Usually exclusion criteria indicate a priority for how diagnoses are to be made and so the DSM-IV rules are generally stratified through exclusion criteria. For instance, most diagnoses in the class of Mood Disorders require the exclusion of Substance Abuse or Bereavement. In other cases, diagnoses may be non-stratified through exclusion criteria. In the case of dissimilar diagnoses, the non-stratification may be considered an error in DSM-IV; however in several cases the lack of stratification reflects a lack of consensus about how to differentiate the diagnoses. We consider each of the non-stratified classes in turn.

Two diagnoses, Adjustment Disorder and Alzheimer's Dementia illustrate the first class, which may constitute "errors" in DSM-IV. Both may be considered to be "default" diagnoses, that are to be made only if no other diagnoses are reasonable; exclusion rules for these diagnoses are very broad and can be cyclic. For instance, within the criteria of Cognitive Disorders, a diagnosis of Alzheimer's Dementia should be made only if no other cognitive disorder is more likely for the patient; accordingly, the exclusion rule for Alzheimer's Dementia states

– The disturbance is not better accounted for by another Axis I disorder (e.g. Major Depression, or Schizophrenia).[1]

Adjustment Disorder, which can also be considered as a default diagnosis, has a similarly broad exclusion. Interpreting DSM-IV rules strictly logically, it is possible to have a set of positive criteria that are met such that that a patient has Adjustment Disorder if his symptoms are not better met by Alzheimer's Dementia and that a patient has Alzheimer's Dementia if his symptoms are not better met by Adjustment Disorder. However, this sort of loop through exclusion

---

[1] An Axis I disorder is any mental disorder that is not a personality disorder or mental retardation.

criteria is not expected to occur in practice, as it is not likely that a given patient would meet positive criteria for both diagnoses at the same time.

To understand the second class of mutually exclusive diagnoses, consider again the exclusion criterion (5) of Asperger's Disorder. Other Pervasive Development Disorders, such as Autism or Childhood Development Disorder contain similar exclusion rules, so that choosing among the three disorders may be indeterminate according to a logical interpretation of the DSM-IV rules. In the case of the Pervasive Development Disorders, the lack of stratification reflects not only the practical clinical problem of distinguishing Asperger's Disorder from, say, Autism, but also the fact that researchers continue to debate the validity of Asperger's Disorder as a distinct diagnosis altogether (see e.g. [12, 17]). The diagnoses of Asperger's Disorder and Autism is not a unique example of this type of stratification. The diagnoses Adjustment Disorder with Disturbance of Emotions and Conduct, Adjustment Disorder, and Attention Deficit/Hyperactivity Disorder are also linked through exclusion criteria and can be difficult to differentiate [8, 9, 6], as can several other sets of diagnoses.

Thus, while most diagnoses are stratified via exclusion rules, many are not. In many cases, the lack of stratification is accountable by the informality of the DSM-IV rules as with Alzheimer's Dementia and Adjustment Disorder. In these cases the DSM-IV rules should arguably be tightened to avoid inadvertent mistakes caused by exclusion rules that are too broad. However in other cases, such as Asperger's Disorder and Autism the lack of stratification has a deeper nature and reflects the similarity of the disorders themselves.

Incomplete Knowledge: If there are no indications that a patient has an uncommon symptom or case history, certain criteria may be ruled out by default. For instance, the diagnosis of Dissociative Fugue disorder depends on determining that the patient has no medical condition that could also account for the observed symptoms, a determination that may be difficult, if not impossible, to make with absolute certainty. Similarly, many diagnoses depend on a history of the patient that may be impossible to obtain, or may be unreliable from patients or their significant others (e.g. criterion 4 for Asperger's Disorder). For instance,

- A 5-year old child in foster care speaks normally. The physician has no way of obtaining a reliable case history, so that the physician concludes by default that there is no evidence of a significant delay in language acquisition.
- A case history is taken from the child's parents and it is explicitly determined that there was no significant delay in language acquisition.

In the first case, the diagnosis may need to be made on less than perfect information, and there is a need to distinguish information that is assumed false because there is no evidence to support it from information that is explicitly known to be false.

Hypothetical Reasoning: Diagnoses sometimes rely on hypothetical reasoning by the physician, particularly with regard to time. An instance of this is Adjustment Disorder, which has the criterion

- Once the stressor (or its consequences) has terminated, the symptoms do not persist for more than an additional 6 months.

Taken literally, this criterion implies that a physician cannot diagnose a patient as undergoing Adjustment Disorder, while the patient is undergoing it. Similarly, hypothetical reasoning about the expected duration of symptoms may be used to differentiate between the diagnoses of Schizophrenia or Schizophreniform Disorder.

Temporal Reasoning: DSM-IV often requires sophisticated temporal reasoning to represent the duration and occurrence of various symptoms. Indeed, certain closely related diagnoses be distinguished primarily through the duration of the symptoms. An example are the diagnoses Brief Psychotic Disorders, in which delusional symptoms last less than one month, Schizophreniform Disorder (symptoms last at least one month but less than six), and Schizophrenia (in which symptoms have lasted more than six months). Furthermore, temporal reasoning also may be used to determine whether a patient is diagnosed with single or multiple disorders. For instance, if a patient is both depressed and anxious, he will be diagnosed for an anxiety-related disorder only if the symptoms of an anxiety disorder preceded those of the depression — otherwise the anxiety is taken to be a symptom of a depression disorder.

3   Representing DSM-IV as a Logic Program

From the discussion above, it is apparent that modeling DSM-IV as a logic program requires the use of non-traditional techniques. The first three of the factors mentioned above: DSM-IV Exclusion Criteria, Incomplete Information, and Hypothetical Reasoning have been formalized and partially implemented. However, a determination has not yet been made of the best way to model time in DSM-IV among the many techniques in the literature.

3.1   Exclusion Criteria

In order to explain our approach to handling exclusion criteria, we first discuss the actions that should be taken when diagnoses are linked through mutual exclusion rules. First, there are certain diagnoses that are not considered to be similar, but that logically may have loops through exclusion criteria: for instance Alzheimer's Dementia and Adjustment Disorder. Positive criteria should not be satisfied for both of these disorders for any patient at a given time; if this happens, it should be considered an error condition. Second, certain diagnoses are known to be similar but mutually exclusive. In the case of Asperger's

and Autism, only one of the diagnoses should be made true: that is, the epi-
demiological theory underlying DSM-IV states that a patient cannot have both
Asperger's and Autism. At the same time if positive criteria are met for both
Diagnoses, the action to take is ambiguous. Some clinicians would prefer Asperger's under the principle that if the diagnosis isn't clearly Autism the lesser
diagnosis of Asperger's should be made. Other clinicians who don't believe that
there is a separate Asperger's disorder separate from Autism would prefer the
diagnosis of Autism. Third, in cases such as Pervasive Development Disorders
and Schizophrenia which are also linked through exclusion rules, the relationship
as specified in DSM-IV is complicated. If a patient has a Pervasive Development
Disorder, the additional diagnosis of Schizophrenia is also made if the patient
has had prominent delusions or hallucinations for over a month. In other words,
Schizophrenia and Pervasive Development Disorders are usually mutually exclusive, but both diagnoses are warranted in certain cases.

Our approach to representing these different kinds of exclusions is based
on modeling the exclusions using default negation augmented by abnormality
conditions and preference rules. The resulting program is then evaluated under
the (extended) well-founded semantics. The three-valued well-founded semantics
will assign the trught value of *undefined* in the cases where all non-exclusion
criteria are met for diagnoses that are mutually exclusive in DSM-IV. In this
way, non-preference rules represent DSM-IV in an informationally sound way.
As will be seen below, a physician can go beyond information in DSM-IV by
creating preference rules to override undefined truth values.

The portion of the diagnostic rule for Asperger's disorder relevant to exclusion criteria is

```
aspergers:-
    exclude(aspergers,retts),
    exclude(aspergers,autism),
    exclude(aspergers,childhood_disintegrative_disorder),
    exclude(aspergers,pervasive_development_disorder_nos),
    exclude(aspergers,schizophrenia).
```

where default negation (not/1) is used to defined exclude/2:

```
exclude(Diag1,Diag2):-
    abnormal_situation(Diag1,Diag2).
exclude(Diag1,Diag2):-
    not Diag2.
```

In the case of Schizophrenia and Pervasive Development disorders, definition of
an abnormal situation allows both diagnoses to be true by allowing the exclusion
criterion to be satisfied by a means other than negation. At the same time, a
set of mutually exclusive diagnoses will be undefined under the well-founded
semantics if the positive criteria are met for each diagnosis in the set and if no
abnormality conditions are defined. Such a situation is useful for representing
cycles through exclusion criteria such as occurs with Alzheimer's Dementia and

Adjustment Disorder, as the truth-value *undefined* can explicitly represent an error that is taken to occur when positive criteria are simultaneously met for both diagnoses.

Both exclusion criteria and abnormality rules model conditions that occur explicitly in DSM IV. However, as discussed previously, there may be similar, mutually exclusive diagnoses, such as Asperger's and Autism for which it should not be an absolute error if positive criteria are simultaneously satisfied for both. In these cases, other criteria, unspecified in DSM-IV may be brought to bear, and it is useful to allow the clinician to state the conditions under which she prefers one diagnosis to another. She would do so by a *preference rule* of the form:

```
prefer(Diagnosis1,Diagnosis2):- Body.
```

A semantics of such preference rules, based on a transformation into normal programs that can be evaluated under the well-founded semantics, is discussed in Section 4. Here, we note that our framework for preference logic is quite general, in that it allows the truth value of preferences (i.e. atoms formed over the predicate *prefer/2*) to depend on the truth value of literals that depend on other preferences, allows preferences to be defined about other preferences, and assigns cyclic preferences the truth value of *undefined*.

Example 1. The following programs illustrate, at a highly abstract level, the actions of Preference Logic Programs on some of the psychiatric diagnoses discussed so far. Let P_1 contain the rules.

```
aspergers :- not autism.
autism :- not aspergers.

major_depression_disorder.
alzheimers.
```

P_1 abstracts DSM IV diagnosis rules, discussed previously, for Asperger's Disorder and Autism, which are related through exclusion rules, and for Major Depression Disorder and Alzheimer's which are not related through exclusion rules. Suppose a psychiatric practice did not believe in the validity of the Asperger's diagnosis and preferred to diagnose patients with Autism. Suppose further that they believed that DSM-IV diagnostic criteria for Major Depressive Disorder and Alzheimer's were too coarse, and wanted to flag an error in the case when a diagnosis might be ambiguous [2]. In this case the practice could add the following preference rules:

```
prefer(autism,aspergers).

prefer(major_depression_disorder, alzheimers).
prefer(alzheimers,major_depression_disorder).
```

---

[2] The psychiatric literature, in fact, offers support for this view. See [13] for a survey of recent literature.

In this case, P_1 together with the preference rules has `autism` true, `aspergers` false, and both `major_depression_disorder` and `alzheimers` undefined.

Next suppose that a particular psychiatrist in a practice wishes to diagnose patients to have Major Depression Disorder rather than Alzheimer's in all cases where non-exclusion criteria for both were met (perhaps because he is part of a study about the efficacy of an experimental medication for depression). The psychiatrist would add the preference rule.

```
prefer(prefer(major_depression_disorder, alzheimers),
       prefer(alzheimers,major_depression_disorder)).
```

We summarize our treatment of exclusion rules in DSM-IV. Representation of DSM-IV knowledge is kept in the diagnosis rules themselves, including the `exclude/2` and `abnormal_situation/2` predicates. Preference rules allow the user to adjust how exclusion rules are interpreted using knowledge not contained in DSM-IV and, as mentioned above, both cyclic preferences and preferences about preferences may make sense in certain situations. Indeed preference rules could be used in place of the predicate `abnormal_situation/2`; the predicate `abnormal_situation/2` was introduced in order to maintain a distinction between DSM-IV knowledge and that represented by the user.

3.2   Incomplete Information

It is well-known from knowledge representation literature that information that is assumed false because there is no evidence to support it can be represented by default negation; while information that is explicitly known to be false can be represented by explicit negation. The well-founded semantics with explicit negation [1], provides a semantics for adding explicit negation to the well-founded semantics. This semantics can be evaluated using a linear transformation of rules with explicit negation into normal logic program rules.

3.3   Speculative Information

Speculative information, such as that needed to conclude an Adjustment Disorder can be represented using abduction, which allows a form of hypothetical reasoning. Since preference rules can be transformed into normal program rules (Section 4) and evaluated with the well founded semantics (with explicit negation) no special semantics for abduction is needed beyond what is present in the literature: e.g. the three-valued abductive frameworks for extended logic programs of [5]. Because preference logic programs are translated into normal programs, preferences are treated no differently than any other predicate in a program. As a result, the truth value of preferences may depend on particular abductive scenarios, and abductive integrity rules may call preferences just as they may call goals with any other predicates. Furthermore, Definition 1 of Section 4 ensures that any abductive dependency of a preference is propagated to literals whose truth depends on these preferences. Evaluation of this framework, which requires abduction over the well-founded semantics, is discussed in Section 4.

Abduction plays a larger role in psychiatric diagnosis beyond what is needed to model hypothetical reasoning in DSM-IV, a topic to which we now turn.

Abduction and Differential Diagnoses. As has been discussed above, clinicians often need to distinguish between closely related diagnoses. Often this is done through exclusion rules, but other times there are wording differences between positive criteria for similar diagnoses that can be used to as a *differential* between the diagnoses. Indeed, understanding differentials for related diagnoses is a fundamental element of clinical training; and applying these differentials is a fundamental element of clinical practice. Providing dynamic differentials for diagnoses can easily be done through abduction. The idea is that, if the differential is required between diagnosis D_1 and diagnosis D_2 then D_1 should be abduced in the presence of the integrity constraint $\perp$:- D_2 which, produces the conditions for failing D_2. The abductive context will then provide the differential for the diagnoses.

In order for abduction to be practical for constructing differentials several conditions must hold. First the differential should be as specific as possible, which requires abducibles to be specific and to have an easily understood relationship with one another. In particular, abducibles should be drawn from atomic propositions that represent the *symptom state* of a patient, and restricted to those atoms of the symptom state that are not known to be true or explicitly false. The most obvious representation of a symptom state makes use of DSM-IV base criteria. Alternatively, the symptom state may consist of elements of other assessment methodologies, such as the World Health Organization's Schedules for Clinical Assessment in Neuropsychiatry [15], which are mapped into DSM-IV base criteria. Adding structure to representation of symptom states benefits the abduction routines: for example if two elements are known to be inconsistent, perhaps because they are antonyms, the inconsistency constraints can be used to restrict abductive solutions.

At the same time, the number of abductive solutions generated should not overwhelm the user. For instance, if criteria 1.a—1.d and 2.a—2.d of Asperger's Disorder in Figure 1 were set as abducibles, then there may be as many as 24 different minimal abductive solutions to the goal ?- **aspergers**. To reduce the number of solutions the abduction routines make use of special presentation routines. For instance, when abducing through a criterion in which at least n of a list of base criteria must be true, and for which k of the base criteria are true and l are explicitly false in the symptom state, the abductive solutions are grouped so that the user is presented with a statement of the form at least $(n - k)$ of a revised list (i.e. excluding the explicitly false base criteria) must be present. When abducing base criteria through exclusion rules, a large number of abductive solutions may similarly be derived. Thus, abduction is not allowed within exclusion rules: rather the exclusion rule itself is returned to the user, after ensuring that the excluded rule is not enforced by the symptom state and presently abduced abducibles.

4   Three-Valued Preference Logic Programs

We now define the Preference Logic Programs upon which the representation of DSM-IV is based.

Definition 1. *A* Preference Logic Program (PLP) *[P, Pref] is a set of extended rules* P *and* Pref *where the set* Pref *of preference rules (or preferences) has the form*

$$prefer(Term_1, Term_2) :- Body.$$

Arguments of prefer/2 *are restricted to be objective literals of [P, Pref] and are called* preference atoms.

   Assume that [P, Pref] does not contain the predicate symbols overridden/2, pnot/1 *or* trans_prefer/2. *The extended embedding of [P, Pref], [P, Pref]_{norm}, is the smallest program containing*

1. *The rules* r' *defined as follows. An objective literal A is* potentially overridden *(resp. potentially preferred) if there is a preference rule* $prefer(A_1, A_2)$:- *Body and A unifies with* A_2 *with mgu* θ *(resp. A unifies with* A_1 *with mgu* θ). *Let r be a rule* H :- $A_1, \ldots, A_n, not\ B_1, \ldots, not\ B_m$ *in P.*
   (a) If H is potentially overridden, then $r' = H$:- $A_1, \ldots, A_n, B'_1, \ldots, B'_m,$ $not\ overridden(H)$.
   (b) Otherwise, $r' = H$:- $A_1, \ldots, A_n, B'_1), \ldots, B'_m$.
   In either case, for $0 \leq i \leq m$, $B'_i = pnot(H, B_i)$ *if* B_i *is potentially preferred, and* $B'_i = B_i$ *otherwise.*
2. *The rules*

   $$overridden(A_1) :- prefer(A_2, A_1), A_2.$$
   $$overridden(A_1) :- prefer(A_2, A_1), overridden(A_2).$$

   $$pnot(A_1, A_2) : -trans\_prefer(A_1, A_2).$$
   $$pnot(A_1, A_2) : -not\ A_2.$$

   $$trans\_prefer(A_1, A_2) : -trans\_prefer(A_1, A_2).$$
   $$trans\_prefer(A_1, A_2) : -trans\_prefer(A_1, A_3), prefer(A_3, A_2).$$

Because the extended embedding is based on potentially overridden and potentially preferred atoms, if the set of preference rules in a PLP [P, Pref] is empty, the normal embedding will have no effect on P beyond adding the rules in clause 2. Definition 1 allows preferences to be dynamic in the sense that their truth-value may depend on the truth value of other parts of the program, including other preferences. In addition, preferences can be declared on preferences themselves.

Since $[P, Pref]_{norm}$ is an extended program, it can be evaluated under any semantics for extended programs. For the purposes of this paper, we restrict our attention to the well-founded semantics with explicit negation [1]. It is immediate from Definition 1 that an objective literal that depends on cyclic preferences (i.e. an objective literal A such that $prefer(A, A)$ is true) will either be false or undefined in the extended well-founded model of $[P, Pref]$, $WFM([P, Pref])$.

4.1   Relation to Other Preference Formalisms

The semantics above extends the possible worlds semantics for PLPs as described in [11] which is concerned with what may be termed *static* PLPs [3].

Definition 2. *Let* $[P, Pref]$ *be a definite PLP, that is a PLP in which P and Pref are restricted to be definite programs. We say that a ground atom* A_1 *depends on a ground atom* A_2 *if there is a path from* A_1 *to* A_2 *in the dependency graph of P. A* derived *atom in* $[P, Pref]$ *is one that depends on a preference atom. A* base *atom is an atom that is neither a preference atom nor a derived atom. Preferences in* $[P, Pref]$ *are* static *if all atoms in the bodies of rules in Pref are base atoms.*

For a static PLP $[P, Pref]$, the semantics of $Pref$ is taken as its minimal model, together with that of the base atoms of P. Based on these observations, we can compute preferences, as it were, apart from P and define a relation $<_{pref}$ between atoms such that $A_1 <_{pref} A_2$ if A_2 is transitively preferred to A_1 (using the relation $prefer/2$ in the minimal model of $Pref$). We say that $<_{pref}$ is *well-behaved* if it is a strict partial order, and well-founded in the sense that there is no infinite chain of atoms $A_1 <_{pref} A_2 <_{pref} \cdots$.

The possible worlds semantics of preference logic programs is based on *strongly optimal worlds*.

Definition 3. *Let* $[P, Pref]$ *be a definite PLP whose preferences are static. A set W of derived and preference atoms over P is* reduced *if there is no* $A_1, A_2 \in W$ *such that* $A_1 <_{pref} A_2$. *If W is also a subset of the minimal model of P, then it is called a* world. *A world* W_1 *is reflexively preferred to a world* W_2 *(denoted* $W_2 \leq_{sp} W_1$*) if for each preference atom* $A_2 \in W_2$ *there is a preference atom* $A_1 \in W_1$ *such that* $A_2 = A_1$ *or* $A_2 <_{pref} A_1$. *A world W is* strongly optimal *if for any other world* W, $W \leq_{sp} W_1 \Rightarrow W_1 \subseteq W$.

The operator T_P *denotes the standard inference operator for definite programs. A world W is* supported *if* $W \subseteq T_P(W)$. *A program* $[P, Pref]$ *has the* optimal subproblem property *if every strongly optimal world for* $[P, Pref]$ *is supported.*

---

[3] In [11], both P and $Pref$ may be locally stratified: for simplicity of presentation, we restrict P and $Pref$ to definite programs while comparing to the semantics of [11].

Example 2. Consider the PLP P_2:

```
prefer(p(a),p(d)).        prefer(p(b),p(d)).
p(a):- p(d).              p(b).            p(d).
```

There are five worlds for P_2: $\{p(a), p(b)\}$, $\{p(a)\}$, $\{p(b)\}$, $\{p(d)\}$ and $\emptyset$. The world $\{p(a), p(b)\}$ is strongly optimal. However $T_P(\{p(a), p(b)\}) = \{p(b), p(d)\}$ so that P_2 does not have the optimal subproblem property.

Theorem 1. *Let $[P, Pref]$ be a simple PLP, and $[P, Pref]_{norm}$ be the normal embedding of P. Then*

1. *There is a unique strongly optimal world, $\mathcal{W}$ for $[P, Pref]$.*
2. *$WFM([P, Pref]_{norm})$ is two-valued;*
3. *A is true in $WFM([P, Pref]_{norm})$ iff $A \in \mathcal{W}$[4].*

While a full comparison with other preference frameworks is beyond the scope of this paper, we note a few comparisons in passing. The atom-based approach to preferences presented above is distinct from those of [3, 4, 10] all of which define preferences on rules rather than on atoms. Finally, [14] present an atom-based approach to preferences, in which statically defined relations among atoms are used to represent priorities in generalized extended disjunctive programs.

4.2 Abductive Frameworks for Preference Logic Programs

Definition 1 indicates how a preference logic program can be translated into an extended program. The resulting abductive framework for the translated program $[P, Pref]_{norm}$ has the form

$$\langle [P, Pref]_{norm}, A, I \rangle$$

in which A is a set of abducibles and I a set of integrity rules. This framework, in which P and I are extended programs that may include non-stratified negation, can then be directly evaluated by the Abdual method (See [2] for details of Abdual and of the frameworks it evaluates)[5]. If A is empty, Abdual reduces to an evaluation of a query under the well-founded semantics with explicit negation and has polynomial data complexity. Using the terminology of [2], this result can easily be extended to preference logic programs:

Proposition 1. *Let $[P, Pref]$ be a PLP whose ground instantiation is finite, and $[P, Pref]_{norm}$ be its normal embedding (Definition 1). Then Abdual evaluation of a query to the abductive framework $\langle [P, Pref]_{norm}, \emptyset, I \rangle$ has a complexity that is polynomial in the size of those rules in $P \cup Pref \cup I$ whose body is empty.*

---

[4] The proof of this theorem can be found in the paper *Preference Logic Grammars: Semantics, Implementation, and Application to Data Standardization* available at http://www.cs.sunysb.edu/~tswift.

[5] In addition, calls to the exclude/2 must also be unfolded in order for the extended embedding to work properly on the psychiatric rules and preferences described in Section 3.

Proof. Straightforward from Theorem 3.3 of [2] and Definition 1 which ensures that the size of $[P, Pref]_{norm}$ is polynomial in the size of $P \cup Pref$.

5 Discussion

Investigation into the logical representation of DSM-IV was sparked by the desire to automate DSM-IV in a commercial system, Diagnostica, a beta version of which is available (see http://medicinerules.com). Full implementation of Diagnostica, using the techniques of Section 3 and using XSB (cf. http://xsb.sourceforge.net) is not yet complete. The current user interface for Diagnostica thus uses abduction in a simple, but clinically relevant way. True differentials for diagnoses are not yet available to the user, nor are screens for adding or manipulating preferences. The inclusion of these features is planned for future versions.

Non-stratified programs are sometimes considered to be of little use for practical problems. However, translation of DSM-IV diagnostic rules into logical rules shows that sets of closely related diagnoses form non-stratified recursive components, so that non-stratified negation is semantically meaningful. Indeed, it is difficult to see how DSM-IV could be adequately coded without non-stratified negation. The well-founded semantics is used as a basis of our semantics for DSM-IV rather than, say, stable models for several reasons. It is convenient to use the *undefined* truth value to represent error conditions for diagnoses such as Alzheimer's Dementia and Adjustment Disorder. At the same time, multiple diagnoses can be obtained by the predicate abnormal_situation/2 in cases where this information is explicit in DSM-IV. The addition of preference rules under the well-founded semantics allows a user-based resolution of non-stratified loops while retaining a polynomial complexity of evaluation when abduction is not required. On the other hand, the addition of abduction to well-founded preference logic programs allows representation of hypotheses used in diagnoses as well as a means of constructing differentials for diagnoses.

The need to implement these aspects of DSM-IV in Diagnostica has helped spur the development of the Abdual evaluation method [2] as well as the Preference Logic presented here. At the same time, development of these formalisms has been necessary in order to understand how to implement abduction and preferences in Diagnostica. Experience gained as Diagnostica becomes fielded will be invaluable in testing the practical usefulness of this framework.

Acknowledgements

The authors thank C.R. Ramakrishnan and David S. Warren for their work on a preliminary version of Diagnostica; Michael Gelfond for a discussion on knowledge representation in psychiatry; and Bharat Jayaraman for a discussion on the possible-worlds semantics of preference logic programs. A U.S. Patent is pending for the use of several of the described techniques for medical reasoning.

Carlos Damásio and Luis Pereira were partially supported by PRAXIS XXI project MENTAL (Mental Agents Architecture in Logic) and FLAD-NSF project REAP. Terrance Swift was partially supported by NSF grants CCR-9702581, EIA-97-5998, and INT-96-00598.

References

1. J. Alferes, C. Damásio, and L. M. Pereira. A logic programming system for non-monotonic reasoning. *Journal of Automated Reasoning*, 14(1):93–147, 1995.
2. J. Alferes, L. M. Pereira, and T. Swift. Well-founded abduction via tabled dual programs. In *Int. Conf. on Logic Programming*, pages 426–440, 1999.
3. G. Brewka. Well-founded semantics for extended logic programs with dynamic preferences. *Journal of Artificial Intelligence Research*, 4:19–36, 1996.
4. G. Brewka and T. Eiter. Preferred answer sets. In *Proceedings of the 6th Conference on Principles of Knowledge Representation and Reasoning*, pages 86–97. Morgan Kaufmann, 1998.
5. C. Damásio and L. M. Pereira. Abduction over 3-valued extended logic programs. In *International Conference on Logic Programming and Non-Monotonic Reasoning*, pages 29–42. Springer-Verlag, 1995. LNAI 1265.
6. P. B. de Mesquita; W. S. Gilliam. Differential diagnosis of childhood depression: using comorbidity and symptom overlap to generate multiple hypotheses. *Child Psychiatry Hum Dev*, 24:157–172, 1994.
7. *Diagnostic and Statistical Manual of Mental Disorders*. American Psychiatric Association, Washington,DC, 4th edition, 1994. Prepared by the Task Force on DSM-IV and other committees and work groups of the American Psychiatric Association.
8. R. Famularo, R. Kinscherff, and T. Fenton. Psychiatric diagnoses of maltreated children: preliminary findings. *J Am Acad Child Adolesc Psych*, 31:863–867, 1996.
9. J. Ford, R. Racusin, W. Daviss, C. Ellis, and J. Thomas. Trauma exposure among children with oppositional defiant disorder and attention deficit-hyperactivity disorder. *J Consult Clin Psychol*, 67:786–789, 1999.
10. M. Gelfond and T. C. Son. Reasoning with prioritized defaults. In *Logic Programming and Knowledge Representation*, pages 164–223. Springer-Verlag, 1997.
11. K. Govindarajan, B. Jayaraman, and S. Mantha. Preference logic programming. In *Int. Conf. on Logic Programming*, pages 731–746, 1995.
12. M. Prior, R. Eisenmajer, S. Leekam, L. Wing, J. Gould, B. Ong, and D. Dowe. Are there subgroups within the autistic spectrum? a cluster analysis of a group of children with autistic spectrum disorders. *Can J Psych*, 43(6):589–595, 1998.
13. L. Rosenstein. Differential diagnosis of the major progressive dementias and = depression in middle and late adulthood: a summary of the literature of the early 1990s. *Neuropsychol Rev*, 8:109–167, 1998.
14. C. Sakama and K. Inoue. Representing priorities in logic programs. In *JICSLP*, pages 82–96, 1996.
15. *Schedules for Clinical Assesment in Neuropsychiatry*. World Health Organization, 1996. Version 2.1.
16. A. van Gelder, K. Ross, and J. Schlipf. Unfounded sets and well-founded semantics for general logic programs. *JACM*, 38(3):620–650, 1991.
17. F. Volkmar, A. Klin, and D. Pauls. Nosological and genetic aspects of asperger syndrome. *J Child Psychol Psychiatry*, 39(6):893–902, September 1998.

Author Index

Lecture Notes in Artificial Intelligence (LNAI)

Vol. 1705: H. Ganzinger, D. McAllester, A. Voronkov(Eds.), Logic for Programming and Automated Reasoning. Proceedings, 1999. XII, 397 pages. 1999.

Vol. 1711: N. Zhong, A. Skowron, S. Ohsuga (Eds.), New Directions in Rough Sets, Data Mining, and Granular-Soft Computing. Proceedings, 1999. XIV, 558 pages. 1999.

Vol. 1712: H. Boley, A Tight, Practical Integration of Relations and Functions. XI, 169 pages. 1999.

Vol. 1714: M.T. Pazienza (Eds.), Information Extraction. IX, 165 pages. 1999.

Vol. 1715: P. Perner, M. Petrou (Eds.), Machine Learning and Data Mining in Pattern Recognition. Proceedings, 1999. VIII, 217 pages. 1999.

Vol. 1720: O. Watanabe, T. Yokomori (Eds.), Algorithmic Learning Theory. Proceedings, 1999. XI, 365 pages. 1999.

Vol. 1721: S. Arikawa, K. Furukawa (Eds.), Discovery Science. Proceedings, 1999. XI, 374 pages. 1999.

Vol. 1724: H.I. Christensen, H. Bunke, H. Noltemeier (Eds.), Sensor Based Intelligent Robots. Proceedings, 1998. VIII, 327 pages. 1999.

Vol. 1730: M. Gelfond, N. Leone, G. Pfeifer (Eds.), Logic Programming and Nonmonotonic Reasoning. Proceedings, 1999. XI, 391 pages. 1999.

Vol. 1733: H. Nakashima, C. Zhang (Eds.), Approaches to Intelligent Agents. Proceedings, 1999. XII, 241 pages. 1999.

Vol. 1735: J.W. Amtrup, Incremental Speech Translation. XV, 200 pages. 1999.

Vol. 1739: A. Braffort, R. Gherbi, S. Gibet, J. Richardson, D. Teil (Eds.), Gesture-Based Communication in Human-Computer Interaction. Proceedings, 1999. XI, 333 pages. 1999.

Vol. 1744: S. Staab, Grading Knowledge: Extracting Degree Information from Texts. X, 187 pages. 1999.

Vol. 1747: N. Foo (Ed.), Adavanced Topics in Artificial Intelligence. Proceedings, 1999. XV, 500 pages. 1999.

Vol. 1757: N.R. Jennings, Y. Lespérance (Eds.), Intelligent Agents VI. Proceedings, 1999. XII, 380 pages. 2000.

Vol. 1759: M.J. Zaki, C.-T. Ho (Eds.), Large-Scale Parallel Data Mining. VIII, 261 pages. 2000.

Vol. 1760: J.-J. Ch. Meyer, P.-Y. Schobbens (Eds.), Formal Models of Agents. Poceedings. VIII, 253 pages. 1999.

Vol. 1761: R. Caferra, G. Salzer (Eds.), Automated Deduction in Classical and Non-Classical Logics. Proceedings. VIII, 299 pages. 2000.

Vol. 1771: P. Lambrix, Part-Whole Reasoning in an Object-Centered Framework. XII, 195 pages. 2000.

Vol. 1772: M. Beetz, Concurrent Reactive Plans. XVI, 213 pages. 2000.

Vol. 1775: M. Thielscher, Challenges for Action Theories. XIII, 138 pages. 2000.

Vol. 1778: S. Wermter, R. Sun (Eds.), Hybrid Neural Systems. IX, 403 pages. 2000.

Vol. 1792: E. Lamma, P. Mello (Eds.), AI*IA 99: Advances in Artificial Intelligence. Proceedings, 1999. XI, 392 pages. 2000.

Vol. 1793: O. Cairo, L.E. Sucar, F.J. Cantu (Eds.), MICAI 2000: Advances in Artificial Intelligence. Proceedings, 2000. XIV, 750 pages. 2000.

Vol. 1794: H. Kirchner, C. Ringeissen (Eds.), Frontiers of Combining Systems. Proceedings, 2000. X, 291 pages. 2000.

Vol. 1805: T. Terano, H. Liu, A.L.P. Chen (Eds.), Knowledge Discovery and Data Mining. Proceedings, 2000. XIV, 460 pages. 2000.

Vol. 1810: R. López de Mántaras, E. Plaza (Eds.), Machine Learning: ECML 2000. Proceedings, 2000. XII, 460 pages. 2000.

Vol. 1813: P.L. Lanzi, W. Stolzmann, S.W. Wilson (Eds.), Learning Classifier Systems. X, 349 pages. 2000.

Vol. 1821: R. Loganantharaj, G. Palm, M. Ali (Eds.), Intelligent Problem Solving. Proceedings, 2000. XVII, 751 pages. 2000.

Vol. 1822: H.H. Hamilton, Advances in Artificial Intelligence. Proceedings, 2000. XII, 450 pages. 2000.

Vol. 1831: D. McAllester (Ed.), Automated Deduction – CADE-17. Proceedings, 2000. XIII, 519 pages. 2000.

Vol. 1834: J.-C. Heudin (Ed.), Virtual Worlds. Proceedings, 2000. XI, 314 pages. 2000.

Vol. 1835: D. N. Christodoulakis (Ed.), Natural Language Processing – NLP 2000. Proceedings, 2000. XII, 438 pages. 2000.

Vol. 1847: R. Dyckhoff (Ed.), Automated Reasoning with Analytic Tableaux and Related Methods. Proceedings, 2000. X, 441 pages. 2000.

Vol. 1849: C. Freksa, W. Brauer, C. Habel, K.F. Wender (Eds.), Spatial Cognition II. XI, 420 pages. 2000.

Vol. 1860: M. Klusch, L. Kerschberg (Eds.), Cooperative Information Agents IV. Proceedings, 2000. XI, 285 pages. 2000.

Vol. 1861: J. Lloyd, V. Dahl, U. Furbach, M. Kerber, K.-K. Lau, C. Palamidessi, L. Moniz Pereira, Y. Sagiv, P.J. Stuckey (Eds.), Computational Logic – CL 2000. Proceedings, 2000. XIX, 1379 pages.

Vol. 1866: J. Cussens, A. Frisch (Eds.), Inductive Logic Programming. Proceedings, 2000. X, 265 pages. 2000.

Lecture Notes in Computer Science